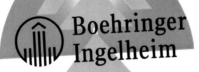

Compliments of/
Gracieuseté de

Boehringer
Ingelheim

Fraser and Paré's

Diagnosis of Diseases *of the* CHEST

Fraser and Paré's

Diagnosis of
Diseases
of the
CHEST
Fourth Edition

Volume I

R. S. Fraser, M.D.
Professor of Pathology
McGill University Health Centre
Royal Victoria Hospital
Montreal, Quebec

Neil Colman, M.D.
Associate Professor of Medicine
McGill University Health Centre
Montreal General Hospital
Montreal, Quebec

Nestor L. Müller, M.D., Ph.D.
Professor of Radiology
University of British Columbia
Vancouver Hospital and Health
  Sciences Centre
Vancouver, British Columbia

P. D. Paré, M.D.
Professor of Medicine
University of British Columbia
St. Paul's Hospital
Vancouver, British Columbia

W.B. SAUNDERS COMPANY
A Division of Harcourt Brace & Company
Philadelphia   London   Toronto   Montreal   Sydney   Tokyo

W.B. SAUNDERS COMPANY
A Division of Harcourt Brace & Company

The Curtis Center
Independence Square West
Philadelphia, Pennsylvania 19106

Library of Congress Cataloging-in-Publication Data

Fraser and Paré's Diagnosis of diseases of the chest / Richard S. Fraser . . . [et al.].—4th ed.

p.   cm.

ISBN 0–7216–6194–7

1. Chest—Diseases—Diagnosis.   I. Fraser, Richard S.
   [DNLM: 1. Thoracic Diseases—diagnosis.   2. Diagnostic Imaging.
   WF 975D536 1999]

RC941.D52   1999   617.5′4075—dc21

DNLM/DLC   98–36145

ISBN 0–7216–6194–7 (set)
ISBN 0–7216–6195–5 (vol. I)
ISBN 0–7216–6196–3 (vol. II)
ISBN 0–7216–6197–1 (vol. III)
ISBN 0–7216–6198–X (vol. IV)

FRASER AND PARÉ'S DIAGNOSIS OF DISEASES OF THE CHEST

Printed in the United States of America.

Last digit is the print number: 9   8   7   6   5   4   3   2   1

This book is dedicated to

ROBERT G. FRASER AND J. A. PETER PARÉ

who had the inspiration to recognize the importance of radiologic findings in
the diagnosis of chest disease, the dedication and perseverance to document
these and other findings in the initial editions of this book, and the grace to
teach us the value of both

and to

OUR WIVES AND CHILDREN

without whose encouragement and patience during our many hours of
reading, writing, and editing this edition would not have been completed.

Preface to the Fourth Edition

Previous editions of this book were based on the principle that the radiograph is the "focal point" or "first step" in the diagnosis of chest disease. We agree with the fundamental importance of the radiograph in this respect; however, we feel that it is best considered as one of two "pillars" of diagnosis, the other being the clinical history. Although it is of course possible to render an opinion about the nature of a patient's illness on the basis of only one of these pillars, this is fraught with potential error and should be avoided in most cases. Instead, it is our belief that the combination of a good clinical history and high-quality posteroanterior and lateral chest radiographs provides the respiratory physician or radiologist with sufficient information to significantly limit the differential diagnosis in the vast majority of patients who have chest disease and to enable a specific (and often correct) diagnosis in many. Additional information derived from ancillary radiologic procedures, laboratory tests, pulmonary function tests, and pathologic examination enables further refinement of differential diagnosis and a confident diagnosis in almost all patients. Of these additional tests, one that has undergone significant advance in the recent past is computed tomography (CT), particularly with the advent of high-resolution (HRCT) and spiral CT. The former has enabled much clearer delineation of the location and extent of disease in the lungs, pleura, and mediastinum, and the latter has greatly improved the ability to image the airways and vessels. The current edition of this book has changed to reflect the increased availability and diagnostic accuracy of these procedures; in addition, numerous figures have been added to illustrate the various abnormalities that they can identify.

Some might argue that a knowledge of the etiology, pathogenesis, and pathologic characteristics of disease is unnecessary for the clinician or radiologist to diagnose chest disease. It is our belief, however, that a thorough understanding of the overall nature of such disease will result in improved diagnostic skill. This potential refinement may be apparent in several areas, including better appreciation of the nature of radiologic abnormalities (*e.g.*, via a knowledge of gross pathologic findings), improved knowledge of the potential value of new diagnostic tests (*e.g.*, via an understanding of the molecular and genetic abnormalities associated with certain diseases and with the techniques by which these are identified), and a more thorough understanding of the associations between certain diseases or disease processes (*e.g.*, viral infection and neoplasia). For these reasons, we have included a significant amount of material that is not directly relevant to diagnosis. We recognize the limitations of this approach, particularly with respect to a consideration of disease pathogenesis—the remarkable amount of research in chest disease, especially that related to cellular and molecular mechanisms, is difficult to summarize accurately, particularly since three of us have limited involvement in fundamental research. Moreover, it is inevitable that the progress that is currently being made in this research is such that some of the material in the text will be outdated at the time it is published. Despite these limitations, we consider an understanding of the etiology and pathogenesis of chest disease to be of sufficient importance to describe them to the best of our ability.

The organization of this book is based on a fairly consistent consideration of specific diseases under the headings of epidemiology, etiology and pathogenesis, pathologic characteristics, radiologic manifestations, clinical manifestations, laboratory findings (including pulmonary function tests), and prognosis and natural history. As with previous editions, a discussion of treatment has been omitted because of the rapidity with which therapeutic strategies may change and the implications that this may have. The scope of the book is such that it is meant primarily for specialists in chest disease, including pneumologists, thoracic surgeons, chest radiologists, and pathologists whose interest lies in this field. However, we believe that residents in training for these specialties will also find the text useful.

What will our readers find that is different from previous editions? Allusion has already been made to the extensive expansion of the discussion of HRCT and the addition of numerous new illustrations. Many new pathologic illustrations, both gross and microscopic, have also been included in an attempt to better explain the anatomic basis of disease. In addition to extensive updating of the material in previous editions, new sections have been written on CT of the normal lung, pulmonary transplantation, the effects on the chest of human immunodeficiency virus (HIV) infection, and pulmonary hemorrhage syndromes. The discussion of pulmonary neoplasia has been reorganized to conform more closely to the latest World Health Organization Classification of Lung Tumors. The Tables of Differential Diagnosis have been simplified to include primarily those diseases that are likely to be encountered by most pulmonary physicians; along with an increase in the number of illustrative examples, it is hoped that this version will provide a more simple and practical guide to differential diagnosis of the commonly enountered radiographic patterns of chest disease.

To make the text more accessible to the reader, the 21 chapters of the previous three editions have been expanded to 79. The subdivision is somewhat arbitrary and has necessitated repetition of material in some areas; for example, the inclusion of a chapter on chest disease in HIV infection necessarily involves a discussion of pulmonary infections and neoplasms that are also included in other, more comprehensive chapters on these subjects. As much as possible, we have tried to limit discussion of a particular topic to one place in the text; nevertheless, we have sometimes repeated material in order to minimize the necessity for the reader to refer to other sections of the book. We have also grouped chapters into larger categories based on anatomic location or presumed etiology and pathogenesis of disease; such grouping is again somewhat arbitrary, but hopefully will provide the reader easier access to appropriate information.

The reference list of the previous editions has been culled in an attempt to include those articles that are most relevant to the points we have chosen to emphasize; however, numerous reports published before 1990 have been retained. As might be expected, many references to articles published in the 1990s have also been added in an attempt to bring the text as up to date as possible. The resulting reference list contains a somewhat daunting total of approximately 31,000 citations! The inclusion of a list such as this might be questioned in light of the relatively easy availability of personal computers and electronic reference archives. However, we feel it is useful to have such references accessible to those who wish quick access to literature sources in book form. In addition, and perhaps more important in a book compiled by only four authors, we wish to provide a "factual" basis for our assertions as much as possible. As will be appreciated by those who publish in medical journals, it is inevitable that there are errors in our reference list, sometimes with respect to omission of an author or the spelling of his or her name and sometimes with respect to inappropriate attribution of statements or to omission of a key article. We apologize for these errors in advance and ask for our readers' understanding and the feedback to correct them. (Correspondence may be sent to [DDC@pathology.lan.mcgill.ca].)

The last edition of this book included a quotation from Ecclesiastes concerning the passage of time. We would also like to offer a quote of general philosophic interest, although one that is perhaps more directly related to the subject matter of this book. It derives from Maimonides, the great twelfth century scholar and physician:

> *Do not consider a thing as proof because you find it written in books: . . . there are fools who accept a thing as (such), because it is in writing.*

What we offer in the following pages are a concept of disease of the chest and an approach to its diagnosis based on the combined experience and knowledge of reported observations of four individuals. As in our everyday practice, we have attempted to be as open-minded to new ideas and as unbiased in our selection of material as possible. Despite this, such bias is to some extent inevitable and errors of commission or omission must be present. We do not, of course, advocate the unequivocal acceptance of Maimonides' aphorism; however, we trust that our readers will take his words to heart and consider the following pages and indeed the entire subject of chest disease with a questioning and open mind.

RSF

NLM

NC

PDP

Acknowledgments

The production of a book such as *Fraser and Paré's Diagnosis of Diseases of the Chest* is a huge task, and we have been fortunate in having the support and encouragement of many colleagues and friends in our endeavor. The availability and efficiency of modern computers have meant that much writing and editing have been performed directly by us; nevertheless, we could not have accomplished our task without secretarial help from Laura Fiorita, Stella Totilo, and Andrea Sanders at the McGill University Health Centre (MUHC); Catherine Goyette and Tamara Eigendorf at St. Paul's Hospital and the University of British Columbia; and Jenny Silver at the Vancouver Hospital and Health Sciences Centre. The diligence with which these individuals carried out their tasks shows in the final product and is deeply appreciated.

The majority of the case histories and radiologic illustrations reproduced in the text are derived from patients of staff members of the MUHC (particularly the Royal Victoria Hospital, the Montreal General Hospital, and the Montreal Chest Hospital Institute) and the Vancouver Hospital and Health Sciences Centre. Almost all illustrations of pathology are related to patients from the MUHC. We are indebted to our colleagues who cared for these patients, not only for their generosity in permitting us to publish the illustrations of various diseases but also for the benefit of their experience and guidance over the years. A number of these colleagues deserve particular mention for their comments and help on selected topics; these include Drs. Richard Menzies and John Kosiuk at the MUHC; Drs. Pearce Wilcox, John Fleetham, Brad Munt, and Hugh Chaun and Ms. Elisabeth Baile at the University of British Columbia; and Drs. A. Jean Buckley, John Aldrich, John Mayo, and Daniel Worsley at the Vancouver Hospital and Health Sciences Centre.

The photographic work throughout these volumes was the accomplishment of many individuals. Illustrations from former editions were provided by members of the Department of Visual Aids of the Royal Victoria Hospital; Susie Gray at the Department of Radiology, University of Alabama; Joseph Donohue, Anthony Graham, and Michael Paré of Montreal; and Sally Osborne at St. Paul's Hospital, Vancouver. Those involved in the production of new illustrations for this edition include Marcus Arts and Helmut Bernhard at the Montreal Neurological Institute Photography Department; Diane Minshall and Stuart Greene at St. Paul's Hospital, University of British Columbia; and Janis Franklin and Michael Robertson at the Vancouver Hospital Sciences Centre.

Throughout our writing and editing, we received support and cooperation from several individuals at W.B. Saunders, notably our Chief Editor, Lisette Bralow, our developmental editors Janice Gaillard and Melissa Messersmith, and our copy editors Sue Reilly and Lee Ann Draud, all of whom helped us overcome a number of the obstacles we encountered at various times. Finally, we acknowledge and thank our wives and children, without whose patience and encouragement this book would not have been completed.

RSF
NLM
NC
PDP

Contents

VOLUME ONE

Part *I*

THE NORMAL CHEST. 1

1 The Airways and Pulmonary Ventilation. 3

2 The Pulmonary and Bronchial Vascular Systems 71

3 Pulmonary Defense and Other Nonrespiratory Functions 126

4 Development and Growth of the Lung. 136

5 Innervation of the Lung 145

6 The Pleura. 151

7 The Lymphatic System of the Lungs, Pleura, and Mediastinum 172

8 The Mediastinum. 196

9 The Control of Breathing 235

10 The Respiratory Muscles and Chest Wall 246

11 The Normal Lung: Radiography 269

12 The Normal Lung: Computed Tomography . . . 281

Part *II*

INVESTIGATIVE METHODS IN CHEST DISEASE. 297

13 Methods of Radiologic Investigation. 299

14 Methods of Pathologic Investigation. 339

15 Endoscopy and Diagnostic Biopsy Procedures 366

16 The Clinical History and Physical Examination 379

17 Methods of Functional Investigation. 404

Part *III*

RADIOLOGIC SIGNS OF CHEST DISEASE 431

18 Increased Lung Density. 433

19 Decreased Lung Density 493

20 Atelectasis 513

21 Pleural Abnormalities. 563

Part *IV*

DEVELOPMENTAL LUNG DISEASE 595

22 Developmental Anomalies Affecting the Airways and Lung Parenchyma 597

23 Developmental Anomalies Affecting the Pulmonary Vessels 637

24 Hereditary Abnormalities of Pulmonary Connective Tissue 676

VOLUME TWO

Part *V*

PULMONARY INFECTION. 695

25 General Features of Pulmonary Infection 697

26 Bacteria Other than Mycobacteria 734

27 Mycobacteria. 798

28 Fungi and Actinomyces 875

29 Viruses, Mycoplasmas, Chlamydiae, and Rickettsiae 979

30 Protozoa, Helminths, Arthropods, and Leeches 1033

Part *VI*

PULMONARY NEOPLASMS 1067

31 Pulmonary Carcinoma. 1069

32 Neuroendocrine Neoplasms 1229

33 Neoplasms of Tracheobronchial Glands 1251

34 Miscellaneous Epithelial Tumors 1262

35 Lymphoproliferative Disorders and Leukemia.................................1269

36 Mesenchymal Neoplasms...................1331

37 Neoplasms of Uncertain Histogenesis and Nonneoplastic Tumors 1363

38 Secondary Neoplasms 1381

VOLUME THREE

Part VII
IMMUNOLOGIC LUNG DISEASE 1419

39 Connective Tissue Diseases................1421

40 Vasculitis 1489

41 Sarcoidosis.............................1533

42 Interstitial Pneumonitis and Fibrosis 1584

43 Langerhans' Cell Histiocytosis 1627

44 The Pulmonary Manifestations of Human Immunodeficiency Virus Infection..........1641

45 Transplantation.........................1698

46 Eosinophilic Lung Disease 1743

47 Goodpasture's Syndrome and Idiopathic Pulmonary Hemorrhage 1757

Part VIII
EMBOLIC LUNG DISEASE 1771

48 Thrombosis and Thromboembolism 1773

49 Emboli of Extravascular Tissue and Foreign Material..........................1845

Part IX
PULMONARY HYPERTENSION AND EDEMA.............................1877

50 Pulmonary Hypertension 1879

51 Pulmonary Edema 1946

Part X
DISEASE OF THE AIRWAYS 2019

52 Upper Airway Obstruction 2021

53 Obstructive Sleep Apnea 2054

54 Asthma 2077

55 Chronic Obstructive Pulmonary Disease......2168

56 Bronchiectasis and Other Bronchial Abnormalities 2265

57 Cystic Fibrosis 2298

58 Bronchiolitis 2321

VOLUME FOUR

Part XI
PULMONARY DISEASE CAUSED BY INHALATION OR ASPIRATION OF PARTICULATES, SOLIDS, OR LIQUIDS 2359

59 Inhalation of Organic Dust................2361

60 Inhalation of Inorganic Dust (Pneumoconiosis).......................2386

61 Aspiration of Solid Foreign Material and Liquids 2485

Part XII
PULMONARY DISEASE CAUSED BY TOXINS, DRUGS, AND IRRADIATION.......2517

62 Inhaled Toxic Gases, Fumes, and Aerosols 2519

63 Drugs.................................2537

64 Poisons 2584

65 Irradiation.............................2592

Part XIII
TRAUMATIC CHEST DISEASE 2609

66 Penetrating and Nonpenetrating Chest Trauma 2611

67 Complications of Therapeutic, Biopsy, and Monitoring Procedures 2659

Part XIV
METABOLIC PULMONARY DISEASE 2697

68 Metabolic Pulmonary Disease 2699

Part *XV*

PLEURAL DISEASE 2737

69 Pleural Effusion 2739

70 Pneumothorax 2781

71 Pleural Fibrosis 2795

72 Pleural Neoplasms 2807

Part *XVI*

MEDIASTINAL DISEASE 2849

73 Mediastinitis, Pneumomediastinum, and
Mediastinal Hemorrhage 2851

74 Masses Situated Predominantly in the
Anterior Mediastinal Compartment 2875

75 Masses Situated Predominantly in the
Middle-Posterior Mediastinal Compartment . . . 2938

76 Masses Situated Predominantly
in the Paravertebral Region 2974

Part *XVII*

DISEASE OF THE DIAPHRAGM AND
CHEST WALL 2985

77 The Diaphragm 2987

78 The Chest Wall 3011

Part *XVIII*

PULMONARY DISEASE ASSOCIATED
WITH A NORMAL CHEST RADIOGRAPH 3043

79 Respiratory Disease Associated with a Normal
Chest Radiograph 3045

Appendix 3077

Index I–1

Glossary of Terms and Symbols in Chest Medicine and Radiology

"Then you should say what you mean," the March Hare went on.

"I do," Alice hastily replied; "at least—at least, I mean what I say—that's the same thing, you know."

"Not the same thing a bit!" said the Hatter. "Why, you might just as well say that 'I see what I eat' is the same thing as 'I eat what I see!'"

This well-known excerpt from Lewis Carroll's *Alice's Adventures in Wonderland* points out a problem that affects many physicians confronted by today's constantly expanding scientific knowledge—the use of words and terms that mean different things to different people. Although this problem has possibly diminished since the last edition of this text, examples of inappropriate usage or conflicting terminology can still be identified in the radiologic and general medical literature. In an attempt to address this problem, a joint committee of the American College of Chest Physicians and the American Thoracic Society published in 1975 a glossary of pulmonary terms and symbols* pertinent to the medical and physiologic aspects of chest disease. Since this glossary omitted words that specifically related to chest radiology, the Fleischner Society formed a Committee on Nomenclature to draw up a glossary of radiologic words and terms that was published in 1984.† In 1996, a second committee of the Fleischner Society published a glossary of terms specifically related to computed tomography of the lungs.‡ We list herewith the terms and symbols selected from these publications that we hope our readers will refer to.

---

*Pulmonary Terms and Symbols: A Report of the ACCP/ATS Joint Committee on Pulmonary Nomenclature. Chest 67:583, 1975.

†Glossary of Terms for Thoracic Radiology: Recommendations of the Nomenclature Committee of the Fleischner Society. Am J Roentgenol 143:509, 1984.

‡Austin JHM, Müller NL, Friedman PJ, et al: Glossary of terms for CT of the lungs: Recommendations of the Nomenclature Committee of the Fleischner Society. Radiology 200:327, 1996.

TERMS USED IN CHEST RADIOLOGY

TERM	COMMENTS

abscess *n., pl.* -es. 1. (pathol.) An inflammatory mass, the central part of which has undergone purulent liquefaction necrosis. It may communicate with the bronchial tree. 2. (radiol.) Within the lung, a mass presumed to be caused by infection. The presence of gas within the mass, with or without a fluid level, represents a cavity *(q.v.)* and implies a communication with the bronchial tree. Otherwise, a pulmonary mass can be considered to represent an abscess in the morphologic sense only by inference. *Qualifiers:* Expressing clinical course: acute, chronic. Expressing etiology: bacterial, fungal, etc. Expressing site of involvement: lung, mediastinum, etc.

Should be used only with reference to masses of presumed infectious etiology. The word is not synonymous with cavity *(q.v.).*

acinar pattern *n.* (radiol.) A collection of round or elliptic, ill defined, discrete or partly confluent opacities in the lung, each measuring 4 to 8 mm in diameter and together producing an extended, inhomogeneous shadow.

Synonyms: Rosette pattern; acinonodose pattern (used specifically with reference to endobronchial spread of tuberculosis); alveolar pattern.

An inferred conclusion usually used as a descriptor. An acceptable term, preferred to cited synonyms (especially "alveolar pattern," which is an inaccurate descriptor).

acinar shadow *n.* (radiol.) A round or slightly elliptic pulmonary opacity 4 to 8 mm in diameter presumed to represent an anatomic acinus rendered opaque by consolidation. Usually employed in the presence of many such opacities *(see* acinar pattern).

An inferred conclusion sometimes applicable as a radiologic descriptor.

acinus *n.* (anat.) The portion of lung parenchyma distal to the terminal bronchiole and consisting of respiratory bronchioles, alveolar ducts, alveolar sacs, and alveoli *(see* acinar shadow, acinar pattern).

A specific feature of pulmonary anatomy.

aeration *n.* (physiol./radiol.) 1. The state of containing air. 2. The state or process of being filled or inflated with air. *Qualifiers:* overaeration (preferred) or hyperaeration; underaeration (preferred) or hypoaeration.

Synonym: Inflation.

An acceptable term with reference to the inspiratory phase of respiration. Inflation is preferred in sense 2.

air *n.* (radiol.) Inspired atmospheric gas. The word is sometimes used to describe gas within the body regardless of its composition or site.

With reference to pneumothorax, subcutaneous emphysema, or the content of the stomach, colon, etc., gas is the more accurate term and is preferred.

air bronchiologram *n.* (radiol.) The equivalent of air bronchogram, but in airways assumed to be bronchioles because of their peripheral location and diameter.

An acceptable term.

air bronchogram *n.* (radiol.) The radiographic shadow of an air-containing bronchus peripheral to the hilum and surrounded by airless lung (whether by virtue of absorption of air, replacement of air, or both), a finding generally regarded as evidence of the patency of the more proximal airway. Hence, any bandlike tapering and/or branching lucency within opacified lung corresponding in size and distribution to a bronchus or bronchi and presumed to represent an air-containing segment of the bronchial tree.

A specific feature of radiologic anatomy whose identity is often inferred. A useful and recommended term.

air-fluid level *n.* (radiol.) A local collection of gas and liquid that, when traversed by a horizontal x-ray beam, creates a shadow characterized by a sharp horizontal interface between gas density above and liquid density below.

A useful radiologic descriptor. Since with rare exception (*e.g.,* fat-fluid level) the upper of the two absorbant media is "air" (gas), it is sufficient to describe such an appearance as a "fluid level."

air space *n.* (*adj.* air-space) (anat./radiol.) The gas-containing portion of lung paren-chyma, including the acini and excluding the interstitium and purely conductive portions of the lung.

Synonyms: Acinar consolidation, alveolar consolidation (when used as an adjective in relation to air-space consolidation).

An inferred conclusion usually used as a radiologic descriptor. An acceptable term whose use as an adjective is also appropriate.

air-trapping *n.* (pathophysiol./radiol.) The retention of excess gas in all or part of the lung at any stage of expiration.

A specific radiologic sign to be employed only if excess air retention is demonstrated by a dynamic study, *e.g.,* inspiration-expiration radiography or fluoroscopy. *Not* to be used with reference to overinflation of the lung at full inspiration (total lung capacity).

airway *n., adj.* (anat./radiol.) A collective term for the air-conducting passages from the larynx to and including the respiratory bronchioles.

Synonyms: Conducting airway; tracheobronchial tree.

A useful anatomic term. May be used as an adjective in relation to disease or abnormality. Note that the respiratory bronchioles are both conducting and gas-exchanging airways and thus constitute the transitory zone.

alveolarization *n.* (radiol.) The opacification of groups of alveoli by a contrast medium.

A misnomer whose use is to be deplored. Excessive filling of peripheral lung structure by contrast media usually employed for bronchography may opacify respiratory bronchioles but not alveoli. Thus, the correct term is "bronchiolar filling or opacification."

anterior junction line *n.* (radiol.) A vertically oriented linear or curvilinear opacity approximately 1 to 2 mm wide, commonly projected on the tracheal air shadow. It is produced by the shadows of the right and left pleurae in intimate contact between the aerated lungs anterior to the great vessels (and sometimes the heart); hence, it never extends above the suprasternal notch (*cf.* posterior junction line).

Synonyms: Anterior mediastinal septum, line, or stripe.

A specific feature of radiologic anatomy; to be preferred to cited synonyms.

aortopulmonary window *n.* 1. (anat.) A mediastinal space bounded anteriorly by the posterior surface of the ascending aorta; posteriorly by the anterior surface of the descending aorta; superiorly by the inferior surface of the aortic arch; inferiorly by the superior surface of the left pulmonary artery; medially by the left side of the trachea, left main bronchus, and esophagus; and laterally by the left lung. Within it are situated fat, the ductus ligament, the left recurrent laryngeal nerve, and lymph nodes. 2. (radiol.) A zone of relative lucency in the mediastinal shadow that is seen to best advantage in the left anterior oblique or lateral projection and that corresponds to the anatomic space defined above. On a posteroanterior radiograph of the chest, the lateral margin of the space constitutes the aortopulmonary window interface.

Synonym: Aortic-pulmonic window.

A specific feature of radiologic anatomy.

atelectasis *n.* (pathophysiol./radiol.) Less than normal inflation of all or a portion of the lung with corresponding diminution in volume. *Qualifiers* may be employed to indicate severity (mild, moderate, severe), mechanism (resorption, relaxation, cicatrization, adhesive), or distribution (*e.g.,* lobar, platelike [*q.v.*], discoid).

Synonyms: Collapse, loss of volume, anectasis.

Generally this term is preferable to "collapse" in describing loss of volume. The word "collapse" connotes total atelectasis in which lung tissue has been reduced to its smallest volume. "Anectasis" is usually used in reference to failure of lung expansion in the neonate.

azygoesophageal recess *n.* 1. (anat.) A space or recess in the right side of the mediastinum into which the medial edge of the right lower lobe (crista pulmonis) extends. It is limited superiorly by the arch of the azygos vein, inferiorly by the diaphragm, posteriorly by the azygos vein in front of the vertebral column, and medially by the esophagus and its adjacent structures. (The exact relationship between the medial edge of the lung and the mediastinal structures is variable.) 2. (radiol.) In a frontal chest radiograph, a vertically oriented interface between air in the right lower lobe and the adjacent mediastinum that represents the medial limit of the anatomic azygoesophageal recess.

Synonyms: Infra-azygos recess; right pleuroesophageal line or stripe; right paraesophageal line or stripe.

A specific feature of radiologic anatomy. The use of the term "recess" to identify an interface is inappropriate; thus, azygoesophageal recess interface is preferred.

bat's-wing distribution *n.* (radiol.) A spatial arrangement of radiographic opacities in a frontal radiograph that bears a vague resemblance to the shape of a bat in flight; said of coalescent, ill-defined opacities that are approximately bilaterally symmetric and that are confined to the medulla of the lungs *(q.v.)*.

Synonym: Butterfly distribution.

A radiologic descriptor of limited usefulness.

bleb *n.* 1. (pathol.) A gas-containing space within or contiguous to the visceral pleura of the lung. 2. (radiol.) A local, thin-walled lucency contiguous with the pleura, usually at the lung apex.

Synonyms: Type I bulla (pathol.); bulla; a form of pulmonary air cyst (radiol.)

An inferred conclusion seldom justifiable by radiography alone. Bulla or air cyst is preferred.

bronchiole *n.* (anat./radiol.) An airway that contains no cartilage in its wall. A bronchiole may be purely conducting (up to and including the terminal bronchiole) or transitory (the respiratory bronchioles that carry out both conduction and gas exchange).

A specific feature of pulmonary anatomy.

bronchocele *n. See* mucoid impaction.

bronchus *n.* (anat./radiol.) A conducting airway distal to the tracheal bifurcation that contains cartilage in its wall.

A specific feature of pulmonary anatomy.

bulla *n., pl.* -lae. 1. (pathol.) A sharply demarcated region of emphysema; a gas-containing space that may contain nothing but gas or may contain overdistended and ruptured alveolar septa and blood vessels. 2. (radiol.) Sharply demarcated hyperlucent area of avascularity within the lung, measuring 1 cm or more in diameter and possessing a wall less than 1 mm in thickness. *Qualifiers:* small, medium, large.

The preferred term to describe all thin-walled air-containing spaces in the lung with the exception of pneumatocele *(q.v.)*.

butterfly distribution *n.* (radiol.) *See* bat's-wing distribution.

To be distinguished from the use of this term in general medicine to describe the distribution of certain cutaneous lesions.

calcification *n.* 1. (pathophysiol.) (a) The process by which one or more deposits of calcium salts are formed within lung tissue or within a pulmonary lesion. (b) Such a deposit of calcium salts. 2. (radiol.) A calcific opacity within the lung that may be organized (*e.g.,* concentric lamination), but that does not display the trabecular organization of true bone. *Qualifiers:* "eggshell," "popcorn," target, laminated, flocculent, nodular, etc.

An explicit conclusion; may be used as a descriptor. To be distinguished from ossification *(q.v.)*.

carina *n.* (anat./radiol.) The keel-shaped ridge that separates the right and left main bronchi at the tracheal bifurcation.

A specific feature of pulmonary anatomy.

carinal angle *n.* (anat./radiol.) The angle formed by the right and left main bronchi at the tracheal bifurcation.

Synonyms: Bifurcation angle; angle of tracheal bifurcation.

A definitive anatomic and radiologic measurement.

cavity *n.* 1. (pathol.) A mass within lung parenchyma, the central portion of which has undergone liquefaction necrosis and has been expelled via the bronchial tree, leaving a gas-containing space, with or without associated fluid. 2. (radiol.) A gas-containing space within the lung surrounded by a wall whose thickness is greater than 1 mm and usually irregular in contour.

A useful descriptor without etiologic connotation. The word must not be used interchangeably with abscess *(q.v.)*, which may exist without bronchial communication and therefore without cavitation.

circumscribed *adj.* (radiol.) Possessing a complete or nearly complete visible border.

An acceptable descriptor.

clot *n.* (pathol.) A semisolidified mass of blood elements.

Cf. thrombus.

coalescence *n.* (radiol.) The joining together of a number of opacities into a single opacity; confluence *(q.v.)*.

An acceptable descriptor.

coin lesion *n.* (radiol.) A sharply defined, circular opacity within the lung suggestive of the appearance of a coin and usually representing a spherical or nodular lesion.

Synonyms: Pulmonary nodule, pulmonary mass.

A radiologic descriptor, the use of which is to be condemned. The term "coin" may be descriptive of the shadow, but certainly not of the lesion producing it.

collapse *n.* (radiol.) A state in which lung tissue has undergone complete atelectasis.

The term is acceptable when employed strictly as defined, but "atelectasis" is preferred, since the degree of loss of lung volume can be qualified by mild, moderate, or severe.

collateral ventilation *n.* (physiol./radiol.) The process by which gas passes from one lung unit (acinus, lobule, segment, or lobe) to a contiguous unit via alveolar pores (pores of Kohn), canals of Lambert, or direct airway anastomoses.

Synonym: Collateral air drift.

An inferred conclusion usually based on fairly reliable signs. A useful term. The channels of peripheral airway communication also function as a mechanism for transmission of liquid from one unit to another (*e.g.*, in acute air-space pneumonia).

confluence *n.* (radiol.) The nature of opacities that are contiguous with or adjacent to one another.

Antonym: Discrete *(q.v.)*.

A useful descriptor; confluence is to be distinguished from coalescence *(q.v.)*, which is the act of becoming confluent.

consolidation *n.* 1. (pathophysiol.) The process by which air in the lung is replaced by the products of disease, rendering the lung solid (as in pneumonia). 2. (radiol.) An essentially homogeneous opacity in the lung characterized by little or no loss of volume, by effacement of pulmonary blood vessels, and sometimes by the presence of an air bronchogram *(q.v.)*.

An inferred conclusion, applicable only in an appropriate clinical setting when the opacity can with reasonable certainty be attributed to replacement of alveolar air by exudate, transudate, or tissue. Not to be used with reference to all homogeneous opacities.

corona radiata *n.* (radiol.) A circumferential pattern of fine linear spicules, approximately 5 mm long, extending outward from the margin of a solitary pulmonary nodule through a zone of relative lucency.

A sign of limited usefulness in the differentiation of benign and malignant nodules.

cor pulmonale *n.* 1. (pathol./clin.) Right ventricular hypertrophy and/or dilation occurring as a result of an abnormality of lung structure or function. 2. (radiol.) The combination of pulmonary arterial hypertension and chronic lung disease, with or without evidence of enlargement of right heart chambers. *Qualifiers:* acute, chronic.

An inferred radiologic conclusion based on usually reliable signs. An acceptable descriptor. Despite the pathologic definition, radiologic evidence of cardiomegaly need not be present.

cortex *n.* (radiol.) The peripheral 2 to 3 cm of lung parenchyma adjacent to the visceral pleura, either over the convexity of the thorax or in the interlobar fissures. (*See* medulla and hilum.)

The peripheral part of an arbitrary subdivision of the lung into three zones from the hilum to the visceral pleura. Of limited usefulness.

CT number *n.* (radiol./physics) In computed tomography, a quantitative numerical statement of the relative attenuation of the x-ray beam at a specified point; loosely, the relative attenuation of a specified tissue absorber, usually expressed in Hounsfield units (HU).

cyst *n.* 1. (pathol.) A circumscribed space whose contents may be liquid or gaseous and whose wall is generally thin and well defined and lined by epithelium. 2. (radiol.) A gas-containing space of any size possessing a thin wall. *Qualifiers:* foregut (bronchogenic, esophageal duplication); postinfectious.

This term is entirely nonspecific and should not possess inferred conclusion as to etiology. It is the preferred term to describe any thin-walled gas-containing space in the lung possessing a wall thickness greater than 1 mm.

defined *adj.* (radiol.) The character of the border of a shadow. *Qualifiers:* well, sharply, poorly, distinctly.

An acceptable descriptor.

demarcated *adj.* (radiol.) Distinct from adjacent structures. *Qualifiers:* well, sharply, poorly.

An acceptable descriptor. (*Cf.* defined.)

dense *adj.* (radiol.) Possessing density *(q.v.).* Usually used in describing or comparing radiographic shadows with respect to their light transmission.

A recommended term in the context defined. Should not be used in referring to the opacity of an absorber of x-radiation. (*See* opaque, opacity.)

density *n.* 1. (physics) The mass of a substance per unit volume. 2. (photometry/radiol.) The opacity of a radiographic shadow to visible light; film blackening. 3. (radiol.) The shadow of an absorber more opaque to x-rays than its surroundings; an opacity or radiopacity. 4. The degree of opacity of an absorber to x-rays, usually expressed in terms of the nature of the absorber (*e.g.,* bone, water, or fat density).

In sense 2, the term refers to a fundamental characteristic of the radiograph, and its use is recommended. In senses 3 and 4, it refers to the character of the absorber and has an exactly opposite connotation with respect to film blackening. Because of this potential confusion, the term should *never* be used to mean an "opacity" or "radiopacity."

diffuse *adj.* 1. (pathophysiol.) Widely distributed through an organ or type of tissue. 2. (radiol.) Widespread and continuous (said of shadows and by inference of the states or processes producing them).

Synonyms: Disseminated, generalized, systemic, widespread.

A useful and acceptable term. In the context of chest radiology, "diffuse" connotes widespread, anatomically continuous but not necessarily complete involvement of the lung or other thoracic structure or tissue; "disseminated" connotes widespread but anatomically discontinuous involvement; and "generalized" connotes complete or nearly complete involvement, whereas "systemic" connotes involvement of a thoracic structure or tissue as part of a process involving the entire body.

discrete *adj.* (radiol.) Separate, individually distinct; hence, with respect to opacities, usually circumscribed.

Antonyms: Confluent, coalescent.

An acceptable descriptor.

disseminated *adj.* 1. (pathophysiol.) Widely but discontinuously distributed through an organ or type of tissue. 2. (radiol.) Widespread but anatomically discontinuous (said of shadows and by inference of the states or processes producing them).

Synonyms: Diffuse *(q.v.)*, generalized, systemic.

A useful and acceptable term.

doubling time *n.* (radiol.) The time span over which a pulmonary nodule or mass doubles in volume (increases its diameter by a factor of 1.25).

An acceptable term. The concept should be used with caution as a criterion for distinguishing benign from malignant nodules.

embolus *n.* 1. (pathol.) A clot or mass of foreign material that has been carried by the bloodstream to occlude partly or completely the lumen of a blood vessel. 2. (radiol.) (a) A lucent defect or obstruction within an opacified blood vessel presumed to represent an embolus in the pathologic sense. (b) An acutely dilated pulmonary artery presumed to represent the presence of blood clot or other embolic material. *Qualifiers:* acute, chronic; air, fat, amniotic fluid, parasitic, neoplastic, tissue, foreign material (*e.g.,* iodized oil, mercury, talc); septic, therapeutic, paradoxic.

In sense 2(a), an inferred conclusion based on reliable evidence (arteriography); in sense 2(b), based on highly suggestive evidence (conventional radiography) in the appropriate clinical setting. A useful descriptor, particularly in arteriography.

emphysema *n.* 1. (pathol.) (a) A morbid condition of the lung characterized by abnormally expanded air spaces distal to the terminal bronchiole, with or without destruction of the air-space walls (per Ciba Conference, 1959). (b) As above, but "with destruction of the walls of involved air spaces" specified (per World Health Organization, 1961, and American Thoracic Society [ATS], 1962). 2. (radiol.) Overinflation of all or a portion of one or both lungs, with or without associated oligemia *(q.v.),* presumed to represent morphologic emphysema.

In radiology, an inferred conclusion based on usually reliable signs (if the disease is moderate or advanced). Applicable only in an appropriate clinical setting and, in the sense of the ATS definition, not applicable to spasmodic asthma or compensatory overinflation.

fibrocalcific *adj.* (radiol.) Of or pertaining to sharply defined, linear, and/or nodular opacities containing cacification(s) *(q.v.),* usually occurring in the upper lobes and presumed to represent old granulomatous lesions.

A widely used and acceptable radiologic descriptor.

fibronodular *adj.* (radiol.) Of or pertaining to sharply defined, approximately circular opacities occurring singly or in clusters, usually in the upper lobes, and associated with linear opacities and distortion (retraction) of adjacent structures. A finding usually presumed to represent old granulomatous disease.

An inferred conclusion usually employed as a radiologic descriptor. Its use is not recommended.

fibrosis *n.* 1. (pathol.) (a) Cellular fibrous tissue or dense acellular collagenous tissue. (b) The process of proliferation of fibroblasts leading to the formation of fibrous or collagenous tissue. 2. (radiol.) Any opacity presumed to represent fibrous or collagenous tissue; applicable to linear, nodular, or stellate opacities that are sharply defined, that are associated with evidence of loss of volume in the affected portion of the lung and/or with deformity of adjacent structures, and that show no change over a period of months or years. Also applicable with caution to a diffuse pattern of opacity if there is evidence of progressive loss of lung volume or if the pattern of opacity is unchanged over time.

In radiology, an inferred conclusion often used as a descriptor. An acceptable term if used in strict accordance with the criteria cited.

fissure *n.* 1. (anat.) The infolding of visceral pleura that separates one lobe or a portion of a lobe from another. 2. (radiol.) A linear opacity normally 1 mm or less in width that corresponds in position and extent to the anatomic separation of pulmonary lobes or portions of lobes. *Qualifiers:* minor, major, horizontal, oblique, accessory, anomalous, azygos, inferior accessory.

Synonym: Interlobar septum.

A specific feature of anatomy.

Fleischner's line(s) *n.* (radiol.) A straight, curved, or irregular linear opacity that is visible in multiple projections; is usually situated in the lower half of the lung; is usually approximately horizontal but may be oriented in any direction; and may or may not appear to extend to the pleural surface. Such lines vary markedly in length and width; their exact pathologic significance is unknown.

An acceptable term. However, the term "linear opacity," properly qualified with respect to location, dimensions, and orientation, is preferred. There are no synonyms ("platelike," "discoid," and "platter" atelectasis should *not* be employed as synonyms; in the absence of clear histologic evidence of the significance of Fleischner's lines, the inferred identification of such lines with a form of atelectasis is unwarranted).

fluffy *adj.* (radiol.) In describing opacities: ill-defined, lacking clear-cut margins; resembling down.

Synonyms: Shaggy, poorly defined.

An imprecise descriptor of limited usefulness.

ground-glass pattern *n.* (radiol.) Any extended, finely granular pattern of pulmonary opacity within which normal anatomic details are partly obscured. Term derived from a fancied resemblance to etched or abraded glass.

Synonym: Granular pattern.

A nonspecific radiologic descriptor of limited usefulness; the synonym is preferred.

hernia *n.* (clin./morphol./radiol.) The protrusion of all or part of an organ or tissue through an abnormal opening.

An inferred conclusion to be used only within the precise terms of the definition. Thus, in the thorax the word is appropriate in relation to the diaphragm but should not be used with reference to pulmonary overinflation and mediastinal displacement.

hilum *n., pl.* -la. 1. (anat.) A depression or pit in that part of an organ where the vessels and nerves enter. 2. (radiol.) The composite shadow at the root of each lung composed of bronchi, pulmonary arteries and veins, lymph nodes, nerves, bronchial vessels, and associated areolar tissue.

Synonyms: Lung root; hilus (hili).

A specific element of pulmonary anatomy. Hilum (hila) is preferred to hilus (hili).

homogeneous *adj.* (radiol.) Of uniform opacity or texture throughout.

Antonyms: Inhomogeneous, nonhomogeneous, heterogeneous.

A useful radiologic descriptor. Inhomogeneous is the preferred antonym.

honeycomb pattern *n.* 1. (pathol.) A multitude of irregular cystic spaces in pulmonary tissue that are generally lined with bronchiolar epithelium and have markedly thickened walls composed of dense fibrous tissue, with or without associated chronic inflammation. 2. (radiol.) A number of closely approximated ring shadows representing air spaces 5 to 10 mm in diameter with walls 2 to 3 mm thick that resemble a true honeycomb; a finding whose occurrence implies "end-stage" lung.

It is recommended that on the radiograph the term be used strictly in accordance with the dimensional limits cited, in which case it possesses specific connotation.

hyperemia *n.* 1. (pathol./physiol.) An excess of blood in a part of the body; engorgement. 2. (radiol.) Increased blood flow.

Synonym: Pleonemia *(q.v.)*.

Although semantically correct, this word has come through common usage to mean the increased blood flow that is part of the inflammatory response. We recommend that it be used as a descriptor only in arteriography. The synonym is preferred when indicating increased blood flow to the lungs.

hypertension *n.* (clin./radiol.) Elevation above normal levels of systolic and/or diastolic pressure within the systemic or pulmonary vascular bed. Generally accepted empiric levels of pressure for systemic arterial hypertension are 140 systolic, 90 diastolic; systemic venous hypertension, 12 mm Hg; pulmonary arterial hypertension, 30 mm Hg systolic, 15 diastolic; pulmonary venous hypertension, 12 mm Hg.

Synonym: High blood pressure.

With the exception of systemic arterial hypertension, radiologic assessment of hypertension in each of the four vascular compartments constitutes an inferred conclusion, although based on usually reliable signs.

infarct *n.* (Literally, a portion of tissue stuffed with extravasated blood or serum.) 1. (pathol.) A zone of ischemic necrosis surrounded by hyperemic lung resulting from occlusion of the region's feeding vessel, usually by an embolus. 2. (radiol.) A pulmonary opacity that, by virtue of its temporal development and in the appropriate clinical setting, is considered to result from thromboembolic occlusion of a feeding vessel. The opacity is commonly but not exclusively hump shaped and pleural based when viewed in profile and poorly defined and round when viewed *en face.*

An inferred radiologic conclusion acceptable in the proper clinical setting and with appropriate signs. Subsequent events may establish that the opacity was the result of either hemorrhage or tissue necrosis. The word should not be used in the absence of an opacity (*e.g.,* with oligemia).

infiltrate *n.* 1. (pathophysiol.) Any substance or type of cell that occurs within or spreads through the interstices (interstitium and/or alveoli) of the lung, which is foreign to the lung or which accumulates in greater than normal quantity within it. 2. (radiol.) (a) An ill-defined opacity in the lung that neither destroys nor displaces the gross morphology of the lung and is presumed to represent an infiltrate in the pathophysiologic sense. (b) Any ill-defined opacity in the lung.

An inferred and often unwarranted conclusion used as a descriptor. The term is almost invariably used in sense 2(b), in which it serves no useful purpose, and, lacking a specific connotation, is so variably used as to cause great confusion. The term's use as a descriptor is to be condemned. The preferred word is "opacity," properly qualified with respect to location, dimensions, and definition.

inflation *n.* (physiol./radiol.) The state or process of being expanded or filled with gas; used specifically with reference to the expansion of the lungs with air. *Qualifiers:* overinflation (preferred) or hyperinflation; underinflation (preferred) or hypoinflation.

Synonyms: Aeration, inhalation, inspiration.

"Inflation" connotes expansion with gas or air. "Aeration" connotes the admission of air, exposure to air. "Inhalation" refers specifically to the act of drawing air into the lungs in the process of breathing (as opposed to exhalation); "inspiration," with reference to breathing, is similar in connotation. The word "inflation" is the preferred term, since it avoids the confusion that surrounds the meaning of aeration as a result of common misusage.

interface *n.* (radiol.) The common boundary between the shadows of two juxtaposed structures or tissues of different texture or opacity (*e.g.,* lung and heart).

Synonyms: Edge, border.

A useful radiologic descriptor.

interstitium *n.* (anat./radiol.) A continuum of loose connective tissue throughout the lung consisting of three subdivisions: (a) bronchoarterial (axial), surrounding the bronchoarterial bundles from the hila to the point at which bronchiolar walls become intimately related to lung parenchyma; (b) parenchymal (acinar), situated between alveolar and capillary basement membranes; and (c) subpleural, situated between the pleura and lung parenchyma and continuous with the interlobular septa and perivenous interstitial space that extends from the lung periphery to the hila.

Synonym: Interstitial space.

A useful anatomic term. The interstitium of the lung is not normally visible radiographically and only becomes visible when disease (*e.g.,* edema) increases its volume and attenuation.

Kerley line *n.* (radiol.) A linear opacity, which, depending on its location, extent, and orientation, may be further classified as follows: Kerley A line—an essentially straight linear opacity 2 to 6 cm in length and 1 to 3 mm in width, usually situated in an upper lung zone, that points toward the hilum centrally and is directed toward but does not extend to the pleural surface peripherally. Kerley B line—a straight linear opacity 1.5 to 2 cm in length and 1 to 2 mm in width, usually situated at the lung base, and oriented at right angles to the pleural surface with which it is usually in contact. Kerley C lines—a group of branching, linear opacities producing the appearance of a fine net, situated at the lung base and representing Kerley B lines seen *en face.*

Synonym: Septal line(s).

A specific feature of pathologic/radiologic anatomy. Except when it is essential to distinguish A, B, and C lines, the term "septal line" is preferred. "Lymphatic line" is anatomically inaccurate and should never be used.

line *n.* (radiol.) A longitudinal opacity no greater than 2 mm in width (*cf.* stripe).

A useful word appropriately employed in the description of radiographic shadows within the mediastinum (*e.g.,* anterior junction line) or lung (interlobar fissures).

linear opacity *n.* (radiol.) A shadow resembling a line; hence, any elongated opacity of approximately uniform width.

Synonyms: Line, line shadow, linear shadow, band shadow.

A generic radiologic descriptor of great usefulness. "Band shadow" and "line shadow" have been employed by some to identify elongated shadows more than 2 mm wide and less than 2 mm wide, respectively; "linear opacity," qualified by a statement of specific dimensions, is the preferred term. The length, width, anatomic location, and orientation of such a shadow should be specified.

lobe *n.* (anat./radiol.) One of the principal divisions of the lungs (usually three on the right, two on the left), each of which is enveloped by the visceral pleura except at the hilum and in areas of developmental deficiency where fissures are incomplete. The lobes are separated in whole or in part by pleural fissures.

A specific feature of pulmonary anatomy.

lobule *n.* (anat./radiol.) A unit of lung structure. A subdivision of lung parenchyma that is of two types: (a) primary, arising from the last respiratory bronchiole and consisting of a series of alveolar ducts, atria, alveolar sacs, and alveoli, together with their accompanying blood vessels and nerves; (b) secondary, composed of a variable number of acini (usually 3 to 5) and bounded in most cases by connective tissue septa.

Acinus is the preferred anatomic/physiologic unit of lung structure. Since a primary lobule is not visible radiographically, the use of the term has been largely abandoned. When unmodified, the word "lobule" refers to a secondary lobule. A secondary pulmonary lobule occasionally becomes visible when it is either selectively consolidated or its surrounding connective tissue septa become visible from a process such as edema.

lucency *n.* (radiol.) The shadow of an absorber that attenuates the primary x-ray beam less effectively than do surrounding absorbers. Hence, in a radiograph, any circumscribed area that appears more nearly black (of greater photometric density) than its surround. Usually applied to local shadows of air density whose attenuation is less than that of surrounding lung (*e.g.,* a bulla) or of fat density when surrounded by a more effective absorber such as muscle.

Synonyms: Radiolucency, translucency, transradiancy.

This term employed by analogy with "opacity," is acceptable in American usage, although it is etymologically indefensible. In British usage, "transradiancy" is preferred.

lymphadenopathy *n.* (clin./pathol./radiol.) Any abnormality of lymph nodes; by common usage usually restricted to enlargement of lymph nodes.

Synonym: Lymph node enlargement.

Since "adeno-" specifically relates to a glandular structure and since lymph nodes are not glands, the term is a misnomer and its use is to be condemned in favor of its synonym.

marking(s) *n.* (radiol.) A descriptor variously used with reference to the shadows produced by a combination of normal pulmonary structures (blood vessels, bronchi, etc.). Usually used in the plural and following "lung" or "bronchovascular."

Synonym: Linear opacity.

When used alone, a vague descriptor of little value and not recommended. With proper qualification, the term is acceptable.

mass *n.* (radiol.) Any pulmonary or pleural lesion represented in a radiograph by a discrete opacity greater than 30 mm in diameter (without regard to contour, border characteristics, or homogeneity), but explicitly shown or presumed to be extended in all three dimensions.

Synonym: Tumor *(q.v.).*

A useful and recommended descriptor. Should always be qualified with respect to size, location, contour, definition, homogeneity, opacity, and number. Its use as a qualifier of "lesion" is to be deplored.

medulla *n.* (radiol.) That portion of the lung situated between the hilum and cortex *(q.v.).*

A term and concept of limited usefulness.

miliary pattern *n.* (radiol.) A collection of tiny discrete opacities in the lungs, each measuring 2 mm or less in diameter, and generally uniform in size and widespread in distribution.

Synonym: Micronodular pattern.

An acceptable descriptor without etiologic connotation.

mucoid impaction *n.* (radiol.) A broad I-, Y-, or V-shaped radiographic opacity caused by the presence within a proximal airway (lobar, segmental, or subsegmental bronchus) of thick, tenacious mucus, usually associated with airway dilation. The shape of the opacity depends on the branching pattern of airway involved.

Synonym: Bronchocele *(q.v.).*

An inferred conclusion based on usually reliable signs. A useful descriptor preferred to its synonym.

Mueller maneuver *n.* (physiol.) Inspiration against a closed glottis, usually but not necessarily from a position of residual volume.

A useful technique for producing transient decrease in intrathoracic pressure.

nodular pattern *n.* (radiol.) A collection of innumerable, small discrete opacities ranging in diameter from 2 to 10 mm, generally uniform in size and widespread in distribution, and without marginal spiculation *(cf.* reticulonodular pattern).

An acceptable radiologic descriptor without specific pathologic or etiologic implications. The size of the nodules should be specified, either as a range or as an average.

nodule *n.* (radiol.) Any pulmonary or pleural lesion represented in a radiograph by a sharply defined, discrete, approximately circular opacity 2 to 30 mm in diameter *(cf.* mass).

Synonym: Coin lesion *(q.v.).*

A useful and recommended descriptor to be used in preference to its synonym, which is a colloquial abomination. Should always be qualified with respect to size, location, border characteristics, number, and opacity.

oligemia *n.* 1. (pathol./physiol.) Reduced blood flow to the lungs or a portion thereof. 2. (radiol.) General or local decrease in the apparent width of visible pulmonary vessels, suggesting less than normal blood flow. *Qualifiers:* acute, chronic; local, general.

Synonym: Reduced blood flow.

An inferred conclusion usually used as descriptor and appropriately based on reliable signs. An acceptable term.

opacity *n.* (radiol.) The shadow of an absorber that attenuates the x-ray beam more effectively than do surrounding absorbers. Hence, in a radiograph, any circumscribed area that appears more nearly white (of lesser photometric density) than its surround. Usually applied to the shadows of nonspecific pulmonary collections of fluid, tissue, etc., whose attenuation exceeds that of the surrounding aerated lung.

Synonym: Radiopacity (*cf.* density).

An essential and recommended radiologic descriptor. In the context of radiologic reporting, "radiopaque" is acceptable but seems redundant; however, it is preferred in British usage. "Density" *(q.v.)* should *never* be used in this context.

opaque *adj.* (radiol.) Impervious to x-rays.

Synonym: Radiopaque.

Opaque and radiopaque are both acceptable terms, although the former is preferred (*see* opacity).

ossification *n.* (radiol.) Calcific opacities within the lung that represent trabecular bone; applicable to calcific opacities that either display morphologic characteristics of trabecular bone (trabeculation and defined cortex) or occur in association with a lesion known histologically to produce trabecular bone within lung (*e.g.,* mitral stenosis).

Synonyms: Ossific nodulation, ossific nodule(s).

A useful radiologic term, although usually an inferred conclusion. To be distinguished from "calcification" *(q.v.).*

paraspinal line *n.* (radiol.) A vertically oriented interface usually seen in a frontal chest radiograph to the left (rarely to the right) of the thoracic vertebral column. It extends from the aortic arch to the diaphragm and represents contact between aerated lower lobe and adjacent mediastinal tissues. The anatomic interface is situated posterior to the descending aorta and is seen between the left lateral margin of the aorta and the spine.

Synonyms: Left paraspinal pleural reflection; left paraspinal interface.

A specific feature of radiologic anatomy. Either of the synonyms cited is preferred inasmuch as the shadow represents an interface, not a line.

parenchyma *n.* 1. (anat.) The gas-exchanging portion of the lung consisting of the alveoli and their capillaries, estimated to comprise approximately 90% of total lung volume. 2. (radiol.) All lung tissue exclusive of visible pulmonary vessels and airways.

A useful anatomic concept and an acceptable radiologic descriptor.

perfusion *n.* (physiol./radiol.) The passage of blood into and out of the lung.

Synonym: Pulmonary blood flow.

A useful and recommended term.

phantom tumor *n.* (radiol.) A shadow produced by a local collection of fluid in one of the interlobar fissures (most often the minor fissure), usually possessing an elliptic configuration in one radiographic projection and a rounded configuration in the other, thus resembling a tumor. It is commonly caused by cardiac decompensation and usually disappears with appropriate therapy.

Synonyms: Vanishing tumor, pseudotumor.

An explicit diagnostic conclusion from serial radiographs but only an inferred conclusion from a single examination. An acceptable descriptor.

platelike atelectasis *n.* (radiol.) A linear or planar opacity presumed to represent diminished volume in a portion of the lung; usually situated in lower lung zones.

Synonyms: Platter, linear, or discoid atelectasis.

An inferred conclusion usually not subject to proof and often unwarranted. Its use as a descriptor is not recommended. "Linear opacity" is preferred.

pleonemia *n.* (pathol./physiol./radiol.) Increased blood flow to the lungs or a portion thereof, manifested radiologically by a general or local increase in the width of visible pulmonary vessels.

Synonyms: Increased blood flow, hyperemia.

An inferred conclusion often used as a descriptor and based on usually reliable signs. An acceptable term preferable to hyperemia *(q.v.).*

pneumatocele *n.* (pathol./radiol.) A thin-walled, gas-filled space within the lung usually occurring in association with acute pneumonia (most commonly of staphylococcal etiology) and almost invariably transient.

An inferred conclusion. An acceptable descriptor if used in accordance with the precise definition.

pneumomediastinum *n.* (pathol./radiol.) A state characterized by the presence of gas in mediastinal tissues outside the esophagus, tracheobronchial tree, or pericardium. *Qualifiers:* spontaneous, traumatic, diagnostic.

Synonym: Mediastinal emphysema.

An appropriate descriptor based on radiologic signs alone; preferred to its synonym.

pneumonia *n.* (pathol./radiol.) Infection (or noninfectious inflammation) of the air spaces and/or interstitium of the lung. *Qualifiers* may be employed to indicate temporal course (acute, chronic), predominant anatomic involvement (air-space or lobar, interstitial, bronchial), or etiology (bacterial, viral, fungal).

Synonym: Pneumonitis.

An inferred conclusion based on usually reliable signs. Generally preferred to its synonym, although the latter is sometimes used to designate infection caused by viruses or *Mycoplasma pneumoniae*.

pneumothorax *n.* (pathol./radiol.) A state characterized by the presence of gas within the pleural space. *Qualifiers:* spontaneous, traumatic, diagnostic, tension *(q.v.).*

A diagnostic conclusion appropriately based on radiologic evidence alone.

popcorn calcification *n.* (radiol.) A cluster of sharply defined, irregularly lobulated, calcific opacities, usually within a pulmonary nodule, suggesting the appearance of popcorn.

An acceptable descriptor.

posterior junction line *n.* (radiol.) A vertically oriented, linear or curvilinear opacity approximately 2 mm wide, commonly projected on the tracheal air shadow, and usually slightly concave to the right. It is produced by the shadows of the right and left pleurae in intimate contact between the aerated lungs. It represents the plane of contact between the lungs posterior to the trachea and esophagus and anterior to the spine; hence, in contrast to the anterior junction line, it may project both above and below the suprasternal notch.

Synonyms: Posterior mediastinal septum; posterior mediastinal line; supra-aortic posterior junction line or stripe; mesentery of the esophagus.

A specific feature of radiologic anatomy; to be preferred to cited synonyms.

posterior tracheal stripe *n.* (radiol.) A vertically oriented linear opacity ranging in width from 2 to 5 mm, extending from the thoracic inlet to the bifurcation of the trachea, and visible only on lateral radiographs of the chest. It is situated between the air shadow of the trachea and the right lung and is formed by the posterior tracheal wall and contiguous mediastinal interstitial tissue.

Synonym: Posterior tracheal band.

A specific feature of radiologic anatomy; to be preferred to its synonym.

primary complex *n.* 1. (pathol.) The combination of a focus of pneumonia due to a primary infection (*e.g.,* tuberculosis or histoplasmosis) with granulomas in the draining hilar or mediastinal lymph nodes. 2. (radiol.) (a) One or more irregular opacities of variable extent and location assumed to represent consolidation of lung parenchyma associated with enlargement of hilar or mediastinal lymph nodes, an appearance presumed to represent active infection. (b) One or more small, sharply defined parenchymal opacities (often calcified) associated with calcification of hilar or mediastinal lymph nodes, an appearance usually regarded as evidence of an inactive process.

A useful inferred conclusion. "Primary complex" is to be preferred to "Ranke complex," which is acceptable but rarely used. "Ghon complex" represents an inappropriate use of the eponym and is unacceptable (Ghon described the pulmonary abnormality alone, which thus becomes a Ghon focus or Ghon lesion).

profusion *n.* (radiol.) The number of small opacities per unit area or zone of lung. In the International Labor Association (ILO) classification of radiographs of the pneumoconioses, the qualifiers 0 through 3 subdivide the profusion into 4 categories. The profusion categories may be further subdivided by employing a 12-point scale.

A useful word to describe the number of opacities in any diffuse disease, including the pneumoconioses.

pseudocavity *n.* (radiol.) A state in which a pulmonary nodule or mass possesses a central portion that is more lucent than its periphery (thus suggesting cavitation) but in which subsequent computed tomography or pathologic examination reveals only the presence of necrotic tissue high in lipid content, with no true cavity.

Synonym: Simulated cavity.

An inferred conclusion sometimes used as a descriptor. The term is without etiologic connotation.

pulmonary edema *n.* 1. (pathophysiol.) The accumulation of liquid in the interstitial compartment of the lung with or without associated alveolar filling. Specifically, the accumulation of water, protein, and solutes (transudate), usually due to one or a combination of the following: (a) increased pressure in the microvascular bed, (b) increased microvascular permeability, or (c) impaired lymphatic drainage. Also, the accumulation of water, protein, solutes, and inflammatory cells (exudate) in response to inflammation of any type (*e.g.,* infection, allergy, trauma, or circulating toxins). 2. (radiol.) A pattern of opacity (usually bilaterally symmetrical) believed to represent interstitial thickening or alveolar filling when associated findings and/or history suggest one of the processes enumerated above. *Qualifiers:* interstitial, air-space, alveolar.

Synonyms: Wet, boggy, or moist lung.

An inferred conclusion often employed as a descriptor, based on usually reliable signs. A useful and acceptable term when used in an appropriate clinical setting. The synonyms are colloquialisms to be avoided.

respiratory failure *n.* (physiol.) A state characterized by an arterial P_{O_2} below 60 mm Hg or an arterial P_{CO_2} above 49 mm Hg, at rest at sea level, resulting from impaired respiratory function.

Synonym: Pulmonary insufficiency.

A useful term that should be restricted to clinical and physiologic usage. It is preferred to its synonym.

reticular pattern *n.* (radiol.) A collection of innumerable small linear opacities that together produce an appearance resembling a net. *Qualifiers:* fine, medium, coarse.

Synonym: Small irregular opacities (in the ILO classification of radiographs of the pneumoconioses).

A recommended descriptor that usually indicates predominant abnormality of the pulmonary interstitium. The synonym should be restricted to the radiographic characterization of pneumoconiosis.

reticulonodular pattern *n.* (radiol.) A collection of innumerable small, linear, and nodular opacities that together produce a composite appearance resembling a net with small superimposed nodules. In common usage, the reticular and nodular elements are dimensionally of similar magnitude. *Qualifiers:* fine, medium, coarse.

An acceptable radiologic descriptor that usually indicates predominant abnormality of the pulmonary interstitium.

right tracheal stripe *n.* (radiol.) A vertically oriented linear opacity approximately 2 to 3 mm wide extending from the thoracic inlet to the right tracheobronchial angle. It is situated between the air shadow of the trachea and the right lung and is formed by the right tracheal wall and contiguous mediastinal interstitial tissue and pleura.

Synonym: Right paratracheal stripe or band.

A specific feature of radiologic anatomy; to be preferred to the cited synonym since the opacity is caused chiefly by the tracheal wall itself.

segment *n.* (anat./radiol.) One of the principal anatomic subdivisions of the pulmonary lobes served by a major branch of a lobar bronchus. *Qualifier:* bronchopulmonary.

A useful anatomic and radiologic descriptor.

septal line(s) *n.* (radiol.) Usually used in the plural, a generic term for linear opacities of varied distribution produced when the interstitium between pulmonary lobules is thickened (*e.g.,* by fluid, dust deposition, cellular material).

Synonym: Kerley line (*q.v.*).

A specific feature of radiologic pathology, sometimes inferred. A recommended term. "Kerley line" is acceptable, particularly when seeking to identify a particular type of septal line (*e.g.,* Kerley B line).

shadow *n.* (radiol.) In clinical radiography, any perceptible discontinuity in film blackening (or fluoroscopic image of CRT display) attributed to the attenuation of the x-ray beam by a specific anatomic absorber or lesion on or within the body of the patient; an opacity or lucency. The word should always be qualified as precisely as possible with respect to size, contour, location, opacity, lucency, and so on.

A useful and recommended descriptor to be employed only when more specific identification is not possible.

silhouette sign *n.* (radiol.) 1. The effacement of an anatomic soft tissue border by either a normal anatomic structure (*e.g.,* the inferior border of the heart and left hemidiaphragm) or a pathologic state such as airlessness of adjacent lung or accumulation of fluid in the contiguous pleural space. 2. A sign of conformity, and hence, of the probable adjacency of a pathologic opacity to a known structure.

Useful in detecting and localizing an opacity along the axis of the x-ray beam. Although the physical basis underlying the production of this sign is contentious, the term is a widely accepted and useful descriptor. Despite the fact that the definition implies *loss* of silhouette, the term has acquired such common popularity that its continued use is recommended.

small irregular opacities *n.* (radiol.) A collection of innumerable small linear opacities that together produce an appearance resembling a net. In the ILO 1980 classification of radiographs of the pneumoconioses, the qualifiers s, t, and u subdivide the dimensions of the opacities into three diameter ranges—up to 1.5 mm, 1.5 to 3 mm, and 3 to 10 mm, respectively.

Synonym: Reticular pattern *(q.v.).*

A term to be employed specifically to describe radiographic manifestations of the pneumoconioses; the synonym is preferred for nonpneumoconiotic disease.

small rounded opacities *n.* (radiol.) A collection of innumerable pulmonary nodules ranging in diameter from bare visibility up to 10 mm, usually widespread in distribution. In the ILO 1980 classification of radiographs of the pneumoconioses, the qualifiers p, q, and r subdivide the dimensions of the opacities into three diameter ranges—up to 1.5 mm, 1.5 to 3 mm, and 3 to 10 mm, respectively.

Synonym: Nodular pattern *(q.v.).*

A term to be employed specifically to describe radiographic manifestations of the pneumoconioses; the synonym is preferred for nonpneumoconiotic disease.

stripe *n.* (radiol.) A longitudinal composite opacity measuring 2 to 5 mm in width (*cf.* line).

An acceptable descriptor when limited to anatomic structures within the mediastinum (*e.g.,* right tracheal stripe).

subsegment *n.* (anat./radiol.) A unit of pulmonary tissue supplied by a bronchus of lesser order than a segmental bronchus.

A useful anatomic and radiologic descriptor.

tension *adj.* 1. (physiol./clin.) When used with reference to pneumothorax or hydrothorax, a state characterized by cardiorespiratory functional impairment. 2. (radiol.) The accumulation of gas or fluid in a pleural space in an amount sufficient to cause airlessness of the ipsilateral lung, marked depression of the ipsilateral hemidiaphragm, and displacement of the mediastinum to the opposite side.

An inferred conclusion to be used only in the presence of clinical cardiorespiratory embarrassment. The word should not be employed as in the term "tension cyst," which does not satisfy the criteria cited.

thromboembolism *n.* (pathol./clin./radiol.) Partial or complete occlusion of the lumen of a blood vessel by a thrombus *(q.v.).*

An inferred conclusion sometimes based on reliable signs (in conventional radiography) or a diagnostic conclusion based on radiologic evidence alone (in angiography).

thrombosis *n.* (pathol./radiol.) The state or process of thrombus formation within a blood vessel or heart chamber.

Cf. clot.

thrombus *n.* (pathol./radiol.) A mass of semisolidified blood, composed chiefly of platelets and fibrin with entrapped cellular elements, at the site of its formation in a blood vessel or heart chamber.

A useful descriptor to be employed only in the precise sense of the definition. (*Cf.* embolus.)

tramline shadow *n.* (radiol.) Parallel or slightly convergent linear opacities that suggest the planar projection of tubular structures and that correspond in location and orientation to elements of the bronchial tree. They are generally assumed to represent thickened bronchial walls.

Synonyms: Thickened bronchial wall, tubular shadow *(q.v.).*

A radiologic descriptor that is not recommended in deference to either of the synonyms. Such shadows are of possible pathologic significance only when they occur outside the limits of the hilar shadows where bronchial walls may be seen normally.

tubular shadow *n.* (radiol.) 1. Paired, parallel, or slightly convergent linear opacities presumed to represent the walls of a tubular structure seen *en face (e.g.,* a bronchus). 2. An approximately circular opacity presumed to represent the wall of a tubular structure seen end-on.

Synonyms: Tramline shadow *(q.v.),* thickened bronchial wall.

Acceptable if the anatomic nature of a shadow is obscure; otherwise, the more precise "thickened bronchial wall" is to be preferred.

tumor *n.* (general) 1. A swelling or morbid enlargement. 2. (pathol./radiol.) Literally, a mass *(q.v.),* not differentiated as to its neoplastic or nonneoplastic nature.

Synonym: Mass.

A useful descriptor, although "mass" is preferred. The use of the word as a synonym for neoplasm is to be condemned.

Valsalva maneuver *n.* (physiol.) Forced expiration against a closed glottis, usually but not necessarily from a position of total lung capacity.

A useful technique to produce transient increase in intrathoracic pressure.

vasoconstriction *n.* 1. (physiol.) Narrowing of muscular blood vessels by contraction of their muscle layer. 2. (radiol.) Local or general reduction in the caliber of visible pulmonary vessels (oligemia [*q.v.*]), presumed to result from decreased flow occasioned by contraction of muscular pulmonary arteries. *Qualifiers:* hypoxic, reflex.

An inferred conclusion based on usually reliable signs. The word is not synonymous with oligemia; although the latter is a *sign* of vasoconstriction, it may also occur when vessel narrowing is organic (as in emphysema) rather than functional and potentially reversible.

vasodilation *n.* (radiol.) The local or general increase in the width of visible pulmonary vessels resulting from increased pulmonary blood flow.

Synonym: Vasodilatation.

An inferred conclusion based on usually reliable signs.

ventilation *n.* (physiol./radiol.) The movement of air into and out of the lungs; inspiration and expiration. *Qualifiers:* hyperventilation (preferred), or overventilation; hypoventilation (preferred), or underventilation.

The term always implies a biphasic dynamic process of admission and expulsion; hence, it cannot be assessed from a single static image (*see* inflation).

TERMS FOR CT OF THE LUNGS

air crescent *n.* Air in a crescentic shape in a nodule or mass, in which the air separates the outer wall of the lesion from an inner sequestrum, which most commonly is a fungus ball of *Aspergillus* species.

air trapping *n.* 1. (pathophys.) The retention of excess gas ("air") in all or part of the lung, especially during expiration, either as a result of complete or partial airway obstruction or as a result of local abnormalities in pulmonary compliance. Although not in common usage, the term "gas trapping" is more accurate. 2. (CT.) Decreased attenuation of pulmonary parenchyma, especially manifest as less than normal increase in attenuation during expiration. To be differentiated from the decreased attenuation of hypoperfusion secondary to locally increased pulmonary arterial resistance.

architectural distortion *n.* A manifestation of lung disease in which bronchi, pulmonary vessels, a fissure or fissures, or septa of secondary pulmonary lobules are abnormally displaced.

band *n.* *See* parenchymal band.

beaded septum sign *n.* Irregular septal thickening that suggests the appearance of a row of beads; usually a sign of lymphangitic carcinomatosis, but may also occur rarely in sarcoidosis. Because the thickening usually is more irregular than beaded, the term "irregular septal thickening" generally is preferred.

bronchiectasis *n.* 1. (pathol.) Irreversible dilation of a bronchus or bronchi, often with thickening of the bronchial wall. When mild, the dilation is cylindric (*i.e.,* normal bronchial tapering is absent). When more severe, the dilation is saccular, and irregular constrictions may be present. When very severe, the bronchi may be markedly dilated, especially distally. *See also* traction bronchiectasis. 2. (CT.) Bronchial dilation, often with thickening of the wall.

bronchiolectasis *n.* 1. (pathol.) Dilation of a bronchiole or bronchioles, often with thickening of the bronchiolar wall. 2. (CT.) Bronchiolar dilation. *See also* traction bronchiolectasis.

bulla *n. pl.* -lae 1. (pathol.) A sharply demarcated, dilated air space that measures 1 cm or more in diameter and possesses a thin epithelialized wall, which is usually no greater than 1 mm in thickness. *See also* bullous emphysema, emphysema, and paraseptal emphysema. 2. (CT.) A round, focal air space, 1 cm or more in diameter, demarcated by a thin wall; usually multiple or associated with other signs of pulmonary emphysema.

bullous emphysema *n.* Emphysema characterized by the presence of bullae. *See* emphysema.

centriacinar emphysema *n.* *See* centrilobular emphysema.

centrilobular *adj.* Referring to the region of the bronchioloarteriolar core of a secondary pulmonary lobule. *See* centrilobular structures.

centrilobular emphysema *n.* 1. (pathol.) Emphysema that is characterized by destroyed centrilobular alveolar septa and enlargement of respiratory bronchioles. Usually in the upper lung zones of cigarette smokers. 2. (CT.) Centrilobular decreased attenuation, usually without visible walls, of nonuniform distribution, and predominantly located in upper lung zones.

Synonym: centriacinar emphysema.

centrilobular structures *n.* 1. (anat.) The central tubular structures in a secondary pulmonary lobule (*i.e.,* the centrilobular artery and bronchiole). 2. (CT.) The pulmonary artery and its immediate branches in a secondary lobule; these arteries measure approximately 1 mm and 0.5 to 0.7 mm in diameter, respectively; HRCT depicts these vessels. However, a normal bronchiole supplying a secondary lobule has a wall thickness of approximately 0.15 mm, which is beyond the resolution of HRCT. Therefore, normal airways in secondary pulmonary lobules are not detected at CT examination.

consolidation *n.* 1. (pathol.) Transudate, exudate, or tissue replacing alveolar air. 2. (CT.) Homogeneous increase in pulmonary parenchymal attenuation that obscures the margins of vessels and airway walls. An air bronchogram may be present.

core structures *n.* *See* centrilobular structures.

cyst *n.* 1. (pathol.) A round, circumscribed space that is surrounded by an epithelial or fibrous wall of thickness, which may be uniform or varied, and that in the lung usually contains air but may contain liquid, semisolid, or solid material. 2. (CT.) A round, parenchymal space with a well-defined wall; usually air-containing when in the lung but without associated pulmonary emphysema; commonly used to describe enlarged air spaces in end-stage fibrosis of idiopathic pulmonary fibrosis and sarcoidosis, and also in Langerhans' cell histiocytosis and lymphangiomyomatosis. *See* bulla, cystic air space, and honeycomb cysts.

cystic air space *n.*   Enlarged unit of peripheral air-containing lung, surrounded by a wall of variable thickness, which may be thin as in lymphangiomyomatosis, or thick as in idiopathic pulmonary fibrosis. *See* bulla, cyst, and honeycomb cysts.

dependent increased attenuation *n.*
See dependent opacity.

dependent opacity *n.*   Subpleural increased attenuation in dependent lung. The increased attenuation disappears when the region of lung is nondependent. May also appear as a subpleural line.

distal acinar emphysema *n.*   1. (pathol.) Emphysema characterized by predominant involvement of alveolar ducts and sacs, characteristically in subpleural lung and adjacent to interlobular septa and vessels. 2. (CT.) Emphysema characterized by subpleural regions of low attenuation or bullae separated by intact interlobular septa.
Synonym: paraseptal emphysema.

distortion *n.*   *See* architectural distortion.

emphysema *n.*   1. (pathol.) Permanently enlarged air spaces distal to the terminal bronchiole, accompanied by destroyed alveolar walls. Absence of "obvious fibrosis" historically has been regarded as an additional criterion, but the validity of that criterion recently has been called into question. 2. (CT.) Focal region or regions of low attenuation, usu-

ally without visible walls, resulting from actual or perceived enlarged air spaces and destroyed alveolar walls. May be associated with air trapping. *See also* bulla, bullous emphysema, centrilobular emphysema, cyst, cystic air space, distal acinar emphysema, panlobular emphysema, and paraseptal emphysema.

fungus ball *n.*   A masslike collection of intertwined hyphae, usually *Aspergillus* species, matted together by mucus, fibrin, and cellular debris and colonizing a pulmonary cavity caused by prior disease (*e.g.,* sarcoidosis). May move to a dependent location when the patient changes position. At CT, may show a "spongework" pattern, including foci of high attenuation.
Synonym: mycetoma.

gas trapping *n.*   *See* air trapping.

ground-glass attenuation *n.*   *See* ground-glass opacity.

ground-glass opacity *n.*   Hazy increased attenuation of lung, but with preservation of bronchial and vascular margins; caused by partial filling of air spaces, interstitial thickening, partial collapse of alveoli, normal expiration, or increased capillary blood volume. Not to be confused with "consolidation," in which bronchovascular margins are obscured. May be associated with an air bronchogram.

halo sign *n.*   Ground-glass opacity surrounding the circumference of a nodule or mass. May be a sign of invasive aspergillosis or hemorrhage of various causes.

honeycomb cysts *n.*   Cystic air spaces, usually of comparable diameter and on the order of 0.3 to 1.0 cm in diameter, formed by the honeycombing of interstitial pulmonary fibrosis.

honeycombing *n.*   1. (pathol.) Destroyed, fibrotic, and cystic lung, representing complete loss of acinar and bronchiolar architecture as the end stage of fibrosing lung

disease. 2. (CT.) Clustered cystic air spaces, usually of comparable diameters on the order of 0.3 to 1.0 cm but as much as 2.5 cm, usually subpleural and characterized by well-defined walls, which are often thick. A CT feature of diffuse pulmonary fibrosis. A diagnostic pitfall is that, in the presence of underlying pulmonary emphysema, air-space consolidation can mimic this appearance.

interlobular septal thickening *n.*
See septal line.

intralobular lines *n.*   Fine linear opacities present in a lobule when the intralobular interstitium is thickened. When numerous, they may appear as a fine reticular pattern.

irregular linear opacity *n.*   Any linear opacity or irregular thickness of 1 to 3 mm, distinct from interlobular septa, bronchovascular bundles, and nodular opacities. May be intralobular or extend through several adjacent secondary lobules.

linear opacity *n.*   An elongated, thin line of soft tissue attenuation. Rarely, calcification or foreign material may increase the attenuation. *See also* irregular linear opacity and subpleural line.

lobular core structures *n.*   *See* centrilobular structures.

lobule *n.*   *See* secondary pulmonary lobule.

micronodule *n.*   Discrete, small, round, focal opacity of at least soft tissue attenuation and with a diameter no greater than 7 mm. Some authors have limited use of this term to a diameter of less than 5 mm or less than 3 mm. Other authors simply use the term "small nodule." *See* nodule.

midlung window *n.*   A midlung region, characterized by the absence of large blood vessels and by a paucity of small blood vessels, that corresponds to the minor fissure and adjacent peripheral lung.

mosaic oligemia *n.* *See* mosaic perfusion.

mosaic perfusion *n.* A patchwork of regions of varied attenuation, interpreted as secondary to regional differences in perfusion. A more inclusive term than the originally described "mosaic oligemia." Air trapping secondary to bronchial or bronchiolar obstruction may also produce focal zones of decreased attenuation, an appearance that can be enhanced by using expiratory CT.

mycetoma *n.* *See* fungus ball.

nodule *n.* 1. (pathol.) Small, approximately spherical, circumscribed focus of abnormal tissue. 2. (radiol.) Round opacity, at least moderately well marginated and no greater than 3 cm in maximum diameter. Some authors use the modifier "small" if the maximum diameter of the opacity is less than 1 cm. *See also* micronodule.

opacification *n.* *See* parenchymal opacification.

panacinar emphysema *n.* *See* panlobular emphysema.

panlobular emphysema *n.* 1. (pathol.) Emphysema that involves, more or less uniformly, all portions of the secondary lobules. It tends to predominate in the lower lobes and is the form of emphysema associated with hereditary α_1-protease inhibitor (α_1-antitrypsin) deficiency. 2. (CT.) Emphysema that tends to show rather uniformly decreased parenchymal attenuation and a paucity of vessels. Severe panlobular emphysema may be indistinguishable from severe centrilobular emphysema, except on the basis of zonal distribution.
Synonym: panacinar emphysema.

paraseptal emphysema *n.* *See* distal acinar emphysema.

parenchymal band *n.* Elongated opacity, usually several millimeters wide and up to about 5 cm long, often extending to the pleura, which may be thickened and retracted at the site of contact. Originally described in asbestosis, but also a sign of focal fibrosis of nonspecific cause.

parenchymal opacification *n.* Increase in pulmonary attenuation that may or may not obscure the margins of vessels and airway walls. "Consolidation" indicates that definition of these margins (excepting air bronchograms) is lost, whereas "ground-glass opacity" indicates a lesser increase in attenuation, in which definition of the margins is preserved. Whenever possible, use of the more specific terms "consolidation" or "ground-glass opacity" is preferred.

peripheral *n.* Referring to pulmonary structures within 1 to 2 cm of any visceral pleural surface. *See also* subpleural.

pseudoplaque *n.* An irregular band of peripheral pulmonary opacity adjacent to visceral pleura that simulates the appearance of a pleural plaque and is formed by the coalescence of small nodules (*e.g.,* in coal-worker's pneumoconiosis).

reticular pattern *n.* *See* reticulation.

reticulation *n.* Innumerable, interlacing line shadows that suggest a mesh. A descriptive term usually associated with interstitial lung diseases. May be fine, intermediate, or coarse.
Synonym: reticular pattern.

secondary pulmonary lobule *n.* 1. (anat.) The smallest unit of lung surrounded by connective tissue septa. These septa, known as "interlobular septa," are best developed in the periphery of the anterior, lateral, and juxtamediastinal regions of the upper and middle lobes, and in the periphery of the

anterior and diaphragmatic regions of the lower lobes. The septa tend to be incompletely developed or absent elsewhere in the lungs. Miller's lobule ranges in size from 0.5 to 3.0 cm and may contain 3 to 20 acini. 2. (anat.) The unit of lung subtended by any bronchiole that gives off three to five terminal bronchioles. Connective tissue septa are not part of this definition. A small Miller's lobule (0.5 cm) corresponds to a Reid's lobule. 3. (CT.) Miller's lobule is the secondary lobule that is identified with CT. *See also* centrilobular structures.

septal line *n.* Thin linear opacity that corresponds to an interlobular septum; to be distinguished from centrilobular structures. *See* septal thickening.

septal thickening *n.* Abnormal widening of an interlobular septum or septa, usually caused by edema, cellular infiltration, or fibrosis. May be smooth, irregular, or nodular. *See also* beaded septum sign.

signet-ring sign *n.* A ring of opacity (usually representing a dilated, thick-walled bronchus) in association with a smaller, round, soft tissue opacity (the adjacent pulmonary artery or, rarely, dilated bronchial artery) suggesting a "signet ring." Usually this finding indicates bronchiectasis, but it may also occur in multifocal bronchioloalveolar carcinoma and metastatic adenocarcinoma.

subpleural *adj.* Referring to pulmonary structures that are next to or near visceral pleura.

subpleural line *n.* A thin curvilinear opacity, a few millimeters or less in thickness, usually less than 1 cm from the pleural surface and paralleling the pleura. A nonspecific indicator of atelectasis, edema, fibrosis, or inflammation. *See also* irregular linear opacity.

traction bronchiectasis *n.* Bronchial dilation, which is commonly irregular, in association with juxtabronchial opacification that is interpreted as representing retractile pulmonary fibrosis.

traction bronchiolectasis *n.* Bronchiolar dilation in association with peribronchiolar opacification that is interpreted as representing retractile pulmonary fibrosis.

tree-in-bud sign *n.* Nodular dilation of centrilobular branching structures that resembles a budding tree and represents exudative bronchiolar dilation (*e.g.,* in panbronchiolitis or endobronchial spread of active pulmonary tuberculosis).

TERMS AND SYMBOLS USED IN RESPIRATORY PHYSIOLOGY AND PATHOPHYSIOLOGY

GENERAL SYMBOLS

P	Pressure, in blood or gas.
$\dot{X}$	A time derivative indicated by a dot above the symbol (rate). This symbol is used for both instantaneous flow and volume per unit time.
%X	Percent sign *preceding* a symbol indicates percentage of the predicted normal value.
X/Y%	Percent sign *following* a symbol indicates a ratio function with the ratio expressed as a percentage. Both components of the ratio must be designated; *e.g.,* $FEV_1/FVC\% = 100 \times FEV_1/FVC$.
XA or Xa	A small capital letter or lower case letter on the same line following a primary symbol is a qualifier to further define the primary symbol. When small capital letters are not available, large capital letters may be used as subscripts; e.g., $X_A = XA$.

GAS PHASE SYMBOLS

Primary Symbols (Large Capital Letters)

V	Gas volume. The particular gas as well as its pressure, water vapor conditions, and other special conditions must be specified in text or indicated by appropriate qualifying symbols.
F	Fractional concentration of gas.

Common Qualifying Symbols

I	Inspired.
E	Expired.
A	Alveolar.
T	Tidal.
D	Dead space or wasted ventilation.
B	Barometric.
L	Lung.
STPD	Standard conditions: Temperature 0 degrees Celsius, pressure 760 mm Hg, and dry (0 water vapor).
BTPS	Body conditions: Body temperature, ambient pressure, and saturated with water vapor at these conditions.
ATPD	Ambient temperature and pressure, dry.
ATPS	Ambient temperature and pressure, saturated with water vapor at these conditions.
an	Anatomic.
p	Physiologic.
rb	Rebreathing.
f	Respiratory frequency per minute.
max	Maximal.
t	Time.

BLOOD PHASE SYMBOLS

Primary Symbols (Large Capital Letters)

Q	Blood volume.
$\dot{Q}$	Blood flow, volume units, and time must be specified.
C	Concentration in the blood phase.
S	Saturation in the blood phase.

Qualifying Symbols (Lower Case Letters)

b	Blood in general.

a   Arterial.

c   Capillary.

ć   Pulmonary end-capillary.

v   Venous.

$\bar{v}$ Mixed venous.

VENTILATION AND LUNG MECHANICS TESTS AND SYMBOLS

Lung Volume Compartments*

RV   Residual volume; that volume of air remaining in the lungs after maximal exhalation. The method of measurement should be indicated in the text or, when necessary, by appropriate qualifying symbols.

ERV   Expiratory reserve volume; the maximal volume of air exhaled from the end-expiratory level.

V_T Tidal volume; that volume or air inhaled or exhaled with each breath during quiet breathing, used only to indicate a subdivision of lung volume.

IRV   Inspiratory reserve volume; the maximal volume of air inhaled from the end-inspiratory level.

IC   Inspiratory capacity; the sum of IRV and V_T.

IVC   Inspiratory vital capacity; the maximal volume of air inhaled from the point of maximal expiration.

VC   Vital capacity; the maximal volume of air exhaled from the point of maximal inspiration.

FRC   Functional residual capacity; the sum of RV and ERV (the volume of air remaining in the lungs at the end-expiratory position). The method of measurement should be indicated, as with RV.

TLC   Total lung capacity; the sum of all volume compartments or the volume of air in the lungs after maximal inspiration. The method of measurement should be indicated, as with RV.

RV/ TLC%   Residual volume to total lung capacity ratio, expressed as a percentage.

CV   Closing volume; the volume exhaled after the expired gas concentration is inflected from an alveolar plateau during a controlled breathing maneuver. Since the value obtained is dependent on the specific test technique, the method used must be designated in the text and, when necessary, specified by a qualifying symbol. Closing volume is often expressed as a ratio of the VC, *i.e.,* CV/VC%.

CC   Closing capacity; closing volume plus residual volume, often expressed as a ratio of TLC, i.e., CC/TLC%.

VL   Actual volume of the lung, including the volume of the conducting airways.

V_A Alveolar gas volume.

Forced Spirometry Measurements*

FVC   Forced vital capacity; vital capacity performed with a maximally forced expiratory effort.

FIVC   Forced inspiratory vital capacity; the maximal volume of air inspired with a maximally forced effort from a position of maximal expiration.

FEVt   Forced expiratory volume (timed). The volume of air exhaled in the specified time during the performance of the forced vital capacity; *e.g.,* FEV_1 for the volume of air exhaled during the first second of the FVC.

FEVt/ FVC%   Forced expiratory volume (timed) to forced vital capacity ratio, expressed as a percentage.

FEF_{25-75} Mean forced expiratory flow during the middle of the FVC (formerly called the "maximal midexpiratory flow rate").

PEF   The highest forced expiratory flow measured with a peak flow meter.

$\dot{V}max_X$ Forced expiratory flow, related to the total lung capacity or the vital capacity of the lung at which the measurement is made. *Modifiers refer to the amount of lung volume remaining when the measurement is made.* For example: $\dot{V}max_{75}$ = Instantaneous forced expiratory flow when the lung is at 75% of its TLC.

$\dot{V}max_{50}$ Instantaneous forced expiratory flow when 50% of the vital capacity remains to be exhaled.

$\dot{V}max_{Xp}$ Forced expiratory flow at "X" percentage of vital capacity on a partial flow volume curve, initiated from a volume below TLC.

MVV_x Maximal voluntary ventilation. The volume of air expired in a specified period during repetitive maximal respiratory effort.

---

*Primary components are designated as volumes. When volumes are combined they are designated as capacities. All are considered to be at BTPS unless otherwise specified.

*All values are BTPS unless otherwise specified.

Measurements of Ventilation

$\dot{V}_E$ — Expired volume per minute (BTPS).

$\dot{V}_I$ — Inspired volume per minute (BTPS).

$\dot{V}_{CO_2}$ — Carbon dioxide production per minute (STPD).

$\dot{V}_{O_2}$ — Oxygen consumption per minute (STPD).

$\dot{V}_A$ — Alveolar ventilation per minute (BTPS).

V_D — The physiologic dead space volume defined as $\dot{V}_D/f$.

$\dot{V}_D$ — Ventilation per minute of the physiologic dead space (wasted ventilation), BTPS, defined by the following equation:

$$\dot{V}_D = \dot{V}_E(Pa_{CO_2} - PE_{CO_2})/Pa_{CO_2}$$

V_{DAN} — Volume of the anatomic dead space (BTPS).

$\dot{V}_{DAN}$ — Ventilation per minute of the anatomic dead space, that portion of conducting airway in which no significant gas exchange occurs (BTPS).

V_{DA} — The alveolar dead space volume defined as $\dot{V}_{DA}/f$.

$\dot{V}_{DA}$ — Ventilation of the alveolar dead space (BTPS), defined by the following equation:

$$V_{DA} = V_D - V_{DAN}$$

MEASUREMENTS OF MECHANICS OF BREATHING*

Pressure Terms

Paw — Pressure in the airway, level to be specified.

Pao — Pressure at the airway opening.

Ppl — Intrapleural pressure.

P_A — Alveolar pressure.

P_L — Transpulmonary pressure.

Pbs — Pressure at the body surface.

P(A-ao) — Pressure gradient from alveolus to airway opening.

Pw — Transthoracic pressure.

---

*All pressures are expressed relative to ambient pressure and gases are at BTPS unless otherwise specified.

Ptm — Transmural pressure pertaining to an airway or blood vessel.

Pes — Esophageal pressure used to estimate Ppl.

Pga — Gastric pressure; used to estimate abdominal pressure.

Pdi — Transdiaphragmatic pressure; used to estimate the tension across the diaphragm.

Pdi Max — Maximal transdiaphragmatic pressure; used to measure the strength of diaphragmatic muscle contraction.

PI Max (also MIP) — Maximal inspiratory pressure; measured at the mouth, used to assess the strength of the inspiratory muscles.

PE Max (also MEP) — Maximal expiratory pressure; measured at the mouth, used to assess the strength of the expiratory muscles.

Flow-Pressure Relationships*

R — A general symbol for resistance, pressure per unit flow.

Raw — Airway resistance.

Rti — Tissue resistance.

RL — Total pulmonary resistance, measured by relating flow-dependent transpulmonary pressure to airflow at the mouth.

Rus — Resistance of the airways on the alveolar side (upstream) of the point in the airways where intraluminal pressure equals Ppl, measured under conditions of maximal expiratory flow.

Rds — Resistance of the airways on the oral side (downstream) of the point in the airways where intraluminal pressure equals Ppl, measured under conditions of maximal expiratory flow.

Gaw — Airway conductance, the reciprocal of Raw.

Gaw/VL — Specific conductance, expressed per liter of lung volume at which G is measured (also SGaw).

Volume-Pressure Relationships

C — A general symbol for compliance, volume change per unit of applied pressure.

Cdyn — Dynamic compliance, compliance measured at points of zero gas flow at the mouth during active breathing. The respiratory frequency should be designated; *e.g.,* $Cdyn_{40}$.

---

*Unless otherwise specified, the lung volume at which all resistance measurements are made is assumed to be FRC.

Cst	Static compliance, compliance determined from measurements made during conditions of interruption of air flow.
C/V_L	Specific compliance.
E	Elastance, pressure per unit of volume change, the reciprocal of compliance.
Pst	Static transpulmonary pressure at a specified lung volume; *e.g.*, PstTLC is static recoil pressure measured at TLC (maximal recoil pressure).
PstTLC/ TLC	Coefficient of lung reaction expressed per liter of TLC.
W	A general symbol for mechanical work of breathing, which requires use of appropriate qualifying symbols and description of specific conditions.
k	Exponential constant describing the shape of the lung pressure-volume curve ($V = A - B_e{}^{-kP}$).
A	Theoretical maximal lung volume at infinite transpulmonary pressure in $V = A - B_e{}^{-kP}$).
B	Difference between A and the lung volume at a P of zero in $V = A - B_e{}^{-kP}$).

Breathing Pattern

T_I	Inspiratory time.
T_E	Expiratory time.
T_{Tot}	Total respiratory cycle time.
T_I/T_{Tot}	Ratio of inspiratory to total respiratory cycle time—Duty cycle.
V_T	Tidal volume.
V_T/T_I	Mean inspiratory flow.
V_T/T_E	Mean expiratory flow.
V_E	$\dfrac{V_T \times T_I}{T_I \times T_{Tot}}$

DIFFUSING CAPACITY TESTS AND SYMBOLS

Dx	Diffusing capacity of the lung expressed as volume (STPD) of gas (x) uptake per unit alveolar-capillary pressure difference for the gas used. Unless otherwise stated, carbon monoxide is assumed to be the test gas; i.e., D is Dco. A modifier can be used to designate the technique: *e.g.*, Dsb is single breath carbon monoxide dif-

fusing capacity and Dss is steady state CO diffusing capacity.

D_M	Diffusing capacity of the alveolar capillary membrane (STPD).
θx	Reaction rate coefficient for red blood cells; the volume STPD of gas (x) that will combine per minute with 1 unit volume of blood per unit gas tension. If the specific gas is not stated, θ is assumed to refer to CO and is a function of existing O_2 tension.
Qc	Capillary blood volume (usually expressed as Vc in the literature, a symbol inconsistent with those recommended for blood volumes). When determined from the following equation, Qc represents the effective pulmonary capillary blood volume, *i.e.*, capillary blood volume in intimate association with alveolar gas:

$$\frac{1}{D} = \frac{1}{D_M} + \frac{1}{\theta \cdot Qc}$$

D/V_A	Diffusion per unit of alveolar volume with D expressed STPD and V_A expressed as liters BTPS. This method is preferred to the occasional practice of expressing both values STPD.

BLOOD GAS MEASUREMENTS*

Pa_{CO_2}	Arterial carbon dioxide tension.
Sa_{O_2}	Arterial oxygen saturation.
Cc'_{O_2}	Oxygen content of pulmonary end-capillary blood.
$P(A\text{-}a)_{O_2}$	Alveolar-arterial oxygen pressure difference. The previously used symbol, $A\text{-}aD_{O_2}$ is not recommended.
$C(a\text{-}\bar{v})_{O_2}$	Arteriovenous oxygen content difference.

PULMONARY SHUNTS

$\dot{Q}sp$	Physiologic shunt flow (total venous admixture) defined by the following equation when gas and blood gas data are collected during ambient air breathing:

$$\dot{Q}sp = \frac{Cc'_{O_2} - Ca_{O_2}}{Cc'_{O_2} - C\bar{v}_{O_2}} \cdot \dot{Q}$$

$\dot{Q}san$	A special case of $\dot{Q}sp$ (often called "anatomic shunt flow") defined by the above equation when

*Symbols for these measurements are readily composed by combining the general symbols recommended earlier.

blood and gas data are collected after sufficiently prolonged breathing of 100% O_2 to ensure an alveolar N_2 less than 1%.

$\dot{Q}s/\dot{Q}t$ The ratio $\dot{Q}sp$ or $\dot{Q}san$ to total cardiac output.

BRONCHIAL REACTIVITY

PC_{20} Provocative concentration of an inhaled agonist producing a 20% decrease in FEV_1.

PD_{20} Provocative dose of an inhaled agonist producing a 20% decrease in FEV_1.

$PD_{40}SGaw$ Provocative dose of an inhaled agonist producing a 40% decrease in SGaw.

Isocapnic hyperventilation (eucapnic hyperventilation) = "hyperventilation" with addition of CO_2 to the inspired air to keep end-tidal PCO_2 constant (Iso) and/or normal (Eu-). Used to assess bronchoconstrictive response to cold and/or dry air.

SLEEP STUDIES

Polysomnography	The evaluation during sleep of vital functions and a quantitative evaluation of sleep parameters overnight.
NREM	Nonrapid eye movement sleep.
REM	Rapid eye movement sleep.
Apnea	Cessation of air flow longer than 10 seconds.
Sleep apnea	The presence of 30 or more apneas in an overnight, 7-hour sleep study. (Apnea frequency > 4/hr.)
Obstructive apnea	Apnea with respiratory effort.
Central apnea	Apnea without respiratory effort.
Mixed apnea	Apnea initially without, but later with, respiratory effort.
Hypopnea	Reduced respiratory effort with associated decrease in arterial saturation.
Apnea index	Number of apneas divided by the total sleep time in hours.
Arousal	Short neurologic awakening.

PULMONARY DYSFUNCTION

Terms Related to Altered Breathing

Many terms are in use, such as tachypnea, hyperpnea, hypopnea, and so on. Simple descriptive terms, such as rapid, deep, or shallow, should be used instead.

Dyspnea	A subjective sensation of difficult or labored breathing.
Overventilation	A general term indicating excessive ventilation. When unqualified, it refers to "alveolar overventilation," excessive ventilation of the gas-exchanging areas of the lung manifested by a fall in arterial CO_2 tension. The term "total overventilation" may be used when the minute volume is increased regardless of the alveolar ventilation. (When there is increased wasted ventilation, total overventilation may occur when alveolar ventilation is normal or decreased.)
Underventilation	A general term indicating reduced ventilation. When otherwise unqualified, it refers to alveolar underventilation, decreased effective alveolar ventilation manifested by an increase in arterial CO_2 tension. (Overventilation and underventilation are recommended in place of hyperventilation and hypoventilation to avoid confusion when the words are spoken.)

Terms Describing Blood Gas Findings

Hypoxia	A term for reduced oxygenation.
Hypoxemia	A reduced blood oxygen content or tension.
Hypocarbia	(hypocapnia) A reduced arterial carbon dioxide tension.
Hypercarbia	(hypercapnia) An increased arterial carbon dioxide tension.

Terms Describing Acid-Base Findings

Acidemia	A pH less than normal; the value should always be given.
Alkalemia	A pH greater than normal; the value should always be given.
Hypobasemia	Blood bicarbonate level below normal.
Hyperbasemia	Blood bicarbonate level above normal.
Acidosis	A clinical term indicating a disturbance that can lead to acidemia. It usually is indicated by hypobasemia when metabolic (nonrespiratory) in origin and by hypercarbia when respiratory in origin. There may or may not be accompanying acidemia. The term should always be qualified as metabolic (nonrespiratory) or respiratory.

Alkalo-sis — A clinical term indicating a disturbance that can lead to alkalemia. It usually is indicated by hyperbasemia when metabolic (nonrespiratory) in origin and by hypocarbia when respiratory in origin. There may or may not be accompanying alkalemia. The term should always be qualified as metabolic (nonrespiratory) or respiratory.

Other Terms

Pulmonary insufficiency — Altered function of the lungs that produces clinical symptoms, usually including dyspnea.

Acute respiratory failure — Rapidly occurring hypoxemia or hypercarbia due to a disorder of the respiratory system. The duration of the illness and the values of arterial oxygen tension and arterial carbon dioxide tension used as criteria for this term should be given. The term "acute ventilatory failure" should be used only when the arterial carbon dioxide tension is increased. The term "pulmonary failure" has been used to indicate respiratory failure due specifically to disorders of the lungs.

Chronic respiratory failure — Chronic hypoxemia or hypercarbia due to a disorder of the respiratory system. The duration of the condition and the values of arterial oxygen tension and arterial carbon dioxide tension used as criteria for this term should be given.

Obstructive pattern — (Obstructive ventilatory defect) Slowing of air flow during forced ventilatory maneuvers.

Restrictive pattern — (Restrictive ventilatory defect) Reduction of vital capacity not explainable by airways obstruction.

Impairment — A measurable degree of anatomic or functional abnormality that may or may not have clinical significance. "Permanent impairment" is that which persists after maximal medical rehabilitation has been achieved.

Disability — A legally determined state in which a patient's ability to engage in a specific activity under a particular circumstance is reduced or absent because of physical or mental impairment. "Permanent disability" exists when no substantial improvement of the patient's ability to engage in the specific activity can be expected.

PART I

THE NORMAL CHEST

CHAPTER 1

The Airways and Pulmonary Ventilation

ANATOMY, 3
  The Conducting Zone, 3
    Geometry and Dimensions, 3
    Morphology and Cell Function, 5
      Epithelium, 5
      Submucosa and Lamina Propria, 12
  The Transitional Zone, 17
    Geometry and Dimensions, 17
    Morphology, 17
  The Respiratory Zone, 17
    Morphology and Cell Function, 17
    Geometry and Dimensions, 23
  The Lung Unit, 24
    The Primary Lobule, 24
    The Secondary Lobule, 24
    The Acinus, 26
  Channels of Peripheral Airway and Acinar Communication, 31
RADIOLOGY, 33
  The Trachea and Main Bronchi, 33
  The Lobar Bronchi and Bronchopulmonary Segments, 35
  Bronchial Anatomy on Computed Tomography, 46
FUNCTION, 51
  Pulmonary Ventilation, 51
    Ventilation of the Acinus, 53
    Alveolar-Capillary Gas Exchange, 53
    Mechanics of Acinar Ventilation, 53
    Elastic Recoil of the Lung Parenchyma and Thoracic Cage, 53
    Surface Tension and Surfactant, 54
      Surfactant Morphology, 56
      Surfactant Composition and Synthesis, 56
      Surfactant Function, 58
    Resistance of the Airways, 58
    Tissue Resistance, 59
    Collateral Ventilation, 59
  Respiratory Mucus and Mucous Rheology, 60
    Biochemical Characteristics of Tracheobronchial Secretions, 60
    Control of Tracheobronchial Secretion, 61
    Physical Characteristics of Tracheobronchial Secretions, 62

ANATOMY

The primary function of the airways is to conduct air to the alveolar surface, where gas transfer takes place between inspired air and the blood of the alveolar capillaries.[1-4] The trachea and bronchi (the walls of which contain cartilage) and membranous bronchioles carry out this function. The remainder of the respiratory system, which consists of the large bulk of the lungs, is concerned with both conduction and gas exchange, the terminal unit (the alveolus) being the only structure whose unique function is gas exchange. Thus the lungs can be subdivided into three zones, each with somewhat different but overlapping structural and functional characteristics.

The *conducting zone* is composed of airways whose walls do not contain alveoli and are thick enough that gas cannot diffuse into the adjacent lung parenchyma. It includes the trachea, bronchi, and membranous (nonalveolated) bronchioles, the latter defined structurally by the absence of mural cartilage. These airways, along with the pulmonary arteries and veins, lymphatic vessels, nerves, connective tissues of the peribronchial and perivascular spaces, interlobular septa, and pleura, constitute the nonparenchymal portion of the lung.

The *transitional zone*, as its name implies, carries out both conductive and respiratory functions. It consists of the respiratory bronchioles and alveolar ducts, each of which conducts air to the most peripheral portion of the lung. Alveoli that arise from the walls of these airways also serve in gas exchange.

The *respiratory zone* consists of the alveoli, whose primary function is the exchange of gases between air and blood. Together with the transitional zone, this tissue constitutes the lung *parenchyma*, the spongy respiratory portion of the lung. It has been estimated that approximately 87% of the total lung volume is alveolar, 6% of which is composed of tissue and the remainder of which is gas.[5]

The Conducting Zone

Geometry and Dimensions

The basic branching pattern of the conducting zone is dichotomous (i.e., the parent branch divides into two parts). Because there is variation in both branch diameter and the number of divisions, the system is one of asymmetric dichotomy. Two methods—presented by Strahler[6] and by Horsfield and Cumming[7]—have been used to describe airway geometry by counting proximally from small to larger airways. According to these methods, the terminal bronchiole is considered to be Order 1. When two of these join, they form a single branch (Order 2); when two of Order 2 join, they form an Order 3; and so on. (For the sake of clarity, "generation" is applied to divisions counted distally from the trachea and "order" to divisions counted proximally.) Difficulties in counting arise when branches of two orders join, and it is at this point that the systems differ. In the Strahler system (Fig. 1–1), the larger number continues unchanged when different orders join, thereby providing little information about the total number of branching points; by contrast, in the Horsfield-Cumming system (Fig. 1–1) the larger order number increases by 1. Thus the segment proximal to the junction of the second-order and sixth-order branch would be the sixth order according to the Strahler system and the seventh order according to the Horsfield-Cumming system.

Several investigators have analyzed the geometry and dimensions of the conducting system by inflating the lungs with plastic, polyester resin, or silicone rubber and taking detailed measurements of the resulting casts.[6–12] Although the results of these studies have been extensively used in lung modeling, it is important to note that they come from a very small number of lungs fixed at a single lung volume; for example, the data of Horsfield and Cumming[7] and those of Weibel[10] were derived from the lungs of only one and five subjects, respectively. There is almost certainly considerable variability between individuals, as well as change in dimensions at different lung volumes.

In their study of resin casts of human lungs inflated and fixed at a volume of 5 liters, Horsfield and Cumming[7] measured the length of each branch between two points of bifurcation and the diameter at the midpoint of every structure starting with an arbitrary diameter of 0.7 mm (Table 1–1). One of the interesting findings was a roughly linear relationship between the order number and the logarithm of the number, diameter, and length of airway branches (Fig. 1–2). Thus, by measuring the slope of the line relating the two, the diameter and length of any order can be predicted by dividing the diameter and length of its parent by 1.4 and 1.49, respectively. Similarly, they found the number of branches to be linearly related to the order number (Fig. 1–2), the branching ratio of the conducting zone (average number of daughter branches per parent branch) being 2.8.

Although these "number laws" do not apply precisely at all airway levels—for example, the trachea clearly does not branch 2.8 times—their predictive accuracy over most

Table 1–1. ASYMMETRIC MODEL OF THE AIRWAYS DERIVED FROM MEASUREMENTS OF A CAST

STRUCTURE	GENERATION UP	NO.	DIAMETER (mm)	LENGTH (mm)
Trachea	25	1	16.0	100
	24	1	12.0	40
	23	2	10.3	2
	22	2	8.9	18
	21	2	7.7	14
	20	3	6.6	11
	19	6	5.7	10
	18	8	4.9	10
	17	12	4.2	10
	16	14	3.5	10
	15	20	3.3	9.6
	14	30	3.1	9.1
	13	37	2.9	8.6
	12	46	2.8	8.2
	11	64	2.6	7.8
	10	85	2.4	7.4
	9	114	2.3	7.0
	8	158	2.2	6.7
	7	221	2.0	6.3
	6	341	1.78	5.7
	5	499	1.51	5.0
	4	760	1.29	4.4
	3	1,104	1.10	3.9
	2	1,675	0.93	3.5
	1	2,843	0.79	3.1
Terminal bronchiole	(−2)*	27,992	0.60	
Distal respiratory bronchiole	(−5)*	223,941	0.40	

* Minus values for the terminal bronchiole and distal respiratory bronchiole are included to give an approximate indication of the number of divisions between the structures in a lobule.

(Reprinted slightly modified from Horsfield K, Cumming G: J Appl Physiol 24:373, 1968.)

of the system is quite good. Thus, the branching ratio of 2.8 is followed closely from Orders 6 through 15. Similarly, the diameter law is not applicable throughout the whole airway system; at Order 7 (approximately), diminution in airway diameter ceases and the more distal branches (to Order 1) retain the parent's diameter. Cumming and colleagues postulated functional significance for this change in branching pattern, which occurs at about the point at which conducting flow becomes the lesser property and diffusive mixing becomes the major property.

Counting distally from the trachea, Horsfield and Cumming found the number of generations to a 0.7-mm airway to range from 8 to 25—that is, the lobular branch with the shortest path length was reached after 8 dichotomous branchings and the longest path length was reached after 25. It is likely that local spatial constraints related to the presence of bronchovascular bundles, interlobular septa, and the pleura are most important in determining these lengths. Analysis of the frequency distribution of airway divisions proximal to the lobular branches (Fig. 1–3) showed a stepwise increase from Division 8 to a peak at 14 and a decrease from 15 to 25.[7] Path lengths proximal to branches 0.7 mm in diameter ranged from 7.5 to 21.5 cm; distally, they were very short, ranging from 0.2 to 0.9 cm, thus giving an overall

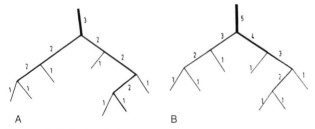

Figure 1–1. Orders Defined by the Methods of Strahler (A) and Horsfield and Cumming (B). The most distal branches (A) are Order 1; two of these join to form an Order 2 branch. Subsequently, the order increases only if branches of like order meet; e.g., two Order 4s produce an Order 5 branch. If two different orders meet, the order of the higher one is continued. In the Horsfield-Cumming method (B), the most distal branches are Order 1; two of these meet to form an Order 2 branch. When any two branches meet, they form a branch one order more than the higher of the two meeting branches. (From Cumming G, Horsfield K, Harding LK, et al: Bull Physiopathol Respir 7:31, 1971.)

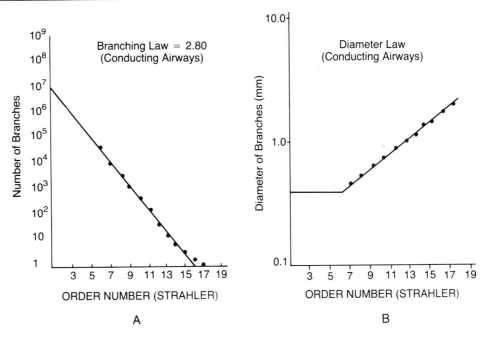

Figure 1–2. Number of Branches *(A)* and Their Diameter *(B)* Plotted Against Their Order Number. In *B*, note that Orders 1 through 7 undergo no diameter change—diminution in caliber ceases at Order 7, chiefly respiratory bronchioles. (From Cumming G, Horsfield K, Harding LK, et al: Bull Physiopathol Respir 7:31, 1971.)

range from carina to distal respiratory bronchioles of 7.7 to 22.4 cm. The volume of airways from the carina to 0.7-mm branches was computed to be 71 ml. This volume, added to that of the upper airways from the mouth to the carina (80 ml), gives a total volume of airways almost identical to the volume of anatomic dead space as determined by physiologic techniques.

As a general rule, the angles made by daughter branches with their parent vary with their diameter:[1] when the branches are of equal size, the angles tend to be equal; when different, the smaller branch usually makes a larger angle with the parent. The branching angle has been found by some observers to be greater in the lower orders.[11]

Morphology and Cell Function

The basic morphology of the trachea, bronchi, and membranous bronchioles is the same and consists of a surface epithelium, composed largely of ciliated and secretory cells, and subepithelial tissue containing supporting connective tissues, inflammatory mediator cells, and glands (Fig. 1–4). The proportion and type of these elements vary at different levels of the conducting system.

Epithelium

The tracheal and proximal bronchial epithelium is composed of tall, columnar ciliated and goblet cells and smaller, somewhat triangular basal cells. All are closely apposed or attached at their bases to a basement membrane; however,

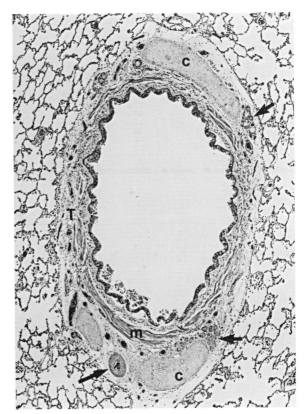

Figure 1–4. Normal Subsegmental Bronchus. C, cartilage plate; T, interstitial connective tissue; M, smooth muscle; *short arrows,* bronchial glands; *long arrow,* bronchial artery. (×30.)

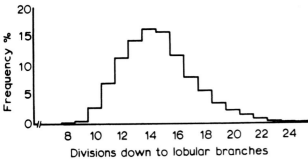

Figure 1–3. Frequency Distribution of the Number of Divisions down to the Lobular Branches. (From Horsfield K, Cumming G: J Appl Physiol 24:373, 1968.)

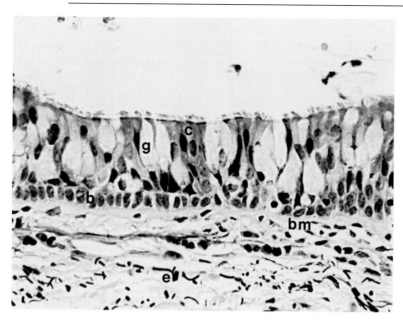

Figure 1–5. Normal Bronchial Epithelium. Ciliated (c), goblet (g), intermediate (i), and basal (b) cells are seen. Note also the thin basement membrane (bm), scattered elastic fibers (e), and inflammatory cells in the lamina propria. (Verhoeff–van Gieson; ×425.)

since not all reach the luminal surface and their nuclei are situated at different levels, the epithelium has a pseudostratified appearance (Fig. 1–5). This characteristic is gradually lost in the distal bronchi and bronchioles as the epithelium becomes low columnar and finally cuboidal. Ciliated and secretory cells—either goblet or Clara in type—constitute the bulk of the epithelium, with basal, intermediate, brush, lymphoreticular, and specialized neuroendocrine cells interspersed in lesser numbers. The morphology and function of these various cell types have been reviewed in detail.[13, 14]

The Ciliated Cell. The ciliated cell, the most prominent cell type in normal epithelium, is four or five times more numerous than goblet cells in the central airways and even greater in proportion peripherally (Fig. 1–6).[15, 16] The cell is roughly columnar in shape, has a thin, tapering base, and extends from the luminal surface to the basement membrane, to which it is attached by a variety of integrin adhesion receptors.[17] The cells are also attached to one another at their apical surface by tight junctions,[18] thus forming a barrier physically impermeable to most substances.[19] Despite this barrier, there is abundant experimental evidence from animals[20] and tissue cultures[21, 22] that transport of particulates can occur across the tracheobronchial epithelium, possibly by means of cytoplasmic vesicles. Although ciliated cells are joined laterally to one another and to basal cells by desmosomes (*see* farther on), prominent intercellular spaces containing numerous microvilli are also seen in this location, especially at the basal aspect of the cell[16, 23] (Fig. 1–7). These spaces and microvilli are important in the transepithelial movement of fluid and electrolytes (*see* page 62).[23, 24]

Emanating from the surface of each ciliated cell are approximately 200 to 250 cilia (Fig. 1–8).[14, 16] In the proximal airways, these measure approximately 6 μm in length and 0.25 to 0.3 μm in diameter;[13, 14] distally, they decrease progressively in height so that at the level of the seventh-generation bronchi they measure only about 3.5 μm in length.[25] In addition to cilia, numerous shorter microvilli are present at the luminal surface; they have been hypothesized to function either in the absorption of secretions emanating from more peripheral airways[26] or in the secretion of a

portion of the sol phase of the surface mucous layer (*see* page 62).[27]

Each cilium is covered by a prolongation of the cell surface membrane and contains a complex structure called

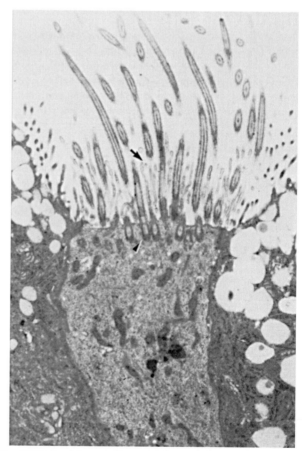

Figure 1–6. Ciliated Cell. Luminal portion showing cilia, surface microvilli *(arrow)*, apical mitochondria, and basal bodies *(arrowhead)*. (Human bronchial epithelium, ×12,500.)

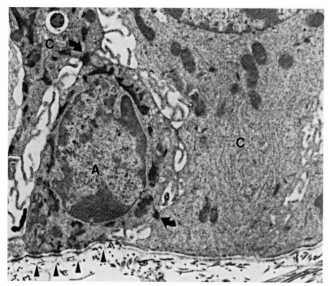

Figure 1–7. Tracheal Epithelium–Ultrastructure. Magnified view of the basal aspect of tracheal epithelium from a sheep shows a basal cell containing relatively little cytoplasm (A) and the inferior portion of several columnar cells (probably ciliated cells) (C). Intercellular spaces containing numerous microvilli are evident. Note also that the basal cell has several hemidesmosomal attachments to the underlying basement membrane *(arrowheads)* whereas the adjacent columnar cell has none. Several desmosome-like attachments are nevertheless present between the basal cell and the columnar cells *(arrows).* ($\times 13,200$.) (Adapted from Evans MJ, Cox RA, Shami SG, et al: The role of basal cells in the attachment of columnar cells to the basal lamina of the trachea. Am J Respir Cell Mol Biol 1:463, 1989.)

the *axoneme* (Fig. 1–9).[28, 29] The axoneme consists of two central microtubules surrounded by nine peripheral doublets, composed in turn of two intimately related microtubules termed *A* and *B subfibers.* Two small arms, which are composed of the energy-producing protein dynein, project from the A subfiber of one doublet to the B subfiber of the next. Also attached to each A subfiber is an axillary-arranged radial spoke that joins it to a central sheath surrounding the inner microtubules.

The apex of the cilium tapers to a fine tip from which arise small, hooklike structures.[28, 30] It is thought that these structures function as anchoring sites within the surface mucous layer to aid in propulsion of mucus. At the base of the cilium, the A and B subfibers continue into the apical cell cytoplasm and are joined by a third, or C, subfiber to form the *basal body.* Along with microtubules and actin filaments adjacent to it, this body serves to anchor the cilium firmly to the cell surface.[28] Although mitochondria are scattered throughout the cell cytoplasm, many are concentrated in a layer just under the basal bodies, presumably to provide an easily accessible energy source for ciliary function. (A discussion of the function of the cilium and the mucociliary escalator is given on page 127.)

Acquired abnormalities of ciliary structure are not uncommon and have been described in a high proportion of cigarette smokers[31–33] and patients who have chronic bronchitis,[34] as well as in some apparently normal individuals who manifest neither acute nor chronic respiratory disease.[33–35] Derangements include compound cilia (multiple axonemes within a single cell membrane), internalized cilia (projecting into cytoplasmic cavities in the cell apex rather than into the

airway), cilia with disorganized axonemes, abnormalities in the ciliary membrane or amount of cytoplasm, transposition of microtubules, radial spoke defects, and a variety of minor microtubular abnormalities.[33, 34, 36] Inherited ciliary abnormalities are much less common than acquired ones but are more important because they affect all cilia and often result in clinically significant bronchiectasis (*see* page 2281).

In addition to roles in transepithelial fluid movement and mucociliary escalator function, there is evidence that ciliated cells (and possibly other airway epithelial cells) may have important effects in the control of local airway inflammatory and immunologic reactions and on smooth muscle function.[37] Thus, airway epithelial cells are capable of producing lysozyme,[37a] a variety of cytokines (such as granulocyte-macrophage colony-stimulating factor),[37, 38] and adhesion molecules (such as intercellular adhesion molecule 1),[39] capable of recruiting and interacting with inflammatory and immune cells. Ciliated cells also express HLA-DR antigens and can therefore theoretically interact directly with intraepithelial immune cells.[40, 41] An influence on fibroblast proliferation and production of extracellular matrix components is also likely to be important in both the normal and injured airway wall.[37, 41a]

The Goblet Cell. The goblet cell accounts for about 20% to 30% of cells in the more proximal airways[15, 16] (almost 7,000/mm² in the normal adult trachea[42]) and decreases in number distally so that only occasional cells are present in normal membranous bronchioles.[43] In conditions associated with either acute or chronic airway irritation, goblet cells often increase in number in the proximal airways and may also appear in bronchioles[42, 44] (Fig. 1–10). Ultrastructurally, the apical portion of the cytoplasm contains numerous membrane-bound, electron-lucent secretory granules (Fig. 1–11); in one detailed study, these granules were located in discrete clusters, each associated with a single Golgi apparatus.[45] Although there may be considerable variation in cell shape,[44] the basal portion tends to become more attenuated as it

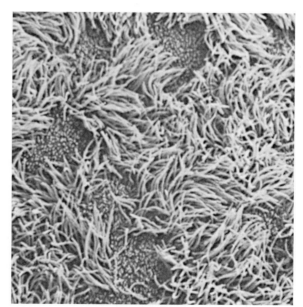

Figure 1–8. Normal Human Bronchial Epithelium. Scanning electron micrograph of the luminal surface showing numerous cilia. (Courtesy of Dr. Nai-San Wang, McGill University, Montreal.)

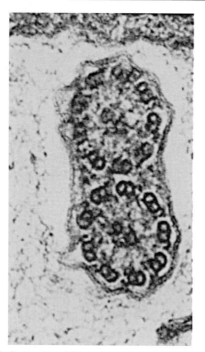
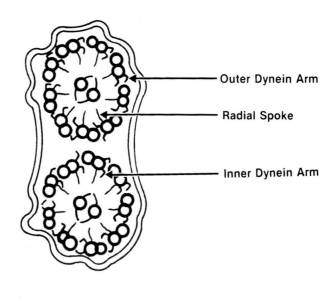

— Outer Dynein Arm

— Radial Spoke

— Inner Dynein Arm

Figure 1–9. Doublet Cilium from Chronic Smoker. Although paired within the same plasma membrane, the individual components of this cilium are normal, with nine peripheral and two central doublets and the typical arrangement of dynein arms and radial spokes.

approaches the basement membrane; the combination of tapered base and expanded apex results in the typical goblet shape from which the name of the cell is derived. A so-called small mucous granule cell has also been described by some investigators;[15] it contains only a few small secretory granules and has been speculated to represent a goblet cell at the beginning or end of its secretory cycle.

The principal function of the goblet cell is mucus secretion.[45a] Histochemical studies have shown strong periodic acid–Schiff positivity[46, 47] and somewhat weaker staining with toluidine blue,[46] alcian blue, and aldehyde fuchsin,[47]

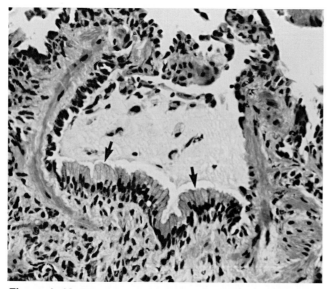

Figure 1–10. Mucous Cell Hyperplasia. A membranous bronchiole from a 60-year-old cigarette smoker shows numerous mucus-secreting cells *(arrows)*; the adjacent airway lumen is virtually completely occluded by mucus. A chronic inflammatory infiltrate is also present in the mucosa.

indicative of a predominantly neutral mucin and sulfomucin content. However, a variation in both ultrastructural and histochemical features has been demonstrated at different sites in the tracheobronchial tree, and cells with a large proportion of nonsulfated sialomucins have also been identified.[48]

Basal and Intermediate Cells. Basal cells (*see* Figs. 1–5, page 6 and 1–7, page 7) are relatively small, somewhat triangular cells whose bases are attached to the basement membrane and whose apices normally do not reach the airway lumen. They are more abundant in the proximal airways, where they form a more or less continuous layer, and gradually diminish in number distally so that they are difficult to identify in bronchioles.[49, 50, 50a] Most of the cell is occupied by its nucleus, and the cytoplasm shows little evidence of cellular specialization; as a result, it is widely believed that the basal cell is a reserve cell from which the epithelium is repopulated, both normally and after airway injury.[50a, 51–53]

Basal cells also appear to function in the attachment of columnar epithelial cells to the basement membrane, particularly in the trachea and proximal bronchi.[54–56] At these sites, basal cells contribute approximately 90% of the epithelial cell surface that makes contact with the basement membrane;[57] by necessity, ciliated and goblet cells are thus indirectly anchored to the basement membrane via intercellular junctions with adjacent basal cells (*see* Fig. 1–7, page 7). There is evidence that basal cells are also metabolically active; for example, they function as a source of extracellular superoxide dismutase.[58]

The nuclei of intermediate cells are located somewhat above the basal cell layer. These cells possess more cytoplasm than do basal cells and show ultrastructural features suggestive of either ciliogenesis or mucous granule accumulation. As their name implies, they are generally believed to

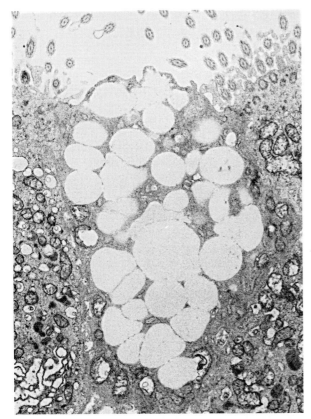

Figure 1–11. Goblet Cell. The apical portion of a goblet cell (flanked by two ciliated cells) contains numerous secretory granules. (×11,500.)

The Brush Cell. First described in animal lungs,[66] the brush cell has been identified rarely in humans.[67, 67a] It can be seen from the trachea to the alveolus and is characterized ultrastructuraly by numerous, fairly regular microvilli on the luminal surface and an abscence of cilia and basal bodies. Although its function is unknown, the prominence of microvilli suggests a role in absorbing airway secretions. The presence of a well-developed Golgi apparatus in the apical cytoplasm also suggests that the cell might itself be secretory.[66]

The Clara Cell. The Clara cell (nonciliated bronchiolar secretory cell) is found primarily in bronchioles, in which it constitutes the majority of the epithelium along with ciliated cells. (Although some nonciliated cells in bronchial epithelium express Clara cell proteins,[68] histologically identifiable Clara cells in this location are uncommon.) The cell shows pronounced interspecies differences in morphology, distribution, and (possibly) function.[69, 70] In humans, it is columnar or (in the more distal airways) cuboidal in shape and bulges somewhat into the airway lumen, slightly projecting above the surrounding ciliated cells (Fig. 1–12). Ultrastructurally, the Clara cell has a prominent Golgi apparatus, abundant granular endoplasmic reticulum and mitochondria, and numerous membrane-bound, electron-dense granules.

Clara cells synthesize a number of lipids and proteins that probably have important functions in the normal lung and may prove useful in the diagnosis of some pulmonary abnormalities.[70–72] One of the more extensively investigated

represent an intermediate stage of differentiation between the basal cell and either the goblet or ciliated cell. It is possible that the secretory form (with early mucous granule accumulation) is important in the repair of injured airway epithelium.[59]

The response of the tracheobronchial epithelium to acute injury is rapid. In one study in which the suprabasal epithelium of rat trachea was mechanically damaged, basal cellular mitotic activity reached a peak between 26 and 30 hours postinjury, and the epithelium was virtually reconstituted with ultrastructurally mature cells by 90 hours.[60] Another scanning electron microscopic investigation of acid-damaged mouse trachea showed complete epithelial recovery by 7 days.[61] According to one group of investigators, healing occurs by a complex sequence of events beginning with migration of basal and "secretory" cells into a wound, followed by their "dedifferentiation," proliferation, and "redifferentiation" into mature epithelial cells.[62] This process is undoubtedly affected by a variety of biochemical mediators such as growth factors and cell adhesion molecules.[63, 63a] The normal epithelial turnover rate has been estimated to be between 7 and 131 days;[14] the normal proliferation fraction has been found to be about 0.75.[64]

The factors that determine the type and rate of cellular differentiation in normal epithelium are incompletely understood and undoubtedly complex. Vitamin A is particularly important in maintaining normal differentiation, its deficiency resulting in squamous metaplasia.[65] Other substances such as insulin, epidermal growth factor, and transforming growth factor β also appear to have important effects.[65]

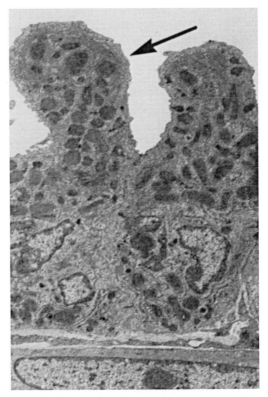

Figure 1–12. Clara Cells. These cells possess tongue-shaped cytoplasmic processes *(arrow)* that project into the airway lumen. Nuclei are basal in position, and the apical cytoplasm contains numerous osmiophilic granules. (×4,500.) (From Wang N-S, Huang SN, Sheldon H, et al: Ultrastructural changes of Clara and type II alveolar cells in adrenalin-induced pulmonary edema in mice. Am J Pathol 62:237, 1971.)

of these substances is a 10-kilodalton protein known as *Clara cell–specific protein* (CC10, CC16, Protein 1). The substance has the ability to inhibit phospholipase A, the rate-limiting enzyme in the production of arachidonic acid, and has been hypothesized to have an important role in the regulation of local inflammatory and immune reactions.[72–75] It can be identified in sputum, bronchoalveolar lavage fluid, and pleural fluid (in the latter, possibly via diffusion across the visceral pleura).[75a] The serum level of the protein has been shown to be increased in a variety of conditions, including pneumonia,[76] cigarette smoking,[77] and silica exposure,[78] which suggests that it might be a useful marker of bronchiolar epithelial damage. Because of its concentration in cell clusters adjacent to neuroepithelial bodies in fetal lung, it has also been proposed that the protein may be involved in the control of airway development.[79] Finally, some investigators have found the protein to be decreased in the amniotic fluid of women whose fetuses have pulmonary hypoplasia, thus suggesting that its measurement might be diagnostically useful.[80]

Clara cells have also been shown to synthesize several surfactant proteins.[72, 81] Both scanning[43] and transmission[82] electron microscopic studies have shown that a surface film covers the bronchiolar epithelium (presumably with a surface tension–lowering function similar to alveolar surfactant), and at least part of the surface film may be composed of these proteins. It is also possible that the Clara cell surfactant proteins are involved in airway antimicrobial defense. Immunohistochemical studies have shown the presence of both a trypsin-like protease and a leukocyte protease inhibitor within Clara cells;[72, 83] although the function of the former is unclear, the latter is presumably involved in maintaining the integrity of the bronchiolar wall.

In addition to these secretory functions, there is evidence that Clara cells act as progenitor cells in the regeneration of damaged bronchiolar[84] and alveolar[85] epithelium. Finally, the presence of abundant smooth endoplasmic reticulum as well as the cytochrome P-450 mono-oxygenase system[72] in a number of animal species suggests that the cells have a detoxification function (although the importance of this function in humans is uncertain).[69, 70]

The Neuroendocrine Cell. Sometimes termed *K cells* because of their similarity to cells described by Kultschitzsky in the gastrointestinal tract, pulmonary neuroendocrine (NE) cells have been the subject of much investigation.[86, 87] The cells have been estimated to constitute 1% to 2% of bronchial epithelial cells in neonates[88] and about 0.4% in adults.[64] Although they have traditionally been thought to be more frequent in peripheral than central airways, some investigators have found no difference in number between the two sites.[64] They have also been demonstrated in bronchial glands and their ducts and, occasionally, in alveoli.[64]

The NE cell has a roughly triangular shape, its base resting on the basement membrane and its somewhat tapering apex extending toward but infrequently reaching the airway surface. Cytoplasmic processes can be seen emanating from the basal aspect and extending laterally between adjacent epithelial cells.[64, 89] Most have no clear association with nerves.[87] Ultrastructurally, the cytoplasm contains abundant smooth endoplasmic reticulum and free ribosomes, a prominent amount of microtubules and microfilaments (at least some of which have been shown immunochemically to

be neurofilaments[90]), and most characteristically, variable numbers of neurosecretory granules (Fig. 1–13).[91, 92] The last are membrane bound and possess a central, electron-dense core surrounded by a thin, lucent halo. The majority range in diameter from 60 to 150 nm. Different subtypes of NE cells have been proposed to account for the ultrastructural differences in granule contents.[93]

NE cells are difficult to recognize at the light microscopic level with routine stains, and a variety of special techniques have been used to identify them. The earliest to be used was based on the ability of the neurosecretory granules to take up and retain silver, a property termed *argyrophilia*. Nowadays, the cells can be identified more easily and specifically by immunohistochemical reactions for several substances contained within the neurosecretory granules, including synaptophysin (a glycoprotein on the granule membrane), chromogranin (a peptide costored with granule hormones), and a variety of peptide hormones, including gastrin-releasing peptide (bombesin), calcitonin, calcitonin gene–related peptide, somatostatin, substance P, endothelin, cholecystokinin, and enkephalin.[87] These peptide hormones appear to be secreted mostly at the basal aspect of the cell; some may also be released in proximinty to other airway epithelial cells (via their lateral cytoplasmic processes) and into the airway lumen itself.

Although the precise functions of pulmonary NE cells are unknown, they are widely believed to be related to the local effects of secreted granule peptides. The cells appear

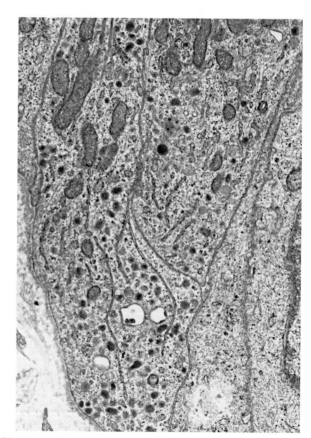

Figure 1–13. Neuroendocrine Cell. Magnified view of the base of a neuroendocrine cell showing lamina propria and thin basal lamina at the bottom left and numerous intracytoplasmic neurosecretory granules. (×31,000.)

as early as 8 weeks in the human fetus and increase in number thereafter,[94] thus suggesting a role in control of airway development.[95] More specifically, it has been proposed that NE cells may influence the migration and growth of intraepithelial nerve fibers in both the developing and regenerating epithelium.[96] It is also possible that the cells function in the regulation of fetal or neonatal circulation. There is evidence that hypoxia may result in an increase in NE cell number[97] and in ultrastructural changes similar to those found in carotid body chief cells;[98] as a consequence, it has also been suggested that NE cells may be involved in mediation of the pulmonary vascular hypoxic response.[91] Finally, a role in the regulation of epithelial growth and repair has been postulated.[87, 99, 100] In addition to their possible functional importance in normal individuals, much attention has been focused on these cells because of a possible association with neuroendocrine-related pulmonary neoplasms such as carcinoid tumor and small cell carcinoma and with airway disease such as is seen in chronic obstructive pulmonary disease.[101]

Neuroepithelial bodies can be seen in the airways of human infants[102] and throughout the tracheobronchial and bronchiolar epithelium,[103] especially near branch points.[92] They consist of fairly well demarcated, ovoid or triangular clusters of 4 to 10 large, columnar cells (Fig. 1–14) individually indistinguishable from the solitary NE cell. The cell apices reach the airway epithelial surface and their bases rest on the basement membrane, often in intimate contact with small nerve fibers[104] and occasionally with fenestrated capillaries.[103] It has been suggested that neuroepithelial bodies function as chemoreceptors, specifically by monitoring oxygen in inspired air and releasing peptides to regulate local airway and/or vascular resistance.[87]

The number of pulmonary NE cells, whether solitary or clustered in neuroepithelial bodies, has been shown experimentally to be increased following fetal and neonatal nicotine exposure,[105] the administration of nitrosamine carcinogens,[106] and bronchial challenge after sensitization with a

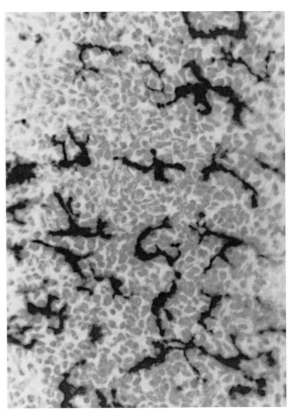

Figure 1–15. Airway Dendritic Cells. A tangential section of rat tracheal epithelium immunostained for Ia antigen shows regularly spaced dendritic cells, each with several irregular processes extending between adjacent epithelial cells. (× 40.) (From Schon-Hegrad MA, Oliver J, McMenamin PG, et al: Studies on the density, distribution, and surface phenotype of intraepithelial class II major histocompatibility complex antigen (Ia)-bearing dendritic cells (DC) in the conducting airways. J Exp Med 173:1345, 1991.)

known antigen.[107] The relevance of these observations to human disease awaits further study.

Lymphoreticular Cells. Cells of the immune system are present within the epithelium of all conducting airways.[14] *Dendritic* and *Langerhans' cells* are structurally similar cells that possess elongated cytoplasmic extensions (Fig. 1–15), highly convoluted nuclei, and an organelle-rich cytoplasm; in addition, Langerhans' cells have characteristic pentalaminar cytoplasmic structures termed *Birbeck granules*.[108] Dendritic cells can be found throughout the lung, including the pleura, alveolar interstitium, peribronchiolar connective tissue, and bronchus-associated lymphoid tissue;[108] Langerhans' cells appear to be present only within airway epithelium. In this location, their number is considerably greater in proximal than in distal branches.[109] In experimental animals, their number has been found to increase with inhalation of inert particles or bacterial lipopolysaccharide.[109] They are also often increased in humans, sometimes in large numbers, in foci of epithelial hyperplasia and some pulmonary carcinomas.

It is believed that dendritic cells are derived from circulating blood monocytes that originate from stem cells in the bone marrow and emigrate from alveolar capillaries into the adjacent interstitium.[108] The cells can then migrate from this location to various sites, including airway epithelium.

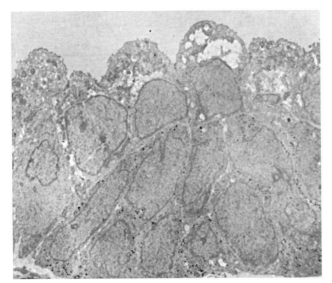

Figure 1–14. Neuroepithelial Body. Bronchiolar epithelium of a neonatal rabbit showing a well-defined aggregate of cells, each containing numerous neurosecretory granules. (Courtesy of Dr. Nai-San Wang, McGill University, Montreal.)

Differentiation into Langerhans' cells may occur in the epithelium itself, possibly as a result of epithelial-derived factors such as granulocyte-macrophage colony-stimulating factor. Immunologic studies show Langerhans' cells to be CD1a positive and to express cell surface receptors for immunoglobulins.[108] It is believed that they act in the initial stage of airway immunologic defense as antigen-processing and antigen-presenting cells and as stimulators of T-cell proliferation.[108, 110, 111] There is evidence that their function is modulated by macrophages in the adjacent lamina propria.[112]

Lymphocytes, including a variety of immunologic and presumably functional subtypes, are present throughout the conducting airway epithelium, usually singly.[113] Greater numbers are occasionally seen in association with lymphoid aggregates in the lamina propria and submucosa (bronchus-associated lymphoid tissue, *see* page 16). *Mast cells* can also be seen within airway epithelium, possibly in increased numbers in cigarette smokers (*see* page 16).[114]

Submucosa and Lamina Propria

The subepithelial tissue can be subdivided into a lamina propria, situated between the basement membrane and muscularis mucosa, and a submucosa, consisting of all the remaining airway tissue. The *lamina propria* is more prominent in the trachea and proximal bronchi than in distal airways. It consists principally of a delicate capillary network, a meshwork of reticulin fibers continuous with the basement membrane, and prominent bundles of elastic tissue. The *submucosa* contains cartilage, muscle, and other supportive connective tissue elements, as well as the major portion of the tracheobronchial glands. Various cells related to airway function and defense are present in both the lamina propria and submucosa.

Since changes in the dimensions and mechanical properties of different tissues of the airway wall may have profoundly different effects on function, a modified nomenclature of airway wall anatomy has been proposed for use in investigative studies.[115] This recommendation is based on the observation that the length of the airway basement membrane is not altered by changes in airway diameter produced by changes in lung volume or smooth muscle contraction (i.e., airway narrowing occurs by mucosal folding). According to the proposed nomenclature, the airway wall can be divided into inner and outer layers, the former from the lumen to the outermost layer of smooth muscle and the latter between the smooth muscle and the airway adventitial-parenchymal boundary.

Basement Membrane. The primary function of the basement membrane is to provide attachment of surface epithelium to the underlying connective tissue (*see* Fig. 1–5, page 6). On the epithelial side, attachment is mediated by adhesion molecules and by hemidesmosomal junctions with basal cells;[116] on the opposite side, anchoring fibrils emanate from the basement membrane and intertwine with collagen fibers in the upper lamina propria. Very thin fibroblast-like cells have been described in intimate contact with the undersurface of the basement membrane in the rat trachea;[116] it has been speculated that they may be involved in maintenance of the basement membrane and in wound healing. Chemical differences in the basement membrane have been described at different airway sites, possibly representing different functional capabilities.[117]

Cartilage. The tracheal cartilage plates consist of a series of 16 to 20 U-shaped structures oriented in a horizontal plane with their open ends directed posteriorly.[118, 119] The spaces between the plates contain smooth muscle, tracheal glands, and collagenous and elastic tissue that is continuous with the perichondrium and binds the plates together. The U shape is maintained in the extrapulmonary main bronchi; however, the plates become quite irregular in shape in lobar and segmental bronchi (Fig. 1–16). At bronchial division

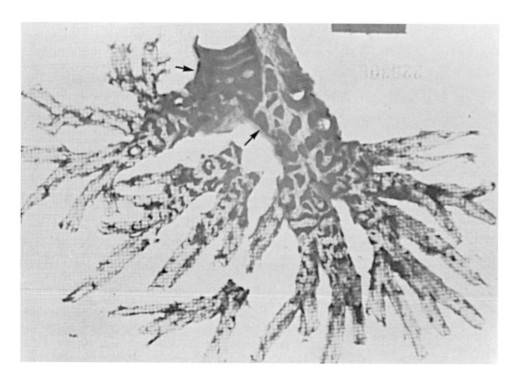

Figure 1–16. Cartilage Distribution in the Bronchial Tree. The bronchial tree of a normal left lung removed at autopsy has been dissected free, laid out on a wire mesh, and stained for cartilage. Note that the cartilage is horseshoe shaped for a short distance in the main bronchus *(upper arrow)* but in the lower lobe bronchus *(lower arrow)* and peripheral bronchi it occurs as irregularly shaped, interconnecting plates.

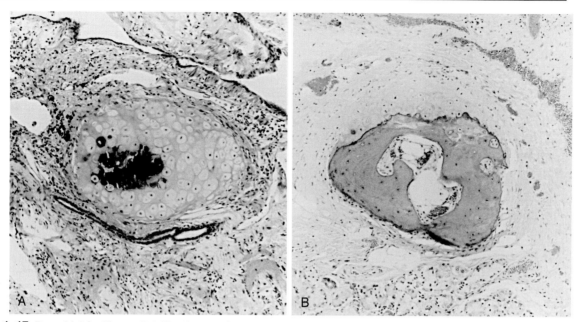

Figure 1–17. Bronchial Cartilage—Calcification and Ossification. Two fragments of bronchial cartilage are illustrated, one with focal calcification *(A)* and one with bone formation *(B)*.

points, the plates frequently take the form of a saddle conforming to the branching angle, thus providing extra support at sites of increased turbulence. As the airways decrease in diameter, cartilage plates become smaller until they finally disappear altogether in airways 1 to 3 mm in diameter (bronchioles). The cartilage is hyaline in type and may become calcified or ossified (Fig. 1–17), particularly in older individuals, in which case it may be visible radiographically.

Elastic Tissue. Elastic tissue in the lamina propria tends to be clustered in bundles oriented primarily in a longitudinal direction. These bundles are especially well developed in the posterior (noncartilaginous) portions of the trachea and main bronchi, where they form well-defined ridges that are visible to the naked eye (Fig. 1–18).[120] Prominent elastic thickening is also present in the lamina propria at bronchial branch points.

The tracheobronchial cartilage plates are tethered together by dense, fibroelastic tissue arranged predominantly in a longitudinal direction. At numerous sites, particularly in smaller airways, elastic fibers pass obliquely from these longitudinally arranged bundles to intermingle with the elastic tissue of the lamina propria.[1, 4] These obliquely arranged fibers are believed to help transmit to the more rigid and stronger cartilaginous-fibrous tissue the tensions that arise in the airway epithelium and lung parenchyma during respiration.[1, 4] The development, structure, and function of the entire pulmonary elastic framework have been reviewed in detail.[121]

Muscle. Tracheal muscle is found predominantly in the membranous portion, where it is oriented in transverse bundles that are attached to the inner perichondrium about 1 mm from the tip of the cartilaginous rings, with the

Figure 1–18. Normal Bronchus and Pulmonary Artery. Longitudinal slice of a small bronchus and adjacent pulmonary artery showing cartilage plates *(long arrows),* more or less circularly oriented smooth muscle bundles, and sparse, relatively thin, longitudinal elastic tissue bundles *(short arrows).* Note the supernumerary artery branches (unassociated with airway branches) (S) and the small focus of mild atherosclerosis *(curved arrow).*

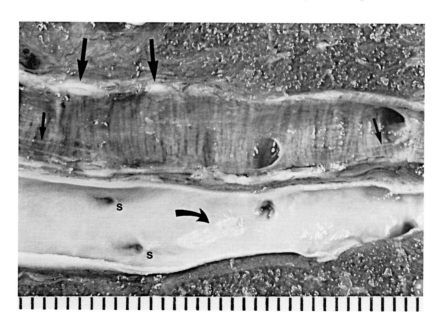

bundles joining each ring posteriorly. Although somewhat less prominent, transverse fibers can also be found between the cartilage rings in the anterior portion.[122] In addition, fairly prominent longitudinally oriented muscle bundles are present in most tracheas (predominantly in the lower half) caudal to the membranous transverse muscle layer.[50]

In the intrapulmonary bronchi, the muscle coat lies close to the epithelium just deep to the lamina propria. In the larger airways, the orientation is mainly circumferential, as in the trachea. In more distal branches, however, the muscle coat becomes obliquely oriented and is arranged in branching and anastomosing bundles that form irregular spirals in the airway wall. Because of this architecture, airway cross sections usually do not show a complete muscle coat, especially in smaller bronchi (Fig. 1–19). The proportion of muscle relative to airway diameter increases as the smaller airways are approached.[123] Airway smooth muscle is well known to undergo hyperplasia in a variety of chronic diseases such as asthma and chronic obstructive pulmonary disease. The mechanism of this hyperplasia is unknown; however, there is evidence that it may be related (at least in part) to physical strain[124] and mediated by endothelin or other growth factors.[125]

The ultrastructural, biophysical, and biochemical characteristics of airway smooth muscle have been reviewed.[126, 127]

Connective Tissue. In addition to cartilage, muscle, and elastic tissue, loose connective tissue consisting of proteoglycans and mature collagen occupies the bulk of the remainder of the submucosa. This loose connective tissue is continuous with adjacent periarterial connective tissue and with perivenous connective tissue near the hilum and thus, by extension,

with interlobular and subpleural interstitial connective tissue. This interdependence of connective tissue is important in maintaining the overall structure of the lung and in providing a scaffold for the more delicate connective tissue of the parenchyma. There is also evidence that extracellular connective tissue, particularly around large airways and vessels, contains superoxide dismutase, an important enzymatic scavenger of the superoxide anion.[128] At all levels of the bronchial tree, adipose tissue, usually small in amount, can be found adjacent to cartilage plates and occasionally in association with mucous glands.

Tracheobronchial Glands. Tracheobronchial glands are specialized extensions of the surface epithelium into the lamina propria and submucosa that are seen exclusively in the trachea and bronchi, roughly paralleling the distribution of cartilage (Fig. 1–20). Both the number and size of the glands are greater in the more proximal airways; according to one study of three normal individuals, total gland volume per unit of airway surface area was greatest between the midtrachea and main bronchi and decreased rapidly thereafter to relatively low levels in the subsegmental bronchi.[129] The number of glands in the trachea has been calculated to range from 3,500 to 6,000 (mean in two studies of 4,750[130] and 3,900[131]). In the cartilaginous portion, the glands are located mainly in horizontal layers in the submucosa between cartilaginous rings, whereas in the membranous portion, they lie both superficial and deep to the transverse muscle layer and in a more craniocaudal orientation.[131] In the bronchi, the glands are more irregularly distributed and can be situated either between the surface epithelium and cartilage or between cartilaginous plates extending into the peribronchial interstitial tissue.

The secretory portion of the gland is connected with the surface by a duct of variable length whose lining contains ciliated cells and goblet cells identical to those of surface airway epithelium. Some investigators have proposed that there is a specialized "collecting duct" interposed between this ciliated epithelium and the secretory portion of the gland;[132] according to these workers, the collecting duct is composed of columnar cells similar to those of the salivary gland intercalated duct[133] and may regulate the water and ion concentration of the final gland secretion.[132]

Multiple secretory tubules, usually branched, arise from the collecting duct. Proximally, these tubules are lined by plump mucus-secreting cells and distally by more basophilic serous cells (Fig. 1–21). The ratio of serous to mucous cells is about 0.5 and is roughly the same from the trachea to medium-sized bronchi.[134] Although these secretory cells form the majority of the glandular tissue, other cells can also be identified. Small clusters of oncocytes—large, eosinophilic cells containing numerous mitochondria—can be found focally in many glands (Fig. 1–21).[135] Their frequency increases with age, which suggests that they may represent a degenerative phenomenon similar to that seen in other secretory organs. Fairly numerous myoepithelial cells are present between the basement membrane and the epithelial cells, from the serous portion of the secretory tubules to the collecting duct;[133] these cells are presumably responsible in part for expulsion of glandular secretions. Occasional neuroendocrine cells similar to those of surface airway epithelium can also be found. Solitary, unmyelinated axons are

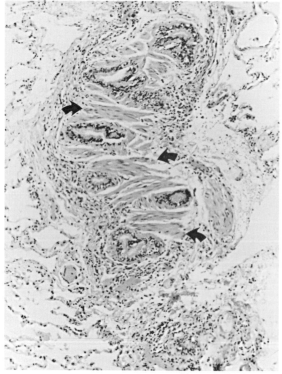

Figure 1–19. Bronchiolar Smooth Muscle. Longitudinal section of a membranous bronchiole showing several bundles of smooth muscle *(arrows)* oriented at a slight angle to the transverse plane.

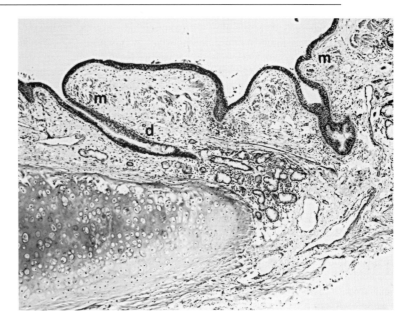

Figure 1–20. Normal Bronchial Wall with Bronchial Gland. Section of lobar bronchus showing a portion of cartilage plate, muscularis mucosa (m), bronchial gland duct (d), and acini (a). (×40.)

frequently seen beneath the basement membrane interdigitating between glandular cells.[133]

Histochemical and autoradiographic studies have shown two types of sulfated mucin and sialomucin within mucous cells.[136] All four varieties are present in older children and adults, but only sulfomucin can be identified in fetuses and children up to the age of 4 years.[137] There is a tendency for the proportion of acid mucosubstance to total glandular tissue to increase from the trachea to more distal airways and to be relatively greater in nonsmokers at all airway levels.[134] Electron microscopic studies show morphologically different secretory granules, consistent with the variety of mucosubstances demonstrated histochemically.[138] (Further discussion of the biochemical characteristics of bronchial gland mucus is given on page 60.) In addition to its function in airway clearance via the mucociliary escalator, there is evidence that mucus has intrinsic antiprotease properties.[139]

The ultrastructural appearance of serous cells, as well as their content of carbonic anhydrase, suggests that their principal secretion is a low-viscosity substance, possibly meant to "flush out" the secretion of the more proximal mucous cells.[48] As in mucous cells, cytoplasmic granules of serous cells show a variable morphology, suggesting that the cells may have different functions. Serous cells have been shown to be a potential source of lysozyme, lactoferrin,[141] transferrin,[141a] and a low-molecular-weight protease inhibitor,[140, 142] substances that are involved in local airway defense. There is also evidence that serous cells may function both in the manufacture of secretory component and in its coupling with and ultimate secretion of dimeric IgA.[143]

Mucous glands frequently increase in size in airway diseases such as chronic bronchitis and asthma.[144, 145] Although the pathogenesis of this increase is uncertain, it appears to be a true hyperplasia rather than simple hypertro-

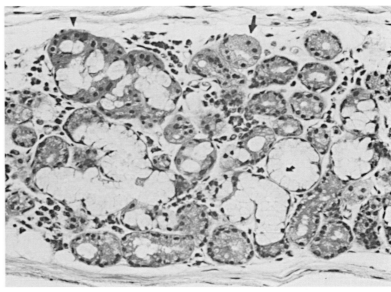

Figure 1–21. Bronchial Gland. Note the mucous *(small arrow)*, serous *(arrowhead)*, and oncocytic *(large arrow)* cells. Plasma cells can also be seen in the insterstitial tissue between the lobules. (×240.)

phy of glandular cells.[146] Interaction with extracellular matrix components such as integrins may be important in this process.[147] It is not known why mucus secretion is divided between mucous glands and goblet cells, but since the volume of glands is estimated to be roughly 40 times that of the total goblet cell mass,[144] mucous gland secretion is regarded as the more significant. The control and function of tracheobronchial gland secretion are discussed on page 60.

Lymphoid Tissue. Many cells concerned with airway defense are found in the airway lamina propria and submucosa. Lymphocytes can be identified either singly or in clusters, the latter being variously termed *lymphoid nodules, lymphoid aggregates,* or *bronchus-associated lymphoid tissue (BALT).*[148, 149] Although a well-established component of the normal airway mucosa in some animal species, the extent of BALT in humans is less clear. Some investigators have found lymphoid clusters to be absent at birth, appear during the neonatal period, and progressively increase in number so that they are found in almost all lungs by the age of 5 years.[150] Others have indentified BALT only rarely[151] or not at all[152] in normal lungs, but frequently in those exposed to cigarette smoke,[151] thus suggesting that the degree of BALT development is related to the presence of inhaled noxious material.

Histologically, airway lymphoid aggregates are composed of well-defined, but unencapsulated clusters of mature lymphocytes and occasional, larger immunoblastic cells (Fig. 1–22). Germinal centers and cells with plasmacytoid differentiation are infrequent.[148] The cells extend into the overlying epithelium, which is often flattened and lacks mucous or ciliary differentiation. The basement membrane adjacent to the lymphoid cells is frequently discontinuous.[148] Small, thin-walled blood vessels are present within the lymphoid aggregates, possibly serving as a site for cell migration to and from the circulation.

Plasma cells, primarily IgA and IgG in type, are common in the tracheobronchial wall, particularly in association with tracheobronchial glands (*see* Fig. 1–21, page 15) and in the lamina propria close to the basement membrane.[153] They are most frequent in proximal bronchi.[153]

Isolated *macrophages* can be found throughout the lamina propria and submucosa and are especially prominent in heavy smokers and in individuals with occupational dust exposure. In the latter situation, they can be so numerous and can contain so much carbon pigment that they impart a gray or black appearance to the epithelium that can be seen with the naked eye. There is evidence that macrophages in the lamina propria can modulate the activity of other lymphoreticular cells in the airway epithelium[112] and can migrate across the epithelium to the airway surface to phagocytose inhaled particulate material.[154]

Mast Cells. Mast cells are round to oval, medium-sized cells with centrally placed nuclei found throughout the lung in airway, alveolar, pleural, and interlobular interstitial tissue, as well as in airway epithelium.[155, 156] Ultrastructurally, they contain numerous cytoplasmic granules with a variable, but highly characteristic internal structure.[157] The cells are rich in heparin, histamine, eosinophil chemotactic factors, and several enzymes, including tryptase and chymase.[156] They are also able to synthesize and release leukotrienes, prostaglandins, platelet activating factor, and a variety of proinflammatory cytokines, including interleukin 4 (IL-4), IL-5, IL-6, IL-8, and tumor necrosis factor α.[158–160]

Human lung mast cells show phenotypic heterogeneity: approximately 80% are sensitive to formalin (losing their characteristic alcian blue staining when fixed), and 20% are formalin resistant.[161] There are differences in both mediator content and release between the two types of cells. They can also be categorized on the basis of their proteolytic enzyme content: one group (MTCT cells) contains tryptase, chymase, cathepsin G, and carboxypeptidases, whereas the other (MCT cells) contains tryptase but lacks the other neutral proteases.[162, 163] Different patterns of cytokine secretion may occur in the different protease-secreting cell types.[159, 160] The functional significance of this mast cell heterogeneity is unclear, although some differences in function have been demonstrated in cells isolated from the upper respiratory epithelium as compared with the interstitium.[164] Possible functions of mast cells in the normal lung include regulation of neuropeptide activity, bronchomotor tone, fibroblast mitogenesis, and tracheobronchial gland secretion.[156]

Mast cells have been implicated in both the pathogenesis and prevention of pulmonary disease. Because they produce numerous substances affecting the inflammatory reac-

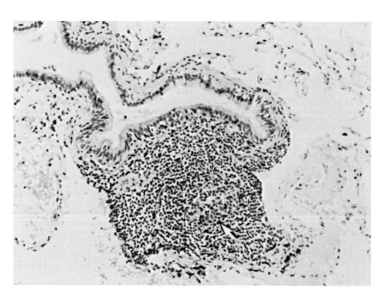

Figure 1–22. Peribronchiolar Lymphoid Tissue. A poorly defined nodule containing a mixture of mature and apparently stimulated lymphoid cells, as well as scattered macrophages, is present adjacent to and partly within bronchiolar epithelium.

tion, abnormalities such as asthma and pneumonitis are the most frequently associated. The cells also undergo hyperplasia in a variety of abnormalities in which fibrosis occurs,[165] and it has been speculated that they may be involved in the genesis of fibrous tissue.[166] Since heparin, an antithromboplastin and antithrombin agent, inhibits fibrin formation, one of its main roles within the lung is to promote blood fluidity. In addition, heparin inhibits hyaluronidase, has an antihistaminic effect, and may have an anti-inflammatory action,[167] perhaps by binding potentially harmful cationic proteins released from activated eosinophils.

The Transitional Zone

Geometry and Dimensions

Detailed three-dimensional studies of the anatomy of the pulmonary parenchyma have shown that the geometry of the transitional airways is much more complex than is usually appreciated by examining two-dimensional histologic sections.[7, 168–172] Although branching can occur in a more or less symmetric dichotomous fashion, trichotomous and even quadrivial (sometimes asymmetric) divisions of the respiratory bronchioles are not uncommon. In addition, the number and length of airway generations from the terminal bronchiole to the alveolar sac are variable, both within the same acinus and between acini. This variability may be related in part to different techniques of examination[170] and the rather limited number of acini that have been investigated. However, some of the irregularity appears to be real, possibly as a result of spatial constraints imposed by pleura, interlobular septa, and larger airways and vessels.

The number of airway generations from the terminal bronchiole to the alveolar sac may be as many as 12; on average, however, there are probably about 2 to 3 respiratory bronchioles and 4 to 6 alveolar ducts per pathway. The length and diameter of respiratory bronchioles and alveolar ducts have been found by some investigators to decrease progressively with generation number;[170] however, others have found the diameter to remain relatively constant despite a diminution in length.[7, 168, 171]

The number of alveoli present in alveolar ducts is also quite variable, with estimates ranging from as few as 4[171] to as many as 40;[173] the figures representing the norm are probably 10 to 20.[7, 170, 172] As with the other structural features of the transitional airways, this variation in number is probably related to a combination of different techniques of examination and real differences caused by local spatial constraints.

Morphology

Respiratory bronchioles have a low columnar to cuboidal epithelium that gradually decreases in extent as the number of alveoli increases. In first- and second-order bronchioles, the epithelium is usually complete on one side, where it overlies a lamina propria and submucosa continuous with that of the terminal bronchiole and is associated with a pulmonary artery branch (Fig. 1–23). As the number of alveoli increases, the submucosa disappears, but the muscle

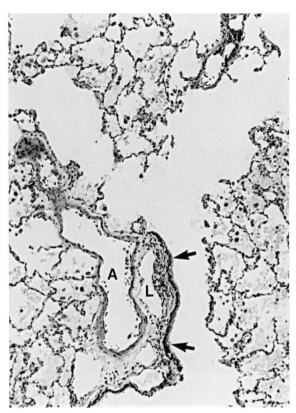

Figure 1–23. Respiratory Bronchioles. One wall of a proximal respiratory bronchiole is completely lined by low columnar epithelium *(arrows).* Adjacent to this is a small amount of interstitial tissue, a dilated lymphatic channel (L), and a branch of the pulmonary artery (A). The walls of the distal bronchiolar branches are almost completely alveolated. (× 80.)

and elastic tissue continue in fairly prominent bundles in a spiral fashion surrounding the alveolar mouths.[174, 175] When the alveolar duct is reached, bronchiolar epithelium and lamina propria are lost altogether and only scanty alveolar interstitial tissue is present in the airway wall. Alveolar ducts terminate in a series of rounded enclosures called *alveolar sacs,* from which arise approximately four to seven alveoli.

The contribution of transitional airways to gas exchange is probably substantial; in one investigation, approximately 35% to 40% of all alveoli in three acini were found to be located in these structures.[168]

The Respiratory Zone

Morphology and Cell Function

Alveoli are small outpouchings of respiratory bronchioles, alveolar ducts, and alveolar sacs that are demarcated by septa (walls) and are lined by a continuous layer of flattened epithelial cells covering a thin interstitium (Fig. 1–24). In humans, the epithelium consists primarily of two morphologically distinct cells, Type I and Type II, with occasional interspersed neuroendocrine cells; alveolar macrophages are also present on the epithelial surface. The interstitium contains capillaries involved in gas exchange, as

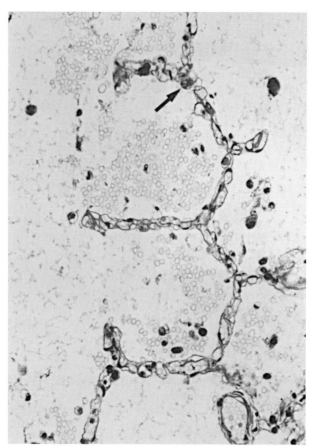

Figure 1–24. Normal Alveoli. Note the minute amount of tissue interposed between air spaces and capillary lumens. The nucleus of a Type II cell, or macrophage, is present at the junction of two septa *(arrow)*; Type I cells are not clearly evident. (×350.)

well as connective tissue and a variety of cells responsible for maintaining alveolar shape and defense.

The Type I Alveolar Cell. Although the Type I alveolar cell (membranous pneumocyte, Type A epithelial cell) represents only 8% of all parenchymal lung cells and is inconspicuous by light microscopy, it covers approximately 95% of the alveolar surface and has a total volume twice that of the histologically more obvious Type II cell.[176] Its nucleus is small and covered by a thin rim of cytoplasm containing few organelles (Fig. 1–25). The rest of the cytoplasm forms a broad sheet or plate that measures only 0.3 to 0.4 μm in thickness and extends in all directions for 50 μm or more over the alveolar surface, covering approximately 5,000 μm².[176] Sheets of adjacent Type I cells interdigitate, and individual plates may reach into neighboring alveoli, either by winding around the septal tip or by extending through alveolar pores.[177] The plates are joined firmly to one another and to Type II cells by occluding or tight junctions *(see* Figs. 1–25, and 2–4, page 76) that are believed to represent a more or less complete barrier to the diffusion of fluid and water-soluble substances into the alveolar lumen.[178, 179] Localized gap junctions have also been identified between adjacent Type I cells and between Type I and Type II cells, usually in association with an occluding junction;[178, 180] it is possible that these junctions act as sites for intercellular communication, as in other epithelia.

Although the paucity of organelles suggests a purely passive role of the Type I cell in lung function, the cell contains pinocytotic vesicles that can theoretically transport material in either direction across the air-blood barrier. Although relatively few in the normal cell, their number appears to increase in response to injury.[181] The vesicles have been hypothesized to be involved in the resorption of alveolar fluid,[182, 183] in the formation of alveolar exudate in some cases of interstitial pneumonitis,[184] and in the production of a part of the hypophase of alveolar surfactant.[179] Type I cells have also been shown to have the ability to take up intra-alveolar particulate material,[185] possibly in association with actin-containing microfilaments.[186] Although the quantitative significance of this uptake with respect to alveolar clearance is not known, it is probably small in comparison with that of the alveolar macrophages and the mucociliary escalator.

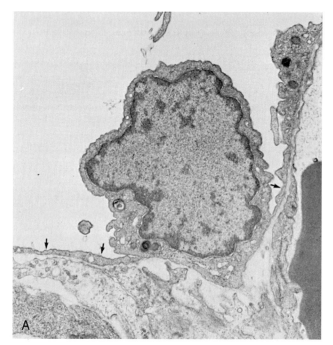

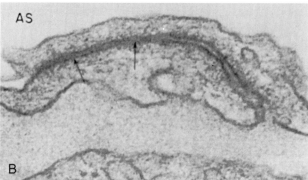

Figure 1–25. Type I Alveolar Epithelial Cell. Low magnification *(A)* showing a large nucleus and scanty cytoplasm that is attenuated on both sides over the alveolar surface *(arrows)*. High magnification *(B)* of the junction between two Type I cells showing a cleft extending roughly horizontally inward from the alveolar space (AS). In several areas *(arrows)* the outer leaflets of the plasma membranes appear fused. (*A,* courtesy of Dr. Nai-San Wang, McGill University, Montreal; *B,* from Schneeberger-Kelley EE, Karnovsky MJ: *J Cell Biol* 37:781, 1968. Reproduced from the *Journal of Cell Biology,* by copyright permission of the Rockefeller University Press.)

It has been speculated, however, that transport of materials into the alveolar interstitium via these cells may be the mechanism by which particles are deposited in regional lymph nodes[187] and may be important in the pathogenesis of some interstitial lung diseases.[186]

The Type II Alveolar Cell. The Type II epithelial cell (granular pneumocyte, Type B epithelial cell) (Fig. 1–26) is usually solitary and located near corners where adjacent alveoli meet.[188] Ultrastructurally, it has a roughly cuboidal shape and lacks the lateral extensions of the Type I cell.[189] The cytoplasm is rich in organelles, including a well-developed endoplasmic reticulum with many ribosomes, prominent Golgi complex, mitochondria, and numerous membrane-bound, osmiophilic granules. The latter range in size from 0.2 to 1.0 μm and contain characteristic stacked, lamellar inclusions that are somewhat irregular in shape when seen by transmission electron microscopy but are highly uniform when viewed on freeze-etched specimens, with a spacing of about 5 nm.[190] There is evidence that the number and volume of such granules may decrease with age.[191]

Type II cells are the source of alveolar surfactant, the substance responsible for modifying alveolar surface tension (*see* page 56).[81, 189, 192, 193] Osmiophilic granules appear to function primarily as a storage depot for the material, although synthesis of some of its components may also occur within them.[194] Release of granule contents into the alveolar lumen has been shown to occur by exocytosis,[195, 196] but the possibility of an additional holocrine type of secretion involving disintegration of the cell similar to that seen in epidermal sebaceous glands has also been proposed.[197] The biochemical composition and morphologic features of surfactant and the factors involved in its synthesis and release are discussed on page 56.

A second major function of the Type II cell is related to its ability to replicate. The Type I cell is thought to be incapable of division; by contrast, about 1% of the Type II cell population is normally mitotically active and repopulates the surface as Type I cells die.[198] In addition, the relative cytoplasmic simplicity and large surface area of Type I cells make them susceptible to damage from a wide variety of noxious agents.[199–202] Following Type I cell death, Type II cells proliferate and migrate over the alveolar surface, temporarily providing epithelial integrity. With time, they differentiate into Type I cells[199] and completely restore normal alveolar structure, provided that significant interstitial fibrosis has not occurred. The molecular events controlling Type II cell proliferation and differentiation are not well understood; however, there is evidence that several growth factors (some presumably derived from alveolar macrophages[203]) may be involved.[204, 205] It is also possible that there are important interactions with interstitial myofibroblasts (*see* farther on).[206]

Type II cells have several other potential functions. Experimental studies of tissue cultures,[207] as well as the presence of surface anionic binding sites[208] and microvilli, suggest that they may act in the resorption of fluid or

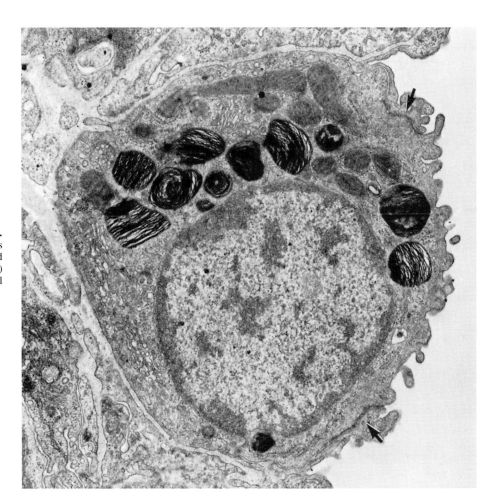

Figure 1–26. Type II Pneumocyte. Note the short surface microvilli, junctions with Type I cells *(arrows)*, and lamellated inclusion bodies. (Mouse lung, ×20,000.) (Courtesy of Dr. Nai-San Wang, McGill University, Montreal.)

other substances from the alveolar lumen, possibly including surfactant itself.[209] There is also evidence that Type II cells may synthesize fibronectin and collagen for use in the basement membrane,[210] as well as substances such as superoxide dismutase[58] and alpha$_1$-antitrypsin[210a] that are involved in maintenance of local alveolar structure. Some surfactant proteins have been shown to have the capacity to bind to bacteria and to alveolar macrophages, which suggests a role in antimicrobial defense.[211] A similar but less potent role in opsonization and phagocytosis of nonbacterial particulate material has also been found.[212] Finally, there is evidence that the cells have the capacity to modulate alveolar airspace defense by suppressing lymphocyte proliferation[213] (an effect again mediated by surfactant[214]) and by enhancing macrophage function.[215]

The Alveolar Interstitium. A more or less continuous basement membrane underlies both Type I and Type II cells. Over about 50% of its surface, it is intimately apposed to the underlying endothelial basement membrane. Interstitial cells and connective tissue, as well as endothelial and epithelial cell nuclei, tend to be absent from this region of apposition, so the thickness of the air-blood barrier in this area is determined only by the thin Type I cell plate, the endothelial

cell, and the fused basement membranes, which together measure about 0.4 to 0.5 μm in thickness (Fig. 1–27). Elsewhere, endothelial and epithelial basement membranes are separated by an interstitial space of variable width. The alveolar interstitium can thus be considered to form two distinct anatomic compartments,[216] the first relatively thin and involved with gas transfer and the second thicker and functioning as mechanical support for the alveolus, a compartment for fluid transfer, and a site for various cells that contribute to alveolar function.

The thick portion of the interstitium contains connective tissue and several cell types. The former consists of a proteoglycan matrix in which are embedded elastic fibers and small bundles of collagen that provide support for the capillaries. These fibers are continuous with the fibroelastic tissue of the pleura, airways, and interlobular septa, thus forming a complex, three-dimensional connective tissue framework that connects the different anatomic compartments of the lung.[216] Elastin makes up about 30% of dry lung weight[217] and collagen about 15%.[218] Immunofluorescent analyses of collagen within the alveolar interstitium have shown the presence of both Types I and III in an irregular pattern, the latter being somewhat more prominent.[219, 220] Types IV and

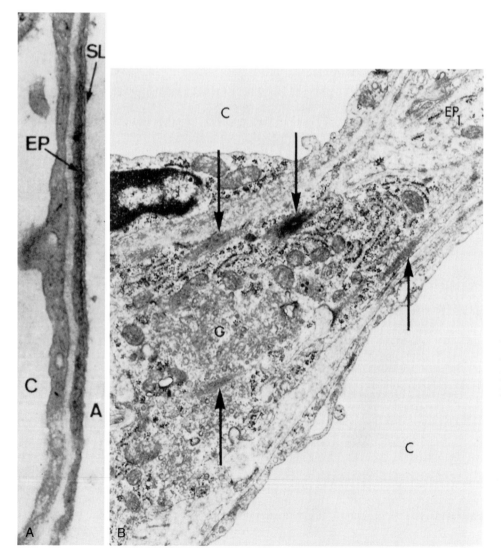

Figure 1–27. The Air-Blood Barrier. Thin portion *(A)*. A capillary (C) is present on the *left* and alveolar space (A) is on the right. A Type I alveolar epithelial cell (EP) is covered by a clearly extracellular osmiophilic layer (SL). (transmission electron microscopy [TEM], ×48,420.) *B*, Thick portion. Capillaries (C) and epithelial cells (EP$_1$) are separated by collagen fibers and a prominent interstitial cell containing a Golgi apparatus (G) and numerous bundles of microfilaments *(arrows)*. (Rat lung; TEM, ×24,000.) (*A*, From Gil J, Weibel ER: Respir Physiol 8:13, 1969; *B*, from Kapanci Y, Assimacopoulos A, Irle C, et al: J Cell Biol 60:375, 1974. Copyright The Rockefeller University Press.)

V are also seen in a linear distribution, which corresponds to their presence in alveolar and endothelial basement membranes.[219, 220] Fibronectin is also present in relation to both alveolar and capillary basement membrane, as well as interstitial collagen fibers.[221]

Although present in much of the alveolar wall, interstitial connective tissue is focally absent. Many of these foci are associated with alveolar pores or fenestrae; however, some show only the absence of connective tissue, the potential space being covered by normal-appearing Type I cell processes.[222] The origin and significance of these connective tissue discontinuities are unclear.

The most prominent cell in the interstitium is the *myofibroblast* (contractile interstitial cell).[223] Ultrastructurally, it contains a well-developed Golgi complex and abundant endoplasmic reticulum and free ribosomes suggestive of fibroblastic differentiation; in addition, there are prominent bundles of microfilaments resembling those found in smooth muscle (*see* Fig. 1–27). In some regions, the cells appear to cross the interstitial space and attach to the basement membrane of epithelial and endothelial cells.[216, 223] Immunofluorescent studies have revealed the presence of actin within the cytoplasm, and pharmacologic investigations have shown hypoxia- and epinephrine-mediated contraction of strips of lung parenchyma, thus providing evidence for a contractile function.[223]

Interstitial myofibroblasts have several potential functions. It has been suggested that their contraction may result in a reduction in capillary blood flow and that this may be the mechanism by which hypoxia causes decreased alveolar perfusion—a possible means for local alveolar $\dot{V}/\dot{Q}$ regulation.[223] It has also been proposed that interstitial myofibroblasts may act to increase resistance to expansion of the interstitial space by edema fluid, thus propelling such fluid from the alveolar interstitium toward peribronchovascular lymphatics, where it may be effectively removed.[216] Finally, it is likely that these cells are responsible for the production of alveolar connective tissue, both in the normal state and in pathologic alveolar fibrosis.[224]

Mast cells can be seen within the alveolar interstitium, alveolar epithelial lining, and lumen,[225, 226] and it has been suggested that they may function in local control of the pulmonary vasculature.[225] A reversible increase in the number of alveolar septal and perivascular mast cells has been found in rats experiencing chronic hypoxia;[227] this increase has been correlated with an increase in right ventricular weight. It has also been speculated that the increase in mast cells may be *secondary* to pulmonary hypertension and in fact is a protective response.[228]

Lymphoreticular cells, including lymphocytes, macrophages (*see* farther on), and CD4+, Ia+ dendritic cells,[229] are present in variable numbers throughout the alveolar interstitium, where they are responsible for local defense.

The Alveolar Macrophage. Numerically, the alveolar macrophage is by far the most important nonepithelial cell in the alveolar lumen. Bronchoalveolar lavage of normal human air spaces yields a cell population composed of approximately 95% macrophages; dendritic cells (0.5%), lymphocytes (1% to 2%), monocyte-like cells of uncertain nature (2%), and polymorphonuclear leukocytes (less than 1%) account for the remainder.[229]

Pulmonary macrophages have been divided into several groups on the basis of their anatomic location:[230] (1) the *airway* macrophage, situated on or beneath the epithelial lining of conducting airways; (2) the *interstitial* macrophage, found either as isolated cells or associated with lymphoid tissue within interstitial connective tissue throughout the lung; (3) the *alveolar* macrophage, situated on the alveolar surface; and (4) the *intravascular* macrophage, located adjacent to the capillary endothelial cell.[231] Although all these cells are morphologically similar, it is likely that they represent subpopulations with different functional capabilities. For example, there is evidence that the intravascular macrophage acts in some animals as a reticuloendothelial cell similar to that in the liver and spleen[232] and that the interstitial form has a role in defense against blood-borne substances such as endotoxin.[233] However, because of its easy accessibility by bronchoalveolar lavage, the alveolar macrophage has been the most extensively studied and the following discussion deals principally with that cell.

As seen by light microscopy, the alveolar macrophage ranges from 15 to 50 μm in diameter, is more or less round in shape, and has a foamy or finely granular cytoplasm. Nuclei may be central or eccentric, and are occasionally multiple. Ultrastructurally (Fig. 1–28), the cells have prominent surface cytoplasmic projections that appear as microvillus-like structures on transmission electron microscopy and as ruffled folds on scanning electron microscopy.[234] The cytoplasm contains a well-developed Golgi apparatus; scattered mitochondria, endoplasmic reticulum, and microfilaments; and an abundance of membrane-bound granules of variable appearance representing primary and secondary lysosomes.[235] The last are especially prominent in the macrophages of cigarette smokers, where they may contain either "fibrillar" or "platelike" foreign material[235, 236] or lamellated lipid material ("sea-blue" granules).[235, 237] The former has been shown to consist of kaolinite (an aluminum silicate found in cigarette smoke),[236, 238] and the latter has been hypothesized to be ingested alveolar surfactant. In addition to an increase in lysosome number, macrophages themselves typically increase in both size and number and show several structural alterations as a result of chronic exposure to either cigarette smoke or inorganic particles such as silica.[239, 240] An age-related increase in alveolar macrophage number in nonsmoking individuals has also been documented.[241]

Pulmonary alveolar macrophages differ from other body macrophages by having predominantly aerobic energy production, an increased number of mitochondria and mitochondrial enzymes, and more numerous and larger lysosomes.[242] These features are believed to be adaptations to its location within the alveolar air spaces, where they are more or less continuously exposed to environmental toxins and a high oxygen concentration.

Many investigators have shown that alveolar macrophages are ultimately derived from bone marrow precursors, presumably by way of the peripheral blood monocyte.[243] Proliferation within the alveolar air space is important in maintaining the normal population.[244] In addition, there is evidence that alveolar interstitial macrophages are capable of division and replenishment or augmentation of the alveolar macrophage population, either in the absence of functioning bone marrow[245, 246] or in times of increased need.[247] The control of proliferation at both these sites may be related to the local production of colony-stimulating factor.[248] The

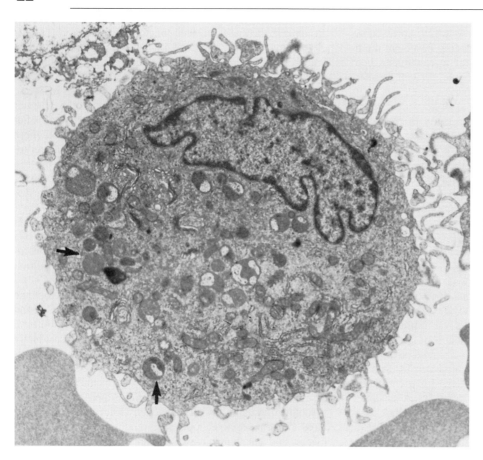

Figure 1–28. Alveolar Macrophage. Note the numerous microvilli and lysosomes *(arrows)*. (Human alveolar air space, ×8,500.)

average life span of the macrophage within the air space has been estimated to be about 80 days.[249]

Various inhaled foreign materials have a deleterious effect on macrophage activity. For example, particulates such as silicon dioxide can rupture the lysosomal membrane and thereby release enzymes into the cytoplasm and cause cell damage. A variety of insoluble compounds such as nitrogen dioxide, ozone, and a number of substances present in cigarette smoke are also toxic. They are not absorbed by the mucous layer of the tracheobronchial tree and penetrate directly to the alveoli, where they damage the macrophage through lipid peroxidation or by chemical combination of the oxidant gas with susceptible enzymes on the cell membrane.[250] Cigarette smoke has also been reported to affect alveolar macrophages by inhibiting metabolic activity and phagocytosis.[251, 252]

The functions of the alveolar macrophage are numerous and complex, and only a brief overview is given here. They can be considered under three headings: (1) phagocytosis and clearance of unwanted intra-alveolar material; (2) immunologic interactions; and (3) production of inflammatory and other chemical mediators. There is evidence that different subpopulations of macrophages may have different capacities for one or more of these functions.[253] This subject has been discussed in greater detail in several reviews.[249, 254, 255]

Phagocytosis and Clearance. Alveolar macrophages are motile and, in response to appropriate chemical stimuli, actively accumulate at the site of foreign material deposition. Their surface possesses receptors for C3 as well as the Fc portion of various immunoglobulins. In association with these and other opsonins such as fibronectin,[256] active phago-

cytosis of foreign material occurs. The latter may be particulate, such as silicates or asbestos, and may remain largely unaltered within secondary lysosomes. On the other hand, ingested microorganisms are subjected to the full battery of lysosomal enzymes and in most cases are completely destroyed. The precise means of microbial killing is not understood but is believed to be predominantly oxygen dependent and to be considerably more effective in activated macrophages; possible mechanisms include a hydrogen peroxidase (catalase) system, superoxide anion, and lysosomal cationic proteins and other enzymes.[255] In addition to inhaled foreign substances, alveolar macrophages ingest and eliminate endogenous pulmonary material, including the small number of dead Type I and Type II epithelial cells, alveolar surfactant,[257, 257a] and any inflammatory exudate that may be produced during pneumonitis.

Although some macrophages containing foreign material enter the alveolar interstitium and either remain there or are transported via lymphatics to regional lymph nodes, there is evidence that few follow this route.[187] Instead, the majority either die within the alveoli or make their way to the terminal bronchioles where they enter the mucociliary escalator and are carried to the larynx and swallowed along with their ingested material.[257b] Migration from the alveolar air spaces to the bronchioles may be partly due to inherent macrophage motility; the continual production of surfactant and its tendency to remain as a monolayer, and respiratory movement[258, 259] may also be important.

Immunologic Interactions. Alveolar macrophages have important immunologic functions, particularly in afferent immunologic mechanisms.[255] Although there are exceptions,[260] alveolar macrophages appear to be relatively poor antigen-presenting cells, and inhaled immunogens are probably phagocytosed and presented to T lymphocytes predominantly by dendritic cells.[261] Subsequent antigen presentation stimulates the T cells, which in time leads to both T- and B-cell and T-cell and macrophage interaction. The latter, mediated via lymphokines, results in macrophage activation, which is manifested by the production of a variety of immune mediators and by an increase in the number of surface receptors, amount of lysosomal enzymes, and microbicidal activity. The importance of these interactions is illustrated by the frequency and severity of pulmonary infections in immunocompromised individuals.

Production of Mediators. In addition to immune mediators,[261a] alveolar macrophages synthesize and secrete a variety of substances in both resting and activated conditions.[254, 255] Many of these undoubtedly have important effects on local pulmonary defense and structural integrity. *Fibronectin* is present in fluid derived from bronchoalveolar lavage and has been shown immunohistochemically to be present in alveolar macrophages.[256] α_1-*Antitrypsin* has also been shown to be synthesized by alveolar macrophages and may serve as a local antiproteolytic agent.[262, 262a] Macrophages studied *in vitro* have been shown to release a factor that modulates polymorphonuclear leukocyte function.[263] The cells are capable of producing other highly active inflammatory mediators such as *prostaglandins*[264] and *leukotrienes;*[265] they also synthesize *lysozyme* and *interferon,*[266] substances that contribute to defense against bacterial and viral infection.

Geometry and Dimensions

Although the shape of alveoli has been likened to that of a honeycomb,[10] on routine light microscopic examination of formalin-fixed tissue their size and shape vary considerably more than those of typical honeycomb cells,[267] the appearance more closely resembling that of closely packed bubbles of soap foam (i.e., an irregular polyhedral configuration). The vast majority of alveolar junctions are formed by the intersection of three septa.

Under dynamic conditions, the shape of the various components of the alveolar septum can be affected by three mechanical factors, each of which can vary in the normal respiratory cycle:[216] (1) tissue force caused by tension on the interstitial connective tissue transmitted through the connective tissue of the visceral pleura; (2) capillary distending pressure; and (3) alveolar air-fluid surface forces. Scanning and transmission electron microscopic studies have demonstrated an irregularity of the alveolar surface produced by deep pleats or folds that project into the inner portion of the septa; these pleats divide it into intercommunicating chambers and give the alveolus a crumpled appearance (Fig. 1–29).[216, 268] Folds are present in most alveoli at lower lung volumes (including those at which tidal breathing takes place) and tend to be obliterated at higher lung volumes as the alveolus expands. The alveolus has thus been likened to a nonelastic "double-walled paper bag" that expands by unfolding its septal pleats rather than by stretching its wall.[268] The folds often contain small pools of surface-lining fluid at the alveolar surface, and their bases are usually adjacent to the thick portion of the interstitium (Fig. 1–30).

The precise forces leading to this arrangement are not clear. In addition to mechanical factors, interstitial myofibroblasts tend to be located at the bases of the folds and it is possible that they have an influence on the localization of folds at these sites. Some investigators have found an ordered structure in connective tissue in these areas, with

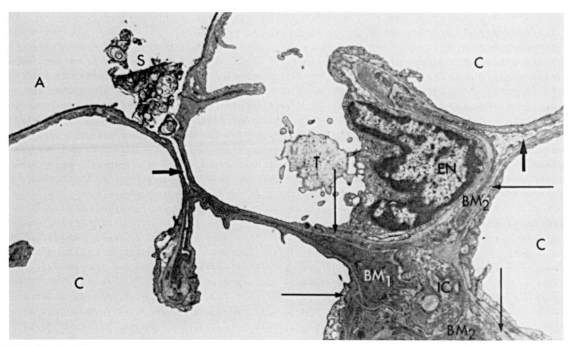

Figure 1–29. Alveolar Pleats or Folds. Folding of the thin portion of the air-blood tissue barrier over the thick portion, which appears to be shifted into the capillary lumen. Two collapsed alveolar lumens *(thick arrows)* are visible, one of which joins an open alveolus (A). The basement membranes (BM$_1$ and BM$_2$) of the two alveoli converge toward a contractile interstitial cell (IC) located at the thick portion of the barrier (the membrane portions seen at the *bottom* belong to the same collapsed alveolus as the one recognizable at the *upper right*). The alveolar and capillary basement membranes fuse with each other at the borders of the cell *(thin arrows)*. S, surfactant; T, thrombocytes; EN, endothelial cell; C, capillary. (Rat lung, fixation at 10 cm H_2O airway pressure, ×8,600.) (From Assimacopoulos A, Guggenheim R, Kapanci Y: Lab Invest 34:10, 1976. Copyright US-Canadian Division of IAP.)

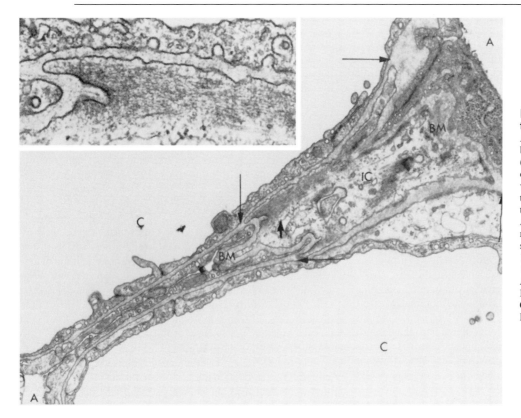

Figure 1–30. The Thick Portion of the Air-Blood Barrier. A contractile interstitial cell (IC) bridges across the capillary space (C). The basement membrane (BM) of the two adjacent alveoli (A) converges toward the cell and fuses with the capillary basement membrane at the borders of this cell *(thin arrows).* A high magnification of a bundle of microfilaments *(thick arrow)* is shown *(inset).* (Rat lung, fixation at 15 cm H_2O airway pressure, $\times 20,000$; inset, $\times 67,000$.) (From Assimacopoulos A, Guggenheim R, Kapanci Y: Lab Invest 34:10, 1976. Copyright US-Canadian Division of IAP.)

collagen and elastic tissue passing in a curved arrangement from one side of the septum to the other suggestive of a possible tethering effect of the connective tissue.[269]

Theoretically, the pleated arrangement has a number of important consequences. First is the tendency to isolate the thick portion of the interstitium to the interior of the septum and leave the thin air-blood barrier exposed to the alveolar gas, thus maximizing surface area contact between gas and blood. Second, pools of surface-active material within the folds may create localized areas of negative pressure concentrated at the thick portion of the septum; it has been hypothesized that this process may be important in determining drainage of the small amount of fluid that normally leaks from alveolar capillaries into the interstitium.[216] Finally, it has been suggested that the intercapillary folds may act in a purely mechanical fashion to impede capillary blood flow; because the folds are greatest in extent in the more collapsed alveoli, this would have the effect of matching ventilation with perfusion.[268]

The number of alveoli in the adult human lung[9, 10, 270] has been estimated to be about 300×10^6. However, one group documented considerable variation in this figure among different individuals, with computed values ranging from 212×10^6 to 605×10^6.[271] Of some interest was the observation in this study of a positive correlation between alveolar number and body length.

In adults, both maximal diameter and depth of the alveolus (measured from the opening at the alveolar duct or sac to the base) are about 250 to 300 μm.[10] Total alveolar surface area at total lung capacity (TLC) has been estimated by several methods to be approximately 70 to 80 m^2,[10] although these figures appear to vary considerably depending on body size.[272] As might be expected, alveolar volume and surface area increase as total lung volume increases.[273, 274] There appears to be a linear decrease in alveolar surface area with increasing age.[275]

The Lung Unit

Of the subdivisions of lung parenchyma that have been proposed as the fundamental "unit" of lung structure, the primary and secondary lobules of Miller[3] and the pulmonary acinus have gained the widest acceptance. The question of which most accurately represents the anatomic basis of normal and pathologic processes is controversial, since each possesses characteristics that suit one set of circumstances better than another. In our opinion, however, the one most acceptable for diagnostic purposes, particularly from the point of view of the radiologist, is the secondary lobule.

The Primary Lobule

The primary lobule (Fig. 1–31) consists of all alveolar ducts, alveolar sacs, and alveoli, together with their accompanying blood vessels, nerves, and connective tissue distal to the last respiratory bronchiole. Because the human lung contains as many as 20 to 25 million primary lobules,[7] it is clear that this unit is too small to be identified radiologically and is thus of no practical significance from the point of view of this diagnostic technique.

The Secondary Lobule

The secondary lobule is defined as the smallest discrete portion of the lung that is surrounded by connective tissue

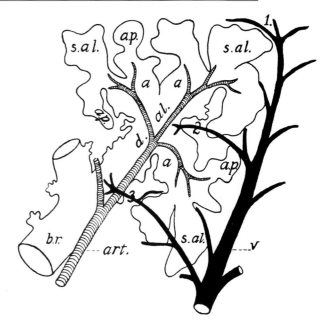

Figure 1–31. Schematic Representation of a Primary Lobule. b.r., respiratory bronchiole; d.al., alveolar duct; a, atrium; s.al., alveolar sac; a.p., alveolus; art., arteriole with branches to the atria and alveolar sacs; v, pulmonary venule with branches from the pleura (1), the alveolar ducts (2), and the respiratory bronchiole (3). (From Miller WS: The Lung. Springfield, IL, Charles C Thomas, 1937.)

septa.[3] It is irregularly polyhedral in shape and generally 1 to 2.5 cm in diameter. Interlobular septa are most well developed in the periphery of the lung, where they are continuous with the vascular layer of the pleura (Fig. 1–32).

They contain pulmonary veins and lymphatic vessels that drain the adjacent lobular tissue and are delimited on both sides by a thin layer of elastic tissue continuous with the pleural internal elastic lamina. Septa are most numerous in

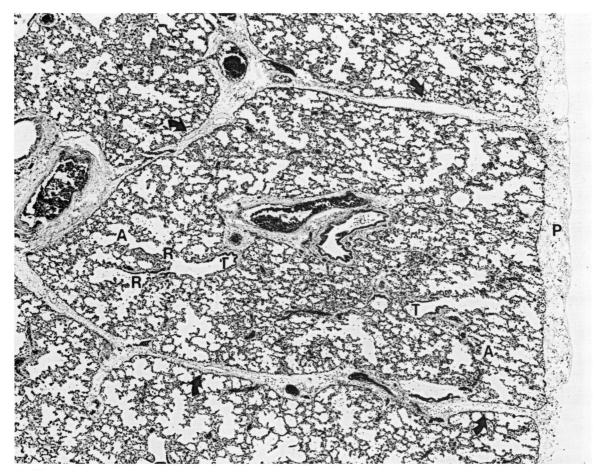

Figure 1–32. Secondary Lobule—Histologic Appearance. A, alveolar duct; *arrows*, interlobular septum; P, pleura; R, respiratory bronchiole; S, alveolar sac; T, terminal bronchiole. (× 6.)

the apical, anterior, and lateral aspects of the upper lobe and in the lateral and anterior regions of the right middle lobe, lingula, and lower lobe (Fig. 1–33).[276] In these areas they measure approximately 100 μm in thickness and can be identified on visual inspection of the pleural or cut surfaces of the lung (Fig. 1–34) and on high-resolution computed tomography (HRCT).[277] In the more central regions of the lung, septa may be difficult to identify and are commonly absent altogether.

The functional significance of interlobular septa is uncertain, particularly since there are considerable differences between animal species and between individual humans in the extent of their development. In some instances, they appear to limit the spread of infection by confining it to one or more lobules (Fig. 1–35). Since many infections related to inhalation of microorganisms appear to begin in the lung periphery, it is possible that this is the reason for the relative prominence of interlobular septa in this location.

Because of the inconstancy of interlobular septa, the distribution of secondary lobules is not uniform within the lung. Reid proposed an alternative definition for the lobule that would be applicable to areas of lung with poorly developed septa.[278] According to this definition, the secondary lobule consists of pulmonary parenchyma supplied by a cluster of three to five terminal bronchioles. A secondary lobule of Miller measuring 5 to 10 mm in diameter corresponds to a lobule as defined by Reid; however, larger Miller's lobules contain several Reid's lobules.[279, 280] Because Reid's lobule cannot be identified radiologically, we consider the secondary lobule as defined by Miller a more useful unit of lung structure for diagnostic and descriptive purposes.

The normal secondary lobule cannot be identified on the chest radiograph. Only when the interlobular septa are rendered visible as septal lines as a result of thickening by fluid or tissue (such as edema or carcinoma) can the volume of lung between two lines be recognized as a secondary lobule. By contrast, normal interlobular septa are easily identified on HRCT, most commonly in the lateral aspect of the lung as straight lines 1 to 2.5 cm in length. Although less well visualized in the more central regions of the lungs, they can be identified in both gross specimens and on HRCT when they are thickened by edema or inflammatory or neoplastic tissue (Fig. 1–36).[277, 281, 282, 282a, 282b] The secondary lobule itself can also be identified on HRCT when it is consolidated by blood or inflammatory exudate (*see* Fig. 1–35).

The preterminal (lobular) bronchiole and accompanying pulmonary artery that supply the secondary lobule measure approximately 1 mm in diameter. The lobular artery can often be visualized on HRCT as a small rounded or branching linear attenuation near the center (core) of the lobule. The smallest arteries that can be identified extend within 3 to 5 mm of the edge of the lobule.[284] Because the wall of the normal lobular bronchiole measures less than 0.1 mm in thickness, it cannot be visualized on computed tomography (CT). The lobular bronchiole divides into terminal bronchioles, which in turn subdivide into respiratory bronchioles and alveolar ducts that occupy progressively more peripheral portions of the lobule (*see* Fig. 1–32).

There are two major reasons for considering the secondary lobule of Miller the fundamental unit of lung structure from a radiologic point of view: (1) it is the smallest anatomic unit that can be clearly identified on HRCT; and (2) assessment of the distribution of abnormalities within it can be helpful in the differential diagnosis of lung disease.[283–285] For example, pathologic processes related to the terminal or respiratory bronchioles are characterized on HRCT by predominant distribution near the center of the lobule.[285a] Specific abnormalities include localized areas of low attenuation in centrilobular emphysema and areas of increased attenuation in tuberculosis, hypersensitivity pneumonitis, sarcoidosis, asbestosis, and silicosis (Fig. 1–37).[284, 286, 287] In addition, various forms of bronchiolitis are characterized on HRCT by the presence of nodular areas of attenuation or branching lines near the center of the lobule (Fig. 1–38) or by decreased attenuation of the lobule because of air trapping or vasoconstriction (Fig. 1–39).[285a, 287–290]

The Acinus

The pulmonary acinus is defined as the portion of lung distal to the terminal bronchiole and is composed of the respiratory bronchioles, alveolar ducts, alveolar sacs, alveoli, and their accompanying vessels and connective tissue (Fig. 1–40).[291, 292] Reported measurements of acinar diameter vary between 6 and 10 mm, depending to some extent on the technique and pressure at which the lung is inflated.[168, 293, 294] Acinar volume has been estimated to be about 180 mm³ at three-quarters TLC.[267]

In one investigation of two acini from a 32-year-old woman, approximately 3,200 and 4,000 alveoli were identified;[168] based on these findings, it has been estimated that the lungs of that particular individual contained a total of approximately 80,000 acini.[169] However, other estimates of alveolar number per acinus have been higher (from 7,100[170] to 20,000[295]), which suggests that the actual number of acini per lung may be considerably less.

In view of the size of the acinus, it is reasonable to assume that it should be visible radiologically when completely or partially filled with contrast material or inflammatory exudate. In fact, experimental studies using a special tantalum suspension have shown that progressive filling of a single acinus initially produces a rosette appearance and eventually a spherical image (Fig. 1–41).[293] In conditions such as pulmonary edema, acute air-space pneumonia, and pulmonary hemorrhage, recognition of this distinctive "alveolar filling" pattern can help the radiologist narrow the differential diagnosis to the relatively few diseases capable of consolidating parenchymal air spaces.[296, 297]

Despite these considerations, we believe that the concept of the acinus is of limited value in assessment of the chest radiograph or CT for several reasons. First, normal acini cannot be identified on the chest radiograph or with HRCT. Second, small nodular areas of consolidation cannot be assumed to represent acinar shadows radiologically. For example, in one radiologic-pathologic investigation, fluffy nodules corresponding to an acinar pattern in bronchopneumonia, "acinonodose" tuberculosis, and bronchiolitis were found to be caused predominantly by inflammation around terminal and respiratory bronchioles, with the distal air spaces usually being spared.[298] Finally, consolidation caused by pneumonia or hemorrhage is seldom limited to the acinus but rather tends to coalesce and have a lobular, segmental, or lobar distribution.

Text continued on page 31

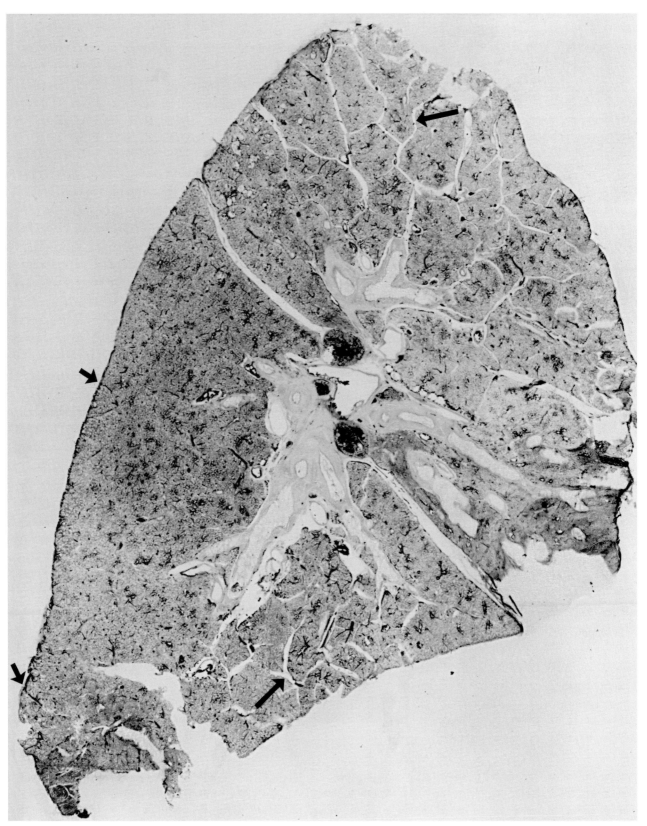

Figure 1–33. Interlobular Septa. A paper-mounted section of a sagittal slice of the right lung shows moderately distended interlobular septa in the anterior and apical portions of the upper lobe and the basal aspect of the lower lobe *(long arrows)*. Some nondistended septa are also evident as thin black lines at the pleural surface of the lower lobe *(short arrows)*.

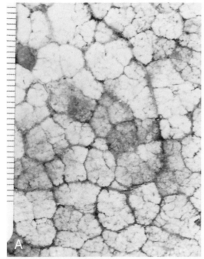

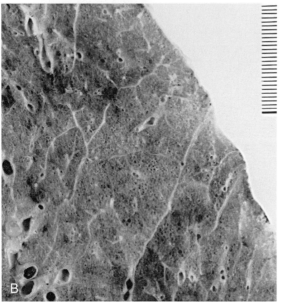

Figure 1–34. Secondary Lobule. A close-up view of the lower lobe visceral pleura *(A)* shows the bases of numerous, irregularly shaped secondary lobules measuring from 0.5 to 1.5 cm in greatest dimension. *B,* A magnified view of a midsagittal section of an upper lobe shows an irregular array of thin septa demarcating secondary lobules of variable shape and size.

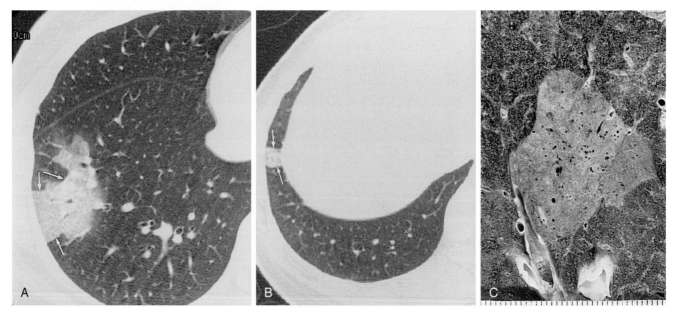

Figure 1–35. Consolidation of Secondary Pulmonary Lobules. HRCT scans demonstrate consolidation of secondary pulmonary lobules, multiple in *A* and solitary in *B*. Note the sharp demarcation between the consolidated lobules outlined by the interlobular septa *(arrows)* and the normal adjacent lung parenchyma. A magnified view of lung from another patient *(C)* shows homogeneous consolidation of a portion of parenchyma demarcated by interlobular septa and the wall of a small bronchus. Histologic sections showed organizing pneumonia of uncertain etiology. The appearance in each of these three cases suggests that the initial pathologic process was limited in its spread within the lung by the presence of the septa.

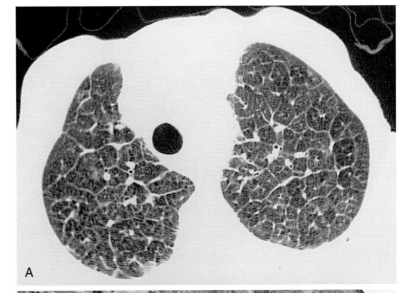

Figure 1–36. Interlobular Septal Thickening. HRCT (1-mm collimation) scan in a patient with interstitial pulmonary edema *(A)* demonstrates thickening of the interlobular septa. Secondary pulmonary lobules are variable in size and have an irregular polyhedral shape. The patient was a 77-year-old woman with congestive heart failure. Incidental note is made of unrelated anterior mediastinal lymphadenopathy. A magnified view of a slice of upper lobe from another patient *(B)* shows mild-to-moderate interlobular septal thickening as a result of lymphangitic carcinomatosis. The architecture is similar to that of the HRCT image.

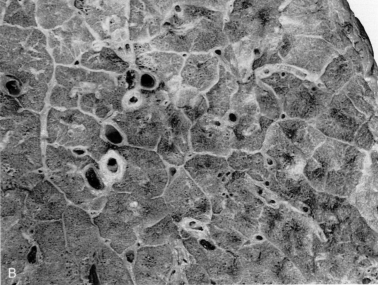

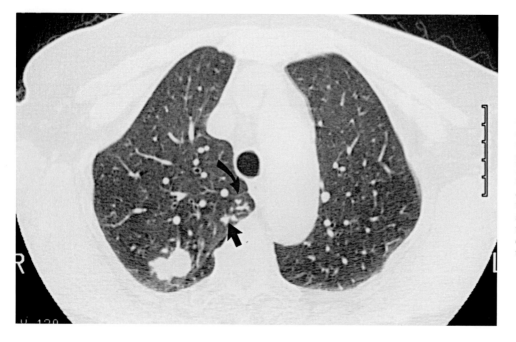

Figure 1–37. Centrilobular Nodules in Tuberculosis. HRCT (1-mm collimation) scan at the level of the aortic arch demonstrates a lobulated, 2-cm-diameter nodule in the posterior segment of the right upper lobe. Note the centrilobular distribution of smaller nodules *(straight arrow)* and normal interlobular septum *(curved arrow)*. The patient was an 80-year-old woman with reactivation tuberculosis (large nodule) and endobronchial spread (smaller nodules).

Figure 1–38. Centrilobular Nodules Caused by Bronchiolitis. HRCT (1.5-mm collimation) scan demonstrates small nodules and branching structures *(arrows)*. These abnormalities are situated approximately 5 mm away from vessels that are too large to be within the secondary pulmonary lobule and therefore represent borders of secondary pulmonary lobules. Structures and abnormalities located 5 mm away from these borders must be centrilobular in location. The patient was a 28-year-old man with bronchiolitis related to inhalation of foreign material.

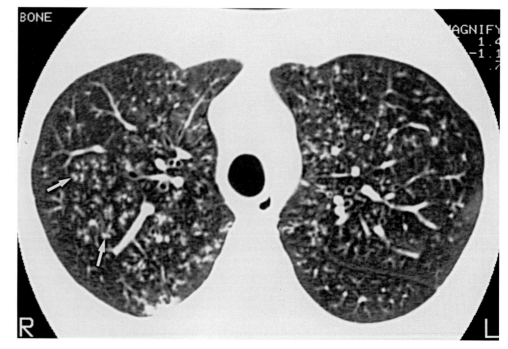

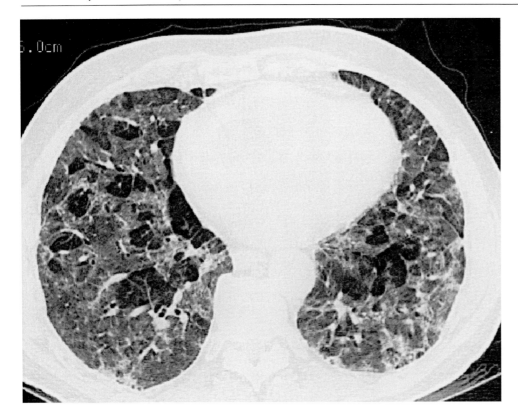

Figure 1–39. Decreased Perfusion Caused by Bronchiolitis. HRCT (1-mm collimation) scan through the lower lung zones demonstrates extensive areas of ground-glass attenuation. Note the localized polyhedral areas of decreased attenuation and small central vessels corresponding to secondary pulmonary lobules with decreased perfusion. The patient was a 74-year-old man with extrinsic allergic alveolitis and severe bronchiolitis. The areas of ground-glass attenuation correspond to alveolitis. The decreased perfusion of some of the secondary pulmonary lobules is presumably related to small airway obstruction.

There has also been some debate concerning whether the acinus can be considered the fundamental unit of lung tissue from a functional point of view. Most physiologists describe the alveolus as the unit of the lung. In so doing, however, they equate this not with the anatomic alveolus, but with a hypothetical unit that cannot be precisely defined morphologically. In fact, it would be unrealistic to consider the alveolus a physiologic unit since each one is part of a family of alveoli that arise from a common alveolar sac, alveolar duct, or respiratory bronchiole and that receive capillaries from a common arteriole.[299] In normal circumstances, it is unlikely that the behavior of any one alveolus differs from that of its "siblings." Thus it is possible that Miller's primary lobule, which consists of the alveolar duct and its ramifications that arise from a last-order respiratory bronchiole, is the smallest portion that can be considered in the concept of a physiologic unit of lung function.

Farther up the airways, at the level of the terminal bronchiole, a greater portion of the lung is included as a unit of function because some 400 alveolar duct units are located distal to this point. Do all the alveoli that make up this acinus behave similarly? This question cannot be answered yet, although accumulating evidence in the areas of both structure and physiology suggests that they do. For this reason, the basic functioning unit of the lung is taken to be the acinus, i.e., all lung parenchyma distal to the terminal bronchiole. If future studies provide evidence that acini within a secondary lobule behave similarly, it would allow a concordance of radiologic and functional units.

Channels of Peripheral Airway and Acinar Communication

The first and probably the most studied of these structures are *alveolar pores* (Fig. 1–42). Although first described by Adriani in 1847, these small discontinuities have come to be known as *pores of Kohn* after the latter's observation of fibrin strands traversing alveolar walls in cases of acute pneumonia. They are present in the lungs of most mammals[300] in numbers varying with the species and with the technique of fixation and examination.[301] They tend to be more numerous in older animals and in the apical and subpleural regions of the lung.[191, 302] The size of the aperture is usually between 2 and 10 μm, although the upper limit is somewhat arbitrary (*see* farther on). Just as the width of the alveolar wall is dependent on lung volume and the degree of capillary engorgement, the width of the pores can also vary with these factors.

Scanning electron microscopy of human lungs shows approximately 5 to 20 pores per alveolus,[303, 304] and the

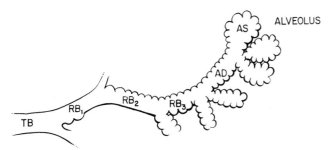

Figure 1–40. Component Parts of the Acinus. TB, terminal bronchiole; RB, respiratory bronchiole; AD, alveolar duct; AS, alveolar sac. (From Thurlbeck WM: *In* Sommers SC [ed]: Pathology Annual. New York, Appleton-Century-Crofts, 1968, p 377.)

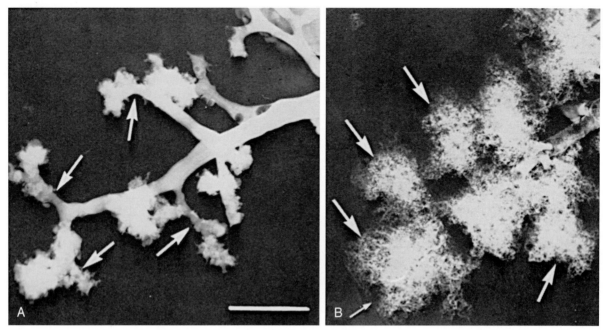

Figure 1–41. Bronchographic Morphology of the Peripheral Airways and Acinus. *A* shows a selected area from the periphery of a bronchogram on a normal human lung removed at autopsy and opacified with a tantalum suspension. *Arrows* indicate terminal bronchioles. *B*, Radiograph after air-drying of the lung. Further opacification of the intra-acinar airways has taken place. *Arrows* indicate partially opacified acini that can be related to the terminal bronchioles in *A*. The *bar* in *A* represents 5 mm. (From Gamsu G, Thurlbeck WM, Macklem PT, et al: Invest Radiol 6:171, 1971.)

number is usually considerably less in lungs fixed via the vasculature than via the airways.[303] The pores are generally round and appear to be fairly evenly distributed over the entire alveolar wall.[304] Their edges are lined by Type I epithelial cells.[305] By transmission electron microscopy, the aperture is usually free of cellular or other material in airway-fixed material; however, in vascular-perfused tissue the pore is typically occluded by a thin film of alveolar surfactant.[213, 303] Since it is probable that vascular-perfused tissue more closely represents the normal state within the alveolar air space, the presence of surfactant occlusion casts some doubt on the significance of alveolar pores as a mechanism

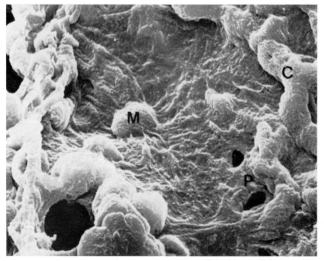

Figure 1–42. Surface of an Alveolus. Note the capillaries (C), a macrophage (M), and alveolar pores (P). (Scanning electron microscopy, ×3,650.) (Courtesy of Dr. Nai-San Wang, McGill University, Montreal.)

for collateral ventilation. It has been suggested, however, that "ventilation" can occur by diffusion across the fluid.[217] It is also possible that the pores represent an interacinar pathway for the spread of edema fluid, with or without pathogenic microorganisms.

The origin of the pores is unknown; however, because of their rarity in young children it is likely that they are acquired.[302] It has been suggested that they result from the desquamation of alveolar epithelial cells[306] or from the action of ventilatory stress on alveolar walls.[302] It has also been hypothesized that the initial event might be loss of interstitial connective tissue,[222] possibly as a result of the release of proteases from macrophages or neutrophils.[222, 307]

The relationship of *alveolar fenestrae* (alveolar discontinuities measuring 20 to 100 μm in diameter) to alveolar pores is unclear.[308] They are thought by most investigators to represent a pathologic state of the alveolar wall, some believing them to be the earliest stage of pulmonary emphysema.[222, 301, 308] It has also been speculated that alveolar pores may themselves be the precursors of fenestrae.[301, 308] Whatever their relationship, it is possible that these larger discontinuities are of greater significance than alveolar pores in providing a pathway for interacinar communication.

Direct communications between alveoli and respiratory, terminal, and preterminal bronchioles were first described by Lambert,[309, 310] and their presence confirmed by others.[311, 312] These *canals of Lambert* consist of epithelial-lined tubular structures that in lungs fixed in deflation range in diameter from practically "closed" to 30 μm;[309] in one study of a lung fixed in full inflation, a single communication measuring 150 μm in diameter was identified.[170] It is not known whether these "airways" provide solely intra-acinar accessory communication or whether interacinar connections capable of subserving collateral ventilation occur as well.

In both animals and humans, particles considerably larger than either alveolar pores or most canals of Lambert are able to pass through collateral channels in lung parenchyma. For example, polystyrene spheres 120 μm in diameter have been passed through collateral channels in dogs' lungs,[313] and spheres up to 64 μm have been passed in excised human lungs.[314] Several investigators have attempted to localize and characterize these channels anatomically. In one investigation in which insufflated India ink aerosols were passed from one segment of a dog's lobe into an adjacent segment, the particles were found to be deposited on collateral channels that resembled respiratory bronchioles.[313] In a micropuncture injection study of cleared human lung, interacinar and, occasionally, interlobular flow of silicon rubber was identified through short, tubular channels approximately 200 μm in diameter that were not further characterized.[315] In another study using bronchial corrosion casts, intersegmental connections were identified in the form of small airways that resembled first-order respiratory bronchioles with a diameter of 80 to 150 μm.[316] Histologic evidence of direct communication between two acini at the level of their alveolar sacs has also been presented.[169]

In summary, it is apparent that collateral ventilation between adjacent acini, lobules, or segments may occur by several anatomic pathways. In addition to being poorly characterized, however, the frequency of these channels within an individual lung and their variation between different regions of the same lung are virtually unknown. The importance and mechanisms of collateral ventilation are thus more easily understood from a knowledge of physiologic data, discussed on page 59.

RADIOLOGY

In 1943, Jackson and Huber published a nomenclature of the bronchial segments that was widely adopted and remains the generally accepted terminology in North America (Table 1–2).[317] In 1955, Boyden proposed a numerical system for identification of bronchial segments;[318] although this system is used by some physicians, the Jackson-Huber nomenclature is used exclusively throughout this book.

No official nomenclature exists for the major bronchi interposed between the trachea and the segmental bronchi of the five pulmonary lobes. Through common usage, however, the designation *main bronchi* is applied to the bronchi arising at the bifurcation of the trachea and extending to the origin of the upper lobe bronchus on each side; the terms *upper, middle,* and *lower lobe bronchi* are used for the corresponding bronchi supplying individual lobes; and *intermediate bronchus* is applied to the airway segment between the right upper lobe bronchus and the origins of the right middle and lower lobe bronchi.

The Trachea and Main Bronchi

With respect to the coronal plane, the trachea is for all intents and purposes a midline structure; a slight deviation to the right at the level of the aortic arch is a normal finding and should not be misinterpreted as evidence of

Table 1–2. NOMENCLATURE OF BRONCHOPULMONARY ANATOMY

JACKSON-HUBER	BOYDEN
Upper lobe	
Apical	B¹
Anterior	B²
Posterior	B₃
Right middle lobe	
Lateral	B⁴
Medial	B⁵
Right lower lobe	
Superior	B⁶
Medial basal	B⁷
Anterior basal	B⁸
Lateral basal	B⁹
Posterior basal	B¹⁰
Left upper lobe	
Upper division	
Apical-posterior	B¹&³
Anterior	B²
Lingular/division	
Superior	B⁴
Inferior	B⁵
Left lower lobe	
Superior	B⁶
Anteromedial	B⁷&⁸
Lateral basal	B⁹
Posterior basal	B¹⁰

displacement. The location of the trachea in the anteroposterior (AP) axis is somewhat more variable; although commonly situated more or less midway between the sternum and spine, it may rest against the vertebral bodies posteriorly or may be positioned more anteriorly than expected and mimic forward displacement.[319] On posteroanterior radiographs, the tracheal walls are parallel except on the left side just above the bifurcation, where the aorta commonly impresses a smooth indentation. The air columns of the trachea and main bronchi have a smoothly serrated contour created by indentations of the horseshoe-shaped cartilage rings at regular intervals within their walls.

There is considerable variation in the cross-sectional shape of the trachea on CT.[319, 320] In one study of 50 subjects without tracheal or mediastinal abnormalities, the most common shapes were round or oval;[320] a horseshoe shape with a flat posterior wall was seen in only 12 of 50 subjects, an inverted pear shape in 6, and an almost square configuration in 2. Twenty-two of the 50 subjects had more than one distinct shape at different levels. The most inferior 1 to 2 cm assumed an oval shape, the azygos arch usually being visible to the right of the trachea at this level.

The length of the normal intrathoracic trachea as measured on CT ranges from 6 to 9 cm (mean, 7.5 ± 0.8 cm).[320] Its caliber has been determined from measurements of coronal and sagittal diameters of the tracheal air column on posteroanterior and lateral chest radiographs of approximately 800 patients with no clinical or radiologic evidence of respiratory disease.[321] Assuming a normative range that encompasses 3 SD from the mean (99.7% of the normal population), in men aged 20 to 79 years the upper limits of normal for coronal and sagittal diameters are 25 and 27 mm, respectively; in women of the same age, they are 21 and 23 mm. Values greater than these figures should be considered to reflect pathologic widening of the tracheal air column. According to the same study, the lower limit of normal for both dimensions is 13 mm in men and 10 mm in women. Of interest was the observation that no statistically significant correlation was found between tracheal caliber and body height.

The pressure-area behavior of the extrathoracic trachea can be measured by performing CT scans during graded Valsalva and Müller maneuvers (Fig. 1–43). In one study performed at functional residual capacity (FRC) in which extrathoracic tracheal transmural pressure was obtained by subtracting atmospheric pressure from airway opening pressure, the pressure-area curves demonstrated a plateau or an increase in tracheal cross-sectional area with extrathoracic transmural pressure lower than -15 cm H_2O.[322] By contrast, pressure-area curves obtained by using extrathoracic esopha-

geal pressure as tracheal external pressure instead of atmospheric pressure did not show a plateau or an increased cross-sectional area with the Müller maneuver. These results demonstrate that extrathoracic tracheal external pressure is not atmospheric, probably as a result of the combination of transmission of pleural pressure to the cervical interstitial tissue and contraction of cervical accessory inspiratory muscles; otherwise, the Müller maneuver should have resulted in a decrease in tracheal cross-sectional area rather than a plateau or an increase.

The intrathoracic trachea, as distinct from the extrathoracic portion, shows no appreciable change in diameter with changes in pleural pressure at a fixed lung volume. In a study in which CT was used to examine the tracheas of two healthy adults at FRC, first at an intratracheal pressure of $+20$ cm H_2O and then at -20 cm H_2O, the intrathoracic

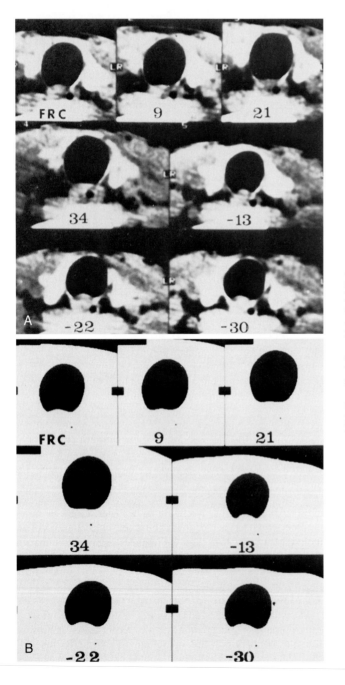

Figure 1–43. Pressure/Area Behavior of the Extrathoracic Trachea. These 5-mm CT cuts (*A* and *B* at different window settings) were made in a plane perpendicular to the long axis of the trachea 3 cm below the larynx. A normal subject performed graded Valsalva maneuvers, which resulted in positive intratracheal (and therefore transmural) pressures of 9, 21, and 34 cm H_2O, as well as graded Müller's maneuvers, which resulted in negative intratracheal (and therefore transmural) pressures of -13, -22, and -30 cm H_2O. It is apparent that with positive transmural pressure the tracheal area increases and the posterior membranous portion flattens. With negative transmural pressure there is an initial decrease in cross-sectional area and inward displacement of the posterior membranous portion of the trachea.

However, with progressively negative pressures, further decrease in cross-sectional area does not occur. The extrathoracic esophageal pressure, presumably representing extratracheal pressure, becomes negative during the Müller's maneuver and prevents further collapse.

portions of the tracheas showed little change in cross-sectional area between the two pressures;[323] by contrast, the cross-sectional area of the cervical trachea decreased by about one third from the higher pressure to the lower, the membranous posterior wall tending to bulge backward strikingly at the higher pressure and to draw well into the tracheal lumen at the lower pressure. The two tracheas were 6% and 12% shorter at the lower pressure.

The diameters of the intrathoracic trachea are influenced by changes in lung volume. In one study, 10 normal subjects ranging in age from 24 to 31 years were assessed by performing 100-msec dynamic scans at 500-msec intervals during a 6-second period as the patient performed a forced inspiratory and expiratory vital capacity maneuver.[324] The mean cross-sectional area of the intrathoracic trachea at the level of the aortic arch decreased from 280 mm² at end inspiration (range, 221 to 388 mm²; SD, 50) to 178 mm² at end expiration (range, 115 to 236 mm²; SD, 40) (mean ± SD of 35% ± 18% decrease between inspiration and expiration). This decrease in cross-sectional area correlated well with the decrease in tracheal AP and coronal diameters from maximum inspiration to maximum expiration.

The dimensions of the growing trachea in relation to age and gender were assessed in one study of CT scans on 130 subjects in the first two decades of life.[325] Measurements included the length, AP and transverse diameters, cross-sectional areas, and gas volumes of the trachea. No differences were found between boys and girls under the age of 14 years, at which time girls' tracheas stopped growing; by contrast, the tracheas of boys continued to enlarge (but not lengthen) for a time after growth in height ceased. The mean transverse diameter tended to be greater than the mean AP diameter up to the age of 6 years; thereafter, the diameters were nearly identical until the age of 18 years, when the AP diameter usually became slightly larger.

The trachea divides into the left and right main bronchi at the carina. Two methods of measuring the angle of bifurcation are available: the interbronchial angle (defined as the angle between the central axis of each of the main bronchi) and the subcarinal angle (the angle of divergence of the right and left main bronchi measured along their inferior borders). The latter seems to us to be the more practical. Two radiologic studies have been performed to assess the angle in adults. In one study performed in 58 subjects aged 16 to 83 years, the carinal angle ranged from 41 to 71 degrees in men (mean, 56) and from 41 to 74 degrees in women (mean, 58).[326] In a second study of 100 normal adults, the range of values was considerably wider—35 to 91 degrees, with a mean of 61 degrees (SD, 12 degrees).[327] In the latter study, age and gender had no relationship with the bifurcation angle. However, there was a weak inverse correlation between the shape of the thorax and the angle of tracheal bifurcation: as the chest became longer and narrower (i.e., the patient was more asthenic), the angle became more acute. It is clear from these figures that there is such a wide range of normal values for the bifurcation angle that even gross deviation from the 55- to 60-degree average should not be interpreted as abnormal.

In adults, the course of the right main bronchus distally is more direct than that of the left. However, measurement of bronchial angles of 50 children and adolescents ranging in age from birth to 18 years has shown symmetry of right and left angles in virtually all subjects up to the age of 15 years.[328] This finding explains the relatively equal incidence of right- and left-sided aspiration of foreign bodies in children.

The transverse diameter of the right main bronchus at TLC is greater than that of the left (15.3 mm as compared with 13.0 mm),[329] although its length before the origin of the upper lobe bronchus as measured at autopsy is shorter (average, 2.2 cm as compared with 5 cm on the left).[330, 331]

The Lobar Bronchi and Bronchopulmonary Segments

The pattern of bronchial branching shows considerable variation, particularly in subsegmental airways but also to some extent in the lobar and segmental branches.[332–338] In the great majority of cases, these variations are of no clinical significance and are discovered only during bronchoscopy or autopsy. In addition, despite the anatomic variation of segmental bronchi, the location of the bronchopulmonary segments is more or less constant; since recognition of these zones is more important radiologically than the identification of specific bronchi, anatomic differences in the latter are relatively unimportant in radiologic diagnosis. The exception is when surgery is being contemplated, in which case knowledge of any deviation may be important in determining the approach to pulmonary resection. For example, a tracheal bronchus or "mirror-image" bronchial tree (bronchial isomerism) may be associated with cardiovascular anomalies or situs inversus, and their presence should be brought to the attention of the surgeon.

On this and the following pages, the anatomic distribution of the pulmonary segments and their feeding bronchi is described and illustrated. Each bronchus is considered separately, preceded by reproductions of a right bronchogram and corresponding drawings in AP (Fig. 1–44) and lateral (Fig. 1–45) projections; left bronchograms are similarly depicted (Figs. 1–46 and 1–47).

Right Upper Lobe. The bronchus to the right upper lobe arises from the lateral aspect of the main bronchus, approximately 2 cm from the tracheal carina. It divides slightly more than 1 cm from its origin, most commonly into three branches designated anterior, posterior, and apical (Figs. 1–48 to 1–50). The branching pattern is particularly variable in relation to the axillary portion of the lobe. Infrequently, the upper lobe bronchus or one of its branches (usually the apical) arises directly from the lateral wall of the trachea (the "tracheal bronchus").

Right Middle Lobe. The intermediate bronchus (bronchus intermedius) continues distally for 3 to 4 cm from the takeoff of the right upper lobe bronchus and then bifurcates to become the bronchi to the middle and lower lobes. The middle lobe bronchus arises from the anterolateral wall of the intermediate bronchus, almost opposite the origin of the superior segmental bronchus of the lower lobe; 1 to 2 cm beyond its origin, it bifurcates into lateral and medial branches (Figs. 1–51 and 1–52).

Right Lower Lobe. The superior segmental bronchus (Fig. 1–53) arises from the posterior aspect of the lower lobe bronchus immediately beyond its origin, as indicated by its position almost opposite the takeoff of the middle lobe bronchus. The four basal segments of the lower lobe can be

Text continued on page 46

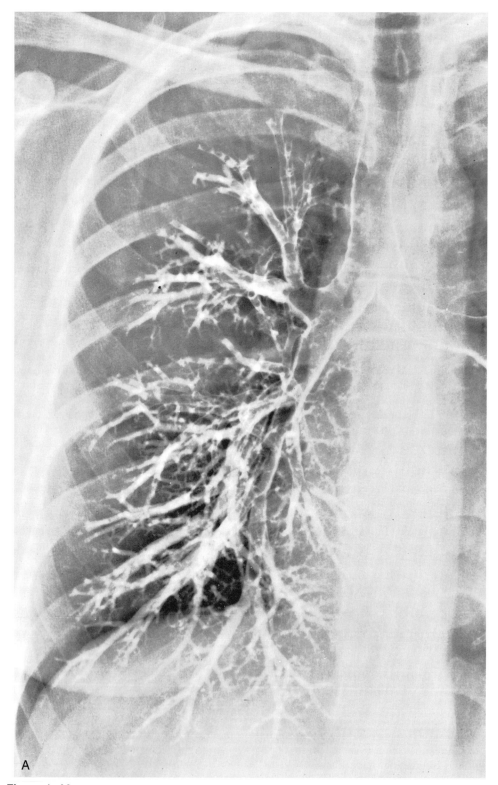

Figure 1–44. Right Bronchial Tree (Frontal Projection). Normal bronchogram *(A)* of a 39-year-old woman.

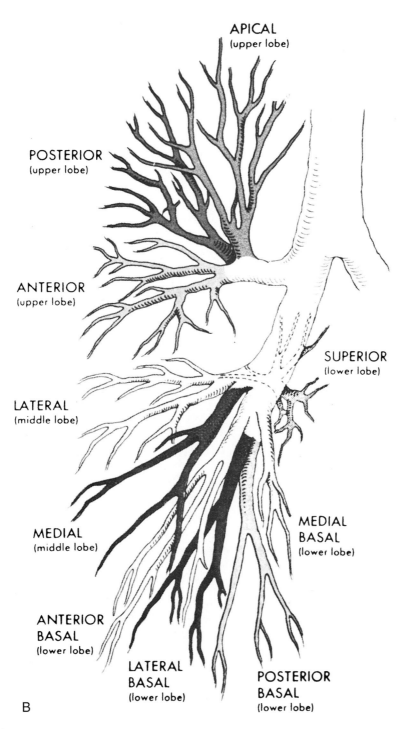

Figure 1–44 *Continued. B,* The normal segments of the right bronchial tree in frontal projection. (*B* from Lehman JS, Crellin JA: Med Radiogr Photogr 31:81, 1955. Reprinted courtesy Eastman Kodak Company.)

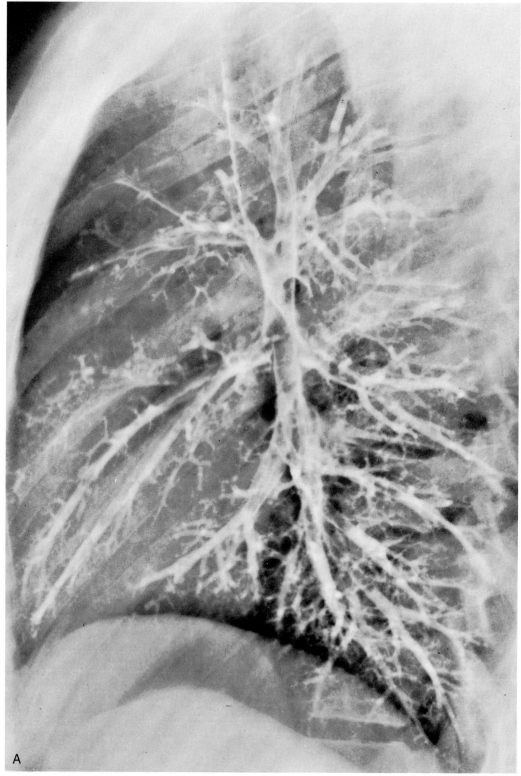

Figure 1–45. Right Bronchial Tree (Lateral Projection). Normal bronchogram *(A)* of a 39-year-old woman.

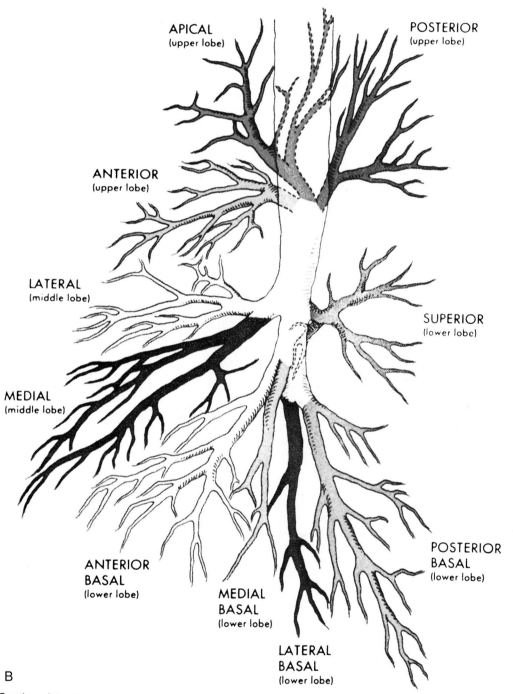

APICAL
(upper lobe)

POSTERIOR
(upper lobe)

ANTERIOR
(upper lobe)

LATERAL
(middle lobe)

SUPERIOR
(lower lobe)

MEDIAL
(middle lobe)

ANTERIOR
BASAL
(lower lobe)

MEDIAL
BASAL
(lower lobe)

POSTERIOR
BASAL
(lower lobe)

LATERAL
BASAL
(lower lobe)

B

Figure 1–45 *Continued. B,* The normal segments of the right bronchial tree in lateral projection. (*B* from Lehman JS, Crellin JA: Med Radiogr Photogr 31:81, 1995. Reprinted courtesy Eastman Kodak Company.)

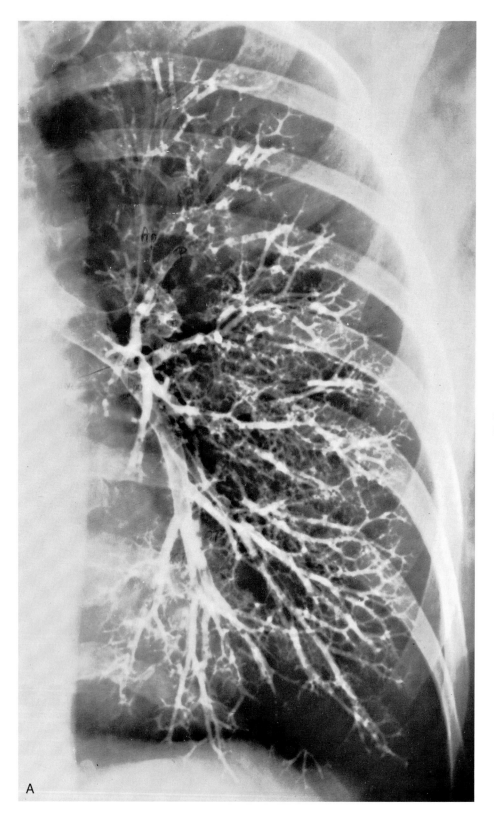

A

Figure 1–46. Left Bronchial Tree (Frontal Projection). Normal bronchogram *(A)* of a 39-year-old woman.

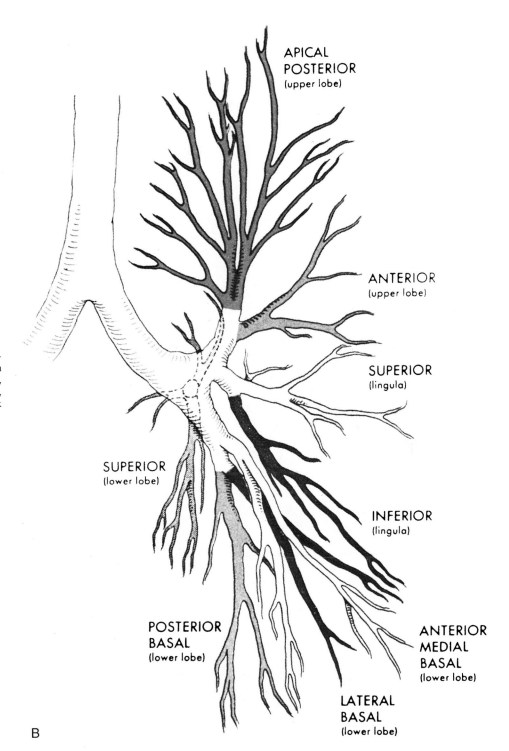

Figure 1–46 *Continued. B*, The normal segments of the left bronchial tree in frontal projection. (*B* from Lehman JS, Crellin JA: Med Radiogr Photogr 31:81, 1955. Reprinted courtesy Eastman Kodak Company.)

APICAL
POSTERIOR
(upper lobe)

ANTERIOR
(upper lobe)

SUPERIOR
(lingula)

INFERIOR
(lingula)

SUPERIOR
(lower lobe)

POSTERIOR
BASAL
(lower lobe)

ANTERIOR
MEDIAL
BASAL
(lower lobe)

LATERAL
BASAL
(lower lobe)

B

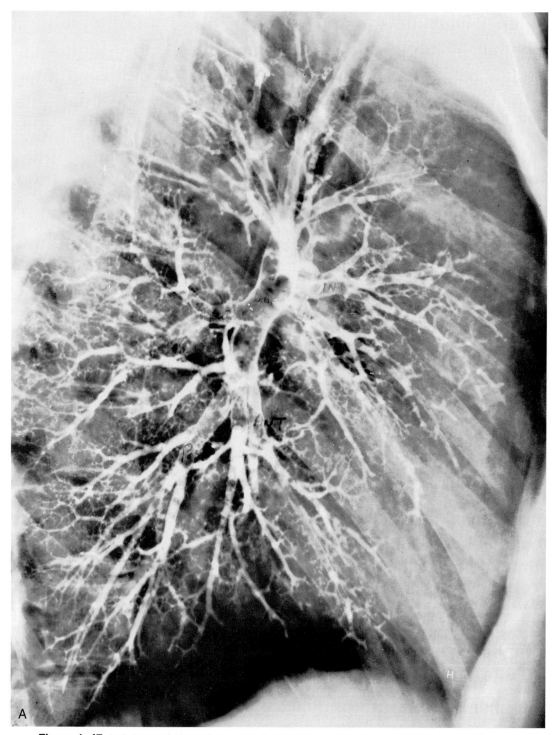

Figure 1–47. Left Bronchial Tree (Lateral Projection). Normal bronchogram *(A)* of a 39-year-old woman.

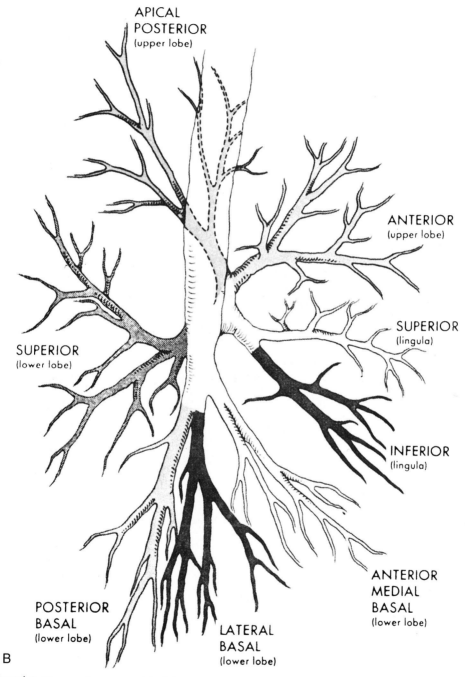

APICAL
POSTERIOR
(upper lobe)

ANTERIOR
(upper lobe)

SUPERIOR
(lingula)

SUPERIOR
(lower lobe)

INFERIOR
(lingula)

POSTERIOR
BASAL
(lower lobe)

LATERAL
BASAL
(lower lobe)

ANTERIOR
MEDIAL
BASAL
(lower lobe)

B

Figure 1–47 *Continued. B,* The normal segments of the left bronchial tree in lateral projection. (*B* from Lehman JS, Crellin JA: Med Radiogr Photogr 31:81, 1955. Reprinted courtesy Eastman Kodak Company.)

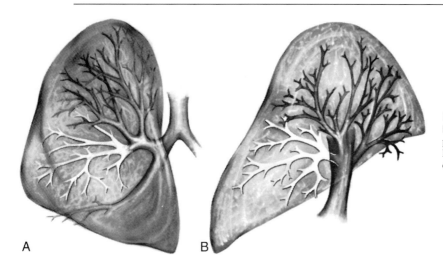

Figure 1–48. Anterior Segmental Bronchus, Right Upper Lobe. Frontal projection *(A)*; lateral projection *(B)*. This airway is directed anteriorly and laterally to supply the portion of the upper lobe contiguous to the minor fissure.

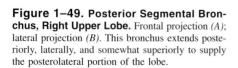

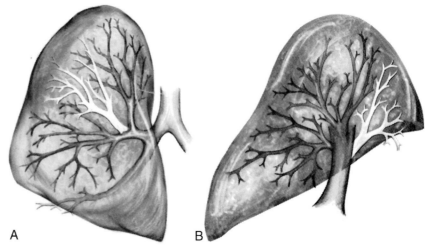

Figure 1–49. Posterior Segmental Bronchus, Right Upper Lobe. Frontal projection *(A)*; lateral projection *(B)*. This bronchus extends posteriorly, laterally, and somewhat superiorly to supply the posterolateral portion of the lobe.

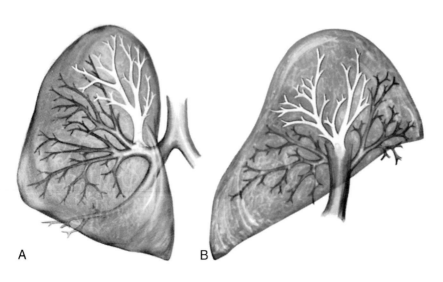

Figure 1–50. Apical Segmental Bronchus, Right Upper Lobe. Frontal projection *(A)*; lateral projection *(B)*. This bronchus supplies the superior paramediastinal zone, including the lung apex.

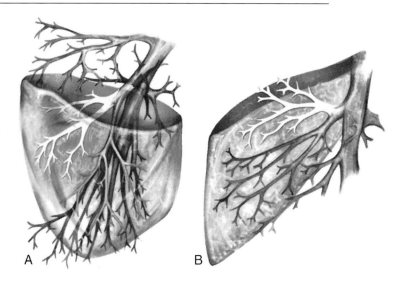

Figure 1–51. Lateral Segmental Bronchus, Right Middle Lobe. Frontal projection *(A)*; lateral projection *(B)*. This segment extends anterolaterally to supply the portion of the middle lobe that lies contiguous to the minor fissure and the anterior segment of the right upper lobe; its extreme lateral portion abuts against the major fissure.

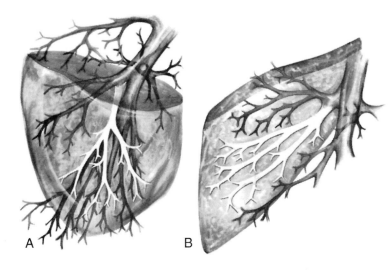

Figure 1–52. Medial Segmental Bronchus, Right Middle Lobe. Frontal projection *(A)*; lateral projection *(B)*. This bronchus extends anteromedially to supply the portion of the middle lobe that is contiguous to the heart and the lower portion of the major fissure.

Figure 1–53. Superior Segmental Bronchus, Right Lower Lobe. Frontal projection *(A)*; lateral projection *(B)*. Usually this bronchus has three subsegments that extend superiorly, laterally, and inferiorly to supply the apical region of the lower lobe.

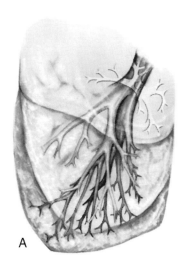
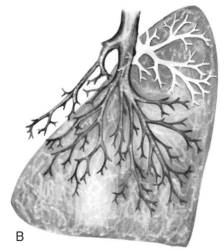

readily identified radiologically by applying a few basic principles of anatomy. Reference to Figures 1–54 to 1–57 shows that in the frontal projection of a well-filled broncho-gram, the order of the basal bronchi from the lateral to the medial aspect of the hemithorax is *anterior-lateral-posterior-medial*. In the lateral projection, the relationship anterior-lateral-posterior is maintained—hence the mnemonic *ALP*.[339] The relationship of one basal segment to another is easily recognized by use of the ALP designation, the medial basal segment being projected between the anterior and lateral segments in the lateral projection.

Left Upper Lobe. About 1 cm beyond its origin from the anterolateral aspect of the main bronchus, the bronchus to the left upper lobe either bifurcates or trifurcates, usually the former. In the bifurcation pattern, the upper division almost immediately divides again into two segmental branches, the apical posterior and anterior (Figs. 1–58 and 1–59). The lower division is the lingular bronchus, which is roughly analogous to the middle lobe bronchus of the right lung. When trifurcation of the left upper lobe bronchus occurs, the apical posterior, anterior, and lingular bronchi originate simultaneously. The lingular bronchus extends anteroinferiorly for 2 to 3 cm before bifurcating into superior and inferior divisions (Figs. 1–60 and 1–61).

Left Lower Lobe. The divisions of the left lower lobe bronchus are almost identical in name and anatomic distribution to those of the right lower lobe (Figs. 1–62 to 1–65). The exception lies in the absence of a separate medial basal bronchus, the anterior and medial portions of the lobe being supplied by a single anteromedial bronchus. The mnemonic ALP applies as well to the left lower lobe as to the right for identification of the order of basilar bronchi and their relationship to one another in frontal, oblique, and lateral projections.

Bronchial Anatomy on Computed Tomography

Visualization of bronchi by CT is influenced by the technique used and by the size and orientation of the bronchus. On conventional 10-mm collimation scans, about 70% of segmental bronchi can be identified;[340] a greater number

can be visualized by using thinner sections. The most common protocol for assessment of the central airways involves the use of contiguous 5-mm-thick sections obtained by dynamic incremental or spiral CT technique during a single breath-hold.[341] Assessment of smaller bronchi requires the use of high-resolution, 1- to 2-mm sections reconstructed by using a high–spatial resolution (edge) enhancing algorithm. Airways with a diameter less than 1.5 to 2 mm cannot be visualized because their walls are less than 0.1 mm in thickness.[342]

Bronchi coursing horizontally within the plane of CT section are seen along their long axes (Fig. 1–66). These bronchi include the right and left upper lobe bronchi, the anterior segmental bronchi of the upper lobes, the middle lobe bronchus, and the superior segmental bronchi of the lower lobes. Bronchi coursing vertically are cut in cross section and are therefore seen as circular lucencies. These bronchi include the apical segmental bronchus of the right upper lobe, the apical posterior segmental bronchus of the left upper lobe, the bronchus intermedius, the lower lobe bronchi, and the basal segmental bronchi. Bronchi coursing obliquely are seen as oval lucencies and are less well visualized on CT. These include the lingular bronchus, the superior and inferior segmental lingular bronchi, and the medial and lateral segmental bronchi of the right middle lobe.

Spiral (volumetric) CT allows acquisition of multiplanar and three-dimensional image reconstructions that provide better depiction of obliquely oriented bronchi than conventional cross-sectional CT images.[342a–d] The use of special reconstruction techniques, such as volume rendering, produces images similar to those obtained by bronchography.[342e]

Upper Lobes. Because they are cut in cross section, the apical segmental bronchus of the right upper lobe and the apical posterior segmental bronchus of the left upper lobe, or their proximal subsegmental branches, are seen as circular lucencies on CT scan at a level immediately above the tracheal carina (*see* Fig. 1–66).

The right main bronchus extends for approximately 2 cm before it divides into the right upper lobe bronchus and the bronchus intermedius. The right upper lobe bronchus usually courses horizontally and divides 1 to 2 cm from its origin into the apical segmental bronchus, which courses

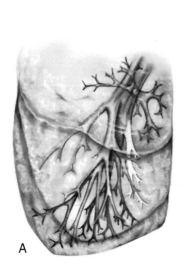
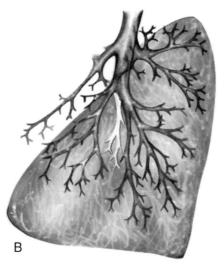

A   B

Figure 1–54. Medial Basal Bronchus, Right Lower Lobe. Frontal projection *(A)*; lateral projection *(B)*. This branch of the lower lobe bronchus is the first beyond the superior segmental bronchus; it supplies the smallest of the basal segments and is the most medial in frontal projection. It arises from the medial aspect of the lower lobe bronchus to supply the anteromedial portion of the lower lobe contiguous to the posterior portion of the heart and the lower end of the major fissure.

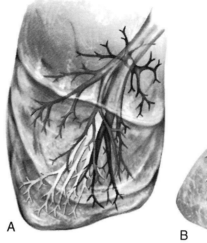
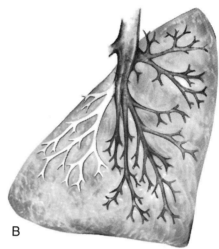

Figure 1–55. Anterior Basal Bronchus, Right Lower Lobe. Frontal projection *(A)*; lateral projection *(B)*. This bronchus, the most lateral of the basal bronchi, extends anterolaterally into the costophrenic sulcus.

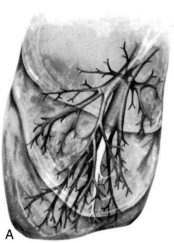
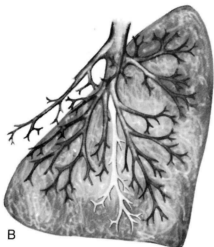

Figure 1–56. Lateral Basal Bronchus, Right Lower Lobe. Frontal projection *(A)*; lateral projection *(B)*. In frontal projection this bronchus is projected just medial to the anterior basal bronchus; it extends laterally and slightly posteriorly to supply the portion of the lower lobe that lies behind the anterior basal segment.

Figure 1–57. Posterior Basal Bronchus, Right Lower Lobe. Frontal projection *(A)*; lateral projection *(B)*. In frontal projection this bronchus appears between the lateral and medial basal bronchi; it supplies the posteroinferior portion of the lower lobe and extends into the posterior costophrenic gutter.

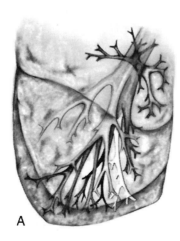
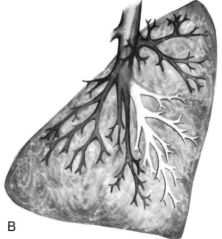

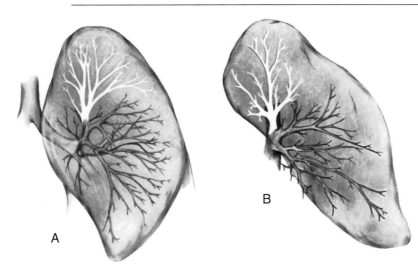

Figure 1–58. Apical Posterior Bronchus, Left Upper Lobe. Frontal projection *(A)*; lateral projection *(B)*. This bronchus bifurcates into apical and posterior segments that supply areas of the left upper lobe in a pattern similar to that of corresponding bronchi in the right upper lobe.

Figure 1–59. Anterior Segmental Bronchus, Left Upper Lobe. Frontal projection *(A)*; lateral projection *(B)*. The distribution is the same as in the right upper lobe.

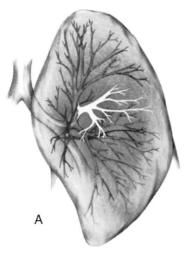
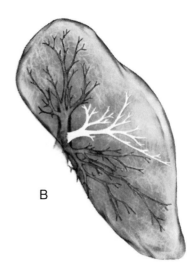

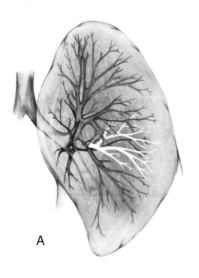
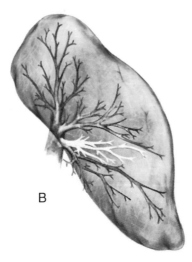

Figure 1–60. Superior Segmental Bronchus, Lingula. Frontal projection *(A)*; lateral projection *(B)*. This bronchus supplies the anterolateral portion of the lingula.

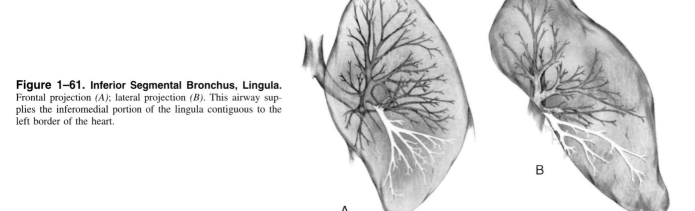

Figure 1–61. Inferior Segmental Bronchus, Lingula.
Frontal projection *(A)*; lateral projection *(B)*. This airway supplies the inferomedial portion of the lingula contiguous to the left border of the heart.

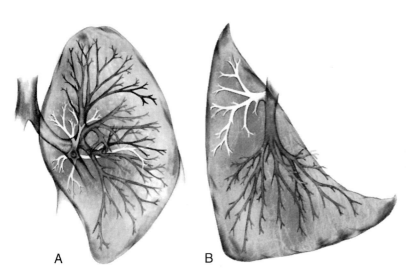

Figure 1–62. Superior Segmental Bronchus, Left Lower Lobe. Frontal projection *(A)*; lateral projection *(B)*. The distribution of this segment is similar to that of the corresponding segment of the right lower lobe.

Figure 1–63. Anterior Basal Bronchus, Left Lower Lobe. Frontal projection *(A)*; lateral projection *(B)*. Distribution is similar to that of the corresponding segment of the right lower lobe. *See* the text regarding the medial basal bronchus.

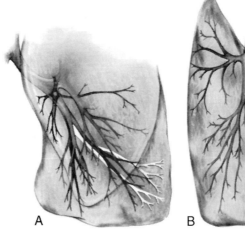
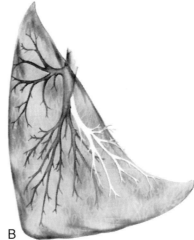

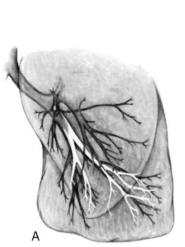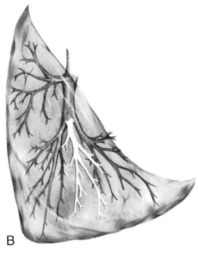

Figure 1–64. Lateral Basal Bronchus, Left Lower Lobe. Frontal projection *(A)*; lateral projection *(B)*. Distribution is similar to that of the corresponding segment of the right lower lobe.

vertically, and the horizontally oriented anterior and posterior segmental bronchi (*see* Fig. 1–66). Immediately lateral to the carina between the anterior and posterior segmental right upper lobe bronchi lies a branch of the right superior pulmonary vein.

The left main bronchus is longer than the right main bronchus and therefore divides into left upper and lower lobe bronchi at a more caudad level than does the corresponding right bronchus. As indicated previously, the divisions of the left upper lobe bronchus are more variable than those of the right upper lobe. In approximately 75% of individuals, the left upper lobe divides into an upper division and a lingular bronchus; in the remaining 25% it trifurcates, in which case the apical posterior and anterior and the lingular bronchi originate simultaneously.

HRCT allows the identification of patterns of branching down to the level of proximal subsegmental bronchi of the upper lobes.[343]

Lingular and Middle Lobe Bronchi. The lingular bronchus arises from the inferior aspect of the left upper lobe bronchus and courses caudally at an oblique angle (*see* Fig. 1–66). It originates 1 to 2 cm cephalad to the right middle lobe bronchus. The bronchus intermedius courses vertically for 3

to 4 cm before it gives off the right middle lobe bronchus. The latter extends anteriorly and slightly inferiorly and bifurcates 1 to 2 cm from its origin into lateral and medial branches.

Because of its oblique cephalocaudal course, the lingular bronchus and its segmental branches are not usually well seen on conventional transverse section CT. Even with HRCT, the complete branching patterns of these airways can be identified in only about 50% of cases.[344] Improved visualization of conventional cross-sectional CT images of the lingular bronchus and its segmental branches, as well as the middle lobe segmental bronchi, can be obtained by the use of 20-degree cranial angulation of the CT gantry.[345]

Lower Lobe Bronchi. The superior segmental bronchi originate at approximately the same level as the corresponding middle lobe and lingular bronchi. The superior segmental bronchus of the left lower lobe is located cephalad to that on the right side. Both airways course horizontally and posteriorly (*see* Fig. 1–66).

The basal segmental bronchi originate at variable levels from each other, either separately or from common trunks. In one study of 31 patients in which both 1.5- and 5-mm-thick sections were used, considerable variation in their

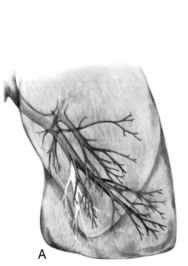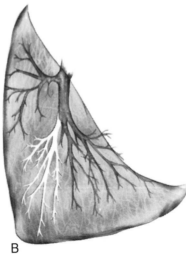

Figure 1–65. Posterior Basal Bronchus, Left Lower Lobe. Frontal projection *(A)*; lateral projection *(B)*. Distribution is similar to that of the corresponding segment of the right lower lobe.

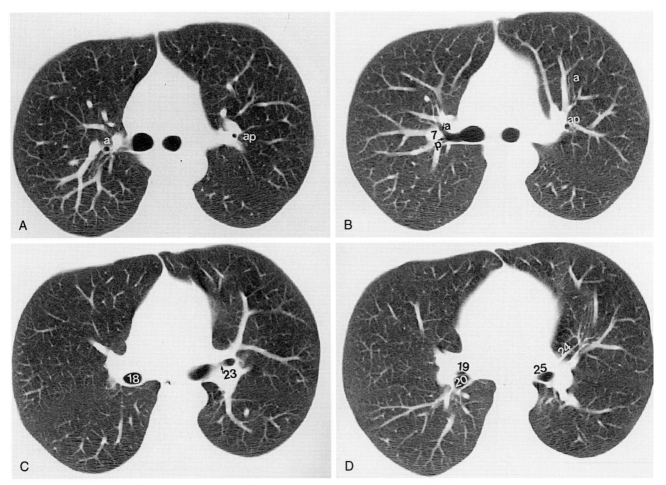

Figure 1–66. Bronchial Anatomy on CT Scan. *A*, CT scan at a level immediately below the tracheal carina demonstrates the apical segmental bronchus of the right upper lobe (a) and the apical posterior segmental bronchus (ap) of the left upper lobe. *B*, CT scan at the level of the anterior (a) and posterior (p) segmental bronchi of the right upper lobe. Between them lies a branch of the right superior pulmonary vein (7). Also seen are right and left main bronchi and apicoposterior (ap) and anterior (a) segmental bronchi of the left upper lobe. *C*, Slightly more caudad, the apicoposterior segmental bronchus joins the left upper lobe bronchus (23). Note the local anterior and posterior indentations of the left upper lobe bronchus by the pulmonary artery. On the right, the intermediate bronchus (18) is seen in cross section. *D*, CT scan at the level of the lingular (24) and left lower lobe (25) bronchi and the carina between the right lower lobe (20) and middle lobe (19) bronchi.

Illustration continued on following page

division was demonstrated, six patterns being seen in the right lower lobe and five in the left.[346] As on standard radiographs, these airways can usually be clearly identified by their location in relation to each other (i.e., medial, anterior, lateral, and posterior). HRCT allows identification of all segmental bronchi of the lower lobes and about 45% of their proximal subsegmental branches.[346]

FUNCTION

Pulmonary Ventilation

The purpose of respiration is to supply oxygen for the metabolic needs of cells and to remove carbon dioxide, one of the waste products of cellular metabolism. In a unicellular organism, respiration is achieved simply by diffusion of these gases across the cell membrane. Although the basic purpose is the same in humans, a much more complex mechanism is necessary that involves two convective transport systems (ventilation and circulation) and two diffusive

systems. The convective ventilatory system brings O_2 to the alveolar air spaces, from which it diffuses across the alveolocapillary membrane into pulmonary capillary blood; the convective circulatory system distributes the O_2 throughout the body, following which it diffuses out of the capillaries and into the mitochondria of tissue cells. Elimination of carbon dioxide is accomplished by the same procedure in reverse: diffusion from tissues into blood, followed by convection to lung capillaries where the gas diffuses from blood to alveolar air spaces and is exhaled via the conducting airways.

Normal lung function requires the provision at the alveoli of sufficient oxygen to satisfy the demands of the tissues and sufficient movement of gas in the tracheobronchial tree to eliminate carbon dioxide. The needs of the tissues for oxygen—and consequently the quantity of carbon dioxide that requires elimination—vary considerably, mainly because of muscle activity. At rest, the oxygen requirement may be 200 to 250 ml/min, whereas during maximal exercise it may increase to 20 times this amount. To satisfy this variation in oxygen need, a similar increase in ventilation is necessary.

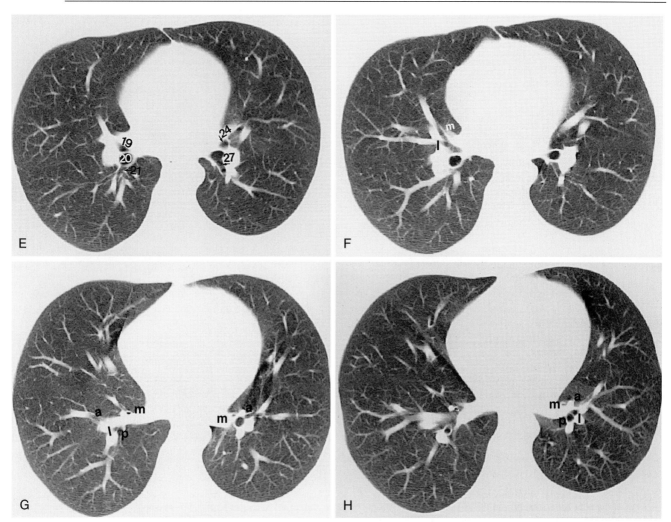

Figure 1–66 *Continued. E,* CT scan slightly more caudad demonstrates the superior segmental bronchus (27) of the left lower lobe, the inferior lingular bronchus (24), and the right superior segmental (21), lower lobe (20), and middle lobe bronchi (19). *F,* CT scan at the level in which the right middle lobe bronchus divides into medial (m) and lateral (l) segmental bronchi. Also seen are the lobar bronchi in cross section with the interlobar pulmonary arteries lateral to them. *G,* CT scan at the level in which the inferior pulmonary veins join the left atrium demonstrates right medial (m) and anterior (a) segmental bronchi anterior to the right inferior pulmonary vein and posterior segmental (p) and lateral segmental (l) bronchi posterior to the vein. On the *left* side the medial segmental (m) and anterior segmental (a) bronchi can be seen, as well as a common trunk between the posterior and lateral segmental bronchi. More commonly the anterior and medial bronchi originate as a common trunk to ventilate the anteromedial segmental bronchus of the left lower lobe. *H,* At a slightly lower level the medial (m) and anterior (a) segmental bronchi of the left lower lobe can be seen anterior to the inferior pulmonary vein whereas the lateral (l) and posterior (p) bronchi are posterior to the vein.

This increase is mediated by stimuli from various sources, the origin depending on the circumstances of the need: oxygen lack or carbon dioxide excess in the blood, stimuli from blood vessel chemoreceptors, reflexes from somatic and visceral tissues, nervous reflexes from the lungs themselves, and input from the cerebral cortex act directly or indirectly on the respiratory center to induce movement of the diaphragm and intercostal muscles and thus an appropriate increase in ventilation.

It is logical that an increase in ventilation sufficient to satisfy the need for oxygen will be to no avail if there is not a parallel increase in circulating blood within the lungs to carry oxygen to the tissues. Accordingly, cardiac rate and stroke volume parallel the increase in ventilation. For example, during exercise, cardiac output may increase from about 5 liters per minute to 25 to 30 liters per minute. (An additional compensation for an increase in tissue O_2 demand is an augmentation in the O_2 extraction ratio [the fraction of

O_2 removed from systemic blood], which may increase from 25% to 75% or greater during maximal exercise.)

Keeping in mind the chemical, nervous, and mechanical stimuli that act directly or indirectly on the respiratory center, cardiac muscle, airways, and pulmonary vessels to vary the amount of gas and blood delivered to the lung, it is useful to focus attention on the acinar unit because it is here that the lung fulfills its role in respiration. To do this, it is necessary to consider: (1) alveolar gas and its composition; (2) the mechanism by which this gas is moved in and out of the acinus; (3) perfusion of the acinus; (4) the process of diffusion of gas in the acinar unit and across the alveolocapillary membrane to red blood cells; (5) the matching of blood flow with ventilation in the acinar unit; and (6) the end result of these processes, blood gas and hydrogen ion concentration. The second of these is discussed in Chapter 10 (see page 246) and the last four in Chapter 2 (see page 104); here we are concerned primarily with the first.

The composition of gas in the alveolar air space depends on the rate and amount of oxygen removed and carbon dioxide added by capillary blood (which in turn depends on aerobic metabolism of tissues) and the quantity and quality of the gas that reaches the acinus via the conducting and transitional airways.

Ventilation of the Acinus

Air contains approximately 21% oxygen and 79% nitrogen and at sea level has an atmospheric pressure of 760 mm Hg; the amount of carbon dioxide and other gases is negligible and can be disregarded. The partial pressures of these gases are approximately 159 mm Hg for oxygen (P_{O_2} = [21 ÷ 100] × 760) and 601 mm Hg for nitrogen (P_{N_2} = [79 ÷ 100] × 760). As air is inhaled into the tracheobronchial tree, it becomes fully saturated with water vapor at body temperature and a partial pressure of 47 mm Hg, and the partial pressure of oxygen drops to 149 mm Hg ([760 − 47] × 21 ÷ 100). At sea level, therefore, ventilation of the acinus depends on the quantity of gas containing oxygen, at a P_{O_2} of 149 mm Hg, that the thoracic "bellows" moves per minute into the acinus.

The amount of gas reaching the alveoli (alveolar ventilation [$\dot{V}_A$]) depends on the depth of inspiration (tidal volume [V_T]), the volume of the conducting airways (the anatomic dead space [V_D]), and the number of breaths per minute (f).

$$\dot{V}_A \ (l/min) = (V_T - V_D) \times f$$

If an individual inhales 15 times per minute, 450 ml with each breath, and has an anatomic dead space of 150 ml, total minute ventilation ($\dot{V}_E$) will be 15 × 450 = 6,750 ml/min and alveolar ventilation will be (450 − 150) × 15 = 4,500 ml/min. (Anatomic dead space ventilation is not considered alveolar ventilation because at the end of expiration it is filled not with atmospheric air but with expired air having a composition equivalent to that of gas in the acinus.)

The $\dot{V}_A$ portion of each breath (ΔV) is added to the residual alveolar gas (V_O), and rapid diffusive mixing occurs so that gas tensions approach a uniform alveolar concentration. Failure of complete diffusive mixing within the air spaces may occur with acinar enlargement (emphysema) and with a decreased time for mixing; this condition is termed *series inhomogeneity*.[347] The ratios of V_D/V_T and $\Delta V/V_O$ vary between different lung regions (interregional) and between closely located acini (intraregional), even in normal lungs; the resulting variation in alveolar gas composition is termed *parallel inhomogeneity*.[347] Parallel inhomogeneity may also be related to diffusive pendelluft* at branch points subtending different-sized parallel units within the acinus; this process can be shown by model analysis to result in inhomogeneity despite proportionate and synchronous emptying and filling of units.[348, 349]

---

*Pendelluft is a process by which gas passes from one portion of the lung to another without exiting the lung (e.g., if gas leaving the right lower lobe during expiration inflated the right upper lobe rather than being exhaled). Such a process is usually convective as a result of marked inhomogeneity of regional airway resistance or lung compliance; however, retrograde "flow" can occur by diffusion at branch points.

Alveolar-Capillary Gas Exchange

In addition to the effect of ventilation on the composition of gas in the acinus, blood flow in the pulmonary capillaries alters the composition by continuous removal of oxygen and addition of carbon dioxide. The ratio of alveolar ventilation to perfusion ($\dot{V}_A/\dot{Q}$) varies within the lung, and the interaction of these two dynamic processes results in fluctuation in alveolar gas tensions not only throughout the respiratory cycle but also from breath to breath, lobe to lobe, and even acinus to acinus (*see* $\dot{V}_A/\dot{Q}$ mismatch, page 108). In a hypothetical example in which perfusion is matched evenly with ventilation (100 ml $\dot{Q}$ for each 100 ml $\dot{V}_A$), alveolar and mixed venous and arterial gas tensions will reach steady-state values (Fig. 1–67). With normal resting mixed venous gas tensions, every 100 ml of blood delivers to the alveolar gas approximately 5.6 ml of CO_2 and at the same time carries away from it 7 ml of O_2. Therefore, the partial pressure of carbon dioxide in the acinus is 40 mm Hg—(5.6 ÷ 100) × 713. The removal of O_2 decreases the fractional concentration from 21% to 14% to yield a P_{O_2} of 100 mm Hg—(21 − 7 ÷ 100) × 713.

Mechanics of Acinar Ventilation

The movement of atmospheric air down the conducting system to the acinar unit requires force, measured as pressure (P), to overcome the elastic recoil of the lung parenchyma and chest wall (Pel), the frictional resistance of pulmonary tissues and the chest wall (Pvis), the frictional resistance to air flow through the tracheobronchial tree (Pfr), and the inertia of the gas. Because air has very little mass, its inertial effect is negligible with normal breathing frequencies; the elastic recoil of the lung and chest wall and the frictional resistance to air flow in the tracheobronchial tree represent the major portion of the work of breathing and are chiefly affected in lung disease.[350]

The force necessary to inflate the lung is provided by contraction of the inspiratory muscles, mainly the diaphragm, to a lesser extent the external intercostal muscles, and in circumstances requiring greatly increased ventilation, the accessory respiratory muscles (*see* page 246). The accessory respiratory muscles are also recruited when the diaphragm is weak, even in the absence of increased ventilatory demand. Normally, expiration is a passive phenomenon associated with relaxation of the inspiratory muscles; in fact, inspiratory muscle electrical activity may extend well into expiration to "brake" expiratory flow, especially during hyperinflation.[351] In patients who have obstructive airway disease and in normal individuals during periods of increased ventilation produced by exercise or CO_2 rebreathing, expiratory muscles (especially the abdominals) may be recruited. Expiratory muscles are also required to breathe out from FRC to residual volume (RV).

Elastic Recoil of the Lung Parenchyma and Thoracic Cage

The static pressure-volume relationships of the lung and thoracic cage are depicted pictorially and graphically in Figure 1–68. At FRC, the chest wall recoils outward and exerts a force that is equal and opposite to the force exerted by the lung recoiling inward. These balanced forces result

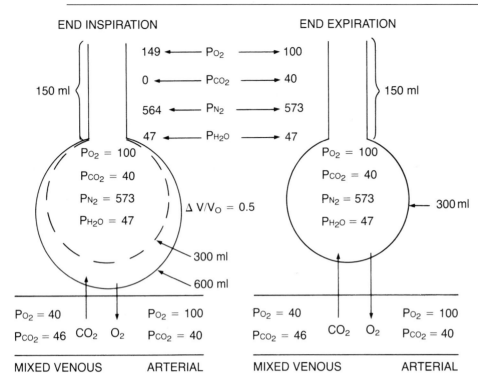

Figure 1–67. Diagram Portraying the Conducting System and Alveolar Space. At the end of an inspiration of 450 ml of air, 150 ml of fresh air (saturated with water vapor) is situated within the conducting system, and the remaining 300 ml has entered and mixed with alveolar gas *(left panel)*. At end expiration, the conducting system (dead space) is filled with alveolar air. The ventilation of the lung in this example is given by the $\Delta V/V_0$ ratio of 0.5.

in a negative pleural pressure of approximately 4 to 5 cm H_2O. FRC is therefore determined by the balance of static recoil forces exerted by the lung and chest wall. On inspiration, the respiratory muscles act initially to overcome the elastic recoil of the lungs only; the chest wall and thoracic cage actually aid inflation by their outward recoil until a volume of about 70% TLC is reached, at which point the chest wall is inflated beyond its resting position and the force of muscle contraction is then exerted against the recoil of both the lung and chest wall. TLC is reached when the inspiratory forces achieved by the muscles are equal and opposite to the combined recoil force of the lung and chest wall. It is apparent from Figure 1–68 that as lung volume increases, the elastic recoil of the lung parenchyma increases in a nonlinear fashion.

During deflation of the lung from FRC toward RV, the expiratory muscles are aided by the elastic recoil of the lung until its resting volume is reached. The chest wall pressure-volume relationship becomes progressively nonlinear near RV as the chest wall becomes more difficult to distort; RV is reached at the point at which outward recoil of the chest wall equals the force exerted by the expiratory muscles. In older subjects and in patients with chronic obstructive pulmonary disease, this point may not be attained because the airways may narrow and limit expiration at higher lung volumes and thereby cause gas trapping.[352, 353] When air is introduced into the pleural space, the visceral and parietal pleurae separate, and the lung and chest wall move along their respective pressure-volume curves, each assuming its resting volume (Points D and D_1 in Fig. 1–68).

The relationship between volume and pressure (V/P, compliance) can be calculated for the lung and chest wall either separately or together (respiratory system compliance). In normal subjects, respiratory system elastance (the inverse of compliance, P/V) is the major determinant of the work of

breathing; in disease states, work of breathing can be altered by increases or decreases in elastance of the lung or chest wall (Fig. 1–69). As the normal lung becomes more inflated, it becomes less compliant; for this reason it is more informative to express compliance as the change in intrapleural pressure required to produce a volume change at a specific degree of lung inflation, usually FRC. To correct for differences in lung size, specific compliance can also be calculated; the latter is defined as the change in lung volume per change in transpulmonary pressure divided by the absolute lung volume at FRC. Interstitial edema, fibrosis, or cellular infiltration renders the lungs stiffer and less compliant so that more pressure is required to move a given volume of gas; that is, a given pressure moves a smaller volume. When the architecture of the elastic tissue of the lung is altered, as in emphysema, a given pressure may actually produce a greater volume change than in the normal lung; in this case, compliance is increased.

During periods of no inspiratory or expiratory flow, the relationship between lung volume and lung elastic recoil pressure (P_L) and lung volume and chest wall recoil pressure (Pcw) is static; during flow, extra pressure must be exerted to overcome flow resistance. This pressure is measurable because it is reflected in the degree of change in intrapleural pressure. Such measurement is made most conveniently with the use of an intraesophageal balloon that reflects changes in intrapleural pressure.

Surface Tension and Surfactant

"Elastic" recoil of the lung has been attributed in part to the peculiar arrangement of collagen and elastic fibers,[354, 355] the helical structure of their arrangement resulting in the lungs having a behavior similar to that of a coil spring. However, tissue elasticity is not the only compo-

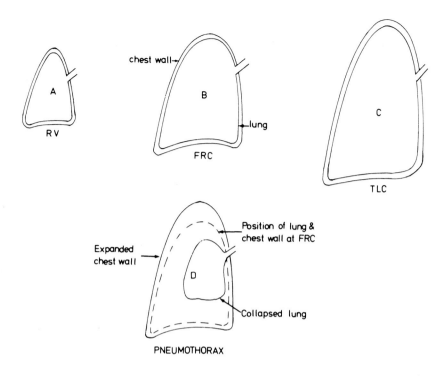

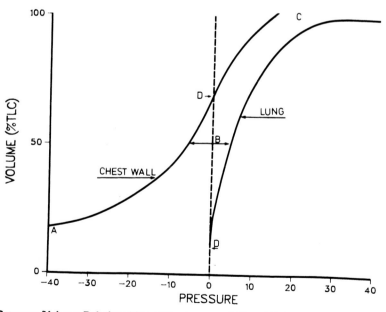

Figure 1–68. Static Pressure/Volume Relationships of the Lung and Chest Wall (Illustrated schematically and graphically). In the *lower* panel, lung and chest wall volumes are plotted against pressure. Transpulmonary pressure (pleural pressure − alveolar pressure) is the appropriate pressure for the lung, whereas transthoracic pressure (pleural pressure − atmospheric pressure) is the appropriate pressure for the chest wall. In the *upper* panel, drawing *B* shows the relationship of the lung and chest wall at functional residual capacity (FRC); point *B below* shows that at FRC the transpulmonary and transthoracic pressures are equal and opposite in sign. At residual volume (RV) (*A above* and *below*), transpulmonary pressure is near zero as the lung deflates toward its resting position, whereas transthoracic pressure is very negative since the chest wall becomes stiffer at low lung volumes. At total lung capacity (TLC) (*C above* and *below*), both the lung and chest wall are expanded beyond their resting position and both exert recoil favoring deflation. With development of a complete pneumothorax, transpulmonary and transthoracic pressures become zero, and the lung and chest wall assume their unstressed and relaxed positions *(D)*.

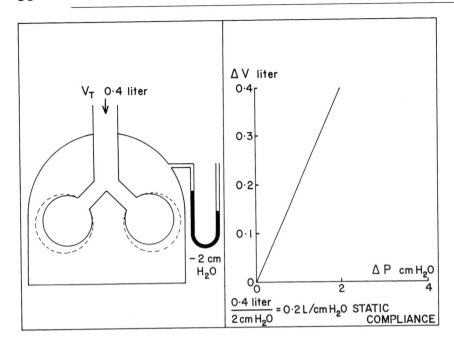

Figure 1–69. Pressure-Volume Relationships. A change of 2 cm H_2O in pleural pressure (ΔP) results in a volume change (ΔV) of 0.4 liter of tidal air (V_T) in two hypothetical acini. The diagram on the *right* depicts the change in volume of 0.4 liter and the change in pressure of 2 cm H_2O. The static compliance in this example is 0.2 liter per cm H_2O.

nent of elastic recoil of the lungs. This point was first indicated by the work of von Neergaard in 1929,[356] who measured the pressure-volume relationships of a fluid-distended lung and an air-distended lung and found that less pressure change was required to fully distend the former than the latter. Von Neergaard deduced that surface tension exists in each alveolus between its wall and its contained gas and results in a force that tends to contract the air space and resist its expansion. He suggested that this surface tension accounts for most of the lung's elastic recoil and that it is eliminated when gas is replaced by liquid.

In contrast to their polyhedral shape after conventional methods of tissue preparation, alveoli appear spherical after rapid freezing, when fixed by vascular perfusion, or when viewed through the pleura of living animals. The common denominator of these three methods of inspection is the presence of air in the alveoli, which molds the epithelium, capillaries, and alveolar lining fluid into a continuous curved surface that probably represents the configuration consistent with the lowest surface energy.[357] When the alveolar spaces are filled with fluid fixative, surface forces are eliminated and alveolar topography becomes dependent on tissue organization and mechanical properties.

Surfactant Morphology

The anatomic basis for this surface force is an extremely thin (4-nm) layer of osmiophilic material that covers the entire alveolar epithelial surface (*see* Fig. 1–27A, page 20).[358, 359] This acellular layer consists of two functionally different components:[360] (1) a film facing the alveolar air space, which is composed of densely spaced, highly surface-active phospholipids; and (2) deep to this film, a layer containing surface-active phospholipids in a different physicochemical configuration, linked to proteins. This deep, or "base," layer of the surface lining material represents the hypophase described by the physiologist.[361] Components of the superficial layer are thought to be recruited from the

deeper hypophase during expansion of the lung and may reenter the base layer at low lung volumes. The hypophase contains aggregates of lipid that are termed *tubular myelin*. These aggregates are particularly evident in the thickest portions of the hypophase and on section exhibit a characteristic fingerprint-like pattern (Fig. 1–70); this material is believed to be a degeneration or breakdown product of surfactant. The lipids in the hypophase include: (1) newly secreted lamellar bodies derived from Type II cells *en route* to the surface film; (2) lipid molecules that have temporarily entered the hypophase from the surface film as the surface area of an alveolus decreases; and (3) aggregates of lipid and protein that are going to be removed by alveolar macrophages or recycled into Type II pneumocytes.[362]

Surfactant Composition and Synthesis

Phospholipids make up 90% of surfactant. Surfactant's main component is dipalmitoyl phosphatidylcholine (dipalmitoyl lecithin [DPPC]), 45% of which is saturated and 25% unsaturated. Phosphatidylglycerol contributes 5%, phosphatidylethanolamine 3%, and neutral lipids 10%. DPPC is largely responsible for the high surface activity.[363] As indicated previously (*see* page 19), surfactant is synthesized and secreted by alveolar Type II cells. Phospholipids are synthesized within the endoplasmic reticulum, are formed into storage or lamellar bodies in the Golgi–endoplasmic reticulum complex, and are eventually discharged into the alveolar air space by classic secretory exocytosis; this latter process can be blocked by anticytochalasin B, a drug that disrupts filamentous actin.[362, 364]

Surfactant contains four proteins designated SP-A, SP-B, SP-C, and SP-D. SP-A and SP-D are glycoproteins of approximately 30,000 to 40,000 daltons, whereas SP-B and SP-C are smaller hydrophilic molecules 5,000 to 18,000 daltons in size. These proteins have several functions. SP-A, SP-B, and SP-C combine to transform the lamellar bodies to tubular myelin and promote rapid spread of the phospho-

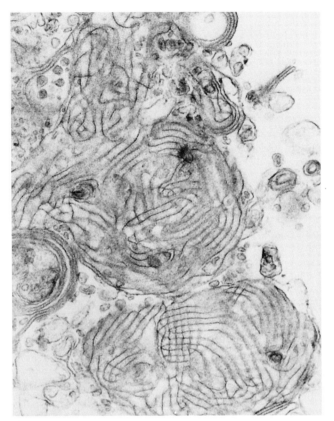

Figure 1–70. Surfactant. Transmission electron micrograph of free alveolar surfactant showing tubular myelin figures. (Courtesy of Dr. David Walker, University of British Columbia, Vancouver.)

lipid film to facilitate the reduction in surface tension.[365] SP-A may also provide negative feedback for further surfactant secretion[366] and can interact with alveolar macrophages to enhance their phagocytic capacity.[367] SP-B and SP-C greatly increase the surface tension–lowering capability of surfactant phospholipids by promoting the adsorption of surfactant phospholipids to the air-liquid interface.[365] SP-D may primarily serve a host defense function by binding to bacteria and enhancing their phagocytosis.[368] Although pure phospholipid and the complex of surfactant proteins and phospholipids have similar capabilities for lowering surface tension, the lipoprotein complex absorbs and spreads much more readily over the air-liquid interface. This quality explains the greater rapidity of onset of the beneficial effects of naturally occurring surfactants that has been observed in studies of exogenous replacement therapy (*see* farther on).[369, 370]

The synthesis of DPPC in Type II cells can be accomplished by two independent pathways: a *de novo* pathway that involves direct synthesis from dipalmitoyl diglyceride and cytidine-diphosphate-choline and a *deacetylation and reacetylation* or *remodeling* pathway that represents conversion of unsaturated phosphatidylcholine molecules to DPPC through acetylation of 1-palmitoyl-2-lysophosphatidylcholine by palmitoyl–coenzyme A. It is likely that the contribution of each pathway varies with substrate availability.[362] Studies on several vertebrate species have shown that the amounts of surfactant and saturated phosphatidylcholine in the lung are related to alveolar surface area.[371]

Surfactant has a very rapid rate of turnover; in studies with dipalmitoyl lecithin labeled with radioactive palmitic acid, its half-life in normal adults has been reported as ranging from 14 hours[372] to somewhat less than 2 days.[373] Its ultimate metabolic fate is complex. The majority is taken up by Type II cells and "recycled" into lamellar bodies or degraded intracellularly and the products used to synthesize new lipids.[193, 374] A small amount moves directly up the airways on the mucociliary escalator or is phagocytosed and degraded by alveolar macrophages.[257, 257a]

Surfactant secretion is under complex neural, hormonal, and chemical control. Its concentration is higher in neonates than adults,[375] the rate of phospholipid synthesis reaching a peak at term and declining rapidly to normal adult levels shortly thereafter.[376] The explanations for this variation are probably related to the necessity for surfactant to be present in abundance at the moment of birth; otherwise, every breath would necessarily resemble the first breath.[377] The burst of phospholipid synthesis shortly before birth is associated with the rapid appearance of phosphatidylglycerol in amniotic fluid and an increase above 2.0 in the ratio of lethicin to sphingomyelin. Both these measurements have proved invaluable in the assessment of fetal lung maturation and the likelihood of the development of neonatal respiratory distress syndrome (RDS).[378, 379] The ratio of surfactant to albumin in amniotic fluid has a predictive value for the development of RDS similar to the lecithin-sphingomyelin ratio.[380]

Acceleration of lung maturation with stimulation of Type II cells and the production of a mature pattern of phospholipid secretion can be induced by the administration of corticosteroids to the fetus or mother.[381, 382] The increased phosphatidylcholine synthesis stimulated by glucocorticosteroids appears to be due to an increase in the fatty acid synthase enzyme,[383] which by increasing the fatty acid pool stimulates the activation of the rate-limiting enzyme cholinephosphate cytidyltransferase.[384] There is evidence that thyroxine, estrogens, β-adrenergic agonists, prolactin, and other pharmacologic agents (including heroin) can also stimulate maturation of the surfactant system; by contrast, insulin, phenobarbital, and metyrapone may retard fetal lung maturation.[362, 385, 386]

β-Adrenergic and cholinergic agonists also increase surfactant secretion. In adult animals, the effects of both agents can be demonstrated *in vivo*, although the latter is not demonstrable with isolated Type II cells.[362, 387, 388] The *in vivo* cholinergic stimulation is attenuated by β-blockers or indomethacin, which suggests that the cholinergic effect acts through the β-adrenergic or prostaglandin system.[388] A_2 and P_2 purinoreceptor agonists such as adenosine, adenosine triphosphate, and uridine triphosphate are also surfactant phospholipid secretagogues. The cell surface receptors are coupled to intracellular adenylate cyclase via G proteins.[363]

Surfactant production in the lung is stimulated by an increase in either ventilation or tidal volume, an effect that has been demonstrated in animals by measurement of phospholipids[387] and by morphologic evidence of a decrease in lamellar body density and identifiable Type II cells.[389] Breathing at low lung volumes results not only in decreased surfactant secretion but also in altered function as a result of diminished alveolar stability and the accumulation of large phospholipid aggregates; the formation of these aggregates is in turn diminished by a deep breath.[390] This ventilation- and sigh-induced secretion of phospholipids appears to be mediated through the β-adrenergic system, since the effect of mechanical stimulation can be blocked by propranolol.[387, 391] Vagotomy has also been reported to alter surface-active properties in rat lungs.[392]

Surfactant Function

Functions of surfactant include the prevention of alveolar collapse, decrease in the work of breathing, an antisticking action that prevents adherence of alveolar walls, and an antiwetting action that may aid in keeping the alveolar lining layer dry.[393–395] The forces that tend to decrease alveolar size are surface tension and tissue elasticity. The force generated by tissue elasticity is roughly proportional to lung volume but constitutes only one third of total lung elastic recoil at TLC. The pressure stemming from surface factors can be calculated from the Young-Laplace relationship:

$$P = 2\ \gamma/r$$

where γ is the surface tension of the alveolar air-liquid interface and r is the alveolar radius. Opposed to the lung elastic recoil and surface tension forces that tend to collapse alveoli is transpulmonary pressure. Mechanical balance is achieved when transpulmonary pressure equals the pressures generated by tissue elastic recoil and surface tension. With lung deflation, transpulmonary pressure decreases at the same time that the alveolar radius is decreasing, a situation that favors alveolar collapse. This is why a substance with the surface tension–lowering ability of surfactant is necessary to achieve alveolar stability.[393] Surfactant lowers the surface tension in the liquid at the alveolar air-liquid interface to values much smaller than if plasma or interstitial fluid lined the surface. In addition, in the presence of surfactant the surface tension decreases even more as the surface layer is compressed during lung deflation.

A second major role of surfactant is to decrease the work of breathing. The compliance of a lung with deficient or denatured surfactant is considerably reduced and the pressures necessary to achieve tidal ventilation are increased.[393] Surfactant's potential role in reducing adhesion between alveolar walls where they come in contact has not been experimentally evaluated.[393]

The reduction in surface tension imparted by surfactant may have an important role in fluid balance in the lung distinct from its role in the mechanics of breathing. The reduced surface tension counteracts the tendency for fluid to be sucked into alveolar spaces from the capillary lumen.[396] The mechanism by which surfactant acts to decrease the driving force for the development of pulmonary edema is related to its ability to lower surface tension; because the pressure drop across a curved interface is proportional to the surface tension and inversely proportional to the radius of curvature, by decreasing surface tension, lung surfactant decreases the pressure drop across the alveolar-interstitial compartment and leads to less-negative tissue pressures.[397] It has also been suggested that the strong hydrophobic nature of cationic surfactants induces a nonwettable alveolar surface that further aids in decreasing transepithelial fluid movement.[398, 399]

In addition to these mechanical functions, there is evidence that the alveolar lining layer has other important roles in the normal lung. For example, it has been reported to contain a protective factor (possibly dipalmitoyl lecithin[400]) that inhibits the lysis of alveolar macrophages. Many environmental toxins such as ozone may exert their effects by inhibiting this protective factor, the resulting damage to alveolar macrophages decreasing their effectiveness in eliminating inhaled microorganisms or particulate matter.[400] As discussed previously, there is evidence that surfactant protein D may function in antimicrobial defense by acting as an adhesion molecule. Surfactant also aids alveolar macrophage migration and has been shown to be chemotactic for these cells, factors that could aid in their clearance from the air spaces up the mucociliary escalator.[401]

Disorders of surfactant metabolism are important in a number of diseases, including pulmonary thromboembolism, adult respiratory distress syndrome (ARDS), alveolar proteinosis, oxygen toxicity, and atelectasis.[402] One disease in which deficient and ineffective surfactant plays a particularly prominent role is neonatal RDS (formerly termed hyaline membrane disease). Although the great majority of infants in whom this abnormality develops have phospholipid profiles on lung lavage or amniotic fluid analysis that accurately predict the immaturity of the lung, in some the syndrome results from the presence of protein inhibitors of surfactant function.[403, 404] In rabbits in whom RDS is induced by repeated lung lavage, transferrin saturated with iron has been found to fulfill this inhibitory function.[405] The procedures with the biggest impact on the natural history of RDS have been prenatal stimulation of surfactant production by glucocorticosteroids[381, 382] and postnatal instillation of exogenous synthetic or natural surfactants;[406–409] both therapies offer an approximate 40% reduction in incidence of the disease. The combined use of prenatal steroids and postnatal surfactant instillation may have an additive benefit.[410]

In the dog, a lobe rendered atelectatic by bronchial ligation will show abnormalities of surface-active material within 24 hours;[411] re-expansion of the lobe up to 24 hours after ligation will restore surface-active properties to normal, but after that time, surface activity remains abnormal in both collapsed and re-expanded lobes. Oxygen toxicity also disrupts the surfactant system, both in susceptible animals and in humans;[412, 413] for example, the results of two studies have indicated that lung compliance decreases after exposure to 100% inspired oxygen.[414, 415] Experimental studies in dogs undergoing cardiopulmonary bypass have shown a decrease in lung compliance thought to be caused by atelectasis. Although light microscopic examination revealed no consistent differences in the number of Type II pneumocytes in bypass and sham-operated dogs, inclusions in these cells were decreased in the former, which suggests early surfactant loss.[416, 417]

Besides acting to decrease surface tension as lung volume decreases, surfactant imparts hysteresis to the lung's pressure-volume behavior. Thus at any given lung volume, surface tension and therefore lung elastic recoil are greater during inflation than during deflation. It has been suggested that in addition to alteration in surface forces, lung hysteresis is due partly to a different sequence of recruitment and derecruitment of alveoli during inflation and deflation.[418, 419]

Resistance of the Airways

The second major factor in the work of breathing is the force necessary to overcome the frictional resistance to air flow through the conducting airways. Resistance is the relationship of pressure to flow ($P/\dot{V}$) and can also be expressed as its reciprocal, conductance ($\dot{V}/P$). The pressure necessary to produce laminar flow through a tube is directly related to the length of the tube and the viscosity and flow rate of the gas and inversely related to the tube radius to the 4th power (r^4).

$$Pressure\ required \sim \frac{Length \times Viscosity \times \dot{V}}{r^4}$$

It is apparent from this equation that airway radius is the dominant variable in determining resistance; a doubling of airway length would only double the pressure necessary to produce a given flow (i.e., double resistance), whereas a halving of the radius would lead to a 16-fold increase in resistance. Under conditions of laminar flow, the flow rate is linearly related to pressure—that is, a doubling of pressure is required for a doubling of flow. However, with the development of turbulence, the relationship becomes nonlinear so that a greater increase in pressure is required to produce a given increment in flow. In addition, with turbulent conditions, gas density begins to play a role, resistance decreasing with gases of low density (e.g., helium-oxygen). In this somewhat more complex situation, the equation becomes

$$Pressure\ required \sim$$
$$\frac{(Length \times Viscosity \times \dot{V}) + (Density \times \dot{V})}{r^4}$$

During quiet breathing through the mouth in normal individuals, the flow status is almost laminar and the importance of this added term is negligible.[420] However, when breathing through the nose, through narrowed airways, or during the increased flow rates of exercise, substantial turbulence may occur[421] and result in an increasing proportion of the work of breathing going to overcoming resistance. In fact, in normal individuals during quiet breathing, nasal resistance constitutes up to two thirds of total airway resistance. Nasal and upper airway resistance is inversely related to lung volume, and the site of major nasal resistance cycles spontaneously between the right and left nasal passages.[422, 423]

Since airway resistance is normally measured during mouth breathing, it represents the combined resistance of the various levels of the airway from the larynx to the respiratory bronchioles. In fact, measurements show that in normal individuals the majority of the resistance is in large airways.[424, 425] The small resistance of smaller airways is partly related to their large cross-sectional area. In addition, the low linear velocity of flow through peripheral airways results in a more laminar flow situation, whereas turbulent flow conditions occur in the larger airways and across the larynx. Although relatively recent studies of excised normal human lungs have shown significantly higher peripheral resistance than that originally reported,[426] there is agreement that the site of increased resistance in disease is the small airways. The larynx also contributes substantially to total airway resistance, and its narrowing probably accounts for the higher resistance during expiration.[427]

Airway caliber and therefore resistance are not static phenomena inasmuch as they are influenced by mechanical factors as well as by complex neurohumoral controls. Both intrathoracic and extrathoracic airways respond to changes in lung volume and transpulmonary pressure, with resistance increasing at low lung volume and at very high lung volume.[428] In addition to these passive forces, a variety of active stimuli act to cause both bronchodilation and bronchoconstriction. As discussed later (*see* page 145), airway caliber is under reflex control through afferent lung receptors and efferent autonomic cholinergic, adrenergic, and "peptidergic" nerves. Local changes in gas tensions, either hypoxia or hypocapnia,[429] can cause airway narrowing. The resulting decrease in ventilation to areas of low P_{O_2} and high P_{CO_2} represents a compensatory mechanism that serves to promote a better match between ventilation and perfusion; as such, it is analogous to, although less important than hypoxic vasoconstriction.

In patients with pulmonary disease, increased airway resistance is the most common cause of increased work of breathing. The processes that narrow airways and increase resistance are both acute and reversible and chronic and irreversible. They include reflex and humorally mediated smooth muscle constriction, degeneration of the supporting structures of both large and small airways, and peripheral airway obstruction caused by mucous plugging, inflammatory cell infiltration, and scarring.

Tissue Resistance

During flow of gas in and out of the lungs, both pulmonary and chest wall tissue move. Although their major impedance during this movement is elastic, they do provide some frictional resistance. This "tissue resistance" or "viscance" has been estimated to be between 5% and 40% of the total pulmonary resistance and can increase in disease.[430–432] Lung tissue resistance can be measured in excised human lungs by using an alveolar capsule technique (which estimates alveolar pressure swings during ventilation) or in intact humans by using a rapid airway occlusion technique.[432a] Unlike airway resistance, lung tissue resistance increases as lung volume and tidal volume increase and decreases as frequency increases. Tissue resistance is a reflection of the mechanical properties of the lung tissue itself and can increase in response to bronchoconstricting stimuli such as methacholine, which suggests that smooth muscle tone is an important contributor to the development of resistance.[432b]

Collateral Ventilation

Acini beyond a completely obstructed airway can be ventilated through collateral channels. Such collateral air flow may be important in preserving gas exchange and in matching ventilation and perfusion. The effectiveness of this ventilation in maintaining alveolar gas tension depends on three variables: (1) the tidal volume of the collaterally ventilated space, which is related to the time constant of the space (resistance × compliance) and the respiratory frequency; (2) the completeness of gaseous diffusion between normally and collaterally ventilated units; and (3) the gas tensions in the collaterally delivered tidal volume. This last factor is intimately dependent on the anatomic site of the collateral channels; if an obstructed unit is ventilated via a collateral respiratory bronchiole, the P_{O_2} will be higher than if collateral ventilation occurs via more distal parenchymal tissue in which inspired air has been in contact with capillaries and has already undergone gas exchange.[433]

Collateral resistance (Rcoll) can be measured by using an ingenious technique in excised or intact lungs.[434, 435] By this method, gas is passed through a catheter that completely obstructs an airway, and the flow rate as well as the pressure within the obstructed segment is measured. The gas passes into the obstructed segment, inflates it, and exits via collateral channels. By relating the pressure to the flow within the obstructed segment, Rcoll can be calculated. Collateral resistance in the human lung is intermediate between that of the dog, whose collateral resistance is low, and the pig, whose collateral resistance is high—in fact, virtually infinite.[436]

The degree of collateral ventilation in a portion of lung depends on several factors. Collateral channels respond to alterations in inspired gas tension:[435] increasing the PCO_2 in inspired gas lowers collateral resistance, whereas the response is opposite with a decrease in inspired PO_2. The effect of lung volume on Rcoll has been measured in animals[436] and in normal human volunteers *in vivo*.[437, 438] Rcoll decreases with lung inflation in a manner similar to the decrease in airway resistance that occurs with lung inflation—and to a comparable degree. In normal lungs, however, collateral flow resistance at FRC is some 50 times greater than resistance to flow through the normal airways.[437] Rcoll is increased in dependent lung regions, presumably as a result of the decrease in regional lung volume secondary to the pleural pressure gradient.[439] Interestingly, it is 5 to 6 times higher in the middle lobe than in upper or lower lobes, an observation that may be important in explaining the pathophysiology of middle lobe syndrome.[440]

Collateral flow resistance is increased by pulmonary vascular congestion[435] and by inhalation of cigarette smoke,[441, 442] histamine,[443] and ozone (1.0 ppm).[444] Exposure to ozone also results in an enhancement of the collateral resistance response to nebulized histamine reminiscent of the increased nonspecific airway reactivity seen in humans after ozone inhalation.[445] Part of these responses is related to a vagal reflex and part is a direct effect.[444] Collateral flow resistance in the lung probably also decreases with age; in one study of human lungs, investigators were unable to demonstrate any collateral flow in the pediatric age group.[446]

Resistance to air flow through collateral channels is much lower in emphysematous than normal lungs; in fact, in excised and *in vivo* emphysematous lungs, air-flow resistance may be much less through collateral channels than through regular conducting airways.[447, 448] This marked drop in collateral air-flow resistance with even minor grades of emphysema may be related to the presence of alveolar fenestrae. These alveolar wall discontinuities are relatively common in emphysema and offer less resistance to collateral flow than is provided by the other channels of collateral ventilation.[448] The obliteration and narrowing of small airways in emphysema contribute to the freer movement of air via alveolar fenestrae and other collateral channels than via the conducting system itself.

Although the channels of collateral ventilation can be thought of as being analogous to collateral perfusion channels in vascular beds, their contribution to ventilation homogeneity in the normal lung is probably small when compared

with perfusion[448a] because the lobar and segmental alveolar gas composition behind an occluded airway rapidly approaches mixed venous concentration. In patients with emphysema, however, collateral channels are probably more important.[449]

Respiratory Mucus and Mucous Rheology

Respiratory mucus has several important roles in pulmonary homeostasis:[450–454, 454a] (1) as a medium for the clearance of particulate matter deposited within the respiratory tract; (2) as an agent in microbial defense as a result of the presence within it of immunoglobulins and a variety of other antibacterial proteins; (3) as a humidifier of inspired air; (4) as a deterrent of excessive fluid loss from the airway surface because of its hydrophilic nature;[453] and (5) (possibly) as a protector of airway epithelium from proteolytic damage.[455]

Respiratory mucus is produced by the tracheobronchial glands and surface epithelial goblet cells. Although the proportion derived from each is not precisely known, it has been estimated that in humans the volume of submucosal glands is approximately 40 times that of goblet cells,[144, 452] so it is generally assumed that the glands are the more important source. Both mucous glands and goblet cells can be stimulated by chronic irritation to increase their size, number, and mucus production.[456] In normal subjects, the volume of cleared respiratory tract secretions has been estimated to range from 0.1 to 0.3 ml/kg of body weight, or up to about 10 ml/day.[452]

The precise definitions of mucus, tracheobronchial secretions, and sputum are sometimes confused. Mucus represents the products derived from the secretion of glands and goblet cells, whereas tracheobronchial (respiratory) secretions include mucus plus fluid and solutes derived from the alveolar and bronchiolar surfaces (surfactant and Clara cell secretions) and the surface epithelium of the conducting airways (transudate from the underlying bronchial vessels). Sputum is a pathologic substance consisting of tracheobronchial secretions contaminated by saliva and inflammatory and desquamated epithelial cells.[452] Purulent sputum contains a substantial number of polymorphonuclear leukocytes, as well as polymerized DNA from degenerated neutrophils.[457]

Biochemical Characteristics of Tracheobronchial Secretions

It has been difficult to characterize the biochemical composition of normal tracheobronchial secretions since they are not expectorated. Nevertheless, small quantities of normal respiratory secretions have been obtained by fiberoptic bronchoscopy and have been examined biochemically.[458–460] The constituents can be divided into two portions: a glycoprotein fraction that gives the mucus its characteristic viscoelastic and rheologic properties and a sol-phase fraction consisting of fluid and proteins that are derived by local production and by transudation from the serum.

Mucous glycoproteins are large (molecular weight, 3 to 7 million[461]) hydrophilic molecules consisting of a core polypeptide chain and numerous sugar side chains that make up the bulk of their molecular weight. The polypeptide cores are synthesized in the rough endoplasmic reticulum of the mucous or goblet cell, and the carbohydrate side chains are attached as they pass through the Golgi apparatus. At least four different core proteins coded by different genes have been identified.[462, 463] The oligosaccharide side chains contain six different sugars: D-galactose, D-glucose, L-fructose, D-xylose, *N*-acetyl-D-glucosamine, and *N*-acetyl-D-galactosamine. Each side chain contains an average of 8 to 10 sugars.[461] Intramolecular and intermolecular bonds, including disulfide linkages and ionic and sugar-sugar interactions, result in gelation of the mucus and account for its viscoelastic properties.

The protein and nonmucous glycoprotein content of the sol-phase fraction of respiratory secretions has been characterized in sputum from patients and in bronchial lavage fluid from normal subjects.[141, 451, 459, 464] Although it has been difficult to quantify the amount of protein in airway secretions that is related to local production in comparison to that resulting from transudation from serum,[460] an estimate of local production can be obtained by assuming that the albumin content of tracheobronchial secretions is neither secreted nor locally produced and then correcting the concentrations of the other proteins for the content of albumin and the known plasma-lymph concentration ratio of the other molecules. By using these correction factors, it has been estimated that there is approximately 35% to 40% more IgG, 85% to 800% more IgA, 45% more transferrin, 15% more α_1-antitrypsin, 100% more α_1-antichymotrypsin, and 15% more ceruloplasmin than should be present if transudation alone is the mechanism for their presence.[141, 460]

Neutral lipids, phospholipids, and glycolipids contribute up to one third of the total macromolecular material of normal airway mucus and can be increased in disease. The major source is probably alveolar surfactant, with contributions from lipid precursors of prostaglandins and from tissue fluid transudate and desquamated cells from the tracheobronchial tree. Their function in airway mucus is not known, although some investigators have shown that surfactant-like lipids may increase mucociliary clearance rates.[465, 466]

The excess immunoglobulins are synthesized by plasma cells in the airway mucosa and released into the airway lumen. IgA forms a dimer that combines with a secretory component before it is released. The secretory component is a protein that is synthesized in airway epithelial or bronchial gland serous cells and secreted in an unbound form; it protects the IgA molecule from enzymatic digestion by proteolytic enzymes[464] and can be identified immunohistochemically in the serous, mucous, and ciliated cells of bronchi, bronchioles, and tracheobronchial glands.[467] Tracheobronchial secretions are also relatively enriched with lysozyme and lactoferrin; these proteins are secreted by submucosal serous cells of the tracheobronchial glands, and both have antimicrobial properties.[464] α_1-Antitrypsin and α_1-antichymotrypsin are important in inhibiting neutral protease originating from leukocyte degeneration.[451] Bronchial mucus also contains locally produced antiproteases. Secretory leukocyte proteinase inhibitor (antileukoprotease) and an elastase-specific antiprotease are probably produced by the bronchiolar Clara cells, and their expression may increase during acute episodes of inflammation to protect the airways from proteolytic damage.[468] Mucins themselves also may exert an antiprotease activity.[445]

Water constitutes 95% to 98% of the weight of normal mucus.[451] The electrolyte composition of the fluid phase of airway secretions is similar to that of serum, but with important differences; for example, the relative concentration of chloride and the absolute concentration of potassium are significantly higher than in serum. Relatively recent investigations also show that airway surface fluid is hypo-osmolar relative to plasma.[469, 470] Regional differences in airway surface liquid ion composition have been reported and suggest local differences in ion transport.[471] Measurements of the pH of tracheobronchial secretions have produced conflicting results,[451] although there is good evidence that the pH of the proximal airway surface liquid is slightly acidic (pH 6.8 to 7.0).[470]

Control of Tracheobronchial Secretion

Tracheobronchial secretion is a two-phase fluid made up of a mucous fraction and a more liquid sol fraction. Studies in which the control of tracheobronchial secretions has been investigated can be divided into those examining factors affecting the secretion of mucous glycoproteins (which form the major structural component of the mucous phase) and those examining the secretion of water and ions in the sol phase.

Mucous Phase. A number of techniques have been developed to characterize the mechanisms that control secretion of the mucous component of tracheobronchial secretions. These techniques include the insertion of a micropipette into individual gland ducts with analysis and quantification of the collected fluid,[472] incorporation of tritium-labeled glucosamine into mucous glycoproteins in cultured human airway tissue,[473] incorporation of labeled sulfate (^{35}S) into the luminal secretions of cultured airway epithelium,[474] quantification of hillocks on the airway surface after tantalum coating,[475, 476] and the development of an enzyme-linked immunosorbent assay to measure glycoprotein production.[477] Combined use of these techniques has yielded an increasingly clear picture of how mucous glycoprotein secretion is controlled.

Since atropine or vagal blockade decreases the basal secretion rate of tracheobronchial glands to approximately 60%,[472, 475] normal secretion appears to be under tonic cholinergic stimulation. There also appears to be both β- and α-adrenergic stimulatory influences,[472, 475, 478] the latter increasing secretion predominantly from serous cells and the former chiefly from mucous cells. Cholinergic stimulation increases secretion from both cell types equally.[475] Specific situations associated with increased mucous gland secretion include hypoxia (apparently related to carotid body and superior laryngeal nerve reflexes[479]), stimulation of mechanoreceptors in the stomach,[480] stimulation of cough receptors in the trachea and bronchi with chemical agents (an effect that is mediated by parasympathetic efferent pathways and also accompanies irritation of the nose, pharynx, or larynx), and inhalation of a wide variety of irritants such as ammonia, cigarette smoke, sulfur dioxide, and organic vapors. Many of the stimuli that elicit cough also result in enhanced mucous secretion, thus suggesting that these two defense mechanisms are linked.[476]

Numerous inflammatory mediators act to stimulate airway mucous production, including histamine (a relatively weak stimulator that acts via an H_2 receptor); many of the prostaglandins (the exception being prostaglandin E, which decreases secretion); the leukotrienes (including leukotriene D_4 and C_4 and hydroxyeicosatetraenoic acids, with leukotriene D_4 being the most potent[473, 481]); vasoactive intestinal peptide;[482] the neurally released polypeptide substance P;[483, 484] bradykinin;[485] platelet-activating factor;[486] and eosinophilic cationic protein.[487]

Sol Phase. Optimal mucociliary clearance by respiratory tract cilia depends on a proper balance between the volume of the mucous layer and the more fluid and less viscous sol phase through which the rapid recovery stroke of the cilia occurs.[450] Water transport—and therefore the periciliary sol phase of tracheobronchial mucus—is controlled by active ion transport across the epithelium.[488, 489] The details of human airway ion and water transport have been recently reviewed[470, 490, 491] and are derived from (1) studies of the ion content of airway surface fluid (ASL); (2) direct measurement of the *in vivo* transepithelial electrical potential difference; (3) *in vitro* transepithelial bioelectrical and ion flow studies;[488, 492] (4) intracellular microelectrode studies of freshly excised and cultured epithelial cells; and (5) patch clamp techniques in which the electrical activity of individual epithelial ion channels can be measured.

The results of these studies show that there is a ouabain-sensitive, sodium-potassium adenosine triphosphatase pump located on the basal lateral surface of the airway epithelial cells. This pump generates an electrochemical gradient that produces a potential difference across the epithelium, the luminal fluid being approximately 30 mV negative relative to the submucosa.[493] The potential difference decreases distally in the tracheobronchial tree to a lumen-negative value of 14 mV in segmental airways.[494] The gradient causes a net movement of Na^+ from the lumen into the cell via a 5-hydroxytryptamine and amiloride-sensitive Na^+ channel in the apical (luminal) membrane.[495] The combination of the apical Na^+ channel and the basal lateral pump generates transcellular Na^+ absorption. Chloride and water are also normally absorbed by the airway epithelium by following Na^+ passively through paracellular pathways and across a number of apical Cl^- channels, one of which is the cystic fibrosis transmembrane regulator (CFTR). The necessity for the airway epithelium to be a net absorber of Na^+, Cl^-, and water is appreciated by calculations based on the average depth of ASL and the surface area of the tracheobronchial tree at different levels. Because of the marked decrease in airway surface area between the bronchioles and the trachea, the airways would quickly become occluded if net fluid absorption did not occur as the ASL moved proximally.

Although the dominant movement of Na^+, Cl^-, and H_2O is from the airway lumen to the lamina propria, airway epithelium can also be stimulated to secrete Cl^- and H_2O, especially if the apical sodium channel is blocked with amiloride. Chloride and water secretion can be stimulated by activation of the cyclic adenosine monophosphate (AMP)-dependent apical membrane conductance channels (β-agonists, adenosine); by stimulation of a K^+ channel, which results in hyperpolarization of the cell and passive outward movement of Cl^- (histamine, bradykinin); or by a non-cyclic AMP–dependent opening of apical Cl^- channels that is stimulated by adenosine or uridine triphosphate.[496]

The interest in airway epithelial ion transport and Cl^- transport in particular has been fueled by the discovery that the mutant protein that leads to cystic fibrosis, CFTR, is an epithelial chloride channel. The biophysical hallmark of this disease is a raised transepithelial potential difference; this condition is caused by accelerated transcellular Na^+ absorption, which in turn is stimulated by failure of the apical Cl^- conductance channel to open.[490, 497] Increased Na^+ absorption and decreased Cl^- secretion result in a net depletion of H_2O from the ASL; it is this dehydration that impedes normal clearance mechanisms and presumably leads to the chronic airway infection that underlies the clinical manifestations of pulmonary disease.

Physical Characteristics of Tracheobronchial Secretions

Adequate mucociliary clearance depends not only on the quantity and biochemical composition of the mucous layer and the periciliary sol layer but also on the viscoelastic properties of the mucus. The rheologic properties of mucus cannot be described by measurements of viscosity alone. A true "Newtonian" liquid has only viscosity and no elasticity; respiratory mucus, however, has characteristics of both a liquid and a solid and has been described as exhibiting "pseudoplastic behavior." Respiratory mucus also shows another unique physical-chemical characteristic known as *thixotropy,* which is a transient decrease in viscosity after exposure to high shear rates.[454, 498] The viscoelastic properties of mucus are related to the molecular-molecular interaction that results in gelation; the bonds that join the molecules into a gel matrix include covalent disulfide bonds, ionic bonds, hydrogen bonds, van der Waal's forces (which consist of weak bonds between methyl groups), and the physical intermingling or entangling of the long molecules themselves.[499] The viscoelastic properties of airway mucus are best quantified by using oscillatory methods to establish dynamic stress-strain relationships; with these techniques, two parameters—elastic modulus and dynamic viscosity—can be determined.[498-500] Given a depth of the mucous and periciliary sol layer and a constant ciliary beat frequency, mucus transport on a ciliated surface relates in a complex fashion to both the elasticity and dynamic viscosity of mucus or sputum.[454] An optimal combination of elasticity and dynamic viscosity results in optimal mucus transportability; therefore, pathologic states can theoretically decrease mucociliary clearance by altering either of these properties.[454, 499, 500]

Despite accurate measurements of elasticity and dynamic viscosity, discrepancies between these physical characteristics and the mucus transport rate have been observed; an additional mechanical characteristic of bronchial mucus, *spinnability,* has been described and may help explain these discrepancies. Spinnability is the ability of mucus to stretch to a long thin thread; it has been shown that the degree to which it can do this correlates closely with its transportability on a ciliated surface.[501] (Spinnability has been extensively studied in mucus from the human cervix; the time of maximal spinnability for cervical mucus is also the time of maximal fertility when spermatozoa can move through highly spinnable mucus with the greatest of ease.[501])

Few data exist on the controlling mechanisms that optimize or disrupt tracheobronchial mucus elasticity and dynamic viscosity. It is known, however, that both vary considerably, not only from day to day but even during the same day.[502] The rate of secretion of mucous glycoprotein and periciliary fluid presumably influences these variations; changes in the biochemical composition of the secreted mucus and the sol-phase proteins undoubtedly play a role as well. Vagal stimulation and methacholine inhalation tend to increase elasticity and dynamic viscosity at low stimulation frequencies and dose, whereas both viscoelastic characteristics decrease at higher frequencies and concentrations.[454, 503] β-Adrenergic stimulation imparts a selective stimulation of mucous cells and leads to increased elasticity and dynamic viscosity; by contrast, α-adrenergic stimulation selectively stimulates serous cells and results in a more watery, less viscous mucus.[454] Inhalation of prostaglandin $F_{2\alpha}$, histamine, or acetylcholine has also been shown to produce alterations in the viscoelastic properties of mucus, probably by altering epithelial permeability and increasing the transudation of serum proteins.[504]

In addition to cystic fibrosis, several pulmonary diseases are associated with altered mucus viscoelasticity. A hereditary deficiency of the lysosomal enzyme α-L-fucosidase impairs the glycosylation of mucin proteins, causes a decrease in mucus viscoelasticity, and is associated with repeated respiratory tract infections.[505] A much more commonly encountered abnormality is purulent sputum, which is more viscous and less elastic than mucoid sputum.[502] At least part of these differences are related to the presence of DNA from necrotic polymorphonuclear leukocytes. The viscosity of such purulent secretions can be decreased *in vitro* and *in vivo* by using recombinant human DNase, a therapeutic intervention that has shown some benefit in patients with cystic fibrosis.[506, 507] Studies have also indicated that viscosity is decreased in association with increased humidity;[508] by the application of water-mist aerosol,[502] L-acetylcysteine, or dithiothreitol;[509] and by the oral administration of guaifenesin, a glycerol ether of glycol.[510] Acetylcysteine directly affects glycoproteins, whereas the water mist and guaifenesin appear to increase the width of the sol layer in which the cilia beat, thereby improving mucus mobility without appreciably changing sputum viscosity.

REFERENCES

1. von Hayek H: The Human Lung. New York, Hafer, 1960.
2. Nagaishi C: Functional Anatomy and Histology of the Lung. Baltimore, University Park Press, 1972.
3. Miller WS: The Lung. Springfield, IL Charles C Thomas, 1937.
4. Krahl VE: Anatomy of the mammalian lung. *In* Fenn WO, Rahn H (eds): Handbook of Physiology. Section 3. Respiration. Vol 1. Washington, DC, American Physiological Society, 1964, pp 213–284.
5. Stone KC, Mercer RR, Freeman BA, et al: Distribution of lung cell numbers and volumes between alveolar and nonalveolar tissue. Am Rev Respir Dis 146:454, 1992.
6. Strahler AN: Equilibrium theory of erosional slopes approached by frequency distribution analysis. Am J Sci 248:673, 1950.
7. Horsfield K, Cumming G: Morphology of the bronchial tree in man. J Appl Physiol 24:373, 1968.
8. Cumming G, Horsfield K, Harding LK, et al: Biological branching systems with special reference to the lung airways. Bull Physiopathol Respir 7:31, 1971.
9. Cumming G: Airway morphology and its consequences. Bull Physiopathol Respir 8:527, 1972.
10. Weibel ER: Morphometry of the Human Lung. New York, Academic Press, 1963.
11. Thurlbeck A, Horsfield K: Branching angles in the bronchial tree related to order of branching. Respir Physiol 41:173, 1980.
12. Phalen RF, Yeh HC, Schum GM, et al: Application of an idealized model to morphometry of the mammalian tracheobronchial tree. Anat Rec 190:167, 1978.
13. Gail DB, Lenfant CJM: State of the art—cells of the lung: Biology and clinical implications. Am Rev Respir Dis 127:366, 1983.
14. Breeze RG, Wheeldon EB: The cells of the pulmonary airways: State of the art. Am Rev Respir Dis 116:705, 1977.
15. McDowell EM, Barrett LA, Glavin F, et al: The respiratory epithelium: I. Human bronchus. J Natl Cancer Inst 61:539, 1978.
16. Rhodin JAG: The ciliated cell: Ultrastructure and function of the human tracheal mucosa. Am Rev Respir Dis 93:1, 1966.
17. Mette SA, Pilewski J, Buck CA, et al: Distribution of integrin cell adhesion receptors on normal bronchial epithelial cells and lung cancer cells *in vitro* and *in vivo*. Am J Respir Cell Mol Biol 8:562, 1993.
18. Godfrey RWA, Severs NJ, Jeffrey PK: Freeze-fracture morphology and quantification of human bronchial epithelial tight junctions. Am J Respir Cell Mol Biol 6:453, 1992.
19. Herard AL, Zahm JM, Pierrot D, et al: Epithelial barrier integrity during *in vitro* wound repair of the airway epithelium. Am J Respir Cell Mol Biol 15:624, 1996.
20. Bhalla DK, Crocker TT: Tracheal permeability in rats exposed to ozone. Am Rev Respir Dis 134:572, 1986.
21. Churg A, Hobson J, Wright J: Effects of cigarette smoke dose and time after smoke exposure on uptake of asbestos fibers by rat tracheal epithelial cells. Am J Respir Cell Mol Biol 3:265, 1990.
22. Keeling B, Li KY, Churg A: Iron enhances uptake of mineral particles and increases lipid peroxidation in tracheal epithelial cells. Am J Respir Cell Mol Biol 10:683, 1994.
23. Nathanson I, Nadel JA: Movement of electrolytes and fluid across airways. Lung 162:125, 1984.
24. Widdicombe JH, Gashi AA, Basbaum CB, et al: Structural changes associated with fluid absorption by dog tracheal epithelium. Exp Lung Res 10:57, 1986.
25. Serafini SM, Michaelson ED: Length and distribution of cilia in human and canine airways. Bull Eur Physiopathol Respir 13:551, 1977.
26. Kilburn KH: A hypothesis for pulmonary clearance and its implications. Am Rev Respir Dis 98:449, 1968.
27. Respiratory Tract Mucus. *In* Ciba Foundation Symposium 54 (New Series). New York, Excerpta Medica, 1978.
28. Kuhn C: Ciliated and Clara cells. *In* Bouhuys A (ed): Lung Cells in Disease. New York, Elsevier, 1976, p 91.
29. Satir P: How cilia move. Sci Am 231:45, 1974.
30. Jeffrey PK, Reid L: New observations of rat airway epithelium: A quantitative and electron microscopic study. J Anat 120:295, 1975.
31. McDowell EM, Barrett LA, Harris CC, et al: Abnormal cilia in human bronchial epithelium. Arch Pathol Lab Med 100:429, 1976.
32. Ailsby RL, Ghadially FN: Atypical cilia in human bronchial mucosa. J Pathol 109:75, 1973.
33. Smallman LA, Gregory J: Ultrastructural abnormalities of cilia in the human respiratory tract. Hum Pathol 17:848, 1986.
34. Lungarella G, Fonzi L, Ermini G: Abnormalities of bronchial cilia in patients with chronic bronchitis. An ultrastructural and quantitative analysis. Lung 161:147, 1983.
35. Wisseman CL, Simel DL, Spock A, et al: The prevalence of abnormal cilia in normal pediatric lungs. Arch Pathol Lab Med 105:552, 1981.
36. Fox B, Bull TB, Makey AR, et al: The significance of ultrastructural abnormalities of human cilia. Chest 80:796, 1981.
37. Rennard SI, Romberger DJ, Robbins RA, et al: Is asthma an epithelial disease? Chest 107(Suppl):127, 1995.
37a. Emery N, Place GA, Dodd S, et al: Mucus and serous secretions of human bronchial epithelial cells in secondary culture. Am J Respir Cell Mol Biol 12:130, 1995.
38. Smith SM, Lee DKP, Lacy J, et al: Rat tracheal epithelial cells produce granulocyte/macrophage colony-stimulating factor. Am J Respir Cell Mol Biol 2:59, 1990.
39. Robbins RA, Koyama S, Spurzem JR, et al: Modulation of neutrophil and mononuclear cell adherence to bronchial epithelial cells. Am J Respir Cell Mol Biol 7:19, 1992.
40. Glanville AR, Tazelaar HD, Theodore J, et al: The distribution of MHC class I and II antigens on bronchial epithelium. Am Rev Respir Dis 139:330, 1989.
41. Rossi GA, Sacco O, Balbi B, et al: Human ciliated bronchial epithelial cells: Expression of the HLA-DR antigens and of the HLA-DR alpha gene, modulation of the HLA-DR antigens by gamma-interferon and antigen-presenting function in the mixed leukocyte reaction. Am J Respir Cell Mol Biol 3:431, 1990.
41a. Yao PM, Delclaux C, d'Ortho MP, et al: Cell-matrix interactions modulate 92-kD gelatinase expression by human bronchial epithelial cells. Am J Respir Cell Mol Biol 18:813, 1998.
42. Tos M: Mucous elements in the airways. Acta Otolaryngol 82:249, 1976.
43. Ebert RV, Terracio MJ: The bronchiolar epithelium in cigarette smokers: Observations with the scanning electron microscope. Am Rev Respir Dis 111:4, 1975.
44. Lumsden AB, McLean A, Lamb D: Goblet and Clara cells of human distal airways: Evidence for smoking-induced changes in their members. Thorax 39:844, 1984.
45. Adler KB, Hardwick DH, Craighead JE: Porcine tracheal goblet cell ultrastructure: A three-dimensional reconstruction. Exp Lung Res 3:69, 1982.
45a. Kim KC, McCracken K, Lee BC, et al: Airway goblet cell mucin: Its structure and regulation of excretion. Eur Respir J 10:2644, 1997.
46. Korhonen LK, Holopainen E, Paavolainen M: Some histochemical characteristics of tracheobronchial tree and pulmonary neoplasms. Acta Histochem Suppl 32:57, 1969.
47. Marsan C, Cava E, Roujeau J, et al: Cytochemical and histochemical characterization of epithelial mucins in human bronchi. Acta Cytol 22:562, 1978.
48. Spicer SS, Schulte BA, Chakrin LW: Ultrastructural and histochemical observations of respiratory epithelium and gland. Exp Lung Res 4:137, 1983.
49. Tamai S: Basal cells of the human bronchiole. Acta Pathol Jpn 33:125, 1983.
50. Wailoo M, Emery JL: Structure of the membranous trachea in children. Acta Anat 106:254, 1980.
50a. Boers JE, Ambergen AW, Thunnissen FBJM: Number and proliferation of basal and parabasal cells in normal human airway epithelium. Am J Respir Crit Care Med 157:2000, 1998.
51. Wang C-Z, Evans MJ, Cox RA, et al: Morphologic changes in basal cells during repair of tracheal epithelium. Am J Pathol 141:753, 1992.
52. Inayama Y, Hook GE, Brody AR, et al: *In vitro* and *in vivo* growth and differentiation of clones of tracheal basal cells. Am J Pathol 134:539, 1989.
53. Breuer R, Zajicek G, Christensen TG, et al: Cell kinetics of normal adult hamster bronchial epithelium in the steady state. Am J Respir Cell Mol Biol 2:51, 1990.
54. Evans MJ, Cox RA, Shami SG, et al: The role of basal cells in attachment of columnar cells to the basal lamina of the trachea. Am J Respir Cell Mol Biol 1:463, 1989.
55. Evans MJ, Cox RA, Shami SG, et al: Junctional adhesion mechanisms in airway basal cells. Am J Respir Cell Mol Biol 3:341, 1990.
56. Baldwin F: Basal cells in human bronchial epithelium. Anat Rec 238:360, 1994.
57. Mercer RR, Russell ML, Roggli VL, et al: Cell number and distribution in human and rat airways. Am J Respir Cell Mol Biol 10:613, 1994.
58. Su WY, Folz R, Chen JS, et al: Extracellular superoxide dismutase mRNA expressions in the human lung by *in situ* hybridization. Am J Respir Cell Mol Biol 16:162, 1997.
59. Inayama Y, Hook GER, Brody AR, et al: The differentiation potential of tracheal basal cells. Lab Invest 58:706, 1988.
60. Lane BP, Gordon R: Regeneration of rat tracheal epithelium after mechanical injury: I. The relationship between mitotic activity and cellular differentiation. Proc Soc Exp Biol Med 145:1139, 1974.
61. Wynne JW, Ramphal R, Hood CI: Tracheal mucosal damage after aspiration: A scanning electron microscope study. Am Rev Respir Dis 124:728, 1981.
62. Shimizu T, Nishihara M, Kawaguchi S, et al: Expression of phenotypic markers during regeneration of rat tracheal epithelium following mechanical injury. Am J Respir Cell Mol Biol 11:85, 1994.
63. Wang A, Yokosaki Y, Ferrando R, et al: Differential regulation of airway epithelial integrins by growth factors. Am J Respir Cell Mol Biol 16:664, 1996.
63a. Kim JS, McKinnis VS, Nawrocki A, et al: Stimulation of migration and wound repair of guinea pig airway epithelial cells in response to epidermal growth factor. Am J Respir Cell Mol Biol 18:66, 1998.
64. Boers JE, den Brok JL, Koudstaal J, et al: Number and proliferation of neuroendocrine cells in normal human airway epithelium. Am J Respir Crit Care Med 154:758, 1996.
65. Floyd EE, Jetten AM: Retinoids, growth factors, and the tracheobronchial epithelium. Lab Invest 59:1, 1988.
66. Meyrick B, Reid L: The alveolar brush cell in rat lung—a third pneumocyte. J Ultrastruct Res 23:71, 1968.
67. DiMaio MF, Kattan M, Ciurea D, et al: Brush cells in the human fetal trachea. Pediatr Pulmonol 8:40, 1990.
67a. Gordon RE, Kattan M: Absence of cilia and basal bodies with a predominance of brush cells in the respiratory mucosa from a patient with immotile cilia syndrome. Ultrastruct Pathol 6:45, 1984.

68. Broers JLV, Jensen SM, Travis WD, et al: Expression of surfactant-associated protein A and Clara cell 10-kilodalton mRNA in neoplastic and non-neoplastic human lung tissue as detected by *in situ* hybridization. Lab Invest 66:337, 1992.

69. Plopper CG: Comparative morphologic features of bronchiolar epithelial cells—the Clara cell. Am Rev Respir Dis 128(suppl):S37, 1983.

70. Widdicombe JG, Pack RJ: The Clara cell. Eur J Respir Dis 63:202, 1982.

71. Patton SE, Gilmore LB, Jetten AM, et al: Biosynthesis and release of proteins by isolated pulmonary Clara cells. Exp Lung Res 11:227, 1986.

72. Massaro GD, Singh G, Mason R, et al: Biology of the Clara cell. Am J Physiol 266:L101, 1994.

73. Jorens PG, Sibille Y, Goulding NJ, et al: Potential role of Clara cell protein, an endogenous phospholipase A$_2$ inhibitor, in acute lung injury. Eur Respir J 8:1647, 1995.

74. Lesur O, Bernard A, Arsalane K, et al: Clara cell protein (CC-16) induces a phospholipase A2–mediated inhibition of fibroblast migration *in vitro*. Am J Respir Crit Care Med 152:290, 1995.

75. Hay JG, Danel C, Chu CS, et al: Human CC10 gene expression in airway epithelium and subchromosomal locus suggest linkage to airway disease. Am J Physiol 268:L565, 1995.

75a. Hermans C, Lesur D, Weynand B, et al: Clara cell protein (CC16) in pleural fluids: A marker of leakage through the visceral pleura. Am J Respir Crit Care Med 157:962, 1998.

76. Nomori H, Horio H, Fuyuno G, et al: Protein 1 (Clara cell protein) serum levels in healthy subjects and patients with bacterial pneumonia. Am J Respir Crit Care Med 152:746, 1995.

77. Bernard AM, Roels HA, Buchet JP, et al: Serum Clara cell protein: An indicator of bronchial cell dysfunction caused by tobacco smoking. Environ Res 66:96, 1994.

78. Bernard AM, Gonzalez-Lorenzo JM, Siles E, et al: Early decrease of serum Clara cell protein in silica-exposed workers. Eur Respir J 7:1932, 1994.

79. Khoor A, Gray ME, Singh G, et al: Ontogeny of Clara cell–specific protein and its mRNA: Their association with neuroepithelial bodies in human fetal lung and in bronchopulmonary dysplasia. J Histochem Cytochem 44:1429, 1996.

80. Bernard A, Thielemans N, Lauwerys R, et al: Clara cell protein in human amniotic fluid: A potential marker of fetal lung growth. Pediatr Res 36:771, 1994.

81. Phelps DS, Floros J: Localization of pulmonary surfactant proteins using immunohistochemistry and tissue *in situ* hybridization. Exp Lung Res 17:985, 1991.

82. Gil J, Weibel ER: Extracellular lining of bronchioles after perfusion-fixation of rat lungs for electron microscopy. Anat Rec 169:185, 1975.

83. DeWater R, Willems LNA, Van Muijen GNP, et al: Ultrastructural localization of bronchial antileukoprotease in central and peripheral human airways by a gold-labeling technique using monoclonal antibodies. Am Rev Respir Dis 133:882, 1986.

84. Evans MJ, Cabral-Anderson LJ, Freeman G: Role of the Clara cell in renewal of the bronchiolar epithelium. Lab Invest 38:648, 1978.

85. Castleman WL, Dungworth DL, Schwartz LW, et al: Acute respiratory bronchiolitis—an ultrastructural and autoradiographic study of epithelial cell injury and renewal in rhesus monkeys exposed to ozone. Am J Pathol 98:811, 1980.

86. Sorokin SP, Hoyt RF Jr: Workshop on pulmonary neuroendocrine cells in health and disease. Anat Rec 236:213, 1993.

87. Becker KL: The coming of age of a bronchial epithelial cell. Am Rev Respir Dis 148:1166, 1993.

88. Ito T, Nakatani Y, Nagahara N, et al: Quantitative study of pulmonary endocrine cells in anencephaly. Lung 165:297, 1987.

89. McDougall J: Endocrine-like cells in the terminal bronchioles and saccules of human fetal lung—an ultrastructural study. Thorax 33:43, 1978.

90. Torikata C, Mukai M, Kawakita H, et al: Neurofilaments of Kultschitsky cells in human lung. Acta Pathol Jpn 36:93, 1986.

91. Pack RJ, Widdicombe JG: Amine-containing cells of the lung. Eur J Respir Dis 65:559, 1984.

92. Cutz E: Neuroendocrine cells of the lung: An overview of morphologic characteristics and development. Exp Lung Res 3:185, 1982.

93. Hage E: Electron microscopic identification of several types of endocrine cells in the bronchial epithelium of human foetuses. Z Zellforsch 141:401, 1973.

94. Watanabe H: Pathological studies of neuroendocrine cells in human embryonic and fetal lung: Light microscopical, immunohistochemical and electron microscopical approaches. Acta Pathol Jpn 38:59, 1988.

95. King KA, Torday JS, Sunday ME: Bombesin and [Leu8]phyllolitorin promote fetal mouse lung branching morphogenesis via a receptor-mediated mechanism. Proc Natl Acad Sci U S A 92:4357, 1995.

96. Stahlman MT, Gray ME: Ontogeny of neuroendocrine cells in human fetal lung: I. An electron microscopic study. Lab Invest 51:449, 1984.

97. Keith IM, Will JA: Hypoxia and the neonatal rabbit lung: Neuroendocrine cell numbers, 5-HT fluorescence intensity and the relationship to arterial thickness. Thorax 34:767, 1981.

98. Moosavi H, Smith P, Heath D: The Feyrter cell in hypoxia. Thorax 28:729, 1973.

99. Sanghavi JN, Rabe KF, Kim JS, et al: Migration of human and guinea pig airway epithelial cells in response to calcitonin gene–related peptide. Am J Respir Cell Mol Biol 11:181, 1994.

100. DeMichele MA, Davis ALG, Hunt JD, et al: Expression of mRNA for three bombesin receptor subtypes in human bronchial epithelial cells. Am J Respir Cell Mol Biol 11:66, 1994.

101. Miller YE: The pulmonary neuroendocrine cell: A role in adult lung disease? Am Rev Respir Dis 140:283, 1989.

102. Lauweryns JM, Peuskens JC: Neuro-epithelial bodies (neuroreceptor or secretory organs?) in human infant bronchial and bronchiolar epithelium. Anat Rec 172:471, 1972.

103. Lauweryns JM, Goddeeris P: Neuroepithelial bodies in the human child and adult lung. Am Rev Respir Dis 111:469, 1975.

104. Lauweryns JM, Cokelaere M, Theunynck P: Neuro-epithelial bodies in the respiratory mucosa of various mammals: A light optical, histochemical and ultrastructural investigation. Z Zellforsch 135:569, 1972.

105. Wan N-S, Chen M-F, Schraufnagel DE, et al: The cumulative scanning electron microscopic changes in baby mouse lungs following prenatal and postnatal exposures to nicotine. J Pathol 144:89, 1984.

106. Kleinerman J, Marchevsky A: Quantitative studies of argyrophilic APUD cells in airways: II. The effects of transplacental diethylnitrosamine. Rev Respir Dis 126:152, 1982.

107. Marchevsky AM, Keller S, Fogel JR, et al: Quantitative studies of argyrophilic APUD cells in airways: The effects of sensitization on anaphylactic shock. Am Rev Respir Dis 129:477, 1984.

108. Hance AJ: Pulmonary immune cells in health and disease: Dendritic cells and Langerhans' cells. Eur Respir J 6:1213, 1993.

109. Schon-Hegrad MA, Oliver J, McMenamin PG, et al: Studies on the density, distribution, and surface phenotype of intraepithelial class II major histocompatibility complex antigen (Ia)-bearing dendritic cells (DC) in the conducting airways. J Exp Med 173:1345, 1991.

110. Toews GB: Pulmonary dendritic cells: Sentinels of lung-associated lymphoid tissues. Am J Respir Cell Mol Biol 4:204, 1991.

111. van Haarst JM, Verhoeven GT, de Wit HJ, et al: CD1a+ and CD1a− accessory cells from bronchoalveolar lavage differ in allostimulatory potential and cytokine production. Am J Respir Cell Mol Biol 15:752, 1996.

112. Holt PG, Oliver J, Bilyk N, et al: Downregulation of the antigen presenting cell function(s) of pulmonary dendritic cells *in vivo* by resident alveolar macrophages. J Exp Med 177:397, 1993.

113. Richmond I, Pritchard GE, Ashcroft T, et al: Distribution of γ, δ T-cells in the bronchial tree of smokers and nonsmokers. J Clin Pathol 46:926, 1993.

114. Lamb D, Lumsden A: Intraepithelial mast cells in human airway epithelium: Evidence for smoking-induced changes in their frequency. Thorax 37:334, 1982.

115. Bai A, Eidelman DH, Hogg JC, et al: Proposed nomenclature for quantifying subdivisions of the bronchial wall. J Appl Physiol 77:1011, 1994.

116. Evans MJ, Guha SC, Cox RA, et al: Attenuated fibroblast sheath around the basement membrane zone in the trachea. Am J Respir Cell Mol Biol 8:188, 1993.

117. Khosla J, Correa MT, Sannes PL: Heterogeneity of sulfated microdomains within basement membranes of pulmonary airway epithelium. Am J Respir Cell Mol Biol 10:462, 1994.

118. Vanpeperstraete F: The cartilaginous skeleton of the bronchial tree. Adv Anat Embryol Cell Biol 48:1, 1974.

119. Reid L: Visceral cartilage. J Anat 122:349, 1976.

120. Monkhouse WS, Whimster WF: An account of the longitudinal mucosal corrugations of the human tracheo-bronchial tree, with observations on those of some animals. J Anat 122:681, 1986.

121. Starcher BC: Elastin and the lung [review article]. Thorax 41:577, 1986.

122. Hakansson CH, Mercke U, Sonesson B, et al: Functional anatomy of the musculature of the trachea. Acta Morphol Neerl Scand 14:291, 1976.

123. Matsuba K, Thurlbeck WM: A morphometric study of bronchial and bronchiolar walls in children. Am Rev Respir Dis 105:908, 1972.

124. Smith PG, Janiga KE, Bruce MC: Strain increases airway smooth muscle cell proliferation. Am J Respir Cell Mol Biol 10:85, 1994.

125. Glassberg MK, Ergul A, Wanner A, et al: Endothelin 1 promotes mitogenesis in airway smooth muscle cells. Am J Respir Cell Mol Biol 10:316, 1994.

126. Stephens NL, Kroeger EA: Ultrastructure, biophysics, and biochemistry of airway smooth muscle. *In* Nadel JA (ed): Physiology and Pharmacology of the Airways. New York, Marcel Dekker, 1980, p 81.

127. Stephens NL: Airway smooth muscle. Am Rev Respir Dis 135:960, 1987.

128. Oury TD, Chang LY, Marklund SL, et al: Immunocytochemical localization of extracellular superoxide dismutase in human lung. Lab Invest 70:889, 1994.

129. Whimster WF, Lord P, Biles B: Tracheobronchial gland profiles in four segmental airways. Am Rev Respir Dis 129:985, 1984.

130. Thurlbeck WM, Benjamin B, Reid L: Development and distribution of mucous glands in the foetal human trachea. Br J Dis Chest 55:54, 1961.

131. Tos M: Anatomy of the tracheal mucous glands in man. Arch Otolaryngol 92:132, 1970.

132. Meyrick B, Sturgess JM, Reid L: A reconstruction of the duct system and secretory tubules of the human bronchial submucosal gland. Thorax 24:729, 1969.

133. Meyrick B, Reid L: Ultrastructure of cells in the human bronchial submucosal glands. J Anat 107:281, 1970.

134. De Poitiers W, Lord PW, Biles B, et al: Bronchial gland histochemistry in lungs removed for cancer. Thorax 35:546, 1980.

135. Matsuba K, Takizawa T, Thurlbeck WM: Oncocytes in human bronchial mucous glands. Thorax 27:181, 1972.

136. Lamb D, Reid L: Histochemical types of acidic glycoprotein produced by mucous cells of the tracheobronchial glands in man. J Pathol 98:213, 1969.

137. Reid L: Evaluation of model systems for study of airway epithelium, cilia, and mucus. Arch Intern Med 126:428, 1970.

138. Spicer SS, Schulte BA, Chakrin LW: Ultrastructural and histochemical observations of respiratory epithelium and gland. Exp Lung Res 4:137, 1983.

139. Nadziejko C, Finkelstein I: Inhibition of neutrophil elastase by mucus glycoprotein. Am J Respir Cell Mol Biol 10:103, 1994.

140. Mooren HWD, Meyer CJLM, Kramps JA, et al: Ultrastructural localization of the low-molecular-weight protease inhibitor in human bronchial glands. J Histochem Cytochem 30:1130, 1982.

141. Wiggins J, Hill SL, Stockley RA: Lung secretion sol-phase proteins: Comparison of sputum with secretions obtained by direct sampling. Thorax 38:102, 1983.

141a. Vogel L, Schoonbrood D, Geluk F, et al: Iron-binding proteins in sputum of chronic bronchitis patients with *Haemophilus influenzae* infections. Eur Respir J 10:2327, 1997.

142. De Water R, Willems LNA, Van Muijen GNP, et al: Ultrastructural localization of bronchial antileukoprotease in central and peripheral human airways by a gold-labelling technique using monoclonal antibodies. Am Rev Respir Dis 133:882, 1986.

143. Goodman MR, Link DW, Brown WR, et al: Ultrastructural evidence of transport of secretory IgA across bronchial epithelium. Am Rev Respir Dis 123:115, 1981.

144. Reid L: Measurement of the bronchial mucous gland layer: A diagnostic yardstick in chronic bronchitis. Thorax 15:132, 1960.

145. Dunnill MS, Massarella GR, Anderson JA: A comparison of the quantitative anatomy of the bronchi in normal subjects in status asthmaticus in chronic bronchitis and in emphysema. Thorax 24:176, 1979.

146. Douglas AN: Quantitative study of bronchial mucous gland enlargement. Thorax 35:198, 1980.

147. Tournier J-M, Goldstein GA, Hall DE, et al: Extracellular matrix proteins regulate morphologic and biochemical properties of tracheal gland serous cells through integrins. Am J Respir Cell Mol Biol 6:461, 1992.

148. Bienenstock J, Clancy RL, Perey DYE: Bronchus-associated lymphoid tissue (BALT): Its relationship to mucosal immunity. *In* Kirkpatrick CH, Reynolds HY (eds): Immunologic and Infections Reactions in the Lung. New York, Marcel Dekker, 1976, p 29.

149. Holt PG: Development of bronchus associated lymphoid tissue (BALT) in human lung disease: A normal host defense mechanism awaiting therapeutic exploitation? Thorax 48:1097, 1993.

150. Emery JL, Dinsdale F: The postnatal development of lymphoreticular aggregates and lymph nodes in infants' lungs. J Clin Pathol 26:539, 1973.

151. Richmond I, Pritchard GE, Ashcroft T, et al: Bronchus-associated lymphoid tissue (BALT) in human lung: Its distribution in smokers and non-smokers. Thorax 48:1130, 1993.

152. Pabst R, Gehrke I: Is the bronchus-associated lymphoid tissue (BALT) an integral structure of the lung in normal mammals including humans? Am J Respir Cell Mol Biol 3:131, 1990.

153. Soutar CA: Distribution of plasma cells and other cells containing immunoglobulin in the respiratory tract of normal man and class of immunoglobulin contained therein. Thorax 31:158, 1976.

154. Geiser M, Baumann M, Cruz-Orive LM, et al: The effect of particle inhalation on macrophage number and phagocytic activity in the intrapulmonary conducting airways of hamsters. Am J Respir Cell Mol Biol 10:594, 1994.

155. Brinkman GL: The mast cell in normal bronchus and lung. J Ultrastruct Res 23:115, 1968.

156. Caughey, GH: The structure and airway biology of mast cell proteinases. Am J Respir Cell Mol Biol 4:387, 1991

157. Orr TSC: Mast cells and allergic asthma. Br J Dis Chem 67:87, 1973.

158. Raible DG, Schulman ES, DiMuzio J, et al: Mast cell mediators prostaglandin D₂ and histamine activate human eosinophils. J Immunol 148:3536, 1992.

159. Bradding P, Feather IH, Howarth PH, et al: Interlukin 4 is localized to and released by human mast cells. J Exp Med 176:1381, 1992.

160. Bradding P, Okayama Y, Howart PH, et al: Heterogeneity of human mast cells based on cytokine content. J Immunol 155:297, 1995.

161. Van Overveld FJ, Houben LA, Schmitz du Moulin FE, et al: Mast cell heterogeneity in human lung tissue. Clin Sci 77:297, 1989.

162. Irani AM, Schwartz LB: Human mast cell heterogeneity. Allergy Proc 15:303, 1994.

163. Caughey GH: Serine proteinases of mast cell and leukocyte granules. A league of their own. Am J Respir Crit Care Med 150:S138, 1994.

164. Finotto S, Dolovich J, Denburg JA, et al: Functional heterogeneity of mast cells isolated from different microenvironments within nasal polyp tissue. Clin Exp Immunol 95:343, 1994.

165. Chanez P, Lacoste J-Y, Guillot B, et al: Mast cells' contribution to the fibrosing alveolitis of the scleroderma lung. Am Rev Respir Dis 147:1497, 1993.

166. Jordana M: Mast cells and fibrosis—who's on first? Am J Respir Cell Mol Biol 8:7, 1993.

167. Page CP: An explanation of the asthma paradox. Am Rev Respir Dis 147(suppl):S29, 1993.

168. Pump KK: Morphology of the acinus of the human lung. Dis Chest 56:126, 1969.

169. Boyden EA: The structure of the pulmonary acinus in a child of six years and eight months. Am J Anat 132:275, 1971.

170. Schreider JP, Raabe OG: Structure of the human respiratory acinus. Am J Anat 162:221, 1981.

171. Hansen JE, Ampaya EP, Bryant GH, et al: Branching pattern of airways and air spaces of a single human terminal bronchiole. J Appl Physiol 38:983, 1975.

172. Parker H, Horsfield K, Cumming G: Morphology of distal airways in the human lung. J Appl Physiol 31:386, 1971.

173. Whimster WF: The microanatomy of the alveolar duct system. Thorax 25:141, 1970.

174. Oderr C: Architecture of the lung parenchyma. Studies with a specially designed x-ray microscope. Am Rev Respir Dis 90:401, 1964.

175. Young CD, Moore GW, Hutchins GM: Connective tissue arrangement in respiratory airways. Anat Rec 198:245, 1980.

176. Crapo JD, Barry BE, Gehr P, et al: Cell number and cell characteristics of the normal human lung. Am Rev Respir Dis 125:332, 1982.

177. Weibel ER, Gehr P, Haies D, et al: The cell population of the normal lung. *In* Bouhuys A (ed): Lung Cells in Disease. New York, North-Holland Biomedical Press, 1976, p 3.

178. Bartels H: The air-blood barrier in the human lung: A freeze-fracture study. Cell Tissue Res 198:269, 1979.

179. Schneeberger EE: Barrier function of intercellular junctions in adult and fetal lungs. *In* Fishman AP, Renkin EM (eds): Pulmonary Edema. Bethesda, MD, American Physiological Society, 1979, p 21.

180. Bartels H, Oestern H-J, Voss-Wermbter G: Communicating-occluding junction complexes in the alveolar epithelium: A freeze-fracture study. Am Rev Respir Dis 121:1017, 1980.

181. Gordon RE: The effects of NO₂ on ionic surface charge on type I pneumocytes of hamster lungs. Am J Pathol 121:291, 1985.

182. Schneeberger EE: The integrity of the air-blood barrier. *In* Brain JD, Proctor DF, Reid LM (eds): Respiratory Defense Mechanisms. New York, Marcel Dekker, 1977, p 687.

183. Matthay MA, Wiener-Kronish JP: Intact epithelial barrier function is critical for the resolution of alveolar edema in humans. Am Rev Respir Dis 142:1250, 1990.

184. Brody AR, Kelleher PC, Craighead JE: A mechanism of exudation through intact alveolar epithelial cells in the lungs of cytomegalovirus-infected mice. Lab Invest 39:281, 1978.

185. Heppleston AG, Young AE: Uptake of inert particulate matter by alveolar cells: An ultrastructural study. J Pathol 111:159, 1973.

186. Brody AR, Hill LH, Stirewalt WS, et al: Actin-containing microfilaments of pulmonary epithelial cells provide a mechanism for translocating asbestos to the interstitium. Chest 83(Suppl):11, 1983.

187. Lehnert BE, Valdez YE, Stewart CC: Translocation of particles to the tracheobronchial lymph nodes after lung deposition: Kinetics and particle-cell relationships. Exp Lung Res 10:245, 1986.

188. Parra SC, Burnette R, Rice HP, et al: Zonal distribution of alveolar macrophages, type II pneumocytes, and alveolar septal connective tissue gaps in adult human lungs. Am Rev Respir Dis 133:908, 1986.

189. Kikkawa Y, Smith F: Biology of disease: Cellular and biochemical aspects of pulmonary surfactant in health and disease. Lab Invest 49:122, 1983.

190. Weibel ER: Morphological basis of alveolar-capillary gas exchange. Physiol Rev 53:419, 1973.

191. Shimura S, Boatman ES, Martin CJ: Effects of aging on the alveolar pores of Kohn and on the cytoplasmic components of alveolar type II cells in monkey lungs. J Pathol 148:1, 1986.

192. Bakewell WE, Viviano CJ, Dixon D, et al: Confocal laser scanning immunofluorescence microscopy of lamellar bodies and pulmonary surfactant protein A in isolated alveolar type II cells. Lab Invest 65:87, 1991.

193. Rooney SA, Young SL, Mendelson CR: Molecular and cellular processing of lung surfactant. FASEB J 8:957, 1994.

194. Rooney SA: Function of type II cell lamellar inclusions in surfactant production. *In* Bouhuys A (ed): Lung Cells in Disease. New York, North-Holland Biomedical Press, 1976, p. 147.

195. Sorokin SP: A morphologic and cytochemical study on the great alveolar cell. J Histochem Cytochem 14:884, 1986.

196. Ahmed A, Chiswick ML: Origin of osmophilic inclusion bodies in type II pneumocytes. J Pathol 113:161, 1974.

197. Johnson NF: Release of lamellar bodies from alveolar type 2 cells. Thorax 35:192, 1980.

198. Crystal RG: Biochemical processes in the normal lung. *In* Bouhuys A (ed): Lung Cells in Disease. New York, North-Holland Biomedical Press, 1976, p 17.

199. Evans MJ, Cabral LJ, Stephens RJ, et al: Renewal of alveolar epithelium in the rat following exposure in NO₂. Am J Pathol 70:175, 1973.

200. Kapanci Y, Weibel ER, Kaplan HT, et al: Pathogenesis and reversibility of the pulmonary lesions of oxygen toxicity in monkeys: II. Ultrastructural and morphometric studies. Lab Invest 20:101, 1969.

201. Adamson IYR, Bowden DH: Origin of ciliated alveolar epithelial cells in bleomycin-induced lung injury. Am J Pathol 87:569, 1977.

202. Huang TW, Carlson JR, Bray TM, et al: Three-methylindole–induced pulmonary injury in goats. Am J Pathol 87:647, 1977.

203. Melloni B, Lesur O, Bouhadiba T, et al: Effect of exposure to silica on human alveolar macrophages in supporting growth activity in type II epithelial cells. Thorax 51:781, 1996.

204. Mason RJ, McCormick-Shannon K, Rubin JS, et al: Hepatocyte growth factor is a mitogen for alveolar type II cells in rat lavage fluid. Am J Physiol 271:L46, 1996.

205. Lesur O, Arsalane K, Lane D: Lung alveolar epithelial cell migration *in vitro*: Modulators and regulation processes. Am J Physiol 270:L311, 1996.

206. Griffin M, Bhandari R, Hamilton G, et al: Alveolar type II cell–fibroblast interactions, synthesis and secretion of surfactant and type I collagen. J Cell Sci 105:423, 1993

207. Mason RJ, Williams MC, Widdicombe JH: Secretion and fluid transport by alveolar type II epithelial cells. Chest 81:615, 1982.

208. Simionescu D, Simionescu M: Differentiated distribution of the cell surface charge on the alveolar-capillary unit: Characteristic paucity of anionic sites on the air-blood barrier. Microvasc Res 25:85, 1983.

209. Kuroki Y, Mason RJ, Voelker DR: Alveolar type II cells express a high-affinity receptor for pulmonary surfactant protein A. Proc Natl Acad Sci U S A 85:5566, 1988.

210. Crouch EC, Moxley MA, Longmore W: Synthesis of collagenous proteins by pulmonary type II epithelial cells. Am Rev Respir Dis 135:1118, 1987.

210a. Boutten A, Venembre P, Seta N, et al: Oncostatin M is a potent stimulator of α₁-antitrypsin secretion in lung epithelial cells: Modulation by transforming growth factor-β and interferon-γ. Am J Respir Cell Mol Biol 18:511, 1998.

211. Kuan S-F, Persson A, Parghi D, et al: Lectin-mediated interactions of surfactant protein D with alveolar macrophages. Am J Respir Cell Mol Biol 10:430, 1994.

212. Stringer B, Kobzik L: Alveolar macrophage uptake of the environmental particulate titanium dioxide: Role of surfactant components. Am J Respir Cell Mol Biol 14:155, 1996.

213. Paine R III, Mody CH, Chavis A, et al: Alveolar-epithelial cells block lymphocyte proliferation *in vitro* without inhibiting activation. Am J Respir Cell Mol Biol 5:221, 1991.

214. Boron P, Veldhuizen RA, Lewis JF, et al: Surfactant-associated protein A inhibits human lymphocyte proliferation and IL-2 production. Am J Respir Cell Mol Biol 15:115, 1996.

215. Van Iwaarden F, Welmers B, Verhoef J, et al: Pulmonary surfactant protein A enhances the host-defense mechanism of rat alveolar macrophages. Am J Respir Cell Mol Biol 2:91, 1990.

216. Weibel ER, Bachofen H: Structural design of the alveolar septum and fluid exchange. *In* Fishman AP, Renkin EM (eds): Pulmonary Edema. Bethesda, MD, American Physiological Society, 1979, p 1.

217. Starcher BC: Elastin and the lung. Thorax 41:577, 1986.

218. Laurent GJ: Lung collagen: More than scaffolding. Thorax 41:418, 1986.

219. Raghu G, Striker LJ, Hudson LD, et al: Extracellular matrix in normal and fibrotic human lungs. Am Rev Respir Dis 131:281, 1985.

220. Madri JA, Furthmayr H: Collagen polymorphism in the lung: An immunochemical study of pulmonary fibrosis. Hum Pathol 11:353, 1980.

221. Torikata C, Villiger B, Kuhn C III, et al: Ultrastructural distribution of fibronectin in normal and fibrotic human lung. Lab Invest 52:399, 1985.

222. Takaro T, Gaddy LR, Parra S: Thin alveolar epithelial partitions across connective tissue gaps in the alveolar wall of the human lung: Ultrastructural observations. Am Rev Respir Dis 126:326, 1982.

223. Kapanci Y, Assimacopoulos A, Irle C, et al: "Contractile interstitial cells" in pulmonary alveolar septa: A possible regulator of ventilation/perfusion ratio? J Cell Biol 60:375, 1974.

224. Vyalov SL, Gabbiani G, Kapanci Y: Rat alveolar myofibroblasts acquire α-smooth muscle actin expression during bleomycin-induced pulmonary fibrosis. Am J Pathol 143:1754, 1993.

225. Fox B, Bull TB, Gut A: Mast cells in the human alveolar wall: An electron microscopic study. J Clin Pathol 34:1333, 1981.

226. Kawanami O, Ferrans VJ, Fulmer JD, et al: Ultrastructure of pulmonary mast cells in patients with fibrotic lung disorders. Lab Invest 40:717, 1979.

227. Haas F, Bergofsky EH: Role of the mast cell in the pulmonary pressor response to hypoxia. J Clin Invest 51:3154, 1972.

228. Williams A, Heath D, Kav JM, et al: Lung mast cells in rats exposed to acute hypoxia and chronic hypoxia with recovery. Thorax 72:287, 1977.

229. Van Haarst JMW, Hoogsteden HC, De Wit HJ, et al: Dendritic cells and their precursors isolated from human bronchoalveolar lavage: Immunocytologic and functional properties. Am J Respir Cell Mol Biol 11:344, 1994.

230. Brain JD, Sorokin SP, Godleski JJ: Quantification, origin, and fate of pulmonary macrophages. *In* Brain JD, Proctor DF, Reid LM (eds): Respiratory Defense Mechanisms. New York, Marcel Dekker, 1977, p 849.

231. Dehring DJ, Wismar BL: Intravascular macrophages in pulmonary capillaries of humans. Am Rev Respir Dis 139:1027, 1989.

232. Warner AE, Barry BE, Brain JD: Pulmonary intravascular macrophages in sheep. Lab Invest 55:276, 1986.

233. Wizemann TM, Laskin DL: Enhanced phagocytosis, chemotaxis, and production of reactive oxygen intermediates by interstitial lung macrophages following acute endotoxemia. Am J Respir Cell Mol Biol 11:358, 1994.

234. Quan SG, Golde DW: Surface morphology of the human alveolar macrophage. Exp Cell Res 109:71, 1977.

235. Pratt SA, Smith MH, Ladman AJ, et al: The ultrastructure of alveolar macrophages from human cigarette smokers and nonsmokers. Lab Invest 24:331, 1971.

236. Brody AR, Craighead JE: Cytoplasmic inclusions in pulmonary macrophages of cigarette smokers. Lab Invest 32:125, 1975.

237. Plowman PN, Flemans RJ: Human pulmonary macrophages: The relationship of smoking to the presence of sea-blue granules and surfactant turnover. J Clin Pathol 33:738, 1980.

238. Matulionis DH, Traurig HH: *In situ* response of lung macrophages and hydrolase activities to cigarette smoke. Lab Invest 37:314, 1977.

239. Takemura T, Rom WN, Ferrans VJ, et al: Morphologic characterization of alveolar macrophages from subjects with occupational exposure to inorganic particles. Am Rev Respir Dis 140:1674, 1989.

240. Wallace WAH, Gillooly M, Lamb D: Intra-alveolar macrophage numbers in current smokers and nonsmokers: A morphometric study of tissue sections. Thorax 47:437, 1992.

241. Wallace WAH, Gillooly M, Lamb D: Age-related increase in the intra-alveolar macrophage population of non-smokers. Thorax 48:668, 1993.

242. Lasser A: The mononuclear phagocyte system: A review. Hum Pathol 14:108, 1983.

243. Bowden DH: Macrophages, dust, and pulmonary diseases. Exp Lung Res 12:89, 1987.

244. Evans MJ, Sherman MP, Campbell LA, et al: Proliferation of pulmonary alveolar macrophages during postnatal development of rabbit lungs. Am Rev Respir Dis 136:384, 1987.

245. Golde DW, Finley RN, Cline MJ: The pulmonary macrophage in acute leukemia. N Engl J Med 290:875, 1974.

246. Lin H-S, Kuhn C III, Chen D-M: Effects of hydrocortisone acetate on pulmonary alveolar macrophage colony-forming cells. Am Rev Respir Dis 125:712, 1982.

247. Adamson IYR, Bowden DH: Role of monocytes and interstitial cells in the generation of alveolar macrophages: II. Kinetic studies after carbon loading. Lab Invest 42:518, 1980.

248. Rose RM, Kobzik L, Filderman AE, et al: Characterization of colony stimulating factor activity in the human respiratory tract: Comparison of healthy smokers and nonsmokers. Am Rev Respir Dis 145:394, 1992.

249. du Bois RM: The alveolar macrophage (editorial). Thorax 40:321, 1985.

250. Green GM: Lung defense mechanisms. Med Clin North Am 57:547, 1973.

251. Kennedy JR, Elliott AM: Cigarette smoke: The effect of residue on mitochondrial structure. Science 168:1097, 1970.

252. Green GM, Carolin D: The depressant effect of cigarette smoke on the *in vitro* antibacterial activity of alveolar macrophages. N Engl J Med 276:421, 1967.

253. Shellito J, Kaltreider HB: Heterogeneity of immunologic function among subfractions of normal rat alveolar macrophages. Am Rev Respir Dis 131:678, 1985.

254. Fantone JC, Feltner DE, Brieland JK, et al: Phagocytic cell–derived inflammatory mediators and lung disease. Chest 91:428, 1987.

255. Sibille Y, Reynolds HY: Macrophages and polymorphonuclear neutrophils in lung defense and injury. Am Rev Respir Dis 141:471, 1990.

256. Villiger B, Broekelmann T, Kelley D, et al: Bronchoalveolar fibronectin in smokers and nonsmokers. Am Rev Respir Dis 124:652, 1981.

257. Eckert H, Lux M, Lachmann B: The role of alveolar macrophages in surfactant turnover: An experimental study with metabolite VIII of bromhexine (Ambroxol). Lung 161:213, 1983.

257a. Bates SR, Fisher AB: Surfactant protein A is degraded by alveolar macrophages. Am J Physiol 271:258, 1996.

257b. Lay JC, Bennett WD, Kim CS, et al: Retention and intracellular distribution of instilled iron oxide particles in human alveolar macrophages. Am J Respir Cell Mol Biol 18:687, 1998.

258. Brain JD: Free cells in the lungs. Arch Intern Med 126:477, 1970.

259. Green GM: The J. Burns Amberson Lecture: In defense of the lung. Am Rev Respir Dis 102:691, 1970.

260. Vecchiarelli A, Dottorini M, Pietrella D, et al: Role of human alveolar macrophages as antigen-presenting cells in *Cryptococcus neoformans* infection. Am J Respir Cell Mol Biol 11:130, 1994.

261. Lipscomb MF, Lyons CR, Nunez G, et al: Human alveolar macrophages: HLA-DR–positive macrophages that are poor stimulators of a primary mixed leukocyte reaction. J Immunol 136:497, 1986.

261a. Hancock A, Armstrong L, Gama R, et al: Production of interleukin 13 by alveolar macrophages from normal and fibrotic lung. Am J Respir Cell Mol Biol 18:60, 1998.

262. Gupta PK, Frost JK, Geddes S, et al: Morphological identification of alpha₁-antitrypsin in pulmonary macrophages. Hum Pathol 10:345, 1979.

262a. Perlmutter DH, May LT, Sehgal PB: Interferon β₂ interleuken 6 modulates synthesis of α₁ antitrypsin in human mononuclear phagocytes and in human hepatoma cells. J Clin Invest 84:139, 1989.

263. Sibille Y, Merrill WW, Naegel GP, et al: Human alveolar macrophages release a factor that inhibits phagocyte function. Am J Respir Cell Mol Biol 1:407, 1989.

264. Hsueh W: Prostaglandin biosynthesis in pulmonary macrophages. Am J Pathol 97:137, 1979.

265. Martin TR, Altman LC, Albert RK, et al: Leukotriene B₄ production by the human alveolar macrophage: A potential mechanism for amplifying inflammation in the lung. Am Rev Respir Dis 129:106, 1984.

266. Nugent KM, Glazier J, Monick MM, et al: Stimulated human alveolar macrophages secrete interferon. Am Rev Respir Dis 131:714, 1985.

267. Hansen JE, Ampaya EP: Human air space shapes, sizes, areas, and volumes. J Appl Physiol 38:990, 1975.

268. Assimacopoulos A, Guggenheim R, Kapanci Y: Changes in alveolar capillary configuration at different levels of lung inflation in the rat: An ultrastructural and morphometric study. Lab Invest 34:10, 1976.

269. Rosenquist TH, Bernick S, Sobin SS, et al: The structure of the pulmonary interalveolar microvascular sheet. Microvasc Res 5:199, 1973.

270. Weibel ER, Gomez DM: Architecture of the human lung. Science 137:577, 1962.

271. Angus GE, Thurlbeck WM: Number of alveoli in the human lung. J Appl Physiol 32:483, 1972.

272. Thurlbeck WM: The internal surface area of nonemphysematous lungs. Am Rev Respir Dis 95:765, 1967.

273. Forrest JB: The effect of change in lung volume on the size and shape of alveoli. J Physiol 210:533, 1970.

274. Dunnill MS: Effect of lung inflation on alveolar surface area in dog. Nature 214:1013, 1967.

275. Gillooly M, Lamb D: Airspace size in lungs of lifelong non-smokers: Effect of age and sex. Thorax 48:39, 1993.

276. Reid L, Rubino M: The connective tissue septa in the foetal human lung. Thorax 14:3, 1959.

277. Webb WR, Stein MG, Finkbeiner WE, et al: Normal and diseased isolated lungs: High-resolution CT. Radiology 166:81, 1988.

278. Reid L: The secondary lobule in the adult human lung, with special reference to its appearance in bronchograms. Thorax 13:110, 1968.

279. Nishimura K, Itoh H: Normal peripheral structures of the lung. Kekkaku 64:55, 1989.

280. Itoh H, Murata K, Konishi J, et al: Diffuse lung disease: Pathologic basis for the high-resolution computed tomography findings. J Thorac Imaging 8:176, 1993.

281. Stein MG, Mayo J, Müller N, et al: Pulmonary lymphangitic spread of carcinoma: Appearance on CT scans. Radiology 162:371, 1987.

282. Munk PL, Müller NL, Miller RR, et al: Pulmonary lymphangitic carcinomatosis: CT and pathologic findings. Radiology 166:705, 1988.

282a. Primack SL, Müller NL, Mayo JR, et al: Pulmonary parenchymal abnormalities of vascular origin: High-resolution CT findings. Radiographics 14:739, 1994.

282b. Storto ML, Kee ST, Golden JA, et al: Hydrostatic pulmonary edema: High-resolution CT findings. Am J Roentgenol 165:817, 1995.

283. Bergin C, Roggli V, Coblentz C, et al: The secondary pulmonary lobule: Normal and abnormal CT appearances. Am J Roentgenol 151:21, 1988.

284. Murata K, Khan A, Herman PG: Pulmonary parenchymal disease: Evaluation with high-resolution CT. Radiology 170:629, 1989.

285. Bessis L, Callard P, Gotheil C, et al: High-resolution CT of parenchymal lung disease: Precise correlation with histologic findings. Radiographics 12:45, 1992.

285a. Müller NL, Miller RR: Diseases of the bronchioles: CT and histopathologic findings. Radiology 196:3, 1995.

286. Remy-Jardin M, Remy J, Wallaert B, et al: Subacute and chronic bird breeder hypersensitivity pneumonitis: Sequential evaluation with CT and correlation with lung function tests and bronchoalveolar lavage. Radiology 189:111, 1993.

287. Gruden JF, Webb WR, Warnock M: Centrilobular opacities in the lung on high-resolution CT: Diagnostic considerations and pathologic correlation. Am J Roentgenol 162:569, 1994.

288. Padley SPG, Adler BD, Hansell DM, et al: Bronchiolitis obliterans: High-resolution CT findings and correlation with pulmonary function tests. Clin Radiol 47:236, 1993.

289. Nishimura K, Kitaichi M, Izumi T, et al: Diffuse panbronchiolitis: Correlation of high-resolution CT and pathologic findings. Radiology 184:779, 1992.

290. Hartman TE, Primack SL, Lee KS, et al: CT of bronchial and bronchiolar diseases. Radiographics 14:991, 1994.

291. Pump KK: The morphology of the finer branches of the bronchial tree of the human lung. Dis Chest 46:379, 1964.

292. Raskin SP: The pulmonary acinus: Historical notes. Radiology 144:31, 1982.

293. Gamsu G, Thurlbeck WM, Macklem PT, et al: Roentgenographic appearance of the human pulmonary acinus. Invest Radiol 6:171, 1971.

294. Lui YM, Taylor JR, Zylak CJ: Roentgen-anatomical correlation of the individual human pulmonary acinus. Radiology 109:1, 1973.

295. Hansen JE, Ampaya EP, Bryant GH, et al: Branching pattern of airways and air spaces of a single human terminal bronchiole. J Appl Pathol 38:983, 1975.

296. Ziskind MM, Weill H, Payzant AR: The recognition and significance of acinus-filling processes of the lungs. Am Rev Respir Dis 87:551, 1963.

297. Ziskind MM, Weill H, Buechner HA, et al: Recognition of distinctive radiologic patterns in diffuse pulmonary disease. Arch Intern Med 114:108, 1964.

298. Itoh H, Tokunaga S, Asamoto H, et al: Radiologic-pathologic correlations of small lung nodules, with special reference to peribronchiolar nodules. Am J Roentgenol 130:223, 1978.

299. Staub NC: The interdependence of pulmonary structure and function. Anesthesiology 24:831, 1963.

300. Loosli CG: Interalveolar communications in normal and in pathologic mammalian lungs: Review of the literature. Arch Pathol 24:743, 1937.

301. Parra SC, Gaddy LR, Takaro T: Ultrastructural studies of canine interalveolar pores (of Kohn). Lab Invest 38:8, 1978.

302. Desplechain C, Foliguet B, Barrat E, et al: Les pores de Kohn des alveoles pulmonaires (the pores of Kohn in pulmonary alveoli). Bull Eur Physiopathol Respir 19:59, 1983.

303. Takaro T, Price HP, Parra SC: Ultrastructural studies of apertures in the interalveolar septum of the adult human lung. Am Rev Respir Dis 119:425, 1979.

304. Kawakami M, Takizawa T: Distribution of pores within alveoli in the human lung. J Appl Physiol 63:1866, 1987.

305. Boatman ES, Martin HB: Electron microscopy of the alveolar pores of Kohn. Am Rev Respir Dis 88:779, 1963.

306. Lindskog GE: Collateral respiration in the normal and diseases lung. Yale J Biol Med 23:311, 1950.

307. Martin HB: The effect of aging on the alveolar pores of Kohn in the dog. Am Rev Respir Dis 88:773, 1963.

308. Pump KK: Fenestrae in the alveolar membrane of the human lung. Chest 65:431, 1974.

309. Lambert MW: Accessory bronchiole-alveolar communications. J Pathol Bacteriol 70:311, 1955.

310. Duguid JB, Lambert MW: The pathogenesis of coal miner's pneumoconiosis. J Pathol Bacteriol 88:389, 1964.

311. Krahl VE: Microscopic anatomy of the lungs. Am Rev Respir Dis 80:24, 1959.

312. Boyden EA: Notes on the development of the lung in infancy and early childhood. Am J Anat 121:749, 1967.

313. Martin HB: Respiratory bronchioles as the pathway for collateral ventilation. J Appl Physiol 21:1443, 1966.

314. Henderson R, Horsfield K, Cumming G: Intersegmental collateral ventilation in the human lung. Respir Physiol 6:128, 1969.

315. Raskin SP, Herman PG: Interacinar pathways in the human lung. Am Rev Respir Dis 111:489, 1975.

316. Anderson JB, Jespersen W: Demonstration of intersegmental respiratory bronchioles in normal human lungs. Eur J Respir Dis 61:337, 1980.

317. Jackson CL, Huber JF: Correlated applied anatomy of the bronchial tree and lungs with system of nomenclature. Dis Chest 9:319, 1943.

318. Boyden EA: Segmental Anatomy of the Lungs. New York, McGraw-Hill, 1955.

319. Kittredge RD: Computed tomography of the trachea: A review. CT 5:44, 1981.

320. Gamsu G, Webb WR: Computed tomography of the trachea: Normal and abnormal. Am J Roentgenol 139:321, 1982.

321. Breatnach E, Abbott GC, Fraser RG: Dimensions of the normal human trachea. Am J Roentgenol 141:903, 1984.

322. Moreno R, Taylor R, Müller N, et al: *In vivo* human tracheal pressure-area curves using computerized tomographic scans: Correlation with maximal expiratory flow rates. Am Rev Respir Dis 134:585, 1986.

323. Griscom NT, Wohl MEB: Tracheal size and shape: Effects of change in intraluminal pressure. Radiology 149:27, 1983.

324. Stern EJ, Graham CM, Webb WR, et al: Normal trachea during forced expiration: Dynamic CT measurements. Radiology 187:27, 1993.

325. Griscom NT, Wohl ME: Dimensions of the growing trachea related to age and gender. Am J Roentgenol 146:233, 1986.

326. Alavi SM, Keats TE, O'Brien WM: The angle of tracheal bifurcation: Its normal mensuration. Am J Roentgenol 108:546, 1970.

327. Haskin PH, Goodman LR: Normal tracheal bifurcation angle: A reassessment. Am J Radiol 139:879, 1982.

328. Cleveland RH: Symmetry of bronchial angles in children. Radiology 133:89, 1979.

329. Fraser RG: Measurements of the caliber of human bronchi in three phases of respiration by cinebronchography. J Can Assoc Radiol 12:102, 1961.

330. Merendino KA, Kiriluk LB: Human measurements involved in tracheobronchial resection and reconstruction procedures: Report of case of bronchial adenoma. Surgery 35:590, 1954.

331. Jesseph JE, Merendino KA: The dimensional interrelationships of the major components of the human tracheobronchial tree. Surg Gynecol Obstet 105:210, 1957.

332. Boyden EA, Hartmann JF: An analysis of variations in the bronchopulmonary segments of the left upper lobes of fifty lungs. Am J Anat 79:321, 1946.

333. Boyden EA, Scannell JG: An analysis of variations in the bronchovascular pattern of the right upper lobe of fifty lungs. Am J Anat 82:27, 1948.

334. Scannell JG: A study of variations of the bronchopulmonary segments in the left upper lobe. J Thorac Surg 16:530, 1947.

335. Scannell JG, Boyden EA: A study of variations of the bronchopulmonary segments of the right upper lobe. J Thorac Surg 17:232, 1948.

336. Smith FR, Boyden EA: An analysis of variations of the segmental bronchi of the right lower lobe of fifty injected lungs. J Thorac Surg 18:195, 1949.

337. Boyden EA, Hamre CJ: An analysis of variations in the bronchovascular patterns of the middle lobe in fifty dissected and twenty injected lungs. J Thorac Surg 21:172, 1951.

338. Atwell SW: Major anomalies of the tracheobronchial tree with a list of the minor anomalies. Dis Chest 52:611, 1967.

339. Nelson S: Personal communication, 1965.

340. Osborne D, Vock P, Godwin JD, et al: CT identification of broncho-pulmonary segments: 50 normal subjects. Am J Roentgenol 142:47, 1984.

341. Naidich DP, Harkin TJ: Airways and lung: Correlation of CT with fiberoptic bronchoscopy. Radiology 197:1, 1995.

342. Murata K, Itoh H, Todo G, et al: Centrilobular lesions of the lung: Demonstration by high-resolution CT and pathologic correlation. Radiology 161:641, 1986.

342a. Naidich DP: Helical computed tomography of the thorax: Clinical applications. Radiol Clin North Am 32:759, 1994.

342b. Rubin GD, Napel S, Leung AN: Volumetric analysis of volumetric data: Achieving a paradigm shift. Radiology 200:312, 1996.

342c. Lee KS, Yoon JH, Kim TK, et al: Evaluation of tracheobronchial disease with helical CT with multiplanar and three-dimensional reconstruction: Correlation with bronchoscopy. Radiographics 17:555, 1997.

342d. Ney DR, Kuhlman JE, Hruban RH, et al: Three-dimensional CT volumetric reconstruction and display of the bronchial tree. Invest Radiol 25:736, 1990.

342e. Remy-Jardin M, Remy J, Artaud D, et al: Tracheobronchial tree—assessment with volume rendering: Technical aspects. Radiology 208:393, 1998.

343. Lee KS, Bae WK, Lee BH, et al: Bronchovascular anatomy of the upper lobes: Evaluation with thin-section CT. Radiology 181:765, 1991.

344. Lee KS, Im JG, Bae WK, et al: CT anatomy of the lingular segmental bronchi. J Comput Assist Tomogr 15:86, 1991.

345. Remy-Jardin M, Remy J: Comparison of vertical and oblique CT in evaluation of the bronchial tree. J Comput Assist Tomogr 12:956, 1988.

346. Naidich DP, Zinn WL, Ettenger NA, et al: Basilar segmental bronchi: Thin-section CT evaluation. Radiology 169:11, 1988.

347. Engel LA, Macklem PT: Gas mixing and distribution in the lung. Int Rev Physiol Respir Physiol 14:37, 1977.

348. Engel LA, Paiva M: Analyses of sequential filling and emptying of the lung. Respir Physiol 45:309, 1981.

349. Paiva M, Engel LA: The anatomical basis for the sloping N_2 plateau. Respir Physiol 44:325, 1981.

350. Mead J: Mechanical properties of lungs. Physiol Rev 41:281, 1961.

351. Martin JG, Habib M, Engle LA: Inspiratory muscle activity during induced hyperinflation. Respir Physiol 39:303, 1980.

352. Leith DE, Mead J: Mechanisms determining residual volume of the lungs in normal subjects. J Appl Physiol 23:221, 1967.

353. Islam MS: Mechanism of controlling residual volume and emptying rate of the lung in young and elderly healthy subjects. Respiration 40:1, 1980.

354. Pierce JA, Ebert RV: Fibrous network of the lung and its change with age. Thorax 20:469, 1965.

355. Oderr C: Architecture of the lung parenchyma: Studies with a specially designed x-ray microscope. Am Rev Respir Dis 90:401, 1964.

356. von Neergaard K: Neue Auffassungen uber einen Grundbegriff der Atemmechanik: Die Retraktionskraft der Lunge, abhängig von der Oberflächenspannung in den Alveolen. Z Ges Exp Med 66:373, 1929.

357. Kuhn C III, Finke EH: The topography of the pulmonary alveolus: Scanning electron microscopy using different fixations. J Ultrastruct Res 38:161, 1972.

358. Kikkawa Y: Morphology of alveolar lining layer. Anat Rec 167:389, 1970.

359. Manabe H: Freeze-fracture study of alveolar lining layer in adult rat lungs. J Ultrastruct Res 69:86, 1979.

360. Gil J, Weibel ER: Improvements in demonstration of lining layer of lung alveoli by electron microscopy. Respir Physiol 8:13, 1969.

361. Scarpelli EM: Lung surfactant: Dynamic properties, metabolic pathways and possible significance in the pathogenesis of the respiratory distress syndrome. Bull N Y Acad Med 44:431, 1968.

362. Kikkawa Y, Smith F: Cellular and biochemical aspects of pulmonary surfactant in health and disease. Lab Invest 49:122, 1983.

363. Rooney SA, Young SL, Mendelson CR: Molecular and cellular processing of lung surfactant. FASEB J 8:957, 1994.

364. Tsilibary EC, Williams MC: Actin and secretion of surfactant. J Histochem Cytochem 31:1298, 1983.

365. Hawgood S, Shiffer K: Structures and properties of the surfactant-associated proteins. Annu Rev Physiol 53:375, 1991.

366. Wright JR, Dobbs LG: Regulation of pulmonary surfactant secretion and clearance. Annu Rev Physiol 53:395, 1991.

367. Tenner AJ, Robinson SL, Borchelt J, et al: Human pulmonary surfactant protein (sp-A), a protein structurally homologous to C1q, can enhance FcR- and CRI-mediated phagocytosis. J Biol Chem 264:13923, 1989.

368. Kuan SF, Rust K, Crouch E: Interactions of surfactant protein D with bacterial lipopolysaccharides—surfactant protein D is an *Escherichia coli*–binding protein in bronchoalveolar lavage. J Clin Invest 90:97, 1992.

369. Wiseman LR, Bryson HM: Porcine-derived lung surfactant: A review of the therapeutic efficacy and clinical tolerability of a natural surfactant preparation (Curosurf) in neonatal respiratory distress syndrome. Drugs 48:386, 1994.

370. Johansson J, Curstedt T, Robertson B: The proteins of the surfactant system. Eur Respir J 7:372, 1994.

371. Clements JA: Comparative lipid chemistry of lungs. Arch Intern Med 127:387, 1971.

372. Morgan TE: Pulmonary surfactant. N Engl J Med 284:1185, 1971.

373. Clements JA: Pulmonary surfactant. Am Rev Respir Dis 101:984, 1970.

374. Wright JR: Clearance and recycling of pulmonary surfactant. Am J Physiol 259:L1, 1990.

375. Brumley GW, Chernick V, Hodson WA, et al: Correlations of mechanical stability, morphology, pulmonary surfactant, and phospholipid content in the developing lamb lung. J Clin Invest 46:863, 1967.

376. Brumley GW: Lung development and lecithin metabolism. Arch Intern Med 127:413, 1971.

377. Avery ME: The J. Burns Amberson Lecture: In pursuit of understanding the first breath. Am Rev Respir Dis 100:295, 1969.

378. Beppu OS, Clements JA, Georke J: Phosphatidylglycerol-deficient lung surfactant has normal properties. J Appl Physiol 55:496, 1983.

379. Gluck L, Kulovich MV, Borer RC, et al: The interpretation and significance of the lecithin/sphingomyelin ratio in amniotic fluid. Am J Obstet Gynecol 120:142, 1974.

380. Bender TM, Stone LR, Amenta JS: Diagnostic power of lecithin/sphingomyelin ratio and fluorescence polarization assays for respiratory distress syndrome compared by relative operating characteristic curves. Clin Chem 40:541, 1994.

381. Crowley P, Chalmers I, Keirse MJNC: The effects of corticosteroid administration before protein delivery: An overview of the evidence from controlled trials. Br J Obstet Gynaecol 97:11, 1990.

382. Robertson B: Corticosteroids and surfactant for prevention of neonatal RDS. Ann Med 25:285, 1993.

383. Rooney SA: Fatty acid biosynthesis in developing fetal lung. Am J Physiol 257:L195, 1989.

384. Rooney SA: Regulation of surfactant associated phospholipid synthesis and secretion. *In* Polin RA, Fox WW (eds): Fetal and Neonatal Physiology. Philadelphia, WB Saunders, 1992, pp 971–985.

385. Avery ME: Pharmacological approaches to the acceleration of fetal lung maturation. Br Med Bull 31:13, 1975.

386. Mendelson CR, Boggaram V: Hormonal control of the surfactant system in fetal lung. Annu Rev Physiol 53:415, 1991.

387. Oyarzun MJ, Clements JA: Control of lung surfactant by ventilation, adrenergic mediators, and prostaglandins in the rabbit. Am Rev Respir Dis 117:879, 1978.

388. Massaro D, Clerch L, Massaro GD: Surfactant secretion: Evidence that cholinergic stimulation of secretion is indirect. Am J Physiol 243:C39, 1982.

389. Massaro GD, Massaro D: Morphologic evidence that large inflations of the lung stimulate secretion of surfactant. Am Rev Respir Dis 127:235, 1983.

390. Massaro D, Clerch L, Temple D, et al: Surfactant deficiency in rats without a decreased amount of extracellular surfactant. J Clin Invest 71:1536, 1983.

391. Corbet A, Cregan J, Frink J, et al: Distention-produced phospholipid secretion in postmortem *in situ* lungs of newborn rabbits: Inhibition by specific beta-adrenergic blockade. Am Rev Respir Dis 128:695, 1983.

392. Kunc L, Kuncova M, Holusa R, et al: Physical properties and biochemistry of lung surfactant following vagotomy. Respiration 35:192, 1978.

393. King RJ: Pulmonary surfactant. J Appl Physiol 53:1, 1982.

394. Schurch S: Surface tension at low volumes: Dependence on time and alveolar size. Respir Physiol 48:339, 1982.

395. Hills BA: The role of lung surfactant. Br J Anaesth 65:13, 1990.

396. Albert RK, Lakshminarayan S, Hildebrandt J, et al: Increased surface tension favors pulmonary edema formation in anesthetized dogs' lungs. J Clin Invest 63:115, 1979.

397. Notter RH, Shapiro DL: Lung surfactant in an era of replacement therapy. Pediatrics 68:781, 1981.

398. Hills BA: What is the true role of surfactant in the lung? Thorax 36:1, 1981.

399. Hills BA: Contact-angle hysteresis induced by pulmonary surfactants. J Appl Physiol 54:420, 1983.

400. Gardner DE, Pfitzer EA, Christian RT, et al: Loss of protective factor for alveolar macrophages when exposed to ozone. Arch Intern Med 127:1078, 1971.

401. Schwartz LW, Christman CA: Alveolar macrophage migration: Influence of lung lining material and acute lung insult. Am Rev Respir Dis 120:429, 1979.

402. Smith FB: Role of the pulmonary surfactant system in lung diseases of adults. N Y State J Med 83:851, 1983.

403. Kankaanpaa K, Hallman M: Respiratory distress syndrome in very-low-birth-weight infants with occasionally normal surfactant phospholipids. Eur J Pediatr 139:31, 1982.

404. Hallman M, Merritt TA, Akino T, et al: Surfactant protein A, phosphatidylcholine, and surfactant inhibitors in epithelial lining fluid: Correlation with surface activity, severity of respiratory distress syndrome, and outcome in small premature infants. Am Rev Respir Dis 144:1376, 1991.

405. Hallman M, Sarnesto A, Bry K: Interaction of transferrin saturated with iron with lung surfactant in respiratory failure. J Appl Physiol 77:757, 1994.

406. Soll RF, Lucey JF: Surfactant replacement therapy. Pediatr Rev 12:261, 1991.

407. Ikegami M, Jobe AH: Surfactant metabolism. Semin Perinatol 17:233, 1993.

408. Corbet A: Clinical trials of synthetic surfactant in the respiratory distress syndrome of premature infants. Clin Perinatol 20:737, 1993.

409. Mauskopf JA, Backhouse ME, Jones D, et al: Synthetic surfactant for rescue treatment of respiratory distress syndrome in premature infants weighing from 700 to 1350 grams: Impact on hospital resource use and charges. J Pediatr 126:94, 1995.

410. Kari MA, Hallman M, Eronen M, et al: Prenatal dexamethasone treatment in conjunction with rescue therapy of human surfactant: A randomized, placebo-controlled, multicenter study. Pediatrics 93:730, 1994.

411. Sutnick AI, Soloff LA, Sethi RS: Influence of alveolar collapse upon surface activity of lung extracts. Dis Chest 53:257, 1968.

412. Morgan TE, Finley TN, Huber GL, et al: Alterations in pulmonary surface active lipids during exposure to increased oxygen tension. J Clin Invest 44:1737, 1965.

413. Clements JA, Fisher HK: The oxygen dilemma. N Engl J Med 282:976, 1970.

414. Burger EJ Jr, Mead J: Static properties of lungs after oxygen exposure. J Appl Physiol 27:191, 1969.

415. Barber RE, Lee J, Hamilton WK: Oxygen toxicity in man: A prospective study in patients with irreversible brain damage. N Engl J Med 283:1478, 1970.

416. Sobonya RE, Kleinerman J, Primiano F, et al: Pulmonary changes in cardiopulmonary bypass: Short-term effects on granular pneumocytes. Chest 61:154, 1972.

417. Balis JU, Cox WD, Pifarré R, et al: The role of pulmonary hypoperfusion and hypoxia in the postperfusion lung syndrome. Ann Thorac Surg 8:263, 1969.

418. Smaldone GC, Mitzner W, Itoh H: Role of alveolar recruitment in lung inflation: Influence on pressure-volume hysteresis. J Appl Physiol 55:1321, 1983.

419. Nielson D, Olsen DB: The role of alveolar recruitment and decruitment in pressure-volume hysteresis in lungs. Respir Physiol 32:63, 1978.

420. Lisboa C, Ross WRD, Jardim J, et al: Pulmonary pressure-flow curves measured by a data-averaging circuit. J Appl Physiol 47:621, 1979.

421. Anch AM, Remmers JE, Bunce H III: Supraglottic airway resistance in normal subjects and patients with occlusive sleep apnea. J Appl Physiol 53:1158, 1982.

422. Series F, Cormier Y, Desmeules M: Influence of passive changes of lung volume on upper airways. J Appl Physiol 68:2159, 1990.

423. Preece M, Eccles R: The relationship of skin temperature to the nasal cycle in normal subjects. Rhinology 32:20, 1994.

424. Macklem PT, Mead J: Resistance of central and peripheral airways measured by a retrograde catheter. J Appl Physiol 22:395, 1967.

425. Hogg JC, Macklem PT, Thurlbeck WM: Site and nature of airway obstruction in chronic obstructive lung disease. N Engl J Med 273:1355, 1963.

426. Van Brabandt H, Cauberghs M, Verbeken E, et al: Partitioning of pulmonary impedance in excised human and canine lungs. J Appl Physiol 55:1733, 1983.

427. England SJ, Bartlett D Jr, Daubenspeck JA: Influence of human vocal cord movements on airflow resistance during eupnea. J Appl Physiol 52:773, 1982.

428. Vincet NJ, Knudson R, Leith DE, et al: Factors influencing pulmonary resistance. J Appl Physiol 29:236, 1970.

429. Saunders NA, Betts MF, Pengelly LD, et al: Changes in lung mechanics induced by acute isocapnic hypoxia. J Appl Physiol 42:413, 1977.

430. Ferris BG, Mead J, Opie LH: Partitioning of respiratory flow resistance in man. J Appl Physiol 19:653, 1964.

431. Kariya ST, Thompson LM, Ingenito EP, et al: Effects of lung volume, volume history, and methacholine on tissue viscance. J Appl Physiol 62:977, 1989.

432. Verbeken EK, Cauberghs M, Mertens I, et al: Tissue and airway impedance of excised normal, senile, and emphysematous lungs. J Appl Physiol 72:2343, 1992.

432a. Calderini E, Tavola M, Bono D, et al: Pulmonary and chest wall mechanics in anesthetized paralyzed humans. J Appl Physiol 70:2602, 1991.

432b. Romero PV, Robatto FM, Simard S, et al: Lung tissue behaviour during methacholine challenge in rabbits *in vivo*. J Appl Physiol 73:207, 1992.

433. Macklem PT: Airway obstruction and collateral ventilation. Physiol Rev 51:368, 1971.

434. Hilpert P: Collaterale Ventilationhabilitations-schrift aus der Medizinischen (thesis). Tübingen, Germany, Tübingen Universitätklinik, 1970.

435. Menkes HA, Traystman RJ: Collateral ventilation, lung disease. *In* Murray J (ed): Lung Disease—State of the Art. New York, American Lung Association, 1978, p 87.

436. Woolcock AJ, Macklem PT: Mechanical factors influencing collateral ventilation in human, dog, and pig lungs. J Appl Physiol 30:99, 1971.

437. Inners CR, Terry PB, Traystman RJ, et al: Effects of lung volume on collateral and airways resistance in man. J Appl Physiol 46:67, 1979.

438. Kikuchi R, Hildebrandt J, Sekizawa K, et al: Influence of lung volume history and increased surface forces on collateral resistance. Respir Physiol 89:15, 1992.

439. Batra G, Traystman R, Rudnick H, et al: Effects of body position and cholinergic blockade on mechanics of collateral ventilation. J Appl Physiol 50:358, 1981.

440. Inners CR, Terry PB, Traystman RJ, et al: Collateral ventilation and the middle lobe syndrome. Am Rev Respir Dis 118:305, 1978.

441. Nakamura M, Hildebrandt J: Cigarette smoke acutely increases collateral resistance in excised dog lobes. J Appl Physiol 56:166, 1984.

442. Gertner A, Bromberger B, Traystman R, et al: Histamine and pulmonary responses to cigarette smoke in the periphery of the lung. J Appl Physiol 53:582, 1982.

443. Kaplan J, Smaldone GC, Menkes HA, et al: Response of collateral channels to histamine: Lack of vagal effect. J Appl Physiol 51:1314, 1981.

444. Gertner A, Bromberger-Barnea B, Dannenberg AM, et al: Responses of the lung periphery to 1.0 ppm ozone. J Appl Physiol 55:770, 1983.

445. Gertner A, Bromberger-Barnea B, Traystman R, et al: Effects of ozone on peripheral lung reactivity. J Appl Physiol 55:777, 1983.

446. Rosenberg DE, Lyons HA: Collateral ventilation in excised human lungs. Respiration 37:125, 1979.

447. Terry PB, Traystman RJ, Newball HH, et al: Collateral ventilation in man. N Engl J Med 298:10, 1978.

448. Hogg JC, Macklem PT, Thurlbeck WM: The resistance of collateral channels in excised human lungs. J Clin Invest 48:421, 1969.

448a. Morell WW, Roberts CM, Biggs T, et al: Collateral ventilation and gas exchange during airway occlusion in the normal human lung. Am Rev Respir Dis 147:535, 1993.

449. Morrell NW, Wignall BK, Biggs T, et al: Collateral ventilation and gas exchange in emphysema. Am J Respir Crit Care Med 150:635, 1994.

450. Sleigh MA: The nature and action of respiratory tract cilia. In Brain JD, Proctor DF, Reid LM (eds): Respiratory Defense Mechanisms. Part I. Lung Biology in Health and Disease. Vol 5. New York, Marcel Dekker, 1977, pp 247–288.

451. Lopez-Vidriero MT, Das I, Reid LM: Airway secretion: Source, biochemical and rheological properties. In Brain JD, Proctor DF, Reid LM (eds): Respiratory Defense Mechanisms. Part I. Lung Biology in Health and Disease. Vol 5. New York, Marcel Dekker, 1977, pp 289–356.

452. Keal EE: Physiological and pharmacological control of airway secretion. In Brain JD, Proctor DF, Reid LM (eds): Respiratory Defense Mechanisms. Part I. Lung Biology in Health and Disease. Vol 5. New York, Marcel Dekker, 1977, pp 357–401.

453. Gallagher JT, Richardson PS: Respiratory mucus: Structure, metabolism, and control of secretion. Adv Exp Med Biol 2:335, 1982.

454. King M: Mucus and mucociliary clearance. Basics Respir Dis 11:1, 1982.

454a. Wanner A, Salathe M, O'Riordan TG: Mucociliary clearance in the airways. Am J Respir Crit Care Med 154:1868, 1996.

455. Nadziejko C, Finkelstein I: Inhibition of neutrophil elastase by mucus glycoprotein. Am J Respir Cell Mol Biol 11:103, 1994.

456. Yamaya M, Ohrui T, Finkbeiner WE, et al: Calcium-dependent chloride secretion across cultures of human tracheal surface epithelium and glands. Am J Physiol 265:L170, 1993.

457. Fahy JV, Steiger DJ, Liu J, et al: Markers of mucus secretion and DNA levels in induced sputum from asthmatic and from healthy subjects. Am Rev Respir Dis 147:1132, 1993.

458. Williams IP, Hall RL, Miller RJ, et al: Analyses of human tracheobronchial mucus from healthy subjects. Eur J Respir Dis 63:510, 1982.

459. Low RB, Davis GS, Giancola MS: Biochemical analyses of bronchoalveolar lavage fluids of healthy human volunteer smokers and nonsmokers. Am Rev Respir Dis 118:863, 1978.

460. Szabo S, Barbu Z, Lakatos L, et al: Local production of proteins in normal human bronchial secretion. Respiration 39:172, 1980.

461. Lopez-Vidriero MT: Airway mucus production and composition. Chest 80:799, 1981.

462. Rose MC: Mucins: Structure, function, and role in pulmonary diseases. Am J Physiol 263:L413, 1992.

463. Porchet N, Dufosse J, Audie JP, et al: Structural features of the core proteins of human airway mucins ascertained by cDNA cloning. Am Rev Respir Dis 144(suppl):S15, 1991.

464. Boat TF, Cheng PW: Biochemistry of airway mucus secretions. Fed Proc 39:3067, 1980.

465. Girod de Bentzmann S, Pierrot D, Fuchey C, et al: Distearoyl phosphatidylglycerol liposomes improve surface and transport properties of CF mucus. Eur Respir J 6:1156, 1993.

466. Girod S, Galabert C, Pierrot D, et al: Role of phospholipid lining on respiratory mucus clearance by cough. J Appl Physiol 71:2262, 1991.

467. Burnett D, Crocker J, Stockley RA: Cells containing IgA subclasses in bronchi of subjects with and without chronic obstructive lung disease. J Clin Pathol 40:1217, 1987.

468. Sallenave JM, Shulmann J, Crossley J, et al: Regulation of secretory leukocyte proteinase inhibitor (SLPI) and elastase-specific inhibitor (ESI/elafin) in human airway epithelial cells by cytokines and neutrophilic enzymes. Am J Respir Cell Mol Biol 11:733, 1994.

469. Man SFP, Adams GK III, Proctor DF: Effects of temperature, relative humidity, and mode of breathing on canine airway secretions. J Appl Physiol 46:205, 1979.

470. Boucher RC: Human airway ion transport. Part one. Am J Respir Crit Care Med 150:271, 1994.

471. Boucher RC, Stutts MJ, Bromberg PA, et al: Regional differences in airway surface liquid composition. J Appl Physiol 50:613, 1981.

472. Ueki I, German VF, Nadel JA: Micropipette measurement of airway submucosal gland secretion—autonomic effects. Am Rev Respir Dis 121:351, 1980.

473. Shelhamer JH, Marom Z, Sun F, et al: The effects of arachnoids and leukotrienes on the release of mucus from human airways. Chest 81(suppl):36S, 1982.

474. Nadel JA, Davis B: Parasympathetic and sympathetic regulation of secretion from submucosal glands in airways. Fed Proc 39:3075, 1980.

475. Nadel JA: New approaches to regulation of fluid secretion in airways. Chest 80:849, 1981.

476. Nadel JD, Davis B, Phipps RG: Control of mucus secretion and ion transport in airways. Annu Rev Physiol 41:369, 1979.

477. Logun C, Mullol J, Rieves D, et al: Use of a monoclonal antibody enzyme-linked immunosorbent assay to measure human respiratory glycoprotein production in vitro. Am J Respir Cell Mol Biol 5:71, 1991.

478. Phipps RJ, Nadel JA, Davis B: Effect of alpha-adrenergic stimulation on mucus secretion and on ion transport in cat trachea in vitro. Am Rev Respir Dis 121:359, 1980.

479. Davis B, Chinn R, Gold J, et al: Hypoxemia reflexly increases secretion from tracheal submucosal glands in dogs. J Appl Physiol 52:1416, 1982.

480. German VF, Corrales R, Ueki IF, et al: Reflex stimulation of tracheal mucus gland secretion by gastric irritation in cats. J Appl Physiol 52:1153, 1982.

481. Marom Z, Shelhamer JH, Bach MK, et al: Slow-reacting substances, leukotrienes C4 and D4, increase the release of mucus from human airways in vitro. Am Rev Respir Dis 126:449, 1982.

482. Peatfield AC, Barnes PJ, Bratcher C, et al: Vasoactive intestinal peptide stimulates tracheal submucosal gland secretion in the ferret. Am Rev Respir Dis 128:89, 1983.

483. Joos GF, Germonpre PR, Kips JC, et al: Sensory neuropeptides and the human lower airways: Present state and future directions. Eur Respir J 7:1161, 1994.

484. Shimura S, Sasaki T, Ikeda K, et al: Neuropeptides and airway submucosal gland secretion. Am Rev Respir Dis 143:S25, 1991.

485. Barnes PJ: Effects of bradykinin on airway function. Agents Actions Suppl 38:432, 1992.

486. Rieves RD, Goff J, Wu T, et al: Airway epithelial cell mucin release: Immunologic quantitation and response to platelet-activating factor. Am J Respir Cell Mol Biol 6:158, 1992.

487. Lundgren JD, Davey RT Jr, Lundgren B, et al: Eosinophil cationic protein stimulates and major basic protein inhibits airway mucus secretion. J Allergy Clin Immunol 87:689, 1991.

488. Widdicombe JH, Welsh MJ: Ion transport by dog tracheal epithelium. Fed Proc 39:3062, 1980.

489. Widdicombe JH, Ueki IF, Bruderman I, et al: The effects of sodium substitution and ouabain on ion transport by dog tracheal epithelium. Am Rev Respir Dis 120:385, 1979.

490. Boucher RC: Human airway ion transport: II. Am J Respir Crit Care Med 150:581, 1994.

491. Liedtke CM: Electrolyte transport in the epithelium of pulmonary segments of normal and cystic fibrosis lung. FASEB J 6:3076, 1992.

492. Knowles MR, Murray GF, Shallal JA, et al: Ion transport in excised human bronchi and its neurohumoral control. Chest 81(suppl):11S, 1982.

493. Olver RE, Davis B, Marin MG, et al: Active transport of NA^+ and Cl^- across canine tracheal epithelium in vitro. Am Rev Respir Dis 112:811, 1975.

494. Knowles MR, Buntin WH, Bromberg PA, et al: Measurements of transepithelial electric potential differences in the trachea and bronchi of human subjects in vivo. Am Rev Respir Dis 126:108, 1982.

495. Graham A, Alton EW, Geddes DM: Effects of 5-hydroxytryptamine and 5-hydroxytryptamine receptor agonists on ion transport across mammalian airway epithelia. Clin Sci 83:331, 1992.

496. Stuuts MJ, Chinet TC, Mason SJ, et al: Regulation of chloride channels in normal and cystic fibrosis airway epithelial cells by extracellular ATP. Proc Natl Acad Sci U S A 89:1621, 1992.

497. Jiang C, Finkbeiner WE, Widdicombe JH, et al: Altered fluid transport across airway epithelium in cystic fibrosis. Science 262:424, 1993.

498. Marriott C: The viscoelastic nature of mucus secretion. Chest 80(Suppl 6):804, 1981.

499. Giordano AM, Holsclaw D, Litt M: Mucus rheology and mucociliary clearance: Normal physiologic state. Am Rev Respir Dis 118:245, 1978.

500. King M: Viscoelastic properties of airway mucus. Fed Proc 39:3080, 1980.

501. Puchelle E, Zahm JM, Duvivier C: Spinnability of bronchial mucus: Relationship with viscoelasticity and mucous transport and properties. Biorheology 20:239, 1983.

502. Adler K, Wooten O, Philippoff W, et al: Physical properties of sputum: III. Rheologic variability and intrinsic relationships. Am Rev Respir Dis 106:86, 1972.

503. King M, Cohen C, Viires N: Influence of vagal tone on rheology and transportability of canine tracheal mucus. Am Rev Respir Dis 120:1215, 1979.

504. Lopez-Vidriero MT, Das I, Smith AP, et al: Bronchial secretion from normal human airways after inhalation of prostaglandin F_2, acetylcholine, histamine, and citric acid. Thorax 22:734, 1977.

505. Rubin BK, MacLeod PM, Sturgess J, et al: Recurrent respiratory infections in a child with fucosidosis: Is the mucus too thin for effective transport? Pediatr Pulmonol 10:304, 1991.

506. Ramsey BW, Astley SJ, Aitken ML, et al: Efficacy and safety of short-term administration of aerosolized recombinant human deoxyribonuclease in patients with cystic fibrosis. Am Rev Respir Dis 148:145, 1993.

507. Fuchs HJ, Borowitz DS, Christiansen DH, et al: Effect of aerosolized recombinant human DNase on exacerbations of respiratory symptoms and on pulmonary function in patients with cystic fibrosis. N Engl J Med 331:637, 1994.

508. Richards JH, Marriott C: Effect of relative humidity on the rheologic properties of bronchial mucus. Am Rev Respir Dis 109:484, 1974.

509. Barton AD, Lourenco RV: Bronchial secretions and mucociliary clearance. Arch Intern Med 131:140, 1973.

510. Thomson ML, Pavia D, McNicol MW: A preliminary study of the effect of guaiphenesin on mucociliary clearance from the human lung. Thorax 28:742, 1973.

CHAPTER 2

The Pulmonary and Bronchial Vascular Systems

THE PULMONARY ARTERIAL AND VENOUS CIRCULATION, 71
  Anatomy, 71
    Pulmonary Arteries, 71
    Pulmonary Veins, 74
    The Pulmonary Endothelium, 74
    Geometry and Dimensions of the Alveolar Capillary Network, 76
    Intervascular Anastomoses, 77
  Radiology, 77
    Pulmonary Arteries, 77
    Pulmonary Veins, 80
    The Pulmonary Hila, 81
      Conventional Posteroanterior and Lateral Radiography, 81
      Computed Tomography, 87
      Magnetic Resonance Imaging, 96
  Function, 104
    Perfusion of the Acinar Unit, 104
    Factors Influencing the Pulmonary Circulation, 104
      Gravity, 104
      Intrapleural Pressure and Lung Volume, 106
      Neurogenic and Chemical Effects, 106
    Diffusion of Gas from Acini to Red Blood Cells, 107
      Diffusion in the Acini, 107
      Diffusion Across the Alveolocapillary Membrane, 107
      Intravascular Diffusion, 107
      Measurement of Diffusing Capacity, 107
    Matching Capillary Blood Flow with Ventilation in the Acinus, 108
    Measurement of Ventilation/Perfusion Mismatch, 111
    Blood Gases and Acid-Base Balance, 114
      Blood Gases, 114
      Acid-Base Balance, 115
THE BRONCHIAL CIRCULATION, 119
  Anatomy, 119
  Flow and Nervous Control, 120
  Function, 121

THE PULMONARY ARTERIAL AND VENOUS CIRCULATION

Anatomy

Pulmonary Arteries

The pulmonary trunk originates from the base of the right ventricle and extends cranially and slightly to the left for 4 to 5 cm, at which point it divides into the right and left main pulmonary arteries. The latter continues in more or less the same line as the pulmonary trunk until it reaches the hilum, where it arches over the left main bronchus and divides into lobar branches. The right pulmonary artery arises at an angle to the axis of the pulmonary trunk and continues in a horizontal direction posterior to the aorta, superior to the vena cava, and anterior to the right main bronchus.

Although the course of the main pulmonary arteries is fairly constant, the origin and branching pattern of lobar and segmental arteries show considerable variation.[1] Despite this, the pulmonary arterial system is invariably intimately related to the airways and divides with them, a branch always accompanying the adjacent airway down to the level of the distal respiratory bronchioles (Fig. 2–1). In addition to these "conventional" vessels, many "supernumerary" (accessory) branches of the pulmonary artery arise at points other than corresponding airway divisions and directly penetrate the lung parenchyma (*see* Fig. 2–1).[2] These supernumerary branches outnumber the conventional ones and originate throughout the length of the arterial tree, most frequently in a peripheral location. Thus, the branching ratio (average number of daughter branches emanating from one parent branch) increases as vessel size decreases from about 3 proximally to about 3.6 distally.[3]

Detailed measurements of resin and gelatin casts of the human pulmonary arterial system have shown a linear relationship between Strahler order (*see* page 3) and the logarithm of both branch diameter and length.[3, 4] The average number of Strahler orders has been estimated to be about 17, measuring from branches 10 to 15 μm in diameter (Table 2–1).[3]

Histologically, precapillary pulmonary vessels can be conveniently divided into three types: elastic, muscular, and arteriolar. *Elastic arteries* include the main pulmonary artery and its lobar, segmental, and subsegmental branches extending roughly to the junction of bronchi and bronchioles. Histologically, the extrapulmonary vessels contain a multi-layered latticework of elastic fibers similar to that in systemic vessels of equivalent size but that is fragmented, more irregular in shape and size, and has more intervening connective tissue (Fig. 2–2).[5] Within the lung, the elastic laminae become more regular, with prominent external and internal layers and a variable number of less well-developed intervening layers. Despite their name, these vessels contain some muscle and are probably capable of active vasoconstriction.[6] As the vessels decrease in size, the number of elastic laminae diminishes so that at a diameter of 1,000 to

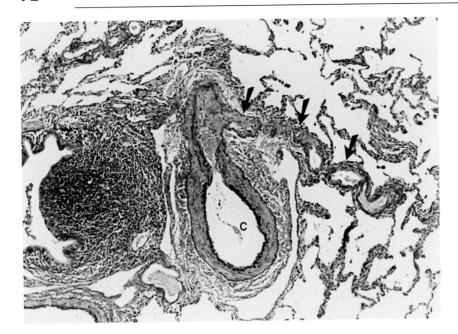

Figure 2–1. Pulmonary Artery—Conventional and Supernumerary Branches. The section shows a "conventional" muscular pulmonary artery (C) adjacent to a bronchiole. A small supernumerary branch _(arrows)_ extends from this vessel into the adjacent lung parenchyma.

500 μm, medial elastic tissue is lost altogether, leaving only well-developed internal and external laminae (at which point the vessels are considered muscular arteries). The internal lamina has been shown to consist of long plates of elastic tissue joined to one another by connecting side branches.[7]

Similar to the aorta, the elastic arteries provide a distensible reservoir for the ventricular ejection fraction. This distensibility has been found to undergo an age-related decrease.[8] Although the results of various studies are somewhat conflicting, most investigators have failed to find either morphologic or chemical changes in elastic tissue that would explain this decrease, and it has been suggested that physical changes in the constituents of the vessel wall may be responsible.[8, 9]

Muscular arteries have an external diameter ranging from about 500 to 100 μm. As indicated earlier, they possess well-developed internal and external elastic laminae, between which are a variable number of circularly arranged smooth muscle cells (_see_ Fig. 2–2). Beginning at a diameter of about 100 μm, arteries gradually lose their medial smooth muscle to become _arterioles_, so that at a diameter of about 70 μm the vessels are composed solely of a thin intima and a single elastic lamina that is continuous with the external elastic lamina of the parent artery. Arterioles of this size or smaller are histologically indistinguishable from pulmonary venules and can be identified only by special injection techniques or by the examination of serial sections. Within the acinus, arterioles continue to divide and accompany their respective bronchiolar and alveolar duct branches. Although some continue to do this to the level of the alveolar sacs, many accessory branches arise that do not precisely follow the transitional airways.[10] These branches, as well as those that terminate around the alveolar sacs, ramify to form the capillary network of the alveoli.

In general, pulmonary arterial and arteriolar vessels have a wide lumen and relatively thin, muscular media compared with systemic arteries of the same size. Morphometric measurements of medial thickness expressed as a percentage of external vessel diameter show a normal range of 3 to 7. No differences have been found between medial thickness of vessels of similar size in different parts of the lung, including apical and basal regions.[11] The ratio between the internal bronchiolar diameter and the external adventitial diameter of the accompanying artery is about 0.6; this appears to be independent of method of inflation and position of the airway/vessel within the lung.[12]

At all levels of the arterial system, the _intima_ is very thin, consisting of an endothelial cell layer and its adjacent basement membrane. With advancing age, alteration in this structure is common. Fatty streaks and atherosclerotic plaques histologically and ultrastructurally similar to those

Table 2–1. INTEGRATED DATA FOR THE TOTAL PULMONARY ARTERIAL SYSTEM WITH REVISED NUMBERS OF BRANCHES FOR THE INTERMEDIATE AND DISTAL ZONES

ORDER	NO. OF BRANCHES	DIAMETER (mm)	LENGTH (mm)
17	1.000	30.000	90.50
16	3.000	14.830	32.00
15	8.000	8.060	10.90
14	2.000×10^6	5.820	20.70
13	6.600×10^6	3.650	17.90
12	2.030×10^2	2.090	10.50
11	6.750×10^2	1.330	6.60
10	2.290×10^3	0.850	4.69
9	6.062×10^3	0.525	3.16
8	1.877×10^4	0.351	2.10
7	5.809×10^4	0.224	1.38
6	1.798×10^5	0.138	0.91
5	5.672×10^5	0.86	0.65
4	1.789×10^6	0.054	0.44
3	5.641×10^6	0.034	0.29
2	2.028×10^7	0.021	0.20
1	7.292×10^7	0.013	0.13

From Horsfield K: Circ Res 42:593, 1978. By permission of the American Heart Association, Inc.

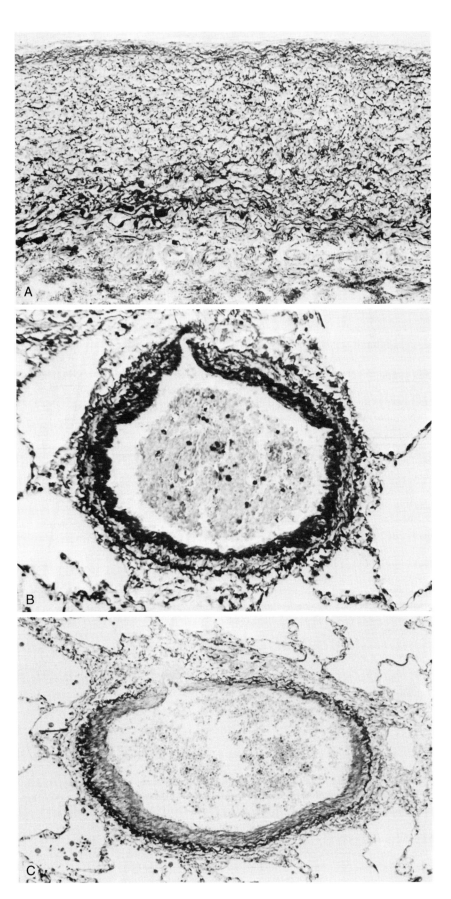

Figure 2–2. Histologic Characteristics of Pulmonary Vessels. Main pulmonary artery *(A)* showing fragmented, multilayered elastic laminae. In *B*, a muscular pulmonary artery with prominent internal and external elastic laminae and thin layer of medial smooth muscle is shown. A pulmonary vein, showing mild intimal thickening and relatively indistinct elastic laminae is shown in *C*. All micrographs are from a 60-year-old man with bronchogenic carcinoma. (Verhoeff-van Gieson; *A*, ×100; *B*, ×240; *C*, ×130.)

seen in the systemic circulation are common in people older than 40 years of age (*see* Fig. 1–18, page 13);[13] in one study, they were noted in 202 of 324 consecutive autopsies.[14] Their presence has been positively correlated with the degree of aortic atherosclerosis, pulmonary hypertension, and thromboembolism.[14] The atheromatous areas are almost always small and are most prominent near branch points in the larger elastic vessels.[15] In the absence of pulmonary hypertension or hyperlipidemia, complicating features (such as the calcification and ulceration) that are so common with systemic atheromas are rare.

Foci of intimal fibrosis without the features of atherosclerosis can also be found at all levels of the arterial tree, especially in the more peripheral muscular branches. Ultrastructurally, they consist of collagen and a cellular population that is composed almost exclusively of smooth muscle cells, apparently derived from the media.[16] Their frequency and thickness increase with age, so that in older people they can comprise as much as one third of the vessel diameter.[17] They are often eccentrically located in the vessel wall, suggesting that they may represent foci of organized thrombi.

In addition to smooth muscle and endothelial cells, several accessory cells can be found scattered within the arterial-arteriolar wall. *Pericytes* are located between the basement membrane and endothelial cells, predominantly in capillaries but also to some extent in arterioles. They have thin microfilament-containing processes that extend toward and attach to the endothelial cell surface.[18, 19] Although the importance and precise function of these cells in the normal lung are not clear, it has been suggested that they may act in either a contractile or phagocytic capacity.[18] A similar cell to the pericyte has been identified in precapillary arterioles between the internal elastic lamina and endothelial basement membrane; it shows ultrastructural features of a smooth muscle cell and has been termed an *intermediate cell*.[19, 20] Although its normal function is also unclear, there is evidence from studies in rats[20] and in children with congenital heart defects[19] that both it and pericytes can develop into mature smooth muscle cells, an observation that may have significance in the pathogenesis of pulmonary hypertension. *Mast cells* are also present in the connective tissue adjacent to pulmonary vessels, where they have been hypothesized to function as mediators of hypoxic vasoconstriction.[21]

Pulmonary Veins

The pulmonary veins arise from capillaries of the alveolar meshwork and from the capillary network of the pleura. Contrary to the pulmonary arteries, they are not associated with the airways. Although their final course is somewhat variable, there are usually two main superior and two main inferior vessels, the former draining the middle and upper lobes on the right side and the upper lobe on the left, and the latter the lower lobes. The right-sided veins course beneath the main pulmonary artery posterior to the superior vena cava and enter the left atrium separately. The left-sided veins pass anterior to the descending aorta and either enter the atrium separately as on the right or join within the pericardial cavity to enter the atrium as a common channel. As in the pulmonary arterial system, numerous supernumerary vessels join the veins as they course through the lung.[22]

Detailed analysis of resin casts of human pulmonary veins, classified by Strahler order, show a 15-order system to the level of the superior and inferior vessels (Table 2–2).[23] As with the conducting airways and pulmonary arteries, there is a roughly linear relationship between the order number and the logarithm of vessel diameter and length.[23]

Histologically, smaller pulmonary venules are indistinguishable from arterioles. With increasing size, occasional smooth muscle cells and an elastic lamina become evident and, at a diameter between 60 and 100 μm, they become clearly recognizable as veins. Larger vessels have a variable number of elastic laminae between which are small, irregular bundles of smooth muscle cells and collagen. In contrast with arteries, there is no well-developed external elastic lamina, the adventitia and media blending together. With advancing age, fragmentation of the elastic laminae and intimal sclerosis similar to that seen in the arterial system are often present.

No valves are present within venous lumina. However, regularly spaced annular constrictions related to local accumulations of smooth muscle have been identified in the veins of some animals.[24] These are capable of active contraction—a process reduced by α-adrenergic antagonists[25]—and have been hypothesized to be important in the control of pulmonary blood flow.[24]

Minute collections of cells intimately associated with pulmonary venules can be identified in some healthy individuals and in patients with several chronic lung diseases associated with alveolar hypoxia or edema.[26] These are histologically similar to intracranial arachnoid villi and have sometimes been termed *minute pulmonary chemodectoma* (*see* page 1374). It has been hypothesized that these structures may have a function similar to that of arachnoid tissue, by reabsorbing and transferring fluid from the air spaces to pulmonary venules.[26]

The Pulmonary Endothelium

Although endothelial cells have been estimated to be the most common cell type in the lung (representing about 35% to 40% of all parenchymal cells[27]), they are relatively inconspicuous at the light microscopic level, being visible only as a series of small intraluminal bumps corresponding to their nuclei. They are arranged in an interlocking mosaic[28] and possess scanty cytoplasm that exists mostly as thin, platelike processes measuring as little as 0.1 μm in thickness.[29] Cellular organelles, including Golgi apparatus, mitochondria, microtubules, Weibel-Palade bodies, and endoplasmic reticulum, are sparse and tend to be concentrated in a perinuclear location. On the cell surface, particularly in arteries, are numerous short, microvillus-like projections.[29, 30] These greatly increase the cell surface area and, along with pinocytotic vesicles (*see* farther on), have been shown to react immunohistochemically for angiotensin-converting enzyme (ACE),[31] implying a role in metabolic function. It has also been proposed that the irregularity and density of these projections may create turbulence in the cell-free plasma layer along the endothelial surface, resulting in slower flow and facilitating metabolite transfer between the blood and the endothelial cells.[30]

A prominent ultrastructural feature of the pulmonary capillary endothelial cell is the presence of numerous small

Table 2–2. MODEL OF THE PULMONARY VENOUS TREE

ORDER	NUMBER	DIAMETER (mm)	LENGTH (mm)	VOLUME (ml)
1	72,920,000	0.013	0.130	1.258
2	23,109,101	0.019	0.192	1.258
3	7,323,513	0.029	0.283	1.369
4	2,320,897	0.043	0.418	1.399
5	735,516	0.064	0.617	1.460
6	233,093	0.096	0.910	1.535
7	73,869	0.14	1.34	1.524
8	23,843	0.22	1.98	1.795
9	7,546	0.39	2.54	2.290
10	1,842	0.61	3.20	1.723
11	496	1.21	11.0	6.274
12	158	1.90	18.5	8.288
13	53	2.90	25.4	8.892
14	14	5.23	39.0	11.730
15	4	13.88	36.7	22.212
TOTALS	106,749,945		142.21	73.762

From Horsfield K, Gordon WI: Lung 159:216, 1981.

pits or vesicles *(caveolae intracellulare)* (Fig. 2–3). These can be seen in the relatively thick, non–gas-exchanging part of the cell, either at the luminal or abluminal surface or free in the cytoplasm.[32] The interior of many luminal surface vesicles is delimited by a thin membrane that appears to have a surrounding electron-dense rim, believed to function as a support.[32] Small electron-dense granules, considered to represent enzyme complexes responsible for various metabolic functions, can be seen at the bases of the vesicles attached to the limiting membrane. Some investigators have found immunochemical and histochemical evidence that enzymes such as 5′-nucleotidase[32] and ACE[31] are present within the granules; however, in one study in which the uptake of substrates such as 5-hydroxytryptamine was traced, no preferential localization was found within vesicles,[33] and

the relative importance of vesicular versus other plasma membrane or cytoplasmic enzymes in endothelial metabolism remains to be clarified. In addition to their metabolic activity, the vesicles are believed to function as a mechanism for transport of fluid and proteins between blood and interstitial tissues and across the air-blood barrier.[34, 35] The transport of specific compounds may depend on localized differences in the charges of different vesicles.[34]

Compared with the vesicular portion, the nonvesicular, gas-exchanging portion of the capillary endothelial cell has been found to have few anionic binding sites.[36] Since red blood cells exhibit a negative surface charge, it has been suggested that this might lead to a slowing of blood flow in the region of the thin portion of the endothelium, thus facilitating gas transfer.[36]

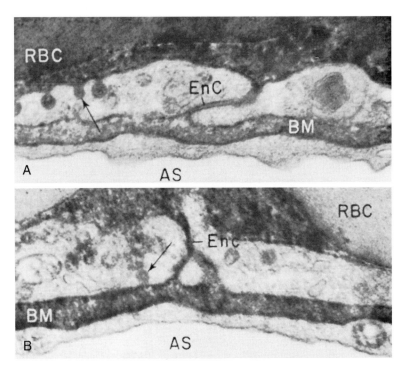

Figure 2–3. Endothelial Intercellular Cleft. Section of alveolar wall from the lung of a mouse sacrificed 90 seconds after horseradish peroxidase injection. Reaction product in the capillary lumen (indicated by RBC) extends through the endothelial intercellular cleft (EnC) into the adjacent basement membrane (BM). In *A*, the staining of horseradish peroxidase is quite light, whereas in *B* the basement membrane is deeply stained. Reaction product is present in endothelial invaginations *(caveolae intracellulare* on both the capillary side *(arrow* in *A)* and the alveolar side *(arrow* in *B)* of the cell. (TEM; ×46,000.) (From Schneeberger-Keeley EE, Karnovsky MJ: J Cell Biol 37:781, 1968.)

Adjacent endothelial cells are joined by tight junctions,[28, 35] which by transmission electron microscopy appear as focal areas of fusion of the outer lamellae of adjacent cell membranes. For the most part these are continuous, although occasional intercellular clefts measuring up to 4 nm in thickness can be observed at the level of the alveolar capillaries.[34, 37] As seen by freeze-fracture techniques, the junctions are less complex than those of the alveolar epithelium (Fig. 2–4); in addition to the presence of intercellular clefts, this suggests that the main site of solute impermeability in the air-blood barrier is the epithelium.[38] The complexity of the endothelial junctions is variable, being greater in arterioles (which are believed to be relatively impermeable) and less in the more permeable venules. As indicated by the number of connecting strands per junction, complexity has also been found to increase from the apex to the base of the lung; it has been hypothesized that this reflects an adaptation of the pulmonary endothelium to regional differences in hydrostatic pressure.[39]

Endothelial cells produce a number of substances, such as cell adhesion molecules, antielastolytic substances, nitric oxide, and endothelin, that likely have important roles in vascular function and pulmonary defense, including vascular repair, vascular tone, the transition from fetal to neonatal circulation, modulation of inflammatory reactions, and even gas exchange itself.[40–45] It is likely that there are metabolic differences between endothelial cells in different regions;[43] for example, endothelial cells of arteries and veins were found by one group of investigators to show evidence of superoxide dismutase production, whereas those of the capillaries did not.[46]

The endothelial cell is capable of division and normally replicates to replenish the endothelial surface at a rate of less than 1% of the total endothelial population daily.[47] A rapid and marked increase in mitotic activity can occur in response to endothelial damage.[48]

Geometry and Dimensions of the Alveolar Capillary Network

The pulmonary capillaries form a dense network of short segments, which schematically can be considered to be short cylindrical tubes, modified at their bases to form "wedges" that allow each segment to join at either end with two adjacent segments (Fig. 2–5).[49, 50] Although junctures of four segments can occur, in most instances only three segments unite, resulting in an average angle of junction of about 120 degrees. Thus, the basic geometric structure of the capillary network is hexagonal, each mesh being surrounded, on average, by six segments. This two-dimensional network becomes three dimensional when three septal facets join, achieved by the rotation of the plane of juncture of three segments by approximately 90 degrees (Fig. 2–6). Although convenient from a conceptual point of view, this description of capillary geometry is highly idealized,[51] particularly when one considers the three-dimensional capillary and alveolar geometry under dynamic conditions.

Weibel found that the external diameter of capillary segments in fresh lung averaged 8.6 μm; allowing 0.3 μm for the average thickness of the capillary endothelium, the average internal capillary diameter was estimated to be 8 μm.[49, 50] As has been shown in rapidly frozen dog lungs, this value may vary substantially with both lung volume and capillary pressure.[52] The axial length of capillary segments

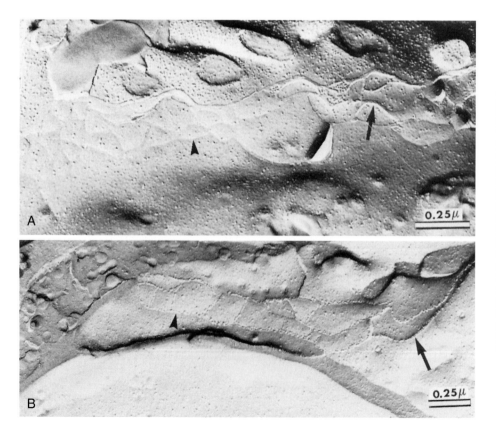

Figure 2–4. Epithelial and Endothelial Cell Junctions. An epithelial tight junction *(A)* between a Type I and a Type II pneumocyte. On the ectoplasmic fracture face, the tight junction is a reticulum of furrows *(arrowhead)*. On the protoplasmic fracture face, the tight junction is a reticulum of continuous fibers *(arrow)*. In *B*, an endothelial tight junction between two alveolar capillary endothelial cells. On ectoplasmic fracture faces, the tight junction is a reticulum of furrows containing particles *(arrowhead)*. On the protoplasmic fracture face, the junctional complex consists of discontinuous particles *(arrow)*. The differences in the complexity of the tight junction structure between endothelial and epithelial cells are believed to relate to the different permeability of these tissues. (Courtesy of Dr. David Walker, University of British Columbia, Vancouver.)

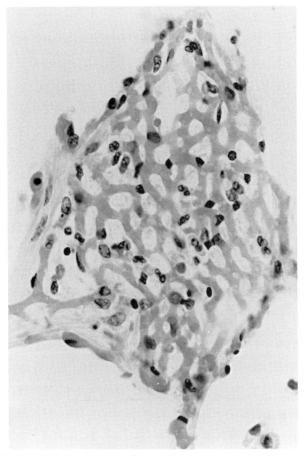

Figure 2–5. Alveolar Capillary Network. *En face* section of an alveolar wall shows numerous short capillary segments interconnecting to form a complex vascular network.

ranges from 9 to 13 μm (average, 10.3). Weibel deduced that each alveolus is surrounded by about 1,800 to 2,000 capillary segments and that the total number of capillary segments in the entire lung averages about 280 billion. He estimated total capillary blood volume to be 140 ml and the total capillary surface area 70 m², only slightly less than that of the alveolar surface. The volume of blood per alveolus was estimated to be 4.7×10^{-7} ml and the capillary surface per alveolus to be 23.4×10^{-4} cm².

Intervascular Anastomoses

Because of the lungs' dual blood supply, several combinations of intervascular anastomoses are theoretically possible. Employing histologic, functional, and corrosion cast techniques, many investigators have attempted to delineate and assess the extent and importance of these combinations.[11]

Anastomoses between bronchial and pulmonary veins are undoubtedly the most common and in fact represent the normal pathway for the bulk of bronchial and bronchiolar venous drainage (*see* page 120). Bronchial artery–pulmonary artery anastomoses have been shown to occur in the normal lung; although their significance in the normal state is uncertain, their number and size can increase appreciably in various disease states, and they can contribute greatly to total pulmonary blood flow. Although investigated exten-

sively, the existence of pulmonary arteriovenous anastomoses is uncertain; some investigators have found evidence for their presence and others have not.[11] Arteriovenous anastomoses in the bronchial circulation have been documented, but are uncommon. In the perinatal period, anastomotic channels from bronchial arteries to alveolar capillaries and from pulmonary arteries to the capillaries of bronchial walls and interstitial tissue can be readily identified; however, under normal circumstances these decrease dramatically in number or disappear altogether during infancy.

With the exception of the bronchial vessels, anastomoses between systemic and pulmonary arteries probably do not occur in the normal lung. However, one group of investigators documented the presence of small arteries originating in the aorta and coursing in the pulmonary ligament to supply a portion of the medial basal pleura;[53] although normally these are not important in terms of flow, it has been suggested that their enlargement might be involved in the pathogenesis of pulmonary sequestration (*see* page 601).[53]

Radiology

Pulmonary Arteries

The main pulmonary artery originates in the mediastinum at the pulmonary valve and passes upward, backward, and to the left before bifurcating within the pericardium into the shorter left and longer right arteries (Figs. 2–7 and 2–8). The right pulmonary artery courses behind the ascending aorta before dividing behind the superior vena cava and in front of the right main bronchus into ascending (truncus anterior) and descending (interlobar) rami (Fig. 2–9). Although somewhat variable, the common pattern is for the ascending artery to subdivide into the segmental branches that supply the right upper lobe and for the descending branch to contribute the segmental arteries to the middle and right lower lobes.[54] In 90% of people, a portion of the

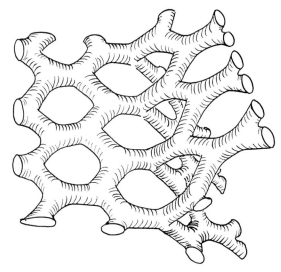

Figure 2–6. Alveolar Capillary Network. Schematic sketch of the capillary network at the juncture of three interalveolar septal facets showing continuity of network. (From Weibel ER: Morphometry of the Human Lung. New York, Academic Press, 1963.)

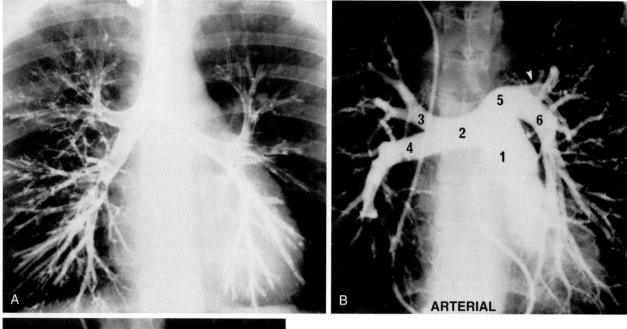

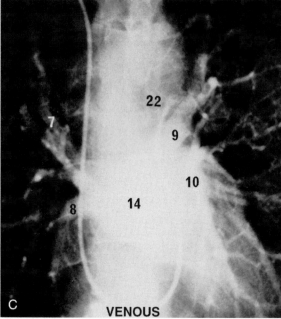

Figure 2–7. Normal Hilar Anatomy in Anteroposterior Projection. An anteroposterior tracheobronchogram *(A)* and anteroposterior angiogram during the arterial *(B)* and venous *(C)* phases for comparison of anatomic relationships. The main pulmonary artery (1) divides into shorter, higher left (5) and longer right (2) branches. In *B*, the right branch divides into ascending (3) and descending (4) arteries within the pericardium, behind the superior vena cava (note course of the catheter), before appearing as hilar vessels. The left pulmonary artery in this patient shows similar divisional features with relatively small ascending *(arrowhead)* and more prominent descending (6) branches. The venous phase of the angiogram *(C)* shows a close relationship between the right (7) and left (9) superior veins as they cross anterior to the hilar arterial vasculature. Note the typical course of the left superior vein in relation to the left main bronchus (22). On the right, three veins drain to the left atrium (14), whereas on the left, superior and inferior veins (10) join to form a common chamber before entering the atrium.

posterior segment of the right upper lobe is supplied by a separate branch that arises from the interlobar artery.[54]

The first portion of the right interlobar artery is horizontal and is interposed between the superior vena cava in front and the intermediate bronchus behind. It then turns sharply downward and backward, assuming a vertical orientation within the major fissure (thus its name) anterolateral to the intermediate and right lower lobe bronchi before giving the segmental branches—one or two to the middle lobe and usually single branches to each of the five bronchopulmonary segments of the lower lobe.

Measurement of the width of the interlobar artery can be useful in the assessment of diseases affecting the pulmonary vessels, and normal limits have been established. In one study of radiographs of more than 1,000 normal adults

taken at full inspiration, the upper limit of the transverse diameter of the artery (measured from its lateral aspect to the air column of the intermediate bronchus) was 16 mm in men and 15 mm in women; these figures decreased by 1 to 3 mm in full expiration.[55]

Another method for estimating changes in arterial caliber is the artery-bronchus index. In a study of 1,200 conventional tomograms of 250 normal subjects in the supine position, the ratio of the transverse diameter of a pulmonary artery to the contiguous bronchus viewed end-on in the perihilar area was found to be independent of age, sex, and body build and to provide a more objective assessment of disturbances in pressure and flow in the pulmonary circulation than was possible with direct measurement of the caliber of the artery itself.[56] The normal mean value of the artery-

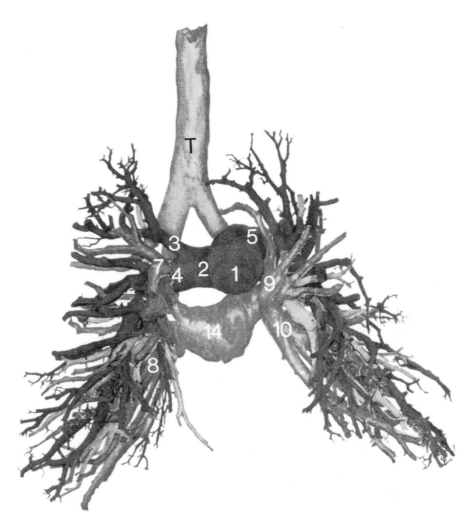

Figure 2–8. Anatomic Features of the Central Pulmonary Vasculature. Anterior cast of the trachea (T), bronchi, pulmonary arteries, and pulmonary veins. The intricate relationship of these structures to one another is apparent. Note that the right (7) and the left (9) superior veins relate most closely to the anterior aspect of the upper hila whereas the right (8) and the left (10) inferior veins are situated posteromedial to the lower lobe bronchi. Numerical anatomic designations are used consistently throughout this section. 1, Main pulmonary artery; 2, right pulmonary artery; 3, truncus anterior; 4, right interlobar artery; 5, left pulmonary artery; 7, right superior pulmonary vein; 8, right inferior pulmonary vein; 9, left superior pulmonary vein; 10, left inferior pulmonary vein; 14, left atrium. (From Genereux GP: Am J Roentgenol 141:1241, 1983.)

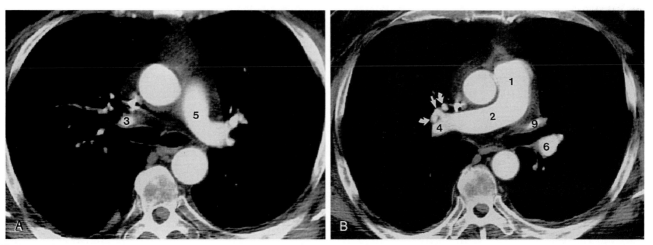

Figure 2–9. Anatomic Features of the Pulmonary Artery and Its Main Branches as Seen on CT Scan. In *A*, CT at the level of the main bronchi demonstrates the ascending branch (3) of the right pulmonary artery and the main left pulmonary artery (5). In *B*, CT at the level of the bronchus intermedius demonstrates the main pulmonary artery (1), right pulmonary artery (2), and right interlobar pulmonary artery (4). Also seen are the anterior segmental arteries of the right upper lobe *(straight arrow)* and right upper lobe pulmonary veins *(curved arrows)*. On the left side, the left interlobar pulmonary artery (6) can be seen behind the left upper lobe bronchus, while the left superior pulmonary vein (9) lies in front of the bronchus.

bronchus index was 1.30 immediately distal to the takeoff of the right upper lobe bronchus and 1.40 immediately beyond the origin of the left upper lobe bronchus.

The pulmonary artery-to-bronchus ratio can also be measured on frontal chest radiographs. In one study of 30 healthy subjects, the ratio was 0.85 ± 0.15 (mean ± SD) above the right hilar angle and 1.34 ± 0.25 below the right hilar angle in the erect position, and 1.01 ± 0.13 above and 1.05 ± 0.13 below the right hilar angle in the supine position.[57] These measurements are particularly helpful in the assessment of pulmonary plethora and congestive heart failure.[58] In 30 patients with pulmonary plethora secondary to volume overload complicating chronic renal failure, the mean artery-to-bronchus ratio in the erect position was 1.62 ± 0.31 above the right hilar angle and 1.56 ± 0.28 below the right hilar angle;[57] in patients with congestive heart failure, the ratio was 1.50 ± 0.25 above and 0.87 ± 0.20 below the hilar angle in the erect position, and 1.49 ± 0.31 above and 0.96 ± 0.31 below the right hilar angle in the supine position.

Normal ranges in size of the pulmonary arteries have also been determined by computed tomography (CT). One group of investigators measured the diameter on routine CT scans photographed on soft tissue windows. Using this method, the mean diameter of the right main pulmonary artery in 25 adult patients with no evidence of pulmonary vascular disease was 13.3 ± 1.5 mm.[59] In a second, theoretically more accurate study, a computer program was used that displayed the density profile of the pulmonary artery and its adjacent tissues in 26 control subjects and 32 patients with cardiopulmonary disease.[60] The widest diameters perpendicular to the long axis of the main and proximal right and left pulmonary arteries were measured at the level of the pulmonary artery bifurcation; the diameter of the right interlobar artery was measured at the level of the origin of the middle lobe bronchus and the diameter of the left descending pulmonary artery at the level of the origin of the superior segmental bronchus. The diameters of the main and right pulmonary arteries gave the best estimates for mean pulmonary artery pressure. The mean ± SD diameter for the main pulmonary artery was 24.2 ± 2.2 mm and for the interlobar artery was 13 ± 1.9 mm. There was no significant difference between measurements in men and women. The results of this study suggest that the maximal normal diameter (mean ± 2 SD) of the main pulmonary artery and the right interlobar artery as measured by CT are 28.6 and 16.8 mm, respectively. The pulmonary artery-to-bronchus ratio has also been measured on high-resolution CT in 30 patients without cardiopulmonary disease.[61] In this study, the mean value ± SD was 0.98 ± 0.14, figures similar to those of 1.04 ± 0.13 reported on chest radiographs of healthy supine subjects.[57]

Although the mean external diameter of the bronchus is similar to the diameter of the accompanying artery, it should be remembered that the normal range (mean ± 2 SD) is wide (0.70 to 1.25). Furthermore, there are significant differences between the artery-to-bronchus ratio of the various lobes and segments.[61]

After passing over the left main bronchus, the *left pulmonary artery* sometimes gives off a short ascending branch that subsequently divides into segmental branches to the upper lobe; more commonly, however, it continues directly into the vertically oriented left interlobar artery, from which the segmental arteries to the upper and lower lobes arise directly.[54] The left interlobar artery lies posterolateral to the lower lobe bronchus (*see* Fig. 2–9).

Pulmonary Veins

As discussed previously, the course of the pulmonary veins is remote from the bronchoarterial bundles, a relationship that commences in the lung periphery where the arterial system is in the center of the secondary lobules and the venous system is located within the interlobular septa. This relationship persists, so that in all areas the arteries and their corresponding veins are separated by air-containing lung. Theoretically, this should permit radiologic distinction of artery from vein, particularly in the medial third of the lung, where the continuity of the artery with its accompanying bronchus may be more readily distinguished and where the typical course of the larger veins on their way to the mediastinum can be recognized. However, in a pulmonary angiographic study of 50 patients in anteroposterior (AP) projection, the upper lobe artery and vein were superimposed in 40% to 50% of subjects, implying that these vessels cannot be distinguished on the chest radiograph.[62] The complex relationship between the central pulmonary arteries and veins is illustrated in Figure 2–8 (*see* page 79).

Segmental veins from the right upper lobe coalesce to form the right superior pulmonary vein (Fig. 2–10; *see also* Fig. 2–7, page 78), which descends medially into the mediastinum before attaching to the upper and posterior aspect of the left atrium as a superior confluence. Along its course caudad, this vessel is intimately associated from above downward with the anterior and posterior upper lobe segmental bronchi, the junction of the horizontal and vertical segments of the right interlobar artery, and the anteromedial aspect of the middle lobe bronchus.[63] After passing under the middle lobe bronchus, the middle lobe vein usually joins the left atrium at the base of the superior pulmonary venous confluence; occasionally, the three veins on the right (superior, middle, and inferior) remain separate.

On the left, the veins from the apicoposterior and anterior segments of the upper lobe join to form the left superior pulmonary vein (*see* Fig. 2–10) which, after uniting with the lingular vein, courses obliquely downward and medially into the mediastinum. Along its course caudad, this vessel lies medial to the apicoposterior bronchoarterial bundle, anterolateral to the left pulmonary artery, and, finally, anterior to the continuum formed by the left main and upper lobe bronchi.[63] It thus separates these airways from the left atrium before it inserts into this chamber.

The horizontally oriented lower lobe segmental veins on both sides coalesce medial to the lower lobe bronchi to form the right and left inferior pulmonary veins (see Fig. 2–10); at the site of their attachment to the left atrium, they form the inferior pulmonary venous confluences.[64, 65] The left inferior pulmonary vein and venous confluence are at the same level as or slightly higher than the right and slightly more posterior; this vein may join with the left superior vein to form a common chamber before entering the left atrium. The normal superior and inferior venous confluences are sometimes prominent enough to simulate a mass on a lateral chest radiograph, particularly on the right.

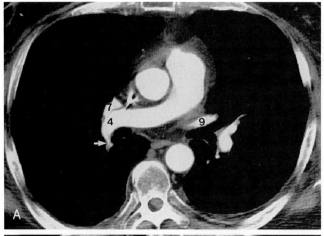
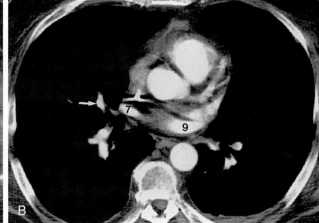
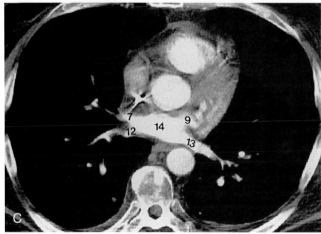

Figure 2–10. Pulmonary Veins on CT Scan. CT scan *(A)* at the level of the bronchus intermedius demonstrates the right superior pulmonary vein (7) immediately anterior to the descending branch of the right pulmonary artery (4). Also seen is the superior segmental artery of the right lower lobe (straight arrow). On the left side, the superior pulmonary vein (9) can be seen anterior to the left main and upper lobe bronchi. At this level, the left interlobar artery can be seen to be bifurcating into lingular and left lower lobe branches. In *B*, a CT scan at the level of the middle lobe bronchus demonstrates right (7) and left (9) superior pulmonary veins converging toward the upper aspect of the left atrium. Also seen are the right middle lobe pulmonary artery *(arrow)* and branches of the right and left lower lobe arteries. A CT scan 5 mm more caudad *(C)* demonstrates the right (7) and left (9) superior pulmonary veins and right (12) and left (13) inferior venous confluences entering the left atrium (14).

The Pulmonary Hila

Although the term *hilum* is widely used in the radiologic literature in reference to the lungs, the anatomic boundaries defining it are vague.[66] Some describe it as lying immediately adjacent to a main bronchus, from the tracheal carina to the origin of the first lobar bronchus.[67] Consensus, however, seems to favor an imprecisely defined area between the mediastinum medially and the substance of the lung laterally, through which pass the bronchi, pulmonary and systemic vessels, and accompanying connective tissue.[66, 68, 69] Consequently, we prefer to define the hila simply as those areas in the center of the thorax that connect the mediastinum to the lungs. The anatomic structures rendering the hila visible are primarily the pulmonary arteries and veins, with lesser contributions from the bronchial walls, surrounding connective tissue, and lymph nodes.[69]

There are three major imaging techniques for examining the hila, each of which possesses distinct advantages and disadvantages: (1) conventional radiography in posteroanterior (PA) and lateral projection, the method that suffices in most cases; (2) CT scanning; and (3) magnetic resonance (MR) imaging.

Conventional Posteroanterior and Lateral Radiography

Posteroanterior Projection. As viewed on a conventional PA radiograph, the hila can be divided into upper and lower components by an imaginary horizontal line transecting the junction of the upper lobe and intermediate bronchi on the right and the upper and lower lobe bronchial dichotomy on the left. On the *right* side, the upper hilar opacity relates to the ascending pulmonary artery and the superior pulmonary vein (Fig. 2–11). The end-on opacity and radiolucency, respectively, of the contiguous anterior (and occasionally posterior) segmental artery and bronchus can be identified in approximately 80% of normal subjects.[70] A short segment of the upper lobe bronchus beneath the ascending right pulmonary artery can sometimes be identified before it trifurcates into the segmental branches serving the upper lobe.

The lower portion of the right hilum (Fig. 2–12) is formed by the vertically oriented interlobar artery, the right superior pulmonary vein superolaterally as it crosses the junction of the horizontal and vertical limbs of the interlobar artery and the respective branches of these vessels. The horizontally oriented inferior pulmonary vein lies more inferiorly. The radiolucent lumen of the intermediate bronchus is invariably identified medial to the interlobar artery. Occasionally, segmental bronchi and arteries in the middle and lower lobes can be seen either in profile or end-on.

On the *left*, the upper hilar opacity is formed by the distal left pulmonary artery, the proximal portion of the left interlobar artery and its segmental arterial branches, and the left superior pulmonary vein and its major tributaries (Fig. 2–13). The proximal left pulmonary artery is almost always higher than the highest point of the right interlobar artery. In one series of 500 normal subjects, this feature was found

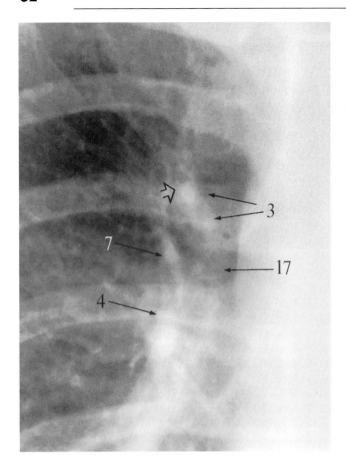

Figure 2–11. Right Upper Hilar Anatomy. A detail view of the right hilum from a conventional posteroanterior radiograph demonstrates the ascending (3) and descending (4) arteries. The right superior pulmonary vein (7) crosses the hilum obliquely to form the typical V configuration. The lumen of the right upper lobe bronchus (17) and of the end-on bronchus and the opaque artery *(open arrow)* of the anterior segment are shown.

Figure 2–12. Right Lower Hilar Anatomy. On this detail view from a conventional posteroanterior radiograph the interlobar (4) artery lies lateral to the intermediate bronchus (18). Note that this vessel dominates the radiographic anatomy of the lower hilum. The horizontally oriented inferior pulmonary vein (8) lies posteroinferior to the hilum.

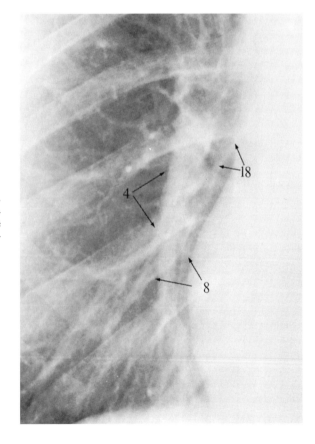

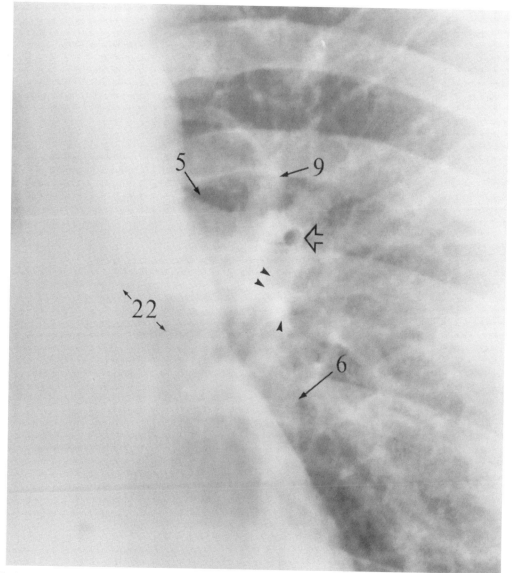

Figure 2–13. Left Hilar Anatomy. A detail view of the left hilum from a posteroanterior chest radiograph shows the left pulmonary artery (5), the interlobar artery (6), and the left superior pulmonary vein (9). The left main bronchus (22) and its superior *(two arrowheads)* and inferior *(single arrowhead)* divisions are overlapped by the hilar vessels. The end-on bronchus and opaque artery *(single open arrowhead)* of the anterior segment are seen.

in 97%, the range of difference in the majority being 0.75 to 2.25 cm;[69] in 3%, the hila were at the same level, and in none was the right hilum higher than the left. The reference point for the determination of this relationship is the site at which the right and left superior pulmonary veins cross their respective pulmonary arteries prior to entering the mediastinum.[71]

The left superior hilum, unlike its counterpart on the right, is often partly or completely covered by mediastinal fat and pleura between the aortic arch and left pulmonary artery, or by a portion of the cardiac silhouette; therefore, it may be largely hidden from view (Fig. 2–14). Frequently, however, the anterior segmental or lingular bronchoarterial bundle can be identified end-on in its upper portion. The air columns of the left upper lobe bronchus and its superior and inferior (lingular) divisions and the left lower lobe bronchus may also be identified. The lower portion of the left hilum is formed by the distal interlobar artery, the lingular artery and vein, and, more caudally, the left inferior pulmonary vein.

Certain normal variations caused by unusual prominence of the hilar vessels can be confused with hilar masses.[63] Most of these vascular pseudotumors are caused by the veins as they cross the hila on their way to the mediastinum, the right and left superior veins and the left superior or common venous confluence (Fig. 2–15) being the most frequent culprits. The right inferior venous confluence is also a well-recognized cause of pseudotumor, particularly in patients with postcapillary pulmonary hypertension as a result of left ventricular failure or mitral valve disease.

The left pulmonary artery normally is oriented roughly in an AP plane as it enters the pleural space; occasionally, it courses more obliquely than usual, thus assuming an unusual prominence that creates an arterial hilar pseudotumor (Fig. 2–16).

Lateral Projection. The radiographic anatomy of the hila in this projection is complex, since the right and left hilar components are, to a large degree, superimposed.[72–74] The carina is projected at the level of the fourth or fifth thoracic vertebra; however, vertebrae are sometimes difficult to count precisely on lateral projection, and more useful landmarks are the left pulmonary artery or the proximal third of the intermediate stem line (*see* farther on), structures that bear a close approximation to the tracheal bifurcation. The air column of the normally more cephalad right upper lobe bronchus can be identified end-on in about 50% of people, whereas that of the more caudad left upper lobe bronchus is seen in about 75% (Fig. 2–17).[73] Occasionally (usually in asthenic people), the uppermost radiolucency represents the right main bronchus and the lowermost radiolucency represents the left main bronchus.

The orifice of the right upper lobe bronchus is seldom as well circumscribed as that of the left. The latter is surrounded by the left pulmonary artery above, the interlobar artery behind, and the mediastinal component of the left superior pulmonary vein in front, whereas the former is devoid of vascular envelopment on its posterior aspect, so that aerated upper or lower lobe parenchyma normally abuts its wall. Consequently, clear identification of the right upper lobe bronchial lumen *en face* constitutes highly suggestive

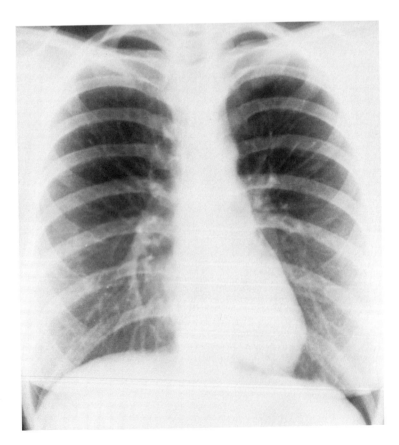

Figure 2–14. Hilar Anatomy on Posteroanterior Radiograph. Note that the inferior portion of the hilum on the left may be overlapped by the cardiac silhouette; this is a normal feature in some subjects and should not be mistaken for bronchial displacement caused by minimal atelectasis of the left lower lobe.

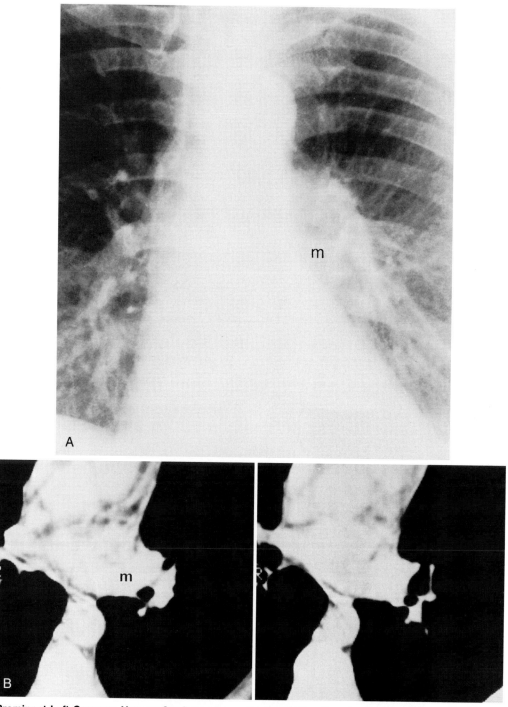

Figure 2–15. Prominent Left Common Venous Confluence as a Cause of Hilar Pseudotumor. A detail view *(A)* of a posteroanterior chest radiograph discloses an unexplained opacity (m) beneath the left main bronchus. Contrast-enhanced CT scans *(B)* demonstrate that the opacity represents a prominent left common venous confluence. (From Genereux GP: Am J Roentgenol 141:1241, 1983. © American Roentgen Ray Society.)

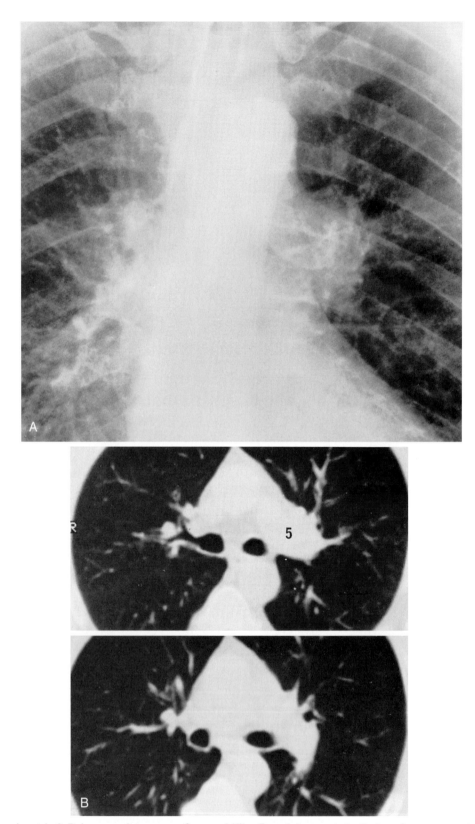

Figure 2–16. Prominent Left Pulmonary Artery as a Cause of Hilar Pseudotumor. A detail view of a posteroanterior chest radiograph *(A)* discloses a prominent left hilum. CT scans through the carina *(B)* reveal an obliquely directed, slightly enlarged left pulmonary artery (5) as the cause.

evidence that the airway is completely surrounded by soft tissue, most likely enlarged lymph nodes (*see* Fig. 2–17).

The posterior wall of the right main and intermediate bronchi form the anatomic foundation for the *intermediate stem line*, a vertically oriented linear opacity measuring up to 3 mm in width[75] that is visible in 95% of people (*see* Fig. 2–17).[73] The posterior wall of these two bronchi is rendered visible by air in their lumen in front and aerated lung parenchyma in the azygoesophageal recess behind. On a well-centered lateral projection, the line transects the mid or posterior third of the circular, radiolucent left upper lobe bronchus; it terminates caudally at the origin of the superior segmental bronchus of the right lower lobe, slightly proximal to or at the same level as the origin of the middle lobe bronchus anteriorly. We have not been able to identify the anterior wall of the intermediate bronchus, although this feature has been reported in one study.[73] We have no explanation for this discrepancy, although it is difficult to understand how the anterior wall of the intermediate bronchus should be visible, considering that it is closely associated with the interlobar artery.

The physical characteristics that render the intermediate stem line visible are also operative to some extent on the left, so that the posterior wall of the left main bronchus and the proximal portion of the left lower lobe bronchus may be profiled as the *left retrobronchial line* (*see* Fig. 2–17).[76] This short, vertical linear opacity measures 3 mm or less in width and terminates caudally at the origin of the superior segmental bronchus of the left lower lobe. The distinction between the intermediate stem line and the left retrobronchial line is not difficult, bearing in mind that the former is both longer and more anteriorly located than the latter.

Occasionally, a convex, lenticular stripe can be identified in the anticipated location of the retrobronchial line, representing the *left retrobronchial stripe*. As shown on correlative conventional lateral radiographic and CT studies, this stripe is invariably delimited posteriorly by a radiolucency representing gas within the esophagus (Fig. 2–18); since the latter structure is closely applied to the left posterior tracheal wall and the posterior wall of the left main bronchus, the stripe represents the combined thickness of the anterior wall of the esophagus, the mediastinal soft tissue, and the posterior wall of the left main bronchus. In essence, the left retrobronchial stripe is a mediastinal opacity, whereas the left retrobronchial line represents a portion of the hilum as defined previously.

The anterior and posterior walls of the right lower lobe bronchus can be identified in about 10% of people, whereas the arcuate configuration of the anterior wall of the left lower lobe bronchus, merging with the orifice of the left upper lobe bronchus, is visible in about 45% (Fig. 2–19).[73] The middle lobe bronchus, the superior segmental bronchi, and the basilar bronchi can be identified in 5% of people.[73, 74]

There has been much confusion concerning the nomenclature of the hilar vasculature. A common misrepresentation has been to depict the right hilar opacity as the "right pulmonary artery." In reality, this vessel divides within the pericardium into ascending and descending (interlobar) branches; it is these branches that emerge from the mediastinum to comprise the true hilar arterial vessels (Fig. 2–20). The right superior pulmonary vein abuts the anterior aspect of the right interlobar artery; consequently, the right hilar complex is composed of the superior vein anteriorly, the ascending and descending arteries posteriorly, and surrounding areolar and nodal tissue. As on PA radiographs, dilation of the right superior pulmonary vein can produce a bulbous configuration of the anterior portion of the hilum, creating a vascular pseudotumor on lateral projection (Fig. 2–21).

The major portion of the left hilar vasculature is visible behind the intermediate stem line. The top of the left pulmonary artery is seen in about 95% of people,[73, 74] usually as a sharply marginated opacity above and behind the radiolucency of the left upper lobe bronchus. Immediately posterior to this bronchus is the left interlobar artery (Fig. 2–22). The left superior pulmonary vein, like its counterpart on the right, is closely associated with the arterial vasculature of the hilum; however, this vein is not a contour-forming vessel on conventional lateral radiographs and thus cannot be identified. Prominence of the left common or superior pulmonary venous confluence can result in impingement on and displacement of the left lower lobe bronchus superiorly and posteriorly both in normal people and when it becomes dilated as a result of postcapillary pulmonary hypertension.

The right and left inferior pulmonary veins are commonly imaged end-on as a result of their horizontal orientation, creating a nodular opacity below and behind the lower portion of the hila. Vessels can usually be identified converging toward the opacity, permitting its distinction from a true parenchymal mass.

Computed Tomography

CT is currently the imaging modality of choice for assessment of the hila. It provides a particularly detailed view, allowing the diagnosis of endobronchial lesions, hilar lymph node enlargement, parahilar masses, and vascular lesions. Optimal assessment requires a thorough understanding of normal cross-sectional anatomy.[77–80] It is also of paramount importance that the radiologist pay meticulous attention to the examination technique. In our opinion, noncontrast-enhanced scans suffice under most clinical circumstances; however, distinction of hilar masses or lymphadenopathy from vascular lesions and assessment of the extent of hilar tumors may require the use of an intravenous contrast agent. Optimal enhancement can be most readily obtained by using power injectors for the administration of the contrast agent and by obtaining multiple contiguous sections during a single breath hold with either dynamic incremental or spiral CT.[81–83] The patient should be examined in the supine position using contiguous 5- to 7-mm collimation scans; occasionally, thinner sections are needed. The scans should always be viewed in continuity; although self-evident, this procedure serves to diminish many of the well-known points of confusion that may arise from the viewing of an isolated scan. The study should be performed under the supervision of a radiologist and viewed with multiple windows and levels. The scans should be photographed using window levels appropriate for assessment of the airways and lung parenchyma (level -600 to -700 Hounsfield units [HU], width 1,000 to 2,000 HU) and for assessment of soft tissues (level 30 to 50 HU, width 350 to 500 HU).[83, 83a, 83b]

Anatomic features of the hila on CT can be conve-

Text continued on page 96

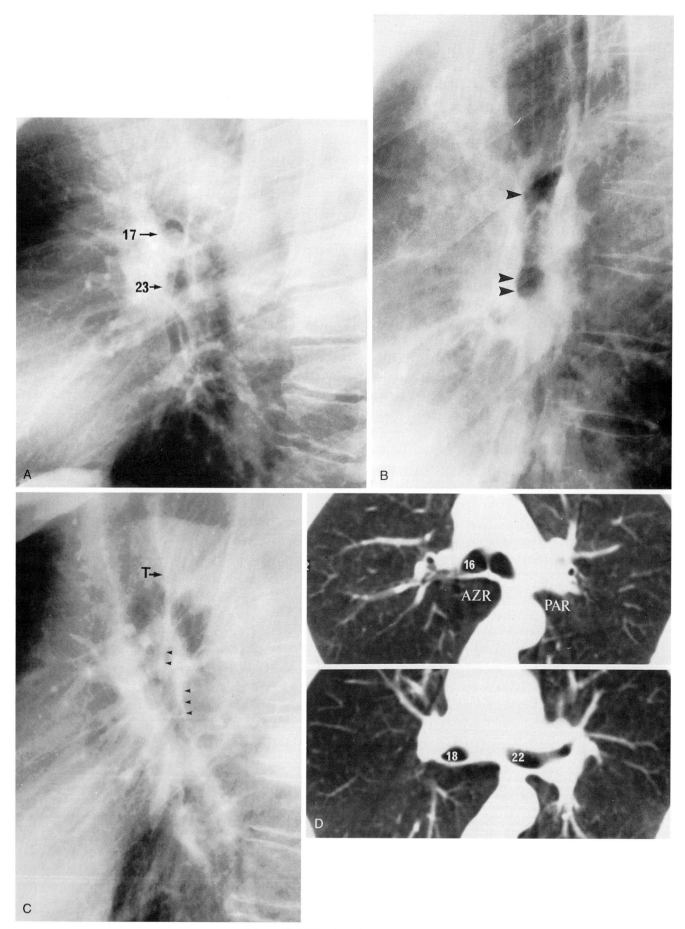

Figure 2–17 *See legend on opposite page*

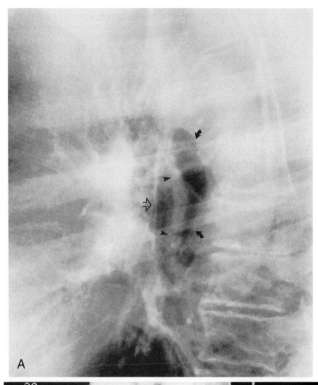

Figure 2–18. Left Retrobronchial Stripe. On this lateral chest radiograph *(A)*, there is a lenticular-shaped opacity *(arrowheads)*, 3- to 4-mm thick, behind the intermediate stem line *(open arrow)* in the anticipated location of the left retrobronchial line. Note the similar-shaped radiolucency *(curved arrows)* posterior to the stripe. Sagittal CT reformation *(B, top)* and transverse CT scans *(bottom)* reveal the anatomic basis for the left retrobronchial stripe. Note that gas within the left main bronchus (22) and esophagus (E) allows for silhouetting of the mediastinal portion of the left main bronchus, mediastinal soft tissue, and anterior wall of the esophagus—the left retrobronchial stripe. Gas in the esophagus accounts for the radiolucency behind the stripe. (The supine position of the patient on the CT scan as opposed to the upright position on the conventional chest radiograph accounts for the fluid level in the esophagus in *B*.)

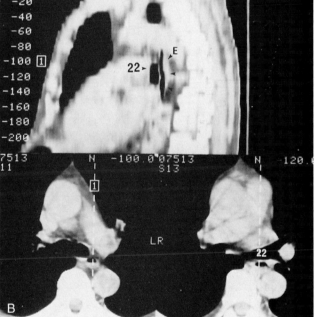

Figure 2–17. Hilar Anatomy on Lateral Chest Radiographs. The end-on orifices of the right (17) and left (23) upper lobe bronchi *(A)* can be easily identified. Although the left hilum is normally located cephalad to the right, the right upper lobe bronchus projects cephalad to its counterpart on the left. A detail view from a conventional lateral chest radiograph *(B)* reveals exceptional clarity of the right *(arrowhead)* and left *(two arrowheads)* upper lobe bronchi. This appearance should suggest an excessive quantity of soft tissue surrounding the respective bronchial lumina, the most common cause of which is hilar node enlargement, as in this patient with Hodgkin's disease. In another subject, a lateral chest radiograph *(C)* demonstrates the posterior tracheal stripe (T), intermediate stem line *(two arrowheads)*, and left retrobronchial line *(three arrowheads)*. On a true lateral view, the intermediate stem line may be straight or gently convex forward and characteristically bisects the orifice of the left upper lobe bronchus. CT scans through the carina *(top)* and 2 cm caudad *(bottom)* *(D)* reveal the anatomic prerequisites underlying the features described in *C*. Aerated lung in the azygoesophageal recess (AZR) and the preaortic recess (PAR) abut the posterior wall of the right main (16) and intermediate (18) bronchi and the posterior wall of the left main bronchus (22), respectively. Essentially, the intermediate stem line and the left retrobronchial line, representing the posterior wall of their respective bronchi, are rendered visible by an intrabronchial and intrapulmonary air envelope.

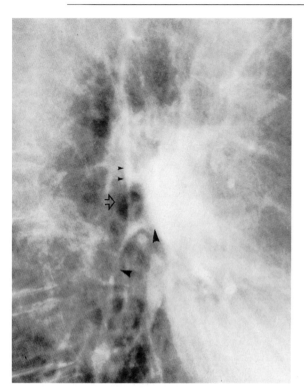

Figure 2–19. Hilar Anatomy in Lateral Projection. On a detail view from a lateral radiograph there is a curvilinear (reversed comma-shaped) opacity *(large arrowheads)* anteroinferior to the end-on orifice of the distal left main or proximal left upper lobe bronchus *(open arrow)*; this opacity represents, in succession, the inferior or anterior wall of the lingular bronchus, the left main bronchus, and the left lower lobe bronchus. The right-sided intermediate stem line *(small arrowheads)* bisects the bronchial lumen.

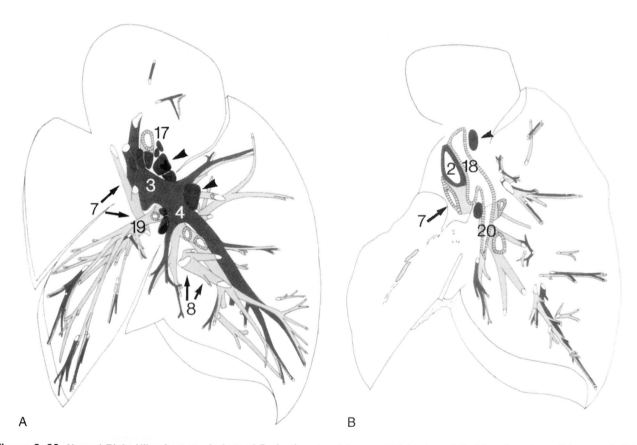

A   B

Figure 2–20. Normal Right Hilar Anatomy in Lateral Projection. *A* and *B* are sagittal drawings of the hilum from the medial aspect, depicting the hilar bronchi (17, 18, 19, 20), pulmonary arteries (2, 3, 4), and pulmonary veins (7, 8). Several small lymph nodes *(arrowheads)* are included in the illustration. The anterior contour of the right hilum is formed by the ascending (3) and the horizontal limb of the interlobar (4) pulmonary arteries; the hilum relates to the front of the intermediate bronchus (18) above and the superior pulmonary vein (7) below. The inferior pulmonary vein (8) relates to the lower lobe bronchi.

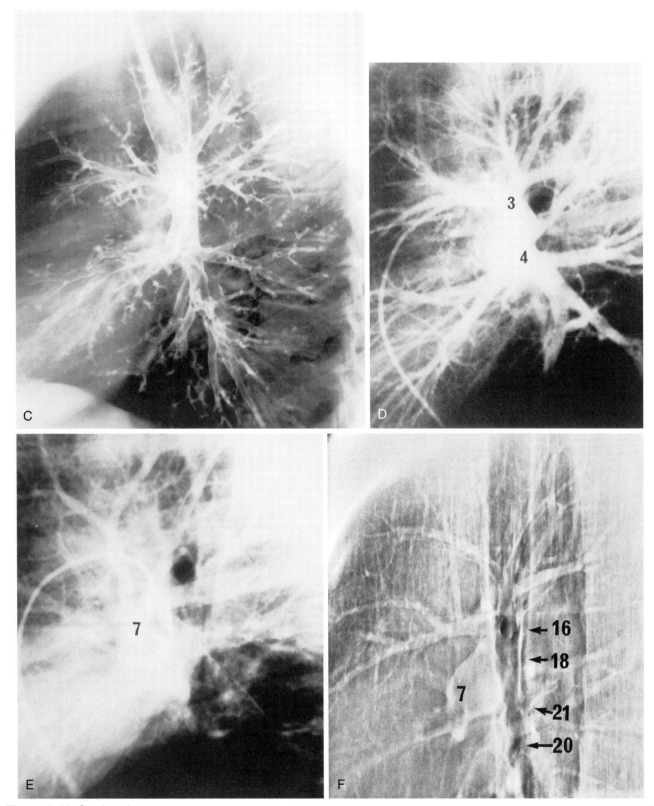

Figure 2–20 *Continued.* A right lateral tracheobronchogram *(C)* and a selective right pulmonary angiogram during the arterial *(D)* and venous *(E)* phases show the right superior vein (7) to lie anterior to the ascending (3) and descending (4) pulmonary arteries. (The catheter is in the right pulmonary artery.) On a right lateral xerotomogram *(F)*, the posterior wall of the right main (16) and intermediate (18) bronchi unite to form the intermediate stem line, which terminates at the origin of the superior segmental bronchus (21) to the lower lobe (20). The right superior pulmonary vein (7) defines the anterior contour of the right hilum. (From Genereux GP: Am J Roentgenol 141:1241, 1983.)

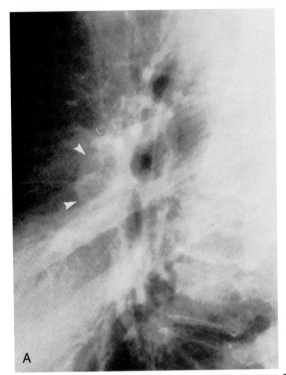

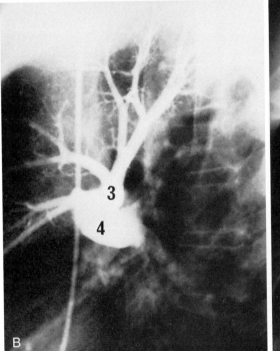

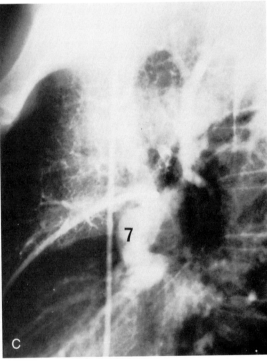

Figure 2–21. Venous Pseudotumor of the Right Hilum. A lateral chest radiograph *(A)* suggests the presence of a small mass *(arrowheads)* in the right hilum. A selective distal right pulmonary angiogram in lateral projection during the arterial *(B)* and venous *(C)* phases shows that the hilar pseudotumor is caused by overlap of the right superior pulmonary vein (7) on the distal right artery (3, 4).

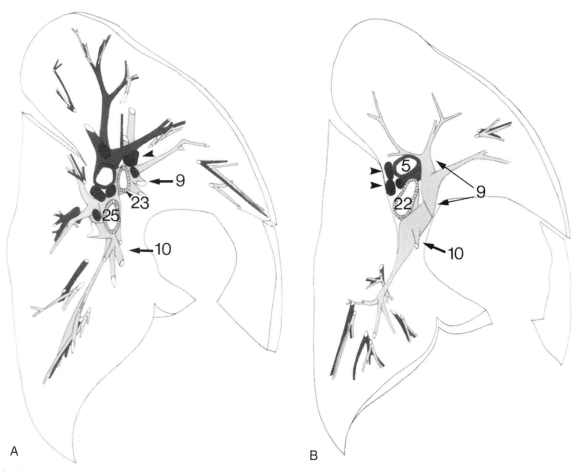

A

B

Figure 2–22. Normal Left Hilar Anatomy in Lateral Projection. Sagittal drawings of the left hilum from the medial aspect *(A and B)* depict the hilar bronchi (22, 25), left pulmonary artery (LPA) (5), and pulmonary veins (9, 10). Several small lymph nodes *(arrowheads)* are included. The entire anterior convexity of the left hilum relates to the superior pulmonary vein (9) in front of the LPA (5) and left main bronchus (22). The relationship of the left inferior vein (10) to the left lower lobe bronchus (25) is shown.

Illustration continued on following page

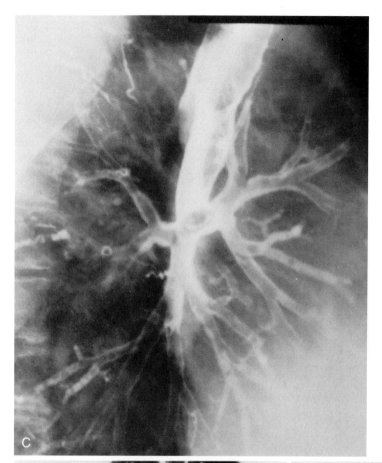

Figure 2–22 *Continued.* A lateral projection of a left tracheobronchogram *(C)* and a selective left pulmonary angiogram during the arterial *(D)* and venous *(E)* phases show that the superoposterior contour of the hilum is formed by the LPA (5) and proximal interlobar (6) artery. In this subject, the left superior (9) and inferior (10) veins coalesce to form a common chamber prior to entering the left atrium (14).

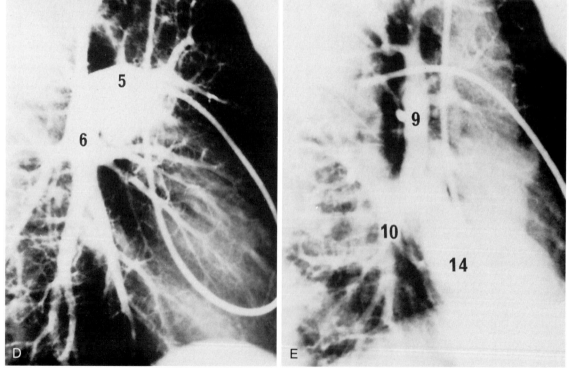

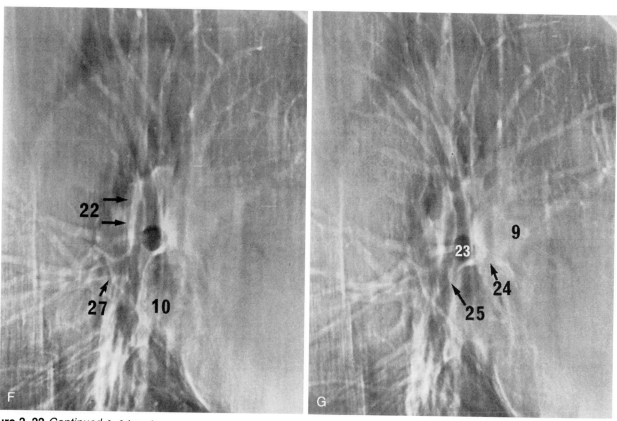

Figure 2–22 *Continued.* Left lateral xerotomograms *(F* and *G)* demonstrate the posterior wall of the left main (22) and lower lobe bronchi terminating at the origin of the superior segmental bronchus (27) of the lower lobe (25). The anteroinferior walls of the lingular (24) and contiguous lower lobe bronchi are devoid of soft tissue. The circular lumen of the left upper lobe bronchus (23) is shown. The left superior (9) and inferior (10) pulmonary veins relate to the anterior hilum and the lower lobe bronchus, respectively. (*A* to *G* from Genereux GP: Am J Roentgenol 141:1241, 1983.)

niently described by examining a series of horizontal planes or levels (Fig. 2–23).[77, 78] When no intravenous contrast agent is used, the anatomy is best assessed on the lung windows by relating the various structures to the bronchi.

Level I (supracarinal trachea, Fig. 2–23*B*). On the *right,* the circular apical pulmonary artery lies medial to the radiolucent end-on apical bronchus; the apical pulmonary vein is situated lateral to this bronchoarterial bundle. On the *left,* the apicoposterior bronchus and artery are seen; the apical and anterior veins lie in front and medial to the bronchus and artery.

Level II (carina/right upper lobe bronchus, Fig. 2–23*C*). On the *right,* the upper lobe bronchus divides into the horizontally oriented anterior and posterior segmental bronchi. In front of the main bronchus and upper lobe bronchus is the ascending branch of the right pulmonary artery; its anterior segmental branch parallels the bronchus medially or superiorly. The right superior pulmonary vein is invariably identified immediately lateral to the site at which the anterior and posterior segmental bronchi divide. In some patients, a small vein from the anterior and apical portion of the upper lobe can be seen in front of the ascending artery.

On the *left,* the circular apicoposterior bronchus and artery are located immediately lateral to the left pulmonary artery. The superior pulmonary vein is situated in front of and medial to the bronchus and artery.

Level III (proximal intermediate bronchus/left upper lobe bronchus, Fig. 2–23*D*). On the *right,* the intermediate bronchus is covered anteriorly by the horizontal limb of the interlobar artery and laterally by the vertical limb of the same vessel. The superior pulmonary vein abuts the junction between the horizontal and vertical components of the interlobar artery, creating a typical "elephant head-and-trunk" configuration.

On the *left,* the distal main and upper lobe bronchial continuum is seen. Frequently, the end-on radiolucency of the superior division of the upper lobe can be identified. The proximal portion of the interlobar artery forms a shallow indentation on the posterior aspect of the upper lobe bronchus. Partial volume averaging through the left pulmonary artery as it crosses cephalad to the left main bronchus frequently causes a subtle "graying" to the normally radiolucent bronchial lumen. Medial to the interlobar artery, air in the superior segment of the left lower lobe may abut the posterior wall of the left main bronchus, creating the CT "retrobronchial stripe."[76]

Level IV (distal intermediate bronchus/lingular bronchus, Fig. 2–23*E*). On the *right,* the anatomic features are similar to those of Level III. On the *left,* the proximal portion of the lingular bronchus is separated from the end-on orifice of the lower lobe bronchus by the lingular carina. The superior segmental bronchus to the lower lobe arises posteriorly. The left interlobar artery is situated lateral to the carina separating the lingular bronchus from the lower lobe bronchus. As it enters the mediastinum, the superior pulmonary vein is joined by the lingular vein in front of and medial to the lingular bronchus.

Level V (middle lobe bronchus, Fig. 2–23*F*). On the *right,* the horizontal middle lobe bronchus courses obliquely into the middle lobe, where it divides after a centimeter or so into the medial and lateral segmental bronchi; posteriorly, the orifice of the lower lobe bronchus can be seen end-on,

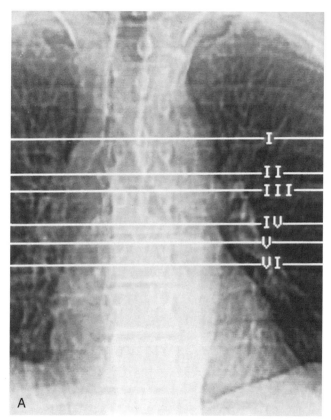

Figure 2–23. Normal CT Hilar Anatomy. On a scoutview of the thorax *(A),* the bars indicate the appropriate levels for *B* through *G.*

divided by a distinct carina or lateral spur. The superior segmental bronchus to the lower lobe arises at or slightly superior to this level and passes posterolaterally for a few millimeters before dividing into two subsegmental bronchi. The vertical part of the interlobar artery is situated posterolateral to the middle lobe bronchus and anterolateral to the lower lobe bronchus as it enters lung parenchyma. The middle lobe artery or vein may be identified lateral to the middle lobe bronchus; the termination of the superior pulmonary vein is located anteromedial to this airway.

On the *left,* the end-on lumen of the lower lobe bronchus is seen medial to the contiguous interlobar artery. Occasionally, a portion of the inferior pulmonary vein can be identified posteromedial to this bronchus.

Level VI (basilar lower lobe bronchi/inferior pulmonary veins, Fig. 2–23*G*). On 10-mm collimation CT images, segmental bronchi in the lower lobes are identified in 60% to 90% of cases on the right and 30% to 80% on the left.[84] On the *right,* the medial segmental bronchus, the first branch to be identified, is characteristically located in front of the horizontal inferior pulmonary vein. The anterior, lateral, and posterior basilar bronchi arise in succession to supply their respective segments. On the *left,* the anteromedial segmental bronchus is located anterior to the inferior pulmonary vein; the lateral and posterior segmental bronchi may be identified behind this vessel.

Magnetic Resonance Imaging

MR imaging differs from CT scanning in several important aspects. Whereas CT evaluates only one tissue

Text continued on page 101

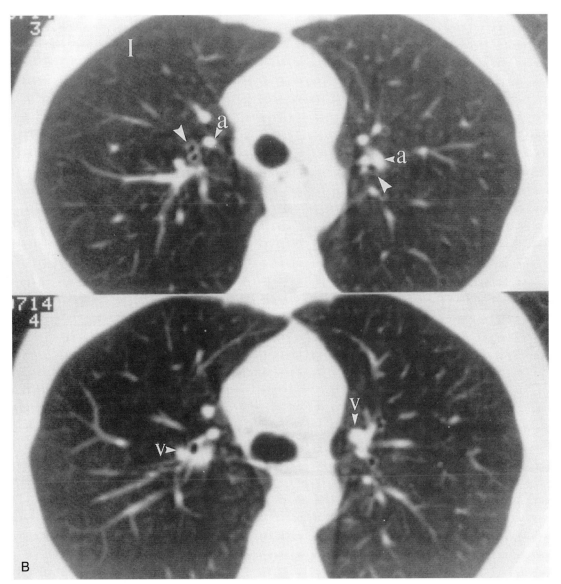

Figure 2–23 *Continued.* In *level I* (supracarinal trachea) *(B)*, the apical bronchus *(arrowhead)*, artery (a), and vein (v) are depicted on the right, and the apicoposterior bronchus *(arrowhead)*, artery (a), and vein (v) are on the left.

Illustration continued on following page

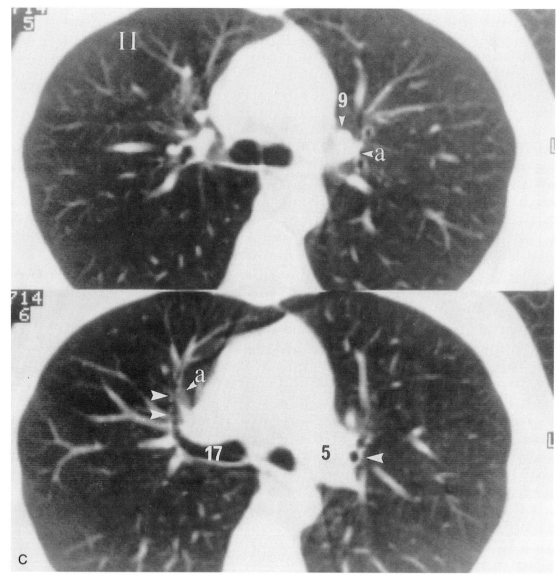

Figure 2–23 _Continued._ In _level II_ (carina/right upper lobe bronchus) _(C)_, the upper lobe bronchus (17), anterior segmental bronchus _(two arrowheads)_, and artery (a) are shown on the right; on the left, the apicoposterior bronchus _(arrowhead)_ and artery (a) are stationed immediately lateral to the left pulmonary artery (5). The left superior pulmonary vein (9) is located anteromedial to the bronchoarterial bundle.

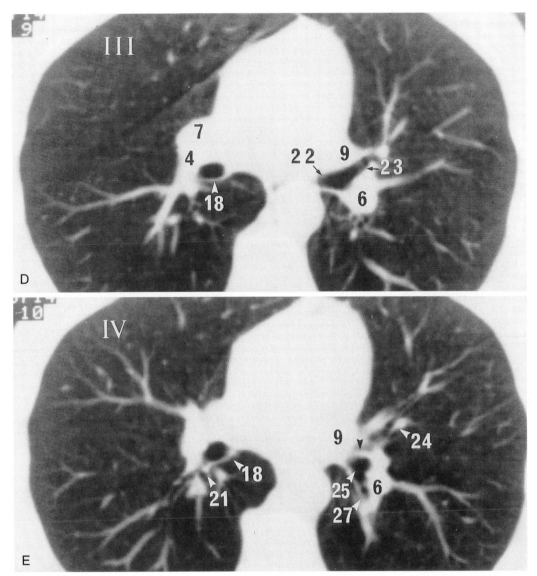

Figure 2–23 *Continued.* In *level III* (proximal intermediate bronchus/left upper lobe bronchus) *(D)*, on the right, the intermediate bronchus (18) is covered anteriorly and laterally by the interlobar artery (4). The right superior pulmonary vein (7) relates closely to the interlobar artery, creating a typical "elephant head-and-trunk" configuration. On the left, the distal main (22) and upper lobe (23) bronchial continuum is seen. Note the shallow indentation on the anterior and posterior wall of the upper lobe bronchus created by the mediastinal component of the left superior vein (9) and the proximal interlobar artery (6). In *level IV* (distal intermediate bronchus/lingular bronchus) *(E)*, the intermediate bronchus (18) and the superior segmental bronchus (21) of the lower lobe can be identified on the right, and the lingular bronchus (24) separated by the lingular spur *(arrowhead)* from the end-on orifice of the lower lobe bronchus (25) is seen on the left. The superior segmental bronchus (27) lies posteriorly, the interlobar artery (6) posterolaterally, and the left superior pulmonary vein (9) anteromedially.

Illustration continued on following page

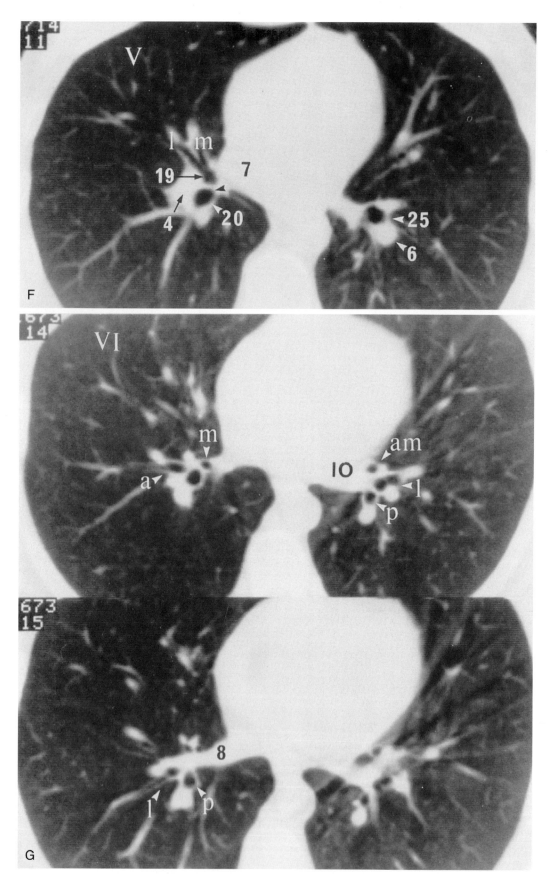

Figure 2–23 *Continued.* In *level V, (F)*, the middle lobe bronchus (19) divides into medial (m) and lateral (l) segmental bronchi. The lower lobe bronchus (20) is separated from the middle lobe bronchus by a distinct spur or carina *(arrowheads)*. The right superior pulmonary vein (7) lies anteromedial to the middle lobe bronchus and the interlobar artery (4) anterolateral to the lower lobe bronchus. On the left, the interlobar artery (6) lies posterolateral to the lower lobe bronchus (25). In *level VI* (basilar lower lobe bronchi/inferior pulmonary veins) *(G)*, on the right, the medial (m), anterior (a), lateral (l), and posterior (p) segmental bronchi relate closely to the inferior pulmonary vein (8). On the left, the anteromedial (am), lateral (l), and posterior (p) segmental bronchi relate to the left inferior pulmonary vein (10).

parameter—electron density—the intensity of the MR image depends on four parameters: nuclear density and motion, and two relaxation times (T1 and T2). Signal intensity within hilar vessels depends on the MR technique being used and on the phase of the cardiac cycle.[85–87] With standard spin-echo technique, rapidly flowing blood produces little or no signal. Thus, a signal void is obtained on MR images gated to cardiac systole (Fig. 2–24).[88] This "flow-void" phenomenon is particularly advantageous in distinguishing a vessel from a mass,[89, 90] such as an enlarged lymph node, which has a high-signal intensity on MR. Such distinction may be difficult on noncontrast CT scan, although it is usually readily made with the use of an intravenous contrast agent and dynamic or spiral scanning. Because the spatial orientation of the image is determined by manipulation of magnetic fields, MR imaging is more adaptable in the display of sagittal and coronal planes without relying on the reformat-

ting of multiple slices, as is necessary with CT scanning (Figs. 2–25 and 2–26).[91, 92]

Pulmonary vessels can also be imaged using specialized flow-sensitive spin-echo or gradient-echo sequences,[86, 93, 94] in which flowing blood produces a signal that is proportional to the mean velocity of pulsatile flow within the pulmonary arteries.[87] In addition to visualizing flowing blood, cine MR imaging using these sequences allows assessment of dynamic flow-related information and dynamic evaluation of hilar vessels. Central pulmonary arteries and veins not only show changes in diameter but also move during the cardiac cycle;[87] for example, during systole the main pulmonary artery increases in diameter, rotates, and moves backward.[87, 94] MR imaging therefore has several potential advantages over CT scanning. The main limitation of MR imaging in the assessment of the hila is its lower spatial resolution when compared with CT. Although CT scanning allows

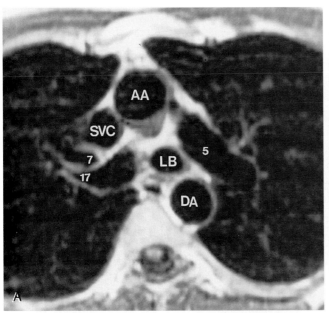

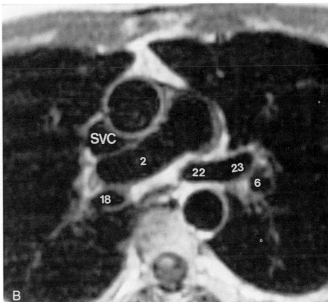

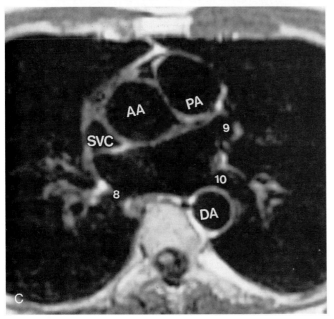

Figure 2–24. Anatomy of the Mediastinum and Hila. Anatomy of the mediastinum and hila on cross-sectional MR images transverse spin-echo (TR 810/TE 15) scans from cephalad *(A)* to caudad *(C)* from a normal subject. Note that blood within vessels has low signal intensity—the "flow-void" phenomenon. Transverse MR image *(A)* is shown at the level of the right upper lobe bronchus (17). The right superior pulmonary vein (7) is situated immediately anterior to the right upper lobe bronchus and posterolateral to the superior vena cava (SVC). The left pulmonary artery (5) is situated superior and lateral to the left main bronchus (LB). Also seen are the ascending (AA) and descending (DA) aorta. At a slightly lower level *(B)*, the right pulmonary artery (2) can be seen between the intermediate bronchus (18) and the superior vena cava (SVC). At this level, the left interlobar pulmonary artery (6) lies behind the distal main (22) and upper lobe (23) bronchial continuum. More caudad *(C)*, the left superior pulmonary vein (9), the left inferior pulmonary vein (10), and right inferior pulmonary vein (8) can be seen entering the left atrium. Also seen are the superior vena cava (SVC), ascending (AA) and descending (DA) aorta, and the main pulmonary artery (PA).

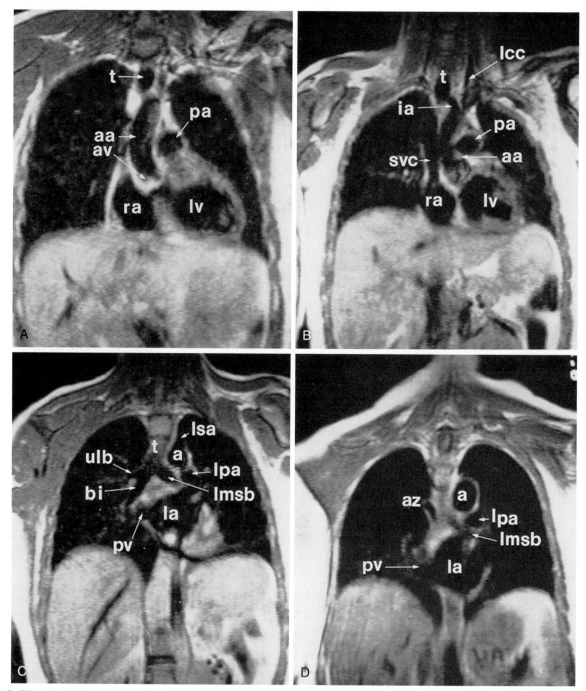

Figure 2–25. Anatomy of the Mediastinum and Hila on Coronal MR Images. Normal coronal SE 1000/30 scans from anterior *(A)* to posterior *(D)*. aa, ascending aorta; t, trachea; av, aortic valve; pa, pulmonary artery; ra, right atrium; lv, left ventricle; svc, superior vena cava; ta, truncus anterior; rpa, right pulmonary artery; lpa, left pulmonary artery; la, left atrium; ivc, inferior vena cava; lsa, left subclavian artery; ulb, upper lobe bronchus; bi, intermediate bronchi; pv, pulmonary vein; lmsb, left main bronchus; az, azygos vein; ia, innominate artery; lcc, left common carotid artery. (From O'Donovan PB, Ross JS, Sivak ED, et al: Am J Roentgenol 143:1183, 1984. © American Roentgen Ray Society.)

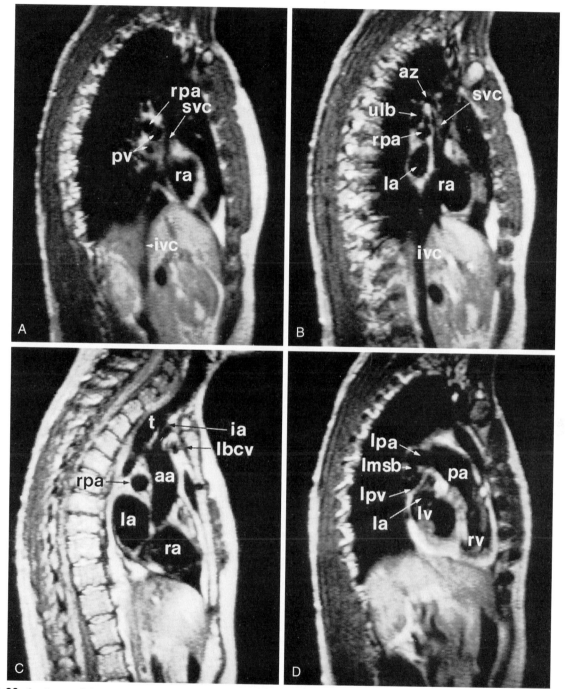

Figure 2–26. Anatomy of the Mediastinum and Hila on Sagittal MR Images. Normal sagittal SE 1000/30 scans of the hila and mediastinum from right *(A)* to left *(D)*. (*See* Figure 2–25 for appropriate anatomic designations.) (From O'Donovan PB, Ross JS, Sivak ED, et al: Am J Roentgenol 143:1183, 1984. © American Roentgen Ray Society.)

routine demonstration of segmental and subsegmental bronchi, identification of these airways is often difficult or impossible on MR images.[95, 96]

Function

Perfusion of the Acinar Unit

Pulmonary blood volume (PBV) is defined as the volume of blood within the pulmonary arteries, pulmonary capillaries, pulmonary veins, and an indeterminate portion of the left atrium. When measured with a dye technique in 15 normal subjects, it ranged from 204 to 314 ml/m² of body surface area (mean, 271 ml/m²),[98] indicating that the amount of blood in the lungs at any one time is about 10% of total blood volume. The capillary blood volume (Vc)—which represents about 20% to 25% of the PBV—is estimated to be 60 to 140 ml in the resting subject, increasing to 150 to 250 ml during exercise.[97–102] These figures, which have been largely calculated by measuring carbon monoxide uptake by intracapillary erythrocytes, closely agree with estimates made by anatomic techniques.[103, 104] This may be interpreted as indicating that the capillary vascular bed, the surface area of which measures 70 to 100 m², is maximally distended during peak exercise.[102]

Despite the fact that the pulmonary vasculature handles the same cardiac output as the systemic circulation, the mean pulmonary arterial pressure is only 14 mm Hg. The caliber of the pulmonary vessels is influenced by the transmural pressure, which is the difference between intravascular pressure and the pressure in the space or tissue surrounding the vessel. The transmural vascular pressure for the large extrapulmonary vessels and cardiac chambers is the intravascular or intracavitary pressure minus intrapleural pressure; for "extra-alveolar" intraparenchymal vessels, it is intravascular minus interstitial pressure; and for the "alveolar" vessels, it is intravascular minus alveolar pressure. In upright subjects at rest, the driving pressure in the pulmonary circulation is the difference between arterial and pulmonary venous pressure in the lower part of the lung (Zone 3, *see* page 105) and the difference between arterial and alveolar pressure in the upper part of the lung (Zones 1 and 2).

The controversial issue of measurement of pulmonary capillary pressure has been extensively reviewed.[105] Although human capillary pressure cannot be measured directly, microvascular pressure has been measured in isolated and *in situ* animal lungs.[106, 107] These studies show that the bulk of the resistance is in small vessels (45% to 70% between arterioles 50 to 60 μm in diameter and venules 20 to 30 μm in diameter) and that as much as 45% of the resistance is in the alveolar wall capillaries themselves. However, controversy exists as to the relative contributions of arterial, capillary, and venous resistance to total pulmonary vascular resistance. When pulmonary vascular resistance is partitioned into arterial, venous, and "middle" (capillary) compartments using a rapid occlusion technique, the "capillary" compartment accounts for only about 15% of total resistance, the rest being shared equally between arterial and venous compartments.[108] Pulmonary capillary pressure can also be estimated in intact humans and animals using a rapid-occlusion technique.[107, 109] This technique involves

back-extrapolation to time 0 of the exponential decline in pulmonary arterial pressure that occurs distal to the obstruction.[110] Pulmonary capillary pressure can be changed by hypoxia, sepsis, cardiac disease, or inflammatory mediators that cause changes in the relative importance of pulmonary arterial and venous resistance.[111]

Whatever the true capillary pressure, it must exceed left atrial pressure for flow to occur. A reasonable normal value is 9 cm H_2O,[107] there being a gradient from the arteriolar to the venous end of the microvessels that is dependent on their resistance. Pulmonary capillary wedge pressure reflects the pressure in large veins or the left atrium rather than that in the capillaries themselves; since flow is transiently interrupted during measurement of the wedge pressure, there is no resistive pressure drop downstream from the point of occlusion.[112]

Since the colloidal osmotic pressure is 25 to 30 mm Hg, under normal resting conditions a considerable force keeps the alveoli dry; even during maximal exercise, when cardiac output increases to 25 to 30 liters per minute in healthy subjects, the hydrostatic pressure does not exceed the osmotic pressure.

The hemodynamics of the pulmonary circulation cannot be deduced on the basis of laws that relate to a rigid tubular system. Like the tracheobronchial tree, the circulatory system is distensible; it branches and bends, is subject to changing pressure on its walls, and has a pressure at each end, either or both of which may vary in degree in certain circumstances. Although flow is pulsatile, it is probably always laminar in small vessels and sometimes turbulent in larger ones. When the left atrial pressure and transpulmonary (alveolar minus intrapleural) pressures are constant, an increase in pulmonary artery pressure causes vessels to distend (transmural pressure increase). As with the airways, doubling or halving the radius causes a 16-fold change in resistance; in this situation, as cardiac output increases, vessels widen and closed capillaries open, leading to a fall in resistance.[113, 114]

The calculation of pulmonary vascular resistance is complicated by the fact that the pressure-flow relationship in the pulmonary vasculature does not have a zero-flow intercept; that is, flow does not immediately increase when pulmonary artery pressure exceeds zero (Fig. 2–27). There is a critical opening pressure in the pulmonary vasculature below which there is no flow. Once this pressure is exceeded, there is progressive opening (recruitment) of pulmonary vessels; when they are fully recruited, the pressure-flow curve is linear. However, the presence of a critical opening pressure makes comparison of pulmonary vascular resistance at different cardiac outputs difficult. As shown in the example in Figure 2–27, there is an apparent decrease in pulmonary vascular resistance as cardiac output is increased from A (∼ 5 liters per minute) to B (∼ 15 liters per minute), although the pressure-flow curve between these two cardiac outputs is linear. This means that a decrease in pulmonary vascular resistance as cardiac output is increased cannot be interpreted as an indication of vascular dilation.

Factors Influencing the Pulmonary Circulation

Gravity

Gravity has an influence on the distribution of blood flow in the lung by altering regional vascular transmural

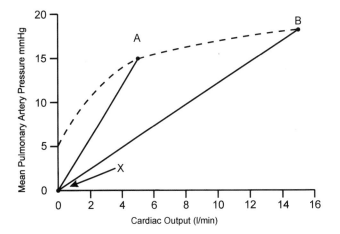

Figure 2–27. Pulmonary Vascular Pressure-Flow Curves. Mean pulmonary artery pressure (PAP) is plotted against cardiac output. The relationship between pressure and flow is curvilinear, as shown by the dashed line. There is a critical pressure that must be achieved before flow is initiated (5 mm Hg in this example). A normal cardiac output of ~5 1/min occurs with a PAP of ~15 mm Hg (Point A), and a large increase in cardiac output beyond this point is associated with only a slight increase in PAP. (Between A and B, cardiac output increases from 5 to 15 1/min, while PAP increases from 15 to 18 mm Hg.) The slope of the lines AX and BX represents pulmonary vascular resistance, which decreases as cardiac output increases.

pressures and therefore vascular diameters. The distribution of flow is largely governed by the relationship among arterial, alveolar, and venous pressures (Fig. 2–28) and can be understood by considering the lungs as a series of zones.[115, 116]

The lung measures approximately 30 cm from apex to base. The pulmonary artery enters the lung at the hilum, which is positioned at about the middle of the lung. Since a column of blood 15-cm high is equivalent to a column of mercury 11-mm high, in the erect subject gravity affects the

intravascular pressure to the extent that systolic, diastolic, and mean pressures are reduced by 11 mm Hg at the apex and are increased by 11 mm Hg at the base. If pulmonary arterial pressure in the hilar vessels is taken as 20/9 mm Hg, it follows that pressure at the extreme apex will be 9/−2 mm Hg and at the base, 31/20 mm Hg. Since the pulmonary veins enter the left atrium at approximately the same level as the arteries, there is a similar and proportional variation in venous pressure.

These gravity-dependent changes in intravascular pressure result in regional differences in the capillary transmural pressure. Since extraluminal capillary pressure averages 0 (atmospheric), apical vessels are virtually closed, at least during diastole; in these regions, the pulmonary vasculature acts as a Starling resistor, in which the pertinent driving pressure is the difference between arterial and alveolar pressures (Zone 1) (*see* Fig. 2–28). Further down the lung, pulmonary artery pressure exceeds alveolar pressure throughout the cardiac cycle, but alveolar pressure still exceeds venous pressure, resulting in a narrowing of capillaries at their downstream venous end (Zone 2). Even further down the lung, both arterial and venous pressures exceed alveolar pressure, and the vasculature progressively dilates as the lung base is approached (Zone 3).

At the base of the lung, blood flow decreases once more—a phenomenon that has led to the concept of Zone 4. This basilar increase in pulmonary vascular resistance has been observed in both intact dogs and humans,[117, 118] but at present there is no adequate explanation for it. Although it was originally postulated that the increased resistance at the base of the lung was caused by a decrease in the diameter of extra-alveolar vessels secondary to the gravity-dependent decrease in lung volume at the base, experiments in dogs relating regional vascular resistance and regional lung volume have cast doubt on this hypothesis.[117] The extent of Zone 4 in humans can be decreased by infusing the pulmonary vasodilator nitroprusside, suggesting a role for vascular tone in the flow reduction.[118]

Figure 2–28. Regional Blood Flow in the Lung as Determined by the Relationship Between Alveolar (A), Pulmonary Arterial (a), and Pulmonary Venous (v) Pressures. At the apex, where pulmonary arterial and venous pressure may be subatmospheric, alveolar pressure will compress alveolar microvessels, increase resistance, and decrease flow (Zone 1). Lower in the lung, pulmonary arterial pressure exceeds alveolar pressure but alveolar pressure still exceeds the subatmospheric venous pressure, and vessel caliber and flow depend on the difference between arterial and alveolar pressure (Zone 2). Nearer the base of the lung, arterial and venous pressures exceed alveolar pressure, dilating microvessels and further increasing flow (Zone 3). At the lung base (Zone 4), a region of decreased flow exists that cannot be simply explained by the relationship of Pa, PA, and Pv.

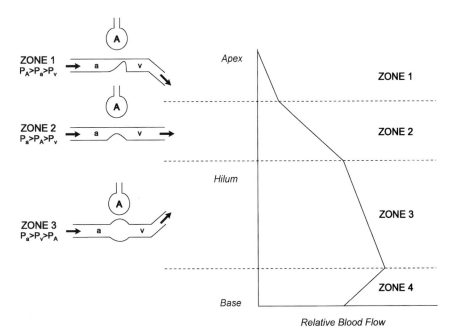

There is also a centrifugal gradient in the distribution of blood flow. When it is expressed as flow per unit of lung tissue, the central portion of the lung is better perfused than the peripheral tissue.[119, 120] However, the gravity-dependent and centrifugal gradients of pulmonary blood flow account for only a small part of the pulmonary blood flow heterogeneity.[119, 121] The spatial distribution of blood flow conforms to a fractal pattern in that lung units close to each other have more similar values for blood flow than more distant units.[122–124] The significance of this nongravitational heterogeneity is unclear. The functionally important heterogeneity is ventilation/perfusion heterogeneity, and in studies where it has been examined, regional $\dot{V}/\dot{Q}$ shows little nongravitational variation, suggesting that the nongravitational heterogeneity of perfusion is matched by a similar heterogeneity of ventilation.[125]

Intrapleural Pressure and Lung Volume

The pulmonary vasculature can be considered in two compartments—extra-alveolar and alveolar—based on its response to changes in lung volume.[126, 127] The former comprises the arteries and veins whose extraluminal pressure consists of pleural and/or interstitial pressure; they respond to such pressure by tending to dilate as lung volume increases. Alveolar vessels are microvessels that respond to alveolar pressure as their extraluminal pressure; they tend to be compressed as the lung is inflated. The interactions between these two compartments with change in lung volume cause complex alterations in the distribution of the PBV and pulmonary vascular resistance. When pulmonary arterial pressure is held constant relative to alveolar pressure (constant zonal conditions), pulmonary vascular resistance initially falls with lung inflation but then rises at high lung volumes, presumably as a result of lengthening of extra-alveolar vessels.[128] When pulmonary artery pressure is not held constant relative to alveolar pressure, the effects on alveolar vessels predominate and pulmonary vascular resistance rises steeply with lung inflation.[129, 130]

It is possible to perfuse the lung slowly even when alveolar pressure substantially exceeds pulmonary artery pressure, because of the patency of the "corner vessels"; these microvessels are situated at the junction of alveolar septa and, although anatomically alveolar, are functionally extra-alveolar.[131, 132]

Neurogenic and Chemical Effects

In addition to the pressure and volume changes that passively influence the pulmonary vasculature, neurogenic, humoral, blood gas, and blood chemistry changes can result in vasomotion that modifies the circulation to acinar units. The alterations in vascular tone and diameter can occur generally throughout the lung or, more important, on a regional basis, altering blood flow distribution and thus affecting regional ventilation/perfusion relationships. In addition, vasoconstriction or dilation may occur upstream (arterial) or downstream (venous) from the capillaries, resulting in varying relationships between regional blood volume and blood flow as well as modification of the hydrostatic pressure in the capillaries.

Hypoxia has important physiologic effects on pulmo-nary vessels. The effect is predominantly local, since the vasoconstrictor response is present in denervated lungs and indeed in excised perfused lungs.[133] The magnitude of hypoxia-induced pulmonary vasoconstriction is influenced by the initial vascular tone, the level of sympathetic stimulation, and the amount of vascular smooth muscle.[134] Despite its obvious importance in both the normal regulation of blood flow and the pathophysiology of pulmonary hypertensive states, the mechanism of hypoxic vasoconstriction has remained elusive. Most evidence suggests that it is the local alveolar PO_2 that provides the major stimulus, although mixed venous PO_2 may also influence the response.[135]

The mystery lies in whether a locally released mediator or hypoxia itself is the important effector. Numerous mediators have been proposed, of which histamine has been a persistent suspect;[134] however, hypoxia causes increased resistance in capillary and precapillary vessels, whereas histamine acts predominantly on the venous side of the capillary bed.[136–138] Endothelin 1, a potent pulmonary vasoconstrictor produced by the vascular endothelium, appears not to be the mediator.[139] Postulated mechanisms for the direct effect of hypoxia on smooth muscle include alterations in membrane permeability to calcium, effects on potassium channels, or direct effects on the energetics of the contractile process itself.[134, 140] Similar to the systemic vascular endothelium, the pulmonary endothelium can synthesize the potent vascular dilator nitric oxide (NO) from L-arginine.[141, 142] NO and the vasodilator prostaglandin I_2 (prostacyclin) are both produced by the pulmonary vascular endothelium and can modulate the degree of hypoxic vasoconstriction.[143, 144] In conditions associated with chronic pulmonary hypoxic vasoconstriction there may be impairment of pulmonary endothelial NO production that contributes to the pulmonary hypertension.[143] Some pulmonary arterial vasodilators such as acetylcholine and vasopressin act by releasing NO from the vascular endothelium.[145]

Increased hydrogen ion concentration, whether induced by hypercapnia or metabolic acidosis, also produces pulmonary vasoconstriction by a separate mechanism and interacts with hypoxia in increasing pulmonary arterial pressure.[146, 147]

The pulmonary vessels receive a rich innervation from the pulmonary plexuses that are formed by a mingling of fibers from the sympathetic trunk and vagus. Appropriate staining techniques show both parasympathetic and catecholamine-containing fibers supplying vessels down to 30 μm in diameter, with relative sparsity on the venous side of the circulation.[148] Although stimulation of sympathetic nerves in intact animals results in increased pulmonary vascular resistance and decreased compliance of large pulmonary vessels, little is known about afferent input that could produce such reflex changes.[148] Parenterally administered neurotransmitters have more pronounced effects on pulmonary vascular resistance: epinephrine, norepinephrine, serotonin, histamine, and prostaglandin F_2 vasoconstrict, whereas β agonists and acetylcholine result in vasodilation.[149] Using the arterial and venous occlusion technique, serotonin, sympathetic stimulation, and prostaglandin F_2 have been shown to act predominantly on precapillary vessels, whereas the vasoconstrictive effects of infused histamine and norepinephrine and of increased cerebrospinal fluid pressure act predominantly on venules.[136, 137]

Diffusion of Gas from Acini to Red Blood Cells

Diffusion in the Acini

Diffusion of a gas occurs passively from an area of higher partial pressure to one of lower partial pressure. The rate of such diffusion is dependent on the medium in which the diffusion takes place. In a gaseous medium, it is related to density, a light gas diffusing faster than a heavier one; in liquid or tissue, it is largely dependent on solubility of the particular gas in that medium. Since oxygen is slightly lighter than carbon dioxide, it diffuses more rapidly in acinar gas. By contrast, in water and tissue, carbon dioxide is more soluble than oxygen and diffuses through both these media 20 times faster than oxygen. Since both gases are able to diffuse many thousands of times more rapidly in a gaseous medium than in water or tissue, resistance to diffusion out of an acinus is primarily related to movement through the alveolocapillary membrane and plasma and into the red blood cell. Because diffusion through these structures is accomplished much more readily by carbon dioxide than by oxygen, diffusion of carbon dioxide from blood to acinar gas is never a clinical problem, and further discussion need concern only the diffusion of oxygen.

Assuming a tidal volume of 450 ml and a dead space of 150 ml, 300 ml of fresh air and 150 ml of dead space alveolar air from the previous expiration enter the acinar units during each inspiration. Since these units already contain seven or eight times this volume (functional residual capacity), the "fresh" air that enters last may fill only the respiratory bronchioles and alveolar ducts. However, because of the rapid diffusion of oxygen in a gaseous medium, complete mixing of this fresh air with intra-acinar gas is probably instantaneous in normal lung. With the breakdown of alveolar septa and the creation of much larger air spaces in emphysema, such mixing may be delayed; in this situation, gaseous diffusion may limit the diffusing capacity.[150]

Diffusion Across the Alveolocapillary Membrane

Since their walls are in close contact with alveolar air,[151] it is probable that some gas transfer occurs at the level of the pulmonary arterioles. Nevertheless, as previously discussed (*see* page 17), the site at which the vast majority of gas diffusion occurs is the thin portion of the alveolar septum, comprising a layer of surface-active liquid, the Type I alveolar epithelial cell, the fused basement membranes of the epithelial cell and the capillary endothelium, and the endothelial cell itself. In normal lung, this "blood-air pathway" is about 0.4- to 0.5-μm thick.[152]

Under resting conditions and at a driving pressure of approximately 60 mm Hg (Po$_2$ of alveolar gas minus Po$_2$ of mixed venous blood [100 − 40 = 60 mm Hg]), oxygen almost fully saturates the blood in one third of the time it takes to traverse the pulmonary capillaries. During moderate exercise, the transit time is reduced as a result of increased cardiac output; nevertheless, aided by the slightly higher Po$_2$ due to increased ventilation, blood is virtually completely saturated by oxygen by the time it reaches the end of the capillary. During maximal exercise, especially in elite athletes, arterial Po$_2$ may decrease owing to a rise in the alveolar-arterial oxygen tension gradient.[153–155] Part of this decrease is caused by a marked reduction in pulmonary

transit time (1.06 to 0.47 seconds in one study[154]); however, most appears to be related to the development of ventilation/perfusion mismatching.[153, 155] Since mild to moderate exercise improves $\dot{V}/\dot{Q}$ mismatch, these results have engendered considerable interest. It has been suggested that heavy exercise results in mild interstitial edema in some subjects and that this explains the worsened $\dot{V}/\dot{Q}$ ratios.[155] In support of this hypothesis is the observation that the pulmonary diffusing capacity (DLCO) can be reduced for a prolonged period ($\leq$ 24 hours) after a bout of heavy exercise.[156–158] This postexercise decrease in DLCO is related to a decrease in its membrane component rather than a reduction in pulmonary capillary blood volume[158] but is unaffected by treatment with furosemide, which argues against pulmonary edema as a mechanism.[157]

With decreased alveolar Po$_2$ (e.g., due to atmospheric conditions at high altitude, respiratory center depression, or neuromuscular disease), the driving pressure of oxygen is reduced; exercise under these conditions results in a shortened transit time, which, together with the reduced driving pressure, may limit diffusion, so that the end-capillary blood may be only partly oxygenated. In situations where intense exercise and low inspired O$_2$ are combined, such as in some mountaineering expeditions, a marked impairment of gas exchange can develop in some people.

The total area over which flowing blood comes in contact with ventilated acinar units also influences the capacity for diffusion, as exemplified by the decrease in diffusion that occurs after pneumonectomy.[159] This factor also may be related in part to the decrease in diffusing capacity that occurs in emphysema, in which a considerable amount of the alveolocapillary membrane may be destroyed. The most common mechanism for a reduced *effective* alveolocapillary membrane area is mismatching of capillary circulation with acinar ventilation (*see* further on). In addition to $\dot{V}/\dot{Q}$ mismatching, an apparent reduction in the alveolocapillary membrane may be caused by mismatching of regional lung perfusion to regional diffusing capacity (DL/Q ratio).[160–162] Since $\dot{V}/\dot{Q}$ and DL/Q mismatch inevitably accompanies diseases that thicken the alveolocapillary membrane, it may be difficult to assess the contribution of diffusion impairment to a reduced DLCO.[163, 164]

Many diseases may involve the acinar unit in such a way as to interfere with diffusion (Fig. 2–29).

Intravascular Diffusion

There is probably little resistance to the diffusion of oxygen across the red blood cell membrane, the important factor affecting intravascular gas transfer being the reaction rate of oxygen with hemoglobin.[165, 166] Differences in the rate of gas exchange in the red blood cell, the final phase of diffusion, are not important in people with normal lungs who breathe air; however, they play a significant role in diffusion impairment in states of low alveolar oxygen tension and in anemia.

Measurement of Diffusing Capacity

The efficiency of the diffusion process for gas uptake by the lung can be quantified in individual subjects or patients by measuring the diffusing capacity. Measurement

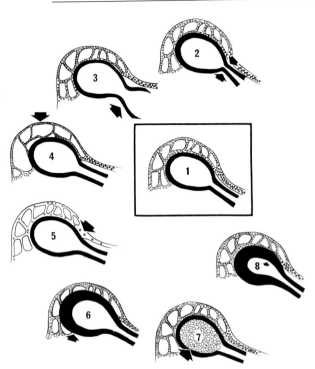

Figure 2–29. Pathophysiology of Diffusion Defect. The structure in the center of the diagram (1) is a normal air-containing acinar unit in which are depicted a conducting system, an alveolar cell lining, a normal amount of tissue between air space and capillary endothelium, and a capillary network containing a normal number of red blood cells. The acinar units around the periphery depict various mechanisms of diffusion defect: (2) obstruction to air entry; (3) dilation and confluence of respiratory bronchioles (resulting in an increased pathway for diffusion, as in centrilobular emphysema); (4) loss of capillaries; (5) anemia; (6) increase in tissue between air space and capillary endothelium; (7) replacement of air in air space by edema, exudate, or blood; and (8) increase in alveolar lining cells.

The three important variables that make up the overall diffusing capacity of the lung (DL) are the alveolocapillary membrane diffusing capacity (DM), the reaction rate of carbon monoxide with hemoglobin (θ), and the pulmonary capillary blood volume (Vc). Since different inhaled oxygen concentrations affect the CO-hemoglobin reaction rate, the two other variables, DM and Vc, can be separated by repeating the measurement with different fractional inspired oxygen (FIO₂).[167] Capillary blood volume and membrane diffusing capacity can also be measured in a one-step test by simultaneous measurement of CO and NO transfer in a single breath-hold method.[158] For research purposes, these techniques allow further dissection of the various causes for a decreased DLCO (*see* Fig. 2–29); however, they are rarely done in patients as a diagnostic test. Estimates of DLCO, DM, and Vc have also been attempted using morphometry; however, unlike physiologic estimates that suggest that Vc and DM are of equal importance, the results of this technique suggest that the capillary blood volume and the CO-hemoglobin reaction rate are the more important diffusing-limiting steps.[168, 169]

The diffusing capacity of the lung is also profoundly influenced by gravity. In zero gravity, the distribution of ventilation and perfusion is much more uniform,[170] and both the Vc and DM components of DLCO increase by about 25%.[171] In younger persons, a similar 25% increase in Vc occurs on going from the upright to the supine position; however, DM does not increase, presumably because of a persistence of V̇/Q̇ mismatching, despite the increased capillary volume.[172] This positional increase in DLCO decreases with advancing age, suggesting a stiffening of the pulmonary vessels.[173] Similarly, the DM and Vc components of DL both decrease with age, the membrane component DM decreasing first.[174, 175]

of the capacity for diffusion of oxygen is a complicated and perhaps unreliable procedure; it is necessary to know the mixed venous PO₂ to determine the driving pressure of oxygen, and the rate of diffusion varies along the capillary as the driving pressure decreases while the PO₂ in capillary blood increases. Because of these problems, carbon monoxide generally is used to measure diffusion; since it has a great affinity for hemoglobin, only a low concentration (0.3%) is required.

The diffusing capacity for carbon monoxide is the amount of this gas taken up per minute divided by the difference between partial pressures of carbon monoxide in the alveolus and in capillary blood. Since there is virtually no carbon monoxide in mixed venous blood under normal conditions, the amount of gas taken up is the difference between the carbon monoxide content of inspired and expired gas.

$$D_L = ml\ CO/min/mm\ Hg$$

The denominator of the equation is equal to the mean alveolar PCO, which can be calculated from an end-tidal sample of expired gas; the mean capillary PCO is so small that it can be ignored. Several techniques have been developed for using this gas, and the advantages of particular methods are discussed elsewhere.[159]

Matching Capillary Blood Flow with Ventilation in the Acinus

Ideally, alveolar ventilation and alveolar perfusion should be uniform; that is, each acinus should receive just the right amount of ventilation to oxygenate the hemoglobin completely and remove the carbon dioxide given off during gas exchange. This would mean that each of the approximately 30,000 acini, with their 400 alveolar ducts and 8000 alveoli, would receive equal portions of the alveolar ventilation (V̇A), which is estimated to average 4.5 liters per minute, and the alveolar perfusion (Q̇), which averages 5 liters per minute. In other words, not only would the ratio of ventilation to perfusion (V̇A/Q̇) be 4.5:5, or 0.9, for each lung, but each acinar unit would have a V̇A/Q̇ ratio of 0.9 as well. Despite the fact that this is not true, even for the normal lung, the concept of an "ideal" V̇A/Q̇ ratio is useful as a point of reference in judging relationships between ventilation and perfusion within acini and the lung.[176] When the V̇A/Q̇ ratio is not ideal (i.e., other than 0.9), it is either because perfusion is reduced relative to ventilation (high V̇A/Q̇) or because ventilation is decreased relative to blood flow (low V̇A/Q̇).

Figure 2–30 shows the theoretical distribution of V̇A/Q̇ ratios in the lung, using a five-compartment model. The central unit (No. 3) corresponds to the "ideal" unit with a V̇A/Q̇ of 0.9. In this acinus, ventilation is sufficient to

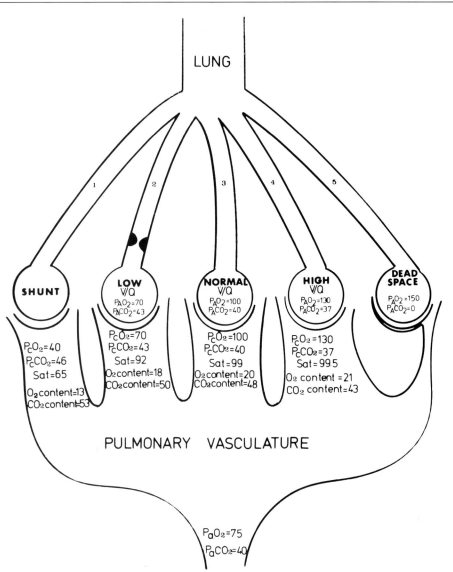

Figure 2–30. Theoretical Distribution of $\dot{V}_A/\dot{Q}$ Ratios in the Lung. Although many possible ventilation/perfusion ratios can exist in a normal or diseased lung, these can be conveniently divided into five compartments. Unit 1 represents pure shunt, an area of lung with a ventilation/perfusion ratio of zero. Blood coming from such a unit will have gas tensions identical to those of mixed venous blood (P_{O_2} = 40 + P_{CO_2} = 46 in this example) and the P_{O_2} of blood from such units will be uninfluenced by changes in inspired O_2. Unit 2 represents a low $\dot{V}/\dot{Q}$ area in which there is insufficient ventilation to completely saturate hemoglobin or lower CO_2 content to normal arterial values. Unit 3 represents the perfect match of ventilation and perfusion, resulting in near 100% saturation of hemoglobin and normal P_{CO_2}, whereas Unit 4 represents an overventilated (high $\dot{V}/\dot{Q}$) area. Blood from the high $\dot{V}/\dot{Q}$ area has a CO_2 content less than normal, which compensates for the higher than normal CO_2 content from Unit 2, but because of the shape of the O_2 dissociation curve, the overventilated unit cannot compensate for the underventilated unit with regard to O_2 transport. Unit 5 represents pure dead space in which the $\dot{V}/\dot{Q}$ ratio is infinity. Ventilation of such units is wasted and does not contribute to gas exchange. Note that although the mean P_{AO_2} of the ventilated units (2, 3, 4, and 5) is greater than 100, the P_{O_2} of the arterialized blood leaving the lung is 75. The $\dot{V}/\dot{Q}$ mismatch has resulted in an A-a gradient for O_2.

achieve an alveolar oxygen tension (P_{AO_2}) of approximately 100 mm Hg. With unimpaired diffusion between alveolar gas and capillary blood, this results in a capillary oxygen tension (P_{CO_2}) of 100 mm Hg in the blood leaving this unit, a level that is sufficient to achieve nearly 100% saturation of the hemoglobin (20 ml O_2 per 100 ml of blood if the hemoglobin concentration is 15 gm/dl). The resulting P_{ACO_2} and P_{CCO_2} is 40 mm Hg, which is sufficient to lower mixed venous carbon dioxide content from 53 to 48 ml/dl.

Unit 1 represents the lowest possible $\dot{V}_A/\dot{Q}$ region, amounting to 0, or true intrapulmonary shunt. Capillary blood emerges from such a unit with gas partial pressures and contents identical to those of mixed venous blood (i.e.,

P_{CO_2} = 40 mm Hg and P_{CCO_2} = 46 mm Hg in our example, for capillary contents of O_2 = 13 ml/dl and CO_2 = 53 ml/dl). Unit 2 has a $\dot{V}_A/\dot{Q}$ ratio somewhere between 0.9 and 0, resulting in alveolar and capillary gas pressures and contents that are less than "ideal" for oxygen and more than ideal for carbon dioxide (i.e., P_{CO_2} = 70 mm Hg and P_{CCO_2} = 44 mm Hg in our example). Unit 5 represents true alveolar dead space, that is, a region of lung that is ventilated but not perfused ($\dot{V}_A/\dot{Q}$ = infinity). The ventilation to such a unit represents completely wasted ventilation, since alveolar gas does not come in contact with capillary blood. Unit 4 has a $\dot{V}_A/\dot{Q}$ ratio between 0.9 and infinity, resulting in alveolar and capillary partial pressures that are greater than ideal for oxygen and less than ideal for carbon dioxide (i.e., PCO_2 = 130 mm Hg and $PCCO_2$ = 37 mm Hg in our example).

Because of the relationships between blood gas content and partial pressure (illustrated in the O_2 and CO_2 dissociation curves (Fig. 2–31), $\dot{V}A/\dot{Q}$ mismatch has quite different effects on the efficiency of the lung to take up oxygen and remove carbon dioxide. As shown in Figure 2–31, the O_2 dissociation curve is relatively flat above PO_2s of 70 to 80 mm Hg, so that the overventilated unit (No. 4) cannot make up for the underventilated unit (No. 2) in terms of oxygen uptake. Although the elevated PO_2 in Unit 4 results in a slight increase in the amount of dissolved oxygen in the capillary blood, hemoglobin is virtually 100% saturated above a PO_2 of 100; since dissolved oxygen can increase only by 0.0003 ml/dl of blood per millimeter of mercury rise in PO_2, little gain is achieved by overventilating units. For carbon dioxide removal, however, overventilated units can compensate for underventilated units: the CO_2 dissociation curve is virtually linear over the range of physiologic PCO_2 values, so that the lowered carbon dioxide content of blood from Unit 4 can compensate for the greater than ideal content in Unit 2.

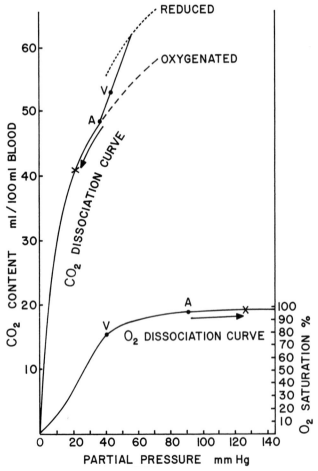

Figure 2–31. Carbon Dioxide and Oxygen Dissociation Curves of Blood. The arrows (A → X) indicate the effect of doubling the ventilation on both CO_2 content and O_2 content (arterial oxygen saturation). The normal values for both arterial (A) and venous (V) oxygen and carbon dioxide are noted. It can be seen that, at any given PCO_2, reduced blood can carry more carbon dioxide than oxygenated blood. *See* text.

When the blood from Units 1, 2, 3, and 4 mix in the pulmonary veins and left atrium, the PaO_2 of this arterial blood will be less than the mean alveolar PO_2 of Units 2, 3, and 4, whereas the $PaCO_2$ will be equal to the mean alveolar PCO_2. Put simply, $\dot{V}A/\dot{Q}$ mismatch decreases the efficiency of oxygen and carbon dioxide uptake and removal; in the case of oxygen, this results in a gradient between mean alveolar PO_2 and arterial PO_2 (P[A-a]O_2). $\dot{V}/\dot{Q}$ mismatch does not result in a gradient for carbon dioxide. If a disease process leads to the development of units with low $\dot{V}A/\dot{Q}$ ratios (No. 2) and to the development of areas of shunt (No. 1), arterial hypoxemia and hypercapnia will result. Since both a lowered PO_2 (indirectly) and an increased PCO_2 (directly) stimulate the respiratory center and increase ventilation, total alveolar ventilation will increase. The alveolar PO_2 in well-ventilated acinar units will rise while the PCO_2 in these units (No. 4) will fall. The excess carbon dioxide retained by blood circulating through the poorly ventilated units (Nos. 1 and 2) will be balanced by the supranormal output from the well-ventilated units. Comparison of the O_2 and CO_2 dissociation curves shows why this compensation can be accomplished for carbon dioxide but not for oxygen. Even if ventilation to an acinar unit is doubled and alveolar PO_2 rises to 130 mm Hg, the curve is so nearly horizontal in this range that a trivial increase in oxygen saturation is accomplished by this increase in PO_2.

Figure 2–30 illustrates a simplified model that spans the entire range of possible $\dot{V}A/\dot{Q}$ ratios in five compartments. In fact, a continuous distribution of ratios occurs, and even in the normal lung substantial regional variation in $\dot{V}A/\dot{Q}$ ratios has been demonstrated, largely in a gravity-dependent fashion. As discussed previously, the effect of gravity is to increase blood flow to the most dependent portions of the lung—in the erect position to the lung base, in the supine posture to the posterior portion of the lung, and in the lateral decubitus position to the dependent lung. These changes in blood flow are the result of alterations in regional pulmonary vascular resistance secondary to gravity-dependent changes in intravascular hydrostatic pressure.[177] In upper lung regions, pulmonary arterial pressure is low relative to alveolar pressure, resulting in compression of the vessels and increased vascular resistance. Descending through the lung, pulmonary artery pressure increases relative to alveolar pressure, causing distention of the pulmonary vasculature, decreasing resistance and increased flow.

The regional distribution of ventilation is also modified by gravity.[178, 179] A vertical gradient in pleural surface pressure results in alterations in regional lung volume:[180] in erect subjects, pleural pressure at the lung apex (or anteriorly in the supine position) is more negative than at the base, and the local pleural pressure increases progressively (i.e., becomes less subatmospheric) as the base of the lung is approached. Since mean alveolar pressure is constant up and down the lung, this means that the local transpulmonary pressure varies in a gravity-dependent fashion. Since the local lung parenchyma responds to the local transpulmonary pressure along its pressure-volume curve, at the end of a quiet expiration acinar units in upper lung regions are more distended and at a higher percentage of their total lung capacity (TLC) value than are the less well-distended units at the base of the lung.[181]

The gravity-dependent pleural pressure gradient averages about 0.25 cm H_2O per centimeter of distance up and down the lung and has been shown to be relatively volume independent;[180, 182] that is, a similar gradient in pleural pressure exists when overall lung volume is at functional residual capacity (FRC), below FRC, or above FRC. Thus, at FRC, pleural pressure may be -7 cm H_2O at the apex and $+1$ cm H_2O at the base, whereas at TLC it may be -37 cm H_2O at the apex and -29 cm H_2O at the base, a gradient of 8 cm H_2O at both lung volumes. As a result of the curvilinear nature of the pressure-volume (PV) curve of the lung, the variation in regional lung volume is substantial at lower lung volumes, whereas near TLC, where the PV curve is relatively flat, the same gradient in applied pressures results in trivial differences in regional lung volume.[180]

Despite the considerable variation in end-expiratory pleural and transpulmonary pressure up and down the lung, the changes in pleural pressure (ΔP) that occur during tidal breathing are similar at different vertical levels. Thus, because of the shape of the PV curve, upper lung units are less well ventilated per unit of lung volume than are those at the lung base, which are on a steeper portion of their PV curve. In summary, the gravity-dependent ΔP gradient results in a regional variation in lung volume (V_0) and regional variation in ventilation ($\Delta V/V_0$).

If the increase in $\Delta V/V_0$ from apex to base were directly proportional to the increase in blood flow from apex to base, the $\dot{V}A/\dot{Q}$ ratio would not vary. However, since the effect of gravity on regional perfusion is greater than that on regional ventilation, blood flow and ventilation are slightly mismatched and regional $\dot{V}A/\dot{Q}$ ratios differ from ideal, even in normal people.[178, 181, 183–187] During quiet breathing in the upright posture, the $\dot{V}A/\dot{Q}$ ratio is between 2 and 3 at the lung apex, decreasing to between 0.5 and 1 at the lung base. This apex-to-base mismatch disappears when the supine position is adopted, being replaced by an anterior-to-posterior gradient in regional ventilation, perfusion, and $\dot{V}A/\dot{Q}$ ratios.[188]

At low lung volumes, ventilation to the lung bases in the upright position or posterior regions in the supine position does not follow the distribution suggested by regional pleural pressure, a phenomenon probably related to airway closure. Airway size, like alveolar size, is dependent on regional transpulmonary pressure; with the relatively positive pressures at the lung base, closure of small airways can occur during a portion of the respiratory cycle. In fact, such airway closure occurs in dependent lung regions during tidal breathing, even in normal people.[189] The overall lung volume at which airways in dependent lung regions first close is termed the *closing volume* and can be measured with the single-breath nitrogen washout curve (*see* page 413). Since FRC decreases on assuming the supine posture while closing volume does not change, a greater number of dependent airways may close during supine tidal breathing, resulting in a paradoxical decrease in ventilation to dependent lung regions. Airway closure at the lung base results in a lower regional alveolar PO_2; this in turn may influence regional perfusion by inducing hypoxic vasoconstriction.[190]

Although the distribution of ventilation during quiet breathing is dependent on regional lung compliance and applied pleural pressure, regional resistance can become important during the increased ventilation of exercise. Ventilation distribution becomes more uniform up and down the

lung with increasing inspiratory flow rates, possibly because of variations in the regional time constant (the product of resistance and compliance). The time constant of a lung unit is a reflection of the rapidity of volume change that occurs in the unit in response to a step change in inflation or deflation pressure. Nondependent lung regions have a lower resistance as a result of their higher regional volume as well as a lower compliance because of the alinear relationship between pressure and volume; the product of a smaller resistance and a lower compliance produces a shorter time constant. During rapid respiratory cycling, this may influence regional ventilation distribution.[191] In addition, the more uniform distribution of ventilation during exercise may come about because of differences in applied pleural pressure up and down the lung as a result of recruitment of different inspiratory muscles during exercise.[191, 192]

During exercise, the vertical gradient in perfusion also diminishes as a result of a slight elevation in pulmonary vascular pressures; this contributes to the decrease in gravity-dependent variations in $\dot{V}A/\dot{Q}$ distribution.[193, 194] Most studies using radioactive gases have been designed to examine interregional variations in gas, blood flow, and $\dot{V}A/\dot{Q}$ distribution, but it is evident that intraregional variations in $\dot{V}A/\dot{Q}$ exist even in normal lungs and that during exercise intraregional mismatch may in fact increase.[153, 194–196]

With the development of lung disease, regional variations in ventilation, perfusion, and $\dot{V}A/\dot{Q}$ ratios increase. In the normal lung, true intrapulmonary shunting (Unit 1) probably does not occur, although some right-to-left flow through channels such as the thebesian vessels does take place. Any pathologic process in which alveolar air spaces are filled with transudate or exudate and in which perfusion persists results in a true shunt. Airway diseases that affect regional resistance and parenchymal diseases that change regional compliance can alter regional time constants and affect ventilation distribution. Abnormalities of the pulmonary vasculature, such as destruction of the capillary bed (as in emphysema) or obstruction of pulmonary vessels (as in thromboembolism), alter regional perfusion distribution; complete vascular obstruction, which may occur with pulmonary thromboemboli, converts affected regions of lung to dead space—ventilated but unperfused units (such as Unit 5).

Measurement of Ventilation/Perfusion Mismatch

A number of methods are available to quantify $\dot{V}A/\dot{Q}$ mismatch, ranging from simple bedside calculations to more elaborate and invasive techniques. Calculation of the physiologic dead space using the Bohr equation provides a useful estimate of overventilated lung units. Ventilation of totally unperfused acinar units (No. 5) and the excess portion of ventilation of high $\dot{V}A/\dot{Q}$ units (No. 4) represent alveolar dead space; the sum of alveolar dead space and anatomic dead space is the physiologic dead space. The ratio of physiologic dead space to tidal volume (VD/VT) can be calculated knowing arterial PCO_2 and mixed expired PCO_2:

$$VD/VT = \frac{Arterial\ PCO_2 - mixed\ expired\ PCO_2}{Arterial\ PCO_2} \quad (1)$$

In this equation, arterial PCO_2 is assumed to reflect mean alveolar PCO_2. With the advent of reliable, relatively low-cost, rapid CO_2 analyzers, this calculation can be made easily, especially in the intensive care unit setting, and can serve as an estimate of $\dot{V}A/\dot{Q}$ mismatch.

The most commonly used and easily calculated estimate of $\dot{V}A/\dot{Q}$ mismatch is the alveolar-arterial gradient for oxygen ($P[A-a]O_2$). Calculation of the $P(A-a)O_2$ requires knowledge of the mean alveolar PO_2, which can be calculated using the alveolar air equation[197]

$$P_{AO_2} = \frac{P_{IO_2}}{R} - P_{ACO_2} + \left[P_{ACO_2} \bullet F_{IO_2} \bullet \frac{1-R}{R} \right] \quad (2)$$

where F_{IO_2} is the fractional concentration of oxygen in the inspired air and R is the respiratory exchange ratio (the ratio of CO_2 production to O_2 consumption).

In practice, calculation of R is somewhat cumbersome, requiring collection and analysis of expired gas, and simplified methods to estimate P_{AO_2} have been advocated.[198] The alveolar air equation may be modified to the form

$$P_{AO_2} = P_{EO_2} - \frac{P_{IO_2} (V_D/V_T)}{(1 - V_D/V_T)} \quad (3)$$

where P_{EO_2} is the partial pressure of oxygen in the expired gas and P_{IO_2} is the partial pressure of oxygen in the inspired gas. Using this equation, a single-breath method for calculation of P_{AO_2} has been described (although the calculation still requires analysis of carbon dioxide and oxygen tensions in expired air).[199]

The simplest and most often used form of the alveolar air equation is

$$P_{AO_2} = \frac{P_{IO_2} - P_{ACO_2}}{R} \quad (4)$$

in which R is assumed to equal 0.8. Since P_{ACO_2} is used for P_{ACO_2} in this equation, all that is required for calculation is knowledge of the arterial PCO_2 and P_{IO_2}. A comparison between calculated P_{AO_2}, assuming a respiratory quotient of 0.8, and the measured value suggests that Equation 4 is adequate for clinical purposes.[200] Once the P_{AO_2} is calculated, the $P(A-a)O_2$ can be obtained by comparing P_{AO_2} with measured arterial PO_2:

$$P(A-a)O_2 = P_{AO_2} - P_{aO_2} \quad (5)$$

Intrapulmonary shunt and $\dot{V}A/\dot{Q}$ mismatch are the major contributors to the $P(A-a)O_2$. A failure of diffusion equilibration of alveolar oxygen with capillary blood may also contribute in three situations: (1) at extreme altitudes; (2) with very short red blood cell transit times through the capillaries, as in extreme exercise; and (3) in certain lung diseases, such as idiopathic pulmonary fibrosis.

The calculation of $P(A-a)O_2$ as a measurement of shunt and $\dot{V}A/\dot{Q}$ mismatch has the disadvantage that it is influenced by the mixed venous PO_2 and inspired PO_2. A given maldistribution of ventilation and perfusion will result in a different P_{aO_2} and calculated $P(A-a)O_2$ with changed mixed venous PO_2. This is most easily understood with shunt: If 25% of the cardiac output is shunted through a completely consolidated lung region, no gas transfer will occur and the shunted

blood will have a PO_2 and PCO_2 equal to that of mixed venous blood; when this is added to blood coming from normally ventilated regions, arterial PO_2 will be decreased and arterial PCO_2 increased. The extent to which the shunted blood alters the arterial blood is determined by the gas tensions in mixed venous blood. With a very low cardiac output, mixed venous PO_2 and oxygen content can reach extremely low values, and a given shunt will be associated with much worse systemic hypoxemia than if the cardiac output were normal or increased.

The calculated $P(A-a)O_2$ is also influenced by the P_{IO_2}, since a given degree of shunt or $\dot{V}A/\dot{Q}$ mismatch will produce a higher calculated $P(A-a)O_2$ as the P_{IO_2} is increased. Again, the easiest example to consider is the situation in which the $\dot{V}A/\dot{Q}$ ratio of a lung region is 0: If a patient is breathing room air and 35% of the cardiac output is being shunted through a consolidated lobe resulting in a P_{aO_2} of 50 mm Hg (calculated $P[A-a]O_2 = 40$), the breathing of 100% oxygen will increase arterial PO_2 only slightly by the addition of small amounts of dissolved oxygen in the normally ventilated areas. Thus, with 100% oxygen, the P_{aO_2} might increase to only 80 mm Hg, with a resultant calculated $P(A-a)O_2$ of more than 500! Shifts of the oxygen dissociation curve due to changes in blood temperature or pH can also influence the calculated $P(A-a)O_2$ without a true effect on the gas-exchanging ability of the lung.[201]

Calculations of venous admixture and shunt provide more accurate estimates of $\dot{V}A/\dot{Q}$ maldistribution and are less affected by mixed venous and inspired gas tension; however, they require a sample of mixed venous blood. The same equation is used for calculation of venous admixture and shunt:

$$\frac{\dot{Q}s}{\dot{Q}t} = \frac{C\acute{c}O_2 - CaO_2}{C\acute{c}O_2 - C\bar{v}O_2} \quad (6)$$

where $\dot{Q}s/\dot{Q}t$ is the venous admixture ratio or shunt if 100% oxygen is breathed, $C\acute{c}O_2$ is the oxygen content of end-capillary blood, CaO_2 is the oxygen content of arterial blood, and $C\bar{v}O_2$ is the oxygen content of mixed venous blood; the equation assumes equilibration between alveolar and capillary PO_2. Ideal capillary PO_2 is calculated using the alveolar air equation (see Equation 2). Content is calculated knowing the hemoglobin concentration and assuming that it is identical in venous, arterial, and capillary blood:

$$\begin{array}{c} O_2 \text{ content (ml/100 blood)} = \\ (Hgb, gm/dl \times 1.39 \times \text{ per cent saturation}) \\ + (PO_2 \times 0.003) \end{array} \quad (7)$$

where PO_2 is the PO_2 of capillary, arterial, or mixed venous blood. The first term in this equation is the oxygen content of hemoglobin, and the second calculates dissolved oxygen. When measurements for this calculation are obtained while the patient is breathing air or a gas mixture containing less than 100% oxygen, the resulting ratio is the venous admixture that is an "as if" shunt, representing the amount of mixed venous blood that would have to be added to capillary blood to result in the observed arterial PO_2 and A-a gradient. As pointed out by West, both the venous admixture and the ratio of dead space to tidal volume (V_D/V_T) are unfortunately influenced by overall ventilation and blood flow and by the FIO_2.[202]

An additional shortcoming in the use of $P(A-a)O_2$ and venous admixture as estimates of $\dot{V}A/\dot{Q}$ mismatch is the fact that both can be altered by diffusion impairment. Whether the partial pressure of capillary blood reaches the alveolar PO_2 during its transit through the pulmonary capillary depends on the red blood cell transit time and the driving pressure for diffusion—the difference between mixed venous and alveolar PO_2. In the normal lung at rest, red blood cell residence time in pulmonary capillaries is approximately 1 second, and the gradient between normal alveolar PO_2 and mixed venous PO_2 is sufficiently large to ensure complete equilibration. With the decreased red blood cell transit time that accompanies increased cardiac output, and especially with lowered PAO_2 secondary to increased altitude or hypoventilation, diffusion impairment may become important by contributing to the calculated $P(A-a)O_2$ and venous admixture.[203]

Only when pure oxygen is breathed for a time sufficient to wash nitrogen out of the lung completely can a measure be obtained of gas exchange uninfluenced by FIO_2 and mixed venous PO_2. The calculation of shunt obtained using Equation 6 gives an estimate of only one compartment in the $\dot{V}A/\dot{Q}$ spectrum. In addition to giving limited information about the spectrum of $\dot{V}A/\dot{Q}$ mismatch, measurement of shunt with 100% oxygen may in fact increase the intrapulmonary shunt. Regions with low $\dot{V}A/\dot{Q}$ ratios may be converted to regions of shunt when gas with higher PO_2 is breathed.[204] In a unit with a sufficiently low $\dot{V}A/\dot{Q}$, oxygen breathing can result in an oxygen uptake by pulmonary capillary blood that exceeds the oxygen delivered by alveolar

ventilation to that unit. When a gas with a lower PO_2 is breathed, nitrogen, being highly insoluble, serves to stabilize these units, preventing their collapse. The critical $\dot{V}A/\dot{Q}$ ratio that results in alveolar instability is dependent on the $\dot{V}A/\dot{Q}$ ratio of the unit and the fraction of oxygen in the inspired gas.[204]

Measurement of regional ventilation/perfusion ratios using radioactive tracers has added greatly to our understanding of topographic $\dot{V}A/\dot{Q}$ variation. However, the techniques used are basically insensitive, in that only relatively large lung regions can be assessed with external counters. Of greater importance in diseased lungs is intraregional, acinar-to-acinar $\dot{V}A/\dot{Q}$ mismatch. The advent of efficient gamma cameras has greatly simplified the qualitative and quantitative assessment of regional $\dot{V}A/\dot{Q}$ inhomogeneity.[205] Their greatest clinical use has been in the search for ventilated but unperfused regions of lung resulting from thromboembolic obstruction of large pulmonary vessels.

Another important advance in the measurement of $\dot{V}A/\dot{Q}$ mismatch is a method to measure the "continuous" distribution of $\dot{V}A/\dot{Q}$ ratios in normal and diseased lungs.[206] The technique involves the intravenous infusion of up to 10 inert gases dissolved in saline; the gases used have a wide range of solubility in blood, and in their passage through the lung enter alveolar gas. The mixed expired and arterial concentration of each gas is measured by gas chromatography when a steady state is achieved; the retention and excretion of each gas can then be calculated and plotted against solubility. From the plot, the distribution of blood flow and ventilation with respect to $\dot{V}A/\dot{Q}$ ratios can be calculated using a computer (Fig. 2–32). The technique allows measurement of absolute shunt as well as alveolar

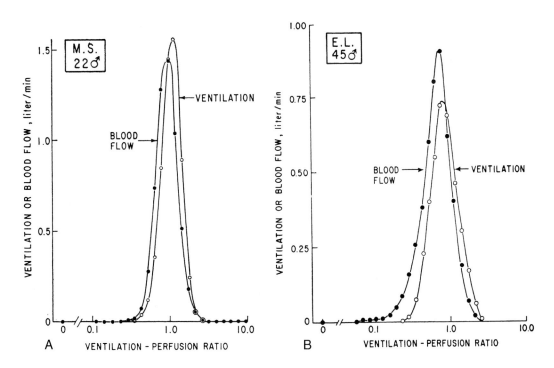

Figure 2–32. Distribution of Blood Flow and Ventilation in Relation to $\dot{V}/\dot{Q}$ Ratios. The distribution of blood flow and ventilation (vertical axis) to units with varying $\dot{V}/\dot{Q}$ ratios (horizontal axis) in a 22-year-old man *(A)* and a 45-year-old man *(B)*. In both normal subjects the bulk of the ventilation and perfusion is well matched, going to units with a $\dot{V}/\dot{Q}$ ratio near 1, and there is no shunt ($\dot{V}/\dot{Q}$ ratio = 0). In the older man a wider range of $\dot{V}/\dot{Q}$ ratios exists. (Reprinted from Wagner PD, Laravuso RB, Uhl RR, et al: J Clin Invest 54:54, 1974. By copyright permission of the American Society for Clinical Investigation and with the permission of the authors.)

dead space and also permits calculation of the proportion of perfusion and ventilation to a large number of normally distributed units of varying $\dot{V}A/\dot{Q}$ ratio.

The advantages of this technique are threefold: (1) it allows a multicompartmental description of the $\dot{V}A/\dot{Q}$ distribution rather than categorizing it into two or three compartments, as do other techniques; (2) it is relatively noninvasive and does not require placement of a central venous line; and (3) no radioactive gases are used. Its disadvantage is that there is no unique solution to the retention and excretion curves: with simple disturbances, the method can adequately describe the $\dot{V}A/\dot{Q}$ relationships, but with complex derangements a number of interpretations of the data are possible.

Blood Gases and Acid-Base Balance

Blood Gases

The ability of the lung to perform its prime function—the exchange of oxygen and carbon dioxide—is readily determined from analysis of a sample of arterial blood. The oxygen carried can be measured as arterial oxygen saturation or as Po_2 (arterial oxygen saturation = O_2 content/O_2 capacity [per cent]). Since each 1.0 gm of hemoglobin can combine with 1.39 ml of oxygen, the oxygen capacity of the blood in a subject with 15 gm of hemoglobin per decaliter of blood is approximately 20. The content is the amount of oxygen that the blood actually contains. In a subject with normal lungs breathing air at sea level, this amounts to 19 ml (or slightly more). Thus, the normal oxygen saturation is 19/20 × 100, or 95%.

The Po_2 may be determined from the oxygen dissociation curve using arterial oxygen saturation; however, this is not completely reliable because of the almost horizontal slope of the upper part of the curve (*see* Fig. 2–31, page 110). The Po_2 can be measured directly by use of an electrode which, as discussed previously, is the only way of determining total oxygen carried by hemoglobin and plasma during the inhalation of 100% oxygen.

In contrast with oxygen, which is carried almost entirely by hemoglobin, approximately 75% of carbon dioxide is contained in plasma. In the resting subject, mixed venous blood holds about 15 ml of oxygen per decaliter of blood at a Po_2 of 40 mm Hg and an oxygen saturation of 75%; its carbon dioxide content is about 52 ml/dl of blood at a Pco_2 of 45 mm Hg. Although the red blood cell carries only 25% of the carbon dioxide, it plays an essential role in the transport of this gas to the lungs; it contains the enzyme carbonic anhydrase, which rapidly hydrates the carbon dioxide passing through the erythrocyte membrane and converts it into carbonic acid, hydrogen ions, and bicarbonate ions (HCO_3^-). The bicarbonate ions quickly permeate the cell membrane and enter the plasma in exchange for chloride ions; thus, most of the carbon dioxide from the tissues is carried as bicarbonate by the blood. Since blood that contains reduced hemoglobin can carry more carbon dioxide than can fully oxygenated blood at the same Pco_2, the circumstances are ideal for the uptake of carbon dioxide in the tissues and for its unloading in the pulmonary capillaries when the hemoglobin has been reoxygenated (*see* Fig. 2–31, page 110).

In anemia, the Po_2 may be normal and hemoglobin may be fully saturated; however, oxygen content and capacity are reduced in direct proportion to the reduction in hemoglobin. When normal hemoglobin is replaced by methemoglobin, sulfhemoglobin, or carboxyhemoglobin, the Po_2 also remains normal, although the oxygen content of blood is decreased and spectrophotometric analysis of the sample reveals reduced oxygen saturation.

Arterial hypoxemia may be caused by one or more of four mechanisms: diffusion defect, shunt, ventilation/perfusion inequality, or hypoventilation. The severity of hypoxemia caused by $\dot{V}/\dot{Q}$ mismatch, shunt, and diffusion impairment is influenced by the mixed venous Po_2. The lower the mixed venous Po_2, the more severe the hypoxemia for a given shunt, $\dot{V}/\dot{Q}$ maldistribution, or diffusion problem. This mechanism is an important contributing factor to gas exchange problems and is often overlooked. For example an increase in cardiac output can improve the hypoxemia associated with shunt simply by increasing the Po_2 in the shunted blood.

Diffusion Defect. A diffusion defect results in hypoxemia if there is failure of equilibration of alveolar and capillary Po_2 during the transit of blood through the pulmonary capillaries. There is continued controversy concerning the importance of this mechanism in the production of arterial hypoxemia in disease; however, it is probable that failure of diffusive equilibration between alveolar gas and capillary blood contributes to the hypoxemia seen in emphysema, the increase in hypoxemia that occurs with exercise in patients with interstitial lung disease, the hypoxemia that develops in some people during severe exercise, and the hypoxemia of altitude. With exercise, the mechanism is probably a decrease in the red blood cell capillary transit time, whereas with altitude it is related to a low alveolar Po_2. Because of the high tissue and blood solubility of carbon dioxide, equilibration times are more rapid than with oxygen, and diffusion limitation does not play a role in the genesis of carbon dioxide retention.

Shunt. A shunt of venous blood to the systemic arterial circulation may be a result of congenital cardiovascular disease, arteriovenous aneurysm of the lung, or, in some diseases that affect the lung parenchyma, precapillary anastomoses between pulmonary arterioles and venules. More commonly, a shunt is caused by pathologic processes that fill the alveolar air spaces with transudate or exudate, producing areas of lung that are unventilated but perfused. This mechanism is the primary cause of hypoxemia in cardiogenic and noncardiogenic pulmonary edema and in other conditions characterized by air-space consolidation, such as pneumonia. The shunted blood never comes in contact with alveolar gas, and for this reason the Po_2 of the arterial blood cannot be raised to a normal value (approximately 600 mm Hg) during inhalation of 100% oxygen. In fact, when the shunt handles 10% or more of the cardiac output, the arterial Po_2 cannot rise above 400 mm Hg. All other mechanisms that produce hypoxemia can be fully corrected by the inspiration of 100% oxygen, which replaces nitrogen in even the most poorly ventilated acini.

In a true shunt, the Pco_2 is usually normal or low, since additional ventilation removes more carbon dioxide from acini that are perfused and ventilated. The inability of this compensatory hyperventilation to improve uptake of oxygen significantly is apparent on study of the oxygen and carbon dioxide dissociation curves (*see* Fig. 2–31). As previously discussed, doubling the ventilation decreases P_{CO_2} from 40 to 20 mm Hg and eliminates considerable amounts of carbon dioxide, whereas the increase in P_{O_2} that results from increase in ventilation insignificantly increases arterial blood oxygen content and saturation.

Ventilation/Perfusion Inequality. $\dot{V}_A/\dot{Q}$ inequality is the commonest cause of the hypoxemia that accompanies pulmonary disease, the clinical conditions most often associated with it being chronic obstructive pulmonary disease, asthma, and interstitial lung disease. In this situation, the capillary blood that perfuses underventilated acinar units is not fully saturated and does not release normal amounts of carbon dioxide since the gradient between the P_{CO_2} of blood and the acinus is reduced. However, because of the differences in the slopes of the dissociation curves, $\dot{V}/\dot{Q}$ mismatching tends to affect oxygen transport and arterial P_{O_2} to a greater extent than carbon dioxide transport and P_{CO_2}. Hyperventilation of well-ventilated acini with consequent reduction in alveolar P_{CO_2} increases the blood-to-acinus gradient and eliminates more carbon dioxide from these areas. Consequently, in patients with $\dot{V}_A/\dot{Q}$ inequality, P_{CO_2} may be low or normal. As with shunt, overventilation of these same units does not make up for the underventilated units in terms of oxygen uptake.

The hypoxemia associated with $\dot{V}_A/\dot{Q}$ inequality can be corrected by breathing 100% oxygen, since oxygen replaces nitrogen in even the most poorly ventilated areas. When carbon dioxide retention is also present, prolonged inhalation of high concentrations of oxygen increases the carbon dioxide concentration in the blood and may lead to confusion and coma. This additional retention of carbon dioxide during oxygen breathing results in part from removal of the carotid body's hypoxic stimulus to ventilation and in part from an increase in physiologic dead space produced by a decrease in hypoxic vasoconstriction in low $\dot{V}/\dot{Q}$ areas.

Hypoxemia associated with a low inspired P_{O_2} occurs on ascending to altitude. This is usually of no clinical significance at moderate elevations, but the exponential decrease in P_{O_2} at higher altitudes can result in significant hypoxemia, especially in people who have pre-existing pulmonary disease.

Hypoventilation. A decrease in overall alveolar ventilation results in both carbon dioxide retention and hypoxemia. Because alveolar P_{O_2} is also reduced, the hypoxemia is not associated with an increased alveolar-arterial gradient for oxygen ($P[A-a]O_2$) and thus differs from that caused by diffusion defects, $\dot{V}_A/\dot{Q}$ inequality, and shunt. Since hypoventilation often occurs in association with these gas exchange abnormalities, calculation of $P(A-a)O_2$ aids in separating the component of hypoxemia related to hypoventilation from that caused by gas exchange problems.

Acid-Base Balance

When combined with clinical information, measurements of Pa_{O_2}, oxygen saturation, Pa_{CO_2}, and the calculated A-a gradient for O_2 allow an assessment of the status of a patient's gas exchange. To make specific diagnoses of disturbances in acid-base balance one needs to examine the arterial hydrogen ion concentration ($[H^+]$), the negative log

of the hydrogen concentration (pH), as well as the Pa_{CO_2}, HCO_3^-, and anion gap in blood and urine. Basic and practical aspects of acid-base regulation have been reviewed in detail, and the interested reader desiring more comprehensive coverage is referred to these sources.[207–210] The section that follows is a simplified account of disturbances in H^+ concentration, with particular reference to the commoner clinical states likely to be encountered by physicians interested in respiratory diseases.

Disturbances of acid-base balance can be divided into those that are respiratory in origin and those that are primarily nonrespiratory (metabolic). The former are the result of overventilation or underventilation associated with excess removal or retention of carbon dioxide and with a decrease or increase in the total carbonic acid pool of the extracellular fluid. Nonrespiratory disturbances are the result of an increase or decrease in noncarbonic acid or a loss or gain of bicarbonate by the extracellular fluid.

Acidosis or alkalosis* may be "simple" (related to a purely respiratory or metabolic disorder) or "mixed" (reflecting physiologic disturbances that cause simultaneous respiratory and nonrespiratory derangements). A variety of mixed disorders seen by chest physicians can cause difficulty in diagnosis. One of the more common is severe acute pulmonary edema, in which acute carbon dioxide retention (respiratory acidosis) combined with tissue hypoxia and anaerobic glycolysis (metabolic lactic acidosis) produces acidemia. Combined respiratory acidosis secondary to alveolar hypoventilation in chronic obstructive pulmonary disease and metabolic alkalosis caused by diuretic administration is another frequently encountered mixed disorder that is usually associated with an arterial pH within the normal range (i.e., acidosis and alkalosis without acidemia or alkalemia). A third important mixed disorder that can cause diagnostic difficulty is the combination of compensated respiratory acidosis and superimposed metabolic acidosis, which may be mistaken for acute respiratory acidosis unless the anion gap is calculated (*see* farther on).

Acids in the body may be derived from processes of cellular metabolism that result in the production of fixed acids (such as phosphates and sulfates) and from hydrogen ion generation by the buffering of CO_2 with bicarbonate. The amount of fixed acid normally produced daily is small ($\sim$40 to 60 mM), whereas the production of CO_2 is large ($\sim$20,000 mM). CO_2 can be excreted rapidly in the lung, whereas the fixed acids must be excreted by the kidney. The two determinants of arterial P_{CO_2} are the CO_2 production and alveolar ventilation:

$$Pa_{CO_2} = \frac{CO_2\ Production}{Alveolar\ Ventilation} \qquad (9)$$

Compensatory Mechanisms. Under normal conditions, values for H^+ concentration ($[H^+]$), pH, bicarbonate concen-

---

*There is often confusion regarding the appropriate use of the terms *acidosis* versus *acidemia* and *alkalosis* versus *alkalemia*. Acidosis can be defined as an abnormal condition or process that would decrease the pH or increase the $[H^+]$ of the blood if there were no secondary compensatory changes. Similarly, alkalosis can be defined as a process that tends to increase the pH or decrease the $[H^+]$ of the blood if there are no secondary changes. The terms *acidemia* and *alkalemia* are best restricted to situations in which arterial pH falls or rises, respectively.

tration ([HCO_3^-]), and $Paco_2$ remain within a relatively narrow range. In arterial blood, the [H^+] may vary from 36 to 44 nM per liter, pH from 7.36 to 7.44, [HCO_3^-] from 22 to 26 mM per liter, and $Paco_2$ from 36 to 44 mm Hg. When the [H^+] moves outside the accepted normal range, the body's homeostatic mechanisms react to restore the balance. The type and magnitude of the mechanisms evoked depend on the degree of disturbance, its duration, and the type of imbalance (carbonic or noncarbonic). For adequate body function, it is more important to maintain near normality of [H^+] than either CO_2 or bicarbonate. In fact, regulation of acid-base balance is often reflected in abnormally high or low levels of carbon dioxide and bicarbonate in the extracellular fluid. Homeostatic mechanisms that operate in acid-base derangements include (1) buffering of an excess H^+ or HCO_3 in intracellular and extracellular fluids; (2) compensatory increase or decrease in alveolar ventilation; and (3) renal response.

The buffer components in extracellular fluids are hemoglobin, plasma proteins, bicarbonate, and phosphate. In the blood itself, buffering of excess H^+ is complete within a few minutes and is largely dependent on the bicarbonate and hemoglobin systems. Bicarbonate moves from the interstitial fluid spaces into the blood in situations of H^+ excess, a process that may take 15 minutes to 2 hours.[211] Within the cells, buffering depends on the presence of protein and phosphate radicals. The respiratory compensatory mechanism is a result of [H^+]-induced stimulation of receptors in the central nervous system and the aortic and carotid bodies. Elimination or retention of carbon dioxide takes minutes to hours.

Shifts of H^+, K^+, and Na^+ from various tissues, particularly muscle, and carbonate from bone are somewhat slower in compensating for disturbances in acid-base balance but are quantitatively of great importance. The movement of H^+ into the cells is reflected in increased [K^+] in the extracellular fluid. The renal response to disturbances in acid-base balance may take up to 1 week; in respiratory acidosis it is well developed in 48 hours and usually maximal within 5 days.[212] Renal compensation for alkalosis depends on the rapidity of development of the alkalosis and, in chronic states, on the volume of extracellular fluid and body stores of sodium, chloride, and potassium.

Despite the many sources of buffering available within the body, in clinical practice one needs only to monitor the carbonic acid-bicarbonate system to assess acid-base homeostasis. The equation governing this buffer system is derived from the law of mass action and is termed the *Henderson equation:*

$$[H^+] = \frac{K[H_2CO_3]}{[HCO_3^-]} \qquad (10)$$

In practice, the measured arterial Pco_2 can be substituted for H_2CO_3 in this equation, and a value of 24 can be used for the constant K. A useful modification of the Henderson equation is

$$H_2O + CO_2 \leftrightarrow H_2CO_3 \leftrightarrow H^+ + HCO_3^- \qquad (11)$$

Respiratory Acidosis. Respiratory acidosis results from the retention of carbon dioxide secondary to alveolar hypo-

ventilation. Intrapulmonary left-to-right shunting and $\dot{V}/\dot{Q}$ inequality do not necessarily result in respiratory acidosis; although these derangements decrease the efficiency of CO_2 elimination by increasing wasted (dead space) ventilation, alveolar ventilation can be maintained by increasing total ventilation (minute ventilation). However, the maintenance of alveolar ventilation in these circumstances requires increased respiratory muscle effort and can cause the sensation of dyspnea.

Several conditions are associated with alveolar hypoventilation and respiratory acidosis. The most common are those related to an increase in the respiratory muscle work necessary to maintain normal alveolar ventilation (such as advanced chronic obstructive pulmonary disease [COPD]). Respiratory acidosis can also develop despite a normal pulmonary gas exchange capacity if there is malfunction of the respiratory center or disease of the efferent neural pathways in the spinal cord, anterior horn cells, or peripheral nerves innervating the diaphragm and intercostal muscles. Myopathy or myositis, and extreme deformity of the thoracic cage, as in kyphoscoliosis, may also impair alveolar ventilation.

Respiratory acidosis may be acute or chronic. The former occurs in severe pulmonary edema, severe asthma, acute respiratory center depression caused by drug intoxication, and neuromuscular disorders such as myasthenia gravis or Guillain-Barré syndrome. Hypoventilation associated with chronic respiratory acidosis occurs in COPD, in diseases in which the anterior horn cells are destroyed, and in the muscular dystrophies. Patients with obesity-hypoventilation syndromes and severe obstructive sleep apnea may also develop chronic respiratory acidosis. The commonest clinical form of respiratory acidosis is seen in patients with COPD who have chronic compensated respiratory acidosis and develop a further acute decrease in alveolar ventilation secondary to lower respiratory infection or drug-precipitated acute respiratory center depression.

Compensatory Mechanisms in Respiratory Acidosis. Sudden alveolar hypoventilation increases the $Paco_2$ (partial pressure of alveolar CO_2) and hence the $Paco_2$ (partial pressure of arterial CO_2); the latter results in the formation of carbonic acid and a shift of the Henderson equation to the right ($H_2O + CO_2 \leftrightarrow H_2CO_3 \leftrightarrow H^+ + HCO_3^-$), thereby increasing both [H^+] and [HCO_3^-]. The increases in [HCO_3^-] and [H^+] that occur with an acute increase in $Paco_2$ can be predicted accurately. For an increase in $Paco_2$ of 10 mm Hg, the [HCO_3^-] increases by 1 mM and the [H^+] by 8 nM (pH decrease of 0.08). If there is a greater or lesser than expected increase in [HCO_3^-] and [H^+], this implies the presence of a more complex acid-base disturbance, such as compensation, or combined primary disturbances.

When carbon dioxide retention is prolonged, there is a renal response, which also helps keep [H^+] within the normal range. This mechanism begins within hours, is well-developed by 48 hours, and is usually maximal within 5 days.[212] The kidney reacts to the acidosis by increasing its ability to reabsorb and generate HCO_3^-. The raised arterial Pco_2 stimulates bicarbonate conservation; the raised Pco_2 in the renal tubule cells increases the formation of carbonic acid (H_2CO_3) and enhances renal intracellular [H^+] and H^+ secretion; the augmented renal tubule H^+ secretion—resulting from carbonic acid dissociation—gives rise to *de novo* generation of HCO_3^- by the renal tubules. The end result of these processes is increased excretion of Cl^- ions, with consequent hypochloremia. The rule of thumb for fully compensated chronic respiratory acidosis is that for an increase of $PaCO_2$ of 10 mm Hg, the $[HCO_3^-]$ will increase by 3 mM and the $[H^+]$ will increase by 3 nM (pH decrease of 0.03). It should be noted that "full compensation" does not mean that the pH returns to the normal range, but rather refers to the maximal physiologic potential for correction *toward* the normal range.

Respiratory Alkalosis. Respiratory alkalosis results from hyperventilation. It is commonest in tension or anxiety states, in which circumstances it is usually acute and rarely prolonged. Some drugs (e.g., salicylic acid, paraldehyde, epinephrine, progesterone, and analeptics) may cause hyperventilation by stimulating the respiratory center. Traumatic, infectious, or vascular lesions of the central nervous system may also produce respiratory alkalosis, presumably by the same mechanism. Fever and gram-negative bacteremia can be associated with alkalosis by inducing hyperventilation (although this is often rapidly balanced by lactic acidosis secondary to tissue hypoperfusion if shock develops). Chronic respiratory alkalosis can be seen in hyperthyroidism, pregnancy, and hepatic failure.

Several pulmonary diseases are associated with mild respiratory alkalosis. In these circumstances, the stimuli to hyperventilation are probably a combination of hypoxemia and reflexes initiated in the lung parenchyma. Some of these diseases are acute (e.g., asthma and pulmonary thromboembolism), and others are chronic (e.g., granulomatous and fibrotic interstitial disorders that cause compensated respiratory alkalosis). Excessive artificial ventilation also may give rise to either acute or chronic respiratory alkalosis.

Compensatory Mechanisms in Respiratory Alkalosis. Hyperventilation decreases $PACO_2$ and hence $PaCO_2$; the decrease in arterial PCO_2 is associated with a shift in the Henderson equation to the left ($H_2O + CO_2 \leftrightarrow H_2CO_3 \leftrightarrow H^+ + HCO_3^-$) and a decrease in both $[H^+]$ and $[HCO_3^-]$. H^+ moves from the intracellular fluid, where it is replaced by sodium and potassium, and increased amounts of lactic acid are produced in the tissues.[213] The decrease in $[HCO_3^-]$ and $[H^+]$ that occurs with an acute decrease in $PaCO_2$ can again be predicted accurately. For a decrease in $PaCO_2$ of 10 mm Hg, the $[HCO_3^-]$ will decrease by 1 mM and the $[H^+]$ will decrease by 7 nM (pH increase of 0.07).

Persistence of the alkalotic state evokes a renal response: the urinary excretion of H^+ decreases and that of HCO_3^- and K^+ increases.[214] The rule of thumb for fully compensated chronic respiratory alkalosis is the following: for a decrease in $PaCO_2$ of 10 mm Hg, the $[HCO_3^-]$ will decrease by 5 mM and the $[H^+]$ will decrease by 2 nM (pH decrease of 0.02).

Metabolic Acidosis. Metabolic (nonrespiratory) acidosis results from an increase in $[H^+]$ from noncarbonic acid or a decrease in $[HCO_3^-]$ in the extracellular fluid. The H^+ excess can result from ingestion or infusion of noncarbonic acid, excess acid metabolic products within the body, or decreased renal excretion of H^+.

Extraneous sources of noncarbonic acid include various drugs and toxic substances, such as salicylates, paraldehyde, phenformin, methyl alcohol, ethylene glycol, ammonium chloride (NH_4Cl), arginine, and lysine hydrochloride. Infused

acid citrate–dextrose added to stored bank blood also may cause metabolic acidosis through anaerobic conversion of dextrose to lactic acid.[215]

Endogenous H^+ formation may result from the accumulation of large quantities of the keto acids—β-hydroxybutyric acid and acetoacetic acid—in uncontrolled diabetes, starvation, and (occasionally) alcoholism. Lactic acid is the other major source of noncarbonic acid within the body. It is produced in situations of tissue hypoxia and diffuses out of the cells in an un-ionized acid form, producing a temporary excess of noncarbonic acid in the extracellular fluid. Clinical situations in which lactic acid is produced include heavy exercise and acute severe tissue hypoxemia or hypoperfusion secondary to arterial hypotension or high levels of circulating catecholamines. Lactic acid may play a major role in increasing the $[H^+]$ in acute pulmonary edema secondary to left ventricular failure, although in some instances there is a superimposed respiratory acidosis. In acute left ventricular failure associated with metabolic acidosis, lactic acid may be produced even in the absence of hypotension or clinical evidence of shock.[216, 217]

Metabolic acidosis can be divided into three categories that can be separated by an analysis of the unmeasured anion gap: anion gap acidosis, nonanion gap acidosis (hyperchloremic acidosis), and combined metabolic acidosis. The anion gap is calculated by subtracting the sum of the concentration serum chloride (Cl^-) and bicarbonate (HCO_3^-) from the serum sodium (Na^+); the normal value is between 10 and 15. The *anion gap acidoses* are those in which an unmeasured acidic anion decreases the bicarbonate concentration. Electrical neutrality is maintained in the serum, but because the anion substituting for bicarbonate is unmeasured, it appears as if there is a deficit in anions. Table 2–3 shows the conditions that result in anion gap acidoses and the associated unmeasured anions.

Nonanion gap acidosis (hyperchloremic acidosis) occurs if there is H^+ loss, a failure of renal H^+ secretion, or an addition of hydrochloric acid (HCl) (Table 2–4). Since the anion accompanying the H^+ in these conditions is Cl^-, which is measured, acidemia and hyperchloremia develop without an anion gap. Nonanion gap acidoses can be further divided into nonrenal causes—characterized by bicarbonate loss and a large negative urinary anion gap—and renal causes—characterized by a failure of urinary H^+ excretion and a small negative or a positive urinary anion gap. The urinary anion gap is calculated as

$$Urinary\ Na^+ + K^+ - urinary\ Cl^- \qquad (12)$$

The normal renal response to metabolic acidosis is to excrete excess H^+ as ammonium (NH_4^+). The latter is a cation that is excreted with Cl^-. Since NH_4^+ is not measured, its presence in the urine is indicated by a negative anion gap (positive cation gap). For example, if urinary $Na^+ = 20$ mEq, $K^+ = 40$ mEq, and $Cl^- = 110$ mEq, the urinary anion gap is negative ($60 - 110 = -50$), indicating a normal renal response to acidosis and therefore a nonrenal cause of the hyperchloremic acidosis. The commonest cause of nonrenal hyperchloremic acidosis is gastrointestinal bicarbonate loss. In renal forms of hyperchloremic acidosis, the sum of urinary Na^+ and K^+ concentrations may exceed the urinary Cl^- concentration, resulting in a positive anion gap. The

Table 2–3. ANION GAP METABOLIC ACIDOSIS

CONDITION	RESPONSIBLE ANION
Renal failure	PO_4, SO_4 acid anions
Diabetic, starvation, or alcoholic ketoacidosis	Acetoacetic and β-hydroxybutyric acid
Tissue hypoperfusion and hypoxia	Lactate
Aspirin overdose	Salicylate
Paraldehyde overdose	Acetate
Ethylene glycol poisoning	Oxalate
Methyl alcohol poisoning	Formate
Total parenteral nutrition	Amino acid anions
High-flux dialysis	Acetate
Bowel disease	D-lactate

most common renal cause of nonanion gap acidosis is distal renal tubular acidosis.

Although the classification of metabolic acidosis into anion gap and nonanion gap forms has proved useful, it is well to remember that certain conditions can result in an increased anion gap in the absence of acidosis or a normal anion gap despite significant acidosis.[218] For example, metabolic alkalosis can cause an increase in the anion gap and methanol intoxication or lactic acidosis can occasionally occur without a significant increase in the anion gap.

Combined metabolic acidosis occurs when there is a combination of retention of an unmeasured anion and loss of HCO_3^-. An important example of this form is chronic renal failure, in which acidosis is the result of retention of fixed acids and failure of ammonium excretion.

Compensatory Mechanisms in Metabolic Acidosis. A rise in $[H^+]$ resulting from noncarbonic acid in the extracellular fluid elicits immediate buffering from hemoglobin, plasma proteins, bicarbonate, and phosphate. This is associated with a shift in the Henderson equation to the left, a decrease in $[HCO_3^-]$, and an increase in carbonic acid (which is dissipated in the lungs as carbon dioxide). The action of the increased $[H^+]$—particularly on brain stem receptors but also on the peripheral aortic and carotid chemoreceptors—augments alveolar ventilation and results in rapid elimination of carbon dioxide produced by the buffering of the excess H^+. Hyperventilation, which develops within minutes, depends on normality of the respiratory center and adequacy of ventilatory mechanics. With normal respiratory control and ventilatory mechanics, the $PaCO_2$ will decrease by approximately 1.1 mm Hg for each 1 mM decrease in HCO_3^-. The degree of compensatory hyperventilation reflects the

Table 2–4. NONANION GAP (HYPERCHLOREMIC) METABOLIC ACIDOSIS

Large Negative Urinary Anion Gap

Gastrointestinal loss of bicarbonate
Carbonic anhydrase inhibitors (e.g., acetazolamide)
Proximal renal tubular acidosis
Infusion of HCl or NH_4Cl
Spuriously low anion gap (e.g., anion gap acidosis with hypoproteinemia)

Positive or Small Negative Urinary Anion Gap

Distal renal tubular acidosis

severity of the metabolic acidosis, but appears to be maximal when the $PaCO_2$ reaches 8 to 12 mm Hg and $[H^+]$ is 80 nM per liter (pH 7.10). In these circumstances, the limiting factor may be the muscular effort required over a prolonged period.[212]

Although intracellular buffering, with the replacement by H^+ of K^+, Na^+, and Ca^{2+} in tissues (including bone), is slower than extracellular buffering, more noncarbonic acid is eventually buffered intracellularly than in the extracellular fluid;[219] carbonate $[CO_3^-]$ is released from bone and combines with some of the extra H^+ to form HCO_3^-. As long as renal function is satisfactory, there is a considerable adaptive increase in H^+ excretion, which may reach 10 times normal. Simultaneously, virtually all HCO_3^- filtered by the kidney is reabsorbed through the renal tubules. This compensatory mechanism, which operates from hours to days, obviously cannot develop when the noncarbonic acid excess is caused by renal failure.

Metabolic Alkalosis. Metabolic alkalosis results when the $[H^+]$ in extracellular fluid is decreased by loss of noncarbonic acid or an increase in alkali. This disturbance in acid-base balance commonly develops in patients with chronic CO_2 retention who are receiving therapy for cardiac and respiratory failure. Therefore, some knowledge of the mechanisms involved is particularly pertinent to the specialist in pulmonary disease.

Metabolic alkalosis can be divided into three types: chloride-responsive metabolic alkalosis, chloride-resistant metabolic alkalosis, and combined metabolic alkalosis. *Chloride-responsive alkalosis* is the most common form and is distinguished by (1) low levels of urinary Na^+ and Cl^-; (2) clinical evidence of intravascular volume depletion; (3) a paradoxical increase in urinary $[H^+]$ (decreased urinary pH); and (4) increased urinary K^+ in the face of decreased serum K^+. A common cause of chloride-responsive metabolic alkalosis is the excessive loss of noncarbonic acid during severe, prolonged vomiting or excessive gastric suction. Hydrochloric acid eliminated in this way depletes not only the H^+ in extracellular fluid but also Na^+, K^+, and Cl^- ions and fluid volume. Faced with decreased extracellular fluid volume, the distal tubules of the kidney retain Na^+ and, to maintain electrical neutrality, HCO_3^-. This type of alkalosis can be corrected by replacing fluid volume with solutions that contain sufficient NaCl and KCl. As volume expansion occurs, Na^+ is absorbed with its preferred anion Cl^-, and the excess bicarbonate is excreted. The metabolic alkalosis that develops as a consequence of chronic diuretic administration and after correction of chronic respiratory acidosis is also chloride responsive.

Chloride-resistant metabolic alkalosis is associated with extracellular fluid expansion and a high level of NaCl in the urine. This variety is caused by abnormal sodium absorption in the distal tubule of the kidney secondary to excessive mineralocorticoid activity; the latter may be related to an endogenous source (as in primary hyperaldosteronism) or an exogenous one (such as drugs and substances such as licorice that have mineralocorticoid activity). *Combined metabolic alkalosis* occurs in situations in which the criteria for the pure chloride-resistant or -responsive forms are absent. These include chronic congestive heart failure, Bartter's syndrome, and milk-alkali syndrome.

The commonest cause of metabolic alkalosis is undoubtedly the treatment of chronic carbon dioxide retention. In this situation, $[HCO_3^-]$ increases to compensate for the increased $[H^+]$; in most cases, this is accompanied by a decrease in chloride ion concentration secondary to increased renal acid excretion that compensates for the chronic respiratory acidosis. In these cases, there may be cardiac as well as respiratory failure, and treatment will be directed toward correcting both decompensated states. If artificial ventilation is used to reduce the P_{CO_2} quickly, the patient is left with excess HCO_3^- and, therefore, with metabolic alkalosis. This will worsen if corticosteroids are also given. The diuretics and low-sodium diet used in the treatment of heart failure deplete the body not only of Na^+ and Cl^- but also of extracellular fluid. As a result, the patient—originally in respiratory acidosis and perhaps still with carbon dioxide retention—now has an excess of HCO_3^- and a lack of Cl^- in a decreased extracellular fluid space, all factors that prolong the alkalosis.

Compensatory Mechanisms in Metabolic Alkalosis. An increased concentration of HCO_3^- is buffered in both extracellular and intracellular compartments. Lactic acid moves from the cells into the extracellular fluid, so that HCO_3^- and other conjugate bases are converted to the conjugate acids. The respiratory system compensates for H^+ depletion or HCO_3^- excess by underventilation,[220, 221] although the metabolic alkalosis resulting from thiazide diuretics and aldosterone may not elicit much compensatory underventilation.[212] As a rule of thumb, one can expect that for every 1 mM per liter increase in serum HCO_3^- the arterial P_{CO_2} will increase approximately 0.5 mm Hg.

The response of the kidney to acute metabolic alkalosis, which is prompt, is increased HCO_3^- excretion. If the cause of the alkalosis is not quickly corrected, however, renal compensation is complicated by such factors as the demand for renal Na^+ reabsorption and the Cl^- concentration in the extracellular fluid. As described earlier, some patients with chronic respiratory acidosis become depleted of Cl^- during therapy; in addition, the extracellular fluid volume decreases, requiring increased Na^+ reabsorption. What is called for in this circumstance is bicarbonate diuresis, but this is impossible because the unavailability of Cl^- and the strong stimulus for Na^+ reabsorption demand reabsorption of bicarbonate. This situation is characteristic of a chloride-responsive alkalosis and can be corrected only by restoring the extracellular fluid volume and by providing Cl^-, K^+, and Na^+; this is readily accomplished by infusion of NaCl supplemented with potassium.[222]

Acid-Base Nomograms. Clinical information is indispensable for the correct interpretation of acid-base disturbances. In addition, nomograms based on *in vivo* studies in humans and animals, delineating 95% confidence bands, may be useful in determining whether the disturbance is "pure" or "mixed."[223] Such confidence bands define the range of acid-base values expected in 95% of cases of a specific acid-base disorder. Values for P_{CO_2}, $[H^+]$, and $[HCO_3^-]$ in response to acute[224, 225] and chronic[214, 226] hypoventilation and hyperventilation have been established. Unlike respiratory disorders, however, acute and chronic metabolic acid-base disturbances do not have such clearly delineated confidence bands.[227]

Most acid-base nomograms suggested for clinical use plot either P_{CO_2} against $[H^+]$ (pH) or P_{CO_2} against $[HCO_3^-]$, with linear isopleths of the third component radiating from the origin.[211, 227–229] Figure 2–33, which depicts such a nomogram, shows 95% confidence bands that define a single respiratory or metabolic acid-base disturbance. Although values outside the bands almost certainly represent "mixed" disturbances, those within the bands do not necessarily represent a single disturbance.[225] For example, as discussed previously, the combination of compensated respiratory acidosis and superimposed metabolic acidosis can result in values for pH, HCO_3^- and P_{CO_2} falling within the expected range for acute respiratory acidosis.

THE BRONCHIAL CIRCULATION

Anatomy

There is considerable variation in the number and origin of human bronchial arteries. In most people, there are two to four arteries, a relatively common pattern being one on the right (originating from the third intercostal artery [the first right intercostal artery that arises directly from the aorta]), and two on the left (arising directly from the aorta on its anterolateral aspect, usually opposite the fifth and sixth thoracic vertebrae).[230–233] Occasionally, they originate elsewhere in the aorta or in extra-aortic vessels such as the subclavian, innominate, internal mammary, or coronary areteries.[234, 235]

The extrapulmonary branches of the bronchial arteries make fairly numerous anastomoses with other mediastinal arteries, including coronary, esophageal, thymic, and pericardial vessels. They then course to the hila, where they form an intercommunicating circular arc around the main bronchi from which the true bronchial arteries radiate.[231] Their diameter at the hilum is about 1 to 1.5 mm.

The intrapulmonary arteries are situated within the peribronchial connective tissue and extend along the bronchial tree, branching with the airways. Generally, two or three major divisions are present with each bronchus, one on each side of the airway wall. These branches have extensive horizontal intercommunications within the bronchial adventitia[236, 237] and also send twigs through the bronchial wall to form a similar intercommunicating vascular plexus in the submucosa. The latter comprises as much as 10% to 20% of the volume of the normal subepithelial tissue, and it has been hypothesized that significant airway narrowing may occur when these vessels become congested.[238] However, in one study of sheep in which the bronchial vascular volume was increased by 50% by inhalation challenge with the vasodilator histamine, most of the airway narrowing was secondary to airway smooth muscle contraction, vascular congestion providing only a minor contribution.[239] The arteries continue as far as the terminal bronchioles; with injection techniques, small arteriolar branches can sometimes be seen to extend to the alveolar ducts and occasionally even into the lung parenchyma around alveolar sacs.[231]

Histologically, the larger bronchial arteries have a well-developed muscular media and a prominent internal elastic lamina. In addition, there is frequently a longitudinal intimal muscle layer that occasionally becomes quite voluminous and appears to occlude the vascular lumen completely. It has been suggested that this layer is the result of airway stretch-

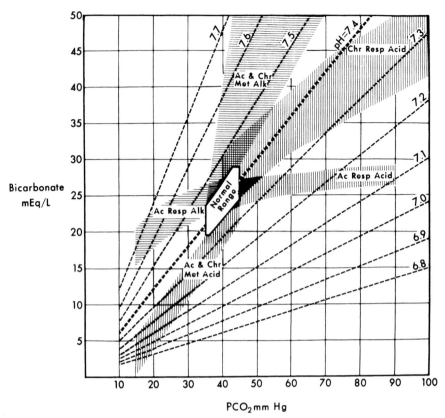

Bicarbonate mEq/L

PCO₂ mm Hg

Figure 2–33. Acid-Base Nomogram. *In vivo* nomogram showing bands for defining a single respiratory or metabolic acid-base disturbance. (From Arbus GS: Can Med Assoc J 109:291, 1973.)

ing during normal respiration;[231] it has also been considered to represent an age-related reparative change.[11] The bronchial capillaries are lined by a continuous layer of endothelial cells joined by tight junctions. These are surrounded almost entirely by basement membrane (the exception being where the vessels are apposed to neuroepithelial bodies, at which point the endothelium is discontinuous).[235]

The bronchial circulation is unique in that it has a dual venous drainage. One portion—related predominantly to the trachea and large bronchi—drains via the bronchial veins to the right side of the heart via the azygos and hemiazygos systems. A second portion, related to the major portion of the intrapulmonary bronchial flow,[235] is derived from extensive anastomoses with the pulmonary circulation at precapillary, capillary, and postcapillary sites and drains into the left atrium via the pulmonary veins (the bronchopulmonary anastomotic flow).[240]

In addition to providing a blood supply to the bronchial and bronchiolar walls, the bronchial arteries supply the peribronchial and perivascular connective tissue; the tracheal wall; the vasa vasorum of the aortic arch, pulmonary arteries, and pulmonary veins; the middle third of the esophagus; at least part of the visceral pleura (*see* page 151); the paratracheal, carinal, hilar, and intrapulmonary lymph nodes and lymphoid tissue; the vagus and bronchopulmonary nerves; and (sometimes) the parietal layer of the pericardium and the thymus.[230]

There are extensive anastomoses between branches of the bronchial arteries and between the bronchial vessels and other systemic intrathoracic arteries (e.g., tracheal and coronary arteries). This may be one explanation of why embolization of the bronchial arteries is often only temporar-

ily effective in stopping hemoptysis. In one study in sheep, embolization of the common bronchial artery by ethanol, sufficient to completely block the vessel by angiographic assessment, caused only a 50% reduction in systemic blood flow to the region of the lung supplied by this vessel as measured with radioactive microspheres.[241]

Flow and Nervous Control

In a study of anesthetized dogs employing a modification of the radioactive-microsphere technique, bronchial blood flow has been partitioned into parenchymal (anastomotic) and large airway fractions;[242] according to this investigation, 55% of the total bronchial blood flow goes to lung parenchyma and 45% to the trachea and bronchi. Approximately 80% of the bronchial blood flow returns to the left heart via anastomotic channels.[243] Measurements of bronchopulmonary anastomotic flow have been made in patients undergoing coronary artery bypass surgery, since during cross-clamping of the aorta bronchopulmonary anastomotic flow is the only blood returning to the left side of the heart. In this circumstance, flow has been found to be highly variable, ranging from 1% to almost 24% of cardiac output; it is increased in patients with cardiac and pulmonary disease.[244]

Bronchial arterial blood flow has been shown to be directly related to changes in systemic blood pressure.[245, 246] An increase in systemic venous pressure or a decrease in left atrial pressure causes a decrease in bronchial venous drainage and preferential drainage to the left side of the heart, whereas the opposite occurs with elevation of the left atrial pressure and a decrease in systemic venous pressure.[245] The bronchial vasculature is compressed with increasing alveolar pressure[246, 247] and is also sensitive to changes in Po_2 and Pco_2, responding to acute changes in gas tensions differently than do either the pulmonary or systemic circulations.[248] Severe hypoxemia causes a significant increase in bronchovascular resistance; hypercapnia causes a decrease in bronchovascular resistance and an increase in bronchial blood flow.

The bronchial vasculature has both parasympathetic and sympathetic innervation.[249] Parasympathetic vagal stimulation causes vasodilation, whereas sympathetic stimulation results in vasoconstriction and a consequent reduction in flow.[250] It has also been shown that dogs have both α- and β-adrenergic receptors;[251] the former predominate and, when stimulated, result in vasoconstriction, whereas β-adrenergic receptors mediate vasodilation. As in other systemic vascular beds, the baseline caliber of the bronchial arteries is controlled by production of the endothelial-derived relaxant nitric oxide (NO).[252] Increased production of NO by these cells may be an important mechanism of bronchial arterial dilation in response to various stimuli.[253]

Function

The bronchial vasculature probably has several functions, although only a few have been examined in any depth. Perhaps the most obvious and certainly one of the most important is the supply of substrate and oxygen to constituents of the airway wall. Bronchial arterial occlusion can cause a reduction in mucociliary transport[254, 255] and, if prolonged, bronchial wall necrosis.[256] The circulation can also serve as a "backup" vascular system for the lungs; in fact, pulmonary infarction rarely occurs after ligation of the main pulmonary artery because of "collateral" bronchial blood flow to the obstructed areas of lung.[257]

The bronchial circulation may also play an important role in the humidification and warming of inspired air.[258] Anatomically, it is ideally suited for this function, since it contains two intercommunicating venous plexuses: one is adjacent to the bronchial epithelium and the other is deep in the peribronchial connective tissue. Studies in dogs have shown that the bronchial vasculature of the trachea and large airways is extremely sensitive to changes in inspired air temperature and humidity: bronchial blood flow increases to more than twice its baseline value in response to the inhalation of cold air and up to 10 times its baseline value in response to the inhalation of warm, dry air.[259] This increase in blood flow is not affected by vagotomy, α- or β-adrenergic blockade, or the inhibition of prostaglandin synthesis.[260] The breathing of dry air has also been shown to increase bronchial blood flow in humans.[261, 262]

Finally, it has been suggested that the bronchial circulation may be important in the production of pulmonary edema when vascular pressure is increased and in the reabsorption of edema fluid from the interstitial space when microvascular pressures decrease.[263]

Although it has long been known that the bronchial circulation contributes to the normal anatomic shunt, its contribution to the gas exchange shunt is small.[264, 265] In one study using the inert gas technique, only about 20% of bronchial blood flow was found to bypass gas-exchanging units;[265] thus, only 20% of less than 1% of the cardiac output is "shunted" by this circulation. The portion that is not shunted from bronchial capillaries to pulmonary veins mixes with blood in the pulmonary arteries and capillaries and takes part in gas exchange. It is important to remember that bronchial vessels have the capacity to proliferate and undergo a marked increase in volume in many pulmonary and cardiac abnormalities, in which case shunting may be much more pronounced: flows of almost 25% of cardiac output have been reported in some patients undergoing cardiopulmonary bypass surgery.[244]

REFERENCES

1. Cory RAS, Valentine EJ: Varying patterns of the lobar branches of the pulmonary artery. Thorax 14:267, 1959.
2. Elliot FM, Reid L: Some new facts about the pulmonary artery and its branching pattern. Clin Radiol 16:193, 1965.
3. Horsfield K: Morphometry of the small pulmonary arteries in man. Circ Res 42:593, 1978.
4. Singhal S, Henderson R, Horsfield K, et al: Morphometry of the human pulmonary arterial tree. Circ Res 33:190, 1973.
5. Heath D, Wood EH, DuShane JW, et al: The structure of the pulmonary trunk at different ages and in cases of pulmonary hypertension and pulmonary stenosis. J Pathol Bacteriol 77:443, 1959.
6. Reid L: Personal communication, 1984.
7. Wilkinson MJ, Gray T: Tissue arrangement in the internal elastic lamina of the rat muscular pulmonary artery. J Pathol 153:177, 1987.
8. MacKay EH, Banks J, Sykes B, et al: Structural basis for the changing physical properties of human pulmonary vessels with age. Thorax 33:335, 1978.
9. Plank L, James J, Wagenvoort CA: Caliber and elastin content of the pulmonary trunk. Arch Pathol Lab Med 104:238, 1980.
10. Pump KK: The circulation in the peripheral parts of the human lung. Dis Chest 49:119, 1966.
11. Wagenvoort CA, Wagenvoort N: Pathology of Pulmonary Hypertension. New York, John Wiley & Sons, 1977.
12. Berend N, Wollcock AJ, Marlin GE: Relationship between bronchial and arterial diameters in normal human lungs. Thorax 34:354, 1979.
13. Brinkman GL: Ultrastructure of atherosclerosis in the human pulmonary artery. Am Rev Respir Dis 105:351, 1972.
14. Moore GW, Smith RRL, Hutchins GM: Pulmonary artery atherosclerosis: Correlation with systemic atherosclerosis and hypertensive pulmonary vascular disease. Arch Pathol Lab Med 106:378, 1982.
15. Brenner O: Pathology of the vessels of the pulmonary circulation: I. Arch Intern Med 56:211, 1935.
16. Balk AG, Dingemans KP, Wagenvoort CA: The ultrastructure of the various forms of pulmonary arterial intimal fibrosis. Virchows Arch [A] Pathol Anat Histol 382:139, 1979.
17. Fernie JM, Lamb D: Effects of age and smoking on intima of muscular pulmonary arteries. J Clin Pathol 39:1204, 1986.
18. Weibel ER: On pericytes, particularly their existence on lung capillaries. Microvasc Res 8:218, 1974.
19. Meyrick B, Reid L: Ultrastructural findings in lung biopsy material from children with congenital heart defects. Am J Pathol 101:527, 1980.
20. Meyrick B, Reid L: The effect of continued hypoxia on rat pulmonary arterial circulation: An ultrastructural study. Lab Invest 38:188, 1978.
21. Nadziejko CE, Loud AV, Kikkawa Y: Effect of alveolar hypoxia on pulmonary mast cells in vivo. Am Rev Respir Dis 140: 743, 1989.
22. Hislop A, Reid L: Fetal and childhood development of the intrapulmonary veins in man: Branching pattern and structure. Thorax 28:313, 1973.
23. Horsfield K, Gordon WI: Morphometry of pulmonary veins in man. Lung 159:211, 1981.
24. Schraufnagel DR, Patel KR: Sphincters in pulmonary veins: An anatomic study in rats. Am Rev Respir Dis 141:721, 1990.
25. Schraufnagel DE, Thakkar MB: Pulmonary venous sphincter constriction is attenuated by α-adrenergic antagonism. Am Rev Respir Dis 148:477, 1993.
26. Heath D, Williams D: Arachnoid nodules in the lungs of high-altitude Indians. Thorax 48:743, 1993.
27. Crapo JD, Barry BE, Gehr P, et al: Cell number and cell characteristics of the normal human lung. Am Rev Respir Dis 125:332, 1982.
28. Heath D, Smith P: The pulmonary endothelial cell. Thorax 34:200, 1979.
29. Ryan JW, Ryan US: Pulmonary endothelial cells. Fed Proc 36:2683, 1977.
30. Smith U, Ryan JW, Michie DD, et al: Endothelial projections as revealed by scanning electron microscopy. Science 173:925, 1971.
31. Ryan US, Ryan JW, Whitaker C, et al: Localization of angiotensin converting enzyme (kininase II): II. Immunocytochemistry and immunofluorescence. Tissue Cell 8:125, 1976.
32. Smith U, Ryan JW: Substructural features of pulmonary endothelial caveolae. Tissue Cell 4:49, 1972.
33. Strum JM, Junod AF: Radioautographic demonstration of 5-hydroxytryptamine-3H uptake by pulmonary endothelial cells. J Cell Biol 54:456, 1972.
34. Pietra GG, Sampson P, Lanken PN, et al: Transcapillary movement of cationized ferritin in the isolated perfused rat lung. Lab Invest 49:54, 1983.
35. Schneeberger EE: Structural basis for some permeability properties of the air-blood barrier. Fed Proc 37:2471, 1978.
36. Simionescu D, Simionescu M: Differentiated distribution of the cell surface charge on the alveolar-capillary unit: Characteristic paucity of anionic sites on the air-blood barrier. Microvasc Res 25:85, 1983.
37. Schneeberger EE: Barrier function of intercellular junctions in adult and fetal lungs. In Fishman AP, Renkin EM (eds): Pulmonary Edema. Bethesda, MD, American Physiological Society, 1979, p 21.
38. Schneeberger-Keeley EE, Karnovsky MJ: The ultrastructural basis of alveolar-capillary membrane permeability to peroxidase used as a tracer. J Cell Biol 37:781, 1968.
39. Yoneda K: Regional differences in the intercellular junctions of the alveolar-capillary membrane in the human lung. Am Rev Respir Dis 126:893, 1982.
40. Hanley ME, Terada LS, Cheronis JC, et al: Endothelial cell associated antielastolytic activity. Inflammation 20:327, 1996.
41. Ziegler JW, Ivy DD, Kinsella JP, et al: The role of nitric oxide, endothelin, and prostaglandins in the transition of the pulmonary circulation. Clin Perinatol 22:387, 1995.
42. Bevilacqua MP, Nelson RM, Mannori G, et al: Endothelial-leukocyte adhesion molecules in human disease. Annu Rev Med 45:361, 1994.
43. Fleming RE, Crouch EC, Ruzicka CA, et al: Pulmonary carbonic anhydrase. IV: Developmental regulation and cell-specific expression in the capillary endothelium. Am J Physiol 265:L627, 1993.
44. Gee MH, Albertine KH: Neutrophil-endothelial cell interactions in the lung. Annu Rev Physiol 55:227, 1993.
45. Kourembanas S, Bernfield M: Hypoxia and endothelial–smooth muscle interactions in the lung. Am J Respir Cell Mol Biol 11:373, 1994.
46. Su WY, Folz R, Chen JS, et al: Extracellular superoxide dismutase mRNA expressions in the human lung by in situ hybridization. Am J Respir Cell Mol Biol 16:162, 1997.
47. Crystal RG: Biochemical processes in the normal lung. In Bouhuys A (ed): Lung Cells in Disease. New York, North Holland Biomedical Press, 1976, p 17.
48. Bowden DH, Adamson IYR: Endothelial regeneration as a marker of the differential vascular responses in oxygen-induced pulmonary edema. Lab Invest 30:350, 1974.
49. Weibel ER: Morphometry of the Human Lung. New York, Academic Press, 1963.
50. Weibel ER, Gomez DM: Architecture of the human lung. Science 137:577, 1962.
51. Kendall MW, Eissman E: Scanning electron microscopic examination of human pulmonary capillaries using a latex replication method. Anat Rec 196:275, 1980.
52. Glazier JB, Hughes JMB, Maloney JE, et al: Measurements of capillary dimensions and blood volume in rapidly frozen lungs. J Appl Physiol 26:65, 1969.
53. Stocker JT, Malczak HT: A study of pulmonary ligament arteries: Relationship to intralobar pulmonary sequestration. Chest 86:611, 1984.
54. Jefferson KE: The normal pulmonary angiogram and some changes seen in chronic nonspecific lung disease: I. The pulmonary vessels in the normal pulmonary angiogram. Proc Roy Soc Med 58:677, 1965.
55. Chang CH (Joseph): The normal roentgenographic measurement of the right descending pulmonary artery in 1,085 cases. Am J Roentgenol 87:929, 1962.
56. Wójtowicz J: Some tomographic criteria for an evaluation of the pulmonary circulation. Acta Radiol (Diagn) 2:215, 1964.
57. Woodring JH: Pulmonary artery–bronchus ratios in patients with normal lungs, pulmonary vascular plethora, and congestive heart failure. Radiology 179:115, 1991.
58. Ravin CE: Gleaning physiologic information from the conventional chest radiograph (editorial). Radiology 179:17, 1991.
59. O'Callaghan JP, Heitzman ER, Somogyi JW, et al: CT evaluation of pulmonary artery size. J Comput Assist Tomogr 6:101, 1982.
60. Kuriyama K, Gamsu G, Stern RG, et al: CT-determined pulmonary artery diameters in predicting pulmonary hypertension. Invest Radiol 19:16, 1984.
61. Kim SJ, Im J-G, Kim IO, et al: Normal bronchial and pulmonary arterial diameters measured by thin-section CT. J Comput Assist Tomogr 19:365, 1995.
62. Burko H, Carwell G, Newman E: Size, location, and gravitational changes of normal upper lobe pulmonary veins. Am J Roentgenol 111:687, 1971.
63. Genereux GP: Conventional tomographic hilar anatomy emphasizing the pulmonary veins. Am J Roentgenol 141:1241, 1983.
64. Heitzman ER: The Mediastinum: Radiologic Correlations with Anatomy and Pathology. St. Louis, CV Mosby, 1977, pp 216–334.
65. Heitzman ER: Radiologic diagnosis of mediastinal lymph node enlargement. J Can Assoc Radiol 29:151, 1978.
66. Yamashita H: Roentgenologic Anatomy of the Lung. Tokyo, Igaku-Shoin, 1978, pp 10–25, 70–107.
67. Shevland JE, Chiu LC, Shapiro RL, et al: The role of conventional tomography and computed tomography in assessing the resectability of primary lung cancer: A preliminary report. J Comput Tomogr 2:1, 1978.
68. Favez G, Willa C, Heinzer F: Posterior oblique tomography at an angle of 55 degrees in chest roentgenology. Am J Roentgenol 120:907, 1974.
69. Felson B: Chest Roentgenology. Philadelphia, WB Saunders, 1973, p 185.
70. Fraser RG, Fraser RS, Renner JW, et al: The roentgenologic diagnosis of chronic bronchitis: A reassessment with emphasis on parahilar bronchi seen end-on. Radiology 120:1, 1976.
71. Simon G: Principles of Chest X-Ray Diagnosis. 3rd ed. London, Butterworth, 1971.
72. Vix VA, Klatte EC: The lateral chest radiograph in the diagnosis of hilar and mediastinal masses. Radiology 96:307, 1970.
73. Proto AV, Speckman JM: The left lateral radiograph of the chest: I. Med Radiogr Photogr 55:30, 1979.
74. Proto AV, Speckman JM: The left lateral radiograph of the chest: II. Med Radiogr Photogr 56:38, 1980.
75. Schnur MJ, Winkler B, Austin JHM: Widening of the posterior wall of the bronchus intermedius: A sign on lateral chest radiographs of congestive heart failure, lymph node enlargement, and neoplastic infiltration. Radiology 139:551, 1981.
76. Webb WR, Gamsu G: Computed tomography of the left retrobronchial stripe. J Comput Assist Tomog 7:65, 1983.

77. Naidich DP, Khouri NF, Scott WW, et al: Computed tomography of the pulmonary hila: Normal anatomy. J Comput Assist Tomogr 5:459, 1981.

78. Webb WR, Glazier G, Gamsu G: Computed tomography of the normal pulmonary hilum. J Comput Assist Tomogr 5:476, 1981.

79. Naidich DP, Khouri NF, Scott WW, et al: Computed tomography of the pulmonary hila: Abnormal anatomy. J Comput Assist Tomogr 5:468, 1981.

80. Webb WR, Glazier G, Gamsu G: Computed tomography of the abnormal pulmonary hilum. J Comput Assist Tomogr 5:485, 1981.

81. Glazer GM, Francis IR, Gebarski K, et al: Dynamic incremental computed tomography in evaluation of the pulmonary hila. J Comput Assist Tomogr 7:59, 1983.

82. Shepard JO, Dedrick CG, Spizarny DL, et al: Technical node: Dynamic incremental computed tomography of the pulmonary hila using a flow-rate injector. J Comput Assist Tomogr 10:369, 1986.

83. Remy-Jardin M, Duyck P, Remy J, et al: Hilar lymph nodes: Identification with spiral CT and histologic correlation. Radiology 196:387, 1995.

83a. Müller NL, Webb WR: Radiographic imaging of the pulmonary hila. Invest Radiol 20:661, 1985.

83b. Primack SL, Lee KS, Logan PM, et al: Bronchogenic carcinoma: Utility of CT in the evaluation of patients with suspected lesions. Radiology 193:795, 1994.

84. Itoh H, Murata K, Todo G, et al: Anatomy of pulmonary lung tissue in the hilum. Jpn J Clin Radiol 29:1459, 1984.

85. Lallemand D, Wesbey GE, Gooding CA: Cardiosynchronous MRI intensity changes of the great vessels and pulmonary circulation: A preliminary report. Ann Radiol 28:299, 1985.

86. Hatabu H, Gefter WB, Kressel HY, et al: Pulmonary vasculature: High-resolution MR imaging—work in progress. Radiology 171:391, 1989.

87. Gefter WB, Hatabu H, Dinsmore BJ, et al: Pulmonary vascular cine MR imaging: A noninvasive approach to dynamic imaging of the pulmonary circulation. Radiology 176:761, 1990.

88. Mazer MJ, Carroll FE, Falke THM: Practical aspects of gated magnetic resonance imaging of the pulmonary artery. J Thorac Imaging 3:73, 1988.

89. Axel L: Blood flow effects in magnetic resonance imaging. Am J Roentgenol 143:1157, 1984.

90. Bradley WG Jr, Waluch V, Lai K-S, et al: The appearance of rapidly flowing blood on magnetic resonance imaging. Am J Roentgenol 143:1167, 1984.

91. O'Donovan PB, Ross JS, Sivak ED, et al: Magnetic resonance imaging of the thorax: The advantages of coronal and sagittal planes. Am J Roentgenol 143:1183, 1984.

92. Webb WR, Jensen BG, Gamsu G, et al: Coronal magnetic resonance imaging of the chest: Normal and abnormal. Radiology 153:729, 1984.

93. Glover GH, Pelc NJ: A rapid-gated cine MRI technique. *In* Kressel HY (ed): Magnetic Resonance Annual 1988. New York, Raven, 1988, p 299.

94. Giovagnoni A, Ercolani P, Misericordia M, et al: Evaluation of the pulmonary artery by cine MRI. J Computer Assist Tomogr 16:553, 1992.

95. Gamsu G, Webb WR, Sheldon P, et al: Nuclear magnetic resonance imaging of the thorax. Radiology 147:473, 1983.

96. Axel L, Kressel HY, Thickman D, et al: NMR imaging of the chest at 0.12 T: Initial clinical experience with a resistive magnet. Am J Roentgenol 141:1157, 1983.

97. Staub NC: The interdependence of pulmonary structure and function. Anesthesiology 24:831, 1963.

98. Yu PN: Pulmonary Blood Volume in Health and Disease. Philadelphia, Lea & Febiger, 1969.

99. Roughton FJW, Forster RE: Relative importance of diffusion and chemical reaction rates in determining rate of exchange of gases in the human lung, with special reference to true diffusing capacity of pulmonary membrane and volume of blood in the lung capillaries. J Appl Physiol 11:290, 1957.

100. Bates DV, Varvis CJ, Donevan RE, et al: Variations in the pulmonary capillary blood volume and membrane diffusion component in health and disease. J Clin Invest 39:1401, 1960.

101. Newman F, Smalley BF, Thomson ML: Effect of exercise, body and lung size on CO diffusion in athletes and nonathletes. J Appl Physiol 17:649, 1962.

102. Johnson RL Jr, Taylor HF, Lawson WH Jr, with the technical assistance of Prengler: Maximal diffusing capacity of the lung for carbon monoxide. J Clin Invest 44:349, 1965.

103. Weibel ER: Morphometrische Analyse von Zahl, Volumen and Oberfläche der Alveolen and Kapillären der menschlichen Lunge. Z Zellforsch Mikrosk Anat 57:648, 1962.

104. Cander L, Forster RE: Determination of pulmonary parenchymal tissue volume and pulmonary capillary blood flow in man. J Appl Physiol 14:541, 1959.

105. Cope DK, Grimbert F, Downey JM, et al: Pulmonary capillary pressure: A review. Crit Care Med 20:1043, 1992.

106. Bhattacharya J, Staub NC: Direct measurement of microvascular pressures in the isolated perfused dog lung. Science 210:327, 1980.

107. Negrini D, Gonano C, Miserocchi G: Microvascular pressure profile in intact *in situ* lung. J Appl Physiol 72:332, 1992.

108. Hakim TS, Michel RP, Chang HK: Partitioning vascular resistance in dogs by arterial and venous occlusion. J Appl Physiol Respir Environ 52:710, 1982.

109. Yamada Y, Komatsu K, Suzukawa M, et al: Pulmonary capillary pressure measured with a pulmonary arterial double-port catheter in surgical patients. Anesth Analg 77:1130, 1993.

110. Baconnier PF, Eberhard A, Grimbert FA: Theoretical analysis of occlusion techniques for measuring pulmonary capillary pressure. J Appl Physiol 73:1351, 1992.

111. Cope DK, Grimbert F, Downey JM, et al: Pulmonary capillary pressure: A review. Crit Care Med 20:1043, 1992.

112. Weed HG: Pulmonary "capillary" wedge pressure not the pressure in the pulmonary capillaries. Chest 100:1138, 1991.

113. Caro CG: Physics of blood flow in the lung. Br Med Bull 19:66, 1963.

114. Means LJ, Hanson WL, Mounts KO, et al: Pulmonary capillary recruitment in neonatal lambs. Pediatr Res 34:596, 1993.

115. West JB, Dollery CT, Naimark A: Distribution of blood flow in isolated lung: Relation to vascular and alveolar pressures. J Appl Physiol 19:713, 1964.

116. West JB: Regional differences in the lung. Chest 74:426, 1978.

117. Maeda H, Itoh H, Ishii Y, et al: Pulmonary blood flow distribution measured by radionuclide computed tomography. J Appl Physiol 54:225, 1983.

118. Nemery B, Wijns W, Piret L, et al: Pulmonary vascular tone is a determinant of basal lung perfusion in normal seated subjects. J Appl Physiol 54:262, 1983.

119. Glenny RW, Lamm WJ, Albert RK, et al: Gravity is a minor determinant of pulmonary blood flow distribution. J Appl Physiol 71:620, 1991.

120. Hakim TS, Lisbona R, Michel RP, et al: Role of vasoconstriction in gravity-nondependent central-peripheral gradient in pulmonary blood flow. J Appl Physiol 74:897, 1993.

121. Glenny RW, Polissar L, Robertson HT: Relative contribution of gravity to pulmonary perfusion heterogeneity. J Appl Physiol 71:2449, 1991.

122. Glenny RW: Spatial correlation of regional pulmonary perfusion. J Appl Physiol 72:2378, 1992.

123. Glenny RW, Robertson HT: Fractal modeling of pulmonary blood flow heterogeneity. J Appl Physiol 70:1024, 1991.

124. Caruthers SD, Harris TR: Effects of pulmonary blood flow on the fractal nature of flow heterogeneity in sheep lungs. J Appl Physiol 77:1474, 1994.

125. Tokics L: Radiospirometry V/Q. Acta Anaesthesiol Scand Suppl 95:97, 1991.

126. Permutt S, Howell JBL, Proctor DF, et al: Effect of lung inflation on static pressure-volume characteristics of pulmonary vessels. J Appl Physiol 16:64, 1961.

127. Howell JBL, Permutt S, Proctor DF, et al: Effect of inflation of the lung on different parts of the pulmonary vascular bed. J Appl Physiol 16:71, 1961.

128. Thomas LJ, Griffo ZJ, Roos A: Effect of negative-pressure inflation of the lung on pulmonary vascular resistance. J Appl Physiol 16:451, 1961.

129. Whittenberger JL, McGregor M, Berglund E, et al: Influence of state of inflation of the lung on pulmonary vascular resistance. J Appl Physiol 15:878, 1960.

130. Hakim TS, Michel RP, Chang HK: Effect of lung inflation on pulmonary vascular resistance by arterial and venous occlusion. J Appl Physiol 53:1110, 1982.

131. Culver BH, Butler J: Mechanical influences on the pulmonary micro-circulation. Annu Rev Physiol 42:187, 1980.

132. Lamm WJ, Kirk KR, Hanson WL, et al: Flow through zone 1 lungs utilizes alveolar corner vessels. J Appl Physiol 70:1518, 1991.

133. Isawa T, Teshima T, Hirano T, et al: Regulation of regional perfusion distribution in the lungs: Effect of regional oxygen concentration. Am Rev Respir Dis 118:55, 1978.

134. Fishman AP: Vasomotor regulation of the pulmonary circulation. Annu Rev Physiol 42:211, 1980.

135. Marshall C, Marshall B: Site and sensitivity for stimulation of hypoxic pulmonary vasoconstriction. J Appl Physiol 55:711, 1983.

136. Hakim TS, Michel RP, Minami H, et al: Site of pulmonary hypoxic vasoconstriction studied with arterial and venous occlusion. J Appl Physiol 54:1298, 1983.

137. Linehan JH, Dawson CA: A three-compartment model of the pulmonary vasculature: Effects of vasoconstriction. J Appl Physiol 55:923, 1983.

138. Sylvester JT, Mitzner W, Ngeow Y, et al: Hypoxic constriction of alveolar and extra-alveolar vessels in isolated pig lungs. J Appl Physiol 54:1660, 1983.

139. Douglas SA, Vickery-Clark LM, Ohlstein EH: Endothelin 1 does not mediate hypoxic vasoconstriction in canine isolated blood vessels: Effect of BQ-123. Br J Pharmacol 108:418, 1993.

140. Dumas JP, Dumas M, Sgro C, et al: Effects of two K^+ channel openers, aprikalim and pinacidil, on hypoxic pulmonary vasoconstriction. Eur J Pharmacol 263:17, 1994.

141. Greenberg B, Kishiyama S: Endothelium-dependent and independent responses to severe hypoxia in rat pulmonary artery. Am J Physiol 265:H1712, 1993.

142. Freden F, Wei SZ, Berglund JE, et al: Nitric oxide modulation of pulmonary blood flow distribution in lobar hypoxia. Anesthesiology 82:1216, 1995.

143. Dinh-Xuan AT: Endothelial modulation of pulmonary vascular tone. Eur Resp J 5:757, 1992.

144. Stewart DJ: Endothelial dysfunction in pulmonary vascular disorders. Arzneimittelforschung 44:451, 1994.

145. Russ RD, Walker BR: Role of nitric oxide in vasopressinergic pulmonary vasodilatation. Am J Physiol 262:H743, 1992.

146. Bergofsky EH, Lehr DE, Fishman AP: The effect of changes in hydrogen ion concentration on the pulmonary circulation. J Clin Invest 41:1492, 1962.

147. Silove ED, Inoue T, Grover RF: Comparison of hypoxia, pH, and sympathomimetic drugs on bovine pulmonary vasculature. J Appl Physiol 24:355, 1968.

148. Downing SE, Lee JC: Nervous control of the pulmonary circulation. Annu Rev Physiol 42:199, 1980.

149. Bergofsky EH: Humoral control of the pulmonary circulation. Annu Rev Physiol 42:221, 1980.

150. Georg J, Lassen NA, Millemgaard K, et al: Diffusion in the gas phase of the lungs in normal and emphysematous subjects. Clin Sci 29:525, 1965.

151. Jameson AG: Diffusion of gases from alveolus to precapillary arteries. Science 139:826, 1963.

152. Nagaishi C: Functional Anatomy and Histology of the Lung. Baltimore, University Park Press, 1972.

153. Hopkins SR, McKenzie DC, Schoene RB, et al: Pulmonary gas exchange during exercise in athletes: I. Ventilation-perfusion mismatch and diffusion limitation. J Appl Physiol 77:912, 1994.

154. Warren GL, Cureton KJ, Middendorf WF, et al: Red blood cell pulmonary capillary transit time during exercise in athletes. Med Sci Sports Exercise 23:1353, 1991.

155. Schaffartzik W, Poole DC, Derion T, et al: $\dot{V}A/\dot{Q}$ distribution during heavy exercise and recovery in humans: Implications for pulmonary edema. J Appl Physiol 72:1657, 1992.

156. Rasmussen J, Hanel B, Saunamaki K, et al: Recovery of pulmonary diffusing capacity after maximal exercise. J Sports Sci 10:525, 1992.

157. Hanel B, Clifford PS, Secher NH: Restricted postexercise pulmonary diffusion capacity does not impair maximal transport for O_2. J Appl Physiol 77:2408, 1994.

158. Manier G, Moinard J, Stoicheff H: Pulmonary diffusing capacity after maximal exercise. J Appl Physiol 75:2580, 1993.

159. Bates DV, Macklem PT, Christie RV: Respiratory Function in Diseases: An Introduction to the Integrated Study of the Lung. 2nd ed. Philadelphia, WB Saunders, 1971.

160. Piiper J: Alveolar-capillary gas transfer in lungs: Development of concepts and current state. Adv Exp Med Biol 345:7, 1994.

161. Piiper J: Diffusion-perfusion inhomogeneity and alveolar-arterial O_2 diffusion limitation: Theory. Respir Physiol 87:349, 1992.

162. Yamaguchi K, Kawai A, Mori M, et al: Distribution of ventilation and of diffusing capacity to perfusion in the lung. Respir Physiol 86:171, 1991.

163. Finley TN, Swenson EW, Comroe JH Jr: The cause of arterial hypoxemia at rest in patients with "alveolar-capillary block syndrome." J Clin Invest 41:618, 1962.

164. Read J, Williams RS: Pulmonary ventilation/blood flow relationships in interstitial disease of the lungs. Am J Med 27:545, 1959.

165. Betticher DC, Geiser J, Tempini A: Lung diffusing capacity and red blood cell volume. Respir Physiol 85:271, 1991.

166. Reeves RB, Park HK: CO uptake kinetics of red cells and CO diffusing capacity. Respir Physiol 88:1, 1992.

167. Roughton FJW, Forster RE: Relative importance of diffusion and chemical reaction rates in determining rate of exchange of gases in the human lung, with special reference to true diffusing capacity of pulmonary membrane and volume of blood in the lung capillaries. J Appl Physiol 11:290, 1957.

168. Crapo JD, Crapo RO: Comparison of total lung diffusion capacity and the membrane component of diffusion capacity as determined by physiologic and morphometric techniques. Respir Physiol 51:183, 1983.

169. Weibel ER, Federspiel WJ, Fryder-Doffey F, et al: Morphometric model for pulmonary diffusing capacity: I. Membrane-diffusing capacity. 93:125, 1993.

170. Engel LA: Effect of microgravity on the respiratory system. J Appl Physiol 70:1907, 1991.

171. Prisk GK, Guy HJ, Elliott AR, et al: Pulmonary diffusing capacity, capillary blood volume, and cardiac output during sustained microgravity. J Appl Physiol 75:15, 1993.

172. Stam H, Kreuzer FJ, Versprille A: Effect of lung volume and positional changes on pulmonary diffusing capacity and its components. J Appl Physiol 71:1477, 1991.

173. Chang SC, Chang HI, Liu SY, et al: Effects of body position and age on membrane diffusing capacity and pulmonary capillary blood volume. Chest 102:139, 1992.

174. Georges R, Sauman G, Loiseau A: The relationship of age to pulmonary membrane conductance and capillary blood volume. Am Rev Respir Dis 117:1069, 1978.

175. Mahajan KK, Mahajan SK, Mishra N: Effect of growth on lung transfer factor and its components. Indian J Chest Dis Allied Sci 34:77, 1992.

176. Riley RL, Cournand A: "Ideal" alveolar air and the analysis of ventilation-perfusion relationships in the lungs. J Appl Physiol 1:825, 1949.

177. Badeer HS: Gravitational effects on the distribution of pulmonary blood flow: Hemodynamic misconceptions. Respiration 43:408, 1982.

178. Milic-Emili J, Henderson JAM, Dolovich MB, et al: Regional distribution of inspired gas in the lung. J Appl Physiol 21:749, 1966.

179. Milic-Emili J: Interregional distribution of inspired gas. Prog Resp Res 16:33, 1981.

180. Milic-Emili J, Mead J, Turner JM: Topography of esophageal pressure as a function of posture in man. J Appl Physiol 19:212, 1964.

181. Glazier JB, Hughes JMB, Maloney JE, et al: Vertical gradient of alveolar size in lungs of dogs frozen intact. J Appl Physiol 23:694, 1967.

182. Mayo JR, MacKay AL, Whittall KP, et al: Measurement of lung water content and pleural pressure gradient with magnetic resonance imaging. J Thorac Imaging 10:73, 1995.

183. Ball WC Jr, Stewart PB, Newsham LGS, et al: Regional pulmonary function studied with xenon 133. J Clin Invest 41:519, 1962.

184. West JB, Dollery CT: Distribution of blood flow and ventilation-perfusion ratio in the lung, measured with radioactive CO_2. J Appl Physiol 15:405, 1960.

185. Glazier JB, DeNardo GL: Pulmonary function studied with the xenon 133 scanning technique: Normal values and a postural study. Am Rev Respir Dis 94:188, 1966.

186. Bentivoglio LG, Beerel F, Stewart PB, et al: Studies of regional ventilation and perfusion in pulmonary emphysema using xenon 133. Am Rev Respir Dis 88:315, 1963.

187. West JB, Dollery CT, Hugh-Jones P: The use of radioactive carbon dioxide to measure regional blood flow in the lungs of patients with pulmonary disease. J Clin Invest 40:1, 1961.

188. Kaneko K, Milic-Emili J, Dolovich MB, et al: Regional distribution of ventilation and perfusion as a function of body position. J Appl Physiol 21:767, 1966.

189. Engel LA, Grassino A, Anthonisen NR: Demonstration of airway closure in man. J Appl Physiol 38:1117, 1975.

190. Prefaut C, Engel LA: Vertical distribution of perfusion and inspired gas in supine man. J Appl Physiol 43:209, 1981.

191. Bake B, Wood L, Murphy B, et al: Effect of inspiratory flow rate on regional distribution of inspired gas. J Appl Physiol 37:8, 1974.

192. Fixley MS, Roussos CS, Murphy B, et al: Flow dependence of gas distribution and the pattern of inspiratory muscle contraction. J Appl Physiol 45:733, 1978.

193. Bake B, Bjure J, Widimsky J: The effects of sitting and graded exercise on the distribution of pulmonary blood flow in healthy subjects studied with the ^{133}Xe technique. Scand J Clin Lab Invest 22:99, 1968.

194. Bryan AC, Bentivoglio LG, Beerel F, et al: Factors affecting regional distribution of ventilation and perfusion in the lung. J Appl Physiol 19:395, 1964.

195. Gledhill N, Froese AB, Buick FJ, et al: $\dot{V}A/\dot{Q}$ inhomogeneity and AaDo$_2$ in man during exercise: Effect of SF_6 breathing. J Appl Physiol 45:512, 1978.

196. Ewan PW, Jones HA, Nosil J, et al: Uneven perfusion and ventilation within lung regions studies with nitrogen 13. Respir Physiol 34:45, 1978.

197. Fenn WO, Rahn H, Otis AB: A theoretical study of the composition of alveolar air at altitude. Am J Physiol 146:637, 1946.

198. Raymond W: The alveolar air equation abbreviated. Chest 74:675, 1978.

199. Minh VD, Patakas DA, Davies PL, et al: A single-breath method of alveolar O_2 determination. Respiration 37:66, 1979.

200. Begin R, Renzetti AD: Alveolar-arterial oxygen pressure gradient: I. Comparison between an assumed and actual respiratory quotient in stable chronic pulmonary disease; II. Relationship to aging and closing volume in normal subjects. Respir Care 22:491, 1977.

201. Turek Z, Kreuzer F: Effects of shifts of the O_2 dissociation curve upon alveolar-arterial O_2 gradients in computer models of the lung with ventilation-perfusion mismatching. Respir Physiol 45:133, 1981.

202. West JB: Ventilation-perfusion inequality and overall gas exchange in computer models of the lung. Respir Physiol 7:88, 1969.

203. Staub NC: Alveolar-arterial oxygen tension gradient due to diffusion. J Appl Physiol 18:673, 1963.

204. Dantzker DR, Wagner PD, West JB: Instability of lung units with low $\dot{V}A/\dot{Q}$ ratios during O_2 breathing. J Appl Physiol 38:886, 1975.

205. Harf A, Pratt T, Hughes JMB: Regional distribution of $\dot{V}A/\dot{Q}$ in man at rest and with exercise measured with krypton 81m. J Appl Physiol 44:115, 1978.

206. Wagner PD, Saltzman HA, West JB: Measurement of continuous distribution of ventilation-perfusion ratios: Theory. J Appl Physiol 36:588, 1974.

207. Halperin ML, Rolleston FS: Clinical Detective Stories: A Problem-Based Approach to Clinical Cases in Energy and Acid-Base Metabolism. London, Portland Press, 1993.

208. Bear RA, Dyck RF: Acid-base disorders: A clinical approach. Med Clin North Am 28:5179, 1988.

209. Fencl V, Leith ED: Stewart's quantitative acid-base chemistry: Applications in biology and medicine. Respir Physiol 91:1, 1993.

210. Preuss HG: Fundamentals of clinical acid-base evaluation. Clin Lab Med 13:103, 1993.

211. Ruch TC, Patton HD (eds): Physiology and Biophysics. Vol II. Circulation, Respiration, and Fluid Balance. Philadelphia, WB Saunders, 1974.

212. Siegel PD: The physiologic approach to acid-base balance. Med Clin North Am 57:863, 1974.

213. Oliva PB: Lactic acidosis. Am J Med 48:209, 1970.

214. Gennari FJ, Goldstein MB, Schwartz WB: The nature of the renal adaptation to chronic hypocapnia. J Clin Invest 51:1722, 1972.

215. Northfield TC, Kirby BJ, Tattersfield AE: Acid-base balance in acute gastrointestinal bleeding. BMJ 2:242, 1971.

216. Fulop M, Horowitz M, Aberman A, et al: Lactic acidosis in pulmonary edema due to left ventricular failure. Ann Intern Med 79:180, 1973.

217. Aberman A, Fulop M: The metabolic and respiratory acidosis of acute pulmonary edema. Ann Intern Med 76:173, 1972.

218. Mahmoud MS, Mujais SK: Gaps in the anion gap. Arch Intern Med 152:1625, 1992.

219. Pitts RF: Physiology of the Kidney and Body Fluids: An Introductory Text. 2nd ed. Chicago, Year Book, 1968.

220. Goldring RM, Cannon PJ, Heinemann HO, et al: Respiratory adjustment to chronic metabolic alkalosis in man. J Clin Invest 47:188, 1968.

221. Lifschitz MD, Brasch R, Cuomo AJ, et al: Marked hypercapnia secondary to severe metabolic alkalosis. Ann Intern Med 77:405, 1972.

222. Goldring RM, Turino GM, Heinemann HO: Respiratory-renal adjustments in chronic hypercapnia in man: Extracellular bicarbonate concentration and the regulation of ventilation. Am J Med 51:772, 1971.

223. Schwartz WB, Brackett NC Jr, Cohen JJ: The response of extracellular hydrogen ion concentration to graded degrees of chronic hypercapnia: The physiologic limits of the defense of pH. J Clin Invest 44:291, 1965.

224. Brackett NC Jr, Cohen JJ, Schwartz WB: Carbon dioxide titration curve of normal man: Effect of increasing degrees of acute hypercapnia on acid-base equilibrium. N Engl J Med 272:6, 1965.

225. Arbus GS, Hebert LA, Levesque PR, et al: Characterization and clinical application of the "significance band" for acute respiratory alkalosis. N Engl J Med 280:117, 1969.

226. Brackett NC Jr, Wingo CF, Muren O, et al: Acid-base response to chronic hypercapnia in man. N Engl J Med 280:124, 1969.

227. Arbus GS: An *in vivo* acid-base nomogram for clinical use. Can Med Assoc J 109:291, 1973.
228. Flenley DC: Another nonlogarithmic acid-base diagram? Lancet 1:961, 1971.
229. Austin WH: Acid-base balance: A review of current approaches and techniques. Am Heart J 69:691, 1965.
230. Botenga ASJ: Selective Bronchial and Intercostal Arteriography. Leiden, HE Stenfert Kroese, NV, 1970.
231. Cudkowicz L: Bronchial arterial circulation in man: Normal anatomy and responses to disease. *In* Moser KM (ed): Pulmonary Vascular Diseases. New York, Marcel Dekker, 1979, p 111.
232. Newton TH, Preger L: Selective bronchial arteriography. Radiology 84:1043, 1965.
233. Liebow AA: Patterns of origin and distribution of the major bronchial arteries in man. Am J Anat 117:19, 1965.
234. Johnsson K-A: Collateral circulation between bronchial and coronary arteries. Acta Radiol [Diagn] (Stockh) 8:393, 1969.
235. Deffebach ME, Charan NB, Lakshminarayan S, et al: The bronchial circulation—small, but a vital attribute of the lung. Am Rev Respir Dis 135:463, 1987.
236. McLaughlin RF, Tyler WS, Canada RO: Subgross pulmonary anatomy in various mammals and man. JAMA 175:694, 1961.
237. Pietra GG, Szidon JP, Leventhal MN, et al: Histamine and interstitial pulmonary edema in the dog. Circ Res 29:323, 1971.
238. Mariassy AT, Gazeroglu H, Wanner A: Morphometry of the subepithelial circulation in sheep airways: Effect of vascular congestion. Am Rev Respir Dis 143:162, 1991.
239. Baile EM, Sotres-Vega A, Paré PD: Airway blood flow and bronchovascular congestion in sheep. Eur Resp J 7:1300, 1994.
240. Murata K, Itoh H, Todo G, et al: Bronchial venous plexus and its communication with pulmonary circulation. Invest Radiol 21:24, 1986.
241. Baile EM, Minshall D, Harrison PB, et al: Systemic blood flow to the lung after bronchial artery occlusion in anesthetized sheep. J Appl Physiol 72:1701, 1992.
242. Baile EM, Nelems JM, Schulzer M, et al: Measurements of regional bronchial arterial blood flow and bronchovascular resistance in dogs. J Appl Physiol 53:1044, 1982.
243. Baile EM, Paré PD, Ernest D, et al: Distribution of blood flow and neutrophil kinetics in bronchial vasculature of sheep. J Appl Physiol 82:1466, 1997.
244. Baile EM, Ling H, Heyworth JR, et al: Bronchopulmonary anastomotic and noncoronary collateral blood flow in humans during cardiopulmonary bypass. Chest 87:749, 1985.
245. Salisbury PF, Weil P, State D: Factors influencing collateral blood flow to the dog's lung. Circ Res 5:303, 1957.
246. Modell HI, Beck K, Butler J: Functional aspects of canine bronchopulmonary vascular communications. J Appl Physiol 50:1045, 1981.
247. Baile EM, Albert RK, Kirk W, et al: Positive end-expiratory pressure decreases bronchial blood flow in the dog. J Appl Physiol 56:1289, 1984.
248. Baile EM, Paré PD: Response of the bronchial circulation to acute hypoxemia and hypocardia in the dog. J Appl Physiol 55:1474, 1983.
249. Brunner HD, Schmidt CF: Blood flow in the bronchial artery of the anesthetized dog. Am J Physiol 148:648, 1947.
250. Martinez L, de Letona J, Castro de la Mata R, et al: Local and reflex effects of bronchial arterial injection of drugs. J Pharmacol Exp Ther 133:295, 1961.
251. Lung MAKY, Wang JCC, Cheng KK: Bronchial circulation: An autoperfusion method for assessing the vasomotor activity and the study of α and β adrenoceptors in the bronchial artery. Life Sci 19:577, 1976.
252. Sasaki F, Paré PD, Ernest D, et al: Endogenous nitric oxide influences acetylcholine-induced bronchovascular dilation in sheep. J Appl Physiol 78:539, 1995.
253. Baile EM, Mayo JR, Sasaki F, et al: Bronchial arterial response to contrast medium. Acad Radiol 2:980, 1995.
254. Herve P, Silbert D, Cerrina J, et al: Impairment of bronchial mucociliary clearance in long-term survivors of heart/lung and double-lung transplantation. Chest 103:59, 1993.
255. Wagner EM, Foster WM: Importance of airway blood flow on particle clearance from the lung. J Appl Physiol 81:1878, 1996.
256. Personal observation.
257. Malik AB, Tracy SE: Bronchovascular adjustments after pulmonary embolism. J Appl Physiol 49:476, 1980.
258. McFadden ET Jr: Respiratory heat and water exchange: Physiological and clinical implications. J Appl Physiol 54:331, 1983.
259. Baile EM, Dahlby RW, Wiggs BJR, et al: Role of tracheal and bronchial circulation in respiratory heat exchange. J Appl Physiol 58:217, 1985.
260. Baile EM, Godden DJ, Paré PD: Mechanism for increase in tracheobronchial blood flow induced by hyperventilation of dry air in dogs. J Appl Physiol 68:105, 1990.
261. Agostoni PG, Arena V, Doria E, et al: Inspired gas relative humidity affects systemic-to-pulmonary bronchial blood flow in humans. Chest 97:1377, 1990.
262. Baile EM, Godden DJ, Paré PD: Effect of cold, dry and warm, humid air hyperventilation on tracheal wall blood flow in humans. Am Rev Respir Dis 139:A63, 1989.
263. Pietra GG, Szidon JP, Leventhal MN, et al: Histamine and interstitial pulmonary edema in the dog. Circ Res 29:323, 1971.
264. Fritts HW Jr, Harris P, Chidsey CA III, et al: Estimation of flow through bronchopulmonary vascular anastomoses with use of T-1824 dye. Circulation 23:390, 1961.
265. Robertson HT, Jindal S, Lakshminarayan S, et al: Gas exchange properties of the bronchial circulation in a dog lobe. Am Rev Respir Dis 129:A229, 1984.

CHAPTER 3

Pulmonary Defense and Other Nonrespiratory Functions

PULMONARY DEFENSE, 126
  Particle Deposition and Clearance, 126
    Deposition of Inhaled Particles, 126
    Clearance of Inhaled Particles, 127
      The Mucociliary Escalator, 127
      Cough, 129
      Clearance of the Alveolar Air Space, 130
      Lymphatic Clearance, 130
  Inflammation and Specific Proteins Involved in
    Pulmonary Defense, 130
  Pulmonary Immune Mechanisms, 130
    Humoral Immunity, 130
    Cell-Mediated Immunity, 131
PULMONARY METABOLISM, 131
THE PULMONARY VASCULAR FILTER, 132

Although the primary role of the lung is respiratory, several additional functions are of considerable importance to the maintenance of well-being of both the lung and the body as a whole. These nonrespiratory functions encompass three general areas: pulmonary defense, pulmonary metabolism, and filtration by the capillaries and precapillary vessels of various cells and tissue fragments.

PULMONARY DEFENSE

The entire surface of the conducting airways and lung parenchyma is normally in contact with the external environment. As a result, there is a constant risk of exposure to a variety of potentially harmful substances, including organic and inorganic particles, toxic gases and fumes, and a bewildering array of microorganisms. The defense mechanisms in response to such inhaled or aspirated substances are numerous and complex and, for convenience of discussion, can be divided into those that are specific (related to the immune system) and those that are nonspecific (including particle clearance, inflammation, and secretion of protective enzymes). The efficiency of many of these defense mechanisms can be impaired by various environmental insults and pathophysiologic conditions, including hypoxia, hyperoxia, acidosis, cigarette smoke, and drugs (particularly corticosteroids and other suppressors of immune or inflammatory reactions).

Particle Deposition and Clearance

The first line of defense against inhaled or aspirated noxious particles* is clearance; obviously, the faster and more effectively the lungs can eliminate such substances, the less the potential for damage. A variety of mechanisms are involved in this process, each of which depends on a number of factors.

Deposition of Inhaled Particles

The lungs of an average adult human are exposed to more than 10,000 liters of air during a 24-hour period. This inhaled air contains innumerable particles of various size, many of which make contact with and remain on the airway or alveolar epithelial surface. Several factors influence such deposition.

Size and Shape of Inhaled Particles. Four physical processes are involved in particle deposition on the pulmonary epithelial surface;[1] these processes are closely related to the size and shape of inhaled particles.

Inertial impaction occurs when the momentum of a particle being carried in an air current causes it to impinge on an airway wall when the direction of air flow changes. Inertial impaction is the principal mechanism by which large particles (ranging in diameter from 2 to 100 μm) are deposited in the respiratory tract.[2] Because of its anatomic complexity, the nose is the most important site for such a mechanism, and in fact, the majority of particles larger than 10 μm in diameter are deposited here.[2] The bend in the nasopharynx and the increased velocity of air flow at this site serve to trap most larger particles that have avoided impaction in the nasal passages.[3, 4] Inertial impaction also occurs at the bifurcation of the trachea, bronchi, and, to a lesser extent, the bronchioles.

Sedimentation is the mechanism by which particles are deposited on airway walls as a result of the influence of gravity. Such deposition depends on the density and diameter of the particle: the larger and denser the particle, the more rapid the settling. Sedimentation is an important mechanism

---

*Strictly speaking, the term *particle* refers to a fragment of inanimate organic or inorganic matter; for purposes of this discussion, however, it includes microorganisms (such as fungal spores or conidia) and liquid droplets (on which bacteria or viruses may be adherent).

of deposition of particles from 0.5 to 2 μm in diameter and occurs mostly in the bronchi and membranous bronchioles.

Diffusion (brownian movement) causes small particles to move randomly as a result of energy transfer from adjacent gas molecules and to impinge by chance on an airway or alveolar wall. Although the vast majority of inhaled particles up to 2 μm in diameter are subsequently exhaled, particles that are retained within the lung are deposited predominantly by diffusion; in fact, diffusion is the major mechanism of deposition of particles 0.5 μm or smaller and the only one for particles smaller than 0.2 μm. Diffusion is most important within the alveolar air spaces, although some particles also settle out in the conducting and transitional airways by this means.

The first three mechanisms of particle deposition relate predominantly to particles that are approximately spherical. As the length-to-diameter ratio of particles increases, they are termed *fibers*, and a fourth mechanism—*interception*—comes into play. (Although the definition varies, a fiber can be defined as a particle larger than 5 μm in length and smaller than 3 μm in diameter whose length-to-diameter ratio is 3:1 or greater.) Some of these particles, especially those with a large real or effective cross-sectional diameter (the latter consisting of fibers such as chrysotile asbestos, which are curled or irregular in shape), are likely to come into contact with and be deposited on a proximal airway wall. By contrast, fibers with a straight configuration and a relatively small diameter can penetrate into the lung periphery.[5]

Rate and Pattern of Breathing. Because the majority of large particles are trapped within the nasal mucosa, a greater concentration of particles tends to reach the lower respiratory tree in habitual mouth breathers or people engaged in heavy labor, in whom there may be excessive mouth breathing. In addition, the increased pulmonary ventilation that accompanies heavy labor may result in a greater number of particles reaching the lung in a given period.

Distribution of Inhaled Particles. Because ventilation in the erect position is relatively greater in lower than in upper lung regions, it might be predicted that the former would be more susceptible to lung damage from inhaled particles. However, this is not always the case, as indicated by the predominant involvement of the upper lung zones in patients with silicosis and coal worker's pneumoconiosis. It is unclear to what extent such anatomic predilection for disease is caused by the initial distribution of particles; theoretically, however, such predilection may be influenced by variations in bronchial branching pattern[6] or size[7] or by the phase of the respiratory cycle at which the particles are inhaled.

Particle size itself may be important in this respect; in one study, investigators showed that relatively large particles (3.5 μm in diameter) were preferentially deposited in the upper lobes as compared with particles 1.1 μm in diameter.[8] As might be expected, intrinsic lung disease such as emphysema can also have an appreciable effect on particle deposition.[9] In addition, particles deposited on both large and small airways can induce bronchospasm, which can itself influence regional particle distribution.[10] This effect is considerably enhanced in the presence of established lung disease because of diversion of inspired gas to unobstructed airways.[11, 12]

Concentration of Inhaled Particles. The ability of the healthy lung to cope with the inhalation of inorganic parti-

cles appears to relate roughly to the concentration of dust inhaled.[13] A concentration of fewer than 10 particles 5 μm or smaller per milliliter can be completely eliminated, whereas only about 90% of a concentration of approximately 1,000 such particles per milliliter is removed; the retained 10% can produce a slowly developing pneumoconiosis. With concentrations as high as 1 million particles per milliliter, a large proportion of particles may be retained and lung disease can develop rapidly.

Clearance of Inhaled Particles

Clearance of inhaled particles is accomplished by several mechanisms, including transport up the mucociliary escalator, cough, phagocytosis and destruction within alveolar macrophages, and lymphatic drainage. Differences in the effectiveness of these mechanisms may partly explain differences in susceptibility to certain diseases between individual patients. For example, particles deposited on the airway mucosa are usually transported in tracheobronchial secretions to the pharynx, where they are either expectorated or swallowed; in healthy subjects, the time to clear the airways may be as little as several hours. However, transport is prolonged in some people as a result of either inherent individual variation in mucus flow rate,[14] ineffective cilia (dyskinetic cilia syndromes), environmental factors such as cigarette smoke[15] and bacterial infection,[16] or intrinsic lung disease such as bronchiectasis;[17] such prolongation may predispose to greater particle retention and an increased risk of pulmonary disease.

The Mucociliary Escalator

The principal function of the mucociliary escalator is to convey inhaled particles from the lung to the larynx, where they are effectively eliminated by swallowing. Efficient functioning of this mechanism depends on the presence of a surface mucous layer of appropriate thickness and chemical composition (*see* page 61) and directed and coordinated ciliary movement sufficient to propel the mucus and entrapped particles toward the larynx. As discussed previously (*see* page 6), each cilium contains an axoneme composed of microtubules arranged in doublets, one centrally and nine peripherally. The latter are linked to the central doublets by radial spokes and to each other by dynein arms (containing an adenosine triphosphatase enzyme responsible for powering microtubule movement).

The most widely accepted theory for the ciliary beating mechanism is the sliding microtubule hypothesis, which is similar to the sliding fiber theory of muscle contraction. According to this theory, ciliary movement occurs by means of the coordinated movement of dynein arms of one doublet along an adjacent doublet, much like going up or down the rungs of a ladder.[18] Since not all doublets move at the same time, this coordinated movement leads to a shortening of some peripheral microtubules relative to those that are either contiguous to or on the opposite side of the cilium. With the internal rigidity that is provided by the radial spokes and the basal anchoring system, the cilium bends in the direction of shortening. The exact means by which the sliding microtubules are coordinated is not well understood.

The ciliary beat itself can be divided into two phases: an

effective (mucus-propulsive) stroke and a slower, recovery stroke. The former occurs perpendicular to the epithelial surface with the cilium almost completely erect and its tip "grasping" the lower portion of the mucous layer with tiny clawlike structures.[19–22] After a short rest at completion of the effective stroke, the cilium swings backward within the less viscous sol layer until it takes up a position compatible with the beginning of a new effective stroke (Fig. 3–1A). During the recovery phase, the backward-swinging cilia push onto cilia in a resting state, the mechanical stimulus causing them to enter their own recovery phase.[21] This mechanical interdependence results in a coordinated wavelike movement of cilia that moves the mucous layer cephalad on the surface of the sol layer like a raft supported and propelled by many hands beneath (Fig. 3–1D). (In fact, the mucous layer is probably not a continuous sheet [at least in the peripheral airways], but rather floating islands of mucus that gradually coalesce as the central airways are reached.)

Studies in humans[24] and animals[25–27] have shown variation in the mucociliary clearance rate of up to 54-fold from the terminal bronchioles to the trachea. The functional basis for this variation is complex and not fully understood. In one investigation in which the mucus clearance rate ranged from 0.4 mm/min in bronchioles to 20 mm/min in the trachea,[27] there was only a 3.7-fold variation in ciliary beat frequency, which ranged from 400 beats per minute in bronchioles to 1,500 beats per minute in the trachea; this finding suggests that factors other than beat frequency contribute to regional variations in clearance rate. Such factors may include an increased number of ciliated cells and an increased length of individual cilia in proximal as compared with distal airways.[28] The influence of ciliary beat frequency itself is somewhat controversial, some authors having documented no difference between central and peripheral airways[29] and others having found a greater[27, 30] or lesser[31] frequency in the central region.

Several techniques have been developed to measure mucociliary clearance:[32] (1) measurement with external counting devices of the clearance rate of radiolabeled, nonabsorbable nebulized particles or molecules inhaled into the lung periphery;[33–35] (2) monitoring of the movement of a single radioactive bolus or radiopaque Teflon disks by fiberoptic bronchoscopy, external counting devices, or fluoroscopic techniques;[36–38] and (3) monitoring by radiographic techniques of the mouthward movement of powdered tantalum following its insufflation into the lung.[39] The major

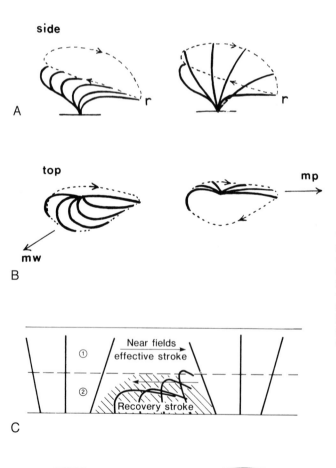

Figure 3–1. Beat Cycle of a Rabbit Tracheal Cilium Seen from the Side and from Above. In the recovery stroke *(A, left)*, the cilium starts from the rest position (r) and unrolls clockwise *(B, left top* view); in the effective stroke *(A, right)*, it remains extended and bends over to reach the rest position at the *right*. Mucus is propelled toward the *right* (mp), and the recovery wave is propagated toward the *lower left* (mw). Cilia move in waves *(C)*, with clusters in their recovery phase bordered by those undergoing their effective stroke. During the effective stroke *(D)*, the ciliary tips extend into the lower portion of the mucous layer and propel it to the *right (D)*. (Adapted from Sleigh MA, Blake JR, Liron N: The propulsion of mucus by cilia. Am Rev Respir Dis 137:726, 1988.)

advantage of the first (aerosol) technique is that it measures mucociliary clearance over the entire ciliated airway surface. However, by necessity this method depends on the initial deposition pattern of the inhaled radioaerosol; since particles are preferentially deposited in central airways, where mucociliary clearance is more rapid, even mild air-flow obstruction can result in an erroneously fast calculated rate of clearance because of reduced peripheral deposition of inhaled radioaerosol.[40] The other two techniques have the disadvantage that only central airway clearance is assessed; in addition, both are invasive since the tracer must be administered through a fiberoptic bronchoscope or an intra-airway catheter.[32]

In one study in which whole-lung clearance as measured by the radioaerosol technique was compared with that measured by central airway clearance techniques, a remarkable correlation of the two was observed.[35] It was concluded that the rate of movement of material from the peripheral to the central airways correlates well with central airway mucus velocity, and it was suggested that discoordination between central and peripheral clearance might occur with disease and be an important pathophysiologic mechanism.[35] On the other hand, considerable variation in central airway mucus transport rates has been observed when different techniques have been employed sequentially.[41] It has been suggested that the faster central airway transport rate observed with radiolabeled particles as compared with Teflon disks is related to a stimulatory effect of local radiation on mucociliary clearance.[36] Simultaneous measurement of the mucociliary clearance of particles averaging 3 μm, 110 μm, and 180 μm has shown no significant difference in clearance rates.[42]

A variety of pharmacologic and other factors influence normal mucociliary clearance. The mechanisms by which they act are complex and probably related to an alteration in ciliary beat frequency, the depth of the periciliary sol layer, the quantity and viscoelastic properties of the mucus, and/or the state of hydration of the secretions. β-Adrenergic agonists have been found to enhance mucociliary transport in normal subjects in some studies,[34, 43] although no benefit has been identified in others.[44] Inhaled atropine delays mucociliary transport, which suggests that basal vagal tone influences the secretion and/or removal of tracheobronchial secretions.[45] Therapeutic levels of aspirin have also been shown to cause a slight reduction in whole-lung and tracheal mucociliary clearance rates in non–aspirin-allergic normal subjects.[46]

In dogs, the use of high-frequency oscillatory ventilation has been shown to impair whole-lung and central airway mucociliary clearance to a marked degree;[47] clearance improves immediately following cessation of the high-frequency oscillatory ventilation, which suggests that the effect is a functional disturbance rather than the production of a structural abnormality of the cilia or an alteration in the viscoelastic or biochemical characteristics of mucus. In contrast to these observations, it has been shown that high-frequency chest wall oscillation results in enhanced central and peripheral mucociliary clearance.[48] The discrepancy in these results is probably related to the different flow rates and air velocity rates in intrathoracic airways during inspiration and expiration when high-frequency oscillatory ventilation is produced at the airway opening or at the chest wall; direct comparison of the two techniques shows that values

for mucociliary clearance are closer when the expiratory flow pattern produced by the two methods is matched, although chest wall oscillation is still more efficient.[49] A difference in expiratory and inspiratory air velocities has been invoked to explain the persistence of some mucociliary clearance in the complete absence of ciliary motility in patients with dyskinetic ciliary syndrome.[50]

Dehydration has been shown to decrease mucociliary clearance and rehydration to improve it.[51] The presence within mucus of surfactant also increases the clearance rate.[52, 53] Disruption of mucociliary clearance in the central airway at the site of flow limitation during forced expiration and cough results in an accumulation of inhaled irritants at the flow-limiting site; it has been hypothesized that such limitation could be responsible for the predominant central location of squamous cell carcinoma.[54]

Cough

Cough is an important mechanism of respiratory defense and an adjuvant to the clearance of tracheobronchial secretions.[55] It can be initiated voluntarily or involuntarily and typically consists of an initial inspiratory maneuver followed by glottic closure. (The latter is not essential, since patients with tracheostomies can develop an effective cough mechanism.[56]) Expiratory muscles then contract to increase pleural, abdominal, and alveolar pressures to a level of 100 mm Hg or more. The glottis is suddenly opened, and expiratory flow begins and peaks in 30 to 50 milliseconds with flows at the mouth as high as 12 liters per second. The initial high-flow transients are related to both collapse of central airways, with displacement of the contained air mouthward, and bulk flow from the parenchyma. After about 0.5 second and the expulsion of approximately 1 liter of air, expiratory flow stops because of glottic closure or expiratory muscle relaxation.

During cough, expiratory flow limitation occurs by the same mechanism that limits maximal flow during forced expiratory maneuvers. An equal pressure point in which intrapleural and intra-airway pressure is the same develops in the central airways; mouthward from this point, dynamic compression of the airways occurs. Cough may be repeated at lower lung volumes and result in progressive peripheral movement of the equal pressure point and progressive collapse of more and more of the intrathoracic airways. The marked collapse of intrathoracic airways leads to gas velocities that reach three quarters of the speed of sound at values of 1,600 to 2,400 cm/sec. These high air velocities produce enormous shear stress on the liquid layer lining the airways and move large amounts of mucus and contained debris proximally. The shear may itself alter the viscoelastic properties of respiratory secretions and enhance the effectiveness of cough.[57] In addition, it has been suggested that cough may increase clearance by stimulating secretion and ciliary beat frequency.[58]

Involuntary cough is initiated by the stimulation of irritant receptors in the larynx, trachea, or large bronchi. These receptors are believed to be fine, nonmyelinated nerve fibers that are present in an extensive network throughout the airway epithelium. Evidence that these fibers subserve the cough mechanism includes the observation that cough is stimulated by irritation of areas where the fibers are most numerous and the fact that single afferent fiber recordings of rapidly adapting receptors in the vagus nerve show a burst of activity when the epithelium is stimulated by events that stimulate cough. It is difficult to provoke cough by stimulating peripheral airways, thus suggesting that irritant receptor density is less in these locations. (Although rapidly adapting receptors are present in the smaller airways, their stimulation results in reflex hyperpnea rather than cough.)

That vagotomy abolishes or greatly reduces the cough reflex indicates that nonvagal pathways must play a minor or no role in the reflex. The stimuli that provoke coughing can also provoke bronchoconstriction via the same afferent reflex pathways. The resulting airway narrowing could aid the cough mechanism by resulting in higher linear flow rates during the cough; in addition, it may stabilize the airway during the vigorous expiratory effort and high transmural pressures of coughing, as has been shown in large airways.[59]

Cough is most effective in clearing secretions from large airways; however, calculations suggest that some clearance can occur down to the 20th generation. The greater the depth of the periciliary sol layer and the less viscous it is, the greater the effectiveness of cough.

Clearance of the Alveolar Air Space

Many particles deposited in the alveoli are phagocytosed by alveolar macrophages, which then migrate to the mucociliary escalator, are transported to the pharynx, and are expectorated or swallowed in the same manner as free particles. When the capacity of these macrophages to clear the air spaces in this manner is overwhelmed by an abundance of particles, disease may ensue. (The function of alveolar macrophages is discussed in greater detail on page 21.)

Inorganic particles such as silicates or asbestos fibers that are not phagocytosed by alveolar macrophages may pass directly across the epithelium into the alveolar or peribronchiolar interstitial tissue. Some of these particles are then transported via peribronchovascular lymphatics to bronchopulmonary and hilar lymph nodes or via lymphatics in the interlobular septa to the pleura. Others, however, remain in the interstitial tissue (particularly peribronchiolar tissue), where they may accumulate and eventually cause fibrosis.

Lymphatic Clearance

The anatomy and function of the pulmonary lymphatics are discussed on page 172. It is only necessary at this point to emphasize the importance of lymph flow in the clearance of particles that penetrate the epithelial barrier and reach the pulmonary interstitial tissue. Histologic studies have shown that the clearance time of particles via lymphatics in peribronchovascular bundles ranges from 1 to 14 days, whereas particles that reach a subpleural location in paraseptal or perivascular lymphatics can remain in the lungs for months.[60] Such regional differences in lymphatic flow have been hypothesized to explain some of the variations in anatomic localization of disease in different pneumoconioses.[61]

Inflammation and Specific Proteins Involved in Pulmonary Defense

Polymorphonuclear leukocytes are normally present both in alveolar air spaces and on the surface of the conduct-

ing airways, albeit in very small numbers. Their role is presumably similar to that of the alveolar macrophage, although the substances that they phagocytose and degrade may differ. In addition to these normally occurring cells, an inflammatory reaction is a common result of particle deposition, particularly if clearance mechanisms are inadequate. Pulmonary macrophages have many important functions in defense and are involved in both inflammatory and immunologic reactions; these functions are discussed in greater detail on page 21.

Several substances secreted by airway and alveolar epithelial cells or by alveolar macrophages, or derived directly from the blood, also have an important role in defense against inhaled microorganisms. These substances include lysozyme, lactoferrin, interferon, fibronectin, surfactant, and various complement components. In addition, epithelial cells produce substances such as leukocyte antiprotease that act to protect the lung from the deleterious side effects of proteolytic enzymes that are probably released normally in small amounts by intrapulmonary inflammatory cells.[62]

Pulmonary Immune Mechanisms

Cells involved in pulmonary immunity are located throughout the lungs and mediastinum and are either grouped in lymph nodes or mucosal lymphoid nodules (bronchus-associated lymphoid tissue, *see* page 16)[64, 65] or occur as isolated cells within the epithelium and adjacent interstitium. Numerous lymph nodes are present in the tissue adjacent to proximal bronchi and trachea, in the mediastinum. They receive lymph containing admixed cells and debris from the parenchyma and conducting airways and function both as a repository for foreign particulate material and as a station for antigen processing.

Humoral Immunity

Although all immunoglobulin classes are found in tracheobronchial secretions, the predominant forms are IgG and IgA.[66] They may be manufactured and secreted locally or derived from the serum by transudation. The former are probably produced mostly by B cells in the lamina propria and the connective tissue immediately adjacent to the tracheobronchial glands. The functions of these antibodies include opsonization and enhanced phagocytosis (particularly IgG), complement activation, toxin neutralization, and microbial agglutination. Their importance to pulmonary defense is indicated by the development of pulmonary disease (usually bronchiectasis or acute bacterial pneumonia[67]) in patients with specific immunoglobulin deficiencies.

IgA is the most abundant immunoglobulin and is present predominantly in its dimeric form, most of which is secretory. Although a proportion of IgA in lung secretions is derived from IgA in the blood, the majority appears to be produced locally.[63, 66] There is evidence that serous cells of the tracheobronchial glands are involved in both the manufacture of secretory component and its coupling with the dimeric form of the molecule.[68] IgG is also produced locally, probably by plasma cells in the lamina propria,[69] although a sizable proportion is also derived from transudation from the blood. All four subclasses of the molecule have been identified in bronchoalveolar lavage specimens, IgG3 and IgG4 apparently being the more abundant.[70]

Experimental evidence suggests that antigen-specific antibody continues to be produced in lung secretions for years after initial immune contact, such antibodies probably being produced by local plasma cells rather than being derived from the blood or cells within lymph nodes.[71]

Cell-Mediated Immunity

Cell-mediated immunity is also clearly important in pulmonary defense, particularly with respect to infection. Bronchoalveolar lavage of normal subjects yields a cellular population composed of about 95% macrophages and 2% lymphocytes,[72] the great majority of which are T cells. Most of the latter cells appear to be derived from a pool of sensitized lymphocytes in the systemic circulation. Such cells emigrate from pulmonary vessels at the site where an appropriate antigen is deposited and participate in either modulation of alveolar macrophage function or cell-mediated cytotoxicity. It is likely that pulmonary dendritic/Langerhans' cells are involved in antigen processing and presentation as well as lymphocyte activation in the initial stage of this process.[74]

PULMONARY METABOLISM

The lungs are involved in the storage, transformation, degradation, and synthesis of a large variety of substances.[75] Since the lung is a very complex organ composed of at least 40 different cell types, it is sometimes difficult to assign specific metabolic functions to a particular cell type.[76] However, studies of metabolic activity, including oxygen consumption, have identified Type II alveolar cells, Clara cells, alveolar macrophages, mast cells, and endothelial cells as the most metabolically active pulmonary cells.[77, 78]

Many cell types in the lung are engaged in lipid metabolism. Perhaps the best known is the Type II alveolar cell, in which lipid synthesis is intimately associated with surfactant production (*see* page 56). The presence of *lipoprotein lipases* within or on the surface of capillary endothelial cells indicates that the lungs have an enormous capacity for lipolysis. Lipids—especially long-chain fatty acids absorbed by the intestinal tract—enter the bloodstream as chylomicrons (glycerides in stable emulsion) and then pass up the thoracic duct and thence through the right side of the heart to the pulmonary vascular bed. The fatty acids released by hydrolysis of lipid ester bonds may be used by various tissues, including the lung, as a substrate for both oxidative metabolism and the formation of complex lipids.

Arachidonic acid, a membrane lipid released by phospholipase A_2, enters the labyrinthine enzymatic cascade that produces prostaglandins and leukotrienes. Various lung cells have the full complement of enzymes for the production of arachidonic acid metabolites, including 5-lipoxygenase (which produces the potent contractile and vasoactive cysteinyl-leukotrienes LTC_4, LTD_4, and LTE_4, as well as the neutrophil chemoattractant LTB_4) and 15-lipoxygenase (which produces 15-hydroxyeicosatetraenoic acid), and the constitutively expressed (COX-1) and inducible (COX-2) cyclooxygenase enzymes that are responsible for prostaglan-

din metabolism.[79–82] Prostaglandin E causes smooth muscle relaxation and is anti-inflammatory, whereas prostaglandin F and thromboxane are contractile agonists.[83] In addition to lipids, both *in vivo* and *in vitro* studies in animals have shown that the lung can synthesize protein[84] and glycoprotein.[85]

Serotonin (5-hydroxytryptamine) is metabolized by the pulmonary vascular endothelium to 5-hydroxyindoleacetic acid in a single passage through the lung.[86] The lung also takes up and metabolizes prostaglandins of the E and F series and norepinephrine, as well as the peptides angiotensin I and bradykinin.[87, 88] Conditions associated with pulmonary endothelial damage such as adult respiratory distress syndrome are associated with impaired pulmonary metabolism of these vasoactive substances; this failure may have clinically important effects on both systemic and pulmonary hemodynamics.[87, 89]

Angiotensin-converting enzyme (ACE) is produced largely by endothelial cells. It inactivates bradykinin, a powerful hypotensive and edematogenic substance, and simultaneously activates angiotensin II, an equally powerful pressor agent.[90] ACE inhibitors not only have a hypotensive effect but may also aggravate lung inflammation and cough because of the unchecked action of bradykinin and related inflammatory peptides. Monitoring of lung ACE content and activity has been advocated as a marker of endothelial cell function.[91–93]

Neutral endopeptidase, an enzyme produced preferentially by airway epithelial cells, can inactivate inflammatory peptides, including bradykinin and the neuropeptides. Administration of inhibitors of neutral endopeptidase by aerosol can aggravate airway obstruction in asthmatic subjects.[94] The tachykinin neuropeptides *substance P* and *neurokinin A* are released from pulmonary afferent and efferent nerves and have effects on vascular and airway smooth muscle, as well as stimulating vascular leak and mucus secretion. They act on three specific neurokinin-type receptors that are differentially expressed on the various target tissues.[95, 96] *Vasoactive intestinal peptide* is a neurally derived peptide that acts as an endogenous bronchodilator.

Nitric oxide (NO) is an extremely important metabolic product that can be produced by a variety of lung cells and has important effects on airway, pulmonary, and bronchial vascular function.[97] It is synthesized by the action of NO synthase (NOS) on the amino acid L-arginine. At least two forms of the enzyme exist in the lung—a constitutively expressed form (c-NOS), which is present in the vascular endothelium, and an inducible form (i-NOS), which is expressed in the airway epithelium. The inducible form is increased in acute and chronic inflammatory airway diseases such as viral respiratory infections,[98] asthma,[99] and bronchiectasis, and its up-regulation can be detected by measuring increased amounts of NO in expired gas. Both chronic and acute cigarette smoking decrease expired NO.[100] In addition to having effects on vascular and airway smooth muscle, NO may have an immunoregulatory role by enhancing the differentiation of T_H2-type T-helper cells and increasing local production of the proinflammatory cytokines interleukin-4 and interleukin-5.[101] There is also good evidence that NO is the neurotransmitter released from nonadrenergic, noncholinergic inhibitory nerves in the human airway (*see* page 148).[102, 103]

Another group of potent, biologically active substances produced by lung cells is the *endothelins*. These substances are a family of small peptides that have potent vasoconstrictor and bronchoconstrictor action, increase vascular permeability, and induce smooth muscle cell proliferation.[104] ET-1 is produced by endothelial cells; other cells such as macrophages and epithelial cells can synthesize ET-2 and ET-3.[105] Three distinct ET receptors (ETA, ETB, and ETC) are also differentially expressed on various target tissues. There is evidence that increased endothelin production and decreased NO synthesis may contribute to pulmonary hypertension in some pulmonary vascular disorders.[106]

The lung is exposed to a wide variety of endogenous and exogenous substances that may exert profound local or systemic toxicologic or pharmacologic effects. Foreign chemicals (xenobiotics) can reach the lung via the pulmonary vessels or airways; the very large surface area of airway and alveolar epithelium and the microvasculature endothelium provide an enormous potential for enzymatic modification of these substances. Foreign chemicals usually undergo stepwise metabolism in the lung. Phase 1 enzymes cause oxidation, reduction, or hydrolysis, whereas Phase 2 reactions usually conjugate the xenobiotic by adding an additional chemical group. The combined effect of Phase 1 and 2 reactions is usually the production of more polar, less lipid-soluble, more readily excretable, and less biologically active compounds.

The classic Phase 1 enzymes are the cytochrome P-450 group, which consists of mixed-function oxidases with broad substrate specificity.[107–109] In the lung, much of the cytochrome P-450 is contained in Clara cells. Phase 2 enzymes can add sulfate, methyl, or acetyl groups or conjugate xenobiotics with glucuronic acids or glutathione. Although generally protective, these reactions may have harmful consequences in some circumstances since certain chemicals require metabolic activation before exerting their toxicity. The high content of enzymes in some cell types makes them vulnerable to damage if the products they produce from the parent compound are toxic. An example of such a reaction is the disastrous pulmonary consequence of the ingestion of paraquat and parathion; these chemicals are converted to more toxic metabolites by P-450 enzymes in Clara cells, and the metabolites cause extensive pulmonary endothelial and epithelial cell damage and pulmonary edema. Another example is the metabolism by human bronchus of polycyclic aromatic hydrocarbons such as benzo[a]pyrene into carcinogenic metabolites that can bind to and damage DNA. As discussed previously, the lungs also contain a variety of enzymes involved in the maintenance of normal structure, such as superoxide dismutase[109a] and antiproteases.[109b]

The lungs also play a role in the excretion of volatile substances other than carbon dioxide, including acetone in diabetes and fasting, methylmercaptan and ammonia in liver failure, methanol of unknown source, allicin following garlic ingestion, a breakdown product of dimethyl sulfoxide that smells like garlic when applied to the skin, paraldehyde, and ethanol (the basis of a test for determining the blood level of alcohol in automobile drivers).

THE PULMONARY VASCULAR FILTER

The pulmonary capillary network is interposed between the systemic venous and arterial circulations and in normal circumstances receives the entire cardiac output. It thus has the capacity to act as a filter protecting vital organs on the systemic side of the circulation from various potentially harmful materials. Probably the most important of these substances is thrombus that originates in peripheral veins. Such thromboemboli are probably common; autopsy studies show anatomic evidence of their presence in as many as two thirds of patients.[110] Most such emboli are small and result in no significant pulmonary damage; however, the potential for harm would be much greater in organs such as the heart or brain. Other substances that may be effectively sieved in the same manner include fat, bone marrow fragments, and exogenous material such as foreign substances injected by drug addicts (*see* page 1845).

Embolism to the lungs of some cells and tissues is so frequent that it can be regarded as normal. For example, the presence of trophoblast cells in the pulmonary vasculature is common during pregnancy; in one autopsy study of 220 women in which a large number of lung sections were examined, trophoblast cells were found in almost 45% of individuals.[111] The greatest number is seen in the peripartum period, a finding probably related to the trauma of labor. In rare cases, the extent of embolism has been such as to suggest a cause of death;[111] in the vast majority of patients, however, the presence of these cells is clearly of no clinical or pathologic significance and they disappear without residua shortly after their appearance in the lungs.[112] In some pregnant women, minute clusters of large eosinophilic cells have also been identified in the pulmonary vasculature and have been considered to be emboli of endometrial decidua.[113, 114]

Megakaryocytes derived from bone marrow are also commonly seen within the lungs (Fig. 3–2).[115, 116] They are more frequent in a hospital-based autopsy population but are also found in lesser numbers in previously healthy people who have died suddenly.[116] They have been estimated to average between 15 and 20 cells per square centimeter in tissue sections 5 to 7 μm thick.[116, 117] There is evidence that their number is increased in association with intravascular coagulation,[116–119] cardiovascular disease,[117] and tumor emboli or metastatic carcinoma to the lungs.[120]

Studies of megakaryocytes in central venous and arterial blood have shown significantly higher numbers in the former,[121–123] thus implying that they are indeed trapped within lung capillaries. Since it has also been shown that the number of platelets is greater in aortic than in pulmonary arterial blood,[123] it has been suggested that a significant proportion of platelet production may normally occur within the lung,[121, 122, 124] possibly by physical fragmentation of megakaryocytes.[124] It has also been suggested that the lung may either remove or add platelets from or to the blood and thus partly regulate the normal blood level of these cells.[75]

The pulmonary capillaries also serve as a storage site for blood leukocytes, resulting in a marginated pool of cells that may be two to three times larger than the number of circulating leukocytes.[23, 125] Rather than remaining in the lung, the sequestered cells are only delayed in their passage, so there is a constant turnover of cells within the pool. This sequestration is probably related to the relatively low perfusion pressure of the pulmonary circulation and the size and deformability of the leukocyte: normal leukocytes are slightly larger than most pulmonary capillaries and thus have to change shape to transit the alveolus; since they are 1,000

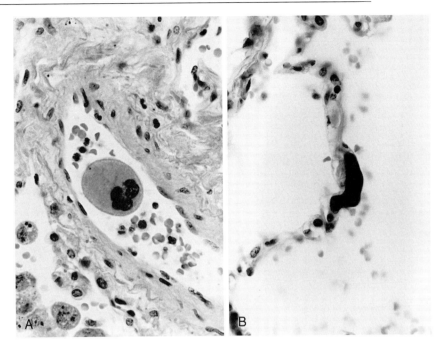

Figure 3–2. Intrapulmonary Megakaryocytes. An intact megakaryocyte is evident within a small pulmonary artery in *A*. A more typical appearance is illustrated in *B*, in which only a distorted nucleus can be discerned within an alveolar capillary, the cytoplasm presumably having been fragmented as the cell was compressed in the microvasculature.

times less deformable than red blood cells, this process is associated with delayed passage through the capillaries. These sequestered leukocytes are presumably important in providing a ready source of cells for migration into the alveolar air spaces to combat inhaled microorganisms.[126] They may also play a role in the pathogenesis of some forms of lung disease such as emphysema and adult respiratory distress syndrome.

REFERENCES

1. Brain JD, Valberg PA: Deposition of aerosol in respiratory tract. Am Rev Respir Dis 120:1325, 1979.
2. Stuart BO: Deposition of inhaled aerosols. Arch Intern Med 131:60, 1973.
3. Proctor DF, Andersen I, Lundqvist G: Clearance of inhaled particles from the human nose. Arch Intern Med 131:132, 1973.
4. Gross P, Detreville RTP: The lung as an embattled domain against inanimate pollutants: A précis of mechanisms. Am Rev Respir Dis 106:684, 1972.
5. Craighead JE, Mossman BT: The pathogenesis of asbestos-associated diseases. N Engl J Med 306:1446, 1982.
6. Pinkerton KE, Plopper CG, Mercer RR, et al: Airway branching patterns influence asbestos fiber location and the extent of tissue injury in the pulmonary parenchyma. Lab Invest 55:688, 1986.
7. Becklake MR, Toyota B, Stewart M, et al: Lung structure as a risk factor in adverse pulmonary responses to asbestos exposure: A case-referent study in Quebec chrysotile miners and millers. Am Rev Respir Dis 128:385, 1983.
8. Pityn P, Chamberlin MJ, Fraser TM, et al: The topography of particle deposition in the human lung. Respir Physiol 78:19, 1989.
9. Sweeny TD, Brain JD, Leavitt SA, et al: Emphysema alters the deposition pattern of inhaled particles in hamsters. Am J Pathol 128:19, 1987.
10. Swartenaren M, Philipson K, Linman L, et al: Regional deposition of particles in human lung after induced bronchoconstriction. Exp Lung Res 10:223, 1986.
11. Macklem PT, Hogg WE, Brunton J: Peripheral airways obstruction and particulate deposition in the lung. Arch Intern Med 131:93, 1973.
12. Goldberg IS, Lourenco RV: Deposition of aerosols in pulmonary disease. Arch Intern Med 131:88, 1973.
13. Davies CN: The handling of particles by the human lungs. Br Med Bull 19:49, 1963.
14. Proctor DF, Andersen I, Lundqvist G: Clearance of inhaled particles from the human nose. Arch Intern Med 131:132, 1973.
15. Bohning DE, Atkins HL, Cohn SH: Long-term particle clearance in man: Normal and impaired. Ann Occup Hyg 26:259, 1982.
16. Seybold ZSV, Abraham WM, Gazeroglu H, et al: Impairment of airway mucociliary transport by *Pseudomonas aeruginosa* products. Am Rev Respir Dis 146:1173, 1992.
17. Veale D, Rodgers AD, Griffiths CJ, et al: Variablility in ciliary beat frequency in normal subjects and in patients with bronchiectasis. Thorax 48:1018, 1993.
18. Kuhn C: Ciliated and Clara cells. *In* Bouhuys A (ed): Lung Cells in Disease. New York, Elsevier, 1976, p 91.
19. Jeffrey PK, Reid L: New observations on rat airway epithelium: A quantitative and electron microscopic study. J Anat 120:295, 1975.
20. Joki S, Toskala E, Saano V, et al: Ciliary ultrastructure and beating activity in rat and guinea pig respiratory mucosa. Clin Exp Pharmacol Physiol 22:619, 1995.
21. Sleigh MA: The nature and action of respiratory tract cilia. *In* Brain JD, Proctor DF, Reid LM (eds): Respiratory Defense Mechanisms—Part I. Lung Biology in Health and Disease. Vol 5. New York, Marcel Dekker, 1977, pp 247–288.
22. King M: Mucus and mucociliary clearance. Basics Respir Dis 11:1, 1982.
23. Gee MH, Albertine KH: Neutrophil-endothelial cell interactions in the lung. Annu Rev Physiol 55:227, 1993.
24. Morrow PE, Gibb FR, Gazioglu KN: A study of particulate clearance from the human lungs. Am Rev Respir Dis 96:1209, 1967.
25. Asmundsson T, Kilburn KH: Mucociliary clearance rates at various levels in dog lungs. Am Rev Respir Dis 102:388, 1970.
26. Ceesay SM, Melville GN, Mills JL, et al: Comparative observations of mucus transport velocity in health and disease. Respiration 44:184, 1983.
27. van As A: Regional variations in mucus clearance in normal and in bronchitic mammalian airways. *In* Chantler EN, Elder JB, Elstein M (eds): Mucus in Health and Disease. No. 2, Advances in Experimental Medicine and Biology. New York, Plenum Press, 1982, p 417.
28. Serafini SM, Michaelson ED: Length and distribution of cilia in human and canine airways. Bull Eur Physiopathol Respir 13:551, 1977.
29. Yager JA, Ellman H, Dulfano MJ: Human ciliary beat frequency at three levels of the tracheobronchial tree. Am Rev Respir Dis 121:661, 1980.
30. Rutland J, Griffin WM, Cole PJ: Human ciliary beat frequency in epithelium from intrathoracic and extrathoracic airways. Am Rev Respir Dis 125:100, 1982.
31. Konietzko N, Nakhosteen JA, Mizera W, et al: Ciliary beat frequency of biopsy samples taken from persons with various lung diseases. Chest 80:855, 1981.
32. Clarke SW, Pavia D: Lung mucus production and mucociliary clearance: Methods of assessment. Br J Clin Pharmacol 9:537, 1980.
33. Pavia D, Sutton PP, Agnew JE, et al: Measurement of bronchial mucociliary clearance. Eur J Respir Dis 64(Suppl 127):41, 1983.
34. Foster WM, Langenback EG, Bersofsky EH: Lung mucociliary function in man: Interdependence of bronchial and tracheal mucus transport velocities with lung clearance in bronchial asthma and healthy subjects. Ann Occup Hyg 26:277, 1982.
35. Yeates DB, Pitt BR, Spektor DM, et al: Coordination of mucociliary transport in human trachea and intrapulmonary airways. J Appl Physiol 51:1057, 1981.
36. Ahmed T, Januszkiewicz AJ, Landa JF, et al: Effect of local radioactivity on tracheal mucous velocity of sheep. Am Rev Respir Dis 120:567, 1979.
37. Chopra SK, Taplin GB, Simmons DH, et al: Measurement of mucociliary transport velocity in the intact mucosa. Chest 71:155, 1977.
38. Toomes H, Vogt-Moykopf I, Heller WD, et al: Measurement of mucociliary clearance in smokers and nonsmokers using a bronchoscopic video-technical method. Lung 159:27, 1981.
39. Forbes AR, Gamsu G: Lung mucociliary clearance after anesthesia with spontaneous and controlled ventilation. Am Rev Respir Dis 120:857, 1979.
40. Agnew JE, Bateman JR, Watts M, et al: The importance of aerosol penetration for lung mucociliary clearance studies. Chest 80(Suppl):843, 1981.
41. Wolff RK, Muggenburg BA: Comparison of two methods of measuring tracheal mucous velocity in anesthetized beagle dogs. Am Rev Respir Dis 120:137, 1979.
42. Connolly TP, Noujaim AA, Man SFP: Simultaneous canine tracheal transport of different particles. Am Rev Respir Dis 118:965, 1978.
43. Mossberg B, Strandbert K, Camner P: Stimulatory effect of beta-adrenergic drugs on mucociliary transport. Scand J Respir Dis Suppl 101:71, 1977.
44. Isawa T, Teshima T, Hirano T, et al: Does a beta$_2$-stimulator really facilitate mucociliary transport in the human lungs in vivo? A study with procaterol. Am Rev Respir Dis 141:715, 1990.
45. Groth ML, Langenback EG, Foster WM: Influence of inhaled atropine on lung mucociliary function in humans. Am Rev Respir Dis 144:1042, 1991.
46. Gerrity TR, Cotromanes E, Garrard CS, et al: The effect of aspirin on lung mucociliary clearance. N Engl J Med 308:139, 1983.
47. McEvoy RD, Davies NJ, Hedenstierna G, et al: Lung mucociliary transport during high-frequency ventilation. Am Rev Respir Dis 126:452, 1982.
48. King M, Phillips DM, Gross D, et al: Enhanced tracheal mucus clearance with high frequency chest wall compression. Am Rev Respir Dis 128:511, 1983.
49. King M, Zidulka A, Phillips DM, et al: Tracheal mucus clearance in high-frequency oscillation: Effect of peak flow-rate bias. Eur Respir J 3:6, 1990.
50. Warwick WJ: Mechanisms of mucus transport. Eur J Respir Dis 64:162, 1983.
51. Chopra SK, Taplin GV, Simmons DH, et al: Effects of hydration and physical therapy on tracheal transport velocity. Am Rev Respir Dis 115:1009, 1977.
52. Rubin BK, Ramirez O, King M: Mucus rheology and transport in neonatal respiratory distress syndrome and the effect of surfactant therapy. Chest 101:1080, 1992.
53. Outzen KE, Svane-Knudsen V: Effect of surface-active substance on nasal mucociliary clearance time: A comparison of saccharin clearance time before and after the use of surface-active substance. Rhinology 31:155, 1993.
54. Smaldone GC, Itoh H, Swift DL, et al: Effect of flow-limiting segments and cough on particle deposition and mucociliary clearance in the lung. Am Rev Respir Dis 120:747, 1979.
55. Bennett WD, Foster WM, Chapman WF: Cough-enhanced mucus clearance in the normal lung. J Appl Physiol 69:1670, 1990.
56. Leith DE: *In* Lenfant C, Brain JD, Proctor DF, et al (eds): Respiratory Defense Mechanisms—Part II. Lung Biology in Health and Disease. Vol 5. New York, Marcel Dekker, 1977, p 545.
57. Hasani A, Pavia D, Agnew JE, et al: Regional mucus transport following unproductive cough and forced expiration technique in patients with airways obstruction. Chest 105:1420, 1994.
58. King M, Zidulka A, Phillips DM, et al: Tracheal mucus clearance in high-frequency oscillation: Effect of peak flow-rate bias. Eur Respir J 3:6, 1990.
59. Widdicombe JG: Mechanisms of cough and regulation. Eur J Respir Dis 61:11, 1980.
60. Green GM: Alveolobronchiolar transport mechanisms. Arch Intern Med 131:109, 1973.
61. Goodwin RA, Des Prez RM: Apical localization of pulmonary tuberculosis, chronic pulmonary histoplasmosis, and progressive massive fibrosis of the lung. Chest 83:801, 1983.
62. Mooren HWD, Meyer CJLM, Kramps JA, et al: Ultrastructural localization of the low-molecular-weight protease inhibitor in human bronchial glands. J Histochem Cytochem 30:1130, 1982.
63. Wiggins J, Hill SL, Stockley RA: Lung secretion sol-phase proteins: Comparison of sputum with secretions obtained by direct sampling. Thorax 38:102, 1983.
64. Bienenstock J, Clancy RL, Perey DYE: Bronchus-associated lymphoid tissue (BALT): Its relationship to mucosal immunity. *In* Kirkpatrick CH, Reynolds HY (eds): Immunologic and Infectious Reactions in the Lung. New York, Marcel Dekker, 1976, p 29.
65. Holt PG: Development of bronchus-associated lymphoid tissue (BALT) in human lung disease: A normal host defense mechanism awaiting therapeutic exploitation? Thorax 48:1097, 1993.
66. Burnett D: Immunoglobulins in the lung. Thorax 41:337, 1986.
67. Heiner DC, Myers A, Beck CS: Deficiency of IgG4: A disorder associated with frequent infections and bronchiectasis may be familial. Clin Rev Allergy 1:259, 1983.
68. Goodman MR, Link DW, Brown WR, et al: Ultrastructural evidence of transport of secretory IgA across bronchial epithelium. Am Rev Respir Dis 123:115, 1981.
69. Soutar CA: Distribution of plasma cells and other cells containing immunoglobulin in the respiratory tract of normal man and class of immunoglobulin contained therein. Thorax 31:158, 1976.
70. Merrill WW, Naegel GP, Ochowski JJ, et al: Immunoglobulin G subclass proteins in serum and lavage fluid of normal subjects: Quantitation and comparison with immunoglobulins A and E. Am Rev Respir Dis 131:584, 1985.
71. Bice DE, Jones SE, Muggenburg BA: Long-term antibody production after lung immunization and challenge: Role of lung and lymphoid tissue. Am J Respir Cell Mol Biol 8:662, 1993.

72. Van Haarst JMW, Hoogsteden HC, De Wit HJ, et al: Dendritic cells and their precursors isolated from human bronchoalveolar lavage: Immunocytologic and functional properties. Am J Respir Cell Mol Biol 11:344, 1994.

73. Raghu G, Striker LJ, Hudson LD, et al: Extracellular matrix in normal and fibrotic human lungs. Am Rev Respir Dis 131:281, 1985.

74. Hance AJ: Pulmonary immune cells in health and disease: Dendritic cells and Langerhans' cells. Eur Respir J 6:1213, 1993.

75. Heinemann HO, Fishman AP: Nonrespiratory functions of mammalian lung. Physiol Rev 49:1, 1969.

76. Sorokin SP: The cells of the lung. *In* Nettesheim P, Hanna MG, Deatherage JW (eds): Morphology of Experimental Respiratory Carcinogenesis. Washington, DC, US Atomic Energy Commission, 1970, pp 3–41.

77. Heinemann HO, Fishman AP: Nonrespiratory functions of mammalian lung. Physiol Rev 49:1, 1969.

78. Said SI: The lung as a metabolic organ. N Engl J Med 279:1330, 1968.

79. Henderson WR Jr: The role of leukotrienes in inflammation. Ann Intern Med 121:684, 1994.

80. Chavis C, Godard P, Crastes de Paulet A, et al: Formation of lipoxins and leukotrienes by human alveolar macrophages incubated with 15(S)-HETE: A model for cellular cooperation between macrophages and airway epithelial cells. Eicosanoids 5:203, 1992.

81. Schellenberg RR, Tsang S, Salari H: Leukotrienes mediate delayed airway effects of 15-HETE. Ann N Y Acad Sci 744:243, 1994.

82. Ellis JL, Undem BJ: Role of cysteinyl-leukotrienes and histamine in mediating intrinsic tone in isolated human bronchi. Am J Respir Crit Care Med 149:118, 1994.

83. Fanburg BL: Prostaglandins and the lung. Am Rev Respir Dis 108:482, 1973.

84. Massaro D, Weiss H, Simon MR: Protein synthesis and secretion by lung. Am Rev Respir Dis 101:198, 1970.

85. Yeager H Jr, Massaro G, Massaro D: Glycoprotein synthesis by the trachea. Am Rev Respir Dis 103:188, 1971.

86. Gillis CN, Cronau LH, Mandel S, et al: Indicator dilution measurement of 5-hydroxytryptamine clearance by human lung. J Appl Physiol 46:1178, 1979.

87. Pitt BR: Metabolic functions of the lung and systemic vasoregulation. Fed Proc 43:2574, 1984.

88. Hammond GL, Cronay LH, Whittaker D, et al: Fate of prostaglandins E_1 and A_1 in the human pulmonary circulation. Surgery 81:716, 1977.

89. Gillis CN, Pitt BR, Wiedemann HP, et al: Depressed prostaglandin E_1 and 5-hydroxytryptamine removal in patients with adult respiratory distress syndrome. Am Rev Respir Dis 134:739, 1986.

90. Trifilieff A, Da Silva A, Gies JP: Kinins and respiratory tract diseases. Eur Respir J 6:576, 1993.

91. Muzykantov VR, Danilov SM: A new approach to the investigation of oxidative injury to the pulmonary endothelium: Use of angiotensin-converting enzyme as a marker. Biomed Sci 2:11, 1991.

92. Block ER, Schoen FJ: Effect of alpha-naphthylthiourea on uptake of 5-hydroxytryptamine from the pulmonary circulation. Am Rev Respir Dis 123:69, 1981.

93. Dobuler KJ, Catravas JD, Gillis CN: Early detection of oxygen-induced lung injury in conscious rabbits—reduced *in vivo* activity of angiotensin-converting enzyme and removal of 5-hydroxytryptamine. Am Rev Respir Dis 126:534, 1982.

94. Crimi N, Polosa R, Pulvirenti G, et al: Effect of an inhaled neutral endopeptidase inhibitor, phosphoramidon, on baseline airway calibre and bronchial responsiveness to bradykinin in asthma. Thorax 50:505, 1995.

95. Lilly CM, Drazen JM, Shore SA: Peptidase modulation of airway effects of neuropeptides. Proc Soc Exp Biol Med 203:388, 1993.

96. Bai TR, Zhou D, Weir T, et al: Substance P (NK_1) and neurokinin A (NK_2) receptor gene expression in inflammatory airway diseases. Am J Physiol 269:L309, 1995.

97. Barnes PJ: Nitric oxide and airway disease. Ann Med 27:389, 1995.

98. Kharitonov SA, Yates D, Barnes PJ: Increased nitric oxide in exhaled air of normal human subjects with upper respiratory tract infections. Eur Respir J 8:295, 1995.

99. Kharitonov SA, Yates D, Springall DR, et al: Exhaled nitric oxide is increased in asthma. Chest 107(Suppl):156, 1995.

100. Kharitonov SA, Robbins RA, Yates D, et al: Acute and chronic effects of cigarette smoking on exhaled nitric oxide. Am J Respir Crit Care Med 152:609, 1995.

101. Barnes PJ, Liew FY: Nitric oxide and asthmatic inflammation. Immunol Today 16:128, 1995.

102. Belvisi MG, Ward JK, Mitchell JA, et al: Nitric oxide as a neurotransmitter in human airways. Arch Int Pharmacodyn Ther 329:97, 1995.

103. Ward JK, Barnes PJ, Springall DR, et al: Distribution of human i-NANC bronchodilator and nitric oxide–immunoreactive nerves. Am J Respir Cell Mol Biol 13:175, 1995.

104. Luscher TF, Wenzel RR: Endothelin and endothelin antagonists: Pharmacology and clinical implications. Agents Actions Suppl 45:237, 1995.

105. Filep JG: Endothelin peptides: Biological actions and pathophysiological significance in the lung. Life Sci 52:119, 1993.

106. Stewart DJ: Endothelial dysfunction in pulmonary vascular disorders. Arzneimittelforschung 44:451, 1994.

107. Cohen GM: Pulmonary metabolism of foreign compounds: Its role in metabolic activation. Environ Health Perspect 85:31, 1990.

108. Krishna DR, Klotz U: Extrahepatic metabolism of drugs in humans. Clin Pharmacokinet 26:144, 1994.

109. Aida S, Takahashi Y, Suzuki E, et al: Electron-microscopic evidence for cytochrome P450 in Clara cells and type I pneumocytes of the rat lung. Respiration 59:201, 1992.

109a. Oury TD, Chang LY, Marklund SL, et al: Immunocytochemical localization of extracellular superoxide dismutase in human lung. Lab Invest 70:889, 1994.

109b. De Water R, Willems LNA, Van Muijen GNP, et al: Ultrastructural localization of bronchial antileukoprotease in central and peripheral human airways by a gold-labelling technique using monoclonal antibodies. Am Rev Respir Dis 133:882, 1986.

110. Freiman DG, Suyemoto J, Wessler S: Frequency of pulmonary thromboembolism in man. N Engl J Med 272:1278, 1965.

111. Attwood HD, Park WW: Embolism to the lungs by trophoblast. J Obstet Gynaecol Br Comm 68:611, 1961.

112. Park WW: Experimental trophoblastic embolism of the lungs. J Pathol Bacteriol 75:257, 1958.

113. Hartz PH: Occurrence of decidua-like tissue in the lung. Am J Clin Pathol 26:48, 1956.

114. Park WW: The occurrence of decidual tissue within the lung: Report of a case. J Pathol Bacteriol 67:503, 1954.

115. Sharnoff JG, Scardino V: Pulmonary megakaryocytes in human fetuses and premature and full-term infants. Arch Pathol 69:27, 139, 1960.

116. Aabo K, Hansen KB: Megakaryocytes in pulmonary blood vessels: I. Incidence at autopsy: Clinicopathologic relations especially to disseminated intravascular coagulation. Acta Pathol Microbiol Scand 86:285, 1978.

117. Sharma GK, Talbot IC: Pulmonary megakaryocytes: "Missing link" between cardiovascular and respiratory disease? J Clin Pathol 39:969, 1986.

118. Wells S, Sissons M, Hasleton PS: Quantitation of pulmonary megakaryocytes and fibrin thrombi in patients dying from burns. Histopathology 8:517, 1984.

119. Hansen KB, Aabo K, Myhre-Jensen O: Response of pulmonary (circulating) megakaryocytes to experimentally induced consumption coagulopathy in rabbits. Acta Pathol Microbiol Scand 87:165, 1979.

120. Soares FA: Increased numbers of pulmonary megakaryocytes in patients with arterial pulmonary tumour embolism and with lung metastases seen at necropsy. J Clin Pathol 45:140, 1992.

121. Kaufman RM, Airo R, Pollack S, et al: Circulating megakaryocytes and platelet release in the lung. Blood 26:720, 1965.

122. Pedersen NT: Occurrence of megakaryocytes in various vessels and their retention in the pulmonary capillaries in man. Scand J Haematol 21:369, 1978.

123. Kallinikos-Maniatis A: Megakaryocytes and platelets in central venous and arterial blood. Acta Haematol 42:330, 1969.

124. Martin JF, Slater DN, Trowbridge EA: Abnormal intrapulmonary platelet production: A possible cause of vascular and lung disease. Lancet 2:793, 1983.

125. Hogg JC: Neutrophil kinetics and lung injury. Physiol Rev 67:1249, 1987.

126. Downey GP, Worthen GS, Henson PM, et al: Neutrophil sequestration and migration in localized pulmonary inflammation. Am Rev Respir Dis 147:168, 1993.

CHAPTER 4

Development and Growth of the Lung

THE CONDUCTING AND TRANSITIONAL AIRWAYS AND
ALVEOLI, 136
   Embryonic Period, 136
   Pseudoglandular Period, 136
   Canalicular Period, 137
   Saccular Period, 137
   Alveolar Period, 138
   Postnatal Period, 138
THE VASCULAR SYSTEM, 139
   Pulmonary Arteries, 139
   Pulmonary Veins, 140
FACTORS INFLUENCING DEVELOPMENT AND
GROWTH, 141

Growth and development of the lung have been divided into intrauterine and postnatal stages, although it is clear that the two overlap and that birth represents only one influence on the whole process. Intrauterine development itself has traditionally been divided into four periods: *embryonic, pseudoglandular, canalicular,* and *saccular.*[1] Some workers have questioned this scheme and suggested either a simplification into three subgroups (embryonic, conducting, and respiratory)[2] or the addition of an intrauterine *alveolar* period.[3]

This subject has been discussed in greater detail in several publications.[4–7] It is important not only because it provides the basis for understanding many of the developmental diseases that affect the lungs but also because there is now increasing evidence that abnormalities in lung growth and development may have a significant influence on the prevalence and severity of adult pulmonary disease.[8–10]

THE CONDUCTING AND TRANSITIONAL AIRWAYS AND ALVEOLI

Embryonic Period

The lung begins to develop at about 26 days of embryonic life as a ventral diverticulum of the foregut near the junction of the occipital and cervical segments (Fig. 4–1A). The outpouching is lined by endodermal epithelium and is invested by splanchnic mesenchyme. During the next 2 or 3 days, it gives rise to right and left lung buds that even at this early stage show a characteristic direction of growth, that on the right being directed caudally and that on the left more transversely (Fig. 4–1B and C).

As the lung buds elongate, the respiratory portion of the gut becomes separated from the esophageal portion by lateral ingrowths of surrounding mesoderm that progressively meet to form the tracheoesophageal septum. By the end of another 2 days (30 to 32 days), the lung buds have elongated into primary lung sacs (Fig. 4–1D), and by days 32 to 34 the five lobar bronchi have appeared as monopodial outgrowths of the primary bronchi (Fig. 4–1E). Thus, by the end of the fifth week, the airways destined to become the five lobar bronchi have begun their development, a point marking the end of the embryonic period.[1] (Some consider this period to include development of the subsegmental bronchi and to extend to about 4½ weeks.[6])

Pseudoglandular Period

The pseudoglandular period extends from the end of the 5th to the 16th week of gestation and is primarily related to development of the bronchial tree (Fig. 4–1F). Following the appearance of the five lobar bronchi, branching occurs quickly and more or less dichotomously. Between the 10th and 14th weeks, 65% to 75% of all bronchial branching has occurred, and by the 16th week virtually all conducting airways are present. During this period the airways are blind tubules lined by columnar or cuboidal epithelium—hence the term *pseudoglandular* (Fig. 4–2).

Epithelial cell differentiation begins in the most proximal bronchi and proceeds distally, a process that occurs throughout the remainder of gestation and, for the transitional airways, continues postnatally. In early development, airway epithelial cells are tall and columnar in shape with abundant clear cytoplasm situated at the abluminal aspect of the airway (Fig. 4–3). Clara cells can be detected by the 15th week of gestation and increase progressively in number thereafter.[11] Members of the forkhead family of transcription factors (e.g., HNF-3α, HNF-3β, and HFH-4), the homeodomain protein TTF-1, and N-*myc* have been hypothesized to play important regulatory roles in specific cellular differentiation.[12]

Cartilage can be seen within the trachea as early as 7 weeks' gestation[13] and develops in the bronchi in a centrifugal direction thereafter (Fig. 4–4). Although some investigators have found all new foci of cartilage to appear by 25 weeks,[13] others have documented evidence for their continued development into neonatal life.[14]

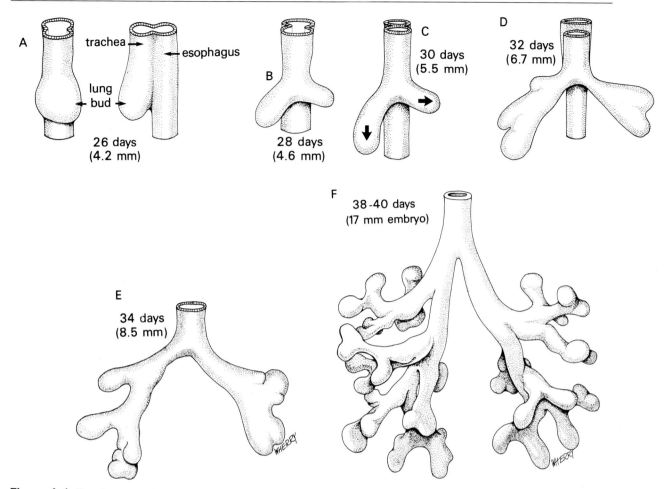

Figure 4–1. Development of the Human Lung. Diagrammatic representation of human lung development in the embryonic and pseudoglandular periods. *A* is depicted from the front and the side; all others are shown from the front only.

Tracheobronchial gland development begins in the middle of the pseudoglandular period and continues into the canalicular phase,[15, 16] so glands in the proximal airway resemble those in the adult by 25 weeks. The glands begin as small cell clusters that grow from the surface epithelium into the lamina propria, a process that appears to be promoted by adjacent fibroblasts.[17] Subsequent development is characterized by elongation and lumen formation of the initial bud, followed by repeated branching and differentiation into serous and mucous cells. There is evidence that the glycoproteins produced during fetal life are different from those after birth.[18]

Canalicular Period

From the 17th to the 24th or 25th week of intrauterine life (28th week, according to some[6]), the peripheral portion of the bronchial tree undergoes further development in the form of primitive canaliculi that represent early stages of the transitional airways (Fig. 4–5). At the same time, the mesenchyme adjacent to the canaliculi becomes vascularized through capillary ingrowth. Throughout this period there is a progressive decrease in the amount of mesenchymal tissue, so the air spaces and newly formed capillaries come to approximate each other.[19] During this time, the airway epithelium progressively decreases in height until the entire acinar pathway is lined by a cuboidal or flattened epithelium. At about 28 weeks, differentiation into Type I and Type II alveolar epithelial cells has clearly begun, and Type II osmiophilic granules can be identified.[5] At this time, a blood-gas barrier exists that is capable of permitting gas exchange.

Saccular Period

By the 24th to 25th week, thin-walled spaces lined by flattened epithelium (saccules) become visible at the ends of the canaliculi. This phase marks the beginning of the terminal sac period, a stage that is traditionally thought to last until birth. Acinar morphology is well developed, and by the 28th week of gestation, several generations of respiratory bronchioles open into so-called transitional ducts, with several generations of saccules arising from them. Further development until birth consists largely of saccular proliferation and a corresponding decrease in mesenchyme and more organized vascularization. At the beginning of this period, small buds (crests) of tissue begin to bulge out at intervals along the saccule walls (Fig. 4–6).[6] As these elongate, they delineate shallow, cuplike structures destined to be the definitive alveoli.

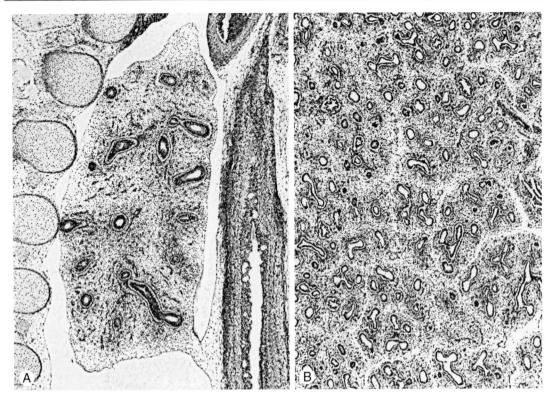

Figure 4–2. Developing Human Lung—Pseudoglandular Period. Early pseudoglandular period *(A)* showing occasional tubular channels within abundant mesenchyme. Thoracic vertebrae are at the *left.* (×40.) Late pseudoglandular period *(B)* shows more numerous branching presumptive airways. (×52.)

Alveolar Period

Structures histologically consistent with alveoli have been demonstrated as early as 30 weeks' gestation; in one study, they were uniformly present by 36 weeks.[3] It has thus been suggested that the final period of normal intrauterine lung development, from 36 weeks to term, be designated the *alveolar phase.*[3] The actual number of alveoli at birth appears to be quite variable, measurements ranging from 10 million to almost 60 million.[3]

Postnatal Period

Although there is variation in their structure,[5] the typical acinus at birth consists of three generations of respiratory bronchioles, one of transitional ducts, and three of saccules that end in a terminal saccule.[1, 20] During early postnatal

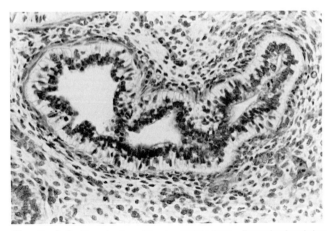

Figure 4–3. Developing Airway Epithelium—Pseudoglandular Period. A magnified view of a presumptive airway illustrated in Figure 4–2B shows tall columnar epithelium with nuclei adjacent to the lumen and abundant clear cytoplasm. (×250.)

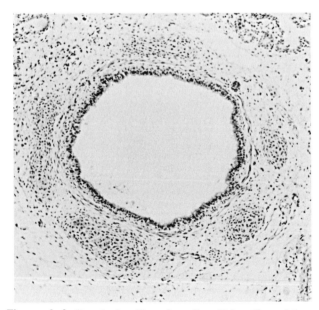

Figure 4–4. Developing Bronchus. Bronchial cartilage plates are clearly evident but still immature in appearance (fetal age about 22 weeks). (×60.)

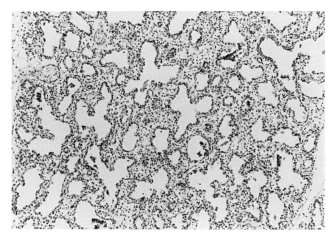

Figure 4–5. Developing Lung—Canalicular Period. A section of lung during the canalicular period shows a more complex pattern, with pulmonary airways now clearly recognizable. (×120.)

development, acinar length increases and its components are remodeled, largely as a result of the appearance of true alveoli. Thus, terminal bronchioles may be transformed into respiratory bronchioles, and distal respiratory bronchioles may become alveolar ducts. The saccules themselves probably develop into both alveolar ducts and sacs. Although there is little true branching after birth, each terminal saccule may generate up to four additional alveolar sacs,[1] probably by budding. Alveoli themselves develop both peripherally in relation to the saccule and more centrally along the walls of the respiratory bronchioles and transitional ducts.

By these processes, a substantial number of alveoli are added after birth. The majority appear during early childhood, probably by 2 years of age.[21] After the age of 1 year, males tend to have somewhat more alveoli than females, an

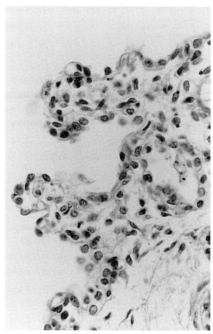

Figure 4–6. Developing Lung—Alveoli. Several presumptive alveoli are illustrated; they are still lined by cuboidal epithelium and contain a moderate amount of mesenchymal tissue in their walls. (×350.)

observation that correlates with a difference in lung volume.[21] The age at which alveolar development is completed is also controversial, although it appears likely that some multiplication occurs until at least 8 years of age.[5] The average area of air-tissue interface increases from 3 to 4 m² at birth[3] to approximately 32 m² at 8 years and 75 m² in the adult, an increase that is related linearly to body surface area.[22]

The acinus increases in length from early gestation to the age of 7 years; however, with increasing body size, acini continue to lengthen and alveoli to enlarge until the adult acinus reaches a diameter of 6 to 10 mm.[1, 23] During this period, the conducting airways also increase in both length and diameter in proportion to body size.[5] Although evidence concerning the relative growth rate of different portions of the bronchial tree is conflicting,[18] several investigators have found that the relative diameter of distal to proximal airways is less in younger children than in adults.[5, 24] This finding supports the observations that peripheral airways contribute a greater proportion of total airway resistance in young children than in adults and that peripheral airway conductance increases significantly at about 5 years of age.[25]

In the neonate the trachea is funnel shaped, the laryngeal end being wider than the carinal.[26] A cylindrical shape gradually becomes evident with increasing age. The rate of growth in relation to crown-to-rump length appears to be greatest between 1 month and 4 years. Tracheal dimensions in relation to age and body height have been described.[27]

The nature of and factors controlling postpneumonectomy compensatory lung growth are poorly understood. On the basis of animal experiments, it appears that such growth is a result of both cellular and connective tissue proliferation (as opposed to simple hypertrophy or alveolar distention)[28] and that stretch is the initial stimulus.[29] As might be expected, there is evidence that a normal complement of hormones is important for growth to occur.[30]

THE VASCULAR SYSTEM

Pulmonary Arteries

The pulmonary artery develops from the sixth aortic arch during the early embryonic period (Fig. 4–7). On both sides, the proximal part of the arch develops into the proximal segment of the right and left pulmonary arteries; on the right side, the distal part loses its connection with the aortic arch whereas on the left it maintains its connection with the aorta as the ductus arteriosus during intrauterine life. Branches from both arches grow toward the developing lung buds and become incorporated with them in the future hila. There is evidence that subsequent vascular development occurs by a combination of budding of new vessels from pre-existing ones proximally and the formation of "blood lakes" in the peripheral mesenchyme.[31]

During the embryonic and pseudoglandular periods, pulmonary arteries develop at approximately the same rate and in the same manner as the airways, so the majority of preacinar branches are present by the end of the 16th week.[32] By 12 weeks, both conventional and supernumerary branches are present in the preacinar region in approximately the same proportion as in the adult. During the latter part of fetal life,

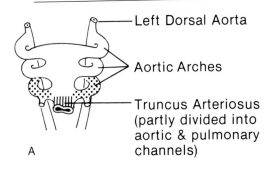

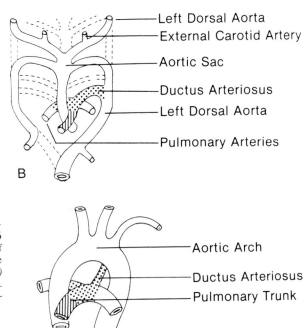

Figure 4–7. Development of the Pulmonary Arteries. Aortic arches (3, 4, and 6) and partly divided truncus arteriosus at 6 weeks *(A)*. Aortic arches at 7 weeks are shown in *B*; the parts of the dorsal aortas and aortic arches that normally disappear are indicated by the *broken lines*. Arterial arrangement at 8 weeks *(C)* shows a well-formed pulmonary trunk and main pulmonary arteries. (Modified from Moore KL: The Developing Human. 3rd ed. Philadelphia, WB Saunders, 1982.)

the main feature of arterial development is an increase in vessel diameter and length. In the postnatal stage, there is a small increase in the development of conventional branches until about 18 months that is related to the small increase in acinar airways that occurs during this period.[5] By contrast, a marked increase in supernumerary branches occurs and corresponds to the prolific alveolar development of early childhood; this increase continues, although at a decreasing rate, until about 8 years of age.[33]

Histologically, the structure of the fetal arterial system differs from that postnatally, a reflection of the different states of intravascular blood flow and pressure. The extrapulmonary arterial wall of the fetus closely resembles that of the aorta in thickness and structure, with fairly uniform and thick medial elastic laminae. As intravascular pressure drops after birth, wall thickness slowly decreases and the elastic laminae become fragmented and fewer in number. This process is clearly evident at about 4 months of age, and the final adult configuration is reached by about 2 years of age.[34]

Muscular arteries are not well developed in early fetal life and contain only thin, poorly staining elastic laminae and muscle cells; however, by the end of the canalicular period they are morphologically mature.[32] At this time, their lumina are small and their media quite thick, representing as much as 15% to 25% of the total external diameter of the vessel,[34] a feature again related to the high pulmonary arterial pressure. Shortly after birth, there is a marked increase in luminal diameter and a corresponding thinning of the media, a process that appears to be related at least in part to a reduction in overlap between adjacent smooth muscle cells.[35] Thinning and other morphologic alterations of endothelial cells also occur rapidly in the neonatal period.[36]

At birth, the pulmonary arteries are readily distensible,[37] a feature seemingly important in ensuring rapid adaptation from fetal to neonatal circulation. It has been hypothesized that this distensibility may be related to the predominance

of Type III collagen in fetal vessels since this form of collagen is itself relatively distensible.[38] In support of this hypothesis is the observation that Type I collagen increases in amount after birth as the vessels become stiffer. It has also been speculated that nerves to the pulmonary vessels, which undergo rapid changes at birth, may be involved in circulatory adaptation.[39]

Pulmonary Veins

In the embryonic stage, pulmonary venous blood drains via the splanchnic plexus into the primordia of the systemic venous system (including the cardinal and umbilicovitteline veins) (Fig. 4–8). Subsequently, caudal and cranial outpouchings of the sinoatrial region of the heart develop and extend toward the lung buds. Normally, the caudal portion regresses and the cranial portion continues to develop as the common pulmonary vein, eventually connecting with that portion of the splanchnic plexus draining the lungs.[40] With time, the common pulmonary vein is incorporated into the left atrial wall and the majority of the splanchnic-pulmonary connections are obliterated, leaving four independent pulmonary veins directly entering the left atrium.

As with the arterial system, the pattern of postacinar venous drainage is complete halfway through fetal life and the intra-acinar pattern is further developed during childhood.[41] With respect to size, number, and branching, the pattern of venous development is generally similar to that of the arteries. However, in contrast to the latter, the veins are less muscular in the fetus than in the adult. In one investigation, a measurable muscle layer was not identified in the walls of the veins before birth, although some small muscle fibers could be seen at 28 weeks' gestation.[41] It is possible that the high resistance within the pulmonary arteries during fetal life may so limit the passage of blood to the venous

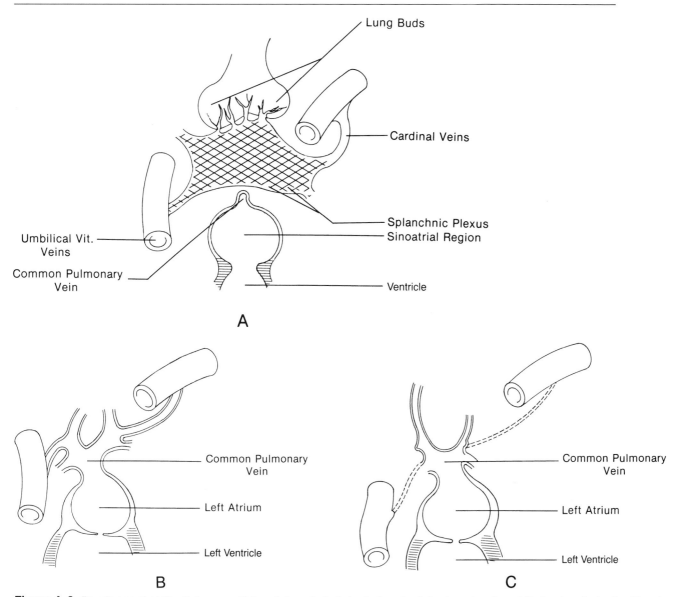

Figure 4–8. Development of the Pulmonary Veins. *A,* Lung buds drain via the splanchnic plexus into the umbilical and cardinal veins. Note the developing common pulmonary vein. *B,* Pulmonary veins, although still draining into the systemic circulation, now also communicate with the left atrium. *C,* Disappearance of the primitive systemic connections results in complete flow into the left atrium.

circulation that venous pressure is too low to stimulate muscle development.

FACTORS INFLUENCING DEVELOPMENT AND GROWTH

The normal and abnormal factors that affect lung growth and development are highly complex and not fully understood.[42] Factors that seem to have some importance include fetal respiration, lung and intrauterine fluid production, systemic and local (paracrine) hormones, interactions between epithelial cells and adjacent mesenchymal cells and connective tissue, and postnatal disease.

Epithelial-Mesenchymal Interaction. As previously discussed, the conducting airways develop by sequential branching of the bilateral lung buds. If the latter are removed from an animal in an early stage of development and then cultured, this branching process continues, but only if the adjacent mesenchyme is included in the culture medium.[43] This epithelial-mesenchymal interaction has both general and highly specific properties; for example, embryonic mesenchyme from one species may have the ability to support branching in another species, but only if it is derived from the lung. On the other hand, significant differences exist between mesenchyme in the same lung—bronchial mesenchyme is able to induce tracheal epithelial branching, whereas tracheal mesenchyme has an inhibitory effect on bronchial branching.[43]

Although the precise mechanisms underlying this interaction are unclear and undoubtedly highly complex, it is likely that both cell surface interactions and the production of locally active soluble mediators are involved.[42, 44] Ultrastructural studies of developing lungs of experimental animals have shown close contacts between epithelial and mesenchymal cells, their number increasing near term.[45, 46] A variety of growth factors—including epidermal growth factor,[47] keratinocyte growth factor,[48] fibroblast growth factor, and platelet-derived growth factor[42]—as well as adhesion molecules such as fibronectin[49] and laminins[50] and their integrin receptors,[51, 52] may be involved in this relationship. It is also likely that the basement membrane itself has an important effect.[53] Regional differences in the expression of specific genes (e.g., homeobox genes)[54] and programmed death (apoptosis) of both epithelial and mesenchymal cells[54a, 54b] are also likely to be important factors affecting morphogenesis.

In addition to local biochemical control, tissue derived from mesenchyme may affect pulmonary morphogenesis by purely physical means. A myofibroblast-like cell that appears to be involved in the synthesis of elastin has been described at the tips of newly formed alveolar septa.[55, 56] It has been hypothesized that this interstitial elastic tissue appears before actual alveolar development and may act as a kind of physical barrier around which the alveoli develop.[57] In support of this hypothesis is the observation that neonatal rats administered β-aminopropionitrile (an inhibitor of lysyl oxidase, the enzyme necessary for elastin cross-linking) have significantly fewer and larger alveoli,[58, 59] thus suggesting that the elastic scaffold may be directly related to alveolar development. A second cell, termed the *lipid-containing interstitial cell,* has been described at the base of the alveolar septa and contains numerous lipid granules as well as fairly prominent microfilaments resembling actin. It has been suggested that this cell, via its microfilaments, may have active contractile properties capable in some way of shaping the alveolar septum.[56]

It has also been suggested that purely physical factors may be responsible for the characteristic dichotomous bronchial branching.[60] According to this hypothesis, the mesenchyme in direct opposition to the tip of a growing bronchial bud becomes more and more compressed; at some point the resistance is great enough that forward growth ceases and new (lateral) branches develop in the region adjacent to the tip where the mesenchyme is not as compact.

Fetal Respiration. Pulmonary hypoplasia develops in animals subjected to intrauterine cervical or phrenic nerve injury;[61–63] it has been speculated that this effect is mediated by abnormalities of respiratory movement as a result of the denervation.[61, 63] Physical abnormalities of the thoracic wall, such as scoliosis and intrathoracic tumors, are also associated with lung hypoplasia (*see* page 598); although this may be related simply to physical constraints on the potential for lung growth, decreased respiratory movements may also be involved.

Pulmonary and Intrauterine Fluid. Oligohydramnios also has an important association with pulmonary hypoplasia.[64] Although it has been suggested that this may be related to compression of the thoracic wall by the closely applied uterus,[64] it appears more likely that an associated decrease in intrapulmonary fluid may be responsible;[65, 66] since such fluid normally exerts positive pressure within the developing lung, its deficiency might result in the loss of a template about which the lung can form. In support of this hypothesis is the observation that fetal airway smooth muscle is capable of spontaneous contraction,[67] possibly resulting in phasic changes in intraluminal pressure.

Hormonal, Paracrine, and Nutritional Factors. The role of hormones in growth and development, although undoubtedly important, is for the most part poorly understood.[7, 68] It has been suggested that there may be a difference between the sexes in biochemical maturation, possibly related to differences in androgenic hormones.[69] Glucocorticoid-related differences in the number of intercellular contacts between the lung cells of male and female fetal rats provide some support for this hypothesis.[45, 46] The influence of glucocorticoids and other hormones on the maturation of alveolar Type II cells has been more extensively investigated and is clearly important (*see* page 56).

As indicated previously, neuroendocrine cells develop first in the proximal airways and can be recognized as early as 8 to 10 weeks' gestation.[70, 71] Several types have been identified on the basis of ultrastructural differences in secretory granules and immunohistochemical characteristics,[72] which suggests the possibility of different functions. Because of their early appearance and prominence in the fetus, it is widely believed that these cells and their peptides may have important effects on local lung development.[73–77]

Although the precise mechanisms are not clear, it is likely that a variety of vitamins (e.g., vitamin A and its derivatives[78, 78a]) and other nutritional substances are essential for normal lung development.

Postnatal Disease. The effects on lung growth of bronchopulmonary or systemic disease acquired in childhood or infancy are not well understood. However, experimental evidence indicates that a variety of conditions, such as viral infection,[79] starvation,[80] obesity,[81] and hypoxia,[82] may have important effects. A reduction in alveolar number and reduced alveolar internal surface area have also been found in the lungs of infants and children with bronchopulmonary dysplasia.[83]

REFERENCES

1. Hislop A, Reid L: Development of the acinus in the human lung. Thorax 29:90, 1974.
2. Have-Opbroek AAWT: The development of the lung in mammals: An analysis of concepts and findings. Am J Anat 162:201, 1981.
3. Langston C, Kida K, Reed M, et al: Human lung growth in late gestation and in the neonate. Am Rev Respir Dis 129:607, 1984.
4. Hodson WA: Development of the lung. In Hodson WA (ed): Development of the Lung. New York, Marcel Dekker, 1977.
5. Thurlbeck WM: Postnatal growth and development of the lung. Am Rev Respir Dis 111:803, 1975.
6. Thurlbeck WM: Lung growth and development. In Churg A, Thurlbeck WM (eds): Pathology of the Lung. New York, Thieme Medical Publishers, 1995.
7. DiFiore JW, Wilson JM: Lung development. Semin Pediatr Surg 3:221, 1994.
8. Helms PJ: Lung growth: Implications for the development of disease. Thorax 49:440, 1994.
9. Shahhen SO, Barker DJ: Early lung growth and chronic airflow obstruction. Thorax 49:533, 1994.
10. Harding R: Sustained alterations in postnatal respiratory function following suboptimal intrauterine conditions. Reprod Fertil Dev 7:431, 1995.
11. Barth PJ, Wolf M, Ramaswamy A: Distribution and number of Clara cells in the normal and disturbed development of the human fetal lung. Pediatr Pathol 14:637, 1994.
12. Hackett BP, Bingle CD, Gitlin JD: Mechanisms of gene expression and cell fate determination in the developing pulmonary epithelium. Annu Rev Physiol 58:51, 1996.
13. Bucher U, Reid L: Development of the intrasegmental bronchial tree: The pattern of branching and development of cartilage at various stages of intrauterine life. Thorax 16:207, 1961.
14. Sinclair-Smith CC, Emery JL, Gadsdon D, et al: Cartilage in children's lungs: A quantitative assessment using the right middle lobe. Thorax 31:40, 1976.
15. Bucher U, Reid L: Development of the mucus-secreting elements in human lung. Thorax 16:219, 1961.
16. Tos M: Development of the tracheal glands in man. Acta Pathol Microbiol Scand 68(Suppl 185):1, 1966.
17. Infeld MD, Brennan JA, Davis PB: Human fetal lung fibroblasts promote invasion of extracellular matrix by normal human tracheobronchial epithelial cells in vitro: A model of early airway gland development. Am J Respir Cell Mol Biol 8:69, 1993.
18. Hislop AA, Haworth SG: Airway size and structure in the normal fetal and infant lung and the effect of premature delivery and artificial ventilation. Am Rev Respir Dis 140:1717, 1989.
19. Lin Y, Lechner AJ: Development of alveolar septa and cellular maturation within the perinatal lung. Am J Respir Cell Mol Biol 4:59, 1991.
20. Boyden EA, Tompsett DH: The changing patterns in the developing lungs of infants. Acta Anat 61:164, 1965.
21. Thurlbeck WM: Postnatal human lung growth. Thorax 37:564, 1982.
22. Dunnill MS: Postnatal growth of the lung. Thorax 17:329, 1962.
23. Osborne DRS, Effmann EL, Hedlund LW: Postnatal growth and size of the pulmonary acinus and secondary lobule in man. Am J Roentgenol 140:449, 1983.
24. Horsfield K, Gordon WI, Kemp W, et al: Growth of the bronchial tree in man. Thorax 42:383, 1987.
25. Hogg JC, Williams J, Richardson JB, et al: Age as a factor in the distribution of lower-airway conductance and in the pathologic anatomy of obstructive lung disease. N Engl J Med 282:1283, 1970.
26. Wailoo MP, Emery JL: Normal growth and development of the trachea. Thorax 37:584, 1982.
27. Griscom NT, Wohl ME: Dimensions of the growing trachea related to age and gender. Am J Roentgenol 146:233, 1986.
28. Koh DW, Roby JD, Starcher B, et al: Postpneumonectomy lung growth: A model of reinitiation of tropoelastin and type I collagen production in a normal pattern in adult rat lung. Am J Respir Cell Mol Biol 15:611, 1996.
29. Cagle PT, Thurlbeck WM: Postpneumonectomy compensatory lung growth. Am Rev Respir Dis 138:1314, 1988.
30. Rannels DE, Stockstill B, Mercer RR, et al: Cellular changes in the lungs of adrenalectomized rats following left pneumonectomy. Am J Respir Cell Mol Biol 5:351, 1991.
31. de Mello DE, Sawyer D, Galvin N, et al: Early fetal development of lung vasculature. Am J Respir Cell Mol Biol 16:568, 1997.
32. Hislop A, Reid LM: Formation of the pulmonary vasculature. In Hodson WA (ed): Development of the Lung. New York, Marcel Dekker, 1977, p 37.
33. Hislop A, Reid L: Pulmonary arterial development during childhood: Branching pattern and structure. Thorax 28:129, 1973.
34. Wagenvoort CA, Wagenvoort N: Pathology of Pulmonary Hypertension. New York, John Wiley & Sons, 1977.
35. Haworth SG, Hall SM, Chew M, et al: Thinning of fetal pulmonary arterial wall and postnatal remodeling: Ultrastructural studies on the respiratory unit arteries of the pig. Virchows Arch 411:161, 1987.
36. Hall SM, Haworth SG: Normal adaptation of pulmonary arterial intima to extra-uterine life in the pig: Ultrastructural studies. J Pathol 149:55, 1986.
37. Hall S, Haworth SG: Conducting pulmonary arteries: Structural adaptation to extrauterine life. Cardiovasc Res 21:208, 1987.
38. Mills AN, Haworth SG: Pattern of connective tissue development in swine pulmonary vasculature by immunolocalization. J Pathol 153:171, 1987.
39. Wharton J, Haworth SG, Polak JM: Postnatal development of the innervation and paraganglia in the porcine pulmonary arterial bed. J Pathol 154:19, 1988.
40. Auer J: The development of the human pulmonary vein and its major variations. Anat Rec 101:581, 1948.
41. Hislop A, Reid L: Fetal and childhood development of the intra-pulmonary veins in man: Branching pattern and structure. Thorax 28:313, 1973.
42. McGowan SE: Extracellular matrix and the regulation of lung development and repair. FASEB J 6:2895, 1992.
43. Smith BT, Fletcher WA: Pulmonary epithelial-mesenchymal interactions: Beyond organogenesis. Hum Pathol 10:248, 1979.
44. Warburton D, Lee M, Berberich MA, et al: Molecular embryology and the study of lung development. Am J Respir Cell Mol Biol 9:5, 1993.
45. Adamson IYR, King GM: Sex differences in development of fetal rat lung: II. Quantitative morphology of epithelial-mesenchymal interactions. Lab Invest 50:461, 1984.
46. Adamson IY, King GM: Epithelial-interstitial cell interactions in fetal rat lung development accelerated by steroids. Lab Invest 55:145, 1986.
47. Johnson MD, Gray ME, Carpenter G, et al: Ontogeny of epidermal growth factor receptor and lipocortin-1 in fetal and neonatal human lungs. Hum Pathol 21:182, 1990.
48. Shiratori M, Oshika E, Ung LP, et al: Keratinocyte growth factor and embryonic rat lung morphogenesis. Am J Respir Cell Mol Biol 15:328, 1996.
49. Roman J, McDonald JA: Expression of fibronectin, the integrin α5, and α-smooth muscle actin in heart and lung development. Am J Respir Cell Mol Biol 6:472, 1992.
50. Virtanen I, Laitinen A, Tani T, et al: Differential expression of laminins and their integrin receptors in developing and adult human lung. Am J Respir Cell Mol Biol 15:184, 1996.
51. Erle DJ, Pytela R: How do integrins integrate? The role of cell adhesion receptors in differentiation and development. Am J Respir Cell Mol Biol 6:459, 1992.
52. Roman J, Little CW, MacDonald JA: Potential role of RGD-binding integrins in mammalian lung branching morphogenesis. Development 112:551, 1991.
53. Kleinman HK, Schnaper HW: Basement membrane matrices in tissue development. Am J Respir Cell Mol Biol 8:238, 1993.
54. Bogue CW, Lou LJ, Vasavada H, et al: Expression of HOXB genes in the developing mouse foregut and lung. Am J Respir Cell Mol Biol 15:163, 1996.
54a. Scavo LM, Ertsey R, Chapin CJ, et al: Apoptosis in the development of rat and human fetal lungs. Am J Respir Cell Mol Biol 18:21, 1998.
54b. Schittny JC, Djonov V, Fine A, et al: Programmed cell death contributes to postnatal lung development. Am J Respir Cell Mol Biol 18:786, 1998.
55. Vaccaro C, Brody JS: Ultrastructure of developing alveoli: I. The role of the interstitial fibroblast. Anat Rec 192:467, 1978.
56. Maksvytis HJ, Vaccaro C, Brody JS: Isolation and characterization of the lipid-containing interstitial cell from the developing rat lung. Lab Invest 45:248, 1981.
57. Emery JL: The postnatal development of the human lung and its implications for lung pathology. Respiration 27(Suppl):41, 1970.
58. Kida K, Thurlbeck WM: The effects of β-aminopropionitrile on the growing rat lung. Am J Pathol 101:693, 1980.
59. Das RM: The effect of β-aminopropionitrile on lung development in the rat. Am J Pathol 101:711, 1980.
60. Hutchins GM, Haupt HM, Moore GW: A proposed mechanism for the early development of the human tracheobronchial tree. Anat Rec 201:635, 1981.
61. Wigglesworth JS, Winston RML, Bartlett K: Influence of the central nervous system on fetal lung development. Arch Dis Child 52:965, 1977.
62. Fewell JE, Lee CC, Kitterman JA: Effects of phrenic nerve section on the respiratory system of fetal lambs. J Appl Physiol 51:293, 1981.
63. Liggins GC, Vilos GA, Campos GA, et al: The effect of spinal cord transection on lung development in fetal sheep. J Dev Physiol 3:267, 1981.
64. Page DV, Stocker JT: Anomalies associated with pulmonary hypoplasia. Am Rev Respir Dis 125:216, 1982.
65. Adzick NS, Harrison MR, Glick PL, et al: Experimental pulmonary hypoplasia and oligohydramnios: Relative contributions of lung fluid and fetal breathing movements. J Pediatr Surg 19:658, 1984.
66. Harding R, Hooper SB: Regulation of lung expansion and lung growth before birth. J Appl Physiol 81:209, 1996.
67. McCray PB: Spontaneous contractility of human fetal airway smooth muscle. Am J Respir Cell Mol Biol 8:573, 1993.
68. Gross I: Regulation of fetal lung maturation. Am J Physiol 259:337, 1990.
69. Torday JS, Nielsen HC, Fencl MDM, et al: Sex differences in fetal lung maturation. Am Rev Respir Dis 123:205, 1981.
70. Stahlman MT, Gray ME: Ontogeny of neuroendocrine cells in human fetal lung. Lab Invest 51:449, 1984.
71. Watanabe H: Pathological studies of neuroendocrine cells in human embryonic and fetal lung: Light microscopical, immunohistochemical and electron microscopical approaches. Acta Pathol Jpn 38:59, 1988.
72. Hage E: Electron microscopic identification of several types of endocrine cells in the bronchial epithelium of human foetuses. Z Zellforsch 141:401, 1973.
73. Aguayo SM, Schuyler WE, Murtag JJ, et al: Regulation of lung branching

morphogenesis by bombesin-like peptides and neutral endopeptidase. Am J Respir Cell Mol Biol 10:635, 1994.

74. Giaid A, Polak JM, Gaitonde V, et al: Distribution of endothelin-like immunoreactivity and mRNA in the developing and adult human lung. Am J Respir Cell Mol Biol 4:50, 1991.

75. Wang D, Yeger H, Cutz E: Expression of gastrin-releasing peptide receptor gene in developing lung. Am J Respir Cell Mol Biol 14:409, 1996.

76. Spindel ER: Roles of bombesin-like peptides in lung development and lung injury. Am J Respir Cell Mol Biol 14:407, 1996.

77. King KA, Torday JS, Sunday ME: Bombesin and [Leu8]phyllolitorin promote fetal mouse lung branching morphogenesis via a receptor-mediated mechanism. Proc Natl Acad Sci U S A 92:4357, 1995.

78. Zachman RD: Role of vitamin A in lung development. J Nutr 125(Suppl):1634, 1995.

78a. Massaro GD, Massaro D: Postnatal treatment with retinoic acid increases the number of pulmonary alveoli in rats. Am J Physiol 272:L792, 1997.

79. Castleman WL: Alterations in pulmonary ultrastructure and morphometric parameters induced by para-influenza (Sendai) virus in rats during postnatal growth. Am J Pathol 114:322, 1984.

80. Das RM: The effects of intermittent starvation on lung development in suckling rats. Am J Pathol 117:326, 1984.

81. Inselman LS, Wapnir RA, Spencer H: Obesity-induced hyperplastic lung growth. Am Rev Respir Dis 135:613, 1987.

82. Weibel ER: Functional morphology of the growing lung. *In* Pathophysiology: I. Prenatal and neonatal anatomy in relation to some pathology in children. Respiration 27(Suppl):27, 1970.

83. Margraf LR, Tomashefski JF Jr, Bruce MC, et al: Morphometric analysis of the lung in bronchopulmonary dysplasia. Am Rev Respir Dis 143:391, 1991.

CHAPTER 5

Innervation of the Lung

The lung is innervated by fibers that travel in the vagus nerve and in nerves derived from the second to fifth thoracic ganglia of the sympathetic trunk.[1–3] These fibers carry afferents and efferents of the parasympathetic and sympathetic autonomic nervous systems. Although these terms are often used interchangeably with cholinergic nervous system (parasympathetic) and adrenergic nervous system (sympathetic), the increasing recognition that additional neurotransmitters can be co-localized in "adrenergic" and "cholinergic" nerve endings has made this classification scheme incomplete. As a result, it has been suggested that the original definitions of parasympathetic and sympathetic systems, which were based on the site of origin of the nerves, be employed.[4,*] In addition, there is pharmacologic and physiologic evidence for a nonadrenergic, noncholinergic, neural inhibitory efferent system that is variously termed the *nonadrenergic inhibitory system* (NAIS) or the *nonadrenergic noncholinergic inhibitory* (NANCi) system; the anatomic pathway for this system has not been well defined.[5, 6] (Innervation of the pleura and respiratory muscles is described in Chapter 10 [*see* page 250]; innervation of the smooth muscle of the airway and vascular smooth muscle has been reviewed in a comprehensive text.[7])

Figure 5–1 is a diagrammatic illustration of pulmonary innervation. The vagus nerve contains preganglionic, parasympathetic efferent fibers and afferent fibers from various lung receptors. The sympathetic fibers are largely postganglionic efferent in type, although in some animals there is physiologic evidence of an afferent component.[9] Small branches of the recurrent laryngeal nerve on the left side and the vagus on the right are distributed directly to the trachea, where they form several plexuses that are most prominent on the posterior wall.[10] After giving off these branches, fibers from the vagus and sympathetic chain enter the hila, join with branches from the cardiac autonomic plexus, and form large posterior and smaller anterior plexuses in the peribronchovascular connective tissue. From these plexuses emanate multiple individual peribronchial and perivascular nerve fibers.

The nerves in the proximal airways number about four to five and contain both thick and thin, myelinated and unmyelinated axons. They are associated with airway ganglia

in which the vagal preganglionic fibers synapse with postganglionic neurons (Fig. 5–2). In addition to acetylcholine, neurons of the airway ganglia contain neurotransmitter peptides such as vasoactive intestinal polypeptide (VIP), neuropeptide Y, galanin, and the enzyme nitric oxide synthase (NOS).[4] There is both anatomic[11] and physiologic[12] evidence for synapses between adrenergic sympathetic fibers and parasympathetic postganglionic neurons within the ganglia. Stimulation of the adrenergic system can modulate cholinergic airway tone. This interaction has clinical importance, as exemplified by the marked bronchoconstriction that can occur in some asthmatic subjects who are treated with adrenergic blocking drugs such as propranolol (an effect that can be blocked with a cholinergic antagonist such as atropine).[13, 14] At numerous points along their course, the airway nerves send out thick and thin fibers into the bronchial submucosa, where they run as bronchial nerves. From these fibers arise numerous thin, unmyelinated parasympathetic and sympathetic efferent fibers that terminate in bronchial muscle and mucous glands and around small blood vessels in the lamina propria and submucosa (Fig. 5–3).

Thicker fibers thought to be largely of an afferent sensory type bypass the ganglia. Some of these fibers from tachykinin-containing, capsaicin-sensitive afferents send side branches that synapse with ganglionic neurons.[15] (Tachykinins are low-molecular-weight neuropeptides that act as neurotransmitters and have additional actions as modulators of inflammation.) The afferent fibers originate from receptors within the airway epithelium, the tracheobronchial smooth muscle, the lamina propria of the airways, the perichondrial region of large airways, the pulmonary parenchyma, and the pulmonary and bronchial arteries and veins.[1, 16] Their endings contain a variety of neurotransmitter peptides, including substance P, neurokinin A, and calcitonin gene–related peptide.[17] These tachykinins can be released on stimulation of the nerve endings and have proinflammatory effects on local structures; they cause mucus hypersecretion, bronchial vasodilation, and increased microvascular permeability and can induce smooth muscle cell hyperplasia *in vitro*. In addition to tachykinin release from a stimulated nerve ending, there may be more diffuse release caused by retrograde activation of branches of the same afferent fiber that innervate adjacent structures; such an "axon reflex" is believed to be responsible for the wheal-and-flare response in the skin. Capsaicin, the active ingredient of hot peppers, excites some afferent nerves directly and, in large concentrations, can deplete neuropeptide stores and damage afferent nerve endings.[18] Tachykinins are metabolized locally by enzymes such as

---

*The parasympathetic nervous system consists of the autonomic nerves carried by the cranial and sacral autonomic outflow and their associated ganglion neurons, whereas the sympathetic nervous system is composed of the autonomic nerves carried by the thoracolumbar autonomic outflow and its associated ganglion neurons.[8]

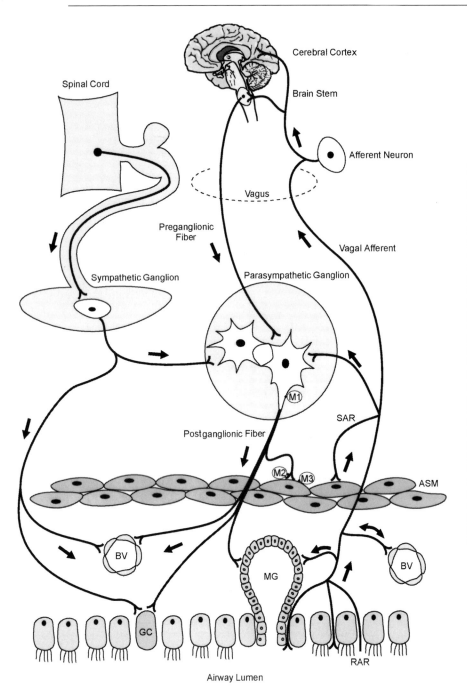

Figure 5–1. Innervation. Schematic diagram of the afferent and efferent innervation of the airways. Afferent nerves arise from rapidly adapting receptors (RAR), which originate as free nerve endings in the airway epithelium, and from slowly adapting receptors (SAR), which originate from nerve endings within the airway smooth muscle (ASM). Branches of the afferent nerves supply mucous glands (MG) and bronchial blood vessels (BV) and synapse with neurons within the parasympathetic airway ganglion. The afferent fibers ascend in the vagus to project to the autonomic ganglion in the brainstem, as well as to the cerebral cortex. Preganglionic efferent parasympathetic nerves descend in the vagus to synapse with postganglionic neurons in the parasympathetic ganglia. Postganglionic fibers supply airway smooth muscle, mucous glands, bronchial blood vessels, and goblet cells (GC) in the airway epithelium. M_1, M_2, and M_3 represent the three subtypes of muscarinic receptor. Acetylcholine (Ach) acts on M_3 receptors to stimulate ASM contraction, on M_2 receptors to decrease further Ach release from the nerve ending, and on M_1 receptors to facilitate transmission of preganglionic impulses through the ganglion. Sympathetic innervation originates as preganglionic fibers in the spinal cord. The preganglionic fibers synapse with postganglionic neuron fibers within the sympathetic ganglion, and the postganglionic fibers supply blood vessels and goblet cells.

angiotensin-converting enzyme and neutral endopeptidase.[19] Although the proinflammatory effects of tachykinins are well documented in rodents, the role of "neural inflammation" in human airway pathophysiology is unclear. In fact, there is indirect evidence that in humans tachykinins may play a protective role by decreasing the damage caused by various stimuli.[20]

Afferent receptors have been divided into three functional groups on the basis of their distribution and physiologic response to various stimuli. The *irritant* or *cough receptors* are located predominantly in the trachea and large bronchi, their number decreasing progressively as the smaller peripheral airways are approached.[21] They are highly arbo-

rized myelinated nerve fibers with numerous free nerve endings that terminate in the airway epithelium immediately below cell junctions. The fibers have also been termed *rapidly adapting stretch receptors* because they show a brief burst of activity with lung inflation or deflation. They also respond to a wide variety of chemical and mechanical stimuli, including inhaled pollutants, inflammatory mediators, and mechanical perturbations of the airway mucosa. Their stimulation results in reflex bronchoconstriction, and their role is probably to inhibit inhalation of toxic material.[9, 22] Other fibers, also presumably of an afferent sensory type, have been identified close to the basement membrane at all levels of the conducting and transitional airways,[23] some in

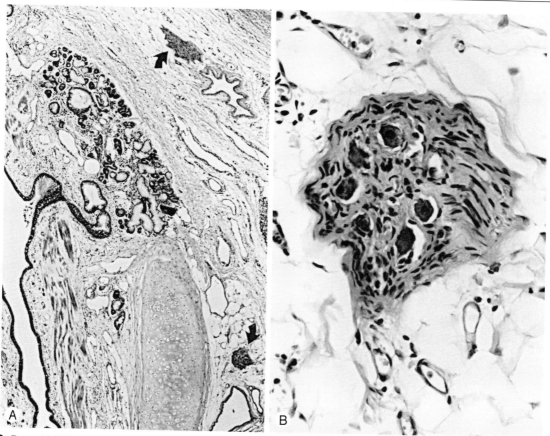

Figure 5–2. Bronchial Wall Nerves. *A,* The adventitia of the wall of a large bronchus contains two small nerves *(arrows),* one of which is associated with a ganglion (magnified in *B*).

relation to neuroepithelial bodies.[24] Their function and the precise course within the lung of fibers derived from them are not known.

The second major group of myelinated lung afferents traveling in the vagus nerve are from *stretch receptors*. Their nerve endings are found in airway smooth muscle, where they appear as tendril-like structures closely applied to the surface of individual muscle cells. They have also been called *slowly responding stretch receptors* since they show prolonged discharge in response to lung inflation. They are responsible for sending information to the respiratory center regarding lung volume; integration of their input results in off-switch activity in the respiratory center. Receptors that can sense changes in the curvature of bronchial cartilage plates are present in the perichondrium of the larger airways.[1]

The third type of lung afferent originates in the *J* (*juxtacapillary,* or *C*) *receptor.*[22, 25, 26] The nerve endings of these small, unmyelinated fibers are situated in lung parenchyma adjacent to alveolar septa and pulmonary capillaries and in the walls of the conducting airways. Although there is evidence from experimental animal studies that the former are sensitive to stretch of the alveolar capillaries and the adjacent interstitial space such as occurs with lung congestion or interstitial edema, the results of studies in humans have put their significance in this regard into question.[27] Pulmonary C fibers have been divided into *bronchial* and *pulmonary* types, based on their accessibility to chemical agents, such as capsaicin, injected into the bronchial or

pulmonary arteries.[28] Ultrastructurally, these fibers are associated with two types of nerve endings: one contains many mitochondria and has been hypothesized to have a sensory function; the other contains numerous neurosecretory-like granules and is situated close to Type II alveolar cells, thus suggesting a possible role in the control of surfactant secretion.[26] Nonmyelinated C fibers in the conducting airways appear to respond more to chemical stimuli than to stretch.[16]

As indicated, efferent innervation of the lung includes preganglionic fibers from vagal nuclei, which descend in the vagus to synapse with postganglionic neurons in the ganglia around the airways, and postganglionic fibers from the cervical sympathetic ganglia, which enter the lung at the hilum. Postganglionic cholinergic fibers supply the mucous glands of the large airways and the goblet cells, their stimulation causing an increase in secretion at both sites. Vagal efferent fibers also supply airway smooth muscle as well as pulmonary and bronchial vascular smooth muscle; stimulation of these cholinergic fibers causes airway smooth muscle contraction (resulting in airway narrowing) and vascular smooth muscle relaxation (leading to pulmonary and bronchial vascular dilation). All these effects are blocked by atropine. A wide variety of stimuli serve to modulate airway caliber via the cholinergic efferent pathway: increased airway smooth muscle tone and airway narrowing are stimulated by hypoxia, hypercapnia, and gastric irritation, as well as by chemical and mechanical irritation of the airway mucosa. Decreased efferent activity and airway dilation can occur

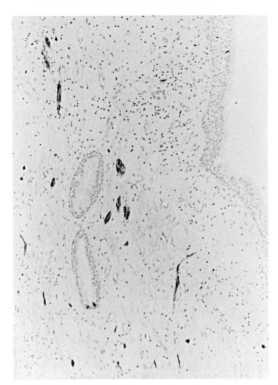

Figure 5–3. Bronchial Wall Nerves. A section of a segmental bronchus incubated with an antibody to protein S-100 shows several positively reacting nerves in the submucosa.

with lung hyperinflation, hypocapnia, stimulation of skeletal muscle and diaphragmatic afferents, and increased carotid sinus pressure.[4]

In addition to its direct stimulatory role in airway smooth muscle contraction, acetylcholine released from cholinergic nerves can act on a variety of receptors. At least three subtypes of muscarinic cholinergic receptors have been characterized pharmacologically:[29] (1) M_1 receptors are expressed on airway ganglion cells; when stimulated, they facilitate the transmission of preganglionic impulses through the ganglion to postganglionic fibers; (2) M_2 receptors are expressed on cholinergic nerve endings; their stimulation by acetylcholine causes a decrease in further acetylcholine release, thus serving a negative-feedback function; and (3) M_3 receptors mediate the contraction of airway smooth muscle, vasodilation, and mucus secretion.

Some (albeit not all[30, 31]) investigators have demonstrated the presence of small numbers of adrenergic nerve fibers in human lung.[32] Although these catecholamine-containing nerves have been demonstrated in human airway smooth muscle,[11] their major innervation appears to be pulmonary and bronchial vascular smooth muscle. Their stimulation causes vasoconstriction, which is mediated by α-adrenergic receptors.[33] Adrenergic nerves may also influence neural transmission via other nerves; for example, α_1-, α_2-, and β_2-adrenoreceptor agonists reduce cholinergic transmission through airway ganglia.[34] In addition to catecholamines, the nerve endings of the sympathetic system contain numerous neuropeptides, including substance P, calcitonin gene–related peptide, neuropeptide Y, and VIP.[35]

Specific receptors for neurotransmitters can also be present on lung cells in the absence of innervation of the

cells. An example can be seen with the endothelial response to acetylcholine, which causes release of the powerful vasodilator nitric oxide (NO) from pulmonary and bronchial vascular endothelial cells via atropine-inhibitable receptors, despite the fact that there is no direct cholinergic innervation of the endothelium.[35] Other circulating endogenous or exogenous catecholamines can also act on a variety of lung cells. For example, radioligand labeling and autoradiographic studies have shown that airway smooth muscle fibers possess numerous adrenergic (largely β_2) receptors,[36] whose density is greatest in the peripheral airways. β_2-receptors are also present on alveolar walls,[37, 38] particularly on Type II pneumocytes; stimulation of these receptors causes surfactant secretion, a reaction that may be particularly important at birth when lung expansion is required.[39, 40] Noninnervated adrenergic receptors located on airway smooth muscle respond to circulating catecholamine and are the reason that therapeutically administered parenteral or aerosols of β_2-adrenergic agonists are so effective in relaxing airway smooth muscle. The density of β_2-receptors on airway smooth muscle is much greater than that of α-receptors, which explains why noradrenaline, which normally stimulates both, has a predominant bronchodilating action.[38] Studies in which the density of cholinergic receptors in airway smooth muscle has been examined have shown that these receptors decrease in peripheral airways (in contrast to the increase in adrenergic receptors).

The third component of the autonomic nervous system, the so-called NAIS or NANC system, has been demonstrated relatively recently.[41, 42] Although both NANC excitatory (NANCe) and inhibitory (NANCi) systems have been demonstrated in rodents, the human lung does not seem to have an excitatory pathway.[19] Initial studies of NANCi innervation were carried out *in vitro* by using electrical field stimulation of isolated airway smooth muscle; subsequently, it has been shown to function *in vivo* in other animals and humans.[43–45] In the cat, the effectiveness of stimulation in terms of bronchial smooth muscle relaxation is equal to that of adrenergic stimulation; in the guinea pig, NANCi innervation is the major bronchodilator system.[46]

The most important neurotransmitter of NANCi neurons is NO.[47, 48] A specific neural form of NO synthetase (NOS) is present in nerves and converts L-arginine to NO and L-citrulline. Stimulation of the nerve causes release of NO, which acts on cyclic guanylyl cyclase within smooth muscle cells to produce relaxation. VIP, a small peptide contained in some vagal nerve endings, may also function as a NANCi neurotransmitter.[45, 49–51] There is evidence that NOS activity is less in nerves located in peripheral as compared with central airways, even though total nerve density is similar in both locations.[52]

Abnormalities of the NANCi system are best documented in the gastrointestinal system; for example, absence of the NANCi system in the colon is associated with Hirschsprung's disease, and a deficiency in the esophagus may be important in the pathogenesis of achalasia. By contrast, the importance of NANCi innervation in the lung and possible alterations in its function in disease are matters of some controversy. It has been suggested that a defect may be important in the production of nonspecific bronchial hyperreactivity, a characteristic feature of asthma and other airway diseases. However, the observation that it is relatively ineffective in producing airway smooth muscle relaxation in excised human bronchi in comparison with β-agonists argues against this hypothesis.[53]

The nerves to the pulmonary arteries run in the perivascular adventitia and interconnect extensively with the peribronchial nerves. They continue along the arterial tree at least as far as parenchymal arterioles. Two plexuses of cholinergic fibers have been identified in larger vessels, one situated in the outer adventitia and the other at the adventitial-medial junction; in smaller vessels only a single (inner) plexus is seen.[54] Some investigators have also described a series of thick fibers extending to the adventitial-medial junction of the larger arteries and ending in a series of tortuous branchings. Their structure and location have led to speculation that they are sensory in type and function as baroreceptors; support for this hypothesis has been provided by physiologic studies that have shown reflex pulmonary arterial vasoconstriction brought about by balloon distention of lobar pulmonary arteries.[55]

Although some nerve fibers in the large pulmonary veins end in the adventitia in a branching complex similar to that in the major pulmonary arteries and possibly possess a similar baroreceptor function, the majority extend into the inner media, where they form a complex subendothelial network. Because of this location, it has been suggested that they may function as chemoreceptors. Other nerves continue as a plexus within the interlobular septa around the venous radicles and eventually end in the deeper layers of the visceral pleura. The bronchial arteries contain a prominent nerve plexus at the medial-adventitial junction, presumably consisting of efferent supply to the smooth muscles of these vessels; this plexus also sends numerous branches to the bronchial mucous glands.

Collections of tissue resembling paraganglionic tissue of the carotid body have been described in association with both the extrapulmonary and intrapulmonary vasculature. One of these, the glomus pulmonale,[56] is situated in the adventitia of the main pulmonary artery adjacent to the aorta. Because of its location, the suggestion has been made that it may function as a receptor for pulmonary arterial oxygen or carbon dioxide. However, the vascular supply of the glomus pulmonale has been shown to originate in the left coronary artery, which makes it an unlikely candidate for this purpose.[57]

REFERENCES

1. Larsell O, Dow RS: The innervation of the human lung. Am J Anat 52:125, 1933.
2. Gaylor JB: The intrinsic nervous mechanism of the human lung. Brain 57:143, 1934.
3. Spencer H, Leof D: The innervation of the human lung. J Anat 98:599, 1964.
4. Canning BJ, Undem BJ: In Raeburn D, Giembycz MA (eds): Airways Smooth Muscle: Structure, Innervation and Neurotransmission. Basel, Birkhäuser-Verlag, 1994, pp 43–78.
5. Richardson J, Beland J: Nonadrenergic inhibitory nervous system in human airways. J Appl Physiol 41:764, 1976.
6. Richardson JB, Ferguson CC: Morphology of the airway. In Nadel JA (ed): Physiology and Pharmacology of the Airways. New York, Marcel Dekker, 1980, p 1.
7. Raeburn D, Giembycz MA (eds): Airways Smooth Muscle: Structure, Innervation and Neurotransmission. Basel, Birkhäuser-Verlag, 1994.
8. Langley JN: The Autonomic Nervous System. Cambridge, England, W Heffer & Sons, 1921.
9. Sant'Ambrogio G: Information arising from the tracheobronchial tree of mammals. Physiol Rev 62:531, 1982.
10. Fisher AWF: The intrinsic innervation of the trachea. J Anat 98:117, 1964.
11. Partanen M, Laitinen A, Hervonen A, et al: Catecholamine- and acetylcholinesterase-containing nerves in human lower respiratory tract. Histochemistry 76:175, 1982.
12. Danser AHJ, Ende RVD, Lorenz RR, et al: Prejunctional β_1-adrenoceptors inhibit cholinergic transmission in canine bronchi. J Appl Physiol 62:785, 1987.
13. Grieco MH, Pierson RN: Mechanism of bronchoconstriction due to beta-adrenergic blockade. J Allergy Clin Immunol 48:143, 1971.
14. Ind PW, Dixon CMS, Fuller RW, et al: Anticholinergic blockade of beta-blocker induced bronchoconstriction. Am Rev Respir Dis 139:1390, 1989.
15. Myers AC, Undem BJ: Electrophysiological effects of tachykinins and capsaicin on guinea pig bronchial parasympathetic ganglion neurones. J Physiol 47:665, 1993.
16. Sant'Ambrogio G: Nervous receptors of the tracheobronchial tree. Annu Rev Physiol 49:611, 1987.
17. Mitzner WA: Leonardo and the physiology of respiration. In Proctor DF (ed): A History of Breathing Physiology. New York, Marcel Dekker, 1995, pp 37–59.
18. Jancsó G, Kiraly E, Jancsó-Garbor A: Pharmacologically induced selective depletion of substance P from primary sensory neurons. Nature 270:741, 1977.
19. Karlsson J-A: Excitatory nonadrenergic, noncholinergic innervation of airway smooth muscle. In Raeburn D, Giembycz MA (eds): Airways Smooth Muscle: Structure, Innervation and Neurotransmission. Basel, Birkhäuser-Verlag, 1994, pp 104–142.
20. Paré PD, Sandford AJ, Bai TR: Pathophysiological processes in chronic obstructive pulmonary disease. In Barnes PJ, Buist AS (eds): The Role of Anticholinergics: COPD and Chronic Asthma. Macclesfield, UK, Gardiner-Caldwell Communications, 1997, pp 19–31.
21. Laitinen A: Ultrastructural organization of intraepithelial nerves in the human airway tract. Thorax 40:488, 1985.
22. Fillenz M, Widdicombe JG: Receptors of the lungs and airways. In Neil E (ed): Enteroceptors. New York, Springer-Verlag, 1972, p 81.
23. Laitinen A: Autonomic innervation of the human respiratory tract as revealed by histochemical and ultrastructural methods. Eur J Respir Dis 140(Suppl):1, 1985.
24. Lauweryns JM, Cokelaere M, Theunynck P: Neuro-epithelial bodies in the respiratory mucosa of various mammals. A light optical, histochemical and ultrastructural investigation. Z Zellforsch 135:569, 1972.
25. Fox B, Bull TB, Guz A: Innervation of alveolar walls in the human lung: An electron microscopic study. J Anat 131:6832, 1980.
26. Hung K-S, Hertweck MS, Hardy JD, et al: Electron microscopic observations of nerve endings in the alveolar walls of mouse lungs. Am Rev Respir Dis 108:328, 1973.
27. Taylor DR, Muir AL, Fleetham JA: Effect of rapid saline infusion on breathing pattern in normal man. Clin Invest Med 7:86, 1984.
28. Coleridge HM, Coleridge JCG: Impulse activity in afferent vagal C-fibres with endings in the intrapulmonary airways of dogs. Respir Physiol 29:125, 1977.
29. Barnes PJ: Modulation of neurotransmitter release from airway nerves. In Raeburn D, Giembycz MA (eds): Airways Smooth Muscle: Structure, Innervation and Neurotransmission. Basel, Birkhäuser-Verlag, 1994, pp 209–259.
30. Richardson JB: State of the art—nerve supply to the lungs. Am Rev Respir Dis 119:785, 1979.
31. Richardson JB: Recent progress in pulmonary innervation. Am Rev Respir Dis 128:65, 1983.
32. Laitinen A, Partanen M, Hervonen A, et al: Electron microscopic study on the innervation of the human lower respiratory tract: Evidence of adrenergic nerves. Eur J Respir Dis 67:209, 1985.
33. Widdicombe JG: Why are the airways so vascular? Thorax 48:290, 1993.
34. Grundström N, Andersson RGG: Inhibition of cholinergic neurotransmission in human airways via prejunctional β_2-adrenoceptors. Acta Physiol Scand 125:513, 1985.
35. Laitenen LA, Laitinen A: Neural elements in human airways. In Raeburn D, Giembycz MA (eds): Airways Smooth Muscle: Structure, Innervation and Neurotransmission. Basel, Birkhäuser-Verlag, 1994, pp 309–324.
36. Nadel JA, Barnes PJ: Automatic regulation of the airways. Annu Rev Med 35:451, 1984.
37. Mak JCW, Nishikawa M, Barnes PJ: Localization of β-adrenoceptor subtype mRNA's in human lung. Am J Respir Crit Care Med 149(Suppl):1027, 1994.
38. Barnes PJ: Localization and function of airway autonomic receptors. Eur J Respir Dis 65:187, 1984.
39. Barnes PJ: Beta-adrenergic receptors and their regulation. Am J Respir Crit Care Med 152:838, 1995.
40. Mak JCW, Shannon JM, Mason R, et al: Glucocorticoid-induced increase in β_2-adrenoceptor gene transcription in rat type II pneumocytes. Am Rev Respir Dis 147:274, 1993.
41. Richardson JB: Nonadrenergic inhibitory innervation of the lung. Lung 195:315, 1981.
42. Barnes PJ: The third nervous system in the lung: Physiology and clinical perspective. Thorax 39:561, 1984.
43. Chesrown SE, Venugopalan CS, Gold WM, et al: In vivo demonstration of nonadrenergic inhibitory innervation of the guinea pig trachea. J Clin Invest 65:314, 1980.
44. Irvin CG, Martin RR, Macklem PT: Nonpurinergic nature and efficacy of nonadrenergic bronchodilatation. J Appl Physiol 52:562, 1982.
45. Michoud MC, Jeanneret-Grosjean A, Cohen A, et al: Reflex decrease of histamine-induced bronchoconstriction after laryngeal stimulation in asthmatic patients. Am Rev Respir Dis 138:1548, 1988.
46. Souhrada JF, Kivity S: The effect of some factors on the inhibitory nervous systems of airway smooth muscle. Respir Physiol 48:297, 1982.
47. Belvisi MG, Stretton CD, Miura M, et al: Inhibitory NANC nerves in human tracheal smooth muscle: A quest for the neurotransmitter. J Appl Physiol 73:2505, 1992.
48. Belvisi MG, Bai TR: Inhibitory nonadrenergic, noncholinergic innervation of airway smooth muscle: Role of nitric oxide. In Raeburn D, Giembycz MA (eds): Airways Smooth Muscle: Structure, Innervation and Neurotransmission. Basel, Birkhäuser-Verlag, 1994, pp 158–187
49. Said SI: Vasoactive peptides in the lung, with special reference to vasoactive intestinal peptide. Exp Lung Res 3:343, 1982.
50. Sheppard MN, Polak JM, Allen JM: Neuropeptide tyrosine (NPY): A newly discovered peptide is present in the mammalian respiratory tract. Thorax 39:326, 1984.
51. Diamond L, Richardson JB: Inhibitory innervation to airway smooth muscle. Exp Lung Res 3:379, 1982.
52. Ward JK, Barnes PJ, Springall DR, et al: Distribution of human i-NANC bronchodilator and nitric oxide–immunoreactive nerves. Am J Respir Cell Mol Biol 13:175, 1995.
53. Taylor SM, Paré PD, Schelenberg RR: Cholinergic and non-adrenergic mechanisms in human and guinea pig airways. J Appl Physiol 56:958, 1984.
54. Amenta F, Cavallotti C, Ferrante F, et al: Cholinergic innervation of the human pulmonary circulation. Acta Anat 117:58, 1983.
55. Osorio J, Russak M: Reflex changes in the pulmonary and systemic pressures elicited by stimulation of baroreceptors in the pulmonary artery. Circ Res 10:664, 1962.
56. Krahl VE: The glomus pulmonale: A preliminary report. Bull School Med Univ MD 45:36, 1960.
57. Becker AE: The glomera in the region of the heart and great vessels: A microscopic-anatomical study. Pathol Eur 1:410, 1966.

CHAPTER 6

The Pleura

ANATOMY, 151
  The Visceral Pleura, 151
  The Parietal Pleura, 151
  The Mesothelial Cell, 151
  Fissures, 153
RADIOLOGY, 154
  Parietal Pleura and Visceral Pleura over the Lung
    Surface, 154
  Fissures, 154
    Normal Interlobar Fissures, 155
    Accessory Fissures, 160
  The Pulmonary Ligament, 165
PHYSIOLOGY, 168
  Pressures, 168
  Fluid Formation and Absorption, 168

ANATOMY

The pleural space is enclosed by the visceral pleura, which covers the lungs, and by the parietal pleura, which lines the chest wall, diaphragm, and mediastinum.[1] The two join at the hila. Although they may contact locally, the left and right parietal pleura are normally separate over most of their surface.[2] Extensions of visceral pleura into the underlying lung form fissures that divide the lung into lobes, which, depending on the fissure's depth, are more or less well developed. Although the left and right pleural spaces are usually separate, there is evidence that they may rarely form a single anatomic compartment.[3]

The Visceral Pleura

The visceral pleura can be considered to consist of three layers (Fig. 6–1). The *endopleura,* which is composed of a continuous layer of mesothelial cells overlying a delicate network of irregularly arranged collagen and elastic fibers, is the most superficial. The second layer (*external elastic lamina,* or *chief layer*) is primarily responsible for pleural mechanical stability and consists of a thin layer of dense collagen and elastic tissue. Whereas the latter is arranged in a more or less haphazard manner in the plane of the pleural surface, the collagen fibers are grouped into well-developed bundles whose orientation varies in different regions.[4] The thickness of the collagen and elastic tissue bundles also varies,[5] possibly as a result of differences in pleural stress during the respiratory cycle.[5, 6] Chemical analysis of the collagen in this layer has shown it to be predominantly Type I.[7]

The third layer (*vascular* or *interstitial*) of visceral pleura lies beneath the chief layer and consists of connective tissue containing lymphatic and blood vessels. It is continuous with the interstitial tissue of the interlobular septa and directly overlies the lobular-limiting membrane (internal elastic lamina). The latter is a thin, elastin-collagen layer that encases almost the entire lung parenchyma and separates alveoli from the pleura, interlobular septa, and bronchovascular bundles. Although delicate collagen bundles connect the pleural chief layer and the limiting membrane, the two are relatively loosely attached and may be readily separated in the connective tissue plane of the vascular layer; thus, in appropriate circumstances, liquid or gas readily accumulates in this region.

The origin of the blood supply of the visceral pleura is contentious. According to some observers,[8] the hilar, apical, mediastinal, and interlobar regions are supplied by vessels derived from the bronchial circulation, the remainder being nourished by the pulmonary arteries; however, others believe that the blood supply of the costal and diaphragmatic portions is also bronchial in origin.[9] With the exception of the hilar regions (which are drained by the bronchial veins), the venous return from the visceral pleural is via the pulmonary veins.[10] Innervation is by branches of the vagus nerve and sympathetic trunks.[1] Lymphatic drainage is described in Chapter 7 (*see* page 172).

The Parietal Pleura

The parietal pleura consists of a layer of connective tissue adjacent to the endothoracic fascia of the chest wall (Fig. 6–2). It is divided into two parts by a layer of fibroelastic tissue, with most of the vessels being located in the part farthest from the pleura. The blood supply is derived from the subclavian, internal mammary, and intercostal arteries.[8] Innervation is by the intercostal nerves.[1]

The Mesothelial Cell

Mesothelial cells form a continuous layer over the whole of the visceral and parietal pleural surfaces. They are normally inconspicuous on light microscopic examination, each cell measuring 15 to 40 μm in diameter and only about 5 to 7 μm in thickness.[2] Their diameter varies with transpulmonary pressure, the cells becoming more flattened as the lung expands.[2] Regional differences in cell shape at

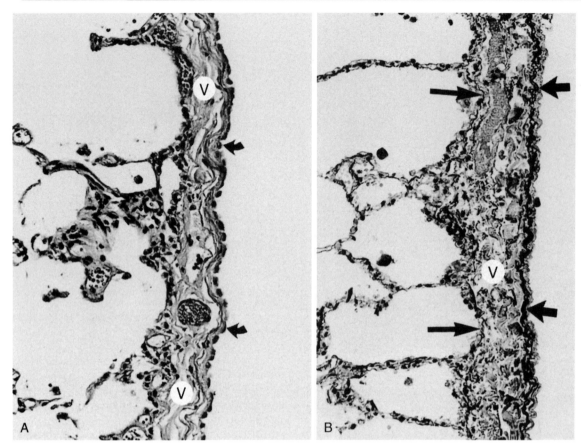

Figure 6–1. Normal Visceral Pleura. *A,* Mesothelial cells *(curved arrows),* vascular layer (V). *B,* Vascular layer (V), internal elastic lamina *(long arrows),* and external elastic lamina *(short arrows).* (*A,* H&E; *B,* Verhoeff–van Gieson; both ×200.)

the same transpulmonary pressure are also apparent, at least in some animals (Fig. 6–3).[11] Mesothelial cells show reactive changes in a variety of conditions, occasionally to a degree that makes cytologic or histologic differentiation from a malignant neoplasm difficult. When stimulated, individual cells enlarge, become cuboidal in shape, and develop large nuclei with prominent nucleoli. Mucous-secreting cells are rarely seen on the pleural surface in patients with cystic fibrosis or with pleural effusion of uncertain etiology; in the latter circumstance, it has been suggested that they may represent metaplastic mesothelial cells.[12]

Ultrastructurally, mesothelial cells are joined to each other by tight junctions and, occasionally, by desmosomes.[2] Within the cytoplasm are moderately abundant mitochondria, microtubules, endoplasmic reticulum, and an occasional Golgi apparatus. A thin basement membrane is usually present, and pinocytotic vesicles are visible on both luminal and basal aspects. Characteristically, the cell surface is covered by microvilli whose number ranges from only a few to more than 600 (Figs. 6–3 and 6–4).[2] These tend to be more numerous on the visceral than on the parietal pleura and are typically long and thin, measuring only about 0.1 μm in diameter and up to 3 μm in length. Fine strands approximately 150 nm in diameter emanate from the surface glycocalyx and extend between the microvilli; it has been suggested that fluid trapped in compartments formed by these strands and by the microvilli themselves protects the mesothelial cells from the trauma of normal pleural movement.[13]

Mesothelial cells are metabolically active and appear to

have several functions. Presumably by means of their microvilli and pinocytotic vesicles, they are responsible, at least in part, for regulating the composition and amount of pleural fluid. However, it is not certain to what extent they actively synthesize substances found in the fluid or simply transport them from underlying connective tissue cells or blood.[2] There is evidence that the cells also have the ability to produce components of the submesothelial connective tissue itself.[14] Mesothelial cells have also been shown to produce prostaglandins[2] and to possess both fibrinolytic[15] and procoagulant[16] activity, features that may be important in repair and in decreasing the development of fibrous adhesions following pleural injury. Surface-active phospholipids similar to alveolar surfactant have been found in the pleural space, where they act as lubricants to facilitate pleural surface movement;[17] although the origin of these substances has not been identified, it seems likely that the mesothelial cell is responsible.[18]

Although the mechanism of repair of damaged mesothelium is controversial, the results of some investigations suggest that it occurs by hyperplasia and migration of mesothelial cells both from the periphery of an area of injury and across fibrin bridges from the opposite pleural surface.[19, 20] Subsequent mesothelial proliferation at the site of injury may be modulated, at least in part, by thrombin[21] and by a macrophage-secreted mitogen.[22] It has also been proposed that submesothelial mesenchymal cells can proliferate and differentiate into mesothelial cells as part of the reparative process.[23] Mesothelial cells themselves can produce a che-

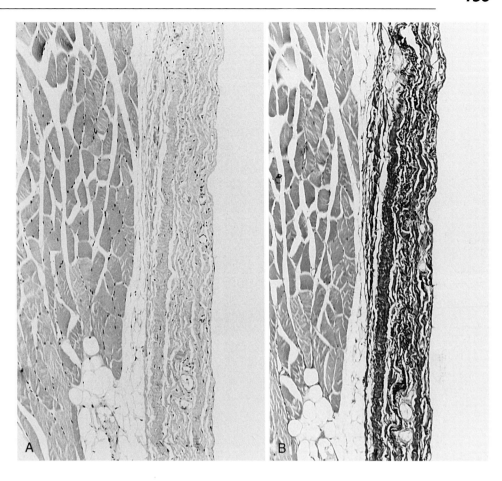

Figure 6–2. Normal Parietal Pleura. Section of pleura overlying the diaphragmatic muscle shows dense collagen *(A)* and numerous elastic fibers *(B)*.

moattractant for fibroblasts and thus may play a role in the regulation of postinjury fibrosis.[24] The origin of the collagen in this situation is probably the mesenchymal cells of the vascular layer.[25]

Fissures

Fissures are clefts that extend from the outer surface of the lung into its substance. They are lined on either side by a layer of pleura that is continuous with the visceral pleura over the convexity of the lung or its mediastinal or diaphragmatic surface. A fissure may extend no more than 1 to 2 cm into the underlying lung or all the way to the hilum, in which case there is complete lobar or segmental isolation. This variability in fissure depth is important: the less complete a fissure, the larger the bridge of lung parenchyma connecting two contiguous lobes or segments. Such parenchymal bridges provide a pathway for collateral air flow or for the spread of disease from one region of lung to another, creating radiographic signs that may give rise to erroneous conclusions (*see* farther on).

Fissures are traditionally considered in two groups: those that separate the lungs into the three right-sided and two left-sided lobes ("normal" fissures) and those that occur within one of the lobes themselves ("accessory" fissures). The normal fissures are the *minor (horizontal) fissure* (located between the right middle and upper lobes), the *right major (oblique) fissure* (between the combined right upper and middle lobes and the right lower lobe), and the *left*

major (oblique) fissure (between the left upper and lower lobes). The most common accessory fissures are the azygous, inferior, and superior (*see* page 160).

As indicated previously, the completeness of fissures is quite variable. In one study of 100 fixed and inflated lung specimens (50 right and 50 left), an incomplete fissure (lobar fusion) was found between the right lower and upper lobes in 70% of cases (Fig. 6–5) and between the right lower and middle lobes in 47%;[26] fusion between the lower and upper lobes was commonly more extensive than between the lower and middle lobes. In the left lung, fusion between the lower and upper lobes was somewhat less frequent than on the right: 40% of cases showed an incomplete fissure between the left lower lobe and the superior part of the upper lobe, and 46% showed an incomplete fissure between the lower lobe and the lingula.

Incompleteness of the minor fissure was far more common than in any portion of either major fissure: of the 50 right lungs examined, extensive fusion was present in 88% of cases, especially medially; thus, fusion is more common and usually more extensive between the middle and upper lobe (across the minor fissure) than between the middle and lower lobe (across the major fissure).

In another investigation of 270 fixed and inflated lungs (140 right and 130 left), a complete right major fissure was seen in 30% of lungs; in an additional 30%, the degree of fusion was minimal.[27] In about 20% of lungs, fusion was present over more than half the surface between the two lobes. Very little fusion was seen between the upper and lower lobes in the central portion of the right lung, most of

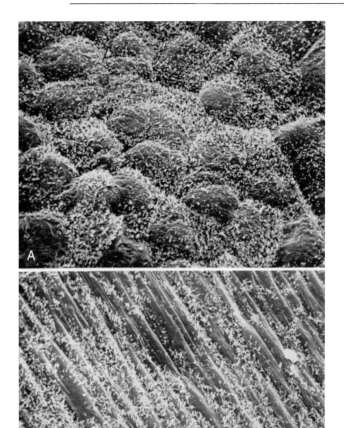

Figure 6–3. Mesothelial Cells. *A,* Note the bumpy appearance, usually indicative of loose and fatty subpleural connective tissue. (Rabbit mediastinal parietal pleura; SEM, ×1950.) *B,* A flattened appearance, implying a more rigid substructure. Note the numerous microvilli in both illustrations. (Rabbit intercostal parietal pleura; SEM, ×1650.) (Courtesy of Dr. Nai-San Wang, McGill University, Montreal.)

it occurring superomedially. On the left, approximately 25% showed complete fissures, the remainder showing fusion that ranged from very minor to almost complete. In this study, 20% of 140 right lungs possessed a complete interlobar fissure between the middle and upper lobes, whereas in approximately 1% there was no fissure; in about 75% of the cases, fusion ranged from slight to that occupying two thirds of the surface area between the two lobes. In all instances of incompleteness, the fusion extended to and involved the perihilar parenchyma.

RADIOLOGY

Parietal Pleura and Visceral Pleura over the Lung Surface

Radiography. Since the combined thickness of the parietal and visceral pleural layers is approximately 0.2 mm, the pleura over the convexity of the lungs and over the

diaphragmatic and mediastinal surfaces is not visible on the chest radiograph in the normal subject. Even when uniformly thickened, the diaphragmatic and mediastinal pleura is not visible on the radiograph, its water density precluding distinction from contiguous diaphragm and mediastinum. By contrast, local thickening, such as occurs with asbestos-related plaques, can be identified because of the alteration it produces in the normally smooth contour of the diaphragm. Over the convexity of the lungs, even slight thickening (1 to 2 mm) can be appreciated because of the greater density of contiguous ribs.

Computed Tomography. As with radiography, the pleura over the convexity of the lungs, diaphragm, and paravertebral regions cannot be distinguished from adjacent structures on conventional CT.[28] Based on a study of a cadaver and 25 normal subjects, the appearance of the costal and paravertebral pleura on high-resolution CT (HRCT) scan has been described in detail.[28] With this technique, a 1- to 2-mm-thick line of soft tissue attenuation is normally seen between the lung and chest wall between the inner edges of the ribs in the intercostal spaces. This line represents the combined thickness of the visceral pleura, normal pleural fluid, parietal pleura, endothoracic fascia, and innermost intercostal muscle (Fig. 6–6).[28] The pleura and endothoracic fascia along the inner aspects of the ribs are normally too thin to be visible on CT scan;[28] however, they may be identified as a thin, smooth line when there is increased extrapleural fat. The latter is most abundant over the posterolateral aspects of the fourth to eighth ribs, where it can be several millimeters thick in normal subjects.[29, 30] The pleura and endothoracic fascia can also be seen when a portion of rib is nearly horizontal, in which case the CT section may include only a portion of the upper and lower rib margins. The rib then appears thinner than normal, with a line representing the pleura and endothoracic fascia internal to it.

The transverse thoracic muscle is usually visible on HRCT as it extends from the end of a rib or its costal cartilage to the lower sternum or xyphoid. This muscle is seen as a 1- to 2-mm-thick line inside the most medial aspect of the ribs (Fig. 6–7). At the same level posteriorly, a thin line internal to the ribs is seen in approximately 15% of normal subjects and represents the combination of subcostalis muscle, endothoracic fascia, and pleura.[28] In the paravertebral region, a 1- to 2-mm-thick line representing pleura, endothoracic fascia, and innermost intercostal muscle is also normally seen on HRCT (*see* Fig. 6–6).[28] Occasionally, it can be identified on conventional 10-mm collimation scans. At one or more levels, the paravertebral portions of the intercostal veins may be visible on both HRCT and conventional CT scans, causing apparent thickening of the pleural line (Fig. 6–8). On both techniques, intercostal veins can be identified as such when they are seen to join the azygos and hemiazygos vein.

Fissures

In the interlobar regions, contiguous layers of visceral pleura are visible on the radiograph because of the presence of air-containing lung on both sides. Interlobar fissures become visible when the x-ray beam passes tangentially along

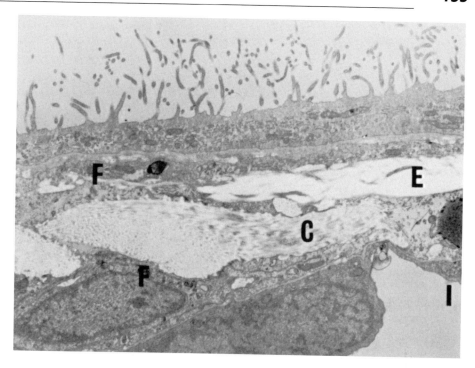

Figure 6–4. Ultrastructure of Mesothelial Cells. Rabbit visceral pleura, showing fibroblasts (F), elastic (E) and collagen (C) fibers, type I pneumocyte (I), and surface mesothelial cell with numerous elongated microvilli. (×12,600.) (From Wang N-S: Am Rev Respir Dis 110:623, 1974.)

their surfaces; their recognition is useful in the assessment of disease of the pulmonary lobes that form them.[31]

Normal Interlobar Fissures

Radiography. As indicated previously, *the major (oblique) fissures* separate the upper (and on the right, the middle lobe) from the lower lobes. They begin at or about the level of the fifth thoracic vertebra and extend obliquely downward and forward, roughly paralleling the sixth rib, ending at the diaphragm a few centimeters behind the anterior pleural gutter (Fig. 6–9). The top of the left lower lobe is usually higher than that of the right, the right major fissure being at the same level as the left in only about 25% of cases.[27] The proportion of upper and lower lobes that contacts the posterior chest wall is 1:4 and 1:5 for the right and left lungs, respectively.

Some variation exists in the orientation of the right and left major fissures. In one study, the anterior surface of the right lower lobe was seen to be divided into upper and lower parts by an interfissural "crest" that separated the area of contact with the upper lobe from the area of contact with the middle lobe.[26] The upper part of this surface almost always faced slightly laterally (Fig. 6–9) and was usually concave; the lower part also faced somewhat laterally (in more than 80% of cases) but was convex rather than concave. The orientation of the left major fissure was somewhat different: whereas the upper part of the fissural surface almost always faced laterally and was usually concave (as on the right), the lower part usually faced medially (although its surface was generally convex). Thus, the lateral orientation of the upper half of the fissure and the medial orientation of the lower half created a twisted appearance similar to that of a propeller, a feature that was not observed on the right side.

In a second study based on 100 consecutive CT scans, the upper part of each major fissure was also shown to be oriented with its lateral aspect posterior to its medial aspect (lateral facing).[32] However, in the lower part of the thorax the lateral aspect of both the right and left major fissures was found to be anterior to the medial aspect (medial facing)

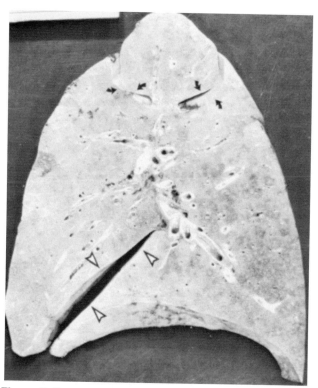

Figure 6–5. Incomplete Pleural Fissures. A sagittal section of an inflated postmortem right lung specimen demonstrates the lower portion of the major fissure *(arrowheads)* to be complete. However, note the complete absence of the upper portion of the major fissure and the whole minor fissure at this level. An azygos lobe fissure *(arrows)* is present at the top of the lung.

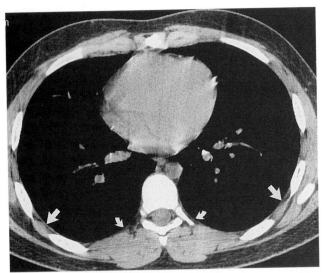

Figure 6–6. Normal Appearance of the Costal Pleura on HRCT Scan. In the intercostal spaces a 1- to 2-mm-thick line is seen *(straight arrows)*. This line represents the combined thickness of the visceral pleura, normal pleural fluid, parietal pleura, endothoracic fascia, and innermost intercostal muscle. The combined thickness of normal visceral and parietal pleura and of endothoracic fascia is too thin to be identified on CT scan over the inner aspect of the ribs, but it can be normally seen in the paravertebral regions as a line measuring 1 mm or less in thickness *(curved arrows).*

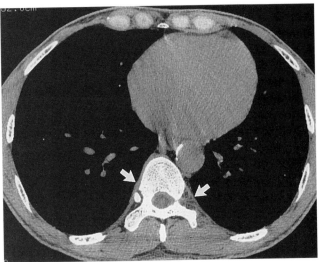

Figure 6–8. Normal Appearance of the Intercostal Veins on HRCT Scan. The intercostal veins are frequently visualized in the paravertebral regions *(arrows)*. They may measure 1 to 3 mm in thickness and can be readily identified when they are seen to join the azygos or hemiazygos vein.

(see Fig. 6–9); at the level of the carina, the lateral and medial aspects of the fissure were in the coronal plane.

The superolateral portion of the major fissures was studied on conventional posteroanterior (PA) chest radiographs of 1,068 normal subjects ranging in age from 18 to 70 years.[33] In about 15% of cases, a shadow was identified in the upper hemithorax that appeared as either a curvilinear opacity or a curving edge; the latter configuration, observed

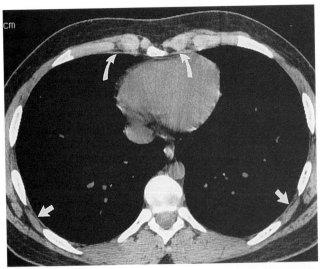

Figure 6–7. Normal Appearance of the Transverse Thoracic Muscle on HRCT Scan. At the level of the lower sternum a 1- to 2-mm-thick line can be seen inside the most medial aspect of the ribs and costal cartilages *(curved arrows)*. This represents the transverse thoracic muscle. Posterolaterally, the thin line seen extending between the inner edges of the ribs *(straight arrows)* represents the combined thickness of visceral pleura, parietal pleura, endothoracic fascia, and innermost intercostal muscle.

in most of the cases, consisted of a ground-glass opacity laterally and a radiolucency medially (Fig. 6–10); a curving line was seen in only a small percentage of cases. These two appearances, whether on the right or left, could be seen close to the lateral chest wall in proximity to the sixth posterior rib. The contours were seen on the right side alone in 4%, on the left alone in 6%, and bilaterally in 4%. When bilateral, the left contour almost always extended slightly higher than the right, occasionally reaching the fourth rib posteriorly. Based on correlative postmortem and CT studies, the curving line appearance was shown to result from orientation of the superolateral portion of the major fissure tangential to the x-ray beam, whereas the curving edge configuration was attributed to extrapleural fat intruding into the major fissure superolaterally (Fig. 6–10).[33]

Not infrequently, a triangular opacity is present at the lower end of the major fissures, its base contiguous with the diaphragm and its apex tapering cephalad into the fissure (Fig. 6–11). This opacity was identified in 39 of 212 CT scans in one study and has been shown to be composed entirely of fat.[34]

The *minor (horizontal) fissure* separates the anterior segment of the right upper lobe from the middle lobe and lies in a roughly horizontal plane at about the level of the fourth rib anteriorly. Its orientation shows considerable variation, the anterior aspect generally being lower than the posterior and the lateral part lower than the medial.[26]

As might be expected, the completeness of identification of the pleural fissures on conventional radiographs is highly variable, considering the normal variation in anatomic development and the observation that the major fissures are curved and are almost always oriented slightly away from the coronal plane. As a result, the major fissures are seldom seen along their entirety on lateral chest radiographs. This variable orientation of the fissural plane implies that the x-ray beam on a lateral chest radiograph is most apt to be tangent to the anterolateral aspect of the major fissures in the lower thorax and the middle or posterolateral surface in

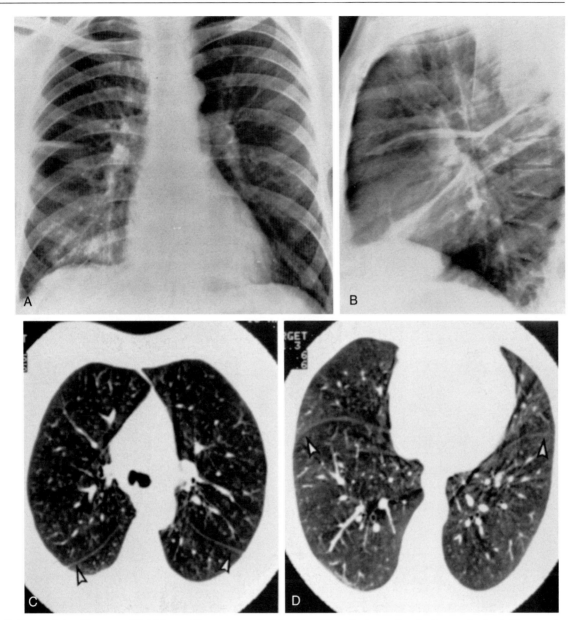

Figure 6–9. Interlobar Fissures, Right Lung. The presence of minimal interlobar effusion renders the fissures clearly visible on posteroanterior *(A)* and lateral *(B)* radiographs. *C,* A CT scan through the upper thorax reveals the lateral portion of the right and left major fissures *(arrowheads)* to be situated posterior to the anteromedial portion of the fissure, so-called lateral facing. *D,* A CT scan through the lower thorax shows that the lateral portion of the major fissures *(arrowheads)* is located anterior to the anteromedial aspect of the major fissures, so-called medial facing.

the upper thorax. Thus, in one study of 300 normal lateral radiographs, a major fissure was identified along its entire length in only 2% of cases, although part of one or both major fissures could be seen in the other 98%.[35]

Similar restrictions apply to visualization of the minor fissure. For example, in the study cited earlier, its entirety was identified in only 6% of the 300 radiographs;[35] part of the fissure was seen in only 44%. Other investigators have identified the fissure in 56% to more than 80% of normal subjects.[36–38] Anatomically, the minor fissure rarely reaches the mediastinum and then only in its anterior portion; despite this, one of the more constant relationships noted on PA radiographs is the fissure's medial termination (or projected termination) at the lateral margin of the interlobar pulmonary artery.[36] A fissure line or interface that projects medial to

this point is almost invariably a downward displaced major fissure, providing strong evidence of volume loss in the right lower lobe.

On a lateral chest radiograph, the posterior extent of the minor fissure is sometimes projected behind the hilum and right major fissure (Fig. 6–12). The probable explanation for this seeming paradox relates to the undulating course of the major and minor fissures, so that in lateral projection the x-ray beam images different areas of each. For instance, the lateral segment of the middle lobe, covered by the posterolateral aspect of the minor fissure, normally resides behind a coronal plane through the hila; it is this particular contour of the minor fissure that can be identified in some patients (Fig. 6–12). If the medial portion of the major fissure is simultaneously displayed, the anatomic conditions

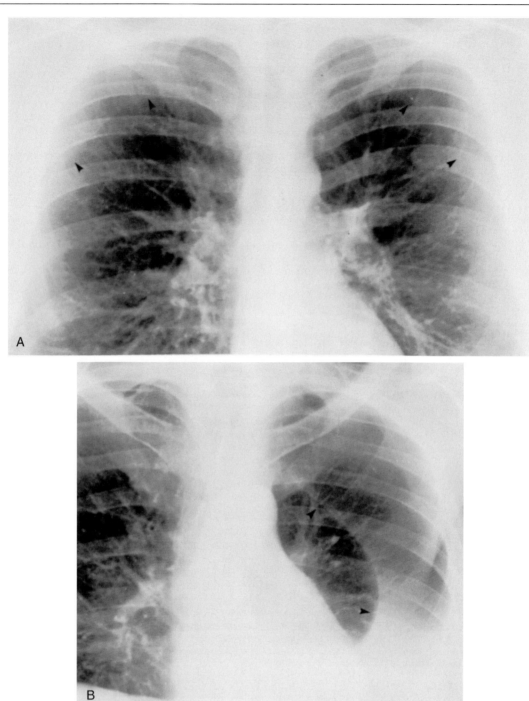

Figure 6–10. Superolateral Major Fissures. *A,* A detail view of a conventional posteroanterior chest radiograph in a normal, young adult man. A curvilinear edge *(arrowheads)* with a ground-glass opacity laterally can be identified bilaterally, representing the superolateral aspect of the major fissures. The left fissure is slightly higher than the right. *B,* A view of the left lung from a conventional posteroanterior chest radiograph in a patient with pleural effusion shows the superolateral aspect of the left major fissure *(arrowheads)* to be accentuated by the interlobar effusion.

that explain the apparent discrepancy just described are more readily understood.

Conventional CT. Using current technology, interlobar fissures can be identified in 100% of cases by conventional CT.[39] Three manifestations of the major fissures may be seen, in decreasing order of frequency: lucent bands, lines, and dense bands. The variable appearance of these fissures is related to the section thickness (collimation) and the plane of the fissure on the cross-sectional image. Thus, a

perpendicular fissure (such as in the upper thorax) is likely to produce a linear configuration, whereas a more oblique orientation causes a well-defined, dense (ground-glass) band. If the upper part of the major fissure is not quite perpendicular to the cross-sectional image, the relative paucity of pulmonary vessels at the periphery of the lobes on both sides of the fissure tends to cause the fissure to be displayed as a relatively avascular lucent band. In one study of 100 consecutive scans, depending on the level of the scan (upper,

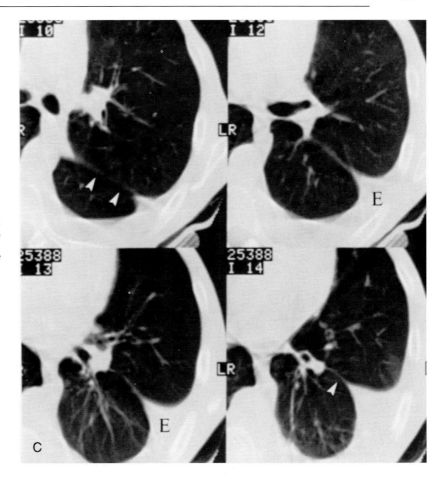

Figure 6–10 *Continued.* In this patient, CT scans *(C)* show a small part of the effusion (E) intruding into the lateral aspect of the fissure *(arrowheads),* accounting for the enhanced visibility. (The appearance in *B* does *not* represent an incomplete fissure.)

middle, or lower thorax), the lucent band form was seen in 60% to 73% of cases on the right and 58% to 74% on the left.[32] The linear manifestation was identified at the three levels in 1% to 10% on the right and 1% to 20% on the left. Dense bands were the least common, being identified in up to 4% on the right and up to 6% on the left.

Since the minor fissure and the plane of the CT scan are more or less tangential to one another, the fissure is typically manifested as a lucent area relatively devoid of vessels when compared with the same region in the left lung. In one study of 100 consecutive patients who underwent 10-mm collimation CT scans, this appearance was identified in 52 patients.[32] In 44% of cases, the region was triangular, with its apex at the hilum; in 8%, it was round or oval, a shape considered to be caused by the domelike configuration of the fissure. The lucent area is generally seen on only one or two scans, usually at the level of the intermediate bronchus. We have occasionally identified the minor fissure as an area of ground-glass attenuation, presumably as a result of fortuitous sectioning through the precise plane of the fissure.

A focal area of vascular deficiency distinct from the lucency described above can also be seen in the region of the minor fissure. In one review of the CT scans of 50 patients, this was identified in the midlung on the right in 46 (92%) and on the left in three (6%). The difference between the right and left lungs was attributed to the arrangement of arteries. On the right, the truncus anterior branch of the pulmonary artery enters the hilum and courses cephalad to supply the right upper lobe; the interlobar artery gives

rise to the middle lobe branch at the level of the minor fissure and then continues caudally to supply the lower lobe. Consequently, the region lateral to the bronchus intermedius is normally devoid of major vessels and hence is perceived as an area of diminished vascularity. By contrast, the pattern of division of the left pulmonary artery displays a more even spatial distribution of major pulmonary vessels within the upper lobe (including the lingula).[40]

HRCT. On HRCT scan, the major fissure can be seen as a single line (Fig. 6–13), two parallel lines, or, less commonly, a band of increased attenuation. The parallel arrangement is the result of motion artefact and occurs because the fissure is thin and relatively long. As a result, significant x-ray attenuation occurs only when the fissure is tangential to the x-ray beam.[41] Motion that occurs between times that the x-ray beam is not tangential is not seen; therefore, rather than blurring or spray artefact resulting from motion (such as is seen with conventional CT), the fissure is seen as two parallel lines. Because this artefact is most commonly the result of cardiac motion, it is seen most frequently between the lingula and the lower lobe.

Visualization of the interlobar fissure as a line allows identification of incomplete fissures (Fig. 6–13); in one study, this was found in 64% of cases on the right side and 52% on the left.[39] In these regions, bronchi and vessels can sometimes be seen to cross between the two fused lobes.[42] In one prospective study of 154 patients assessed with HRCT, incomplete interlobar fissures were seen in 128 (83%) of 154 right lungs and 77 (50%) of 154 left lungs.[42] A pulmo-

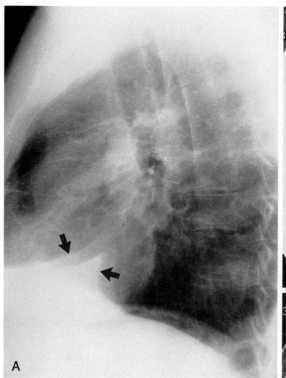

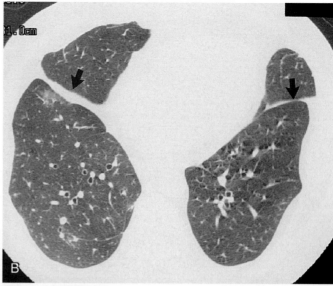

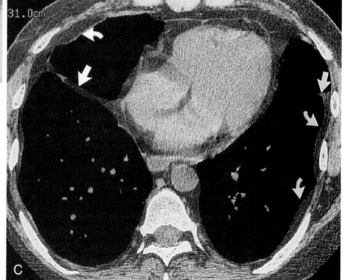

Figure 6–11. Fat in the Major Fissure. *A,* A lateral chest radiograph demonstrates triangular opacities at the lower end of the major fissures *(arrows)*. *B,* HRCT scan of the chest immediately above the level of the diaphragm confirms the presence of thickening of the interlobar fissures *(arrows),* shown in *C* to be caused by fat *(straight arrows)*. Also note the marked accumulation of extrapleural fat *(curved arrows)*.

nary vein was seen crossing the two fused lobes in 87 right lungs (56%) and 20 left lungs (13%) (Fig. 6–14). A pulmonary artery was seen extending across fused lobes in 7 right lungs and 13 left lungs and a bronchus in 3 right lungs. Bronchi and vessels were most commonly seen extending between upper and lower lobes and less commonly between the middle lobe or lingula and lower lobes. No bronchi or vessels were seen extending across incomplete minor fissures.

The minor fissure is usually visualized on HRCT as a curvilinear line or band of increased attenuation that forms a quarter- or semi-circle in its highest aspect (located slightly cephalad to the level of the origin of the middle lobe bronchus).[43] The apparent thickness ranges from 1 to 15 mm and decreases with the steepness of the fissure with respect to the transverse plane of section (Fig. 6–15).[43]

In one study of 40 consecutive patients who underwent HRCT, the minor fissure was not seen in eight (20%).[43] Of the 32 cases in which it was seen, it was incomplete in 23 (72%). In all cases, the upper surface of the middle lobe was convex superiorly. The minor fissure was higher medially than laterally in 84% of cases and its posterior margin was higher than the anterior margin in 81%. As should be expected from the previous discussion of anatomy, it is the medial component that is not identified when the minor fissure is incomplete.[43, 44]

Accessory Fissures

Any segment of lung may be partly or completely separated from adjacent segments by an accessory pleural fissure. The anatomic incidence of such fissures is much higher than is generally appreciated, amounting to about 50% of lungs.[41] Radiologically, they can be identified in approximately 10% of chest radiographs and 20% of conventional CT scans.[45] These fissures vary in their degree of development, from superficial slits in the lung surface not more than 1 or 2 cm deep to complete fissures that extend all the way to the hilum.

Most accessory fissures are of little more than academic

Figure 6–12. Position of the Minor Fissure Relative to the Hilum in Lateral Projection. *A,* A conventional lateral chest radiograph discloses a horizontal curvilinear stripe *(arrowheads)* representing a thickened minor fissure. Note that in this patient the fissure extends well behind the right hilum, overlapping the disc space at T6–7. *B* and *C,* CT scans at the level of the intermediate bronchus reveal an oval lucency representing the dome of the minor fissure (RMF). The fissure is slightly thickened due to pleural effusion *(arrowheads).* Scans show that the component of the minor fissure that is seen behind the hilum relates to the posterolateral aspect of the middle lobe. A small portion of the right major fissure *(arrows)* is shown. If the medial portion of the major fissure and the lateral component of the minor fissure are arranged so that both are tangential to the x-ray beam, the posterior portion of the minor fissure will be depicted behind the medial aspect of the major fissure.

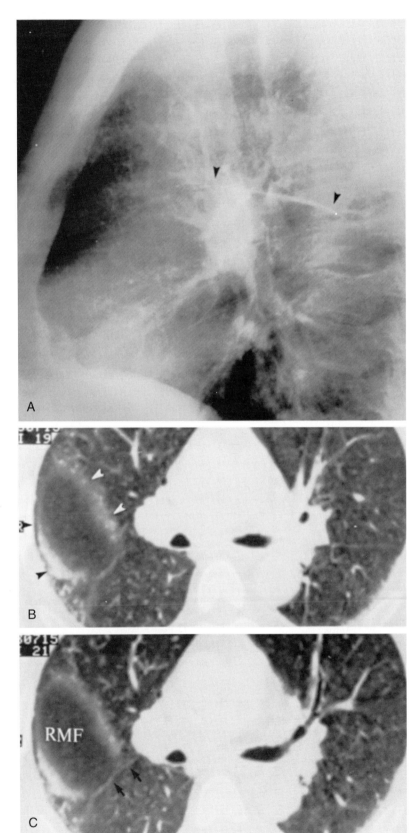

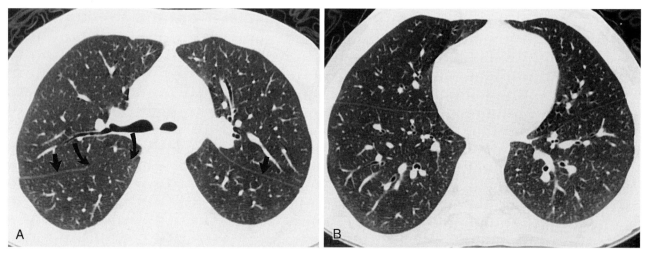

Figure 6–13. Normal Appearance of the Major Fissures on HRCT Scan. *A,* On HRCT, the major fissure is usually seen as a well-defined thin line *(straight arrows).* Note that the medial portion of the upper aspect of the right interlobar fissure is incomplete, resulting in fusion of the lower and upper lobes at this level *(curved arrows). B,* The lower aspect of both interlobar fissures is complete.

interest. However, their presence is sometimes important for three reasons: (1) the segment they subtend may be the only site of disease whose spread is prevented by the fissure; (2) identification of a fissure in a specific anatomic location can create confusion in interpretation (e.g., a fissure between the superior and basal segments of the right lower lobe can be mistaken for the minor fissure between the upper and middle lobes); and (3) the fissures are important components of linear atelectasis *(see* page 554).

Azygos Fissure. The best known of the accessory fissures is the azygos fissure (the mesoazygos), which is created by downward invagination of the azygos vein through the apical portion of the right upper lobe (Fig. 6–16). It is manifested radiographically by a curvilinear shadow that extends

obliquely across the upper portion of the right lung and terminates at a variable distance above the right hilum in a "teardrop" shadow caused by the azygos vein itself. Since the vein runs outside the parietal pleura, the fissure is formed by four pleural layers (two parietal and two visceral). The fissure is visible in about 0.5% of chest radiographs.[31] A 2:1 male preponderance was reported in one study of 100 consecutive cases,[46] and a familial incidence has been described.[47]

In one CT study of 11 patients with an azygos lobe, considerable alteration was observed in the contour of the right side of the mediastinum and in the relation of the lung to the superior vena cava and trachea.[48] In the presence of an azygos lobe, the azygos arch occupies a more cephalad

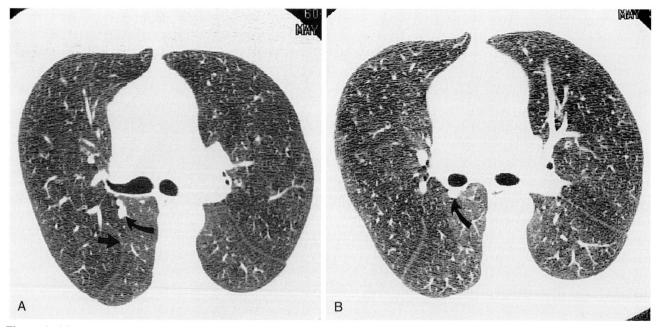

Figure 6–14. Pulmonary Vein Crossing an Interlobar Fissure. *A,* An HRCT scan demonstrates incomplete upper medial aspect of the right major fissure *(straight arrow).* An upper lobe pulmonary vein *(curved arrow)* can be seen crossing the fissure. *B,* At a slightly lower level, the upper lobe vein *(curved arrow)* can be seen posterior to the bronchus intermedius.

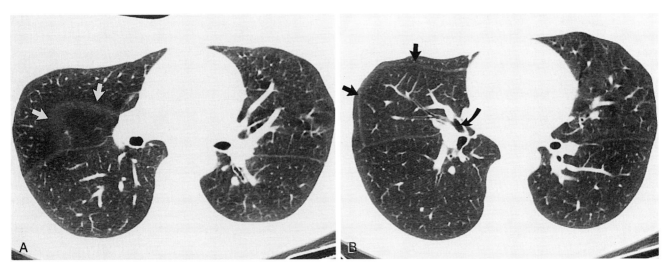

Figure 6–15. Normal Appearance of the Minor Fissure on HRCT Scan. *A,* The upper aspect of the minor fissure is seen as a curvilinear band of increased attenuation *(arrows)*. *B,* The lower and steeper portion of the minor fissure is seen as a thin line *(straight arrows)*. The right middle lobe bronchus can be seen at this level *(curved arrow)*.

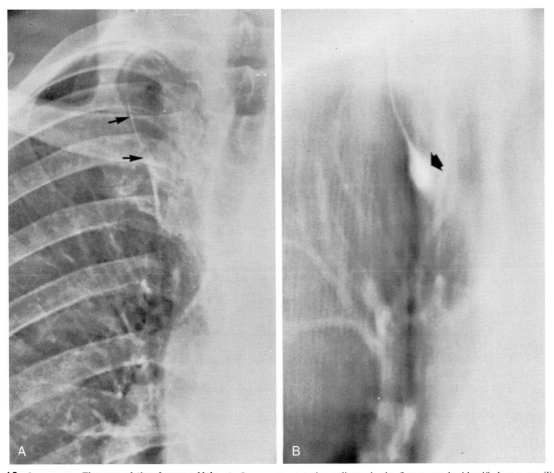

Figure 6–16. Accessory Fissure of the Azygos Vein. *A,* On a posteroanterior radiograph, the fissure can be identified as a curvilinear shadow *(arrows)* extending obliquely across the upper portion of the right lung, its lower end some distance above the right hilum. *B,* A tomographic section with the patient in the supine position permits better perception of the teardrop shadow of the vein *(arrow)* because of distention.

position than normal, ending anteriorly at the junction of the brachiocephalic veins and superior vena cava. Above the azygos vein, the fissure is seen as a curvilinear line. The fissure may also be seen a short distance below the vein.[49] Lung tissue within the azygos lobe intrudes into the pretracheal and retrotracheal mediastinum, contacting the anterior wall and most of the posterior wall of the trachea in most patients (Fig. 6–17). Similarly, lateral displacement of the azygos vein may be associated with intrusion of lung posterior to the superior vena cava, permitting identification of the posterior wall of this structure on the lateral chest radiograph.

Although the bronchial supply of the azygos lobe is variable, either the apical bronchus or its anterior subsegmental branch is always present within the lobe.[50] Larger lobes may contain both these subsegments or only the apical subsegments supplied by the apical and posterior segmental bronchi. The importance of the anomaly radiologically (in addition to the reasons previously stated) lies in the failure of the apical pleural surfaces to separate when pneumothorax is present.

A left upper lobe fissure analogous to the azygos fissure is rare.[51, 52] Like its right-sided counterpart, the left fissure consists of four layers of pleura, with a "trigonum parietale" (triangular opacity) at the apex and a vein at the other end.[51] The malpositioned vein corresponds to the left superior intercostal vein;[52] it drains the second, third, and fourth intercostal veins into the left brachiocephalic vein and usually connects with the accessory hemiazygos vein.[53] The CT appearance in one case was similar to that of a right azygos lobe, except that the left-sided counterpart did not insinuate itself deeply into the mediastinum.[52]

Inferior Accessory Fissure. This fissure separates the medial basal segment from the remainder of the lower lobe; when complete, the isolated lung is termed the *inferior accessory,* or *retrocardiac, lobe* (Fig. 6–18). The fissure extends laterally from a point near the pulmonary ligament and makes a convex arc forward to join the major fissure. On conventional radiographs, the fissure line extends superiorly and slightly medially from the inner third of the right or left hemidiaphragm. As with all normal and accessory fissures, consolidation in contiguous lung parenchyma pro-

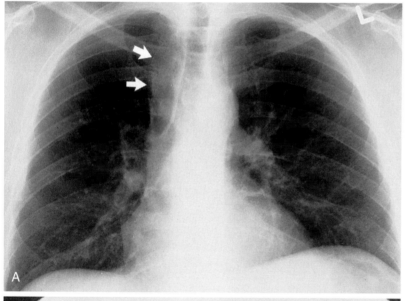

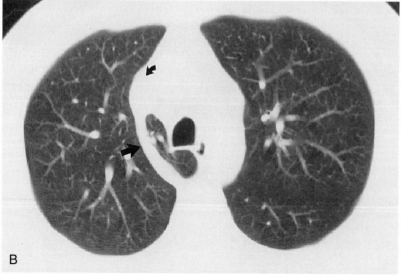

Figure 6–17. Azygos Fissure on CT Scan. *A,* On a standard posteroanterior radiograph the fissure is identified as a curvilinear line *(arrows)* extending obliquely across the upper portion of the right lung. *B,* On CT, the azygos arch *(straight arrow)* can be seen to end at the superior vena cava *(curved arrow).* Lung tissue is visualized between the azygos vein and the trachea.

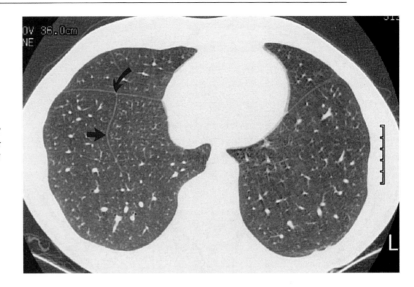

Figure 6–18. Inferior Accessory Fissure. An HRCT scan demonstrates the inferior accessory fissure as a linear arc convex laterally *(straight arrow)* and ending anteriorly at the level of the major fissure *(curved arrow).*

vides a sharp interface between diseased and normal lung parenchyma.

This accessory fissure is fairly common, being seen anatomically in 30% to 45% of lungs.[4, 54] Its incidence radiologically depends on the mode of examination. In one study of 500 radiographs, it was identified in 41 (8%), 33 times on the right, 5 times on the left, and 3 times bilaterally. In another investigation of 50 patients examined by both conventional chest radiographs and CT scan, the latter mode revealed the fissure in 8 cases (16%); of these, only 2 were also visible on the radiograph. On the other hand, chest radiographs showed 3 fissures that were not visible on CT, so that the overall incidence in this series was 22%. The fissure is better seen on HRCT scan than on conventional CT; in the former, it is visible as a linear arc, convex laterally and extending from the mediastinum near the esophagus to the major fissure anteriorly at the lung base (Fig. 6–18).[45]

Superior Accessory Fissure. This fissure separates the superior segment from the basal segments of the lower lobes, more commonly on the right (Fig. 6–19). It varies in length from a complete fissure to a slight notch less than 1 cm; when complete, the separated segment has been termed the *dorsal lobe of Nelson.* Since the fissure commonly lies horizontally at the same level as the minor fissure, the two may be confused on a frontal radiograph; however, their separate anatomic positions can be clearly established on lateral or oblique projections.

Left Minor Fissure. This fissure separates the lingula from the rest of the left upper lobe. Although it is analogous to the minor fissure on the right side, the lingula typically retains its superior and inferior segmental anatomy rather than assuming the medial and lateral segmental anatomy of the right middle lobe.[55] The fissure was observed in 8% of 100 specimens in one anatomic investigation.[55] In another study of 2000 consecutive PA and lateral chest radiographs, it was identified in 32 cases (1.6%);[56] its position was usually more cephalad than the right minor fissure, and its lateral end usually was superior to its medial end.

On conventional CT scan, the left minor fissure is similar to its counterpart on the right and is seen as an area devoid of vessels;[57] with HRCT scan, it appears as a line or narrow band of attenuation (Fig. 6–20).[58]

The Pulmonary Ligament

The pulmonary ligament* consists of a double layer of pleura that tethers the medial aspect of the lower lobe to the adjacent mediastinum and diaphragm.[59–62] It is formed by the mediastinal parietal pleura as it reflects over the main bronchi and pulmonary arteries and veins onto the surface of the lung as the visceral pleura (Fig. 6–21). Although the anterior and posterior layers of this pleural reflection are excluded from one another at the hilum, apposition is possible caudad to the inferior pulmonary vein (rarely cephalad to the pulmonary vein), thus forming the pulmonary ligament. The ligament can terminate in a free falciform border anywhere between the inferior pulmonary vein and the superior aspect of the hemidiaphragm (*incomplete* form), or it can extend inferiorly and cover a portion of the medial aspect of the hemidiaphragm (*complete* form). Thus, the pulmonary ligament divides the mediastinal pleural space below the hilum into either complete or incomplete, anterior and posterior compartments. The bare area of mediastinum thus created contains connective tissue, small systemic vessels,[63] lymphatics, and lymph nodes.

Although the pulmonary ligament is anatomically extra-parenchymal, it is contiguous laterally with a cleavage plane in the parenchyma of the lower lobe known as the *interseg-mental (intersublobar) septum,* which separates the medial from the posterior basal segments.[59–62, 64] The left pulmonary ligament is closely related to the esophagus and is bordered posteriorly by the descending aorta; the shorter right ligament can be situated anywhere along an arc that extends from the inferior vena cava anteriorly to the azygos vein posteriorly.

Although the pulmonary ligaments are never seen on conventional PA or lateral chest radiographs, that on the left can be visualized on CT scan in 60% to 70% of subjects and that on the right in 40% to 60%.[62, 65] The appearance is variable, but usually consists of a small peak or pyramid on the mediastinal surface that represents the ligament and a

---

*Although sometimes termed the *inferior pulmonary ligament,* this structure is more properly designated simply the *pulmonary ligament,* since there is no superior component.

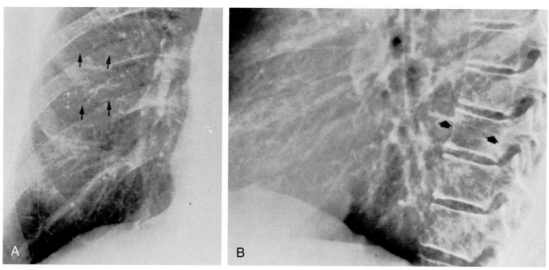

Figure 6–19. Accessory Fissure Between the Superior and Basal Segments of the Right Lower Lobe. *A,* In a posteroanterior projection of the lower half of the right lung, two horizontal fissures can be identified: the superior *(upper arrows),* representing the normal minor fissure, and the inferior *(lower arrows),* representing an accessory fissure between the superior and basal bronchopulmonary segments of the right lower lobe. *B,* In lateral projection, the accessory fissure is well seen *(arrows).*

thin, linear opacity that extends from the apex of the peak to the lung, marking the intersegmental septum (Fig. 6–22).[64] The ligament is most evident on scans obtained at or just above the level of the hemidiaphragm.[60] In about 90% of cases, the course of the ligament on both sides is obliquely posterior.[60] Ordinarily, the right ligament is seen at a level slightly more cephalad than the left, and both ligaments can be appreciated on only one or two slices of a series.

The function of the pulmonary ligament is uncertain, although it may serve as an anchor for the lower lobe in resisting torsion. The ligament plays a role in modifying the radiographic appearance of pneumothorax (Fig. 6–23), lower lobe atelectasis, and medial pleural effusion.[59] Pathologic involvement of the pulmonary ligament by tumors, cysts, varicosities, and fat has also been described.[59, 60]

The subject of gas collections within the ligament is controversial; some investigators consider that air can dissect into the mediastinum from the lung within the ligament, creating a triangular radiolucency in the lower hemithorax on a PA radiograph.[66–69] However, this hypothesis has been challenged by the authors of one investigation, in which six patients were found to have a radiolucency conforming to the shape of the pulmonary ligament in one or other hemithorax on conventional PA and lateral radiographs;[70] long fluid levels, inconsistent with the normal anatomic location of the ligament, were identified in three of the six subjects. CT analysis of the gas collections showed quite clearly that they were located either between pleural layers in front of or behind the ligaments or within the mediastinum outside the parietal pleura altogether.

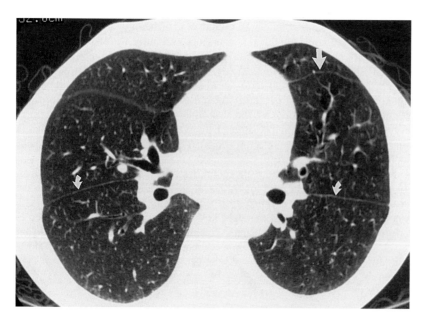

Figure 6–20. Left Minor Fissure. An HRCT scan demonstrates the left minor fissure as a curvilinear area of attenuation *(straight arrow).* The right minor fissure is seen at the same level as a slightly thicker area of attenuation. Also seen are both major interlobar fissures as thin lines of attenuation *(curved arrows).*

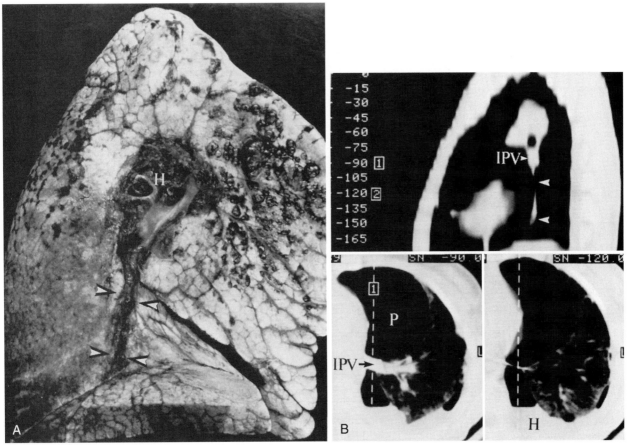

Figure 6–21. The Pulmonary Ligament. *A,* As seen on an inflated postmortem specimen of the left lung viewed from the medial aspect, the mediastinal (parietal) pleura reflects over the hilum superiorly, anteriorly, and posteriorly; caudally these pleural layers are more closely apposed to compose the pulmonary ligament *(arrowheads).* In *B* are a reformatted CT scan *(top)* and representative transverse images *(bottom)* through the plane of the left inferior pulmonary vein (IPV) and 3 cm caudally in a patient with a spontaneous hydropneumothorax (H and P). Note that the vertically oriented septum *(arrowheads)* divides the mediastinal pleural space into anterior and posterior compartments.

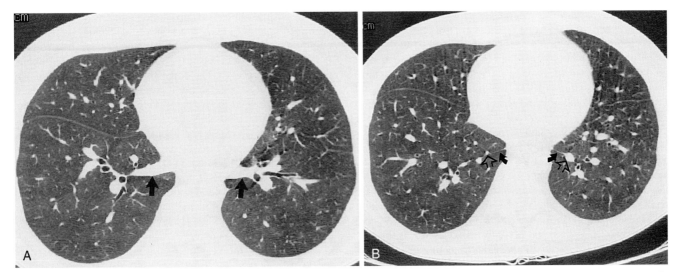

Figure 6–22. Inferior Pulmonary Ligaments and Their Relationship to the Inferior Pulmonary Veins. *A,* An HRCT scan demonstrates the right and left inferior pulmonary veins *(straight arrows). B,* Immediately caudad to the veins, thin lines of attenuation can be seen extending to the mediastinum *(curved arrows).* These represent the intersegmental septa of the lower lobes, which are bounded at the mediastinum by the base of the pulmonary ligament and laterally by a vertically oriented vein *(open arrows).*

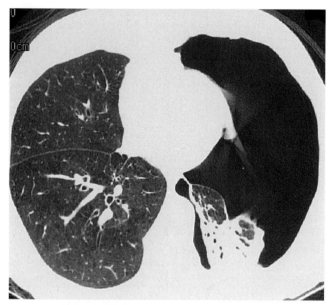

Figure 6–23. Pulmonary Ligament. An HRCT scan in a patient with a large spontaneous pneumothorax reveals passive atelectasis of the left lung. The inferior aspect of the lung remains attached to the mediastinum medially by the pulmonary ligament.

PHYSIOLOGY

The visceral and parietal pleura form smooth membranes that facilitate the movement of the lungs within the pleural space, chiefly by the secretion and absorption of pleural fluid. The discussion that follows about pressures within the pleural cavity and the formation and absorption of pleural fluid is only a brief summary of these complex subjects, and the reader interested in acquiring additional information is directed to more comprehensive reviews.[71–73]

Pressures

Pressure within the pleural cavity is generated by the difference between the elastic forces of the chest wall and of the lungs. At functional residual capacity (FRC), the lung tends to recoil inward while the chest wall and the rib cage tend to recoil outward. Even at the end of a maximal expiration (residual volume [RV]), the lungs continue to recoil inward, a completely relaxed position of a normal lung being achieved only after its removal from the chest or following a pneumothorax. By contrast, the chest wall's resting position is at about 55% of vital capacity (70% of total lung capacity [TLC]); below this volume, the chest wall has a tendency to expand, whereas above it, it tends to recoil inward toward its resting position. At FRC, the outward recoil of the chest wall and the inward recoil of the lung generate a pleural surface pressure (Ppl) of about -5 cm H_2O. However, the pleural pressure is not uniform through the pleural cavity, being more negative at the apex than at the base, with a gradient of about 0.2 cm H_2O per centimeter of vertical height. This gradient is gravity dependent, being reversed in subjects in the head-down position and altered to an anterior-posterior gradient in patients in the supine position.

As a result of this pleural pressure gradient, the upper lung zones are more expanded than the lower zone in subjects in the upright position at all lung volumes other than TLC.[74] In addition, the lower lung zones expand more than the upper zones during inspiration, a process reflected by the greater ventilation of the lower zones in healthy, erect subjects. These regional differences in volume behavior of the lung have been compared with those of an easily extensible coiled spring.[74] If the spring is held at its upper end so that it is acted on only by the force of gravity, the coils will be further apart at the upper than at the lower end; this is analogous to the greater alveolar volume in the upper than in the lower lung zones. If the spring is lengthened by applying a weight at the bottom, the distances between coils will increase until they are equal; the change in distance between the coils is greater at the lower end, corresponding to the greater change in volume at the bottom of the lung during inspiration.

Although Ppl is the pertinent pressure with respect to lung and chest wall mechanics, it is pleural liquid pressure (Pliq) that is pertinent with respect to fluid exchange across the pleura. There is evidence that Pliq is more negative than Ppl and has a gradient nearer to 1 cm H_2O per centimeter down the lung.[73]

Fluid Formation and Absorption

The amount of fluid in a single pleural space in normal humans ranges from less than 1 ml to 20 ml,[75] the average being approximately 2 ml.[76] It is possible to aspirate some fluid in about 30% of healthy subjects at rest and in about 70% after exercise. In one investigation of 120 healthy subjects, 15 were found to have up to 15 ml of pleural fluid using a special radiographic technique (*see* page 563);[77] the smallest amount of fluid that could be identified was 3 to 5 ml. Human pleural fluid has an average protein concentration of 1.77 g/dl (range, 1.38 to 3.35)[75] and contains sodium, potassium, and calcium at concentrations similar to those of interstitial fluid.

In normal subjects, transudation and absorption of fluid within the pleural cavity are believed to follow the Starling equation and to depend on a combination of hydrostatic, colloid osmotic, and tissue pressures, as well as lymphatic drainage (Fig. 6–24). The force that drives fluid out of the parietal pleura results from a combination of the hydrostatic pressure in parietal pleura capillaries ($\sim$30 cm H_2O) and the pressure in the pleural space (~ -5 to -8 cm H_2O at FRC), the net drive being about 35 to 38 cm H_2O. The colloid osmotic pressure in the systemic capillaries is approximately 30 to 34 cm H_2O, and that of the pleura is approximately 8 cm H_2O,[79] yielding a net drive of about 22 to 26 cm H_2O colloid osmotic pressure from the pleural space to the capillaries of the parietal pleura. The balance of these forces ($\sim$9 to 15 cm H_2O) is directed from the parietal pleura to the pleural cavity.

In humans, the visceral pleura is supplied primarily by the bronchial vessels. Since these are part of the systemic circulation, it might be anticipated that the capillary pressure in the visceral pleura would be similar to that in the parietal layer. However, there is an important difference between the two capillary networks: that of the parietal pleural vasculature drains to the right side of the heart, and that of the visceral pleura drains to the left. There are also extensive anastomoses between the bronchial and pulmonary vessels within the lung. As a result of these anatomic and physiologic differences, it is probable that the visceral pleural capillary pressure is less than that of the parietal pleura (i.e., closer to pulmonary capillary pressure). In the example shown in Figure 6–24, we have assigned a value for visceral pleural capillary pressure of 20 cm H_2O (approximately intermediate between expected systemic and pulmonary capillary pressure). Since the other pressures remain constant, the net pressure across the visceral pleura would be between -1 cm H_2O (favoring absorption from the pleural space into the visceral pleural capillaries) and $+5$ cm (favoring the formation of pleural fluid). These calculations suggest that it is most likely that pleural fluid is formed at both parietal and visceral surfaces and is removed primarily by the parietal pleural lymphatics. However, if visceral pleural capillary pressure is closer to that of the pulmonary capillaries, then the hypothesis that fluid forms at the parietal surface and is absorbed at the visceral surface could still be correct. This discussion of the forces governing the formation and absorption of pleural fluid is an oversimplification, since it ignores tissue pressures, the permeability of the mesothelial layer, and pressures within the lymphatics.

Normal pleural fluid has a low-protein content,[75, 80] which limits the rate of its formation at the parietal surface and affords the possibility of absorption at the visceral surface. If an inflammatory or neoplastic process alters the permeability of the parietal or visceral pleural capillaries, fluid with a high-protein content can form. When the protein concentration of pleural fluid rises sufficiently, the effect of colloid osmotic pressure in parietal and visceral pleural capillaries becomes negligible, and the only route of absorption of pleural fluid is by bulk flow via the lymphatics.[82, 83] Similarly, if the parietal or visceral pleural capillary pressure increases or serum osmotic pressure decreases, increased pleural fluid formation and removal by the lymphatics will result. In patients with mild congestive heart failure, the 24-hour clearance of pleural fluid has been estimated to be between 500 and 1,000 ml.[80, 84] If increased pulmonary capillary pressure or permeability results in the accumulation of interstitial pulmonary edema fluid, the primary route for its removal is the intrapulmonary lymphatics; however, there is evidence that increased interstitial pressure in the lung can cause direct pleural transudation, thus providing an accessory route of clearance of pulmonary edema.[81, 85, 86]

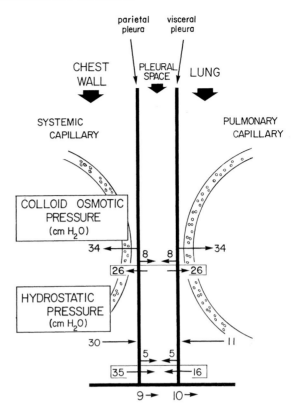

Figure 6–24. Diagrammatic Representation of the Pressures Involved in the Formation and Absorption of Pleural Fluid. *See text for description.*

Lymphatic absorption of fluid from the pleural space takes place on the parietal side.[87] Communication between lymphatics and the pleural cavity is via stomata that form between adjoining mesothelial cells. Since parietal pleural lymphatics pass through the diaphragm and intercostal muscles, movement of the chest wall may increase both the speed of fluid absorption from the pleural space and lymphatic flow, a process that has been shown to occur in unanesthetized dogs.[83] In humans, the rate of absorption of fluid high in protein falls significantly during the night, a finding that may be related to the decreased rate and depth of respiration during sleep.[80] There is also evidence that the lymphatics that drain the pleural space undergo peristaltic activity;[88] it has been suggested that it is this active component of pleural fluid drainage that generates the negative Pliq.[89]

REFERENCES

1. Harley R: Anatomy of the pleura. Sem Respir Med 9:1, 1987.
2. Wang N-S: Anatomy and physiology of the pleural space. Clin Chest Med 6:3, 1985.
3. Gruden JF, Stern EJ: Bilateral pneumothorax after percutaneous transthoracic needle biopsy: Evidence for incomplete pleural fusion. Chest 105:627, 1994.
4. von Hayek H: The Human Lung. New York, Hafner, 1960.
5. Mariassy AT, Wheeldon EB: The pleura: A combined light microscopic, scanning, and transmission electron microscopic study in the sheep: I. Normal pleura. Exp Lung Res 4:293, 1983.
6. Krahl VE: Anatomy of the mammalian lung. In Fenn WO, Rahn H (eds): Handbook of Physiology. Section 3, Respiration. Vol 1. Washington, DC, American Physiological Society, 1964, pp 213–284.
7. Bray BA, Keller S, Mandl I, et al: Collagenous membrane from the surface of human visceral pleura. Lung 163:361, 1985.
8. Pistolesi M, Miniati M, Giuntini C: Pleural liquid and solute exchange. Am Rev Respir Dis 140:825, 1989.
9. McLaughlin RF, Tyler WS, Canada RO: Subgross pulmonary anatomy in various mammals and man. JAMA 175:694, 1961.
10. Agostoni E: Mechanics of the pleural space. Physiol Rev 52:57, 1972.
11. Wang N-S: The regional difference of pleura mesothelial cells in rabbits. Am Rev Respir Dis 110:623, 1974.
12. Bashir MS, Cowen PN: Mucous metaplasia of the pleura. J Clin Pathol 45:1030, 1992.
13. Andrews PM, Porter KR: The ultrastructural morphology and possible functional significance of mesothelial microvilli. Anat Rec 177:409, 1973.
14. Rennard SI, Jaurand M-C, Bignan J, et al: Role of pleural mesothelial cells in the production of the submesothelial connective tissue matrix of lung. Am Rev Respir Dis 130:267, 1984.
15. Whitaker D, Papadimitriou JM, Walters MN-I: The mesothelium: Its fibrinolytic properties. J Pathol 136:291, 1982.
16. Idell S, Zwieb C, Kumar A, et al: Pathways of fibrin turnover of human pleural mesothelial cells in vitro. Am J Respir Cell Mol Biol 7:414, 1992.
17. Hills BA, Butler BD, Barrow RE: Boundary lubrication imparted by pleural surfactants and their identification. J Appl Physiol 53:463, 1982.
18. Hills BA. Graphite-like lubrication of mesothelium by oligolamellar pleural surfactant. J Appl Physiol 73:1034, 1992.
19. Whitaker D, Papadimitriou J: Mesothelial healing: Morphological and kinetic investigations. J Pathol 145:159, 1985.
20. Wheeldon EB, Mariassy AT, McSporran KD: The pleura: A combined light microscopic and scanning and transmission electron microscopic study in the sheep: II. Response to injury. Exp Lung Res 5:125, 1983.
21. Hott JW, Sparks JA, Godbey SW, et al: Mesothelial cell response to pleural injury: Thrombin-induced proliferation and chemotaxis of rat pleural mesothelial cells. Am J Respir Cell Mol Biol 6:421, 1992.
22. Fotev Z, Whitaker D, Papadimitriou JM: Role of macrophages in mesothelial healing. J Pathol 151:209, 1987.
23. Bolen JW, Hammar SP, McNutt MA: Reactive and neoplastic serosal tissue. Am J Surg Pathol 10:34, 1986.
24. Kuwahara M, Kuwahara M, Bijwaard KE, et al: Mesothelial cells produce a chemoattractant for lung fibroblasts: Role of fibronectin. Am J Respir Cell Mol Biol 5:256, 1991.
25. Isoda K, Maeda T, Hamamoto Y: Collagen-producing mesothelial cells in Adriamycin-induced pleuritis in rat: Microautoradiographic study utilizing tritiated proline. Acta Pathol Jpn 37:1305, 1987.
26. Raasch BN, Carsky EW, Lane EJ, et al: Radiographic anatomy of the interlobar fissures: A study of 100 specimens. Am J Roentgenol 138:1043, 1982.
27. Yamashita H: Roentgenologic Anatomy of the Lung. New York, Igaku-Shoin, 1978, pp 46–58.
28. Im J-G, Webb WR, Rosen A, et al: Costal pleura: Appearance at high-resolution CT. Radiology 171:125, 1989.
29. Vix VA: Extrapleural costal fat. Radiology 112:563, 1974.
30. Sargent EN, Boswell WD Jr, Ralls PW, et al: Subpleural fat pads in patients exposed to asbestos: Distinction from non-calcified pleural plaques. Radiology 152:273, 1984.
31. Felson B: The lobes and interlobar pleura: Fundamental roentgen considerations. Am J Med Sci 230:572, 1955.
32. Proto AV, Ball JB: Computed tomography of the major and minor fissures. Am J Roentgenol 140:439, 1983.
33. Proto AV, Ball JB: The superolateral major fissures. Am J Roentgenol 140:431, 1983.
34. Gale ME, Greif WL: Intrafissural fat: CT correlation with chest radiography. Radiology 160:333, 1986.
35. Proto A, Speckman JM: The left lateral radiograph of the chest. Med Radiogr Photogr 55:1, 1979.
36. Felson B: Chest Roentgenology. Philadelphia, WB Saunders, 1973.
37. Ritter H, Eyband M: Der diagnostische Wert eines lageveränderten Ober-Mittellappenspaltes im Lungensagittalbild. [The diagnostic significance, in the sagittal chest film, of a shift in the upper and middle lobe fissures.] Fortschr Roentgenstrahl 86:431, 1957.
38. Simon G: Principles of Chest X-Ray Diagnosis. 3rd ed. London, Butterworth, 1971.
39. Glazer HS, Anderson DJ, DiCroce JJ, et al: Anatomy of the major fissure: Evaluation with standard and thin-section CT. Radiology 180:839, 1991.
40. Goodman LR, Golkow RS, Steiner RM, et al: The right mid-lung window: A potential source of error in computed tomography of the lung. Radiology 143:135, 1982.
41. von Hayek H: The Human Lung. New York, Hafner, 1960.
42. Otsuji H, Uchida H, Maeda M, et al: Incomplete interlobar fissures: Bronchovascular analysis with CT. Radiology 187:541, 1993.
43. Berkmen YM, Auh YH, Davis SD, et al: Anatomy of the minor fissure: Evaluation with thin-section CT. Radiology 170:647, 1989.
44. Frija J, Yana C, Laval-Jeantet M: Anatomy of the minor fissure: Evaluation with thin-section CT (letter to the editor). Radiology 173:571, 1989.
45. Godwin JD, Tarver RD: Accessory fissures of the lung. Am J Roentgenol 144:39, 1985.
46. Fisher MS: Adam's lobe (letter to the editor). Radiology 154:547, 1985.
47. Postmus PE, Kerstjens JM, Breed A, et al: A family with lobus venae azygos. Chest 90:298, 1986.
48. Speckman JM, Gamsu G, Webb WR: Alterations in CT mediastinal anatomy produced by an azygos lobe. Am J Roentgenol 137:47, 1981.
49. Mata J, Cáceres J, Alegret X, et al: Imaging of the azygos lobe: Normal anatomy and variations. Am J Roentgenol 156:931, 1991.
50. Boyden EA: The distribution of bronchi in gross anomalies of the right upper lobe, particularly lobes subdivided by the azygos vein and those containing preeparterial bronchi. Radiology 58:797, 1952.
51. Hanke R: Die vena hemiazygos accessoria im röntgenbild: Gleichzeitig ein beitrag zur frage des "linken azygoslappens." Beitr Klin Erforsch Tuber Lungenkr 135:116, 1967.
52. Takasugi JE, Godwin JD: Left azygos lobe. Radiology 171:133, 1989.
53. Lane EJ, Heitzman ER, Dinn WM: The radiology of the superior intercostal veins. Radiology 120:263, 1976.
54. Schaffner VD: Chest. In Shanks SC, Kereley P (eds): A Textbook of X-Ray Diagnosis. Vol II, 2nd ed. Philadelphia, WB Saunders, 1950–1952, p 241.
55. Boyden EA: Cleft left upper lobes and the split anterior bronchus. Surgery 26:167, 1949.
56. Austin JHM: The left minor fissure. Radiology 161:433, 1986.
57. Godwin JD, Tarver RD: Accessory fissures of the lung. Am J Roentgenol 144:39, 1985.
58. Berkmen T, Berkmen YM, Austin JHM: Accessory fissures of the upper lobe of the left lung: CT and plain film appearance. Am J Roentgenol 162:1287, 1994.
59. Rabinowitz JG, Cohen BA, Mendleson DS: The pulmonary ligament. Radiol Clin North Am 22:659, 1984.
60. Rost RC, Proto AV: Inferior pulmonary ligament: Computed tomographic appearance. Radiology 14:479, 1983.
61. Cooper C, Moss AA, Buy J, et al: CT of the pulmonary ligament. Am J Roentgenol 141:231, 1983.
62. Godwin JD, Bock P, Osborne DR: CT of the pulmonary ligament. Am J Roentgenol 141:231, 1983.
63. Stocker JT, Malczak HT: A study of pulmonary ligament arteries: Relationship to intralobar pulmonary sequestration. Chest 86:611, 1984.
64. Berkmen YM, Drossman SR, Marboe CC: Intersegmental (intersublobar) septum of the lower lobe in relation to the pulmonary ligament: Anatomic, histologic, and CT correlations. Radiology 185:389, 1992.
65. Rost RC, Proto AV: Inferior pulmonary ligament: Computed tomographic appearance. Radiology 148:479, 1983.
66. Hyde I: Traumatic para-mediastinal air cysts. Br J Radiol 44:380, 1971.
67. Fagan CJ, Swischuk LE: Traumatic lung and para-mediastinal pneumatoceles. Radiology 120:11, 1976.
68. Ravin CE, Smith GW, Lester PD, et al: Post-traumatic pneumatocele in the inferior pulmonary ligament. Radiology 121:39, 1976.
69. Friedman PJ: Adult pulmonary ligament pneumatocele: A loculated pneumothorax. Radiology 155:575, 1985.
70. Godwin JD, Merten DF, Baker ME: Paramediastinal pneumatocele: Alternative explanations to gas in the pulmonary ligament. Am J Roentgenol 145:525, 1985.
71. Agostoni E, Taglietti A, Setnikar I: Absorption force of the capillaries of the visceral pleura in determination of the intrapleural pressure. Am J Physiol 191:277, 1957.
72. Black LF: The pleural space and pleural fluid. Mayo Clin Proc 47:493, 1972.
73. Agostoni E, D'Angelo E: Pleural liquid pressure. J Appl Physiol 71:393, 1991.
74. Milic-Emili J, Henderson JAM, Dolovich MB, et al: Regional distribution of inspired gas in the lung. J Appl Physiol 21:749, 1966.
75. Yamada S: Über die seröse Flüssigkeit in der Pleurahöhle der gesunden Menschen. Z Ges Exp Med 90:342, 1933.
76. Rohrer F: Physiologie der Atembewegung. In Bethe A, von Bergmann G, Embden G, et al (eds): Handbuch der Normalen und Pathologischen Physiologie. Vol II. Berlin, Springer, 1925, pp 70–127.
77. Müller R, Löfstedt S: The reaction of the pleura in primary tuberculosis of the lungs. Acta Med Scand 122:105, 1945.
78. Agostoni E, D'Angelo E, Roncoroni G: The thickness of the pleural liquid. Resp Physiol 5:1, 1968.
79. Agostoni E, Mead J: Statics of the respiratory system. In Fenn WO, Rahn H (eds): Handbook of Physiology. Section 3: Respiration. Vol I. Washington, DC, American Physiological Society, 1964, pp 387–409.

80. Stewart PB: The rate of formation and lymphatic removal of fluid in pleural effusions. J Clin Invest 42:258, 1963.
81. Hermans C, Lesur O, Weynand B, et al: Clara cell protein (CC16) in pleural fluids: A marker of leakage through the visceral pleura. Am J Respir Crit Care Med 157:962, 1998.
82. Courtice FC, Simmonds WJ: Absorption from the lungs. J Physiol 109:103, 1949.
83. Burgen ASV, Stewart PB: A method for measuring the turnover of fluid in the pleural and other serous cavities. J Lab Clin Med 52:118, 1958.
84. Leckie WJH, Tothill P: Albumin turnover in pleural effusions. Clin Sci 29:339, 1965.
85. Wiener-Kronish JP, Broaddus VC: Interrelationship of pleural and pulmonary interstitial liquid. Annu Rev Physiol 55:209, 1993.
86. Pearse DB, Wagner EM, Sylvester JT: Edema clearance in isolated sheep lungs. J Appl Physiol 74:126, 1993.
87. Courtice FC, Simmonds WJ: Physiological significance of lymph drainage of the serous cavities and lungs. Physiol Rev 34:419, 1954.
88. Negrini D, Ballard ST, Benoit JN: Contribution of lymphatic myogenic activity and respiratory movements to pleural lymph flow. J Appl Physiol 76:2267, 1994.
89. Miserocchi G, Venturoli D, Negrini D, et al: Model of pleural fluid turnover. J Appl Physiol 75:1798, 1993.

CHAPTER 7

The Lymphatic System of the Lungs, Pleura, and Mediastinum

MORPHOLOGY, 172
FUNCTION, 174
THE THORACIC DUCT AND RIGHT LYMPHATIC
DUCT, 175
LYMPH NODES OF THE MEDIASTINUM, 175
    Parietal and Visceral Groups of Thoracic Lymph
        Nodes, 175
        Parietal Lymph Nodes, 175
        Visceral Lymph Nodes, 176
    Classification of Regional Nodal Stations, 180
    Lymph Node Size, 184
    Magnetic Resonance Imaging Versus Computed
        Tomography in the Assessment of Mediastinal
        Lymph Nodes, 189
LYMPH NODES OF THE HILA, 191
LYMPHATIC DRAINAGE OF THE LUNGS, 192

MORPHOLOGY

Parietal pleural lymphatics are extensively distributed over the costal and diaphragmatic surfaces. In the former region, they run parallel to the intercostal muscle fibers; in the diaphragm, they run perpendicular to the muscular and tendinous fibers. In the mediastinal pleura, the lymphatics are organized in a branching network accompanying the blood vessels.[1] Between the parietal pleural mesothelial cells are numerous pores (stomata) 6 to 8 μm in diameter (Fig. 7–1).[2–4] These stomata are especially well developed over the diaphragmatic surface, where they connect with a network of lymphatics that drains to the mediastinum. The stomata and their connections represent the major pathway for removal of fluid and cells from the pleural space. A similar network of lymphatics on the abdominal side of the diaphragm collects peritoneal fluid and cells.[5]

Visceral pleural lymphatics course within the vascular layer, where they form a plexus of broad channels roughly following the pleural lobular boundaries. Between these channels and joining with them are smaller intercommunicating and blindly ending tributaries that ramify over the pleural surface. Branches occasionally dip into the immediate subpleural lung parenchyma, form a short loop, and then return to the pleural surface. This network is more prominent in neonatal than adult lungs, in which larger channels tend to have a somewhat more irregular, nonlobular distribution.[6] Although lymphatic vessels run over the whole of the pleural

surface, they are more numerous over the lower than the upper lobes (Fig. 7–2). Lymph flows toward the medial aspect of the lung and ultimately drains into hilar lymph nodes.

Within the lung, lymph flows within two major pathways, one in peribronchovascular connective tissue (Fig. 7–3) and the other in interlobular septal connective tissue. In both, it flows centripetally toward the hilum, eventually reaching the peribronchial and hilar lymph nodes. Anastomotic channels connect the interlobular lymphatics with those in the bronchoarterial sheath; they are up to 4 cm long and are particularly evident midway between the hilum and the periphery of the lung. (Distention of these communicating lymphatics and edema in their surrounding connective tissue results in Kerley A lines [*see* farther on]; similar processes in the interlobular lymphatics and connective tissue result in Kerley B lines.) Anastomotic channels also connect the bronchoarterial and pleural plexuses;[6–8] even though fluid from the pleural cavity can theoretically reach the hilum through these connecting vessels,[6] the presence of intralymphatic valves directed toward the pleural surface argues against significant flow in this direction.[7]

Although lymphatic capillaries have not been identified within alveolar interstitial tissue—the bronchoarterial lymphatics begin in the region of the distal respiratory bronchioles[9]—they may be seen in intimate apposition to alveolar air spaces next to interlobular, pleural, peribronchial, and perivascular connective tissue (Fig. 7–4). These channels have been termed *juxta-alveolar* lymphatics[10] because of their close topographic and possible functional relationship to the alveolar air spaces.

When examined under the light microscope, pulmonary lymphatics can be divided into capillaries and collecting channels.[9] In the normal lung, both are relatively inconspicuous and appear only as small spaces lined by a single layer of flattened endothelial cells. Occasionally, the presence of mural smooth muscle cells or valves indicates the presence of a collecting duct. The three-dimensional anatomy of the pulmonary lymphatics has also been described by using casting techniques and scanning electron microscopy.[11–14] With these techniques, three types of vessel can be distinguished: (1) reservoir lymphatics, which are relatively broad, ribbon-like structures that are closely linked to lymphatic capillaries; (2) conduit lymphatics, which are tubular structures that may contain valves and travel long distances

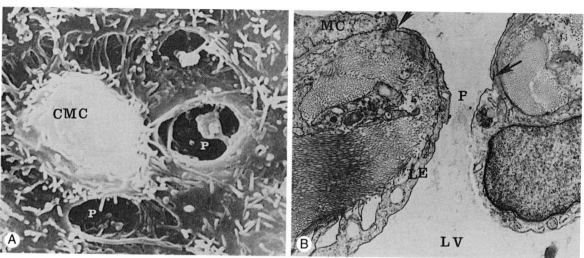

Figure 7–1. Diaphragmatic Pores. A scanning electron micrograph of the diaphragm *(A)* shows a surface cuboidal cell (CMC) (possibly a macrophage) and numerous slender mesothelial microvilli. Two intercellular pores (P) are evident. (×8950). A section through a pore (P) viewed by transmission electron microscopy *(B)* shows processes from two lymphatic endothelial cells (LE) extending onto the peritoneal surface to form intercellular junctions *(arrows)* with the surface mesothelial cells (MC). The close contact between the two cell types provides a direct passageway between the peritoneal cavity and the underlying lymphatic vessels (LV). (×16,200.) (From Leak LV, Rahil K: Am Rev Respir Dis 119[Suppl]:8, 1979. © American Lung Association.)

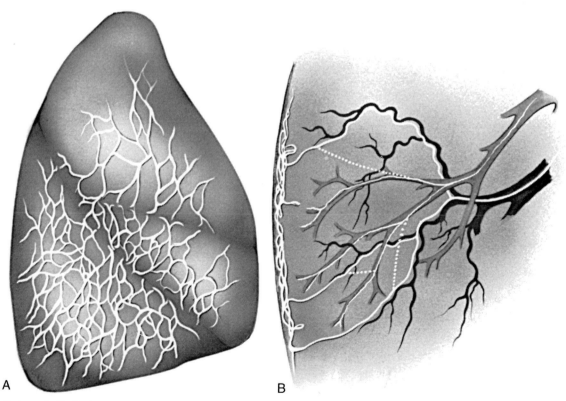

Figure 7–2. Lymphatic Drainage of the Pleura and Lungs. A drawing of the lateral aspect of the right lung *(A)* shows the pleural lymphatics to be much more numerous over the lower half of the lung than over the upper. In a coronal section through the midportion of the lung *(B)*, lymphatic channels from the pleura enter the lung at the interlobular septa and extend medially to the hilum along venous radicles *(dark-shaded vessels)*; lymphatic channels originating in the peripheral parenchyma extend medially in the bronchovascular bundles *(light-shaded vessels)*. Communicating lymphatics *(dotted lines)* extend between the peribronchial and perivenous lymphatics.

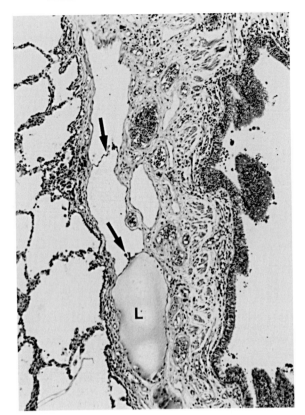

Figure 7–3. Peribronchial Lymphatic Channel. A peribronchiolar lymphatic (L) is distended by fluid (partially lost during tissue processing). Two valves are apparent *(arrows)*. (×72.)

without side branches; and (3) saculotubular lymphatics, which form a plexiform complex surrounding the arteries, veins, and bronchi.[11, 12] Lymphatic channels can hypertrophy and dilate following lung injury[11] or during edematous states.[14]

The lymphatic capillary endothelium rests on a discontinuous basement membrane that can be entirely absent for considerable lengths.[9] In some areas, endothelial cells are joined by intercellular junctions, but in others they are entirely free, with significant gaps left in the vessel wall. Perilymphatic connective tissue fibers are in close contact with endothelial cells and basement membrane and have been regarded as a tethering mechanism that keeps the capillaries open.[9] These features—endothelial and basement membrane discontinuities and connective tissue anchoring system—appear to be ideal for the provision of easy and continuous access of interstitial fluid to the capillary lumen.

Lymphatic endothelial cells possess many irregular cytoplasmic protrusions that extend into the lumen and the perilymphatic connective tissue. The cytoplasm itself contains scattered mitochondria and endoplasmic reticulum, occasional pinocytotic vesicles, and fairly numerous microfilaments, some of which are thought to constitute an actin-like contractile system that regulates opening or closing of the intercellular gaps.[9] Ultrastructurally, the larger (collecting) lymphatics differ from capillaries by having a continuous basement membrane, more regular endothelium, and the presence of muscle in their wall.

Numerous valves 1 to 2 mm apart direct lymph flow in both the pleural and intrapulmonary lymphatics (*see* Fig. 7–3). They consist of a connective tissue core covered by a continuous layer of endothelium and seem to be firmly attached to the adjacent connective tissue.[9] Although these valves appear to be bicuspid in two-dimensional histologic sections, stereomicroscopic studies have shown most to be monocuspid and shaped like a funnel.[9] They are well adapted to unidirectional flow since they cannot be inverted and are easily occluded by flow in an abnormal direction.

FUNCTION

The flow of lymph through pulmonary lymphatic channels appears to depend in part on the "pumping" action of ventilation,[9, 15] and it has been postulated that the "butterfly" pattern of pulmonary edema may be caused by the greater ventilatory excursion of the periphery (cortex) than of the central portion (medulla) of the lung.[16] Evidence for this process is derived from several experimental studies. In anesthetized dogs, cessation of ventilation abruptly diminishes flow in mediastinal lymphatics draining lung lymph.[17] Ethiodized oil injected into the pleural lymphatics of human lungs removed at autopsy can be shown to fill the deep pulmonary lymphatics;[18, 19] subsequent flow within these

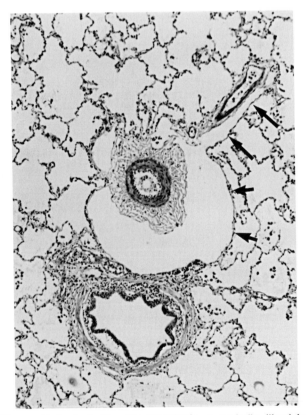

Figure 7–4. Juxta-Alveolar Lymphatic. A markedly dilated lymphatic *(short arrows)* almost completely encircles a pulmonary artery and extends next to one of its smaller branches *(long arrows)*. Note the close proximity of the lymphatic lumen to the adjacent alveolar air spaces. (×70.)

lymphatics occurs only during ventilation. During life, contraction of smooth muscle in the collecting lymphatics also contributes to lymph flow; in fact, pressure as great as 30 cm H_2O has been measured in the major lymphatic vessels.

THE THORACIC DUCT AND RIGHT LYMPHATIC DUCT

The thoracic duct is a continuation of the cisterna chyli, which in turn is formed by the junction of the two lumbar lymphatic trunks on the anterior aspect of the vertebral column at the level of T12 to L2.[18] (In 10% to 15% of people, the cisterna chyli lies at the level of T10.[20]) The duct enters the thorax through the aortic hiatus of the diaphragm. In the majority of subjects, it lies to the right of the aorta and follows its course cephalad; thus, in the lower portion of the thorax it lies roughly in the midline or slightly to one side of the vertebral column. In patients who have a markedly tortuous aorta, the thoracic duct lies to the left of the spine.

At about the level of the carina, the duct crosses the left main bronchus and runs cephalad in a plane parallel to the left lateral wall of the trachea and slightly posterior to it. The distance between the left tracheal wall and the thoracic duct on posteroanterior radiographs does not exceed 10 mm in normal subjects;[18] a measurement greater than 10 mm indicates lateral displacement by a mediastinal mass. The duct leaves the thorax between the esophagus and left subclavian artery and runs posterior to the left innominate vein; much of the cephalic third (the cervical portion) is supraclavicular. The thoracic duct then joins the venous system, most commonly by emptying into the internal jugular vein but sometimes into the subclavian, innominate, or external jugular veins.

The normal diameter of the thoracic duct ranges from 1 to 7 mm.[18] In one study of 390 lymphangiograms, valves were identified within the duct in about 85% of cases, primarily in the upper two thirds; a maximum of 13 valves was found.[18] Several variations in thoracic duct anatomy, presumably congenital, have been observed.[18]

The radiologic anatomy of the right lymphatic duct has been poorly documented since it cannot be easily opacified and it is an inconstant channel.[21] Its three trunks—the right jugular, right subclavian, and right mediastinal—often open separately into the jugular, subclavian, and innominate veins, respectively.

LYMPH NODES OF THE MEDIASTINUM

Although pleuropulmonary lymphatics are not normally visible radiologically, their intrathoracic repository, the hilar and mediastinal lymph nodes, are frequently discernible. Indeed, enlargement of the hilar and mediastinal lymph nodes is a common and often diagnostically important feature of disease arising within the thorax; furthermore, individual patterns of lymph node involvement can supply an important clue to the origin or nature of diseases originating both within and outside the thorax.

Grossly enlarged mediastinal lymph nodes can often be suspected on plain radiographs by increased opacity and alteration of the normal mediastinal contour. Lymph nodes are identified on computed tomographic (CT) scans as round or oval structures of soft tissue attenuation, with or without central or eccentric radiolucent fat, in a location that does not correspond to normal vascular or neural structures. When present, foci of calcification or lymphangiographic contrast medium serve as definitive markers. On magnetic resonance (MR) imaging, lymph nodes have soft tissue intensity and can be readily distinguished from vessels and fat; however, scattered calcifications cannot be identified.

Limited information is available about the number of normal mediastinal lymph nodes. In one investigation of five autopsied patients, the average number was 64;[22] 80% were situated in relation to the trachea, carina, and main bronchi. On the other hand, the general organization of mediastinal and hilar lymph nodes has been thoroughly described by several observers, and various classifications have been proposed.[23-26] The multiplicity of schemes is eloquent testimony to the difficulty that both anatomists and radiologists have had in lymph node classification. In the following section we discuss two of these classifications: a grouping into parietal and visceral compartments (which corresponds most closely to the anatomist's description of nodal groups) and groupings into nodal stations, which reflect an attempt to classify the nodes in a fashion more relevant to radiologists and surgeons.

The range in size of mediastinal lymph nodes accepted as normal on a CT scan varies considerably, the upper limit having been variously reported as 7 mm,[27] 10 mm,[28] 11 mm,[29] and 15 mm.[30] Measurements have included the long-axis nodal diameter as assessed in the transverse plane of the CT image,[26, 28, 31] both long- and short-axis diameters,[32, 33] and cross-sectional area.[34] Careful analysis of CT scans *in vivo* and in autopsy specimens has shown that the normal nodal diameter varies in different regions of the mediastinum.[26, 32] Rather than reviewing all studies, we will focus our attention on the ones most relevant to the understanding of normal anatomy.

Parietal and Visceral Groups of Thoracic Lymph Nodes

Intrathoracic lymph nodes can be considered in *parietal* and *visceral* groups;[35] the former reside outside the parietal pleura in extramediastinal tissue, where they drain the thoracic wall and other extrathoracic structures, whereas the latter are located within the mediastinum between the pleural membranes and are concerned primarily with drainage of intrathoracic tissue.

Parietal Lymph Nodes

Parietal lymph nodes can in turn be subdivided into three groups.

Anterior Parietal (Internal Mammary) Lymph Nodes. These nodes are located in the upper portion of the thorax behind the anterior intercostal spaces bilaterally, either medial or lateral to the internal mammary vessels (Fig. 7–5). They receive afferent channels from the upper anterior abdominal wall, anterior thoracic wall, anterior portion of the diaphragm, and the medial portion of the breasts. They communicate with the visceral group of the anterior medias-

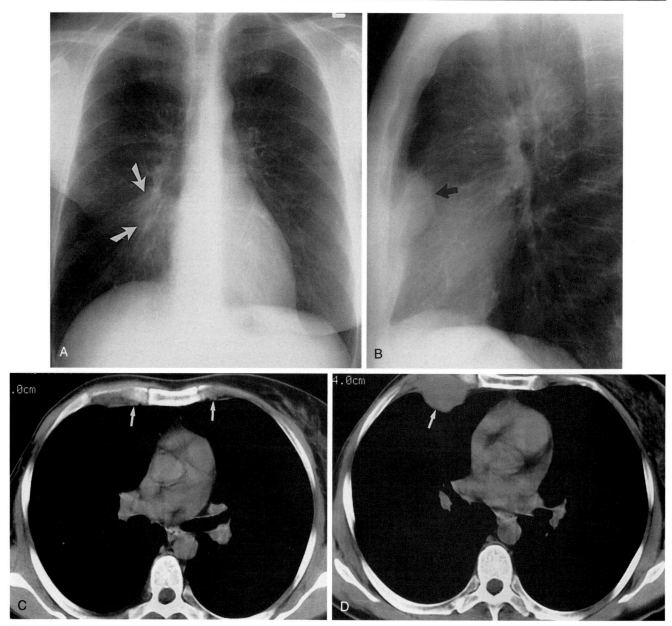

Figure 7–5. Enlargement of Internal Mammary Lymph Nodes. A posteroanterior radiograph *(A)* shows surgical absence of the right breast and poorly defined increased opacity over the right hilum *(arrows)*. A lateral chest radiograph *(B)* demonstrates a smooth, homogeneous soft tissue opacity in the retrosternal area *(arrow)* caused by enlargement of the internal mammary lymph nodes. A CT scan at the level of the bronchus intermedius *(C)* shows the right and left internal mammary artery and vein *(arrows)*; the enlarged internal mammary node is seen at a slightly lower level *(D) (arrow)*. The patient was a 46-year-old woman with metastatic carcinoma of the breast.

tinal nodes and the cervical nodes; their main efferent channel is the right lymphatic duct or thoracic duct.

Posterior Parietal Lymph Nodes. Lymph nodes in this group are found adjacent to the rib heads in the posterior intercostal spaces *(intercostal nodes)* or adjacent to the vertebrae *(juxtavertebral nodes)* (Fig. 7–6). Both groups drain the intercostal spaces, parietal pleura, and vertebral column. They communicate with other posterior mediastinal lymph nodes that relate to the descending aorta and the esophagus. Efferent channels drain to the thoracic duct in the upper part of the thorax and to the cisterna chyli in the lower thoracic area.

Diaphragmatic Lymph Nodes. These nodes are composed of the *anterior (prepericardiac)* group, which is located

immediately behind the xiphoid and to the right and left of the pericardium anteriorly (Fig. 7–7); the *middle (juxtaphrenic)* group, which is in the proximity of the phrenic nerves as they meet the diaphragm; and the *posterior (retrocrural)* nodes, which reside behind the right and left crura of the diaphragm. The diaphragmatic nodes drain the diaphragm and the anterosuperior portion of the liver.

Visceral Lymph Nodes

The visceral lymph nodes are also divided into three groups.

Anterosuperior Mediastinal (Prevascular) Lymph Nodes. These nodes are congregated along the anterior aspect of the

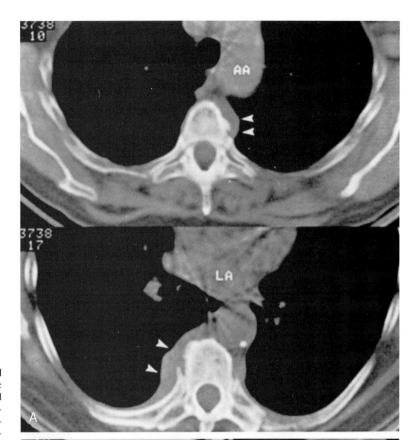

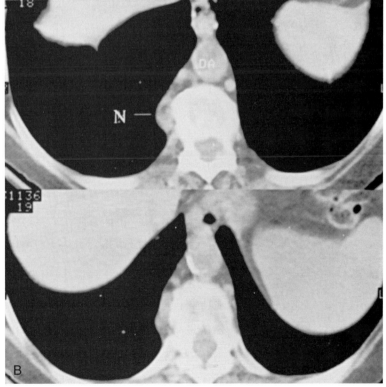

Figure 7–6. Enlargement of Posterior Parietal Lymph Nodes. Transverse CT scans *(A)* through the aortic arch (AA, *top*) and left atrium (LA, *bottom*) show lobulated masses related primarily to the costovertebral junctions *(arrowheads)*. These features represent enlargement of the posterior parietal (intercostal) nodes in this patient with Hodgkin's disease. CT scans *(B)* through the lower portion of the thorax of a patient with non-Hodgkin's lymphoma show enlargement of the juxtavertebral nodes (N). DA, descending aorta.

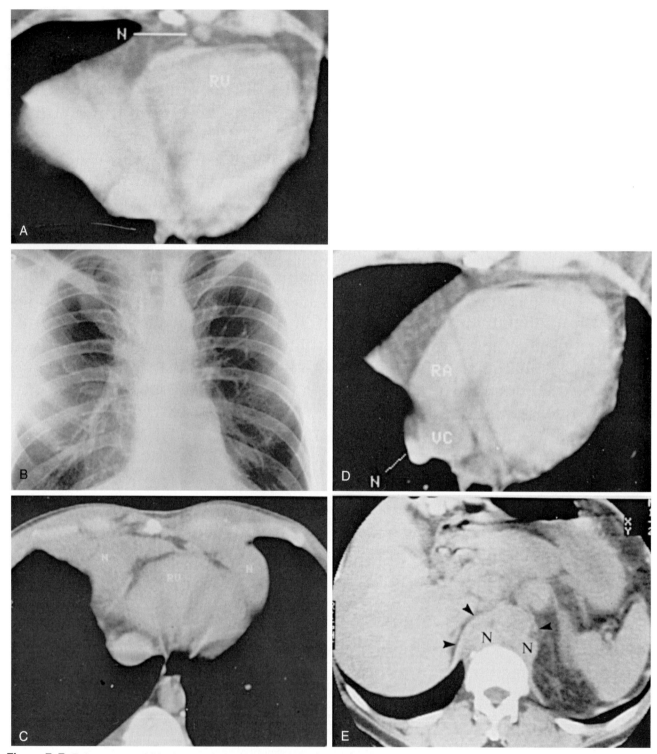

Figure 7–7. Enlargement of Diaphragmatic Lymph Nodes. In this CT scan *(A)* the anterior (prepericardiac) group is located immediately behind the xiphoid and anterior to the right ventricle (RV) and pericardium. There is only slight enlargement of the nodes (N) in this young patient with Hodgkin's disease; even massive involvement of this group is sometimes undetectable on conventional posteroanterior (PA) and lateral chest radiographs. A PA chest radiograph *(B)* of another patient with Hodgkin's disease reveals blunting of the cardiophrenic angles and abnormal contours of the right and left hemidiaphragms suggestive of enlargement of the right and left prepericardiac chains of nodes. However, distinction from prominent epicardial fat pads cannot be determined with certainty without a CT scan. *C,* A CT scan of the patient depicted in *B* confirms the presence of enlarged nodes (N) anterior and lateral to the right ventricle (RV). Note that the enlarged nodes and the heart are isodense. In a 40-year-old man with non-Hodgkin's lymphoma, a CT scan *(D)* through the lower part of the thorax reveals enlargement of the middle (juxtaphrenic) nodes (N). Note the relationship of this nodal group to the inferior vena cava (VC) and right atrium (RA). Posterior (retrocrural) lymph node enlargement (N) is present on the CT scan *(E)* of this 60-year-old man with metastatic adenocarcinoma of the left kidney. The crura *(arrowheads)* are displaced laterally by the enlarged nodes.

superior vena cava, right and left innominate veins, and ascending aorta (Fig. 7–8). Some are situated posterior to the sternum in the lower portion of the thorax, and others reside behind the manubrium anterior to the thymus. They drain most of the structures in the anterior mediastinum, including the pericardium, thymus, diaphragmatic and mediastinal pleurae, part of the heart, and the anterior portion of the hila. Efferent channels drain into the right lymphatic or thoracic duct.

Posterior Mediastinal Lymph Nodes. These nodes are located around the esophagus *(periesophageal nodes)* and along the anterior and lateral aspects of the descending aorta *(periaortic nodes)* (Fig. 7–9); they are most numerous in the lower portion of the thorax. Their afferent channels arise from the posterior portion of the diaphragm, the pericardium, and the esophagus and directly from the lower lobes of the lungs via the right and left pulmonary ligaments. They communicate with the tracheobronchial nodes, particularly the subcarinal group, and drain chiefly via the thoracic duct.

Tracheobronchial Lymph Nodes. Tracheobronchial lymph nodes constitute the most important group of visceral lymph nodes and consist in turn of several subgroups. The *paratracheal* nodes are located in front and to the right and left of the trachea (Fig. 7–10); occasionally, a retrotracheal compo-

nent is present. The right paratracheal chain is usually the best developed; its lowermost member, the azygos node, is situated medial to the azygos vein arch in the pretracheal mediastinal fat. These lymph nodes receive afferent channels from the bronchopulmonary and tracheal bifurcation nodes, the trachea, and the esophagus. They can also receive lymph directly from the right and left lungs without diversion through the bronchopulmonary or tracheal bifurcation nodes. Direct communication also exists with the anterior and posterior visceral mediastinal nodes. The efferent channels are the right lymphatic and thoracic ducts.

The *tracheal bifurcation (carinal)* lymph nodes are situated in the precarinal (Fig. 7–10) and subcarinal (Fig. 7–11) fat, as well as around the circumference of the right and left main bronchi. Those in mediastinal fat between the left pulmonary artery and aortic arch are designated *aortopulmonary window* nodes (Fig. 7–12); they can be divided into medial, lateral (subpleural), and superior groups and merge above with the left prevascular nodes. Carinal lymph nodes receive afferent flow from the bronchopulmonary nodes, anterior and posterior mediastinal nodes, heart, pericardium, esophagus, and lungs. Efferent drainage is to the paratracheal group, particularly the right-sided component.

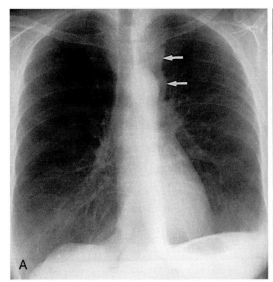
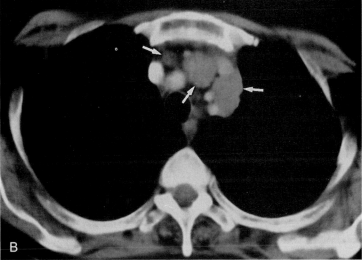
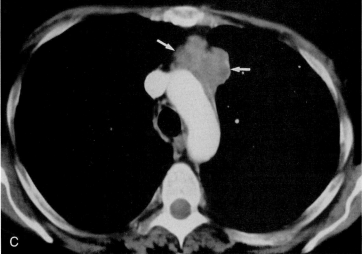

Figure 7–8. Enlargement of the Anterior (Prevascular) Group of Mediastinal Nodes. A conventional posteroanterior radiograph *(A)* shows a widened and lobulated contour of the left upper mediastinal silhouette *(arrows)*. Intravenous contrast–enhanced CT scans through the superior mediastinum *(B* and *C)* confirm the presence of enlarged nodes *(arrows)* and reveal their intimate relationship to the great vessels. The patient was a 64-year-old woman with metastatic pulmonary carcinoma.

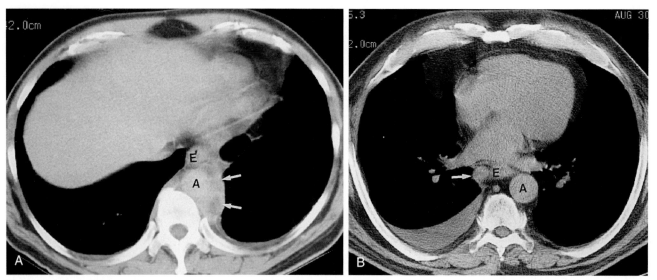

Figure 7–9. CT Scan of Juxtavertebral Nodes (Periesophageal and Periaortic). An intravenous contrast–enhanced CT scan *(A)* demonstrates enlarged periaortic nodes *(arrows)* in a 60-year-old woman with lymphoma. A CT scan without intravenous contrast agent *(B)* demonstrates an enlarged periesophageal node *(arrow)* in a 63-year-old man with pulmonary carcinoma. Also noted is a small right pleural effusion (A, aorta; E, esophagus).

The *bronchopulmonary* or *hilar* lymph nodes (Fig. 7–13) are numerous but are normally too small to be detected on conventional radiographs or unenhanced CT studies. Hilar nodes are well visualized on contrast-enhanced CT (Fig. 7–14) and with MR imaging (Fig. 7–15). They are located around the main bronchi and vessels, particularly at their points of division and receive afferent channels from all lobes of the lungs; their efferent drainage is to the carinal and paratracheal nodes. Lymph nodes located within the right and left inferior pulmonary ligaments are often included as components of the lower hilar lymph node group.

Intraparenchymal lymphoid nodules resembling lymph nodes but not related to airways are sometimes large enough to be visualized macroscopically and radiologically.[36, 37] In one investigation, they were found in 5 of 28 lungs in which the deep lymphatic channels could be outlined.[38] In another study of 26 patients who had a pulmonary nodule less than 1 cm in diameter identified on the chest radiograph, 12 (46%) proved to be intrapulmonary lymph nodes following surgical resection.[38a] It has been suggested that at least some of these nodules represent foci of hyperplastic lymphoid tissue in the interlobular connective tissue.[37]

Classification of Regional Nodal Stations

In 1983, the American Thoracic Society (ATS) published a map of regional pulmonary mediastinal lymph nodes based on their relationship to major anatomic structures.[39] The ATS committee recommended that the terms *mediastinal* and *hilar* be dropped because of a lack of clinical-anatomic specificity and be replaced with carefully defined "nodal stations" (Table 7–1, Fig. 7–16). The latter are based on the relationship of lymph node groups to major anatomic structures that can be readily identified by the radiologist and by the surgeon at mediastinoscopy or thoracotomy. On the right side, these structures include the innominate artery, trachea, azygos vein, right main bronchus, origin of the right upper lobe bronchus, and carina; on the left side, they

include the aorta, left pulmonary artery, ligamentum arteriosum, and left main bronchus (Fig. 7–17). A guide to the ATS nodal map classification on CT has been published and is based on the demonstration of calcified mediastinal nodes.[40]

The 1983 ATS classification was generally well accepted, although several minor modifications were subsequently proposed[41] based on a change in the TNM staging system of lung cancer.[42] Despite this, a different classification scheme continued to be used by the American Joint Committee on Cancer (AJCC).[42a] To overcome this conflict, the AJCC and the Union Internationale Contre le Cancer (UICC) proposed a classification of lymph node stations for lung cancer staging that unifies the two systems (Table 7–2, page 188).[42b]

The main differences between the new regional lymph node classification and the 1983 ATS classification are inclusion of Station 1 and hilar nodes, and modifications in the definition of Stations 4 and 10 nodes. According to the latest classification, Station 1 (highest mediastinal nodes) includes lymph nodes lying above a horizontal line at the upper edge of the brachiocephalic (left innominate) vein where it ascends to the left in front of the trachea at its midline. Stations 10R and 10L comprise hilar nodes, whereas more distal nodes are designated *intrapulmonary*. Station 10 includes all proximal lobar nodes distal to the mediastinal pleural reflection as well as nodes adjacent to the bronchus intermedius on the right; radiographically, the hilar shadow may be created by enlargement of either hilar or interlobar nodes (or both). Station 4R (lower paratracheal nodes) includes all nodes to the right of the midline of the trachea between a horizontal line drawn tangential to the upper margin of the aortic arch and a line extending across the right main bronchus at the upper margin of the upper lobe bronchus, and contained within the mediastinal pleural envelope. Station 4L includes all nodes to the left of the midline of the trachea between a horizontal line drawn tangential to the upper margin of the aortic arch and a line extending across the left main bronchus at the level of the

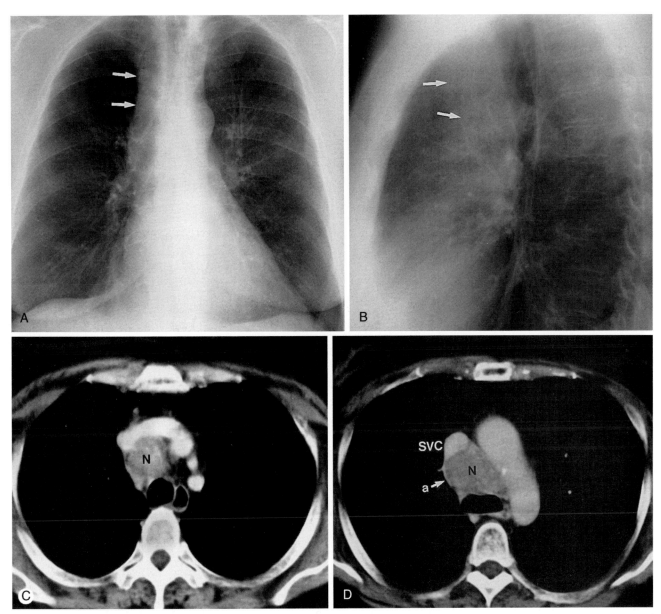

Figure 7–10. Enlargement of the Paratracheal Nodes. Posteroanterior *(A)* and lateral *(B)* chest radiographs demonstrate increased opacity to the right and anterior to the trachea *(arrows).* An intravenous contrast–enhanced CT scan at the level of the great vessels *(C)* demonstrates enlarged paratracheal lymph nodes (N). A CT scan at the level of the tracheal carina *(D)* demonstrates anterior displacement of the superior vena cava (SVC) and lateral displacement of the azygos vein (a) by enlarged precarinal nodes (N). The patient was a 59-year-old woman with metastatic pulmonary carcinoma.

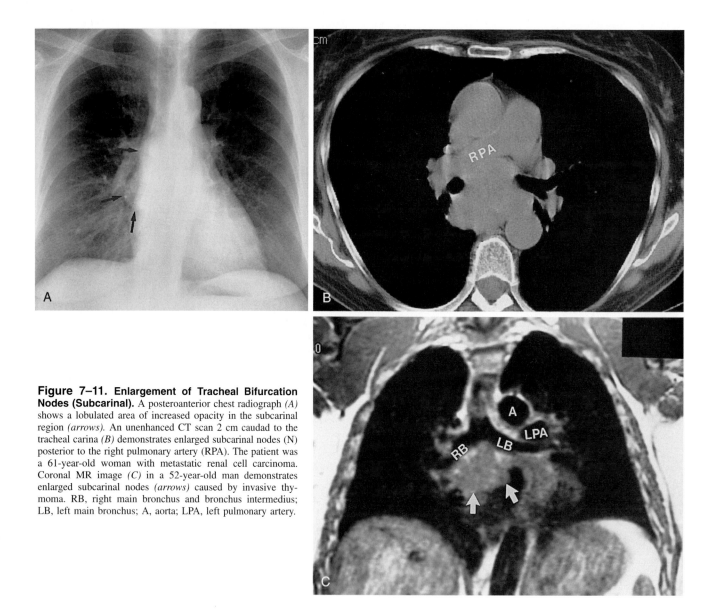

Figure 7–11. Enlargement of Tracheal Bifurcation Nodes (Subcarinal). A posteroanterior chest radiograph *(A)* shows a lobulated area of increased opacity in the subcarinal region *(arrows)*. An unenhanced CT scan 2 cm caudad to the tracheal carina *(B)* demonstrates enlarged subcarinal nodes (N) posterior to the right pulmonary artery (RPA). The patient was a 61-year-old woman with metastatic renal cell carcinoma. Coronal MR image *(C)* in a 52-year-old man demonstrates enlarged subcarinal nodes *(arrows)* caused by invasive thymoma. RB, right main bronchus and bronchus intermedius; LB, left main bronchus; A, aorta; LPA, left pulmonary artery.

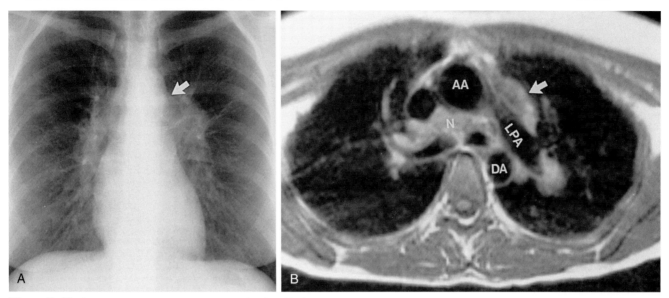

Figure 7–12. Enlargement of Aortopulmonary Window Nodes. A posteroanterior chest radiograph *(A)* demonstrates a localized lateral convexity at the level of the aortopulmonary window *(arrow)*. Enlargement of the hila is also evident. A cardiac-gated MR image *(B)* demonstrates enlarged aortopulmonary window nodes *(arrow)*, as well as enlarged precarinal (N) and hilar nodes. The patient was a 31-year-old woman with sarcoidosis. AA, ascending aorta; DA, descending aorta; LPA, left pulmonary artery.

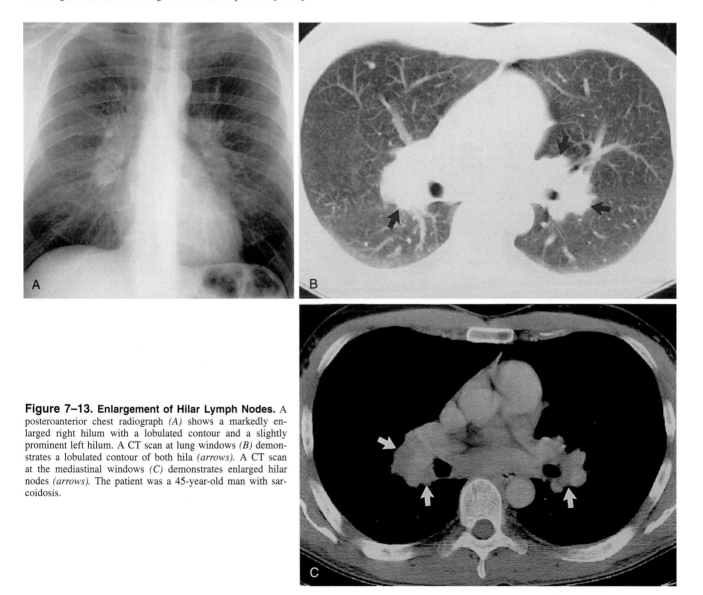

Figure 7–13. Enlargement of Hilar Lymph Nodes. A posteroanterior chest radiograph *(A)* shows a markedly enlarged right hilum with a lobulated contour and a slightly prominent left hilum. A CT scan at lung windows *(B)* demonstrates a lobulated contour of both hila *(arrows)*. A CT scan at the mediastinal windows *(C)* demonstrates enlarged hilar nodes *(arrows)*. The patient was a 45-year-old man with sarcoidosis.

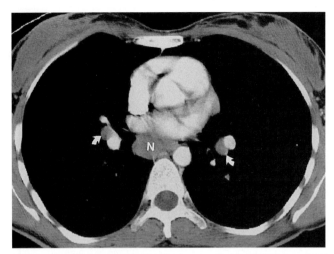

Figure 7–14. Enlarged Hilar Nodes on Contrast-Enhanced CT Scan. A CT scan obtained after intravenous administration of contrast material demonstrates bilateral hilar *(arrows)* and subcarinal adenopathy (N). The patient was a 22-year-old woman with sarcoidosis.

upper margin of the left upper lobe bronchus, medial to the ligamentum arteriosum and contained within the mediastinal pleural envelope.

The 1983 ATS classification has been used in the majority of studies in which the normal number and size of mediastinal lymph nodes have been assessed on CT and MR and in which the accuracy of these imaging modalities in the staging of pulmonary carcinoma has been compared. Therefore, this classification is used in the current chapter. However, since consistent classification of nodal stations is essential in clinical research, we recommend the use of the new classification scheme adopted by the AJCC and the UICC.

Lymph Node Size

A thorough combined autopsy and CT study designed to evaluate the size, number, and location of normal mediastinal lymph nodes was carried out in 1984.[26] The investiga-

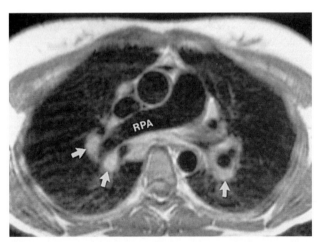

Figure 7–15. Enlarged Hilar Nodes on MR Imaging. A cardiac-gated MR image (TR 750, TE 20) demonstrates bilateral enlarged hilar lymph nodes *(arrows)*. The patient was a 31-year-old woman with sarcoidosis. RPA, right pulmonary artery.

Table 7–1. PROPOSED DEFINITIONS OF REGIONAL NODAL STATIONS FOR PRETHORACOTOMY STAGING

X	Supraclavicular nodes.
2R	Right upper paratracheal (suprainnominate) nodes: nodes to the right of the midline of the trachea between the intersection of the caudal margin of the innominate artery with the trachea, and the apex of the lung. (Includes highest R mediastinal node.) (Radiologists may use the same caudal margin as in 2L.)
2L	Left upper paratracheal (supra-aortic) nodes: nodes to the left of the midline of the trachea between the top of the aortic arch and apex of the lung. (Includes highest L mediastinal node.)
4R	Right lower paratracheal nodes: nodes to the right of the midline of the trachea between the cephalic border of the azygos vein and the intersection of the caudal margin of the brachiocephalic artery with the right side of the trachea. (Includes pretracheal and paracaval nodes.) (Radiologists may use the same cephalic margin as in 4L.)
4L	Left lower paratracheal nodes: nodes to the left of the midline of the trachea between the top of the aortic arch and the level of the carina, medial to the ligamentum arteriosum. (Includes some pretracheal nodes.)
5	Aortopulmonary nodes: subaortic and para-aortic nodes, lateral to the ligamentum arteriosum or the aorta or left pulmonary artery (LPA), proximal to the first branch of the LPA.
6	Anterior mediastinal nodes: nodes anterior to the ascending aorta or the innominate artery. (Includes some pretracheal and preaortic nodes.)
7	Subcarinal nodes: nodes arising caudal to the carina of the trachea but not associated with the lower lobe bronchi or arteries within the lung.
8	Paraesophageal nodes: nodes dorsal to the posterior wall of the trachea and to the right or left of the midline of the esophagus. (Includes retrotracheal, but not subcarinal nodes.)
9	Right or left pulmonary ligament nodes: nodes within the right or left pulmonary ligament.
10R	Right tracheobronchial nodes: nodes to the right of the midline of the trachea from the level of the cephalic border of the azygos vein to the origin of the right upper lobe bronchus.
10L	Left peribronchial nodes: nodes to the left of the midline of the trachea, between the carina and the left upper lobe bronchus, medial to the ligamentum arteriosum.
11	Intrapulmonary nodes: nodes removed in the right or left lung specimen plus those distal to the main stem bronchi or secondary carina. (Includes interlobar, lobar, and segmental nodes.)

From Tisi GM, Friedman PJ, Peters RM, et al: Am Rev Respir Dis 127:659, 1983. Official Statement of the American Thoracic Society. © American Lung Association.

tors divided the mediastinum into four zones. Zone I corresponded to the pretracheal space at the level of the innominate vein (ATS Stations 2R and 2L); Zone II, to the pretracheal space bounded anteriorly by the superior vena cava (ATS Stations 4R and 4L); Zone III, to the precarinal and subcarinal spaces (ATS Stations 10R, 10L, and 7); and Zone IV, to the aortopulmonary window (ATS Station 5).

One or more normal lymph nodes were seen on CT scans in Zones I and II in approximately 90% of patients and in Zones III and IV in 60% of patients.[26] These results are at variance with findings at autopsy, in which 100% of patients had lymph nodes in Zones II, III, and IV; this discrepancy is most likely related to the technique of CT examination used in the study (10-mm collimation, single-slice selection for analysis), which can create apparent "gaps" in lymph node continuity. The autopsy material, however, involved dissection of the entire area, thus eliminating the potential error inherent in the CT methodology.

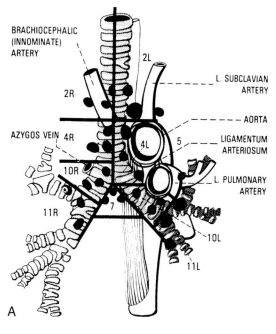

A

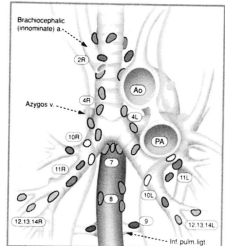

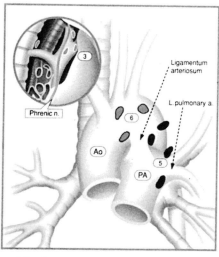

B

Superior Mediastinal Nodes

🔘 **1** Highest Mediastinal

🔘 **2** Upper Paratracheal

🔘 **3** Pre-vascular and Retrotracheal

🔘 **4** Lower Paratracheal
(including Azygos Nodes)

N_2 = single digit. ipsilateral
N_3 = single digit. contralateral or supraclavicular

Aortic Nodes

⚫ **5** Subaortic (A-P window)

🔘 **6** Para-aortic (ascending
aorta or phrenic)

Inferior Mediastinal Nodes

🔘 **7** Subcarinal

🔘 **8** Paraesophageal
(below carina)

🔘 **9** Pulmonary Ligament

N_1 Nodes

⚪ **10** Hilar

🔘 **11** Interlobar

⚪ **12** Lobar

🔘 **13** Segmental

⚪ **14** Subsegmental

Figure 7–16. Classification of Regional Lymph Node Stations. *A,* 1983 American Thoracic Society scheme. *B,* 1997 American Joint Committee on Cancer and the Union Internationale Contre le Cancer scheme. (*A* from Tisi GM, Friedman PJ, Peters RM, et al: Am Rev Respir Dis 127:658, 1983; *B* from Mountain CF, Dresler CM: Chest 111:1718, 1997, © 1996, Mountain and Dresler. Originally adapted from Naruke T, Suemasu K, Ishikawa S: Lymph node mapping and curability of various levels of metastases in resected lung cancer. J Thorac Cardiovasc Surg 76:832–839, 1978, and American Thoracic Society: Clinical staging of primary lung cancer. Am Rev Respir Dis 127:1–6, 1983.)

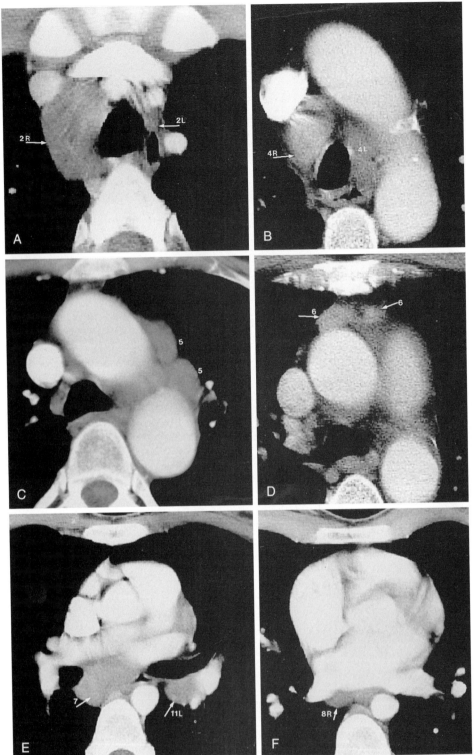

Figure 7–17. American Thoracic Society Nodal Stations. *A,* Upper paratracheal nodes to the right (2R) or left (2L) of the midline of the trachea above the level of the aortic arch. A CT scan *(A)* demonstrates an enlarged right upper paratracheal node (2R) and a normal-sized left upper paratracheal node (2L). *B,* Lower paratracheal nodes to the right (4R) or left (4L) of the midline of the trachea from the level of the aortic arch to the cephalic border of the azygos vein (4R) or to the level of the tracheal carina (4L) medial to the ligamentum arteriosum. A CT scan *(B)* demonstrates enlarged right and left lower paratracheal nodes. *C,* Aortopulmonary nodes lateral to the ligamentum arteriosum, lateral to the aortic arch, or lateral to the left pulmonary artery as far as the first branch of the left pulmonary artery (left upper lobe artery). A CT scan *(C)* demonstrates lymph nodes (ATS station 5) in an enlarged aortopulmonary window. *D,* Anterior mediastinal nodes anterior to the ascending aorta or brachiocephalic artery. A CT scan *(D)* demonstrates enlarged anterior mediastinal (Station 6) nodes. *E,* Subcarinal nodes arising caudal to the tracheal carina but originating within 2 cm of the carina and not associated with lower-lobe bronchi or arteries within the lung. A CT scan *(E)* demonstrates enlarged subcarinal (Station 7) and left intrapulmonary (11L) nodes. *F,* Paraesophageal nodes adjacent to the esophagus, to the right (8R) or left (8L) of the midline of the esophagus, and below Region 7, i.e., at least 3 cm below the level of the carina. A CT scan at the level of the confluence of the inferior pulmonary veins and left atrium *(F)* demonstrates a paraesophageal node (8R).

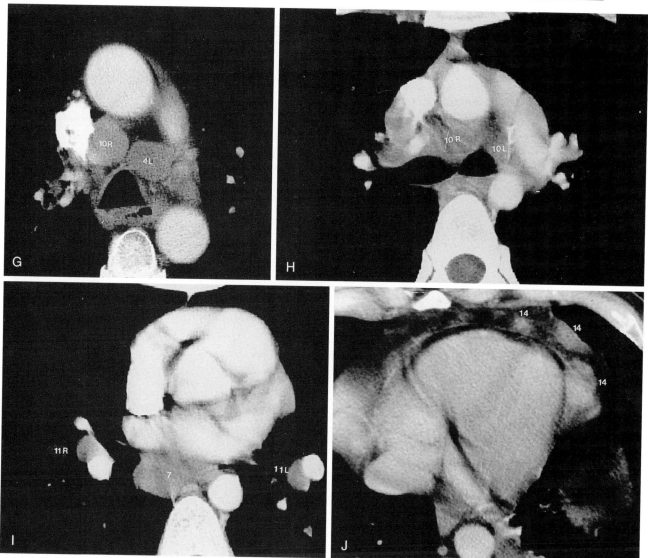

Figure 7–17 *Continued. G,* Tracheobronchial nodes to the right side of the midline of the trachea from the level of the cephalic border of the azygos vein to the origin of the right upper lobe bronchus. A CT scan at the level of the tracheal carina *(G)* demonstrates an enlarged right tracheobronchial (10R) node and left lower paratracheal node (4L). *H,* Left peribronchial nodes to the left of the midline of the trachea and medial to the ligamentum arteriosum, from the tracheal carina, and along the left main bronchus up to the level of the left upper-lobe bronchus takeoff. A CT scan at the level of the proximal main bronchi *(H)* demonstrates enlarged right tracheobronchial (10R) and left peribronchial (10L) lymph nodes. *I,* Intrapulmonary nodes within the lungs along the right (11R) and left (11L) lobar or segmental bronchi. A CT scan *(I)* demonstrates enlarged right (11R) and left (11L) intrapulmonary nodes as well as enlarged subcarinal (7) nodes. *J,* Superior diaphragmatic nodes adjacent to the pericardium within 2 cm of the diaphragm. A CT scan *(J)* demonstrates enlarged nodes adjacent to the diaphragm at the level of the left cardiophrenic angle (14).

There was a distinct tendency for lymph nodes to vary in size according to their location within the mediastinum. Although the overall size of the nodes in cadavers corresponded closely to that measured on the CT scans, lymph nodes were identified at autopsy that were larger than any identified by CT (Fig. 7–18). The probable explanation for this discrepancy is the tendency for lymph nodes to be oriented vertically along their long axis; thus the transverse plane of the CT scan records the width rather than the length of most lymph nodes. On the other hand, the morphologist logically measures the greatest dimension, which is usually the length. In Zone I, only 7% of the nodes measured more than 5 mm in diameter on CT, whereas in Zones II, III, and IV, 55%, 90%, and 67% of the nodes, respectively, were larger than 5 mm. Consequently, the diameter at which a

node should be considered to be enlarged depends on its location in the mediastinum. The authors suggested that the right lower paratracheal nodes (4R) should be considered enlarged when their maximal diameter as measured in the transverse plane of the CT scan is greater than 10 mm.[26] The remaining mediastinal nodes were considered enlarged when their maximal diameter was greater than 15 mm.[26, 31]

On CT or MR images, lymph nodes are usually ovoid in shape. Investigators assessing the role of CT in the evaluation of mediastinal nodes initially measured the largest nodal diameter (long axis) as seen on the transverse CT image. In 1984 it was suggested that the short axis is a more reliable measurement (Fig. 7–19).[34] This proposal was based on the results of preoperative assessment of the mediastinum in 60 patients with non–small cell carcinoma, 49 of whom had

Table 7–2. LYMPH NODE MAP DEFINITIONS—AMERICAN JOINT COMMITTEE ON CANCER AND THE UNION INTERNATIONALE CONTRE LE CANCER

NODAL STATION	ANATOMIC LANDMARKS
N2 nodes—all N2 nodes lie within the mediastinal pleural envelope	
1 Highest mediastinal nodes	Nodes lying above a horizontal line at the upper rim of the brachiocephalic (left innominate) vein where it ascends to the left, crossing in front of the trachea at its midline
2 Upper paratracheal nodes	Nodes lying above a horizontal line drawn tangential to the upper margin of the aortic arch and below the inferior boundary of No. 1 nodes
3 Prevascular and retrotracheal nodes	Prevascular and retrotracheal nodes may be designated 3A and 3P; midline nodes are considered to be ipsilateral
4 Lower paratracheal nodes	The lower paratracheal nodes on the right lie to the right of the midline of the trachea between a horizontal line drawn tangential to the upper margin of the aortic arch and a line extending across the right main bronchus at the upper margin of the upper lobe bronchus, and contained within the mediastinal pleural envelope; the lower paratracheal nodes on the left lie on the left of the midline of the trachea between a horizontal line drawn tangential to the upper margin of the aortic arch and a line extending across the left main bronchus at the level of the upper margin of the left upper lobe bronchus, medial to the ligamentum arteriosum and contained within the mediastinal pleural envelope
	Researchers may wish to designate the lower paratracheal nodes as No. 4s (superior) and No. 4i (inferior) subsets for study purposes; the No. 4s nodes may be defined by a horizontal line extending across the trachea and drawn tangential to the cephalic border of the azygos vein; the No. 4i nodes may be defined by the lower boundary of No. 4s and the lower boundary of No. 4, as described above
5 Subaortic (aortopulmonary window) nodes	Subaortic nodes are lateral to the ligamentum arteriosum or the aorta or left pulmonary artery and proximal to the first branch of the left pulmonary artery and lie within the mediastinal pleural envelope
6 Para-aortic (ascending aorta or phrenic) nodes	Nodes lying anterior and lateral to the ascending aorta and the aortic arch or the innominate artery, beneath a line tangential to the upper margin of the aortic arch
7 Subcarinal nodes	Nodes lying caudal to the carina of the trachea, but not associated with the lower lobe bronchi or arteries within the lung
8 Paraesophageal nodes (below carina)	Nodes lying adjacent to the wall of the esophagus and to the right or left of the midline, excluding subcarinal nodes
9 Pulmonary ligament nodes	Nodes lying within the pulmonary ligament, including those in the posterior wall and lower part of the inferior pulmonary vein
N1 nodes—all N1 nodes lie distal to the mediastinal pleural reflection and within the visceral pleura	
10 Hilar nodes	The proximal lobar nodes, distal to the mediastinal pleural reflection and the nodes adjacent to the bronchus intermedius on the right; radiographically, the hilar shadow may be created by enlargement of both hilar and interlobar nodes
11 Interlobar nodes	Nodes lying between the lobar bronchi
12 Lobar nodes	Nodes adjacent to the distal lobar bronchi
13 Segmental nodes	Nodes adjacent to the segmental bronchi
14 Subsegmental nodes	Nodes around the subsegmental bronchi

From Mountain CF, Dresler CM: Regional lymph node classification for lung cancer staging. Chest 111:1718, 1997.

thorough surgical-pathologic sampling of mediastinal nodes. The study demonstrated much less variability in the short-axis diameter than the long-axis diameter of normal lymph nodes, a result probably related to the fact that the short-axis measurement is less dependent on the spatial orientation of the node relative to the transverse plane of the CT image. These observations have been confirmed in subsequent studies.[43, 44]

The ATS scheme was used to carry out a thorough CT study of the number and size of normal mediastinal lymph nodes at 11 stations in 31 men aged 21 to 75 years and 25 women aged 18 to 82 years (mean age in both groups, approximately 50 years).[32] (Investigators measured both the short- and long-axis diameters of the nodes in the transverse plane [Table 7–3].) The largest nodes were in the subcarinal (Station 7) and right tracheobronchial (10R) regions, where the mean short-axis measurements were 6.2 mm and 5.9 mm, respectively. Upper paratracheal nodes (Station 2) were

smaller than lower paratracheal (Station 4) or tracheobronchial nodes (Station 10). More nodes were located in Station 4 than in Stations 2 and 10. As with the studies cited previously, measurements indicated that the threshold size for nodal enlargement depended on the particular station under scrutiny: in the upper paratracheal region (Station 2), the value of the short-axis measurement above which a lymph node was considered enlarged was 7 mm, whereas for nodes residing in the lower paratracheal region (Station 4) or around the carina (Stations 7 and 10), the figure was 10 to 11 mm.

Other investigators of the ATS nodal classification have used cadavers to compare mediastinal lymph node detection and sizing at CT with anatomic findings. In one of these studies, an excellent correlation was demonstrated for right-sided nodes but poorer correlation for those on the left, particularly in the left lower peribronchial region;[43] 43 of 45 right-sided (2R, 4R, 10R) nodes were detected at CT as

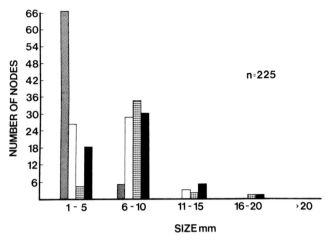

Figure 7–18. Graph Depicting Size of Normal Mediastinal Lymph Nodes by Zone. The *dotted area* represents Zone I; *solid white,* Zone II; *grid,* Zone III; and *solid black,* Zone IV. The total number of nodes *(n)* examined was 225. Note that most of the lymph nodes in Zone I are less than 6 mm in diameter, whereas the majority in Zones II to IV are in the 6- to 10-mm range. (From Genereux GP, Howie JL: Am J Roentgenol 142:1095, 1984. © American Roentgen Ray Society.)

Table 7–3. NUMBER AND SIZE OF NORMAL MEDIASTINAL LYMPH NODES IN 56 PATIENTS

| STATION | NUMBER | | SHORT-AXIS DIAMETER (mm) | | THRESHOLD SIZE* (mm) |
	Mean	± SD	Mean	± SD	
2R	2.1	1.3	3.5	1.3	7
2L	1.9	1.6	3.3	1.6	7
4R	3.2	2.0	5.0	2.0	10
4L	2.1	1.6	4.7	1.9	10
5	1.2	1.1	4.7	2.1	9
6	4.8	3.5	4.1	1.7	8
7	1.7	1.1	6.2	2.2	11
8R	1.0	1.1	4.4	2.6	10
8L	0.8	1.2	3.8	1.7	7
10R	2.8	1.3	5.9	2.1	10
10L	1.0	0.8	4.0	1.2	7

*Short-axis diameter above which a node should be considered enlarged.
Modified after Glazer GM, Gross BH, Quint LE, et al: Am J Roentgenol 144:261, 1985.

compared with only 22 of 39 left-sided nodes (2L, 4L, 10L, and 5). Station 10L showed the poorest CT/dissection correlation, with only 2 of 8 nodes being seen on CT. As the authors pointed out, lack of intravenous contrast may have led to difficulty in differentiating lymph nodes from vascular structures, thus accounting for the apparent poor visualization of the left-sided nodes. Short- and long-axis CT diameters and nodal area were also correlated with autopsy nodal diameters and volume. The best correlation was observed between nodal short-axis diameter at CT and autopsy nodal volume.[43]

In a second cadaver study of 40 adults without intrathoracic malignancy or infection, lymph nodes were identified in 90% to 100% of cadavers in Regions 4, 7, and 10 and in 70% to 85% of cadavers in Regions 2 and 6.[44] The largest nodes on CT measured 6.2 mm in mean diameter and were located in Region 7. The mean diameter was 5.9 mm in Region 10R, 5 mm in Region 4, 4.7 mm in Region 5, and as small as 4.4 to 3.3 mm in other regions. Because the short-axis diameter of the nodes at CT showed the smallest variation, the investigators again concluded that this was a more useful measurement than the long axis.

In summary, since the short-axis measurement shows less variability than the long one, it is recommended in the assessment of lymph node size. The short-axis diameter above which a node should be considered enlarged depends on the nodal location within the mediastinum. Strictly speaking, upper paratracheal (2R and 2L), left peribronchial (10L), and left paraesophageal nodes (8L) should be considered enlarged when the short-axis diameter is greater than 7 mm. The threshold value for anterior mediastinal nodes (6) is 8 mm; for lower paratracheal (4R and 4L), right tracheobronchial (10R), and right paraesophageal (8R) nodes 10 mm; and for subcarinal nodes (7) 11 mm. A more pragmatic and commonly used approach, although less accurate, is to consider all mediastinal lymph nodes as being normal in size unless they exceed 10 mm in short-axis diameter.

Magnetic Resonance Imaging Versus Computed Tomography in the Assessment of Mediastinal Lymph Nodes

Posteroanterior and lateral chest radiographs often suffice for the identification of gross hilar and mediastinal

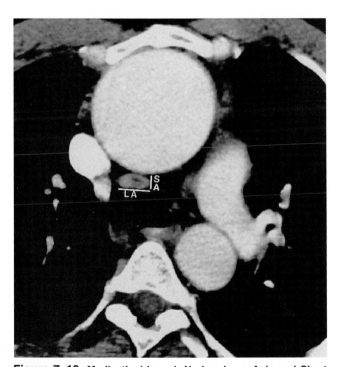

Figure 7–19. Mediastinal Lymph Nodes: Long-Axis and Short-Axis Measurements. An intravenous contrast–enhanced CT scan demonstrates a normal precarinal node in a patient with an aneurysm of the ascending aorta. The node is ovoid rather than round. Initial studies measured the maximal diameter of the node in the cross-sectional image (long axis) (LA). Because there is less variability in the normal range of short-axis (SA) diameters, most authors recommend using the short-axis diameter when measuring mediastinal lymph nodes. The long-axis measurement of the node illustrated is 15 mm and the short-axis measurement is 7 mm.

lymph node enlargement, the main findings being increased opacity and alteration of the normal mediastinal or hilar contour. When enlargement is less pronounced or when more precise understanding of abnormal anatomy is necessary, CT or MR imaging is required[45–49] (*see* Figs. 7–10 to 7–13). Each technique has its own advantages and disadvantages. MR imaging is capable of showing greater soft tissue contrast than CT, has a direct multiplanar imaging capability, and has an intrinsic flow sensitivity that allows easy distinction between vascular structures and soft tissue, including lymph nodes (Fig. 7–20).[50, 51] Despite these advantages, at the present time MR imaging has a lower spatial resolution than CT does; as a result, the MR image of adjacent normal nodes may resemble a single enlarged node.[52] Furthermore, calcification within nodes is not visible on MR images but is readily detected on CT scans.[52]

Perhaps the greatest limitation of both CT and MR imaging is the similarity of the soft tissue signal characteristics of benign and malignant lymph nodes. Preliminary results suggest that these two conditions may be distinguished in the majority of cases by using positron emission tomography (PET) with labeled substances such as 2-(^{18}F)-fluoro-2-deoxy-D-glucose (FDG), which is preferentially accumulated in both primary lung cancers and metastatic deposits in

lymph nodes.[53–55] FDG-PET imaging may detect tumor in normal-sized lymph nodes and exclude tumor in enlarged nodes; in one prospective study of 99 patients who had newly diagnosed or suspected pulmonary carcinoma, FDG-PET imaging had a sensitivity of 83% and a specificity of 94% for the detection of hilar and mediastinal lymph node metastases, whereas CT had a sensitivity of 63% and a specificity of 73%.[54] Similar results have been reported in several other studies.[55–57]

Proper evaluation of mediastinal and hilar lymph nodes on CT scans requires attention to the CT imaging technique and detailed knowledge of mediastinal vascular anatomy. Mediastinal nodes can usually be well visualized on CT scans without a need for intravenous contrast; however, contrast is necessary for optimal assessment of hilar lymph nodes.[58, 59] Scans may be obtained by using 5- to 10-mm collimation, thinner sections allowing more detailed assessment. In one investigation of 79 adult patients, 5-mm-thick sections without intravenous contrast were compared with 10-mm sections with contrast.[60] The thinner sections allowed the identification of more mediastinal nodes than did the 10-mm-thick sections and tended to show slightly (1 to 2 mm) larger nodes than did the 10-mm contrast-enhanced CT scans. For assessment of mediastinal nodes, CT scans are

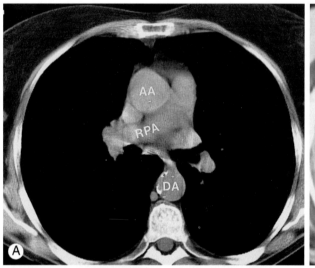
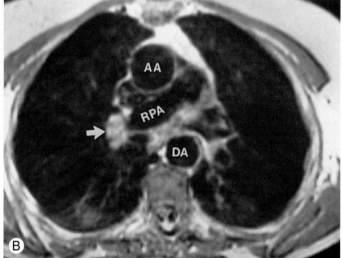
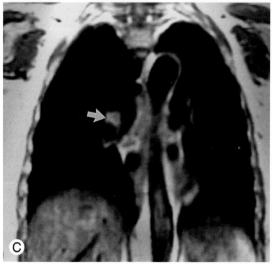

Figure 7–20. Hilar Lymph Node Missed on an Unenhanced CT Scan. A 10-mm-collimation, unenhanced CT scan at the level of the hila *(A)* was interpreted as being normal. A cardiac-gated MR image (TR 857, TE 20) at the same level *(B)* demonstrates right hilar lymphadenopathy *(arrow)*. The enlarged lymph node is also well seen on the coronal MR image *(C) (arrow)*. The patient was a 65-year-old woman with pulmonary carcinoma. RPA, right pulmonary artery; AA, ascending aorta; DA, descending aorta.

usually performed from the suprasternal notch to the top of the diaphragm with the patient in the supine position during suspended full inspiration. A window width of 350 to 500 Hounsfield units (HU) with the window level adjusted to yield the greatest subjective visual clarity (commonly in the 30- to 50-HU range) is appropriate.

Several investigations have been conducted to compare the sensitivity and specificity of MR and CT imaging in the detection of both normal and abnormal mediastinal lymph nodes. In 1985, a preoperative blind comparison of MR and CT imaging was carried out in 20 patients with pulmonary neoplasms.[61] Pathologically, 10 of the 20 had metastatic disease. Using the criterion of 16 mm or more as an abnormal lymph node diameter, false-positive interpretations were made on three CT scans and five MR images; there were no false-negative scans with either modality. The investigators concluded that although the sensitivity of the two imaging techniques was identical, specificity was slightly better for CT, probably as a result of the poor spatial resolution of the MR technique used.

In a second study performed in 1985, investigators compared the findings of MR imaging, CT, and surgery in 33 patients being staged for pulmonary carcinoma.[62] In 29 of the 33 patients, CT and MR imaging provided identical interpretations of lymph nodes being normal (less than 10 mm), suspicious (10 to 15 mm), or abnormal (greater than 15 mm). MR and CT interpretations differed in 4 instances, and pathologic correlation was available in 3 of these patients. In 1 patient, CT suggested a subcarinal mass, differentiation from the left atrium not being possible; by contrast, MR imaging clearly defined the true extent of enlarged nodes. In 2 other patients, the superior resolution of CT permitted the identification of two or more discrete, normal-sized lymph nodes, whereas the impression on MR imaging was of a single, large abnormal mass.

Two studies were performed in the mid-1980s to prospectively assess patients with pulmonary carcinoma by CT and MR imaging. In the first, CT scans were carried out with contrast enhancement, whereas the MR images were not cardiac gated.[50] Nodes were considered enlarged when their short axis in transverse CT or MR section exceeded 10 mm. The investigators found no statistically significant differences between MR and CT images in the evaluation of tumor extent or node involvement. Both CT and MR imaging had a low sensitivity (60% for MR imaging and 53% for CT) and good specificity (93% for MR imaging and 97% for CT) in the detection of nodal metastases.[50] In the second study, MR and CT images were interpreted by three experienced radiologists using a five-point rating scale to permit receiver operating characteristic (ROC) analysis.[63] All MR images were cardiac gated to reduce cardiac motion artifacts and thus optimize visualization of the mediastinum. All three radiologists chose their own threshold value for enlarged nodes. Again, MR imaging and CT performed equally well, as indicated by similar areas under the ROC curves.

In another investigation of 120 patients who had pulmonary carcinoma, findings on MR and CT images were compared with those at mediastinoscopy and thoracotomy.[64] MR imaging had a slightly higher sensitivity than CT scanning (93% versus 79%) in the detection of mediastinal lymph node metastasis but a lower specificity (74% for MR imaging as compared with 82% for CT), which resulted in a similar diagnostic accuracy (81% for both modalities). Similar results were obtained by the Radiologic Diagnostic Oncology Group in a prospective cooperative multicenter study comparing MR and CT imaging in 170 patients with non–small cell pulmonary carcinoma.[65] The MR images were cardiac gated and the CT scans were performed following intravenous administration of contrast material. Analysis of the presence or not of lymph node enlargement was subjective, no specific node diameter being used to distinguish normal from abnormal nodes. The study demonstrated no significant difference between the diagnostic accuracy of MR and CT imaging in the detection of mediastinal lymph node metastasis, the sensitivities being 48% for MR imaging and 52% for CT and the specificities, 64% and 69%, respectively. ROC analysis also showed no difference between MR imaging and CT.

The use of dynamic contrast-enhanced MR imaging to distinguish benign from malignant mediastinal lymph nodes shows some promise. In one study, nine patients with biopsy-proven pulmonary carcinoma underwent dynamic MR imaging after administration of a bolus of gadoterate meglumine;[66] MR images were compared with pathologic specimens obtained at surgical resection. With dynamic contrast-enhanced MR imaging, the nodes containing carcinoma had a peak enhancement at 60 to 80 seconds with a slow decrease until 6 minutes. By comparison, anthracotic lymph nodes and nodes showing granulomatous inflammation displayed less enhancement with no peak within 6 minutes.

Several conclusions can be drawn from these studies.

1. Both CT and MR imaging are capable of identifying normal and abnormal lymph nodes; however, the superior resolution of CT is better suited for the identification and separation of small (usually normal) lymph nodes.

2. Whereas the sensitivity of CT and MR imaging is comparable in the mediastinum, the specificity of CT is greater, probably as a result of inferior MR image resolution.

3. It may be possible in the future to distinguish normal from abnormal lymph nodes on MR imaging by their different enhancement following intravenous administration of contrast agents.

LYMPH NODES OF THE HILA

Normal lymph nodes in the hila are inconspicuous and are not demonstrable as separate units on the chest radiograph or non–contrast-enhanced CT scan. However, with intravenous contrast material and the use of a spiral or dynamic incremental technique, their identification is possible with CT.[58, 59, 67]

The relation of hilar lymph nodes to the bronchi and pulmonary vessels was assessed in 1983 on the basis of transverse scans of four cadavers.[58] Patients were also studied in a clinical setting with dynamic contrast-enhanced CT scans (25 ml contrast medium, four rapid-sequence scans at each level of interest, 4.8-second scan time with a 1.4-second interscan delay). The investigators classified the lymph nodes in the right hilum into four groups—right upper lobe, descending right pulmonary artery, middle lobe, and lower lobe—and in the left hilum into three groups—left upper lobe, descending pulmonary artery, and lower lobe.

A more detailed analysis of the appearance of normal hilar lymph nodes and the adjacent soft tissue was performed in 1995 by using contrast-enhanced spiral CT.[67] Forty-two right and 45 left hila were systemically evaluated in healthy patients. Assessment of the mediastinal and hilar vessels and lymph nodes was performed on 5-mm-thick sections with a table feed of 5 mm/sec (pitch = 1) and reconstruction of overlapped images (3-mm intervals). The images were obtained following intravenous administration of contrast material and during a single breath-hold of 24 seconds, which allowed a scanning length of 12 cm and a total of 52 sections. Hilar lymph nodes were identified as nonenhancing areas of soft tissue attenuation in the anatomic groups described in the 1983 study cited earlier (Fig. 7–21).[58] The nodes measured less than 3 mm in diameter.[67]

On the right side at the level of the upper lobe bronchus, the most frequent site of hypoattenuation (corresponding to normal hilar lymph nodes and seen in 33 of 42 [79%] cases) was usually linear and located lateral to the truncus anterior of the right pulmonary artery. At the level of the right interlobar pulmonary artery, a triangular area of hypoattenuation was seen lateral to the bronchus intermedius in 32 of 42 (76%) cases. At the level of the right middle lobe bronchus, the most frequent sites of attenuation were lateral to the bronchus and medial to the right lower lobe pulmonary artery (30 of 42 [71%] cases). The lower lobe group was seen most commonly at the level of origin of the basilar segmental bronchi (17 of 42 [40%] cases).

On the left side, the upper lobe group was most commonly seen as a focal area of hypoattenuation in close contact with the anterior wall of the left main pulmonary artery (28 of 45 [62%] cases). The descending pulmonary artery group was always identified between the anteromedial wall of the left pulmonary artery and the left upper lobe bronchus and was seen in all 45 cases. The investigators also noted a lingular group of lymph nodes that was seen as a partial or complete rim of hypoattenuation adjacent to the medial border of the pulmonary arteries—a constant finding in all 45 cases. The left lower lobe group of nodes was seen most commonly at the angle of bifurcation of the basal segmental bronchi, usually lateral to the bronchi and medial

to the corresponding pulmonary arteries (18 of 45 [40%] cases). Lymph nodes were also seen with lower frequency at various other levels of the hila.

In five patients, areas of hilar hypoattenuation were selected on preoperative enhanced CT scans and compared with findings at thoracotomy and ipsilateral hilar dissection.[67] In all cases, resected lymph nodes at the level of specific hypoattenuated areas confirmed the CT findings.

LYMPHATIC DRAINAGE OF THE LUNGS

Much of our knowledge of patterns of regional lymph node drainage from the lung derives from Rouvière's treatise on the anatomy of the human lymphatic system, published in 1938; the investigation was based on autopsy studies of 200 fetuses, neonates, and children.[68] Many of his observations have since been confirmed.[69, 70] Rouvière subdivided the lungs into three main drainage areas—superior, middle, and inferior—without correspondence to the pulmonary lobes.

On the right side, lymph drains from the superior area directly into the paratracheal and upper bronchopulmonary nodes. The middle zone drains directly into the paratracheal nodes, the bifurcation nodes, and the central group of bronchopulmonary nodes. The inferior zone drains into the inferior bronchopulmonary and bifurcation nodes and the posterior mediastinal chain. Thus on the right side, all the lymph drains eventually via the right lymphatic duct.

In the left superior area, lymph drains into the prevascular group of anterior mediastinal nodes and directly into the left paratracheal nodes. The middle zone drains mainly into the bifurcation and central group of bronchopulmonary nodes and in part directly into the left paratracheal group. The inferior zone drains into the bifurcation and inferior bronchopulmonary nodes and into the posterior mediastinal chain. Thus according to Rouvière, the superior portion and part of the middle zone drain via the left paratracheal nodes into the thoracic duct, whereas lymph from the remainder of the left lung eventually empties into the right lymphatic duct.

Although this "crossover" phenomenon was long

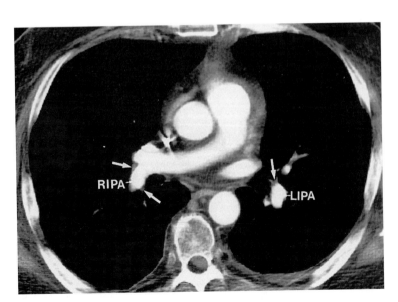

Figure 7–21. Normal Hilar Nodes on Contrast-Enhanced CT. Localized areas of hypoattenuation representing normal hilar lymph nodes can be seen adjacent to the proximal right interlobar pulmonary artery (RIPA) and left interlobar pulmonary artery (LIPA) *(arrows).*

thought to be of diagnostic and therapeutic importance in diseases originating in the middle or lower portion of the left lung, more recent studies have cast some doubt on the validity of the phenomenon in adults. For example, in one study of 17 consecutive autopsies of patients who had primary carcinoma of the left lung, only 1 had contralateral prescalene node metastases;[71] unfortunately, the sites of origin in the left lung were not stated. Similarly, a review of bilateral prescalene node biopsies in 218 patients (110 of whom had pulmonary carcinoma) showed the direction of lymphatic spread within the mediastinum to be cephalad and usually ipsilateral, irrespective of the location of the primary growth.[72] Contralateral spread was uncommon and about equally frequent from either lung.

REFERENCES

1. Masada S, Ichikawa S, Nakamura Y, et al: Structure and distribution of the lymphatic vessels in the parietal pleura of the monkey as studied by enzyme-histochemistry and light and electron microscopy. Arch Histol Cytol 55:525, 1992.
2. Li J: Ultrastructural study on the pleural stomata in human. Funct Dev Morphol 3:277, 1993.
3. Li J, Jiang B: A scanning electron microscopic study on three-dimensional organization of human diaphragmatic lymphatics. Funct Dev Morphol 3:129, 1993.
4. Wang NS: The preformed stomas connecting the pleural cavity and the lymphatics in the parietal pleura. Am Rev Respir Dis 111:12, 1975.
5. Abu-Hijleh MF, Habbal OA, Moqattash ST: The role of the diaphragm in lymphatic absorption from the peritoneal cavity. J Anat 186:453, 1995.
6. Lauweryns JM: The blood and lymphatic microcirculation of the lung. In Sommers SC (ed): Pulmonary Pathology Decennial; 1966–1975. New York, Appleton-Century-Crofts, 1975, p 1.
7. Miller WS: The Lung. Springfield, IL, Charles C Thomas, 1937.
8. Hendin AS, Greenspan RH: Ventilatory pumping of human pulmonary lymphatic vessels. Radiology 108:553, 1973.
9. Lauweryns JM, Baert JH: Alveolar clearance and the role of the pulmonary lymphatics. State of the art. Am Rev Respir Dis 115:625, 1977.
10. Lauweryns JM: The juxta-alveolar lymphatics in the human adult lung. Histologic studies in 15 cases of drowning. Am Rev Respir Dis 102:877, 1970.
11. Scfraufnagel DE: Forms of lung lymphatics: A scanning electron microscopic study of casts. Anat Rec 233:547, 1992.
12. Peao MN, Aguas AP, de Sa CM, et al: Scanning electron microscopy of the deep lymphatic network of the murine lung as viewed in corrosion casts. Lymphology 26:42, 1993.
13. Marchetti C, Poggi P, Clement MG, et al: Lymphatic capillaries of the pig lung: TEM and SEM observations. Anat Rec 238:378, 1994.
14. Hainis KD, Sznajder JI, Schraufnagel DE: Lung lymphatics cast from the airspace. Am J Physiol 267:L199, 1994.
15. Drinker CK: Extravascular protein and the lymphatic system. Ann N Y Acad Sci 46:807, 1946.
16. Fleischner FG: The butterfly pattern of acute pulmonary edema. Am J Cardiol 20:39, 1967.
17. Warren MF, Drinker CK: The flow of lymph from the lungs of the dog. Am J Physiol 136:207, 1942.
18. Rosenberger A, Abrams HL: Radiology of the thoracic duct. Am J Roentgenol 11:807, 1971.
19. Hendin AS: Postmortem demonstration of inspiratory constriction of deep lymphatic vessels of the human lung. Radiology 9:1, 1974.
20. Fuchs WA, Galeazzi RL: The radiographic anatomy of the thoracic duct (in German). Radiologe 10:180, 1970.
21. Abramson DI: Blood Vessels and Lymphatics. New York, Academic Press, 1962, p 703.
22. Beck E, Beattie EJ Jr: The lymph nodes in the mediastinum. J Int Coll Surg 29:247, 1958.
23. Heitzman ER: Royal College Lecture: Radiologic diagnosis of mediastinal lymph node enlargement. J Can Assoc Radiol 29:151, 1978.
24. Yamashita H: Anatomy of hilar lymph nodes. In Roentgenologic Anatomy of the Lung. New York, Igaku-Shoin, 1978.
25. Glazer GM, Gross BH, Quint LE, et al: Normal mediastinal lymph nodes: Number and size according to American Thoracic Society mapping. Am J Roentgenol 144:261, 1985.
26. Genereux GP, Howie JL: Normal mediastinal lymph node size and number: CT and anatomic study. Am J Roentgenol 142:1095, 1984.
27. Osborne DR, Korobkin M, Ravin CE, et al: Comparison of plain radiography, conventional tomography, and computed tomography in detecting intrathoracic lymph node metastases from lung carcinoma. Radiology 142:157, 1982.
28. Baron RL, deVitt RG, Sagel SS, et al: Computed tomography in the preoperative evaluation of bronchogenic carcinoma. Radiology 145:727, 1982.
29. Moak GD, Cockerill EM, Farber MO, et al: Computed tomography vs. standard radiology in the evaluation of mediastinal adenopathy. Chest 82:69, 1982.
30. Faling LJ, Pagatch RD, Jung-Leggy Y, et al: Computed tomographic scanning of the mediastinum in the staging of bronchogenic carcinoma. Am Rev Respir Dis 124:690, 1981.
31. Schnyder PA, Gamsu G: CT of the pretracheal retrocaval space. Am J Roentgenol 136:303, 1981.
32. Glazer GM, Gross BH, Quint LE, et al: Normal mediastinal lymph nodes: Number and size according to American Thoracic Society mapping. Am J Roentgenol 144:261, 1985.
33. Berkman YM, Drossman SR, Marboe CC: Intersegmental (intersublobar) septum of the lower lobe in relation to the pulmonary ligament: Anatomic, histologic, and CT correlations. Radiology 185:389, 1992.
34. Glazer GM, Orringer MB, Gross BH, et al: The mediastinum in non–small cell lung cancer: CT-surgical correlation. Am J Roentgenol 152:1101, 1984.
35. Leigh TF, Weens HS: The Mediastinum. Springfield, IL, Charles C Thomas, 1959, pp 16–27.
36. Greenberg HB: Benign subpleural lymph node appearing as a pulmonary "coin" lesion. Radiology 77:97, 1961.
37. Kradin RL, Spirn PW, Mark EJ: Intrapulmonary lymph nodes—clinical, radiologic, and pathologic findings. Chest 87:662, 1985.
38. Trapnell DH: Recognition and incidence of intrapulmonary lymph nodes. Thorax 19:44, 1964.
38a. Yokomise H, Mizuno H, Ike O, et al: Importance of intrapulmonary lymph nodes in the differential diagnosis of small pulmonary nodular shadows. Chest 113:703, 1998.
39. Tisi GM, Friedman PJ, Peters RM, et al: American Thoracic Society, Medical Section of American Lung Association. Clinical staging of primary lung cancer. Am Rev Respir Dis 127:659, 1983.
40. Glazer HS, Aronberg DJ, Sagel SS, et al: CT demonstration of calcified mediastinal lymph nodes: A guide to the new ATS classification. Am J Roentgenol 147:17, 1986.
41. Friedman PJ: Lung cancer: Update on staging classifications. Am J Roentgenol 150:261, 1988.
42. Mountain CF: A new international staging system for lung cancer. Chest 89(Suppl):225, 1986.
42a. Mountain CF: Revisions in the International System for staging lung cancer. Chest 111:1710, 1997.
42b. Mountain CF, Dresler CM: Regional lymph node classification for lung cancer staging. Chest 111:1718, 1997.
43. Quint LE, Glazer GM, Orringer MB, et al: Mediastinal lymph node detection and sizing at CT and autopsy. Am J Roentgenol 147:469, 1986.
44. Kiyono K, Sone S, Sakai F, et al: The number and size of normal mediastinal lymph nodes: A postmortem study. Am J Roentgenol 150:771, 1988.
45. Müller NL, Webb WR, Gamsu G: Paratracheal lymphadenopathy: Radiographic findings and correlation with CT. Radiology 156:761, 1985.
46. Müller NL, Webb WR, Gamsu G: Subcarinal lymph node enlargement: Radiographic findings and CT correlation. Am J Roentgenol 145:15, 1985.
47. Platt JF, Glazer GM, Orringer MB, et al: Radiologic evaluation of the subcarinal lymph nodes: A comparative study. Am J Roentgenol 151:279, 1988.
48. Müller NL, Nichols DM: Accuracy of the plain radiograph in the detection of aortopulmonary lymphadenopathy. J Can Assoc Radiol 38:82, 1987.
49. Müller NL, Webb WR: Radiographic imaging of the pulmonary hila. Invest Radiol 20:661, 1985.
50. Musset D, Grenier P, Carette MF, et al: Primary lung cancer staging: Prospective comparative study of MR imaging with CT. Radiology 160:607, 1986.
51. Webb WR, Gamsu G, Stark DD, et al: Magnetic resonance imaging of the normal and abnormal pulmonary hila. Radiology 152:89, 1984.
52. Levitt RG, Glazer HS, Roper CL, et al: Magnetic resonance imaging of mediastinal and hilar masses: Comparison with CT. Am J Roentgenol 145:9, 1985.
53. Gupta NC, Frank AR, Dewan NA, et al: Solitary pulmonary nodules: Detection of malignancy with PET with 2-(F-18)-fluoro-2-deoxy-d-glucose. Radiology 184:441, 1992.
54. Valk PE, Pounds TR, Hopkins DM, et al: Staging non–small cell lung cancer by whole-body positron emission tomographic imaging. Ann Thorac Surg 60:1573, 1995.
55. Patz EF Jr, Lowe VJ, Goodman PC, et al: Thoracic nodal staging with PET imaging with [18]FDG in patients with bronchogenic carcinoma. Chest 108:1617, 1995.
56. Wahl RL, Quint LE, Greenough R, et al: Staging of mediastinal non–small cell lung cancer with FDG PET, CT, and fusion images: Preliminary prospective evaluation. Radiology 191:371, 1994.
57. Sazon DAD, Santiago SM, Hoo GWS, et al: Fluorodeoxyglucose–positron emission tomography in the detection and staging of lung cancer. Am J Respir Crit Care Med 153:417, 1996.
58. Sone S, Higashihara T, Morimoto S, et al: CT anatomy of hilar lymphadenopathy. Am J Roentgenol 140:887, 1983.
59. Glazer GM, Francis IR, Gebarski K, et al: Dynamic incremental computed tomography in evaluation of the pulmonary hila. J Comput Assist Tomogr 7:59, 1983.
60. Haramati LB, Cartagena AM, Austin JHM: CT evaluation of mediastinal lymphadenopathy: Noncontrast 5 mm vs postcontrast 10 mm sections. J Comput Assist Tomogr 19:375, 1995.
61. Heelan RT, Martini N, Westcott JW, et al: Carcinomatous involvement of the hilum and mediastinum: Computed tomographic and magnetic resonance evaluation. Radiology 156:111, 1985.
62. Webb WR, Jensen BG, Sollitto R, et al: Bronchogenic carcinoma: Staging with MR compared with staging with CT and surgery. Radiology 156:117, 1985.
63. Poon PY, Bronskill MJ, Henkelman RM, et al: Mediastinal lymph node metastases from bronchogenic carcinoma: Detection with MR imaging and CT. Radiology 162:651, 1987.
64. Laurent F, Drouillard J, Dorcier F, et al: Bronchogenic carcinoma staging: CT vs MR imaging—assessment with surgery. Eur J Cardiothorac Surg 2:31, 1988.
65. Webb WR, Gatsonis C, Zerhouni EA, et al: CT and MR imaging in staging non–small cell bronchogenic carcinoma: Report of the Radiologic Diagnostic Oncology Group. Radiology 178:705, 1991.
66. Laissy JP, Gay-Depassier P, Soyer P, et al: Enlarged mediastinal lymph nodes in bronchogenic carcinoma: Assessment with dynamic contrast-enhanced MR imaging. Radiology 191:263, 1994.

67. Remy-Jardin M, Duyck P, Remy J, et al: Hilar lymph nodes: Identification with spiral CT and histologic correlation. Radiology 196:387, 1995.
68. Rouvière H: Anatomy of the Human Lymphatic System (translated by MJ Tobias). Ann Arbor, MI, Edwards, 1938.
69. Nohl HC: An investigation into the lymphatic and vascular spread of carcinoma of the bronchus. Thorax 11:172, 1956.
70. McCort JJ, Robbins LL: Roentgen diagnosis of intrathoracic lymph node metastases in carcinoma of the lung. Radiology 57:339, 1951.
71. Klingenberg I: Histopathologic findings in the prescalene tissue from 1,000 postmortem cases. Acta Chir Scand 127:57, 1964.
72. Baird JA: The pathways of lymphatic spread of carcinoma of the lung. Br J Surg 52:868, 1965.

CHAPTER 8

The Mediastinum

THORACIC INLET, 197
ANTERIOR MEDIASTINAL AREA, 198
  The Thymus, 198
    Anatomy, 198
    Radiology, 200
  Anterior Junction Anatomy, 201
  Retrosternal Stripe, Parasternal Stripe, and Cardiac
    Incisura, 204
SUPRA-AORTIC AREA, 205
  Left Subclavian Artery, 208
  Left Superior Intercostal Vein, 209
  Other Structures, 211
INFRA-AORTIC AREA, 211
  Aortopulmonary Window and Aortopulmonary
    Line, 211
  Posterior Pleural Reflections, 212
  Preaortic Recess, 216
SUPRA-AZYGOS AREA, 218
  Azygos and Hemiazygos Veins, 218
  Tracheal Interfaces, 219
  Posterior Junction Anatomy, 223
  Right and Left Superior Esophageal Stripes, 223
  Azygos Arch, 223
  Vascular Pedicle, 227
INFRA-AZYGOS AREA, 228
  Azygoesophageal Recess, 228
THE HEART, 229

The mediastinum divides the thorax vertically into two compartments and can thus be defined anatomically as the partition between the lungs.[1] Considerable controversy has raged over the years concerning the most practical and informative method of dividing the mediastinum into compartments radiologically, and several classifications have been proposed.[2–5] This controversy originated in part from the inherent anatomic complexity of the mediastinum and in part from the difficulty in understanding its anatomy from conventional posteroanterior (PA) and lateral chest radiographs. This anatomic understanding has been greatly facilitated with the advent of CT and MR imaging techniques, which allow direct assessment of the location of the various mediastinal structures. Awareness of normal and abnormal mediastinal anatomy as seen on PA and lateral chest radiographs, however, remains essential because mediastinal abnormalities are frequently first suspected on the chest radiograph. Moreover, the need for further investigation and the optimal imaging modality to be used, whether CT, MR imaging, ultrasound, or barium swallow, are often dictated by the location of the abnormality and the tentative diagnosis

made on the radiograph. The following discussion will thus focus on the chest radiograph, with CT and MR imaging being used mainly as an aid in understanding the radiographic features.

According to classic teaching, the mediastinum is separated into superior and inferior compartments by an imaginary line extending from the sternal angle to the fourth intervertebral disk; the inferior compartment is further subdivided into anterior (prevascular), middle (cardiovascular), and posterior (postvascular) compartments.[1, 6] This arrangement has undoubtedly been the most popular and generally accepted classification of the mediastinal compartments over the years. Since each compartment contains anatomic structures almost unique to it, many of the afflictions to which the mediastinum is subject tend to occur *predominantly* in one or another compartment. A modification of this classification, used by us in the second edition of this book, was exclusion of the superior compartment since it contains structures that are for the most part continuous with the compartments below; thus its separation serves little diagnostic purpose.

In this modification of the traditional classification, the *anterior mediastinal compartment* is bounded anteriorly by the sternum and posteriorly by the pericardium, aorta, and brachiocephalic vessels. It is narrowest anteriorly, where the pleura of the right and left upper lobes converges to form the anterior junction line (*see* farther on); it broadens posterosuperiorly in an apex-down triangular configuration to form the anterior mediastinal triangle. The compartment contains the thymus gland, branches of the internal mammary artery and vein, lymph nodes, the inferior sternopericardial ligament, and variable amounts of fat.

The *middle mediastinal compartment* contains the pericardium and its contents, the ascending and transverse portions of the aorta, the superior and inferior vena cava, the brachiocephalic (innominate) arteries and veins, the phrenic nerves and cephalad portion of the vagus nerves, the trachea and main bronchi and their contiguous lymph nodes, and the pulmonary arteries and veins.

The *posterior mediastinal compartment* is bounded anteriorly by the pericardium and the vertical part of the diaphragm, laterally by the mediastinal pleura, and posteriorly by the bodies of the thoracic vertebrae. It contains the descending thoracic aorta, esophagus, thoracic duct, azygos and hemiazygos veins, autonomic nerves, fat, and lymph nodes. Although strictly speaking the paravertebral gutters are not part of the mediastinum, for practical purposes, abnormalities within them are sometimes included in discussion of the posterior mediastinum.

Although Heitzman thinks that this classification contains certain deficiencies and limitations because it is insufficiently based on radiologic anatomy and minimizes detailed anatomic analysis,[3] we believe that it is a reasonable approach, particularly when combined with CT, and use it to describe the location of mediastinal *abnormalities* throughout the book. Nonetheless, because the Heitzman method of classification provides a systematic approach to the description of mediastinal *anatomy* as seen on the chest radiograph, we will be using his outline in this chapter to describe normal radiographic findings. According to the Heitzman classification, the normal mediastinum can be divided into six anatomic regions:[3]

1. *The thoracic inlet*: a region with a narrow cephalocaudad dimension marking the cervicothoracic junction and lying immediately above and below a transverse plane through the first rib.

2. *The anterior mediastinum*: a region extending from the thoracic inlet to the diaphragm in front of the heart, ascending aorta, and superior vena cava.

The remaining four subdivisions reside behind the anterior mediastinum and depend on the relationship of anatomic structures to the arches of the aorta and azygos vein. They include structures in the middle and posterior mediastinum.

3. *The supra-aortic area*: the region above the aortic arch.

4. *The infra-aortic area*: the region below the aortic arch.

5. *The supra-azygos area*: the region above the azygos arch.

6. *The infra-azygos area*: the region below the azygos arch.

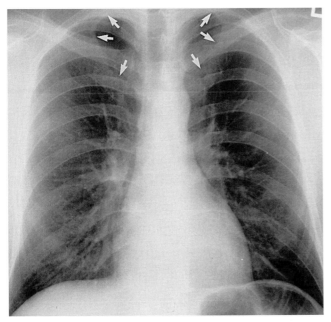

Figure 8–1. Normal Thoracic Inlet. A posteroanterior chest radiograph from a 40-year-old man demonstrates the normal appearance of the thoracic inlet. Because the inlet parallels the first rib *(arrows)*, it is higher posteriorly than anteriorly.

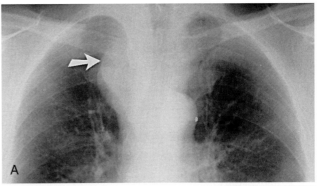

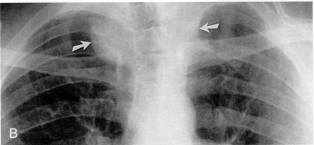

Figure 8–2. Cervicothoracic Sign. A posteroanterior (PA) chest radiograph *(A)* from a 69-year-old man with a thyroid goiter demonstrates a mass in the thoracic inlet *(arrow)* displacing the trachea to the left. The mass is effaced above the level of the clavicle because it is anterior and lateral to the trachea and therefore continuous with the soft tissues of the neck. A PA chest radiograph *(B)* from a 34-year-old patient demonstrates bilateral paraspinal soft tissue opacities *(arrows)* above the level of the clavicles. These are well seen at this level because they are situated posterior to the trachea. The patient had bilateral paraspinal hydatid cysts with involvement of the T3 vertebral body.

The descriptions that follow have been derived from several sources to which reference will be made in the appropriate sections. However, the bulk of the material, including the classification, has come from Heitzman's treatise on the mediastinum.[3] Other reviews have also been published,[7–9] including some with emphasis on CT.[10, 11]

THORACIC INLET

The thoracic inlet, or cervicomediastinal continuum, represents the junction between structures at the base of the neck and those of the thorax. It parallels the first rib and is thus higher posteriorly than anteriorly (Fig. 8–1). On the basis of this anatomic observation, it is evident that an opacity on a PA chest radiograph that is effaced on its superior aspect and that projects at or below the level of the clavicles must be situated anteriorly, whereas one that projects above the clavicles is retrotracheal and posteriorly situated (Fig. 8–2). These characteristic findings have together been termed the *cervicothoracic sign*.[12]

From front to back, structures occupying the thoracic inlet include the upper portion of the thymus gland, the right and left brachiocephalic veins (which join behind the right side of the manubrium to form the superior vena cava), the common carotid arteries (lying immediately anterior to the subclavian arteries and medial to the subclavian veins), the trachea (situated either in the midline or slightly to the right or left immediately behind the great vessels), the esophagus (located behind the trachea and in front of the spine), and the recurrent laryngeal nerves on either side of the esophagus (Figs. 8–3 and 8–4). The lower trunk of the brachial plexus is situated immediately behind the subclavian artery in relation to the first rib; the vagus and phrenic nerves enter the thorax in front of the subclavian arteries and behind the great veins. The thoracic duct is situated along the left side of the esophagus, from which point it arches anteriorly to terminate at the junction of the left internal jugular and subclavian veins.

A fascial envelope, the *deep cervical fascia*, surrounds the deep structures of the neck and divides into three layers that define distinct compartments.

1. The posterior layer *(prevertebral fascia)* delineates the prevertebral space, which extends from the occipital bone to the thorax, where it becomes continuous with the anterior longitudinal ligament of the spine. Pathologic processes within the prevertebral space of the neck (e.g., an abscess secondary to infectious spondylitis) can extend caudally to the thoracic inlet but usually not below this point because of merging of the fascia with the anterior longitudinal ligament.

2. The middle layer *(pretracheal fascia)* lies anterior to the trachea and extends inferiorly from the thyroid gland into the thorax, where it blends with the fascia that surrounds the aorta and pericardium. The pretracheal fascia anteriorly, the prevertebral fascia posteriorly, and the carotid sheaths laterally define a visceral compartment that extends from the neck into the mediastinum (cervicothoracic continuum);[13] this compartment contains the pharynx, larynx, trachea, and esophagus and is continuous with the mediastinum across the thoracic inlet. Pathologic processes arising in this compartment (such as a retropharyngeal abscess) can readily

spread inferiorly into the mediastinum; similarly, various abnormalities originating in the mediastinum (such as abscess or hemorrhage) can extend upward into the neck.

3. At the level of the thyroid gland, the anterior layer of the deep cervical fascia forms the suprasternal space, which encloses the salivary gland, the mastoid process, and the mandible. Infections arising from these structures can enter the suprahyoid space but are generally confined there by the fascial planes and seldom extend into the mediastinum. However, it is by this route that goiters usually extend from the neck inferiorly to become retrosternal. (Occasionally, goiters grow into the mediastinum posteriorly rather than anteriorly and descend along the perivisceral fascia around the trachea and esophagus; this modification is almost invariably right sided and is confined to the supra-azygos area.)

ANTERIOR MEDIASTINAL AREA

The anterior mediastinum is bounded anteriorly by the sternum and posteriorly by the pericardium, aorta, and brachiocephalic vessels. It merges superiorly with the anterior aspect of the thoracic inlet and extends down to the level of the diaphragm.

The Thymus

Anatomy

The thymus gland is located in the anterosuperior portion of the mediastinum and, in adults, generally extends from a point above the manubrium to the fourth costal cartilage. Posteriorly, it relates to the trachea, aortic arch and its branches, and the pericardium covering the ascending aorta and main pulmonary artery (Fig. 8–5). Most glands have a roughly bilobed structure, probably reflecting embryologic derivation from the bilateral third pharyngeal pouches.[3] Nevertheless, variations in gross morphology are not uncommon, and unilobed, trilobed, and irregularly shaped glands have been described.

As a proportion of body weight, the thymus is largest at birth and during infancy. The absolute mean weight tends to increase slightly during the first decade of life and decrease slightly thereafter.[14] However, there is a wide variation in normal thymic weight at different ages,[14, 15] the range of normal probably being 5 to 50 gm. Histologically, the thymus is divided by thin fibrous septa into lobules of variable size.[16, 17] The lobules themselves can be subdivided into cortical and medullary regions (Fig. 8–6). Although both are composed of lymphocytes and epithelial cells, the lymphocytes in the cortical region are less mature and more closely packed than those in the medulla, which gives it a darker appearance on standard light microscopy.

Thymic epithelial cells are variable in morphology and can be subdivided into a variety of types based on their ultrastructural appearance.[18] In the cortical region, these cells separate blood vessels from lymphocytes in a fashion similar to the blood-brain barrier. In the medullary region, small aggregates of keratinized epithelial cells (Hassall's corpuscles) are commonly present. Other epithelial cells may also

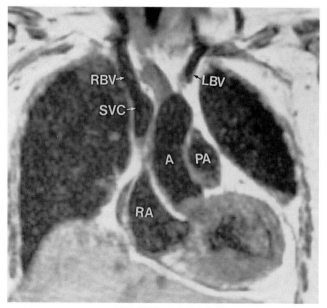

Figure 8–3. Normal MR Image of the Thoracic Inlet. A coronal MR image from a 64-year-old woman demonstrates the right brachiocephalic vein (RBV) joining the superior vena cava (SVC) and forming the lateral margin of the right thoracic inlet. Also seen are the left brachiocephalic vein (LBV) surrounded by fat, ascending aorta (A), right atrium (RA), and main pulmonary artery (PA).

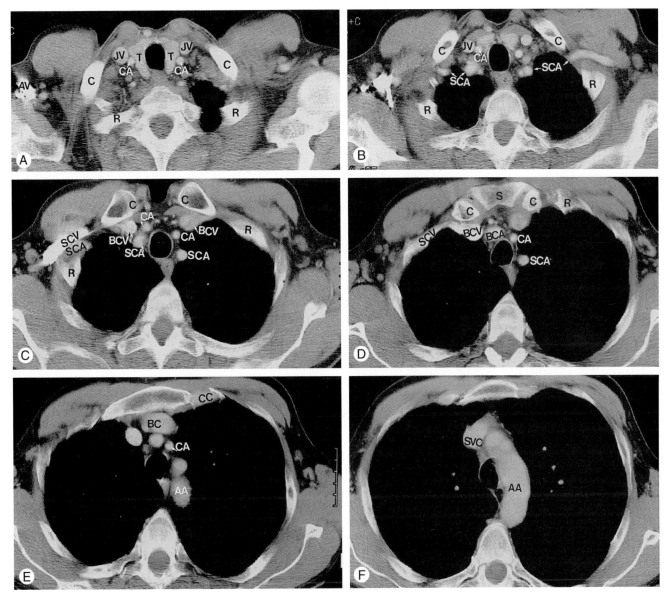

Figure 8–4. Normal CT Scan of the Thoracic Inlet. A contrast-enhanced CT scan in a 51-year-old man illustrates the normal anatomy of the thoracic inlet. *A,* A CT scan at the level of the posterior aspect of the first rib (R) demonstrates the left lung apex, clavicles (C), thyroid gland (T), jugular veins (JV), and carotid arteries (CA). Contrast injected into a right antecubital vein resulted in marked enhancement of the right axillary vein (AV). The thyroid gland surrounds the anterior and lateral aspects of the trachea in the lower part of the neck, whereas the esophagus lies immediately posterior to the trachea. *B,* A CT scan at the level of the lateral aspect of the first ribs demonstrates the subclavian arteries (SCA), carotid arteries, jugular veins, and inferior aspect of the thyroid gland. *C,* A CT scan at the level of the anteromedial aspect of the first ribs demonstrates the right subclavian vein (SCV) lying anterior to the subclavian artery, the proximal portions of the subclavian arteries, and the carotid arteries. The right and left brachiocephalic veins (BCV) can be seen anterior to the carotid arteries. The medial portion of the clavicle anterior to the first ribs outlines the region of the suprasternal notch. The esophagus is situated immediately posterior to the trachea. *D,* A CT scan at the level of the anterior aspect of the first ribs demonstrates the left costochondral junction, the upper aspect of the sternum (S), and the clavicles at the level of the sternoclavicular joint. At this level, the right subclavian vein (SCU) can be seen joining the brachiocephalic vein (anterolateral to the brachiocephalic artery [BCA]). The left brachiocephalic vein is seen anterolateral to the left carotid artery. At this level, as with the higher levels, the left subclavian artery and surrounding fat can be seen to form the left lateral margin of the thoracic inlet. *E,* A CT scan at the level of the first costal cartilage (CC) demonstrates the left brachiocephalic (BC) vein crossing the midline anterior to the brachiocephalic and carotid arteries. Also seen is the left subclavian artery as it originates from the uppermost aspect of the aortic arch (AA). *F,* A CT scan at the level of the aortic arch (AA) demonstrates the origin of the brachiocephalic and left carotid arteries from the aorta. At this level, the left brachiocephalic vein can be seen joining the superior vena cava (SVC).

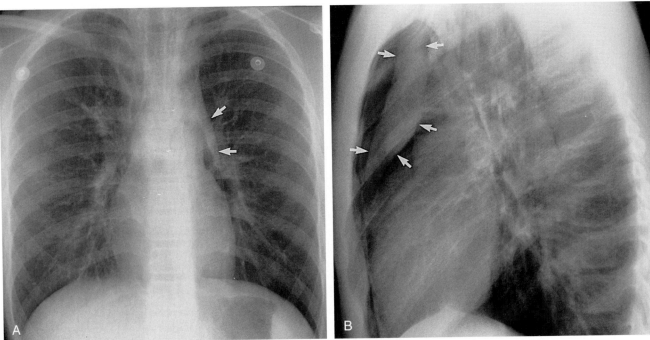

Figure 8–5. Normal Thymus Delineated by Pneumomediastinum. Posteroanterior *(A)* and lateral *(B)* chest radiographs in a 10-year-old boy with pneumomediastinum demonstrate the normal location of the thymus, which is outlined by surrounding air *(arrows)*. Note that the left lobe of the thymus is larger than the right lobe.

be recognized on the basis of antigen expression.[19] These variations in antigenicity and structure presumably reflect functional differences related to antigen processing and lymphocyte differentiation.

Other cells that can be found in the normal thymus include CD1-positive dendritic cells analogous to Langerhans' cells,[20] cells with immunohistochemical evidence of muscle proteins such as myoglobin and actin (myoid cells),[21] and neuroendocrine cells.[22]

Radiology

On conventional radiographs of the chest, the thymus is visible only in infants and young children, in whom it fills much of the anterior mediastinal space. Although the gland attains its maximal weight in people between 12 and 19 years of age,[23] it is inconstantly visible radiographically after the age of 2 or 3 years, an apparent paradox explained by the fact that the body is also growing and the ratio of thymic weight to body weight decreases with age. In addition to its location, three radiographic signs aid identification of the normal thymus gland: the *thymic notch sign*, seen as an indentation in the thymic contour at the junction of the thymus and the heart, either unilaterally or bilaterally; the *sail sign* (present in only 5% of infants), related to the presence of a triangular opacity of thymic tissue that projects to the right or left (or sometimes both);[24] and the *thymic wave sign*, seen as a rippled or undulating contour of the thymic border caused by anterior rib indentation (Fig. 8–7).

In one CT study of the normal thymus of 154 subjects, the gland was recognized in 100% of patients under 30 years of age, in 73% of patients between the ages of 30 and 49 years, and in 17% of patients over 49 years of age.[23] The maximal size was observed in individuals between 12 and 19 years of age, regression occurring between 20 and 60 years and usually associated with fatty replacement of the parenchyma; by the age of 60 years, the thymus was estimated to weigh 50% less than at age 19 years. Sixty-two per cent of normal glands showed an arrowhead configuration, whereas 32% had separate right and left lobes (Fig. 8–7). The shape of the separate lobes was highly variable, being ovoid, elliptical, triangular, or semilunar. In 6% of cases, only a right or left lobe was identified. In a comparison CT study of thymic morphology in 309 normal subjects and 23 patients with clinically or surgically proved thymic abnormality, thymic shape was found to reliably separate normal from abnormal glands; specifically, multilobularity was never a feature of a normal gland at any age and was seen only in patients who had thymic disease.[25]

In the study of 154 subjects mentioned previously, the left lobe was almost invariably larger than the right.[23] The CT width (Fig. 8–8) tended to decrease in older patients, although this was not statistically significant. The mean width of the right and left lobes in the 6- to 19-year-old group was 20 mm (±5.5 mm SD) and 33 mm (±11 mm SD), respectively; in the 40- to 49-year-old group, the width was 14 mm (±6.6 mm SD) and 19 mm (±7.6 mm SD), respectively. By contrast, the thickness (short axis or transverse dimension of a lobe) displayed a statistically significant decrease between the 6- to 19-year-old and the 40- to 49-year-old comparison groups; the thickness of the right and left lobes in these two age categories was 10 mm (±3.9 mm SD) and 11 mm (±4.0 mm SD) and 6 mm (±2.3 mm SD) and 6 mm (±2.0 mm SD), respectively.

The CT attenuation values of the thymus decrease with age: under 19 years, the attenuation value is equal to or higher than that of the chest wall musculature; in the majority of patients over 40 years of age, however, the density approaches that of fat (*see* Fig. 8–7).[23]

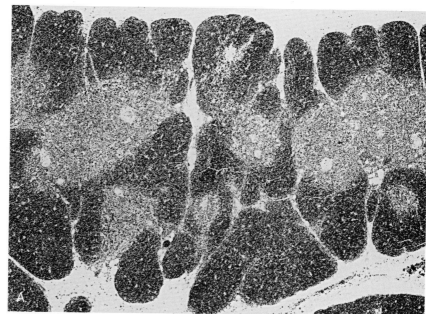

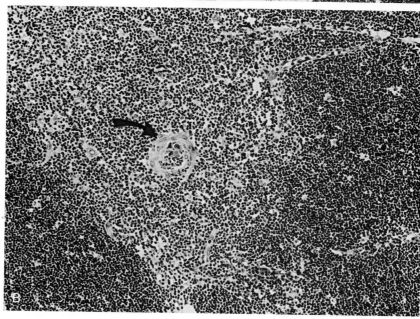

Figure 8–6. Normal Thymus Gland. A portion of a normal thymus *(A)* shows it to be divided by thin fibrous bands into numerous, variably sized lobules. The dark cortex and pale medulla are clearly visible. Magnified view *(B)* showing Hassall's corpuscle *(arrow)* and numerous lymphocytes (more densely packed in the cortex). *(A, ×40; B, ×130.)*

The thymus gland may decrease in size with physical stress, burns, illness, or the administration of corticosteroids and return to normal size or become enlarged secondary to hyperplasia after recovery (*see also* page 2875).[26–28] This size variation is observed most commonly in children, but has also been described in adults following chemotherapy for malignant testicular tumors.[29] In a study of 200 patients who had the latter abnormality, thymic enlargement developed 3 to 14 months after initiation of treatment in 14 of 120 patients (11.6%) who received chemotherapy as compared with only 1 of 80 patients who received no treatment.[29]

It has been suggested that MR imaging may permit more accurate assessment of the thymus gland than CT does.[30–32] In a study of the MR characteristics of the normal thymus in 18 individuals ranging in age from 5 to 77 years and without thymic or other mediastinal pathology, the thymus was visible in all patients regardless of age and

differed from subcutaneous fat in hydrogen density (the average thymus-to-fat hydrogen density ratio was 0.60).[32] Although the T1 relaxation times of the thymus were much longer than those of fat in patients under 30 years of age, this difference decreased with age. The thymus appeared thicker on MR images than on CT scans in patients older than 20 years.

Anterior Junction Anatomy

The pleura at the anteromedial portions of the right and left lungs contact the mediastinum in the retrosternal area to form the anterior junction line,[7] which defines the superior and inferior recesses. All three anatomic features show a typical, although somewhat variable appearance on the radio-

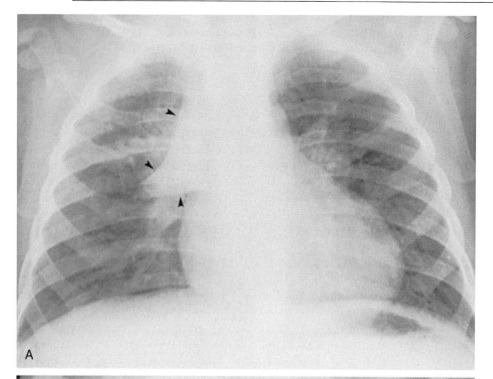

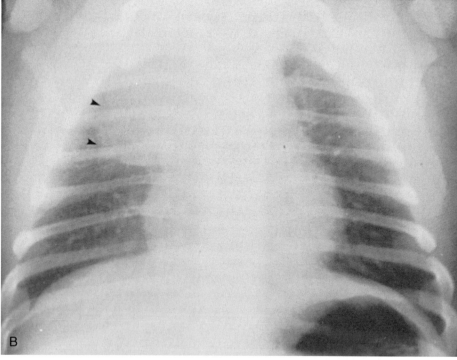

Figure 8–7. Normal Thymus Gland. An anteroposterior radiograph of an infant *(A)* shows a triangular opacity *(arrowheads)* projecting into the right lung and simulating the sail of a boat (the *sail sign*). An anteroposterior chest radiograph in another infant *(B)* shows gentle undulations *(arrowheads)* along the contour of the opacity caused by impression from the anterior ribs (the *thymic wave sign*).

graph that depends largely on the quantity of mediastinal fat and the degree of lung inflation.

Superior Recesses. As viewed on a PA radiograph, the right and left superior recesses are formed by the contact of lung with the retromanubrial mediastinum; typically they marginate a V-shaped area, the *anterior mediastinal triangle,* the apex of which points caudally (Fig. 8–9). The right and left boundaries of this triangle are formed by mediastinal fat in front of or contiguous with the brachiocephalic veins.[7] Displacement of the superior recesses to the right has been

described as a secondary sign of right lower lobe atelectasis caused by intrusion of a hyperinflated left upper lobe into the right hemithorax.[33] We have also seen displacement of the anterior mediastinal triangle into the left hemithorax in association with left lower lobe atelectasis.

Anterior Junction Line. As the two lungs approximate anteromedially, they are separated by four layers of pleura and a variable quantity of intervening mediastinal adipose tissue, thus forming a "septum" of variable thickness (the anterior junction line, anterior mediastinal line) (Fig. 8–9).

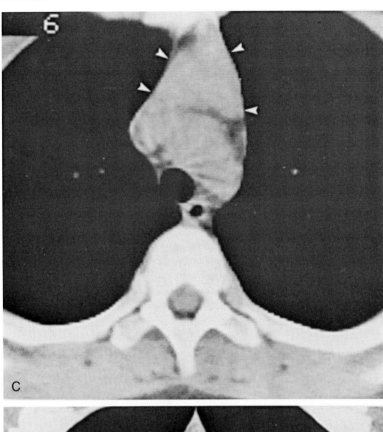

Figure 8–7 *Continued.* A CT scan through the superior mediastinum of a normal 15-year-old boy *(C)* reveals a triangular opacity *(arrowheads)*, the apex of which points forward whereas the base abuts the great vessels. CT density is equivalent to that of the chest wall musculature. CT scans through the superior mediastinum of an elderly man *(D)* disclose a thymus gland *(arrowheads)* composed of isolated nodular opacities and intervening fat (compare the CT density of the gland with that of the subcutaneous fat).

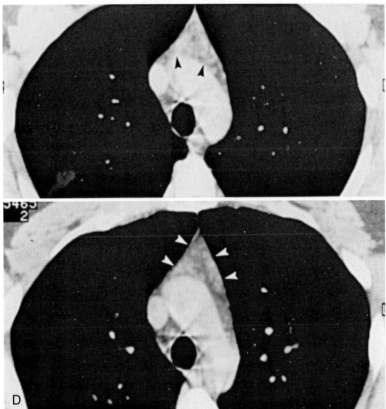

As seen on CT, this septum appears as a curvilinear opacity coursing vertically from front to back, angling to the right or to the left, and ranging in thickness from 1 to more than 3 mm. On a PA chest radiograph, the anterior junction line is typically oriented obliquely from the upper right to the lower left behind the sternum; cephalad, it begins at the apex of the anterior mediastinal triangle and continues caudally for several centimeters before terminating at the apex of the inferior recess. Since the septum dividing the two lungs is variable in thickness, the resulting opacity may be either a

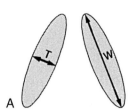

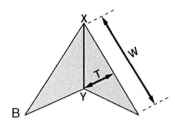

Figure 8–8. Measurement of Thymic Size. The two thymic lobes are measured separately. The width (W) corresponds to the long axis of the lobe as seen on the transverse CT scan, and the thickness (T) corresponds to the short-axis diameter *(A)*. When the two lobes are confluent, the thymus has a triangular or arrowhead shape *(B)*. The thymus is divided in half by a line through the anterior apex of the gland and perpendicular to it (X-Y). The width (W) and thickness (T) of each lobe are then measured.

line or a stripe; if the former, Mach band formation contributes strongly to its visibility. The anterior junction line may be displaced when there is loss of volume or overinflation of a lobe or lung (Fig. 8–10).

Inferior Recesses. Inferiorly, the anteromedial portions of the right and left lungs are further separated from one another by the heart and adjacent mediastinal fat; consequently, those lung surfaces in contact with the lower anterior mediastinum form interfaces that marginate an inverted V-shaped area known as the inferior recesses. On a lateral chest radiograph, the inferior recesses cannot be identified since they are not profiled; however, their posterior contour may be portrayed as components of the right and left cardiac incisuras (*see* farther on).

Retrosternal Stripe, Parasternal Stripe, and Cardiac Incisura

On a true lateral radiograph of the chest, the retrosternal region may be equal in radiolucency to the retrocardiac region as a result of apposition of the right and left lungs, which create little to no discernible shadow,[3] or be increased because of the presence of mediastinal fat.[34] In one study of

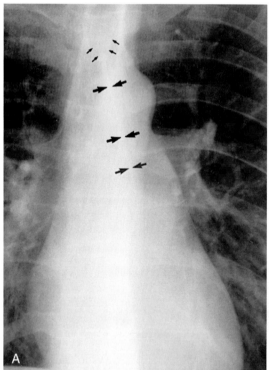

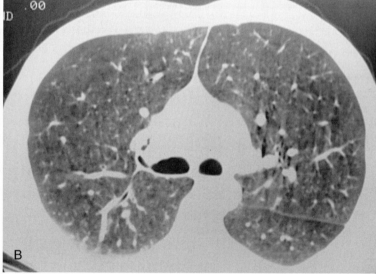

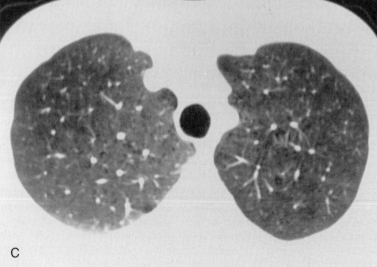

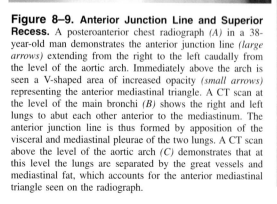

Figure 8–9. Anterior Junction Line and Superior Recess. A posteroanterior chest radiograph *(A)* in a 38-year-old man demonstrates the anterior junction line *(large arrows)* extending from the right to the left caudally from the level of the aortic arch. Immediately above the arch is seen a V-shaped area of increased opacity *(small arrows)* representing the anterior mediastinal triangle. A CT scan at the level of the main bronchi *(B)* shows the right and left lungs to abut each other anterior to the mediastinum. The anterior junction line is thus formed by apposition of the visceral and mediastinal pleurae of the two lungs. A CT scan above the level of the aortic arch *(C)* demonstrates that at this level the lungs are separated by the great vessels and mediastinal fat, which accounts for the anterior mediastinal triangle seen on the radiograph.

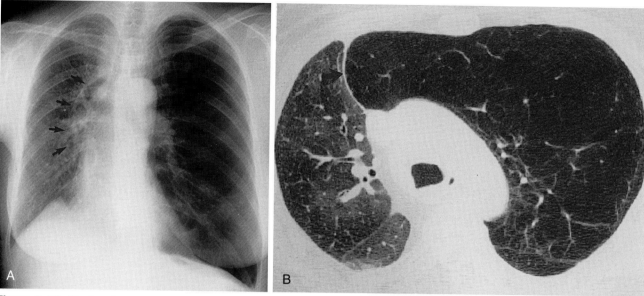

Figure 8–10. Displaced Anterior Junction Line. A posteroanterior chest radiograph *(A)* in a 54-year-old woman demonstrates marked displacement of the anterior junction line *(arrows)* to the right. This displacement is confirmed on the CT scan *(B)*, which shows herniation of the hyperinflated left lung to the right. The patient had undergone right lung transplantation for panacinar emphysema. The native left lung shows severe emphysema whereas the transplanted right lung is normal.

38 patients in which lateral chest radiographs and normal CT scans were reviewed, the retrosternal region had radiolucency equal to that of the retrocardiac region in 50% of patients;[34a] in 42%, it was more opaque than the retrocardiac region, and in 8% it was more radiolucent. The majority of patients with increased retrosternal radiopacity were women, and all 3 patients with increased radiolucency were men. There was no significant correlation between retrosternal opacity on the radiograph and mediastinal fat/thymus volume estimates or chest wall thickness on CT, age, weight-height index, or smoking history. When lung is excluded from the retrosternal space by mediastinal fat, a vertical retrosternal opacity, the *retrosternal stripe* (Fig. 8–11), is often seen.[34] In one investigation of 153 normal subjects, the average thickness of the retrosternal stripe was 2.7 mm (± 1.4 mm SD) and its maximal thickness 6.8 mm (3 SD greater than mean).[35] Although these measurements are occasionally of value in assessment of the upper half of the retrosternal shadow, they are seldom useful for the lower half because of wide variation in the retrosternal stripe in this region.

The lung can also contact the upper two thirds of the anterior chest wall, either to the right or left of the midline, thus outlining the parasternal areas and creating the *parasternal stripe* (Fig. 8–11).[34] This stripe is particularly prominent when the anterior surface of the lung is indented by costal cartilage and ribs, creating a lobulated contour (with each lobulation centered at the level of a rib). A lobulated contour can also be caused by enlargement of the internal mammary lymph nodes, tortuosity of the internal mammary arteries associated with coarctation of the aorta, and extrapleural hematomas associated with anterior rib fractures.

On the left side, as the sternum is followed inferiorly, the lung is normally excluded from the anteromedial chest wall by the cardiac apex, the epicardial fat pad, or both; this "deficiency" is termed the *cardiac incisura*. The interface between it and contiguous left lung has a variable appearance, including straight, angular, or rounded (Fig. 8–11). On the right side, the lung may also profile the lower third of the anteromedial wall of the chest, unless the right cardiophrenic angle fat pad causes separation as on the left (a common occurrence in our experience).

On a lateral projection, the superior limit of the anterior mediastinum behind the manubrium sometimes causes confusion in radiographic interpretation because of a smooth, homogeneous opacity that indents the lungs and simulates an anterior mediastinal mass. In a radiographic-morphologic correlative study of adult cadavers frozen in the erect position and sectioned in horizontal and sagittal planes, it was suggested that this slightly undulating interface is related to a composite of normal anatomic structures, the subclavian arteries causing the superior and posterior indentation and the innominate veins causing the inferior and anterior indentation.[36] These indentations were called the *vascular incisura,* analogous to their counterpart in the lower part of the thorax adjacent to the heart. The authors cautioned that the first costochondral junctions can cause an opacity similar to that formed by the venous indentation; although others have concurred in this interpretation,[34] in our experience the so-called venous vascular incisura is more commonly related to mediastinal fat surrounding the left innominate vein than to the vein itself.

SUPRA-AORTIC AREA

The supra-aortic area comprises that portion of the left side of the mediastinum extending from the aortic arch to the thoracic inlet, behind the anterior mediastinum. Structures included within this area are the left subclavian artery, the left wall of the trachea, the left superior intercostal vein, and mediastinal fat. Most of these structures are situated in the

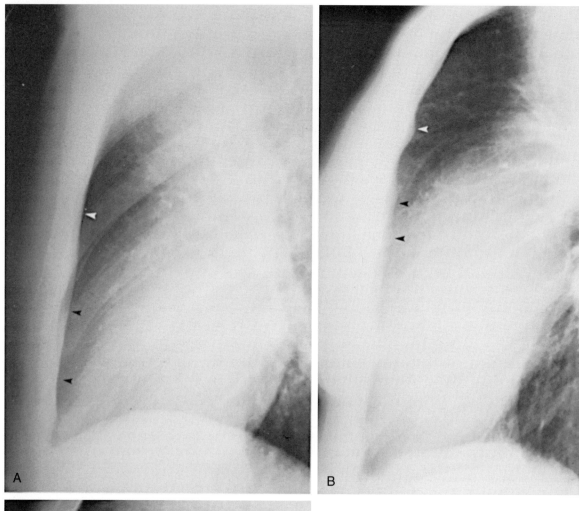

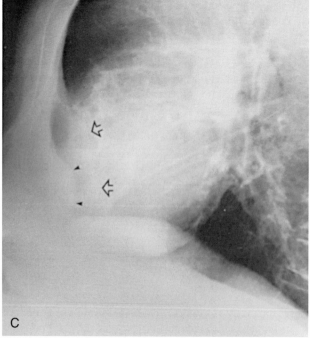

Figure 8–11. Lateral Radiographic Anatomy of the Anterior Mediastinum. A detail view from a lateral chest radiograph *(A)* shows a vertical retrosternal opacity that constitutes the *retrosternal stripe (arrowheads).* The stripe is formed as retrosternal mediastinal fat excludes coalition of the anteromedial portion of the right and left lungs. In another patient, a close-up view of a lateral chest radiograph *(B)* discloses an undulating stripe (the *parasternal stripe, arrowheads)* in which lobulation can be seen to relate to the anterior ribs. In a third patient, a conventional lateral chest radiograph *(C)* reveals a rounded opacity *(arrowheads)* overlying the anteroinferior aspect of the cardiac silhouette (the *cardiac incisura)*; a second curvilinear opacity *(open arrows)* is seen behind the incisura.

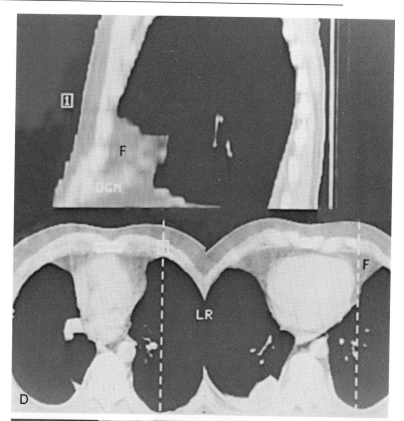

Figure 8–11 *Continued.* In *D,* a sagittal CT reformation slightly to the left of the cardiac apex *(above)* and appropriate transverse images *(below)* show that the more posterior opacity in *C* is formed by paracardiac mediastinal fat (F) contiguous with the cardiac apex. Note that the opacity relates to the epicardial fat pad and not to the cardiac apex. DGM, diaphragm. *E,* Similar features on CT scan were demonstrated on the *right,* thus accounting for the second, more anterior shadow.

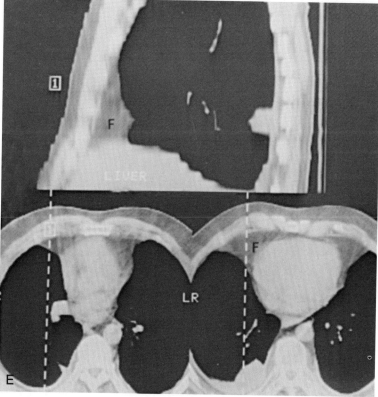

middle mediastinum. The left superior intercostal vein is located in the posterior mediastinum as it courses along the spine and in the middle mediastinum as it arches forward to drain into the left brachiocephalic vein. On a lateral radiograph of the chest, the area bounded by the posterior wall of the trachea, the top of the aortic arch, and the anterior surface of the thoracic vertebral bodies constitutes the *supra-aortic triangle.*

Left Subclavian Artery

The left subclavian artery arises from the aorta behind the left common carotid artery and passes upward lateral to the trachea in contact with the left mediastinal pleura. The subclavian artery and surrounding fat thus form an interface with the superomedial left upper lobe that can be identified on a PA radiograph as an arcuate opacity (concave laterally) extending from the aortic arch to a point at or just above the medial end of the clavicle (Fig. 8–12). At this point the vessel relates posteriorly to the scalenus anterior muscle, where its radiographic visibility depends on the depth of the groove it creates in the apical portion of the left lung. On a lateral radiograph, posteromedial lung can intrude above the aortic arch and in so doing may reveal either the posterior third or two thirds of the aortic arch (in about 75% of individuals); the area of obscuration between the outline of the ascending aorta and the aortic arch represents the sites of origin of the brachiocephalic artery, the left common carotid artery, and the left subclavian artery.[34]

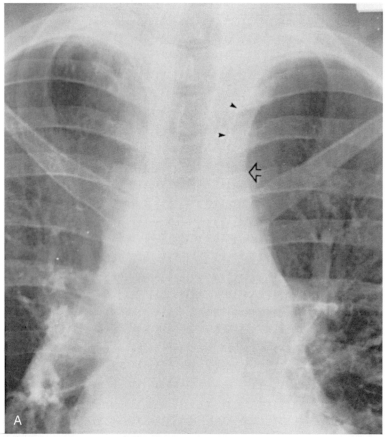

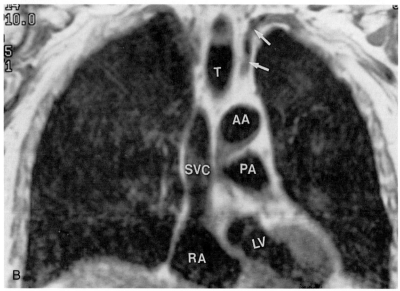

Figure 8–12. Supra-aortic Area. A detailed view from a posteroanterior chest radiograph *(A)* reveals two curvilinear interfaces that extend superiorly and laterally from the aortic arch and trachea. The medially positioned interface *(arrowheads)* represents lung abutting the posterior mediastinum; because it is *concave,* it is illuminated by a positive Mach band. By contrast, the more lateral opacity *(arrow)* is created by the left subclavian artery and is a *convex* surface; consequently, it is highlighted by a negative Mach band. A coronal MR image in an 83-year-old man *(B)* demonstrates the normal course of the left subclavian artery *(arrows).* Note that in this patient there is a considerable amount of fat surrounding the artery. Thus, the interface between the left upper mediastinum in this patient is caused by fat surrounding the subclavian artery. Also seen are the trachea (T), aortic arch (AA), pulmonary artery (PA), left ventricle (LV), and superior vena cava (SVC) joining the right atrium (RA).

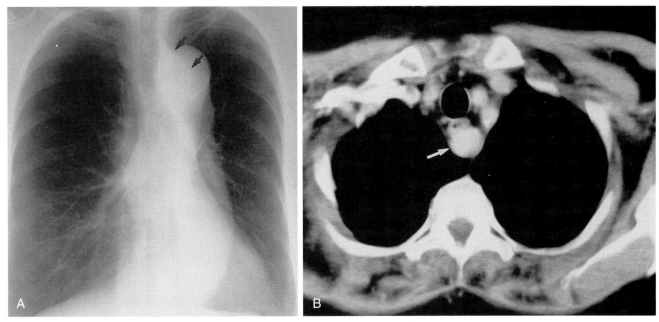

Figure 8–13. Aberrant Right Subclavian Artery. A posteroanterior chest radiograph *(A)* demonstrates an oblique opacity extending superiorly from the aortic arch to the right *(arrows).* A CT scan *(B)* demonstrates an aberrant right subclavian artery *(arrow)* coursing to the right, posterior to the esophagus.

Unlike the left subclavian artery, which is frequently abutted by left upper lobe parenchyma, the brachiocephalic artery and the left common carotid artery are commonly enveloped by mediastinal fat and are therefore unlikely to be contour forming. Consequently, on a lateral chest radiograph the posterior margin of the left subclavian artery may be identified through the posterior portion of the tracheal air column as a relatively straight opacity coursing obliquely upward toward the neck. The posterior margin of the innominate artery/right subclavian artery complex merges with the posterior wall of the right innominate vein/superior vena cava complex to form a sigmoid-shaped interface.[34]

The opacity of an aberrant right subclavian artery can occasionally be identified on PA and lateral radiographs of the chest (Fig. 8–13). In a study in which conventional radiographs were correlated with great vessel angiograms of 12 patients with such aberrant vessels,[37] an oblique opacity ascending from left to right from the superior margin of the aortic arch could be identified in 7 patients on conventional radiographs; in 2, the lateral projection revealed a round shadow contiguous with the superior margin of the aortic arch overlying the tracheal air column.

Left Superior Intercostal Vein

Venous blood from the first left intercostal space drains into the left supreme intercostal vein, whereas that from the second, third, and fourth left intercostal spaces drains into a common vessel, the left superior intercostal vein. In approximately 75% of subjects,[3] the vessel communicates with the accessory hemiazygos vein as it descends along the spine. At T3 or T4, the vein arches forward adjacent to the aortic arch to empty into the posterior aspect of the left brachiocephalic vein (Fig. 8–14).

Three components of the left superior intercostal vein can sometimes be identified radiographically: the "aortic nipple," the paraspinal portion, and the retroaortic portion.[38] The aortic nipple consists of a rounded protuberance adjacent to the aortic arch that is created by the vein seen end-on as it passes anteriorly adjacent to the aortic arch before entering the left brachiocephalic vein.[39] The incidence with which it is seen on PA radiographs of erect normal subjects ranges from about 1% to 10%.[38, 40] In this situation, the nipple ranges in size from a small protuberance up to 4.5 mm in diameter.[40] The position of the nipple in relation to the aortic arch can vary from superomedial to inferolateral (Fig. 8–15). As might be expected, the vein dilates and becomes more prominent when an individual assumes the supine position or performs a Müller maneuver.[38] Dilation also occurs in a variety of disease states that result in increased flow or

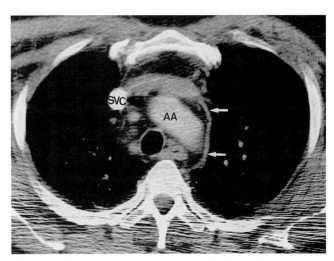

Figure 8–14. Left Superior Intercostal Vein. A CT scan demonstrates the left superior intercostal vein *(arrows)* as it courses from the paraspinal region forward and lateral to the aortic arch (AA) to drain into the left brachiocephalic vein. The latter can be seen coursing to the right to join the superior vena cava (SVC).

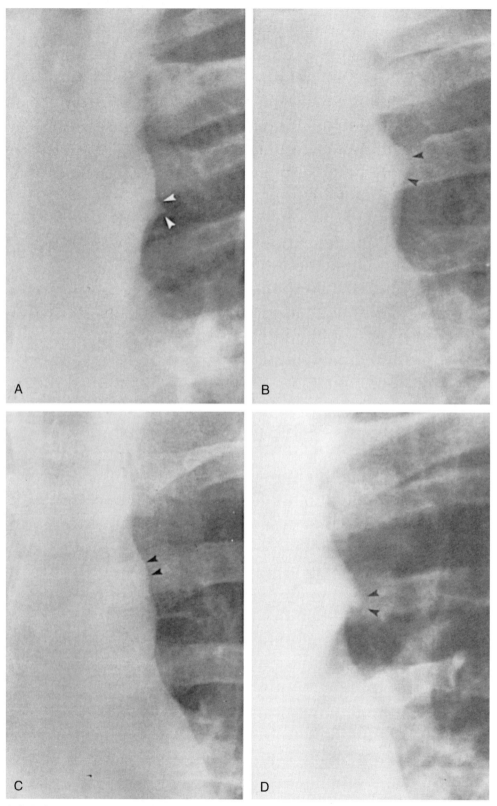

Figure 8–15. Left Superior Intercostal Vein. Detail views from conventional posteroanterior chest radiographs of four normal adults (*A* to *D*) show variations of the "aortic nipple" *(arrowheads)* representing the left superior intercostal vein as it passes anteriorly adjacent to the aortic arch; note that its position can vary from superomedial to inferolateral. In the upright position, the vein appears as a small protuberance along the lateral contour of the aortic arch.

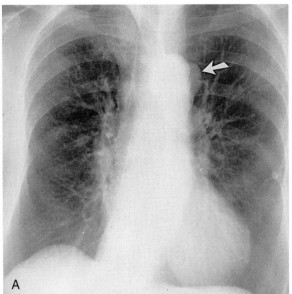 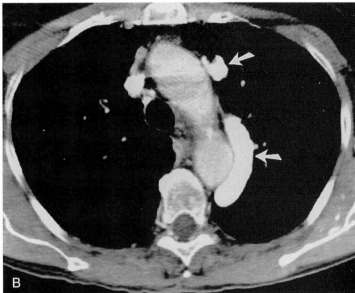

Figure 8–16. Enlarged Left Superior Intercostal Vein. A posteroanterior chest radiograph *(A)* demonstrates a prominent aortic nipple *(arrow)*. (Incidental note is made of a calcified granuloma in the left lung.) A contrast-enhanced CT scan *(B)* demonstrates a dilated left superior intercostal vein *(arrows)* caused by collateral blood flow from the left brachiocephalic vein into the hemiazygos and azygos veins. Also note the collateral blood flow adjacent to the left scapula. The patient was a 77-year-old woman with long-standing superior vena cava obstruction caused by fibrosing mediastinitis (presumably related to histoplasmosis). Note the calcified paratracheal lymph nodes.

pressure (or both) within the systemic venous system and is a useful radiographic sign analogous to abnormal distention of the azygos vein in the presence of systemic venous hypertension (Fig. 8–16).

As the paraspinal portion of the left superior intercostal vein turns anteriorly at the level of T3 or T4, it may abut aerated lung that delineates the top of the left paraspinal interface, thus forming an interface that is radiographically visible.[41] In our experience, however, it is more common for the vein to be surrounded by mediastinal fat and buried deep within the mediastinum so that its presence is only indirectly related to the cephalad portion of the paraspinal interface. Similarly, the retroaortic segment of the intercostal vein—that is, the segment between the aortic nipple and the paraspinal portion—can only rarely be visualized on chest radiographs.[38]

Other Structures

The left lateral wall of the trachea is rarely visible on a PA chest radiograph because of contiguity of the left subclavian artery and mediastinal fat. Similarly, the esophagus, which typically lies immediately posterior to the trachea on its left side, seldom creates a distinct interface with the left lung unless it is distended with gas; in the latter circumstance, a vertical stripe (the *left superior esophagopleural stripe*) is created. Occasionally, the opacity of the left paraspinal line above the aortic arch can be seen medial to the interface formed by the left subclavian artery. The posterior junction line is described in the section on the supra-azygos area.

INFRA-AORTIC AREA

This compartment of the left side of the mediastinum extends from the aortic arch above to the diaphragm below

and from the anterior mediastinal space in front to the paravertebral region behind. The contour of the mediastinum cephalad from the diaphragm includes the left ventricle, the left atrial appendage (seldom if ever identifiable as a separate opacity in normal subjects), the left border of the main pulmonary artery, the pleural reflection from the aorta downward onto the main pulmonary artery, and the aortic arch (Fig. 8–17). General characteristics of the cardiac silhouette are described later. In this section we describe the paraspinal lines, the preaortic recess, and the inferior reflections of pleura off the aortic arch.

Aortopulmonary Window and Aortopulmonary Line

The aortopulmonary window consists of a space situated between the arch of the aorta and the left pulmonary artery and occupied largely by mediastinal fat; its medial boundary is the ductus ligament and its lateral boundary is the mediastinal pleura and visceral pleura over the left lung, thus creating the aortopulmonary window interface (Fig. 8–17). Within this space are situated fat, the left recurrent laryngeal nerve, and lymph nodes. The lateral border (aortopulmonary window interface) is normally concave or straight. A lateral convexity should suggest a mediastinal abnormality, most commonly lymphadenopathy, although it may occasionally be a normal variant caused by the accumulation of fat (Fig. 8–18).

The patterns of pleural reflection in the vicinity of the aortic arch, left pulmonary artery, left hilum, and left heart border on a frontal chest radiograph have been extensively reviewed in three large studies.[42-44] In approximately 60% of individuals, the contour is seen as a continuous opacity with a sharp left border extending caudad from the aortic arch to the level of the left main bronchus, usually as a smooth prolongation of the left heart border. The opacity extending

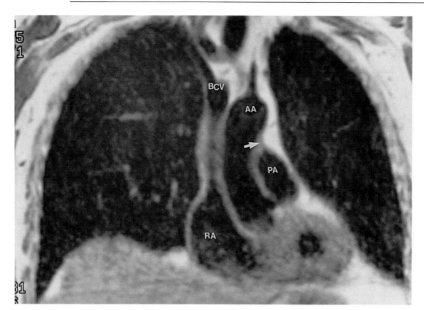

Figure 8–17. Normal Infra-aortic Area. An MR image in an 83-year-old man demonstrates the structures responsible for the left mediastinal border in the infra-aortic area. Fat can be seen lateral to the aortic arch (AA) and main pulmonary artery (PA) and outlines the region of the aortopulmonary window. The ligament of the ductus arteriosus *(arrow)* can be seen to delineate the medial margin of the window. The inferior margin of the infra-aortic area is related to epicardial fat outlining the wall of the left ventricle. Also noted are the left carotid artery, right brachiocephalic vein (BCV), superior vena cava, and right atrium (RA).

from the aortic arch to the left main bronchus represents the aortopulmonary line or interface (Fig. 8–18).[43] In approximately 40% of individuals, no continuous border opacity can be seen; the pleura over the left margin of the aortic arch simply extends inferiorly and merges with the superior margin of the left pulmonary artery.[42] CT correlation indicates that the aortic-pulmonary interface is formed largely by mediastinal fat residing in front and to the left of the transverse portion of the aortic arch, anterolateral to the left pulmonary artery (Fig. 8–18). Displacement of this interface laterally, particularly as revealed by sequential radiographs, should suggest the possibility of mediastinal pathology (Fig. 8–18).

The accuracy of PA and lateral radiographs in the diagnosis of aortopulmonary window pathology was assessed in a retrospective study of 80 patients for whom conventional PA and lateral radiographs and CT images were available for review; in all patients, CT revealed convincing evidence of abnormality in the aortopulmonary window.[45] In 39 patients (49%), there was no detectable abnormality in the window on conventional radiographs, and in 8 patients (10%) the findings were equivocal. Major contributing factors to this low detectability were the size and, more importantly, the location of lesions within the window.[45] A second study suggests that in the absence of obstructive pneumonitis or left upper lobe atelectasis, chest radiography allows detection of the majority of cases with enlarged aortopulmonary window nodes.[46] In this study, a lateral convexity in the aortopulmonary window interface was seen in 21 of 26 patients who had enlarged nodes (sensitivity, 80%) and in only 1 of 49 patients who had normal-sized aortopulmonary window nodes (specificity, 98%).

Posterior Pleural Reflections

Paramount to an understanding of the right and left posterior pleural reflections—that is, the anatomic basis of the paraspinal lines—is knowledge of the distribution of normal mediastinal fat. Since the advent of CT, it has be-

come clear that fat is ubiquitous within the mediastinum of adults (it is absent or small in amount in children) and envelops all important structures to some extent. Unfortunately, anatomy textbooks pay little attention to the distribution and quantity of mediastinal fat; indeed, most anatomic illustrations depict structures with the fat carefully removed.

The quantity and location of mediastinal fat vary considerably depending on the habitus, nutritional state, and age of the patient; the shape of the thorax; and the integrity and position of the vascular structures.[47] Normally, mediastinal fat accumulates in the superior, anterior, and lower posterior mediastinum (Fig. 8–19). Above the level of the aortic arch, the retroesophageal prevertebral space is usually devoid of fat, so the right and left upper lobe pleurae can approximate and form the posterior junction line. The quantity of fat around the esophagus tends to increase at the aortic arch; below this point, the paraesophageal and para-aortic fat diminishes only to increase again in the posterior mediastinum above the diaphragm. The lower thoracic aorta may be prespinal and completely surrounded by mediastinal fat and hence form no contour with the lung. Above the aortic arch, the quantity of fat lateral to the vertebral bodies is usually symmetric, although below this level the left side almost always has more than the right, provided that the aorta descends in the left paraspinal or prespinal location (Fig. 8–19); if it descends on the right, the opposite pertains. Rarely, paravertebral fat is present only on the right or is completely absent.

In the left hemithorax, the pleura reflects off the posterior chest wall and passes forward for a few centimeters in an anteroposterior (AP) plane before deviating over the posterior and lateral wall of the descending aorta; in the transverse plane, the shape of this interface between the retroaortic, paravertebral lung and the mediastinum is usually concave, although at a lower level it may be either straight or slightly convex. The descending aorta normally deviates anteromedially and lies in a more central position before it exits through the aortic hiatus; in so doing, it may lose its contour-forming left border. As the aging aorta unfolds and protrudes into the left hemithorax, fat is deposited posteri-

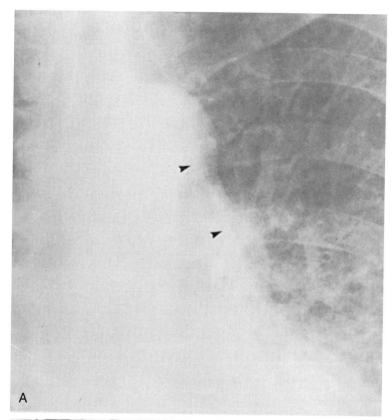

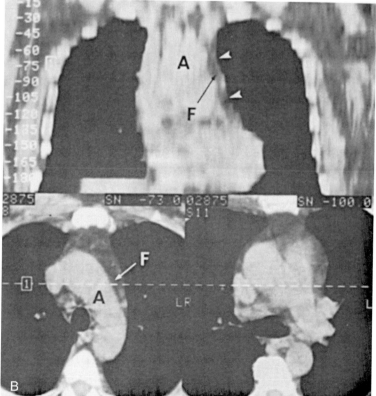

Figure 8–18. Infra-aortic Area. A detail view from a conventional posteroanterior (PA) chest radiograph *(A)* discloses a sharply defined interface that extends caudally from the aortic arch to the level of the left main bronchus *(arrowheads),* defining the *aortopulmonary line* or *interface. B,* A coronal CT reformation *(top)* and representative transverse images *(bottom)* show that the interface *(arrowheads)* represents air-containing lung abutting normal mediastinal fat (F) between the aortic arch (A) and the upper hilum.

Illustration continued on following page

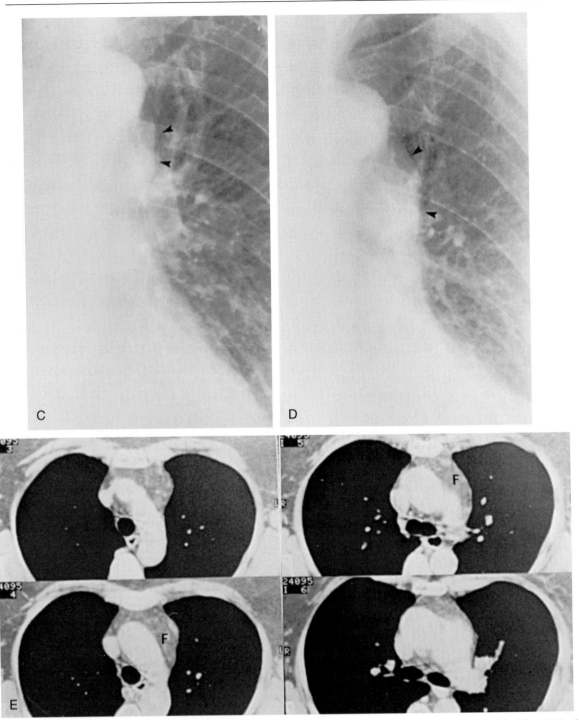

Figure 8–18 *Continued.* Detail views from PA chest radiographs of a middle-aged woman before *(C)* and several months after *(D)* institution of corticosteroid therapy for rheumatoid arthritis show an increasingly lobulated configuration in the contour of the aortopulmonary interface *(arrowheads).* Sequential CT scans *(E)* reveal normal (albeit abundant) mediastinal fat (F) as the cause of the lobulated contour; this unusual fat deposition presumably relates to the corticosteroid therapy.

orly, medially, and anteromedially to it (Fig. 8–20). On the right side, the pleura continues in a posteromedial orientation and is often inseparable from the cortex of the contiguous vertebral bodies; above and below the azygos arch, it usually intrudes medially into the supra- and infra-azygos recesses.

The nature of the right and left posterior pleural reflections was clarified in a study of eight normal adults in which conventional linear tomography, CT, and photodensitometry were used.[47] The right and left paraspinal lines are about 1 mm wide and appear as linear opacities on an AP thoracic spine film or, occasionally, on a conventional chest radiograph. The left line extends from the top or middle of the aortic arch to the level of the 9th to 12th thoracic vertebrae, depending on the degree of lung inflation (Fig. 8–21). When

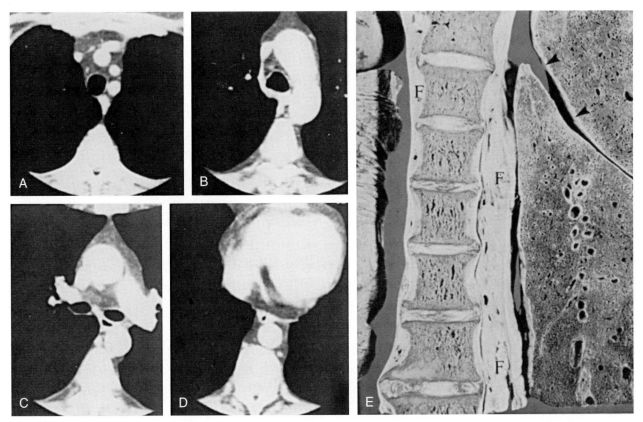

Figure 8–19. Posterior Pleural Reflections. Representative CT scans through the superior mediastinum *(A)*, aortic arch *(B)*, left pulmonary artery *(C)*, and left ventricle *(D)* reveal the normal locations of fat within the mediastinum. The major fat deposits in adults are in the superior, anterior, and lower posterior mediastinum. Above the aortic arch, the retroesophageal prevertebral space is commonly devoid of fat. The quantity of fat around the esophagus tends to increase at the aortic arch, but below this point the paraesophageal and para-aortic fat diminishes but increases again in the posterior mediastinum above the diaphragm. *E,* In a coronal anatomic section through the midthoracic vertebrae, the quantity of paravertebral fat (F) to the right and left of the vertebrae at the level of the aortic arch (medial border of the left major fissure) *(arrowheads)* is equal; below this level, paravertebral fat is much more prominent on the left. *(A to D* from Genereux GP: Am J Roentgenol 141:141, 1983; *E* from Heitzman ER: The Mediastinum: Radiologic Correlations with Anatomy and Pathology. St. Louis, CV Mosby, 1977, pp 33–66.)

mediastinal fat is abundant, the line may be visible above the aortic arch and project through the arch as a smooth curvilinear opacity that extends over the apex of the lung medial to the left subclavian artery. The left line tends to parallel the lateral margin of the vertebral bodies and can lie anywhere medial to the interface formed by the lung and the descending aorta, although commonly its position is midway between the spine and aorta. The lateral relationship of the descending aorta to the left paraspinal line exists throughout most of its course, although as the aorta declines toward the midline inferiorly, it tends to overlap the paraspinal line. Rarely, the left paraspinal line projects outside the plane of the descending aorta and causes the latter to disappear from view.[47] The lung-aorta interface is margined by a 1-mm black line, a feature that serves to distinguish it from the left paraspinal line.

The right paraspinal line is seen less often than the left because the two pleural membranes on the right cross obliquely in front of the vertebrae, thus rendering their orientation inappropriate for the creation of a tangential interface.[48] The right paraspinal line usually extends for only two or four vertebral segments at the T8 to T12 level before it merges below with the right crus of the diaphragm. Normally, the line lies within a few millimeters of the

vertebrae, a reflection of the lesser quantity of paravertebral fat on the right side.

Photodensitometric analysis through the paraspinal and para-aortic lines demonstrates no density increase or decrease corresponding to these respective interfaces (Fig. 8–21).[47] Visualization of the paraspinal and para-aortic lines is therefore not related to the presence of pleural layers. Instead, they represent Mach bands or edge-enhancing phenomena created by the retina in response to strong differences in transmitted illumination.[47] Mach band formation is optimum when differences in transmitted light are created by structures whose surfaces are oriented at angles of less than 90 degrees (i.e., concave or convex surfaces).[49] These two prerequisites are met in the posterior mediastinum (and indeed, elsewhere within the thorax) by the interfaces formed by the lung and mediastinum and the lung and descending aorta. The former interface is usually concave, so the eye enhances it by forming a positive (white) Mach band; the latter is convex, and consequently a negative (black) Mach band marginates its surface. In essence, therefore, it is the *true shape* of the lung-mediastinal interface (as viewed in the transverse plane) that defines the physical conditions for the visual perception of the paraspinal and para-aortic lines and *not* the tissue composition of this interface.

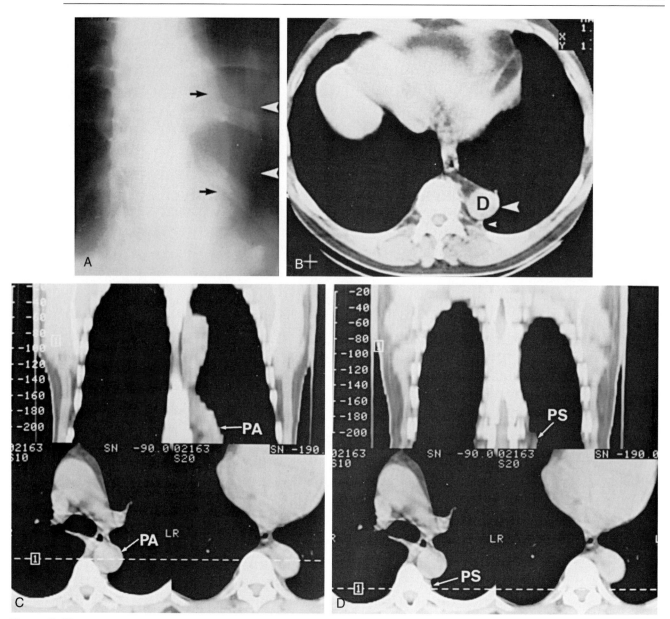

Figure 8–20. Posterior Pleural Reflections. A conventional linear tomogram in anteroposterior (AP) projection through the posterior mediastinum *(A)* shows the left paraspinal line *(arrows)* to be displaced laterally, closely paralleling the course of the elongated descending aorta *(arrowheads)*. An unenhanced transverse CT scan through the lower part of the thorax *(B)* reveals posterior and lateral displacement of the descending aorta (D); the quantity of fat medial to the aorta is increased. The concave interface between lung and mediastinum behind the aorta *(small arrowhead)* is situated medial to the outer edge of the convex descending aorta *(large arrowhead)*. Coronal CT reformations *(top)* and appropriate transverse images *(bottom)* through the descending aorta *(C)* and immediately posterior to it *(D)* permit correlation with the linear tomogram in *A*. Note that in AP projection the paraspinal (PS) and para-aortic (PA) lines are both convex toward the lung, whereas in the transverse plane their true shape is concave and convex, respectively, which accounts for the positive and negative Mach band enhancement that characterizes these interfaces. *(A* and *B* from Genereux GP: Am J Roentgenol 141:141, 1983.)

Preaortic Recess

The left lower lobe can intrude anterior to the descending aorta and medial to the esophagus into the preaortic space (or recess) and form, with the soft tissues of the mediastinum, an interface known as the *preaortic line.*[44] Anatomically, the left-sided recess is analogous to the azygoesophageal recess on the right *(see* farther on), although there are noteworthy differences; in keeping with the nomenclature of the azygoesophageal recess, we believe that the left-sided features are properly termed the *preaortic recess*

and the medial contact of the lungs with the mediastinum, the *preaortic recess interface.*

The preaortic recess extends from the aortic arch above to the left hemidiaphragm below. Usually, only a small amount of lower lobe lung parenchyma invaginates into the preaortic region, thus creating a much narrower and smaller recess than its equivalent on the right. Occasionally—for example, in patients with emphysema or kyphosis—the depth of the preaortic recess (and azygoesophageal recess) can increase greatly and thereby permit recognition of both recess interfaces simultaneously. The left pulmonary artery

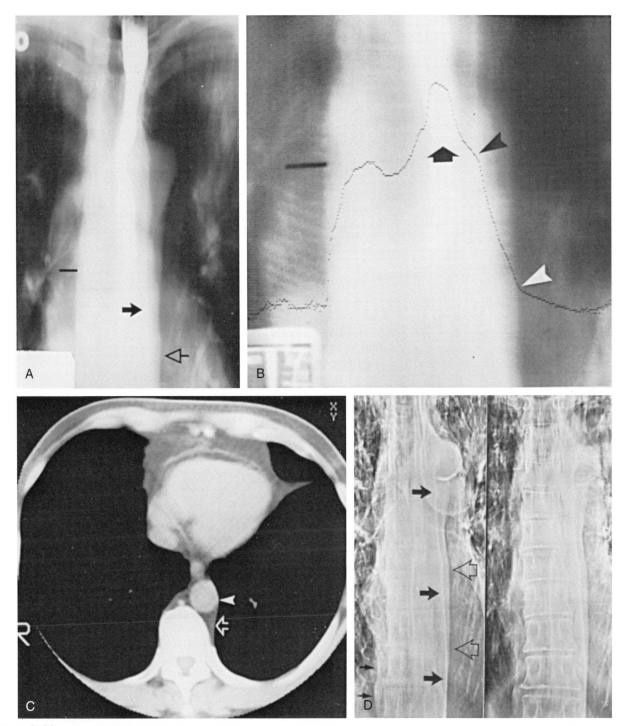

Figure 8–21. Posterior Pleural Reflections. On this anteroposterior radiograph of the thorax with barium in the esophagus *(A)*, the left paraspinal line *(black arrow)* and the aortic interface *(open arrow)* are shown; the paraspinal line is depicted as a *white line* whereas the aortic interface is enhanced by a *black line*. Photodensitometric analysis *(B)* of the lines depicted in *A* at the level of the *horizontal bar* reveals a broad positive plateau over the spine and a focal peak *(broad arrow)* through the barium in the esophagus. There is no similar deflection over the left paraspinal line *(black arrowhead)* or aortic line *(white arrowhead)*. These lines are Mach bands that are related to the shape of the lung-mediastinal interface rather than the composition of tissue interposed between the lung and mediastinum. A transverse CT scan *(C)* through the posterior mediastinum at the level of the *bar* depicted in *A* shows that the paraspinal line *(arrow)* relates to the *concave* interface between the lung and posterior mediastinum behind the aorta; by contrast, the aortic line is caused by the *convex* shape of the descending aorta *(arrowhead)* as it abuts the lung. Anteroposterior xerotomograms *(D)* through the carina *(left)* and 2 cm posterior to the carina *(right)* reveal the 1-mm white, left paraspinal line *(large solid arrows)* extending from the midaortic arch to a point opposite T12 and paralleling the vertebrae. Superiorly, the line is medial to the lateral wall of the descending aorta, the latter marginated by a 1-mm *black line (open arrows)*; inferiorly, the lines converge. Both lines disappear when opaque paper is placed adjacent to them, thus proving their optical properties as Mach bands. A right paraspinal line *(small arrows)* is seen in the lower hemithorax.

passes over the left main bronchus and then extends backward and downward into the interlobar fissure; in so doing, particularly when the depth of the aortopulmonary window is diminished, the artery can "close" the cephalad portion of the recess so that it extends only from the inferior border of the interlobar artery to the diaphragm. Most commonly, the preaortic recess can be identified as a shallow convex-medial, straight, or concave-medial interface. If gas is present in the proximal and middle portion of the infra-aortic esophagus, the interface will be depicted as the *left inferior esophagopleural stripe.*

SUPRA-AZYGOS AREA

The supra-azygos area is that portion of the right side of the mediastinum that extends cephalad from the azygos arch to the thoracic inlet; it is separated from the infra-azygos area by the azygos vein and arch, important landmarks in radiographic interpretation.

Azygos and Hemiazygos Veins

The *azygos vein* originates in the upper lumbar region at the level of the renal veins as a continuation of the right subcostal vein or as an extension of the right ascending lumbar vein. It passes into the thorax through the aortic hiatus medial to the right crus of the diaphragm.[50] In the thorax, the vein pursues a somewhat variable course and can be situated in front, to the right, or rarely to the left of the lower eight thoracic vertebrae (Fig. 8–22); it is joined at the

T8 or T9 level by the hemiazygos vein ascending on the left. At the level of T4 or T5, the azygos vein arches anteriorly and slightly inferiorly and relates intimately to the lateral wall of the esophagus and the right posterior surface of the trachea. It then turns laterally for a short distance before proceeding anteriorly once again and passing over the right main bronchus and truncus anterior and lateral to the right inferior tracheal wall; it finally inserts into the back of the superior vena cava (Fig. 8–22). Along its course, the vein receives tributaries from the 5th to 11th intercostal veins on the right, the right subcostal vein, the right superior intercostal vein (which terminates in the azygos vein as it passes forward from the spine at the T4 or T5 level), the right bronchial veins, and the superior and inferior hemiazygos veins.

The *superior hemiazygos vein* begins at the vertebral end of the fourth left intercostal space as a continuation of the fourth posterior intercostal vein; its upper part is often connected to the left superior intercostal vein. It courses downward and forward in relation to T4 and then descends in close relationship to the left side of the descending aorta as far as the eighth thoracic vertebra. It then bends abruptly to the right and crosses behind the aorta to terminate in the azygos vein.

The *inferior hemiazygos vein* originates from the posterior aspect of the left renal vein or as a continuation of the left subcostal vein or left ascending lumbar vein. It enters the thorax medial to the left crus of the diaphragm and behind the descending aorta and ascends anterolateral to the vertebral column; at the level of T8 or T9, it turns abruptly to the right and joins the azygos vein.

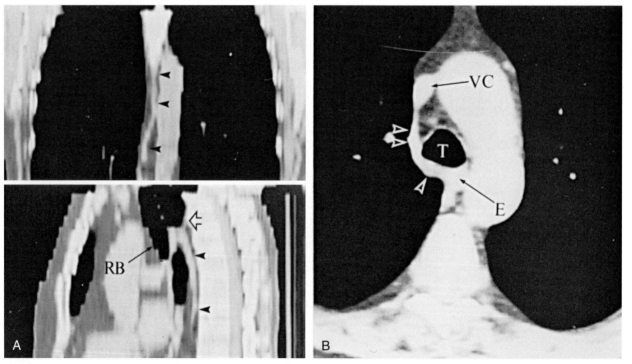

Figure 8–22. The Supra-Azygos Area. *A,* Coronal *(top)* and sagittal *(bottom)* CT reformations demonstrate the course of the azygos vein *(arrowheads).* The azygos arch receives the right superior intercostal vein *(arrow)* and turns forward slightly above the plane of the right upper lobe bronchus (RB). A CT scan *(B)* identifies the transverse course of the azygos vein. Note that before entering the superior vena cava (VC), it relates closely to the esophagus (E), the right posterior tracheal wall (T) *(arrowhead),* and the right upper lobe bronchus *(double arrowheads).*

Tracheal Interfaces

The trachea is normally bordered on its right lateral aspect by pleura covering the right upper lobe; its anterior and posterior aspects are bordered to a variable extent. Contact of the right lung in the supra-azygos area with the right lateral wall of the trachea creates a thin stripe of soft tissue density usually visible on frontal chest radiographs that is designated the *right paratracheal stripe* (Fig. 8–23). This stripe is formed by the right wall of the trachea, contiguous parietal and visceral pleura, and a variable quantity of mediastinal fat (Fig. 8–23).[51] The frequency with which the stripe is identified on PA radiographs varies in different studies from 63% to 94% of normal individuals.[3, 4, 51] Although the significance of an increased paratracheal stripe width has been questioned in view of the variation in the amount of tissue that separates the lung and trachea,[3] its measurement may nevertheless be useful in some circumstances. The thickness of the stripe must be measured above the level of the azygos vein; an increase in width on serial films is a more important sign of abnormality than is a single static measurement. In one series of 1,259 normal subjects, the maximal width of the stripe was 4 mm.[51]

Widening of the paratracheal stripe (≥5 mm) may be

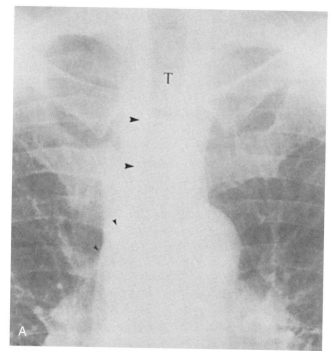

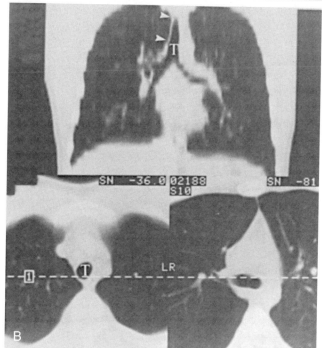

Figure 8–23. Right Paratracheal Interfaces. A detail view from a posteroanterior (PA) chest radiograph *(A)* shows a vertically oriented 2-mm linear opacity *(large arrowheads)* that parallels the tracheal air column (T) and is designated the *right paratracheal stripe.* The ovoid opacity in the right tracheobronchial angle *(small arrowheads)* represents the third portion of the azygos arch as the vein passes over the right main and upper lobe bronchi. *B,* Coronal CT reformation *(top)* and transverse images *(bottom)* through the mid and lower parts of the trachea (T) show minimal areolar tissue between the tracheal wall and the lung *(arrowheads).* The linear opacity identified in *A* is caused primarily by the width of the tracheal wall.

Illustration continued on following page

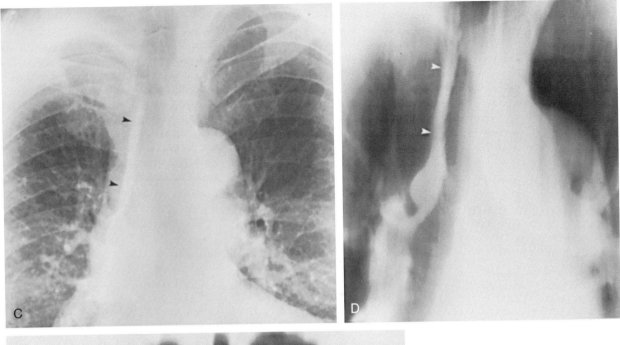

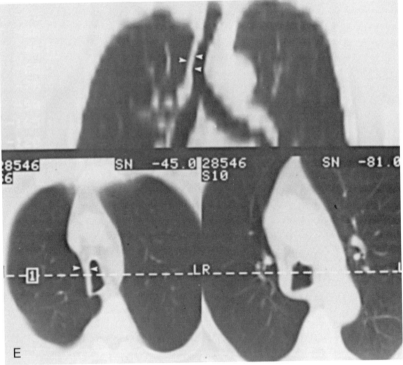

Figure 8–23 *Continued.* In another patient, detail views from a conventional PA chest radiograph *(C)* and an anteroposterior linear tomogram *(D)*, show a tracheal stripe that measures 4 to 5 mm in diameter *(arrowheads). E,* Coronal CT reformation *(top)* with appropriate transverse scans *(bottom)* through the mid and lower parts of the trachea of this patient reveals a small amount of intervening fat between the tracheal wall and aerated right upper lobe parenchyma (between *arrowheads*). Since the amount of mediastinal fat is highly variable, quantitative values for the width of the stripe should not be relied on as the sole determinant of abnormality; an increase in width on serial films is a more important sign of abnormality.

due to paratracheal lymph node enlargement, mediastinal hemorrhage, pleural disease, or thickening of the tracheal wall. It is not a particularly sensitive sign for the detection of paratracheal lymphadenopathy, since it is present in only approximately 30% of patients who have enlarged nodes.[52] This low sensitivity is related to the location of the paratracheal nodes anterior rather than lateral to the trachea; the nodes therefore need to be enlarged considerably to displace the stripe.[52] Widening of the stripe may also be due to mediastinal hemorrhage; in one study of 102 patients with blunt chest trauma, tears of the aorta, brachiocephalic artery, or right subclavian artery were demonstrated by arteriogra-

phy in 11 of 48 (23%) patients whose right paratracheal stripe was greater than 5 mm in thickness.[53] Rarely, the left upper lobe abuts the left lateral wall of the trachea; since the left subclavian artery and contiguous mediastinal fat usually relate to the left side of the trachea, a *left paratracheal stripe* is seldom seen.

The *posterior tracheal stripe* (originally designated the posterior tracheal band[54]) is a vertically oriented opacity formed by the posterior wall of the trachea where it comes in contact with right upper lobe parenchyma. On well-exposed lateral radiographs of the chest, the stripe is frequently seen for the entire length of visible trachea and is often continuous inferiorly with the line or stripe formed by the posterior wall of the right main and intermediate bronchi (Fig. 8–24). The anatomic structures located in the posterior tracheal region include retrotracheal soft tissue (Fig. 8–24) and/or the anterior esophageal wall (rendered visible by a small amount of intraesophageal gas).[55, 56] Thus, the soft tissue stripe behind the tracheal air column should be considered either a *posterior tracheal stripe* or a *tracheoesophageal stripe*, the former being composed of the posterior tracheal wall and any surrounding mediastinal tissue and the latter of the posterior

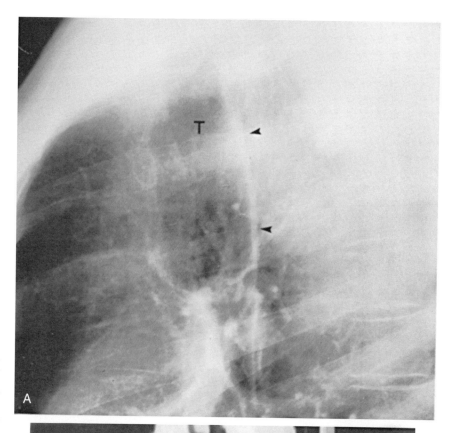

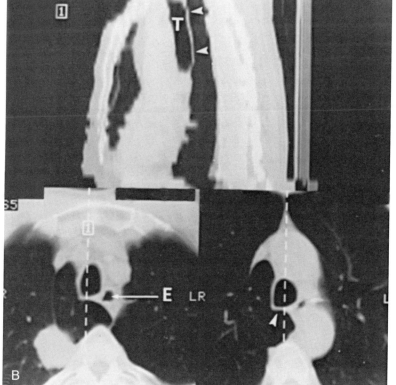

Figure 8–24. Posterior Tracheal Interface. A conventional lateral chest radiograph *(A)* demonstrates a 4-mm-wide stripe *(arrowheads)* that parallels the air column of the trachea (T), the *posterior tracheal stripe. B,* Sagittal CT reformation *(top)* and transverse images *(bottom)* through the trachea (T) at the level of the aortic arch show that the stripe is caused by the posterior wall of the trachea itself *(arrowheads).* Note that in this patient the esophagus (E) is not contour forming in lateral projection and thus does not contribute to the stripe.

Illustration continued on following page

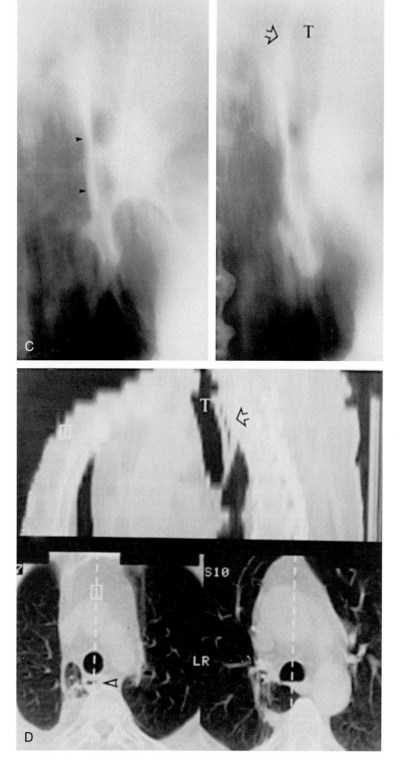

Figure 8–24 *Continued.* Detail views from conventional linear tomograms in lateral projection *(C)* disclose a stripe 5 mm in width that extends along the entire length of the tracheal air column (T) *(arrow) (right)* and intermediate stem line *(arrowheads) (left). D,* Sagittal CT reformation *(top)* and transverse images *(bottom)* show that the linear opacity identified in *C* is caused by a combination of the posterior tracheal wall, mediastinal soft tissue, and gas-containing esophagus *(arrowhead),* thus constituting the *tracheoesophageal stripe (arrow).* A CT scan is needed to distinguish the two appearances with certainty.

tracheal wall, the anterior esophageal wall (the lumen containing a small amount of gas), and any surrounding mediastinal tissue (Fig. 8–24). Distinction between the two varieties of stripes is possible only occasionally on conventional radiographs; however, the tracheoesophageal stripe can be identified as such if a thin vertical radiolucency of fat separates the soft tissue stripe of the trachea from the esophagus

or if the stripe courses through the level of the azygos arch.[56] The incidence of such visibility is slightly less than 50%.[55, 56] The only certain way of distinguishing the two is by CT scan.

As a consequence of the variability in the amount of retrotracheal soft tissue, the position of the esophagus, and the amount of gas within the esophageal lumen, the tracheoesophageal stripe ranges in thickness from 1 to 5.5 mm (mean, 2 mm).[56] There is general agreement that a posterior tracheal stripe or tracheoesophageal stripe that measures more than 5 mm in width should be considered abnormal, most commonly a manifestation of primary or recurrent esophageal carcinoma.[54, 57–60] Regardless of the accuracy of this measurement, CT can be used to clarify the nature of the stripe in an individual case. In a CT study of 100 normal subjects in which the trachea and its surrounding tissues were studied at the level of the sternal notch and 2 cm caudad, the average thickness of the stripe was 8.4 mm (± 3.8 mm SD), whereas at a CT level 2 cm below the sternal notch, the posterolateral tracheal stripe had an average thickness of 6.4 mm (± 1.8 mm SD).[61] The apparent increased thickness of the posterior tracheal or tracheoesophageal stripe on CT may have been related to a difference in patient position or level of inspiration between the radiograph and CT or to the window level and width used to make the CT measurements.

Posterior Junction Anatomy

The apices of the right and left upper lobes contact the mediastinum behind the esophagus anterior to the first and second vertebral bodies. In so doing, they create a V-shaped triangular opacity that constitutes the *posterior mediastinal triangle*; marginating the triangle are the *right* and *left superior recesses* (Fig. 8–25). Caudally, the lungs intrude deeper into a prespinal location posterior to the esophagus and anterior to the third through fifth vertebral bodies where they form a pleural apposition that, along with any intervening mediastinal tissue, forms the *posterior junction line* (Fig. 8–25). On a PA radiograph, the posterior junction line usually projects through the air column of the trachea; it may be straight or slightly convex to the left. When intervening mediastinal tissue is abundant or a narrowed retroesophageal space precludes lung apposition, the posterior junction line can appear as a distinct stripe (Fig. 8–25).[8]

Below the posterior junction line, the lungs are excluded from the midline by the forward arching of the right and left superior intercostal veins and by the posterior portion of the azygos arch on the right and the aortic arch on the left. This divergence defines an inverted V-shaped opacity that is marginated by the *right* and *left inferior recesses,* analogous to the situation superiorly (Fig. 8–25). The former is usually longer and extends more caudad than the left, which is a reflection of the more caudal location of the azygos arch than the aortic arch.

Right and Left Superior Esophageal Stripes

Gas can be seen in the esophagus on PA radiographs of the chest in approximately 35% of normal subjects and in 50% of patients who have abnormal chest radiographs.[62] The most common site for it to be identified relates to the aortic arch and, in decreasing order of frequency, includes the portions of the esophagus immediately below, above, and medial to the arch. The posteromedial portion of the upper lobe abuts the lateral wall of the esophagus on the right side, whereas the posteromedial portion of the left upper lobe

may or may not show a similar relationship, depending on the position of the esophagus, the depth of the retroesophageal mediastinum, and the quantity of mediastinal fat. When gas is present within the upper portion of the esophagus, a vertically oriented soft tissue stripe may be identifiable on the right side, left side, or both, provided that the inner and outer margins of both esophageal walls are tangential to the x-ray beam. Originally designated the *esophagopleural stripe,*[63, 64] this opacity has been renamed the *esophageal stripe* to negate the contribution of the paper-thin pleura (Fig. 8–26).[48, 62]

In its most typical configuration, the right esophageal wall courses obliquely from the upper right to the lower left and is usually convex along its inner border. The left esophageal wall runs parallel to the right, although the two may diverge superiorly and inferiorly in relation to the superior and inferior recesses of the posterior junction.

Azygos Arch

At the level of the aortic arch, the azygos vein is composed of three parts: posterior (paraesophageal), middle (retrotracheal), and anterior (right tracheobronchial angle). The *posterior* part is abutted by the right upper or lower lobe laterally and the esophagus medially. The posterior turn of the azygos vein merges above with that of the right inferior recess and below with the pleura in the cephalad portion of the azygoesophageal recess. The *middle* component is seen through the air column of the trachea as an opacity that is angled slightly downward and to the right; it merges laterally with the oval or elliptical shadow of the *anterior* component viewed end-on as it passes forward in the tracheobronchial angle. Depending on the distention of the vessel and the depth of the supra-azygos and infra-azygos recesses, the vein may be identified on a lateral chest radiograph as a retrotracheal elongated opacity as it passes forward over the right main bronchus (Fig. 8–27). This appearance should not be mistaken for a mass such as enlarged lymph nodes.

Measurement of the anterior portion of the azygos vein is important in some diseases, notably portal hypertension, obstruction of the superior vena cava, and systemic venous hypertension. The only segment that can be measured accurately on conventional radiographs is the point at which the vein is viewed roughly tangentially in the right tracheobronchial angle as it enters the superior vena cava. In this location, it is often visible as a slightly flattened elliptical opacity (Fig. 8–28). In one study in which the vein was measured from its outer border to the contiguous air column of the right main bronchus on erect PA radiographs, a maximal transverse diameter of 6 mm was recorded.[65] In another investigation of 100 men and 100 nonpregnant women, an average diameter of 4.9 mm (range, 3 to 7 mm) was found in the men and 4.8 mm (range, 3 to 7 mm) in the women.[66] Despite these figures, in our experience and that of others, a transverse diameter of 10 mm is observed in many normal subjects.[4, 67]

During the 1970s, for all subjects 30 years of age or older, Fraser routinely performed PA chest radiography at both full inspiration and maximal expiration; this practice showed great variation in the size of the azygos vein shadow,

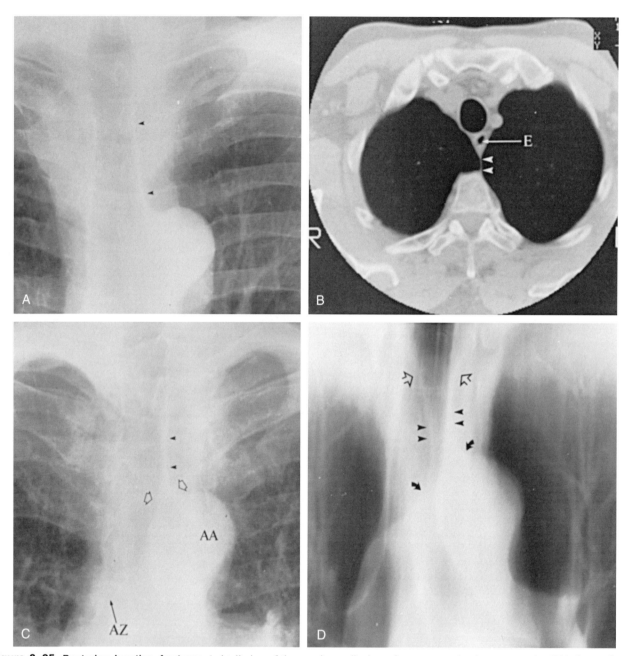

Figure 8–25. Posterior Junction Anatomy. A detail view of the superior mediastinum from a conventional posteroanterior (PA) chest radiograph *(A)* demonstrates a thin linear opacity called the *posterior junction line (arrowheads).* It courses obliquely from above downward, slightly to the left of the midline, and relates to thoracic vertebrae 3 to 5. On a transverse CT scan through the posterior mediastinum above the aortic arch *(B)* the right and left upper lobes can be seen to be almost contiguous with one another behind the esophagus (E), separated only by a small amount of mediastinal soft tissue and four layers of pleura *(arrowheads).* In a different patient, a detail view from a PA chest radiograph *(C)* demonstrates a somewhat thicker posterior junction line *(arrowheads)* that terminates inferiorly in a triangular opacity whose apex points cephalad and whose base abuts the aortic arch (AA). The right and left interfaces *(arrows)* are designated the *right* and *left inferior recesses.* The right recess extends caudally to cover the azygos arch (AZ), whereas the shorter left recess terminates on the medial aspect of the aortic arch. A conventional linear tomogram in anteroposterior (AP) projection *(D)* reveals a thick stripe *(arrowheads)* or septum that connects the superior *(open arrows)* and inferior *(closed arrows)* recesses. This manifestation is caused by a narrow retrotracheal space, increased mediastinal fat, or both.

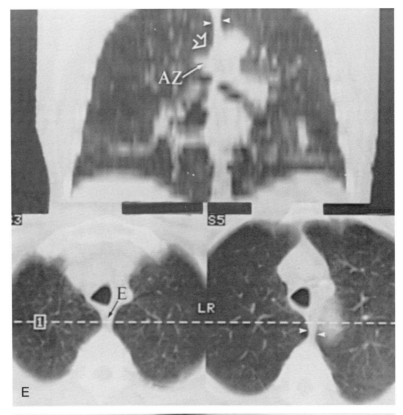

Figure 8–25 *Continued.* In a different patient *(E)*, coronal CT reformation *(top)* with appropriate transverse images *(bottom)* shows the upper lobes behind the esophagus (E) to be separated by a thick septum *(arrowheads)* composed of posterior mediastinal fat, the esophagus, and four layers of pleura; the right inferior recess *(arrow)* extends to the azygos vein arch (AZ). A conventional linear tomogram in AP projection through the posterior mediastinum *(F)* demonstrates the three components of the posterior junction anatomy: (1) the right and left superior recesses *(small arrowheads above)* separated by the superior, posterior triangle (SM); (2) the posterior junction line *(large arrowheads)*; and (3) the right and left inferior recesses *(small arrowheads below)* separated by the inferior, posterior mediastinal triangle (IM).

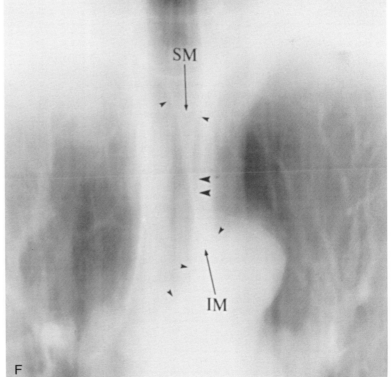

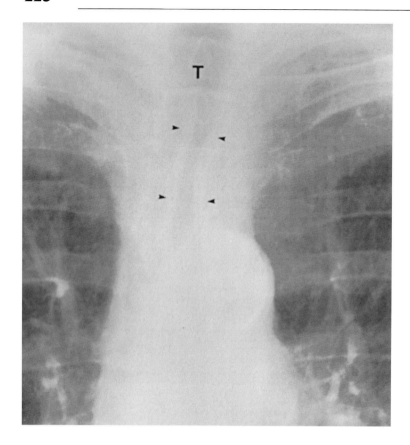

Figure 8–26. Superior Esophageal Stripes. A detail view from a conventional posteroanterior chest radiograph shows two vertical stripes *(arrowheads)* projected through the tracheal air column (T). The linear opacities represent the right and left walls of the gas-distended esophagus, designated the *right* and *left superior esophagopleural* or *esophageal stripes.*

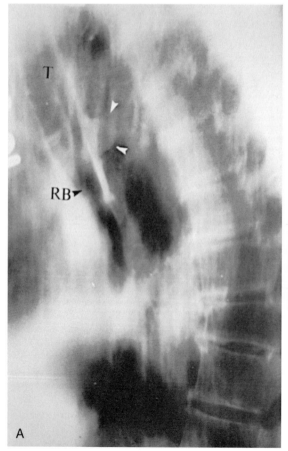

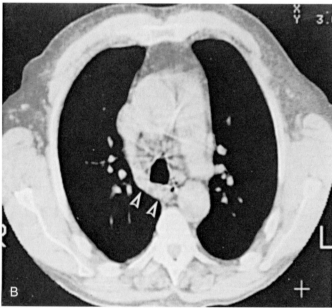

Figure 8–27. Azygos Vein: Retrotracheal Component. A conventional lateral tomogram through the trachea (T) *(A)* reveals a rounded opacity *(arrowheads)* above the right upper lobe bronchus (RB) that represents the retrotracheal component of the azygos arch. Its location and shape serve to differentiate this condition from enlarged lymph nodes. A CT scan at the level of the azygos arch *(B)* demonstrates the retrotracheal component *(arrowheads)* abutted by aerated right upper lobe, which accounts for the visibility of the vein in this location.

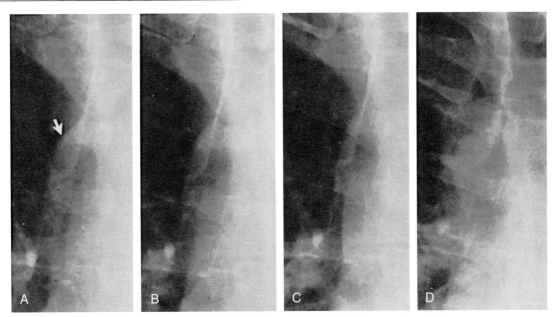

Figure 8–28. Physiologic Variations in Azygos Vein Diameter. Detail views of the region of the right tracheobronchial angle from four posteroanterior radiographs of a healthy 30-year-old man showing variations in size of the azygos vein caused by changes in intrathoracic pressure. At full inspiration with a sustained Müller maneuver *(A)*, vein diameter is 13 mm *(arrow)*; at full inspiration maintained with the glottis open *(B)*, vein diameter is 7 mm; at full inspiration with a sustained Valsalva maneuver *(C)*, vein diameter is 3 mm; at full expiration with a sustained Müller maneuver *(D)*, vein diameter is 17 mm. See the text for discussion.

being larger on inspiration than on expiration in some patients and vice versa in others (Fig. 8–29). Since these patients included a majority of subjects with no suspicion of pulmonary or cardiovascular disease, it is clear that variation in azygos vein diameter is related to intrathoracic pressure phenomena: when the vein is smaller on inspiration than on expiration, patients are probably involuntarily performing the Valsalva maneuver when asked to hold their breath for exposure of the inspiration film, whereas subjects with a larger vein diameter on the inspiratory film are presumably holding their breath with the glottis open.

Of considerable interest is the wide range of measurements and increased average size of the azygos vein observed in a study of 100 pregnant women.[66] The minimal diameter was 3 mm, but the maximal diameter was 15 mm and the average, 7.1 mm. This normal effect of pregnancy, undoubtedly related to hypervolemia, should be borne in mind when considering the differential diagnosis of azygos vein enlargement.

We believe that in normal subjects in the erect position, the upper limit of normal for the diameter of the azygos vein is 10 mm. A diameter exceeding 10 mm should be regarded as pathologic except in pregnant women and in unusual circumstances of very negative intrapleural pressure. Vascular distention caused by change in body position from erect to recumbent also increases the vein's diameter (Fig. 8–30). In one study of 40 healthy subjects, the maximal diameter of the vein in the supine position was measured by using a tomographic technique with a shortened focus-film distance and was correlated with several parameters, including age, sex, weight, height, and body surface area.[68] The only significant correlation was with body weight. Standardization of the diameters to a body weight of 64 kg yielded a mean azygos vein diameter of 14.2 mm; the diameter exceeded 16 mm in only 8 subjects. It seems reasonable to use

these figures to indicate normality or otherwise in patients whose radiographs must be obtained in a supine position at the bedside.

Vascular Pedicle

In an extensive review of the superior mediastinal vascular interfaces, Milne and associates[69] pointed out that a large portion of the mediastinal opacity on both PA and AP chest radiographs is caused by the great systemic vessels and that the heart may be considered to be "hanging" from these vessels; this concept prompted these workers to call this "structure" the *vascular pedicle*. On a frontal chest radiograph, the vascular pedicle extends from the thoracic inlet to the top of the heart. On the right, its boundary is formed by the right brachiocephalic vein above and the superior vena cava below. The left border of the pedicle is formed by the left subclavian artery above the aortic arch. In essence, the right side of the pedicle is situated anteriorly and is entirely venous, whereas the left side lies more posteriorly and is arterial (Fig. 8–31).

The authors measured the width of the vascular pedicle on PA (or AP) chest radiographs from the point at which the superior vena cava crosses the right main bronchus to the point at which the left subclavian artery arises from the aortic arch (Fig. 8–31). Using these landmarks in 83 normal subjects, it was determined that the mean value was 48 mm (±5 mm SD). As anticipated, there was considerable difference in vascular pedicle width between asthenic and nonasthenic subjects; however, 95% of measurements fell within 38 to 58 mm (mean, ±2 SD).

The concept that changes in the width of the vascular pedicle and azygos vein reflect intrathoracic vascular transmural pressure has been applied in an assessment of the

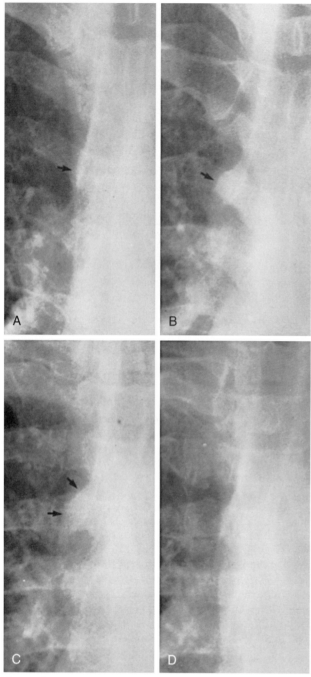

Figure 8–29. Variation in Azygos Vein Diameter from Inspiration to Expiration. Detail view of the region of the right tracheobronchial angle from two normal subjects in the erect position in maximal inspiration (total lung capacity) and full expiration (residual volume). In *A* and *B* the azygos vein *(arrow)* is smaller on inspiration than on expiration, the more common appearance. In *C (arrows)* and *D* the azygos vein is larger on inspiration than on expiration.

hemodynamic status of the systemic circulation in 61 patients with cardiac disease and correlated with total blood volume.[70, 71] A linear correlation between the width of the vascular pedicle and total blood volume was demonstrated. In patients with dilated neck veins, vascular pedicle width was greater than 62 mm, a measurement that also correlated strongly with a change in total blood volume. By contrast, correlation between azygos vein width and total blood vol-

ume was poor, although the correlation between vein width and mean right atrial pressure was stronger.

In an attempt to differentiate between physiologic and pathologic intravascular and extravascular causes for widening of the vascular pedicle, the same group of investigators measured the width of the pedicle and correlated it with visibility of the right tracheal stripe and the azygos vein on the PA radiographs of 158 patients.[71] The widened pedicle was attributed to intravascular causes in 108 patients and to perivascular hemorrhage or the infusion of fluid through inappropriately positioned subclavian lines in 50. An increase in systemic blood volume (or the supine position) resulted in a combination of widening of the vascular pedicle to the right and dilation of the azygos vein (Fig. 8–32); the tracheal stripe and azygos vein were visible in 86% of patients in this group. By contrast, extravascular causes of widening of the mediastinal silhouette (e.g., aortic trauma or extravasation of blood or saline) resulted in widening of the pedicle to either the left or right of the midline (depending on the specific etiology), obliteration of the tracheal stripe, and loss of visibility of the azygos vein. Of 40 patients with post-traumatic bleeding into the vascular pedicle and in 10 with inadvertent extravascular infusion into the pedicle, the tracheal stripe and azygos vein were only visible in 6%.

INFRA-AZYGOS AREA

Azygoesophageal Recess

The azygos vein ascends in the posterior mediastinum in relation to the right side or front of the vertebral column. The esophagus is usually located slightly anterior and to the left of the vein in the prevertebral region, although they are sometimes in contact. The *azygoesophageal recess* is formed by contact of the right lower lobe with the esophagus and the ascending portion of the azygos vein (Fig. 8–33).[72, 73] It is highly variable in depth, depending largely on the degree of lung inflation and the position of the descending aorta.

The recess is frequently identified on well-penetrated PA radiographs as an interface that extends from the diaphragm below to the level of the azygos arch above. Its right side is sharply delineated by aerated right lower lobe parenchyma; its left side is usually of unit density because of contiguity of the azygos vein, esophagus, aorta, and surrounding posterior mediastinal connective tissue. Viewed from above downward on a frontal chest radiograph, the configuration of the azygoesophageal recess interface is variable. Typically, it is seen as a continuous shallow or deep arc concave to the right; however, in young adults, a straight or slightly dextroconvex interface may be seen.[74] Focal right-sided convexity of the azygoesophageal recess interface should raise the suspicion of an underlying pathologic process such as hiatal hernia, esophageal tumor, duplication cyst, dilation of the azygos vein, or subcarinal lymphadenopathy.[73] It should be noted, however, that displacement of the azygoesophageal recess is not a particularly sensitive sign for the detection of subcarinal lymphadenopathy. In one study of radiographic and CT findings in 90 patients, a focal abnormality in the contour of the azygoesophageal recess interface was present on the radiograph in only 7 of 30 patients (23%) with enlarged subcarinal nodes on CT;[75] in

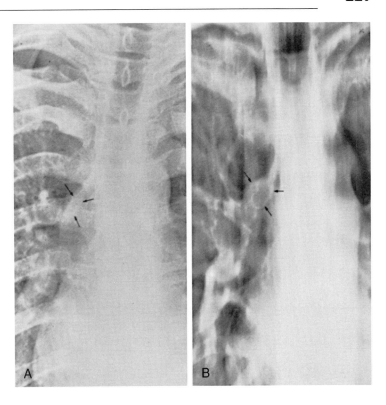

Figure 8–30. Effect of Body Position on Azygos Vein Diameter. A radiograph in the erect position *(A)* shows the azygos vein as an elliptical shadow projected in the right tracheobronchial angle *(arrows)*. In the same subject, a tomographic section of the midmediastinum in the supine position *(B)* demonstrates a much larger vein shadow *(arrows)* owing to distention brought about by the supine body position.

fact, lymphadenopathy was seldom detected on the radiograph unless the subcarinal nodes were greater than 2 cm in diameter.

If gas is present in a distended esophagus, the combined thickness of the right esophageal wall and contiguous pleura can create a vertically oriented linear opacity or stripe known as the *right inferior esophagopleural stripe* (Fig. 8–34). Although the left lung may abut the left wall of the esophagus, it is normally excluded by paraesophageal fat and the descending aorta; when intruding lung does make contact with the gas-distended esophagus, a *left inferior esophagopleural stripe* may be formed. If the right and left lower lobe pleurae meet behind the esophagus (an uncommon situation), a *posteroinferior junction line* may be identified. Although the posterior superior junction line is seen in approximately 40% of normal chest radiographs, the posteroinferior (intra-aortic) line is seen in less than 1%.[75a] The majority of individuals in whom the latter is identified have emphysema, a tortuous aorta, or thoracic kyphosis. In one study of 118 consecutive chest radiographs of patients who had emphysema, a posterior inferior junction line or left inferior esophagopleural stripe was seen in 27 (23%).[75a]

THE HEART

It is beyond the scope of this book to discuss the radiology of the heart in detail. However, it is important to recognize that certain deviations in the normal radiographic anatomy of the cardiovascular silhouette may give rise to confusion in the diagnosis of pleuropulmonary disease.

In a frontal radiograph of the normal chest, the position of the heart in relation to the midline of the thorax depends largely on the patient's build. Assuming radiographic exposure with the lungs fully inflated, the heart shadow is almost exactly midline in position in asthenic individuals, only projecting slightly more to the left; in those of stockier build, it lies a little more to the left of midline (in the range of three quarters to one quarter).[76] In one study of 500 healthy adults the following variations in the heart's position relative to the midline were noted:[77] projection of a small to moderate segment of the heart to the right of the spine (87.5%), extension of the heart to the right almost as far as to the left of the spine (7%), extension more to the right than to the left (0.2%, 1 subject), coincidence of the right border of the heart and spine (3.3%), and (in about 2%) projection of the right heart border over the spine (a common finding in patients with pectus excavatum).

In normal subjects, the transverse diameter of the heart measured on standard PA radiographs is usually in the range of 11.5 to 15.5 cm;[76] it is less than 11.5 cm in approximately 5% and only rarely exceeds 15.5 cm (in very heavy subjects of stocky build). The custom of trying to assess cardiac size by relating it to the transverse diameter of the chest (cardiothoracic ratio), although helpful, has potential pitfalls. On PA radiographs, a cardiothoracic ratio of 50% is widely accepted as the upper limit of normal; however, it exceeds 50% in at least 10% of normal subjects.[76] Measurement of the ratio is especially fallacious in patients who have a small heart: in a person with an 8-cm transverse cardiac diameter in a 24-cm thorax, the heart would have to enlarge 4 cm before the cardiothoracic ratio reaches 50%.[76] In our view, it is preferable to evaluate cardiac size subjectively on the basis of experience; alternatively, it is reasonable to assume that a heart whose transverse diameter exceeds 15.5 to 16 cm is enlarged.

Chiefly as a result of the influence of systole and diastole, both the size and contour of the heart may vary from one examination to another, even when all examinations are made with an identical degree of lung inflation. In

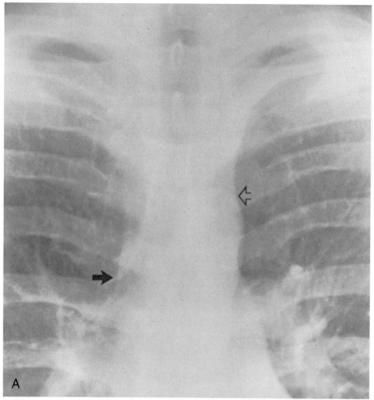

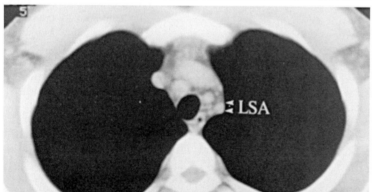

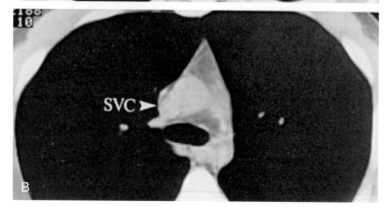

Figure 8–31. Normal Vascular Pedicle. A detail view from a conventional posteroanterior radiograph *(A)* demonstrates the points for measuring the width of the vascular pedicle. The right (venous) border of the vascular pedicle is the point at which the superior vena cava crosses the right main bronchus *(closed arrow)*, whereas the left border is the point of takeoff of the left subclavian artery from the aorta *(open arrow)*. Vascular pedicle width is measured from the superior vena cava to a perpendicular line extended caudally from the left subclavian artery. A CT scan *(B)* through the superior mediastinum at the level of the superior vena cava (SVC) *(single arrowhead)* and left subclavian artery (LSA) *(double arrowheads)* shows that the right border is entirely venous and the left border is entirely arterial.

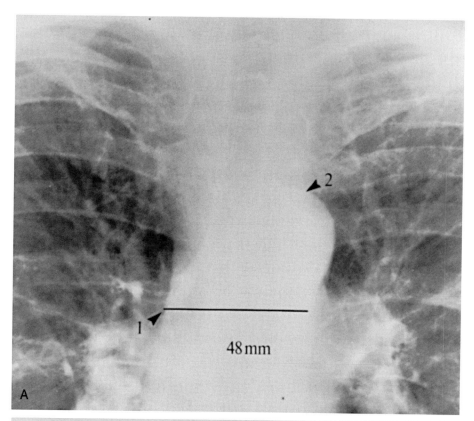

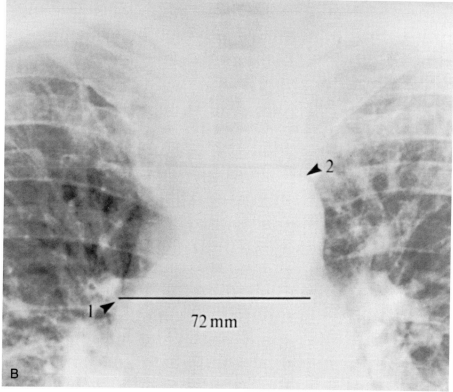

Figure 8–32. Abnormal Vascular Pedicle. A detail view from a conventional posteroanterior chest radiograph *(A)* reveals a vascular pedicle width of 48 mm (measured from Point 1 to a perpendicular dropped from Point 2—*see* Fig. 8–31). *B,* Following the onset of congestive heart failure, the vascular pedicle width has increased to 72 mm (compare the size of the upper lobe vasculature in the two illustrations). Most of the increase in vascular pedicle width is caused by distention of the superior vena cava.

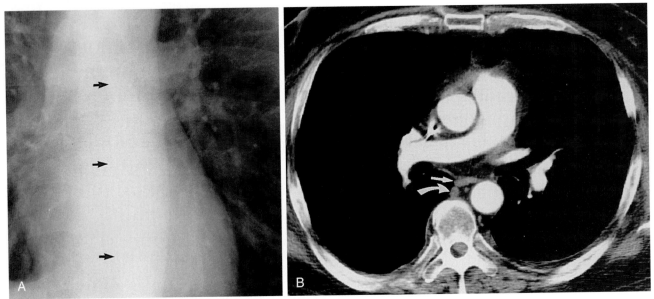

Figure 8–33. Azygoesophageal Recess. A posteroanterior chest radiograph *(A)* in a 36-year-old man demonstrates a normal azygoesophageal recess interface *(arrows)* extending from the level of the tracheal carina to the diaphragm to form a shallow arc convex to the right. A CT scan *(B)* demonstrates that the interface results from contact between the right lung and the posterior mediastinum (more specifically, between the right lung and the esophagus *[straight arrow]* and azygos vein *[curved arrow]*).

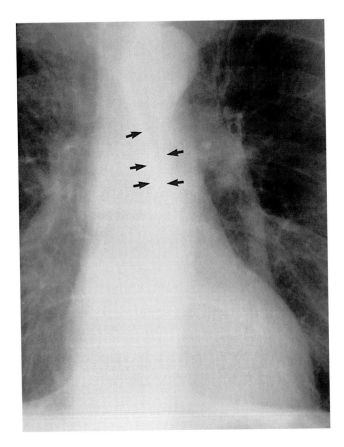

Figure 8–34. Inferior Esophagopleural Stripe. A posteroanterior chest radiograph demonstrates two curvilinear opacities *(arrows)* that extend from the infra-aortic region to the diaphragm; these opacities represent the right and left walls of the gas-distended esophagus. The soft tissue stripe between the gas-filled esophagus and the right lung represents the right inferior esophagopleural stripe.

one study of 324 patients for whom PA radiographs were obtained in both systole and diastole (through electrocardiographic monitoring), the change in transverse cardiac diameter was 0.3 cm or less in 52%, 0.4 to 0.9 cm in 41%, and 1.0 to 1.7 cm in 7%.[78] An addendum to this report states that the researchers had observed a cardiac diameter increase of 2.0 cm or more from systole to diastole in only 5 of about 1,500 patients. In another study of 200 normal individuals, the maximal difference in transverse cardiac diameter on successive examinations was 2 cm (in 1 patient only), and the group average was 0.5 cm.[76]

When the influence of systole and diastole is controlled (by exposure of 1 second or longer), the major influences on cardiac size and contour are threefold: (1) the *height of the diaphragm*, which in turn is influenced by the degree of pulmonary inflation—the lower the position of the diaphragm, the longer and therefore narrower the cardiovascular silhouette; (2) *intrathoracic pressure*, which influences not only cardiac size but also the appearance of the pulmonary vascular pattern; and (3) *body position*—assuming equality of all other factors, the heart is broader when a subject is recumbent than when erect.

Physiologic accumulations of fat are common in the cardiophrenic recesses bilaterally and produce an obtuse angular configuration of the inferior mediastinum at its junction with the diaphragm. Their density may be slightly less than that of the heart and thus allow identification of the approximate position of the cardiac borders. These pleuropericardial fat shadows should not be misinterpreted as cardiac enlargement or as mediastinal or diaphragmatic masses of possible importance; however, as stated earlier, the bilateral cardiophrenic regions contain parietal lymph nodes of the middle mediastinal chain; enlargement of such nodes—for example, in patients with lymphoma—may simulate pleuropericardial fat.[79]

REFERENCES

1. Banister LH: The respiratory system. *In* Williams PL (ed): Gray's Anatomy. New York, Churchill Livingstone, 1995, pp 1627–1682.
2. Leszczynski SZ, Pawlicka L: Purulent and Fibrous Mediastinitis. Radiological Diagnosis. Warsaw, PZWL (Polish Medical Publishers), 1972.
3. Heitzman ER: The Mediastinum. Radiologic Correlations with Anatomy and Pathology. St. Louis, CV Mosby, 1977, pp 216–334.
4. Felson B: Chest Roentgenology. Philadelphia, WB Saunders, 1973.
5. Zylak CJ, Pallie W, Jackson R: Correlative anatomy and computed tomography: A module on the mediastinum. Radiographics 2:555, 1982.
6. Davies DV, Coupland RE (eds): The respiratory system. *In* Gray's Anatomy: Descriptive and Applied. London, Longmans, Green, & Company, 1958.
7. Proto AV, Simmons JD, Zylak CJ: The anterior junction anatomy. CRC Crit Rev Diagn Imaging 19:111, 1983.
8. Proto AV, Simmons JD, Zylak CJ: The posterior junction anatomy. CRC Crit Rev Diagn Imaging 20:121, 1983.
9. Proto AV: Mediastinal anatomy: Emphasis on conventional images with anatomic and computed tomographic correlations. J Thorac Imaging 2:1, 1987.
10. Woodring JH, Daniel TL: Medical analysis emphasizing plain radiographs and computed tomograms. Med Radiogr Photogr 62:1, 1986.
11. Chasen MH, McCarthy MJ, Gilliland JD, et al: Concepts in computed tomography of the thorax. Radiographics 6:793, 1986.
12. Felson B: The mediastinum. Semin Roentgenol 4:31, 1969.
13. Oliphant M, Wiot JF, Whalen JP: The cervicothoracic continuum. Radiology 120:257, 1976.
14. Kendall MD, Johnson HRM, Singh J: The weight of the human thymus gland at necropsy. J Anat 131:485, 1980.
15. Steinmann GG: Changes in the human thymus during aging. Curr Top Pathol 75:43, 1986.
16. von Gaudecker B: Functional histology of the human thymus. Anat Embryol 183:1, 1991.
17. Suster S, Rosai J: Histology of the normal thymus. Am J Surg Pathol 14:284, 1990.
18. van de Wijngaert FP, Kendall MD, Schuurman H-J, et al: Heterogeneity of epithelial cells in the human thymus: An ultrastructural study. Cell Tissue Res 237:227, 1984.
19. Janossy G, Bofill M, Trejdosiewicz LK, et al: Cellular differentiation of lymphoid subpopulations and their microenvironments in the human thymus. Curr Top Pathol 75:89, 1986.
20. Barthelemy H, Pelletier M, Landry D, et al: Demonstration of OKT6 antigen on human thymic dendritic cells in culture. Lab Invest 55:540, 1986.
21. Sato T, Tamaoki N: Myoid cells in the human thymus and thymoma revealed by three different immunohistochemical markers for striated muscle. Acta Pathol Jpn 39:509, 1989.
22. Rosai J, Levine G, Weber WR, et al: Carcinoid tumors and oat cell carcinomas of the thymus. Pathol Annu 11:201, 1976.
23. Baron RL, Lee JKT, Sagel SS, et al: Computed tomography of the normal thymus. Radiology 142:121, 1982.
24. Day DL, Gedgaudas E: The thymus. Radiol Clin North Am 22:519, 1984.
25. Francis IR, Glazer GM, Bookstein FL, et al: The thymus: Reexamination of age-related changes in size and shape. Am J Roentgenol 145:249, 1985.
26. Caffey J, Sibley R: Regrowth and overgrowth of the thymus after atrophy induced by oral administration of corticosteroids to human infants. Pediatrics 26:762, 1960.
27. Gelfand DW, Goldman AS, Law AJ: Thymic hyperplasia in children recovering from thermal burns. J Trauma 12:813, 1972.
28. Cohen M, Hill CA, Cangir A, et al: Thymic rebound after treatment of childhood tumors. Am J Roentgenol 135:152, 1980.
29. Kissin CM, Husband JE, Nicholas D, et al: Benign thymic enlargement in adults after chemotherapy: CT demonstration. Radiology 163:67, 1987.
30. Siegel MJ, Glazer HS, Wiener JI, et al: Normal and abnormal thymus in childhood: MR imaging. Radiology 172:367, 1989.
31. Brown LR, Aughenbaugh GL: Masses of the anterior mediastinum: CT and MR imaging. Am J Roentgenol 157:1171, 1991.
32. de Geer G, Webb WR, Gamsu G: Normal thymus: Assessment with MR and CT. Radiology 158:313, 1986.
33. Kattan KR, Felson B, Holder LE, et al: Superior mediastinal shift in right lower lobe collapse. The "upper triangle sign." Radiology 116:305, 1975.
34. Proto AV, Speckman JM: The left lateral radiograph of the chest. Med Radiogr Photogr 55:2, 1980.
34a. Landay M: Anterior clear space: How clear? How often? How come? Radiology 192:165, 1994.
35. Jemelin C, Candardjis G: Retrosternal soft tissue: Quantitative evaluation and clinical interest. Radiology 109:7, 1973.
36. Whalen JP, Oliphant M, Evans JA: Anterior extrapleural line: Superior extension. Radiology 115:525, 1975.
37. Branscom JJ, Austin JHM: Aberrant right subclavian artery: Findings seen on plain chest roentgenograms. Am J Roentgenol 119:539, 1973.
38. Ball JB Jr, Proto AV: The variable appearance of the left superior intercostal vein. Radiology 144:445, 1982.
39. McDonald CJ, Castellino RA, Blank N: The aortic nipple: The left superior intercostal vein. Radiology 96:533, 1970.
40. Friedman AC, Chambers E, Sprayregen S: The normal and abnormal left superior intercostal vein. Am J Roentgenol 131:599, 1978.
41. Lane EJ, Heitzman ER, Dinn WM: The radiology of the superior intercostal veins. Radiology 120:263, 1976.
42. Blank N, Castellino RA: Patterns of pleural reflections of the left superior mediastinum: Normal anatomy and distortions produced by adenopathy. Radiology 102:585, 1972.
43. Keats TE: The aortic-pulmonary mediastinal stripe. Am J Roentgenol 116:107, 1972.
44. Heitzman ER, Lane EJ, Hammack DB, et al: Radiological evaluation of the aortic-pulmonic window. Radiology 116:513, 1975.
45. Jolles PR, Shin MS, Jones WP: Aortopulmonary window lesions: Detection with chest radiography. Radiology 159:647, 1986.
46. Müller NL, Nichols DM: Accuracy of the plain radiograph in the detection of aortopulmonary lymphadenopathy. J Can Assoc Radiol 38:82, 1987.
47. Genereux GP: The posterior pleural reflections. Am J Roentgenol 141:141, 1983.
48. Heitzman ER: The Mediastinum: Radiologic Correlations with Anatomy and Pathology. St. Louis, CV Mosby, 1977, pp 33–66, 198–206.
49. Lane EJ, Proto AV, Phillips TW: Mach bands and density perception. Radiology 121:9, 1976.
50. Grant JCB: Respiratory system. *In* Brash JC (ed): Cunningham's Textbook of Anatomy. New York, Oxford University Press, 1951, p 1331.
51. Savoca CJ, Austin JHM, Goldberg HI: The right paratracheal stripe. Radiology 122:295, 1977.
52. Müller NL, Webb WR, Gamsu G: Paratracheal lymphadenopathy: Radiographic findings and correlation with CT. Radiology 156:761, 1985.
53. Woodring JH, Pulmano CM, Stevens RK: The right paratracheal stripe in blunt chest trauma. Radiology 143:603, 1982.
54. Bachman AL, Teixidor HS: The posterior tracheal band: Reflector of local superior mediastinal abnormality. Br J Radiol 48:352, 1975.
55. Palayew MJ: The tracheo-esophageal stripe and the posterior tracheal band. Radiology 132:11, 1979.
56. Proto A, Speckman JM: The left lateral radiograph of the chest. Med Radiogr Photogr 55:1, 1979.
57. Yrjana J: The posterior tracheal band and recurrent esophageal carcinoma. Radiology 136:615, 1980.
58. Kormano M, Yrjana J: The posterior tracheal band: Correlation between computed tomography and chest radiography. Radiology 136:689, 1980.
59. Putman CE, Curtis AM, Westfried M, et al: Thickening of the posterior tracheal stripe: A sign of squamous cell carcinoma of the esophagus. Radiology 121:533, 1976.
60. Figley M: Mediastinal minutiae. Semin Roentgenol 4:22, 1969.
61. Kittredge RD: The right posterolateral tracheal band. J Comput Assist Tomogr 3:348, 1979.
62. Proto AV, Lane EJ: Air in the esophagus: A frequent radiographic finding. Am J Roentgenol 129:433, 1977.
63. Cimmino CV: The esophageal-pleural stripe on chest teleroentgenograms. Radiology 67:754, 1956.
64. Cimmino CV: Further notes on the esophageal-pleural stripe. Radiology 77:974, 1961.
65. Fleischner FG, Udis SW: Dilatation of the azygos vein: A roentgen sign of venous engorgement. Am J Roentgenol 67:569, 1952.
66. Keats TE, Lipscomb GE, Betts CS III: Mensuration of the arch of the azygos vein and its application to the study of cardiopulmonary disease. Radiology 90:990, 1968.
67. Felson B: Letter from the editor. Semin Roentgenol 2:323, 1967.
68. Doyle FH, Read AE, Evans KT: The mediastinum in portal hypertension. Clin Radiol 12:114, 1961.
69. Milne ENC, Pistolesi M, Miniati M, et al: The vascular pedicle of the heart and the vena azygos. Part I: The normal subject. Radiology 152:1, 1984.
70. Pistolesi M, Milne ENC, Miniati M, et al: The vascular pedicle of the heart and the vena azygos. Part II: Acquired heart disease. Radiology 152:9, 1984.
71. Milne E, Imray TJ, Pistolesi M, et al: The vascular pedicle and the vena azygos. Part III: In trauma—the "vanishing" azygos. Radiology 153:25, 1984.
72. Heitzman ER, Scrivani JV, Martino J, et al: The azygos vein and its pleural reflections. I. Normal roentgen anatomy. Radiology 101:249, 1971.
73. Heitzman ER, Scrivani JV, Martino J, et al: The azygos vein and its pleural reflections. II. Applications in the radiological diagnosis of mediastinal abnormality. Radiology 101:259, 1971.
74. Onitsuka H, Kuhns LR: Dextroconvexity of the mediastinum in the azygoesophageal recess. Radiology 135:126, 1980.
75. Müller NL, Webb WR, Gamsu G: Subcarinal lymph node enlargement: Radiographic findings and CT correlation. Am J Roentgenol 145:15, 1985.
75a. Curtis BR, Fisher MS: Posterior inferior junction line and left pleuroesophageal stripe: Their association with emphysema. J Thorac Imaging 13:184, 1998.
76. Simon G: Principles of Chest X-ray Diagnosis. 3rd ed. London, Butterworth, 1971.
77. Felson B: Chest Roentgenology. Philadelphia, WB Saunders, 1973.
78. Gammill SL, Krebs C, Meyers P, et al: Cardiac measurements in systole and diastole. Radiology 94:115, 1970.
79. Castellino RA, Blank N: Adenopathy of the cardiophrenic angle (diaphragmatic) lymph nodes. Am J Roentgenol 114:509, 1972.

CHAPTER 9

The Control of Breathing

THE INPUT, 235
    Peripheral Chemoreceptors, 235
    Central Chemoreceptors, 237
    Receptors in the Respiratory Tract and Lungs, 237
    Respiratory Muscle Afferents, 238
THE CENTRAL CONTROLLER, 238
THE OUTPUT, 240
CONTROL OF VENTILATION DURING EXERCISE, 241
COMPENSATION FOR ADDED VENTILATORY
LOADS, 241
CONTROL OF UPPER AIRWAY MUSCLES, 242
CONTROL OF BREATHING DURING SLEEP, 243

The main purpose of breathing is to achieve and maintain alveolar and arterial blood gas homeostasis so that the oxygen demands of the organism are met and the metabolic byproduct, carbon dioxide, is exhaled. For purposes of discussion, the respiratory control system can be divided into four parts: (1) afferent input to the central respiratory controller; (2) the controller and its central integration; (3) output from the respiratory center; and (4) the effectors of the output, the respiratory muscles. In this chapter we consider the first three of these components; the respiratory muscles are discussed separately in Chapter 10 (*see* page 246). The subject of control of breathing has received considerable attention and is well summarized in several reviews.[1–8] Figure 9–1 is an overview of the respiratory control systems.

THE INPUT

Input to the central regulator of respiration conveys information about arterial blood gas tensions, lung mechanics, and respiratory muscle function. The input includes (1) information from the peripheral and central chemoreceptors, which respond to alterations in arterial PO_2, PCO_2, and hydrogen ion concentration; (2) afferents from receptors in the respiratory tract and lungs, which are influenced by lung mechanics; and (3) afferents from muscle spindles and tendon organs in the respiratory muscles, which monitor the effectiveness of the peripheral effector system.

Peripheral Chemoreceptors

The anatomy and physiology of the peripheral chemoreceptors have been extensively reviewed.[9, 10] The carotid body is the major peripheral chemoreceptor.[5, 11] It develops with the third branchial arch and can be recognized in the human embryo as early as 6 weeks of gestation. The adult organ measures approximately $3 \times 1.5 \times 1.5$ mm and is situated in the adventitia of the carotid artery at its bifurcation into internal and external branches. Histologically, it is composed of compact nests of cells (predominantly chief cells with lesser numbers of sustentacular cells) surrounded by a richly vascular stroma. The chief cells are derived from neural crest ectoderm and contain abundant dopamine as well as norepinephrine, 5-hydroxytryptamine, and acetylcholine. Sensory neurons originate in juxtaposition to chief cells, and their axons ascend in the glossopharyngeal nerve to nerve bodies in the glossopharyngeal sensory ganglia. Hypoxia increases dopamine release and synthesis by the chief cells, a process that is presumably followed by stimulation of afferent nerve endings. The central projections of carotid chemoreceptor afferents stimulate respiration during hypoxia by release of substance P.[12]

Although the normal carotid body is very small (weighing only about 5 to 20 mg), the organ has been estimated to receive up to 0.2 liter of blood per minute per gram of tissue (more than 40 times the flow per gram to the brain).[13] This enormous blood flow results in a virtually unchanged PO_2 in the blood during its passage through the carotid body. In the presence of chronic hypoxemia, the carotid body enlarges as a result of hypertrophy and hyperplasia of glomus cells, as well as a proliferation of blood vessels and connective tissue elements. People who live continuously at high altitudes have not only enlarged carotid bodies but also an increased incidence of carotid body tumors.

Receptor activity from the carotid body can be measured by recording afferent nerve impulses in the carotid sinus nerve before it joins the glossopharyngeal nerve or by splitting out individual afferent fibers and recording their response characteristics. There is always some afferent activity from the carotid body, even with a very high PaO_2; the firing frequency increases progressively as the PaO_2 is lowered and increases steeply below a PaO_2 of 200 mm Hg. The response to acute hypoxic challenge is brisk, but with sustained hypoxemia there tends to be adaptation with an attenuation of the hyperpnea.[14, 15] The firing frequency in the carotid chemoreceptor nerves is also increased by hypercapnia and a change in pH. The hypoxic and hypercapnic responses are additive, in that both stimuli together result in enhanced response. In addition to the steady-state responses of the chemoreceptor, enhanced firing appears to accompany

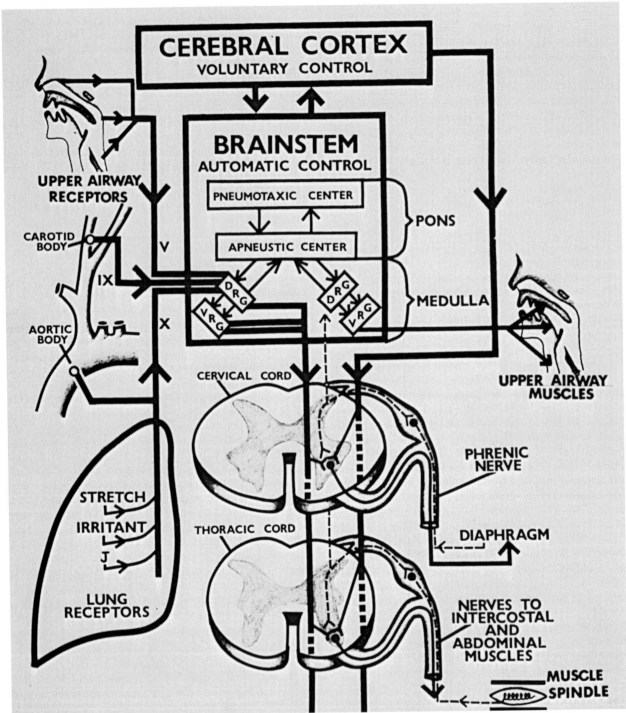

Figure 9–1. Respiratory Control System. Central respiratory control is shared by voluntary (cerebral) and automatic (brainstem) centers. The efferent fibers from each run in distinct spinal cord pathways, as depicted on the left side of the coronally sectioned spinal cord *(right side of drawing).* A variety of interconnections exist between the cortex and the different components of the brainstem. The pontine pneumotaxic (PNC) center and apneustic center (APC) are now termed the *pontine respiratory group* (PRG). Afferent fibers ascending the 5th (V), 9th (IX), and 10th (X) cranial nerves from upper airway receptors, peripheral chemoreceptors, and visceral and lung receptors connect with the ipsilateral dorsal respiratory group of neurons (DRG). In addition, afferents from Golgi tendon organs in the diaphragm and intercostal muscle spindles travel in the phrenic and intercostal nerves and reach the anterior horn cells, as well as ascend to the DRG via the dorsal columns. Respiratory neurons in the DRG are connected with those in the ventral respiratory group (VRG), from which the descending neural output originates. The efferent fibers cross in the brainstem and descend in the spinal cord to supply the diaphragm, intercostal, accessory, and expiratory muscles. Neurons in the VRG also project via the ipsilateral 9th, 10th, and 12th cranial nerves to the upper airways, where they innervate the laryngeal, genioglossal, geniohyoid, and other upper airway muscles.

rapid swings in arterial P_{O_2} and P_{CO_2}, which suggests that the rate of change of arterial blood gas tension is as important a stimulus as the average level. In humans at rest, there are substantial swings in arterial P_{O_2} and P_{CO_2} related to the ventilatory and cardiac cycles; since these swings tend to increase during exercise, rates of change of arterial P_{O_2} and P_{CO_2} may be important in the regulation of exercise ventilation.[9, 10, 16]

The carotid body receives sympathetic and parasympathetic efferent input. Stimulation of either causes increased chemoreceptor activity, which may be produced by redistribution of blood flow within the receptor. Stimulation of the carotid body receptors by hypoxia, hypercapnia, and acidosis results in an increase in ventilation, bronchomotor tone, systemic blood pressure, and pulmonary vascular resistance, as well as a generalized increase in catecholamine secretion; during sleep, it may cause arousal.[17] In the absence of peripheral chemoreceptors, the hypoxic ventilatory response is abolished, and in fact, hypoxemia may cause ventilatory depression; in this circumstance, however, 85% of the ventilatory response to CO_2 is preserved.[18]

Central Chemoreceptors

The exact location and structure of the central chemoreceptors have not been established. However, three areas have been identified in the ventrolateral surface of the medulla oblongata, some 200 to 500 μm below the surface, that respond to alterations in cerebrospinal fluid (CSF) and extracellular hydrogen ion concentration with an increase in ventilation. By magnetic resonance imaging, these areas show increased blood flow during inhalation of hypercarbic gas mixtures.[19] The exact cells involved in the transduction and their connections to the dorsal and ventral respiratory neurons that generate the respiratory rhythm have not been fully elucidated.[20]

As indicated, the stimulus for these receptors is the hydrogen ion concentration of brain extracellular fluid. Since the blood-brain barrier is more permeable to carbon dioxide than to hydrogen ion or bicarbonate ion, hypercapnic acidosis is a more powerful stimulus to central chemoreceptors than is metabolic acidosis. With the increased circulating hydrogen ion concentration associated with the latter condition, there is stimulation of the peripheral chemoreceptors, an increase in ventilation, and a decrease in P_{CO_2}; there can actually be a paradoxical transient decrease in CSF hydrogen ion concentration despite the blood metabolic acidosis. The higher CSF pH tends to attenuate the central ventilatory response to acute metabolic acidosis. Similarly, the acute ventilatory response to hypoxia from the stimulation of peripheral chemoreceptors is partly offset by the resulting hypocapnic alkalosis. With time, changes in CSF pH occur as hydrogen ion concentration equilibrates across the blood-brain barrier over a period of hours. Thus, if acidosis is prolonged, there is a progressive fall in CSF pH to more acid levels that results in progressive stimulation of ventilation so that arterial P_{CO_2} continues to decrease as metabolic acidosis is sustained. The exact mechanism by which the CSF hydrogen ion concentration is regulated remains controversial, and both passive and active transporting mechanisms have been suggested.[18]

Receptors in the Respiratory Tract and Lungs

Afferent input to the respiratory center is derived from receptors at all levels of the respiratory tract and is carried by the 5th, 9th, and 10th cranial nerves. Nasal receptors, which travel in the trigeminal nerve, are responsible for sneezing, reflex bronchodilation, and increased production of mucus; they may be important in initiating the diving reflex (apnea on immersion). When stimulated, rapidly adapting fibers in the nasopharynx cause bronchodilation and increased secretion of mucus; these receptors, whose afferent fibers are carried in the glossopharyngeal nerve, may also be important in modulating the ventilatory response to carbon dioxide and have been shown to result in inhibition of diaphragmatic contraction when stimulated by the passage of cold air through the nasopharynx.[21–23] Nasal afferents also respond to a variety of chemical substances, including aldehyde gases, ammonia, nicotine, and capsaicin.[7]

The larynx is richly supplied with afferent nerve endings, which are carried in both the superior and recurrent laryngeal nerves. Input from superficial receptors situated in the epithelium and subepithelial connective tissue initiates coughing, apnea, expiratory efforts, bronchoconstriction, laryngeal constriction, and increased airway mucus secretion. Specific cold-sensitive receptors are also present that decrease ventilatory drive during the inhalation of cold air and are apparently especially active in infants.[7] Cold air reaching the larynx also depresses laryngeal mechanoreceptors. These important receptors respond to changes in transmural pressure, upper airway air flow, and contraction of the upper airway muscles; the most important stimulus appears to be negative intra-airway pressure.[7, 21, 24] The mechanoreceptor reflexes are important in maintaining upper airway patency, especially during the increased transmural pressure swings associated with upper airway obstruction. Changes in laryngeal surface liquid osmolality and ion concentration can also stimulate ventilation and modulate the response to mechanostimulation.[7]

Tracheobronchial receptors include irritant, stretch, and J receptors (*see* also page 146). Irritant receptors (rapidly adapting stretch or cough receptors) are most numerous in the large airways around the tracheal carina. They consist of free nerve endings located just below the tight junctions between cells in the tracheobronchial epithelium and are the termination of the neural network that extends throughout this epithelium. These receptors respond to mechanical as well as nonspecific chemical irritation by substances such as ammonia, sulfur dioxide, cigarette smoke, and (possibly) carbon dioxide. Histamine is a potent stimulator of irritant receptors and causes reflex bronchoconstriction as well as a direct contractile action on airway smooth muscle. Stimulation of irritant receptors also results in cough, increased mucus production, and rapid shallow breathing, chiefly by shortening the expiratory duration. Irritant receptor stimulation has been implicated in the bronchoconstriction associated with asthma and in alteration of the breathing pattern in patients with chronic airway diseases.

Pulmonary stretch receptors (slowly adapting stretch receptors) are situated within airway smooth muscle. They are responsible for the Hering-Breuer reflex (a period of apnea following lung inflation) and are concentrated in the trachea and large airways; 40% are situated in extrapulmonary airways. Stretch receptors respond by increasing their firing frequency with lung inflation or with an increase in transpulmonary pressure. They have a low threshold, and in animal studies most fire within the tidal volume range; airway smooth muscle constriction increases their responsiveness.

"J" receptors (abbreviated from juxtapulmonary capillary receptors) are small, nonmyelinated, slowly conducting fibers that are located largely in the periphery of the lung in close proximity to pulmonary capillaries, respiratory bronchioles, and alveolar ducts. They respond to a variety of stimuli, including microembolization of the pulmonary circulation, pulmonary edema, irritant gases such as ammonia, volatile anesthetics such as halothane, and drugs such as phenyldiguanide and capsaicin. Although the receptors probably play little role in the normal control of breathing, in the presence of pulmonary pathology such as pneumonia and congestion, their firing frequency may increase and result in reflex rapid shallow breathing, laryngeal constriction, hypotension, and bradycardia. Unlike the other airway receptors, their stimulation does not appear to enhance airway mucus secretion.[21]

Study of patients who have undergone successful lung and heart-lung transplantation has allowed an assessment of the importance of lung and cardiac afferents in the control of breathing. Somewhat surprisingly, there is remarkably little effect of the inevitable denervation on resting ventilation or the response to CO_2; the only change appears to be a slight increase in tidal volume at any level of ventilation, presumably the result of a lack of stretch receptor input.[25, 26]

In addition to afferents from the lung, the vagus nerve carries afferent input from subdiaphragmatic visceral organs that can modify ventilation. For example, stimulation of mechanoreceptors in the gallbladder decreases ipsilateral drive to the diaphragm, decreases tidal volume, and causes a switch from predominantly diaphragmatic to rib cage breathing.[27] This reflex is the probable explanation for the postoperative decrease in diaphragmatic function that is seen following upper, but not lower, abdominal surgery.[28, 29]

Respiratory Muscle Afferents

The respiratory muscle receptors are the least understood of the peripheral inputs to the respiratory center.[30] The major striated muscle receptors are Golgi tendon organs and muscle spindles. In the diaphragm, the chief sensory organ appears to be the former structure, muscle spindles being rare. The Golgi tendon apparatus consists of numerous free nerve endings entwined in the tendinous fibers of muscle origins. They are the afferents to the primary efferent alpha motor neurons in the spinal cord; the importance of central projections of these afferents is unknown.

The muscle spindle is a more complex receptor that is most prominent in the intercostal muscles, both inspiratory and expiratory, and in the accessory muscles of respiration. It consists of a spindle-shaped structure in which an intrafusal muscle fiber is innervated by sensory nerve endings, in addition to a gamma motor efferent. Stimulation of the afferent intrafusal fiber results in the classic gamma loop excitation by alpha motor neurons of extrafusal muscle fibers in the same spinal cord segment (intrasegmental reflex).

Extrasegmental reflexes that presumably originate in the muscle spindles have also been demonstrated by electrical stimulation of afferents in the central cut end of intercostal nerves; stimulation of these reflexes results in contraction of adjacent intercostal muscles. In addition, experiments in which stimulation of the central cut end of lower thoracic intercostal nerves causes reflex excitation of phrenic motor neurons have provided evidence of an intercostal-diaphragmatic reflex.

The precise role of these afferents and their influence on the central respiratory controller is unknown; however, the results of a number of studies suggest that they may be important. For example, cutting the dorsal cervical and thoracic roots can lead to temporary respiratory muscle paralysis in both animals and humans, and stimulation of splanchnic or muscle afferents produced by the trauma of upper abdominal surgery depresses diaphragmatic activity.[30–33] In addition to afferents from tendon organs and spindles that subserve stimulation of ventilation, the phrenic nerve contains nonmyelinated fibers that can cause a prolonged decrease in respiratory motoneuron output. Similar responses are elicited by stimulation of thin fibers from other skeletal muscles; their role could be to prevent respiratory muscle overload and fatigue.[34, 35]

THE CENTRAL CONTROLLER

Central control of respiratory rhythm and pattern can be either voluntary or involuntary. Automatic breathing originates from a highly complex accumulation of interconnected nerve cell groups situated in the brainstem. The most rostral of these aggregations is a group of neurons in the pons, most often designated the pontine respiratory group, but formally termed the *pneumotaxic center* (PNC). This neural complex is believed to be important in influencing the timing of the inspiratory cutoff by providing tonic input to pattern generators located at other sites. By this mechanism, cells in the PNC may modulate the respiratory response to stimuli such as hypercapnia, hypoxia, and lung inflation.[2, 5, 33, 36]

Immediately caudal to the PNC near the pontomedullary border lies the apneustic center (APC) (apneusis being the cessation of rhythmic breathing because of prolonged inspiratory activity). Although little is known about the APC, damage to it results in inactivation of the inspiratory cutoff switch and the production of apneusis when vagal input is also abolished. Removal of signals from the PNC and APC by transecting the brainstem between the medulla and the pons does not abolish respiratory rhythmicity; thus it is believed that the medulla alone is capable of generating a primary respiratory rhythm, the PNC and the APC being modulators of the timing mechanism. However, the rhythm generated from the isolated medulla is slower and of a more gasping nature than that developed when the PNC and the APC are intact. It is possible that multiple rhythm generators exist within the brainstem and that they only function as pacemakers after ablation of higher-order centers—a situation analogous to that in the heart, in which Purkinje fibers and the atrioventricular node serve as backup to the sinoatrial node.

Within the medulla, the respiratory neurons are grouped in two distinct areas: (1) the dorsal respiratory group (DRG), which consists of two bilateral aggregations of neurons located near the nucleus of the tractus solitarius and consisting almost exclusively of inspiratory cells; and (2) the ventral respiratory group (VRG), which lies close to the nucleus ambiguus and the nucleus retroambigualis and contains both inspiratory and expiratory cells. The DRG appears to play an important role in the regulation of respiration, since it is the primary projection site of numerous afferent fibers that travel in the 5th, 9th, and 10th cranial nerves from sensors originating in the upper airway, lungs, peripheral chemoreceptors, and (probably) proprioceptive afferents from the respiratory muscles and the chest wall. It is thought that the DRG is the primary site of rhythm generation, with the axons originating from it descending in the contralateral part of the spinal cord and serving as the principal respiratory rhythmic drive to anterior horn cells that innervate the diaphragm and inspiratory intercostals.

Cells from the DRG also stimulate cells in the VRG, which does not appear to have inherent respiratory rhythmicity or sensory input from peripheral or central chemoreceptors and mechanoreceptors. Axons from the VRG cross and descend in the spinal cord to innervate anterior horn cells in the cervical and thoracic cord; these cells then project to the intercostal inspiratory and expiratory muscles as well as to the abdominal and accessory muscles of respiration. Neurons in the VRG also project via the ipsilateral 9th, 10th, and 12th nerves to the upper airways, where they innervate the laryngeal, genioglossal, geniohyoid, and other muscles. These muscles receive rhythmic respiratory input and are important in maintaining upper airway patency.

Although traditionally considered in two phases, the concept that the respiratory cycle can be divided into three neurologic phases has also been considered. According to this concept, Phase I is initiated by an abrupt termination of inhibition of inspiratory neurons in the brainstem. This results in a sudden onset of inspiratory motor neuron activity, which is followed by slowly increasing activity and terminated by a sudden switchoff. The switchoff is in turn followed by the resurgence of a lesser degree of inspiratory activity termed the *postinspiratory inspiratory activity* (PIIA) or Phase II. Although insufficient to prolong inspiration, the PIIA can brake the rate of exhalation and, in some instances, may be important in setting functional residual capacity at a higher level than the static recoil of the lung and chest would otherwise dictate. The neurons responsible for the PIIA are different from those responsible for the main inspiratory activity. Phase III follows cessation of PIIA and is characterized by neural "quiet" (unless expiratory neurons are recruited). The latter are not stimulated until after the PIIA ceases and are usually recruited only with increased ventilatory drive. The greater the ventilatory drive, the shorter the PIIA and the greater the expiratory neuronal discharge.[37] Respiratory motoneurons can be classified by their timing and pattern of firing relative to the three phases of the cycle; some fire only in early inspiration, some late in inspiration, others only in the early postinspiratory period (PIIA), and some only in expiration.[5]

The pattern of central drive is altered depending on the stimulus. For example, hypoxia exerts a stronger action on inspiratory activity than does hypercapnia, which exerts a stronger action on expiratory muscles when matched for the same level of ventilation. The output to muscles controlling the upper airway is influenced more by peripheral than by central chemoreceptors, and stretch receptor–induced inspiration is accomplished preferentially by inspiratory intercostals rather than the diaphragm. The onset of stimulation of intercostal muscles occurs slightly later than phrenic motor neuron discharge during quiet breathing, although with increased ventilatory drive this difference in timing is lost.

The act of breathing involves control of not only the major pumping muscles of the respiratory system, the diaphragm, and the intercostals but also the muscles of the larynx, pharynx, tongue, and face, which control patency of the upper airway.[38] The pattern of recruitment of the muscles that control upper airway caliber differs strikingly from that of the main inspiratory muscles. Their onset of stimulation is in very early inspiration, and their peak activity coincides with peak inspiratory flow rather than volume. Thus their activity is in phase with flow-related negative pressure in the upper airway, and their contraction counteracts the tendency for the negative pressure to narrow the airway. Laryngeal abductor activation occurs early in expiration and, along with the inspiratory muscles that are still active during PIIA, brakes expiration. The rate of rise of central inspiratory activity—and therefore the discharge rate down the phrenic and intercostal nerves—is dependent on the intensity of the afferent input integrated in the central integrator. The off-switch that terminates the slow increase in inspiratory activity during Phase I is influenced by the input of pulmonary stretch receptors from the vagus.[39]

The classic concept that a basic respiratory rhythm is generated in the brainstem and only modulated by chemoreceptor and other input must be questioned since it appears that chemical and other input is necessary to generate respiratory rhythmicity. Both high-frequency oscillatory ventilation and CO_2 removal from venous blood by means of an extracorporeal circuit result in central apnea and cessation of respiratory rhythm generation. Under those circumstances, apnea can occur despite mean levels of arterial P_{CO_2} that would normally be associated with substantial neural output. It has been suggested that ventilation-related fluctuations in arterial P_{O_2} and P_{CO_2} represent one of the inputs that generate central respiratory rhythmicity, since both extracorporeal CO_2 removal and high-frequency oscillatory ventilation abolish these fluctuations.[40, 41]

Although most of our knowledge of central respiratory control involves the automatic brainstem-controlling mechanisms, it is clear that the cerebral cortex can influence brainstem mechanisms or bypass them completely to accomplish behavior-related respiratory activity like speech, cough, defecation, micturition, singing, and so on. During voluntary activity such as speech, requirements for tone or loudness may override chemical and mechanical input. For example, during speech the response to inhaled carbon dioxide is markedly depressed and the sensation of dyspnea diminished when compared with the response to similar CO_2 levels occurring without speech.[42] Magnetic stimulation of the cerebral cortex while recording diaphragmatic electromyograms has been used to show that cortical pathways project bilaterally to the diaphragm and that contralateral activation of the diaphragm is markedly decreased following cerebral vascular accidents that affect the internal capsule.[19, 43]

Recent research has started to shed light on the neurotransmitters involved in the generation and modulation of respiratory rhythm.[5, 12] Those neurotransmitters involved in rhythm generation are primarily amino acids; they may be excitatory or inhibitory and act on specific receptors. The major excitatory amino acid is glutamate, which acts via *N*-methyl-D-aspartate (NMDA) and non-NMDA receptors. The main inhibitory amino acids are glycine and γ-aminobutyric acid, which act via chloride channels. Neuromodulators are substances released from cells whose axons are within the central respiratory control areas but whose bodies are outside the respiratory center. These neuromodulators include acetylcholine, serotonin, catecholamines, and neuropeptides such as enkephalins, β-endorphins, somatostatin, and substance P. Although these substances are not directly involved in respiratory rhythmogenesis, they can exert powerful effects on respiratory motoneurons by changing their state of excitability.

THE OUTPUT

Knowledge about the central respiratory controller can only be obtained in humans by altering the input and observing changes in output. The three input variables that have been used most commonly in investigation are (1) alterations in the concentration of inhaled O_2 and CO_2 (which stimulate peripheral and central chemoreceptors); (2) added resistive or elastic loads (which stimulate muscle and lung mechanoreceptors); and (3) exercise.

By measuring respiratory center output at various levels of stimulation by these types of input, an assessment of respiratory center integrity can be made. As discussed in greater detail in Chapter 17, there are problems in extrapolating from the measured output back to neuronal drive, since most tests of output are some steps removed from the neural output itself. The most fundamental types of output are minute ventilation and its components tidal volume (V_T) and respiratory frequency (F). Minute ventilation can also be divided into mean inspiratory flow (V_T/Ti) and the ratio of inspiratory time to total respiratory cycle time ($Ti/Ttot$). It has been proposed that V_T/Ti reflects the neural drive whereas $Ti/Ttot$ is a measure of central timing mechanisms;[44] these measures of respiratory pattern have gained wide acceptance.

Until relatively recently, the study of respiratory patterns has been hampered by the necessity of using a mouthpiece and nose clip, which in themselves can alter the breathing pattern in conscious subjects.[45] However, by using a head mask or the respiratory inductance plethysmograph, breathing patterns can be monitored in a more natural state and input-dependent differences in pattern can be observed;[46–49] for example, with CO_2 inhalation, breathing frequency has been found to increase less and tidal volume more than at matched ventilation stimulated by exercise.[49]

The most commonly used inputs by which respiratory control is assessed are increasing levels of inhaled CO_2 and decreasing levels of inhaled O_2. The methods by which hypoxic and hypercapnic ventilatory response curves are generated are described fully in Chapter 17 (*see* page 404). Briefly, although progressive hypercapnia produces a linear increase in ventilation in normal subjects, the slope of the curve can vary widely between individuals. With progressive hypoxemia, a parabolic curve of ventilation against Po_2 is

generated, with little increase in ventilation until Po_2 falls to levels between 50 and 60 mm Hg; the relationship can become linear by plotting ventilation against arterial O_2 saturation. There is also wide variability between individuals in the response to progressive hypoxemia. The CO_2 response curve largely reflects the integrity of central chemoreceptor activity. Studies in which monozygotic and dizygotic twins are compared have shown a genetic influence on both the slopes of the hypoxic and hypercapnic ventilatory response curves and on the pattern of breathing in response to hypoxemia; however, no genetic influence has been observed on the ability to detect added resistive loads.[50–54]

The ventilatory response curves to CO_2 and O_2 are also influenced by various drugs and other extraneous factors. Ethanol decreases the ventilatory response to CO_2 but not low O_2, an effect that is abolished by naloxone, thus suggesting ethanol-induced endorphin release.[55] Almitrine increases peripheral chemoreceptor responsiveness to hypoxia, but has little effect on CO_2 sensitivity or on resting ventilation.[56] Aminophylline increases the slope of the ventilatory response curve to hypoxia and, in some studies, to hypercapnia.[57] Propranolol and other β-blockers have little influence on the ventilatory response to CO_2.[59–61] Halothane markedly decreases the ventilatory response to hypoxia at both sedative and anesthetic levels, although it has little influence on the response to hypercapnia.[62] Semistarvation has been shown to produce a decreased ventilatory response to hypoxia, but not to hypercapnia.[58] As discussed farther on, sleep has an important influence on the control of breathing by decreasing the ventilatory response to CO_2 and hypoxia.

Genetic or acquired alterations in ventilatory response to hypoxia and hypercapnia can have profound influences in disease and may govern the ability of normal individuals to perform various functions. For example, it has been postulated that the genetically determined ventilatory drives to hypoxia and hypercapnia influence the pattern and course of chronic obstructive pulmonary disease (COPD): patients who have a genetically determined brisk response to CO_2 and low O_2 tend to maintain blood gas tensions near normal despite significant airway obstruction, whereas those who have depressed ventilatory responses tend to hypoventilate.[63] This hypothesis is supported by family studies that show that healthy relatives of patients who have hypercapnic COPD have significantly decreased hypoxic ventilatory response curves when compared with relatives of patients who have similar degrees of air-flow obstruction but who do not have hypercapnia. It is interesting that the hypercapnic ventilatory drive in relatives does not separate hypercapnic from nonhypercapnic patients who have COPD despite the fact that there is considerable genetic influence on the hypercapnic response curve.[54, 64]

It is uncertain whether inherited variation in ventilatory drive can also influence exercise capacity in normal individuals. Trained endurance athletes have a significantly reduced ventilatory drive to hypoxemia and hypercapnia when compared with normal controls; by contrast, similarly fit high-altitude mountain climbers have a significantly increased hypercapnic and hypoxic drive when compared with distance runners.[65, 66] Whether these athletes have genetically determined ventilatory responses that facilitate their performance or altered responses secondary to their conditioning programs remains controversial. In one study, the effect of short-term exercise on the ventilatory response to CO_2 showed no change, suggesting that it is the genetic influences that preselect athletes.[67]

Although it is clear that the major receptor mediating hypercapnic hyperpnea is the central chemoreceptor, it is possible that upper airway or intrapulmonary CO_2 receptors also may modulate (increase or decrease) the hypercapnic ventilatory response. The existence of such receptors is based on limited evidence. For example, ventilatory responses to CO_2 are lower when breathing is carried out through the nose rather than mouth, especially when the air is cold.[23, 68] In addition, during separate perfusion of the systemic and pulmonary circuits, increased ventilation has been observed with increased pulmonary CO_2 tensions at constant systemic Pco_2.[69] This observation suggests the presence of intrapulmonary receptors that enhance the ventilatory response to CO_2; however, some investigators have postulated that pulmonary receptors may attenuate the CO_2 response, since blocking of airway slowly adapting stretch receptors with inhaled local anesthetic agents or by blockade of the vagus nerve results in an enhanced ventilatory response to CO_2.[70, 71]

CONTROL OF VENTILATION DURING EXERCISE

The precise control of arterial gas tensions during exercise—when O_2 consumption and CO_2 production can reach 20 times their resting levels—is an impressive phenomenon indeed. The mechanisms by which this control is achieved remain a controversial topic on which several reviews have been published.[6, 72–75]

There appear to be at least four phases in the ventilatory response to exercise. *Phase I* is characterized by an abrupt increase in ventilation that coincides with the start of exercise and may in fact precede it if the subject is cued to the time of beginning of the exercise. This increase in ventilation occurs prior to any alterations in the gas tensions of mixed venous blood and has been termed the *neurogenic component* of the ventilatory response. It is not clear which neurogenic sensation mediates the response, although muscle spindles in the exercising muscles are probably important. At least part may also be related to a central command mechanism that involves neural output from the rostral pontomedullary region, which is capable of stimulating both ventilation and exercise in parallel.[6] The carotid body chemoreceptors are not implicated in the Phase I reaction, since hyperpnea is preserved in patients who have resected carotid bodies.

Phase II begins some 10 or 15 seconds following onset of the hyperpneic response to exercise, coincident with alterations in blood gas tensions in mixed venous blood. The carotid bodies have some role in this phase, since there is a lag in the ventilatory response in patients without these structures; however, the ultimate level of ventilation achieved is not different from that in normal individuals. *Phase III* represents the steady-state response to exercise and is closely linked to CO_2 production. Circulating catecholamines, as well as increased serum concentrations of K^+, adenosine, and blood osmolality, may act as additional drives to ventilation during this phase. The carotid bodies contribute about 20% of the ventilatory response in this phase.[74]

With heavy exercise, a further increase in ventilation occurs coincident with the metabolic production of lactic acid *(Phase IV)*. This stage in progressive exercise is termed the *anaerobic threshold*, since it is at this point that ventilation becomes uncoupled from metabolic CO_2 production. This final lactic acidosis–induced hyperpnea is mediated by peripheral chemoreceptors.[75] Additional contributors to the hyperpnea of heavy exercise are increased body temperature and (in some individuals at extremely high work rates) a decrease in arterial Po_2. Such hypoxemia is the result of an increase in the alveolar-arterial oxygen tension gradient thought to be caused by O_2 diffusion limitation secondary to the rapid red cell pulmonary capillary transit times. The observation that all phases of the ventilatory response to exercise are preserved after heart and heart-lung transplantation indicates that afferent neural input from these organs does not contribute to exercise hyperpnea.[76–78]

It is apparent that the tight control of ventilation during exercise cannot be totally accounted for by known neural, chemoreceptor, and humoral input; although all appear to play a role in the total ventilatory response to exercise, their relative importance and means of integration during the various phases of the response remain a mystery.[72, 73, 79] It is interesting that breathing 100% oxygen during exercise can prolong exercise capacity in normal subjects and patients who have COPD. This finding may be related to the observation that breathing 100% oxygen during exercise results in significantly less catecholamine release, peripheral lactate production, and heart rate response.[80] The fact that hypoxia and exercise are additive in their effect on ventilation, even at levels of arterial Po_2 that do not normally stimulate peripheral chemoreceptors, indicates that exercise in some way may increase chemoreceptor responsiveness to hypoxemia. It has been suggested that stimulation of some peripheral muscle chemoreceptors by low oxygen tension enhances the chemoreceptor response.[81]

COMPENSATION FOR ADDED VENTILATORY LOADS

The impedance that the inspiratory muscles must overcome consists of three components: a resistive load related to the friction of air flow through the tracheobronchial tree, an elastic load related to stretching of the lung and chest wall, and a trivial inertial load related to the acceleration of inspired air.

Small changes in upper airway caliber and alterations in body position produce rapid fluctuation in the resistive and elastic loads against which the respiratory muscles must shorten.[82] The decrease in tidal volume and ventilation that would occur with an added elastic or resistive load can be calculated by the ratio of initial to added impedance. Studies in humans have shown that the decrease in tidal volume that occurs with such added loads is less than would be expected on a purely mechanical basis. This discrepancy indicates that some compensatory mechanisms are brought into play during loaded breathing to protect tidal volume and acinar ventilation.[83]

The first of these compensatory mechanisms is related

to the basic mechanical properties of skeletal muscle. The force generated by skeletal muscle is related to its velocity of shortening: an unloaded muscle shortens rapidly and produces little force; with an added load, shortening is slowed and force generation is increased, which tends to counteract the expected decrease in tidal volume. A second mechanism of load compensation involves reflexes initiated by mechanoreceptors in the lung and chest wall, of which the pulmonary stretch receptors are especially important. With an added elastic or resistive load, inspiration is slowed. Because of the adaptive nature of pulmonary stretch receptors, their level of activity at any volume during inspiration is decreased; this decrease results in prolonged inspiration, which tends to increase tidal volume back toward control levels.[84] Upper airway receptors also respond to the increases in transmural pressure that occur with added external resistive loads and, by causing reflex stimulation of upper airway muscles, aid in compensation.[24, 85]

Muscle spindles represent an additional mechanism by which load compensation is accomplished. As discussed previously, they contain intrafusal fibers that regulate the spindles' stretch and contract in concert with the extrafusal fibers that move the rib cage. Muscle spindle afferent activity increases whenever contraction of the extrafusal fibers is hindered; that is, alpha motor neuron activity is increased via the gamma loop segmental reflex and the activity of the intercostal muscles is thus enhanced. There is a greater response to a given increase in resistance when it is produced by bronchoconstriction with methacholine than by added external resistance, which suggests that mechanical and irritant receptors enhance the response elicited from muscle afferents.[86] A final load compensation is initiated when central and peripheral chemoreceptors detect changes in the arterial blood gas composition.[84]

Closely associated with the topic of load detection and compensation are respiratory sensation and the symptom of dyspnea. Dyspnea, which should be distinguished from hyperventilation or hyperpnea, is the unpleasant awareness of breathing and respiratory distress signaled by proprioceptic information from the lungs and chest wall. Normal breathing is an automatic, unconscious motor act. The mechanism by which the sensation of breathing reaches the conscious level and engenders the sensation of dyspnea is poorly understood. The origin of the afferent input that could theoretically result in such a sensation includes the peripheral and central chemoreceptors, lung receptors, and receptors in the chest wall and respiratory muscles. The fact that most patients with dyspnea do not have sufficient alterations in blood gas tensions to stimulate ventilation is strong evidence against chemoreceptor activation as a major contributor. Moreover, the discomfort of breath-holding can be relieved by breathing a gas mixture that results in further deterioration of blood gas tensions, thus suggesting that some stimulus related to the act of breathing itself rather than arterial P_{O_2} and P_{CO_2} is important in generation of the dyspneic sensation. On the other hand, the sensations of dyspnea and respiratory effort can be dissociated during hypercapnic hyperpnea.[87] Lung receptors do not subserve conscious respiratory sensation, since dyspnea persists after vagal blockade. Although upper airway receptors contribute to load compensation, they are not important for load detection since inhaled

local anesthetics cause no change in the ability to sense added elastic loads.[88]

Strong support for the role of muscle receptors and afferents as the origin of respiratory sensation has been provided by studies showing that respiratory muscle paralysis induced by curare completely abolishes the sensation of dyspnea.[89] Chest wall vibration impairs the respiratory sensation of volume, which suggests that muscle spindles are sensory organs.[90] The balance of evidence favors the hypothesis that dyspnea occurs when afferent input from respiratory muscles in some way signals an inappropriateness of the relationship between the central neurogenic drive to breathe and the resulting displacement of the lung and chest wall (i.e., too little ventilation for a given neural output).[91] The results of experiments assessing the effects of different flow rates, lung volumes, and timing on the ability to detect added loads suggest that it is the relationship between flow and pressure early in inspiration that is the major signal for load detection and the sensation of dyspnea.[92] Load detection is not influenced by increased ventilation during exercise or CO_2 breathing.[93] When the load is sufficiently high, normal subjects can distinguish between a resistive and an elastic load because of the different time sequence in the major impedance.[94] The ability to detect added resistive loads can be expressed quantitatively by the Weber fraction (the ratio of the added load first detected over the initial load). This fraction remains constant over a wide range of baseline resistance values, although the sensitivity of load detection decreases at very low and very high baseline resistance. Resistive loads are probably detected because of a phase difference or delay between respiratory motor neuron output and the rate of change of lung volume; when severe, this signal is interpreted centrally as dyspnea.[95, 96]

CONTROL OF UPPER AIRWAY MUSCLES

With recognition of the importance of obstructive sleep apnea, respiratory center control of the upper airway muscles that are important in maintaining airway patency, especially during sleep, has received considerable attention. Numerous muscles of the pharynx, hypopharynx, larynx, and tongue, including the genioglossals, tensor palatini, medial pterygoids, thyrocricoid, and posterior cricoarytenoids, receive respiratory-related rhythmic neurogenic input.[97] As discussed previously, stimulation of upper airway muscles occurs earlier in the respiratory cycle than stimulation of the diaphragm and intercostals and coincides with the period of peak inspiratory flow and presumably peak negative upper airway pressure. Hypercapnia and hypoxia increase the neural drive to upper airway muscles, although the relationship between phrenic output and hypoglossal output is not linear, the latter increasing steeply at higher drives.[98] The increased drive to upper airway muscles in response to hypoxia and hypercapnia may not relate only to increased input from central or peripheral chemoreceptors, since blockade of pulmonary stretch receptors impairs upper airway muscle contraction during hypoxia and hypercapnia.[99] The genioglossal muscles may be especially important in maintaining upper airway patency during sleep, and ingestion of alcohol results in a selective reduction in genioglossal electromyographic activity in normal subjects.[100, 101]

CONTROL OF BREATHING DURING SLEEP

Alterations in the regulation of respiration that occur during sleep have been the subject of considerable interest and review.[97, 102, 103] As discussed previously, breathing is regulated by two essentially separate control-integrating mechanisms: the automatic (metabolic) control system and the voluntary (behavioral) control system. The major purpose of the former is to maintain acid-base and oxygen homeostasis, whereas the latter is involved in such actions as speech and singing, activities in which the respiratory system is used for nonrespiratory purposes. During wakefulness, control of breathing is constantly being shared by the two systems; however, during sleep, automatic metabolic control predominates, at least during its slow-wave phase. Absence of the volitional control of breathing results in respiratory apraxia, whereas absence of automatic control results in Ondine's curse (cessation of breathing associated with falling asleep).[104]

The profound influences that sleep has on the various performance aspects of the control of breathing are summarized in Table 9–1. Resting ventilation is decreased during slow-wave sleep, with both tidal volume and frequency being less than during wakefulness.[105] During rapid eye movement (REM) sleep, resting ventilation varies as a result of marked irregularity of the breathing pattern; however, on

the whole, hyperventilation rather than hypoventilation is the rule. The hypoventilation of slow-wave sleep is associated with a slight rise in arterial Pco_2 and fall in arterial Po_2, and during REM sleep there is considerable fluctuation in arterial blood gas tensions. During Stages 1 and 2 of slow-wave sleep, periodic breathing reminiscent of Cheyne-Stokes respiration may occur and then change to a regular pattern during the deeper stages (3 and 4) of slow-wave sleep. The pattern of breathing during REM sleep is characterized as irregular rather than periodic: although the mean tidal volume decreases and frequency increases, the characteristic feature is marked breath-to-breath variability. During slow-wave sleep, the automatic control system appears to dominate respiratory control, but during REM sleep, a dissociation occurs between metabolic demands and ventilatory responses. Intercostal and upper airway muscles, which are normally more involved in postural and behavioral activities, are depressed during slow-wave sleep and profoundly depressed during REM sleep, when there appears to be central inhibition of gamma loop neurons; this depression occurs in the respiratory muscles as well as in skeletal muscle generally. The diaphragm, which is virtually devoid of muscle spindles, is immune from this flaccidity, so during REM sleep, maintenance of ventilation is dependent on diaphragmatic activity.

The responsiveness of the respiratory control mechanisms to afferent input is also profoundly altered during sleep; for example, responsiveness to hypercapnia is decreased during slow-wave sleep and further decreased during REM sleep.[106, 107] Although less certain, it has been suggested that hypoxic responses are also depressed in both stages of sleep, more profoundly during REM.[108, 109] The respiratory centers also appear to ignore afferent input from other sources during sleep: pulmonary stretch and irritant receptor discharge, as well as muscle spindle input, is less effective in increasing ventilation and effecting load compensation during sleep. The profound changes that occur during REM sleep make this period one of special vulnerability for patients who have abnormalities of the respiratory control system or the lungs and airways.

The influence of sleep on control of ventilation is not confined to the period of sleep itself; it has been shown in normal individuals that sleep deprivation for 24 hours results in a decreased ventilatory response to carbon dioxide and oxygen. Such an alteration in respiratory control could be important in hospitalized patients whose sleep is disturbed and in patients who have sleep apnea syndromes.[110] Respiratory dysrhythmia is common during sleep and is related to prolonged circulation times, increased receptor gain, and decreased receptor damping. Decreased stability of hypoxic rather than hypercapnic drive is the usual source of respiratory cycling; the instability is caused by the poor damping as a result of the alinearity of the hypoxic response curve and the low O_2 stores.

Table 9–1. EFFECTS OF SLEEP ON BREATHING

RESPIRATORY ACTIVITY	SLOW-WAVE SLEEP	REM SLEEP
Alveolar ventilation	Decreased due to ↓ V_T and ↓ F	Variable
Arterial Pco_2	↑ 4–6 mm Hg	Variable
Arterial Po_2	↓ 4–8 mm Hg	Variable
Breathing pattern	Stages 1 and 2 periodic	Irregular
	Stages 3 and 4 regular	↑ F plus ↓ V_T
Diaphragmatic contraction	No change	No change
Intercostal contraction	↓	↓ ↓
Upper airway muscle contraction	↓	↓ ↓
Ventilatory response to CO_2	↓	↓ ↓
Ventilatory response to hypoxemia	↓	↓ ↓
Response to lung afferents	↓	↓ ↓
Response to respiratory muscle afferents	↓	↓ ↓

REM, rapid eye movement.

REFERENCES

1. Berger AJ, Mitchell RA, Severinghaus JW: Regulation of respiration (first of three parts). N Engl J Med 297:92, 1977.
2. Berger AJ, Mitchell RA, Severinghaus JW: Regulation of respiration (second of three parts). N Engl J Med 297:138, 1977.
3. Berger AJ, Mitchell RA, Severinghaus JW: Regulation of respiration (third of three parts). N Engl J Med 297:194, 1977.
4. Hornbein TF, Lenfant C (eds): Regulation of Breathing, Parts One and Two. Lung Biology in Health and Disease. New York, Marcel Dekker, 1981.
5. Armand BL, Denavit-Saub ié M, Champagnat J: Central control of breathing in mammals: Neuronal circuitry, membrane properties, and neurotransmitters. Physiol Rev 75:1, 1995.
6. Mateika JH, Duffin J: A review of the control of breathing during exercise. Eur J Appl Physiol 71:1, 1995.
7. Sant'Ambrogio G, Tsubone H, Sant'Ambrogio FB: Sensory information from the upper airway: Role in the control of breathing. Respir Physiol 102:1, 1995.
8. Henke KG, Badr MS, Skatrud JB, et al: Load compensation and respiratory muscle function during sleep. J Appl Physiol 72:1221, 1992.
9. McDonald DM: Peripheral chemoreceptors: Structure, function, relationship of the carotid body. *In* Hornbein TF, Lenfant C (eds): Regulation of Breathing, Part One. Lung Biology in Health and Disease. New York, Marcel Dekker, 1981, p 321.
10. Biscoe TJ, Willshaw P: Stimulus-response relationships of the peripheral arterial chemoreceptors. *In* Hornbein TF, Lenfant C (eds): Regulation of Breathing, Part One. Lung Biology in Health and Disease. New York, Marcel Dekker, 1981.
11. Lugliani R, Whipp BJ, Seard C, et al: Effect of bilateral carotid body resection on ventilatory control at rest and during exercise in man. N Engl J Med 285:1105, 1971.
12. Bonham AC: Neurotransmitters in the CNS control of breathing. Respir Physiol 101:219, 1995.
13. Heath D: The human carotid body in health and disease. J Pathol 164:1, 1991.
14. Berkenbosch A, Dahan A, DeGoede J, et al: The ventilatory response to CO_2 of the peripheral and central chemoreflex loop before and after sustained hypoxia in man. J Physiol 456:71, 1992.
15. Okabe S, Hida W, Kikuchi Y, et al: Upper airway muscle activity during sustained hypoxia in awake humans. J Appl Physiol 75:1552, 1993.
16. Poon CS: Potentiation of exercise ventilatory response by airway CO_2 and dead space loading. J Appl Physiol 73:591, 1992.
17. Phillipson EA, Sullivan CE: Arousal: The forgotten response to respiratory stimuli (editorial). Am Rev Respir Dis 118:807, 1978.
18. Pavlin EG, Hornbein TF: Basics of respiratory disease. Am Thorac Soc 7:26, 1979.
19. Gozal D, Hathout GM, Kirlew KA, et al: Localization of putative neural respiratory regions in the human by functional magnetic resonance imaging. J Appl Physiol 76:2076, 1994.
20. Bledsoe SW, Hornbein TF: Central chemosensors and the regulation of their chemical environment. *In* Hornbein TF, Lenfant C (eds): Regulation of Breathing. Part One. Lung Biology in Health and Disease. New York, Marcel Dekker, 1981, p 347.
21. Widdicombe JG: Nervous receptors in the respiratory tract and lungs. *In* Hornbein TF, Lenfant C (eds): Regulation of Breathing, Part One. Lung Biology in Health and Disease. New York, Marcel Dekker, 1981, p 429.
22. McBride B, Whitelaw WA: A physiological stimulus to upper airway receptors in humans. J Appl Physiol 51:1189, 1981.
23. Burgess KR, Whitelaw WA: Reducing ventilatory response to carbon dioxide by breathing cold air. Am Rev Respir Dis 129:687, 1984.
24. Sant'Ambrogio G, Mathew OP, Fisher JT, et al: Laryngeal receptors responding to transmural pressure, airflow and local muscle activity. Respir Physiol 54:317, 1983.
25. Lofaso F: Ventilatory control in lung transplantation. Arch Int Physiol Biochim Biophys 101:A41, 1993.
26. Morales P, Cordero P, Borro JM, et al: Ventilation pattern at rest and respiratory response to hypercapnic stimulation after lung transplantation. Arch Bronconeumol 30:440, 1994.
27. Ford GT, Grant DA, Rideout KS, et al: Inhibition of breathing associated with gallbladder stimulation in dogs. J Appl Physiol 67:72, 1988.
28. Ford GT, Whitelaw WA, Rosenal TW, et al: Diaphragm function after upper abdominal surgery in humans. Am Rev Respir Dis 127:431, 1993.
29. Road JD, Burgess KR, Whitelaw WA, et al: Diaphragm function and respiratory response after upper abdominal surgery in dogs. J Appl Physiol 57:576, 1984.
30. Duron B: Intercostal and diaphragmatic muscle endings and afferents. *In* Hornbein TF, Lenfant C (eds): Regulation of Breathing, Part One. Lung Biology in Health and Disease. New York, Marcel Dekker, 1981, p 473.
31. Ford GT, Whitelaw WA, Rosenal TW, et al: Diaphragm function after upper abdominal surgery in humans. Am Rev Respir Dis 127:431, 1983.
32. Road JD, Burgess KR, Ford GT: Diaphragm function after upper versus lower abdominal surgery in dogs. Physiologist 25:331, 1982.
33. Mitchell RA: Neural regulation of respiration. Clin Chest Med 1:3, 1980.
34. Road JD, Osborne S, Wakai Y: Delayed poststimulus decrease of phrenic motoneuron output produced by phrenic nerve afferent stimulation. J Appl Physiol 74:68, 1993.
35. Hussain SNA, Roussos C: The role of small-fibre phrenic afferents in the control

of breathing. *In* Roussos C (ed): The Thorax. *In* Lenfant C (ed): Lung Biology in Health and Disease. New York, Marcel Dekker, 1995, pp 869–901.
36. Mitchell RA, Berger AJ: Neural regulation of respiration. *In* Hornbein TF, Lenfant C: Regulation of Breathing, Part One. Lung Biology in Health and Disease. New York, Marcel Dekker, 1981, p 541.
37. Martin J, Aubier M, Engel LA: Effects of inspiratory loading on respiratory muscle activity during expiration. Am Rev Respir Dis 125:352, 1982.
38. van Lunteren E, Dick TE: Intrinsic properties of pharyngeal and diaphragmatic respiratory motoneurons and muscles. J Appl Physiol 73:787, 1992.
39. von Euler C: On the central pattern generator for the basic breathing rhythmicity. J Appl Physiol 55:1647, 1983.
40. Fitzgerald RS: The respiratory control system. Chest 85:585, 1984.
41. Phillipson EA, Duffin J, Cooper JD: Critical dependence of respiratory rhythmicity on metabolic CO_2 load. J Appl Physiol 50:45, 1981.
42. Phillipson EA, McClean PA, Sullivan CE, et al: Interaction of metabolic and behavioural respiratory control during hypercapnia and speech. Am Rev Respir Dis 117:903, 1978.
43. Carr LJ, Harrison LM, Stephens JA: Evidence for bilateral innervation of certain homologous motoneurone pools in man. J Physiol 475:217, 1994.
44. Milic-Emili J: Recent advances in clinical assessment of control of breathing. Lung 160:1, 1982.
45. Jammes Y, Auran Y, Gouvernet J, et al: The ventilatory pattern of conscious man according to age and morphology. Bull Eur Physiopathol Respir 15:527, 1979.
46. Tobin MJ, Jenouri G, Sackner MA: Effect of naloxone on change in breathing pattern with smoking. Chest 82:530, 1982.
47. Tobin MJ, Chadha TS, Jenouri G, et al: Breathing patterns. 2. Diseased subjects. Chest 84:286, 1983.
48. Tobin MJ, Chadha TS, Jenouri G, et al: Breathing patterns. 1. Normal Subjects. Chest 84:202, 1983.
49. Askanazi J, Milic-Emili J, Broell JR, et al: Influence of exercise and CO_2 on breathing pattern of normal man. J Appl Physiol 47:192, 1979.
50. Collins DD, Scoggin CH, Zwillich CW, et al: Hereditary aspects of decreased hypoxic response. J Clin Invest 62:105, 1978.
51. Kawakami Y, Yamamoto H, Yoshikawa T, et al: Respiratory chemosensitivity in smokers—studies on monozygotic twins. Am Rev Respir Dis 126:986, 1982.
52. Kawakami Y, Yoshikawa T, Shida A, et al: Control of breathing in young twins. J Appl Physiol 52:537, 1982.
53. Kawakami Y, Yamamoto H, Yoshikawa T, et al: Chemical and behavioural control of breathing in adult twins. Am Rev Respir Dis 129:703, 1984.
54. Kobayashi S, Nishimura M, Yamamoto M, et al: Dyspnea sensation and chemical control of breathing in adult twins. Am Rev Respir Dis 147:1192, 1993.
55. Michiels TM, Light RW, Mahutte CK: Naloxone reverses ethanol-induced depression of hypercapneic drive. Am Rev Respir Dis 128:823, 1983.
56. Stanley NN, Galloway JM, Gordon B, et al: Increased respiratory chemosensitivity induced by infusing almitrine intravenously in healthy man. Thorax 38:200, 1983.
57. Laksminarayan S, Sahn SA, Weil JV: Effect of aminophylline on ventilatory responses in normal man. Am Rev Respir Dis 117:33, 1978.
58. Baier H, Somani P: Ventilatory drive in normal man during semi-starvation. Chest 85:222, 1984.
59. Folgering H, Braakhekke J: Ventilatory response to hypercapnia in normal subjects after propranolol, metoprolol and oxprenolol. Respiration 39:139, 1980.
60. Bosisio E, Sergi M, Sega R, et al: Respiratory response to carbon dioxide after propranolol in normal subjects. Respiration 37:197, 1979.
61. Hutchinson PF, Harrison RN: Effect of acute and chronic beta-blockade on carbon dioxide sensitivity in normal man. Thorax 35:869, 1980.
62. Knill RL, Gelb AW: Ventilatory responses to hypoxia and hypercapnia during halothane sedation and anesthesia in man. Anesthesiology 49:244, 1978.
63. Leitch AG: The hypoxic drive to breathing in man. Lancet 1:428, 1981.
64. Fleetham JA, Arnup ME, Anthonisen NR: Familial aspects of ventilatory control in patients with chronic obstructive pulmonary disease. Am Rev Respir Dis 129:3, 1984.
65. Byrne-Quinn E, Weil JV, Sodal IE, et al: Ventilatory control in the athlete. J Appl Physiol 30:91, 1971.
66. Schoene RB: Control of ventilation in climbers to extreme altitude. J Appl Physiol 53:886, 1982.
67. Bradley BL, Mestas J, Forman J, et al: The effect on respiratory drive of a prolonged physical conditioning program. Am Rev Respir Dis 122:741, 1980.
68. Douglas NJ, White DP, Weill JV, et al: Effect of breathing route on ventilation and ventilatory drive. Respir Physiol 51:209, 1983.
69. Sheldon MI, Green JF: Evidence for pulmonary CO_2 chemosensitivity effects on ventilation. J Appl Physiol 52:1192, 1982.
70. Sullivan TY, Yu P-L: Airway anesthesia effects on hypercapnic breathing pattern in humans. J Appl Physiol Respir Environ 55:368, 1983.
71. Mador MJ: Effect of nebulized lidocaine on ventilatory response to CO_2 in healthy subjects. J Appl Physiol 74:1419, 1993.
72. Whipp J: Ventilatory control during exercise in humans. Annu Rev Physiol 45:393, 1983.
73. Whipp BJ: The control of exercise hyperpnea. *In* Hornbein TF, Lenfant C (eds): Regulation of Breathing, Part Two. Lung Biology in Health and Disease. New York, Marcel Dekker, 1981, p 1069.

74. Whipp B: Peripheral chemoreceptor control of exercise hyperpnea in humans. Med Sci Sports Exerc 26:337, 1994.

75. Ward SA: Peripheral and central chemoreceptor control of ventilation during exercise in humans. Can J Appl Physiol 19:305, 1994.

76. Braith RW, Limacher MC, Staples ED, et al: Blood gas dynamics at the onset of exercise in heart transplant recipients. Chest 103:1692, 1993.

77. Grassi B, Ferretti G, Xi L, et al: Ventilatory response to exercise after heart and lung denervation in humans. Respir Physiol 92:289, 1993.

78. Levy RD: The respiratory system after lung transplantation. *In* Roussos C (ed): The Thorax. *In* Lenfant C (ed): Lung Biology in Health and Disease. New York, Marcel Dekker, 1995, pp 2007–2034.

79. Forster HV, Pan LG: Contribution of acid-base changes to control of breathing during exercise. Can J Appl Physiol 20:380, 1995.

80. Hesse B, Kanstrup I-L, Christensen NJ, et al: Reduced norepinephrine response to dynamic exercise in human subjects during O_2 breathing. J Appl Physiol 51:176, 1981.

81. Flenley DC, Brash H, Clancy L: Ventilatory response to steady-state exercise in hypoxia in humans. J Appl Physiol 46:438, 1979.

82. Banzett RB, Mead J: Reflex compensation for changes in operational length of inspiratory muscles. *In* Roussos C (ed): The Thorax. *In* Lenfant C (ed): Lung Biology in Health and Disease. New York, Marcel Dekker, 1995, pp 987–1003.

83. Daubenspeck JA: Mechanical aspects of loaded breathing. *In* Roussos C (ed): The Thorax. *In* Lenfant C (ed): Lung Biology in Health and Disease. New York, Marcel Dekker, 1995, pp 953–985.

84. Cherniack NS, Altose MD: Respiratory responses in ventilatory loading. *In* Hornbein TF, Lenfant C (eds): Regulation of Breathing, Part Two. Lung Biology in Health and Disease. New York, Marcel Dekker, 1981, p 905.

85. Mathew OP: Upper airway negative-pressure effects on respiratory activity of upper airway muscles. J Appl Physiol 56:500, 1984.

86. Kelsen SG, Prestel TF, Cherniack NS, et al: Comparison of the respiratory responses to external resistive loading and bronchoconstriction. J Clin Invest 67:1761, 1981.

87. Demdiuk BH, Manning H, Lilly J, et al: Dissociation between dyspnea and respiratory effort. Am Rev Respir Dis 146:1222, 1992.

88. Burki NK, Davenport PW, Safdar F, et al: The effects of airway anesthesia on magnitude estimation of added inspiratory resistive and elastic loads. Am Rev Respir Dis 127:2, 1983.

89. Campbell EJM, Guz A: Breathlessness. *In* Hornbein TF, Lenfant C (eds): Regulation of Breathing, Part Two. Lung Biology in Health and Disease. New York, Marcel Dekker, 1981, p 1181.

90. Stubbing DG, Killian KJ, Campbell EJM: The quantification of respiratory sensations by normal subjects. Respir Physiol 55:251, 1981.

91. Killian KJ, Campbell EJM: Dyspnea and exercise. Annu Rev Physiol 45:465, 1983.

92. Killian KJ, Mahutte CK, Howell JBL, et al: Effect of timing, flow, lung volume, and threshold pressures on resistive load detection. J Appl Physiol 49:958, 1980.

93. Killian KJ, Campbell EJM, Howell JBL: The effect of increased ventilation on resistive load discrimination. Am Rev Respir Dis 120:1233, 1979.

94. Zechman FW, Wiley RL, Davenport PW: Ability of healthy men to discriminate between added inspiratory resistive and elastic loads. Respir Physiol 45:111, 1981.

95. Stubbing DG, Killian KJ, Campbell EJM: Weber's law and resistive load detection. Am Rev Respir Dis 127:5, 1983.

96. Mahutte CK, Campbell EJM, Killian KJ: Theory of resistive load detection. Respir Physiol 51:131, 1983.

97. Remmers JE: Control of breathing during sleep. *In* Hornbein TF, Lenfant C (eds): Regulation of Breathing, Part Two. Lung Biology in Health and Disease. New York, Marcel Dekker, 1981, p 1197.

98. Weiner D, Mitra M, Salamone J: Effect of chemical stimuli on nerves supplying upper airway muscles. J Appl Physiol 52:530, 1982.

99. Bartlett D Jr, Knuth SL, Knuth KV: Effects of pulmonary stretch receptor blockade on laryngeal response to hypercapnia and hypoxia. Respir Physiol 45:67, 1981.

100. Brouilette RT, Thach BT: A neuromuscular mechanism maintaining extrathoracic airway patency. J Appl Physiol 46:772, 1979.

101. Korl RC, Knuth SL, Bartlett D: Selective reduction of genioglossal muscle activity by alcohol in normal human subjects. Am Rev Respir Dis 129:247, 1984.

102. Phillipson EA: State of the art—control of breathing during sleep. Am Rev Respir Dis 118:909, 1978.

103. Remmers JE, Anch AM, deGroot WJ: Respiratory disturbances during sleep. Clin Chest Med 1:57, 1980.

104. Cherniack NS: Respiratory dysrhythmias during sleep. N Engl J Med 305:325, 1981.

105. Douglas NJ, White DP, Pickett CK, et al: Respiration during sleep in normal man. Thorax 37:840, 1982.

106. Gothe B, Altose MD, Goldman MD, et al: Effect of quiet sleep on resting and CO_2 stimulated breathing in humans. J Appl Physiol 50:724, 1981.

107. Douglas NG, White DP, Weil JV, et al: Hypercapnic ventilatory response in sleeping adults. Am Rev Respir Dis 126:758, 1982.

108. Douglas J, White P, Weil V, et al: Hypoxic ventilatory response decreases during sleep in normal men. Am Rev Respir Dis 125:286, 1982.

109. Berthon-Jones M, Sullivan CE: Ventilatory and arousal responses to hypoxia in sleeping humans. Am Rev Respir Dis 125:632, 1982.

110. White DP, Douglas NJ, Pickett CK, et al: Sleep deprivation and the control of ventilation. Am Rev Respir Dis 128:948, 1983.

CHAPTER 10

The Respiratory Muscles and Chest Wall

THE RESPIRATORY MUSCLES, 246
  Upper Airway Muscles, 246
  Intercostal and Accessory Muscles, 246
  The Diaphragm, 247
    Development, 247
    Anatomy, 248
      Blood Supply, 250
      Lymphatic Drainage, 250
      Nerve Supply, 250
    Radiology, 251
      Radiographic Appearance, 251
      Computed Tomographic Appearance, 251
      Diaphragmatic Excursion, 254
  The Respiratory Pump, 255
    Contractile Mechanism, 255
    Energy Sources, 257
    Respiratory Muscle Weakness and Fatigue, 257
THE CHEST WALL, 259
  Soft Tissues, 259
  Bones, 260
    The Ribs, 260
    Other Chest Wall Bones, 263

THE RESPIRATORY MUSCLES

The respiratory muscles can be divided into four groups, each with different functions and mechanisms of action—the upper airway muscles, the diaphragm, the intercostal and accessory inspiratory muscles, and the abdominal muscles.[1–3] The structure, function, and pathophysiology of all these groups have been reviewed in a comprehensive text[4] and in several articles.[5, 6]

Upper Airway Muscles

Although respiratory neural input to upper airway muscles has been known to occur for some time, interest in this subject has increased recently because of the relationship between dysfunction of these muscles and obstructive sleep apnea.[1] A variety of muscles are important in this regard. The alae nasi are nasal dilatory muscles that are activated during increased respiratory drive; their action is increased by sensory input from receptors in the nose that detect increased nasal air flow.[7] The nasal versus oral route of breathing is determined by the action of two palatal muscles, the palatoglossus and the levator palatini.[8] The genioglossal and geniohyoid muscles, as well as the muscles of the larynx

and pharynx, display electromyographic (EMG) activity related to the respiratory cycle,[1, 9] their action being to stiffen the airway and prevent collapse.

Receptors in the hypopharynx and larynx respond to negative pressure by reflex activation of the upper airway muscles. The afferent limb of this reflex is carried in the superior laryngeal and the 9th and 10th cranial nerves.[10, 11] Further recruitment of these muscles occurs with increased neural output generated by hypoxia and hypercapnia.[12–14] These muscles contract simultaneously with the inspiratory muscles, although their EMG activity starts somewhat earlier and peaks during maximal inspiratory flow rather than at maximal inspired volume. When phrenic nerve discharge is out of phase with upper airway muscle contraction, there is a tendency for increased resistance of the upper airways or for complete closure.[15] Such incoordination of inspiratory action between the upper airway muscles and the diaphragm probably accounts for the obstruction that develops in patients with electrical pacers of the phrenic nerve.[16] The upper airway muscles are more sensitive than the other respiratory muscles to depression by sleep,[17] anesthesia,[15] partial paralysis with curare,[18] and alcohol consumption.[9] This observation probably explains the increased tendency for upper airway obstruction that occurs during sleep, anesthesia, and sedation.

Intercostal and Accessory Muscles

Muscles involved in respiration may be considered "primary" (those that routinely contract during tidal breathing in normal individuals) and "accessory" (those that are not normally active during tidal breathing but are recruited when the demand for ventilation increases). The diaphragm is the principal primary muscle of inspiration;[19] others include the scalenes, the parasternal, and the external intercostals. The accessory inspiratory muscles include the sternocleidomastoid, pectoralis, serratus anterior, trapezius, and latissimus dorsi.[20, 21] The respiratory function of the rib cage muscles has been reviewed.[22] Tonic inspiratory muscle activity in the parasternal and external intercostal muscles in the upright posture prevents the paradoxical inward movement of the rib cage that can be caused by the negative pleural pressure associated with diaphragmatic descent. During rapid eye movement sleep, anesthesia, or high spinal cord section, this tonic activity is absent and paradoxical inward motion of the chest wall occurs with inspiration.[23, 24]

The expiratory muscles include the abdominals, the internal intercostals, and the triangularis sterni. The abdominal muscles include the rectus and transverse abdominis and the external and internal obliques; although these muscles are generally regarded as expiratory in function, they may also play an active role in inspiration (*see* farther on).[25] The triangularis sterni is an accessory expiratory muscle that originates from the sternum and inserts into the internal surface of the chondrocostal junctions of ribs 3 to 7.[26, 27] In healthy individuals, expiration is largely passive, with expiratory muscle activity becoming manifested only when minute ventilation exceeds about 50% of maximal voluntary ventilation or when the inspiratory muscles are faced with increased loads.[28–30]

The Diaphragm

Development

The precursor of the diaphragm can be first noted in human embryos of 3 weeks' gestation as a mesodermal ridge termed the *septum transversum* that originates between the stalk of the yolk sac and the pericardial cavity (Fig. 10–1). It extends dorsally to divide the coelomic cavity incompletely, leaving two large dorsolateral intracoelomic openings, the pericardioperitoneal canals. The developing lung buds expand within the cranial portion of these canals and extend into the mesenchyme of the dorsolateral body wall. In the process, the mesenchyme is partially eroded except for a midline portion that eventually forms a mesentery for the esophagus and in which develop the diaphragmatic crura. The pericardioperitoneal canals are eventually divided into definitive thoracic and abdominal cavities by mesenchymal folds, the pleuroperitoneal membranes; by the sixth to seventh week, these membranes have grown anteriorly and medially to fuse with the esophageal mesentery and the septum transversum.

During the third month, the developing lungs extend farther into the lateral body walls, at which time a further layer of body wall tissue is split off and incorporated into the peripheral portion of the diaphragm. The definitive diaphragm is thus derived from four structures (*see* Fig. 10–1): (1) the septum transversum, which corresponds to the adult

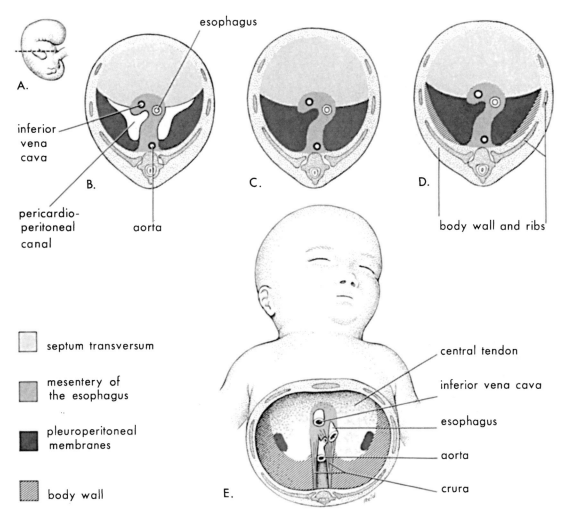

Figure 10–1. Drawings Illustrating Development of the Diaphragm. *A*, Sketch of a lateral view of an embryo at the end of the fifth week (actual size) indicating the level of section. *B* to *E* show the diaphragm as viewed from below. *B*, Transverse section showing the unfused pleuroperitoneal membranes. *C*, Similar section at the end of the sixth week after fusion of the pleuroperitoneal membranes with the other two diaphragmatic components. *D*, Transverse section through a 12-week embryo after ingrowth of the fourth diaphragmatic component from the body wall. *E*, View of the diaphragm of a newborn infant indicating the probable embryologic origin of its components. (From Moore KL: The Developing Human. 3rd ed. Philadelphia, WB Saunders, 1982.)

central tendon; (2) the two pleuroperitoneal membranes, which are thought to represent only a very small portion of the mature diaphragm; (3) the esophageal mesentery with incorporated crura; and (4) the body wall component, which corresponds to the majority of the mature muscular portion. In the later half of gestation, the fetal/neonatal type of myosin is slowly replaced by the adult isoforms.[31]

This rather complex development can be associated with a variety of diaphragmatic anomalies, including failure of formation or fusion of the various diaphragmatic components (resulting in complete or partial absence of the diaphragm or in posterolateral [foramen of Bochdalek] hernia), incomplete muscularization of the lateral or anterior body wall segments (causing eventration of the diaphragm or anterior [foramen of Morgagni] hernia), and defects of the septum transversum (pericardioperitoneal communication). These defects are discussed in more detail in Chapter 77 (*see* page 2995).

Anatomy

The diaphragm is a musculotendinous sheet separating the thoracic and abdominal cavities (Fig. 10–2). It has a complex three-dimensional structure that defies mathematical description. Although its overall shape can be appreciated on posteroanterior and lateral radiographs, more detailed shape analysis has been performed with computed tomography (CT) and magnetic resonance (MR) imaging.[32] The central tendon is a broad sheet of decussating fibers, in shape similar to a broad-bladed boomerang, the point of the boomerang being directed toward the sternum and the concavity toward the spine. The costal muscle fibers arise anteriorly from the xiphoid process and around the convexity of the thorax from ribs 7 to 12; posteriorly, the crural fibers arise from the lateral margins of the first, second, and third lumbar vertebrae on the right side and from the first and second lumbar vertebrae on the left. These fibers converge toward the central tendon and are inserted into it nearly perpendicular to its margin. The muscle fibers are of variable length, from 5 cm anteriorly at the sternal origin to 14 cm posterolaterally where they originate from the 9th, 10th, and 11th ribs.[33] The greatest respiratory excursion occurs in the posterolateral portion of the hemidiaphragms, where the muscle fibers are longest.[33] The fibers that compose the sternal attachment and those that arise from the 7th rib are

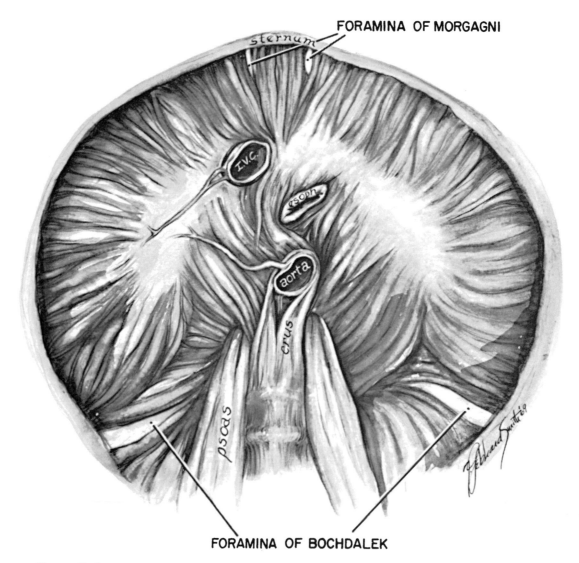

FORAMINA OF MORGAGNI

FORAMINA OF BOCHDALEK

Figure 10–2. Anatomy of the Normal Diaphragm Viewed from Below. *See* the text. I.V.C., inferior vena cava.

separated bilaterally by triangular spaces poor in muscular and tendinous tissue, which may subsequently be the site of herniation or eventration.

Although difficult to discern at first glance, there is evidence that the diaphragm is in fact two distinct muscles with separate nervous and vascular supply as well as function.[34] The costal portion of the diaphragm is mechanically in series with the intercostal and accessory muscles, and its contraction can result in both descent of the diaphragm and elevation of the rib cage; by contrast, the crural portion is in parallel with the costal portion of the diaphragm, and its contraction results in descent of the diaphragm without elevation of the rib cage.[34, 35] The rib cage itself can also be divided into two components, the diaphragm-apposed portion and the lung-apposed portion. Diaphragmatic contraction expands the apposed portion of the rib cage by increasing abdominal pressure and, by lowering pleural pressure, can have an expiratory action on the lung-apposed portion. However, if the linkage between the lung-apposed and diaphragm-apposed portions of the rib cage is stiff, costal diaphragmatic contraction will also lift the rib cage. The link between the two portions of the rib cage is shown in Figure 10–3 as a spring that can be stiff or flaccid depending on the state of contraction of the rib cage muscles.[36]

Like other mammalian skeletal muscles, the human diaphragm is composed of three types of muscle fibers, each with specific physiologic features and corresponding histochemical profiles;[37, 38] all fibers within individual motor units are of the same type. The physiologic and histochemical differences between fiber types are largely determined by the different myosin heavy-chain isotypes expressed by the cells.[39] The three types of muscle fibers are known as (1) slow-twitch oxidative fatigue-resistant units (Type 1); (2) fast-twitch oxidative glycolytic fatigue-resistant units (Type 2a); and (3) fast-twitch glycolytic fatigable units (Type 2b). In the normal human diaphragm, Type 1 represents approximately 50% of the muscle fibers, Type 2a about 20%, and Type 2b about 30%; these percentages could conceivably change with atrophy or training of the respiratory muscles.[40–43] It is likely that the diaphragm behaves like other skeletal muscles, slow-twitch motor units being recruited during low-intensity contractions such as in sustained or quiet breathing and fast-twitch units (both fatigue resistant and fatigue susceptible) playing a greater role with increasing respiratory activity.

The relative proportion of the different types of motor fibers present in the diaphragm may be of great importance in the pathogenesis of muscle fatigue and ventilatory failure

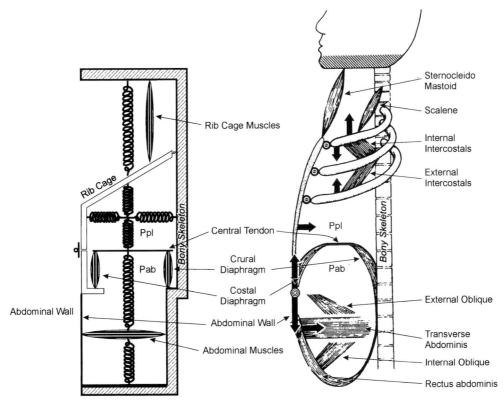

Figure 10–3. Mechanical Model of the Inspiratory Musculature. The diaphragm is composed of crural and costal portions joined by the central tendon. The inverted L-shaped structure represents the rib cage; the latter is divided into a lung-apposed portion and a diaphragm-apposed portion. The coiled springs represent the elastic properties of the rib cage, lung, and abdomen and the hatched area, the bony skeleton. The costal and crural portions of the diaphragm are arranged mechanically in parallel. In this situation, the force applied is the sum of the forces generated by the two muscles; however, the displacement (volume change) is equal to the displacement of either muscle. The costal part of the diaphragm is in series with the intercostal and accessory muscles. In this situation, the displacements of the two muscles can be added but the forces are not summed. The spring linking the two portions of the rib cage indicates that the rib cage may be flexible (i.e., the lung-apposed and diaphragm-apposed portions can move independently in response to applied pressures). The drawing on the *right* represents a more anatomically realistic representation showing separation of costal and crural parts of the diaphragm and lung-apposed portions of the rib cage. Ppl, pleural pressure; Pab, abdominal pressure. (Adapted from Macklem PT, Macklem DM, De Troyer A: J Appl Physiol 55:547, 1983; and Ward ME, Ward JW, Macklem PT: J Appl Physiol 72:1338, 1992.)

(*see* farther on). For example, a paucity of slow-twitch oxidative fibers in premature infants may explain their poor tolerance to respiratory loads and their susceptibility to ventilatory failure.[44] Sufficiently rapid atrophy of fatigue-resistant fibers could also explain the extreme susceptibility to respiratory failure of patients being weaned from artificial ventilation and also offer some hope for efforts being made to restore strength and endurance with respiratory muscle training. The weight (muscle mass) of the diaphragm is closely related to nutritional status and body weight,[45, 46] although in some disease states such as chronic obstructive pulmonary disease (COPD) there is evidence of a loss of muscle, especially Type 2 fibers, with resultant decreased weight that is independent of any change in body weight itself.[45, 47, 48]

Microscopically, the muscular portion comprises multiple muscle fascicles of variable size containing individual muscle fibers with differing ultrastructural and functional characteristics.[49] In addition to numerous blood vessels, there is also an extensive intradiaphragmatic lymphatic network.

Blood Supply

The diaphragm receives its blood supply from the phrenic and intercostal arteries and from branches of the internal thoracic (mammary) arteries. Small phrenic branches generally arise directly from the lower part of the thoracic aorta and sometimes from the renal arteries. They are distributed to the posterior part of the upper surface of the diaphragm and anastomose with the musculophrenic and pericardiacophrenic arteries. The latter two arteries are separate branches from the internal thoracic arteries and approach the diaphragm from a more anterior position.[50] The internal mammary and phrenic arteries anastomose to form an arterial circle around the central tendon. This circle gives off branches that form an arcade; a second arterial circle is formed by the intercostals around the insertion of the diaphragm. This diversity of blood supply may be an important factor in the diaphragm's resistance to fatigue.[51]

Scanning electron microscopic studies have shown individual myofibers to be surrounded by 8 to 10 blood vessels (Fig. 10–4), with an extensive capillary network in close topographic relationship with each myofiber. This intimate arrangement of capillaries and myofibers facilitates diffusion of gases, nutrients, and metabolites along the surface of the sarcolemma. The diaphragm has an abundant blood supply; flow can increase to ~250 ml/min/100 gm of muscle during maximal activation (about half of the maximal blood flow to the heart).[52] The increasing demand for oxygen by the working diaphragm is largely supplied by augmenting blood flow rather than by increasing the extraction of oxygen from the blood.[53] However, blood flow can reach a maximum and be an impediment to further force generation. Like other skeletal muscles, blood flow is impeded by increased intramuscular pressure during contraction, and at high levels of activation, most of the blood supply and gas exchange occur during the expiratory phase of the respiratory cycle. Blood supply limitation is related to the tension-time index of the diaphragm (TTdi): when TTdi is greater than 0.2, blood flow becomes limited and marked postexercise hyperemia becomes apparent;[54] a TTdi of about 0.2 is also the critical value beyond which diaphragmatic fatigue invariably develops (*see* farther on).

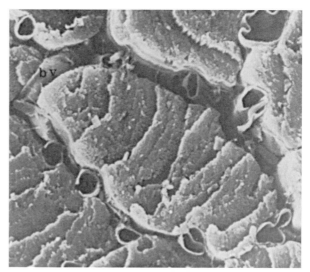

Figure 10–4. Morphologic Characteristics of the Diaphragm. Low-power scanning electron micrograph depicting a cross section of myofibers surrounded by numerous blood vessels (bv). (×3000.) (From Leak LV, Rahil K: Am Rev Respir Dis 119[Suppl]:8, 1979.)

Lymphatic Drainage

An extensive intradiaphragmatic lymphatic network drains via collecting vessels into mediastinal channels.[49] A single layer of mesothelial cells, continuous with the cells lining the wall of the chest and abdominal cavities, covers the peritoneal and pleural surfaces of the diaphragm. These mesothelial cells rest on a loose connective tissue layer containing a rich plexus of lymphatic channels. On the peritoneal surface, small pores 4 to 12 μm in diameter have been demonstrated between mesothelial cells; these pores appear to provide direct communication between the peritoneal cavity and lymphatic spaces.[49, 55] Both particulate and cellular material has been shown to concentrate around and apparently enter these pores,[49] thus providing a direct pathway for the transport of intraperitoneal neoplastic cells or fluid into the mediastinum or pleural space.

Nerve Supply

The phrenic nerve is the sole motor nerve supply to the diaphragm. It arises chiefly from the fourth cervical nerve, but also receives contributions from the third and fifth. At the level of the diaphragm, each phrenic nerve gives off a few small branches that are distributed to the parietal pleura above and the parietal peritoneum below the central part of the diaphragm. They then divide into three motor branches, the anterior (sternal) branch, the anterolateral branch, and the posterior branch, which supplies the crural part of the diaphragm. This branch distribution probably has a significant functional correlation; as has been shown in the dog, the costal and crural parts of the diaphragm can be separately stimulated, the costal branch increasing and the crural branch decreasing the dimensions of the lower rib cage.[34]

There is evidence that in most individuals, hemidiaphragmatic and intercostal muscle activity has a predominantly contralateral cortical representation; for example, in patients with acute hemiplegia secondary to a cerebrovascular accident, diaphragmatic and intercostal EMGs usually show a striking reduction in activity on the side of the paresis.[56] In a minority of patients, however, innervation of the diaphragm appears to be bilaterally symmetric. The conduction velocity in the phrenic nerve is high, reaching a maximum of 78 m/sec; also, the innervation is dense, each nerve fiber subserving a low number of motor units—an anatomic arrangement that is usually seen in muscles performing precise movements, such as those of the eye. The intercostal motor neurons are located between T1 and T12 in the spinal cord and reach the intercostal muscles via the intercostal nerves. Abdominal muscle motor neurons are located between T11 and L1.[57]

A contracting diaphragm can also be sensed,[58, 59] with most people experiencing a "squeezing" sensation in the lower half of the chest during breath-holding. This phenomenon is not abolished by spinal lesions or spinal anesthesia below the level of the C3 to C5 anterior horn cells, but is eliminated by transection of the cord at the C3 level and by curarization;[59, 60] it appears that the afferent limb for this sensation lies in the 9th or 10th cranial nerve.

Radiology

Radiographic Appearance

On the chest radiograph, the upper surface of the dome-shaped diaphragm is normally visualized as it forms an interface with the lung; its inferior surface is obscured by the soft tissues of the abdomen. Although the entire upper surface of the right hemidiaphragm is usually visible on both posteroanterior and lateral radiographs, the heart generally obscures the silhouette of the medial third of the left hemidiaphragm on the posteroanterior radiograph and its anterior portion on the lateral view.[61]

A definitive study of the height and position of the hemidiaphragms on frontal chest radiographs was performed in 500 normal adults, 250 of each sex, over 21 years of age.[62] In 94%, the level of the cupola of the right hemidiaphragm was projected in a plane ranging from the anterior end of the fifth rib to the sixth anterior interspace; 41% were at the level of the sixth rib anteriorly and 4% were at or below the level of the seventh rib. Generally speaking, the height of the right dome was higher in women and in subjects of heavy build and/or over the age of 40 years.

Although the tendency for the plane of the right diaphragmatic dome to be about half an interspace higher than the left is well recognized, both were at the same height or the left was higher than the right in approximately 10% of 500 normal subjects in another study;[63] in 2%, the right hemidiaphragm was more than 3 cm higher than the left. In approximately half of the 10%, gaseous distention of the stomach or colon was noted—a potential cause of left hemidiaphragmatic elevation. In a third investigation of 114 healthy young men, the left hemidiaphragm is higher than the right in 12%.[64]

Although the higher position of the right hemidiaphragm is commonly ascribed to the mass of the liver beneath it, the available evidence suggests that the cardiac mass determines the lower position of the hemidiaphragm that is ipsilateral to the heart. In two studies of 60 and 65 individuals who had various combinations of congenital malposition of thoracic and abdominal viscera, the apex

of the heart was located on the same side as the lower hemidiaphragm.[65, 66]

Scalloping of the diaphragm, in which the normally smooth contour is replaced by smooth, arcuate elevations, is relatively uncommon (Fig. 10–5), being observed in only 5.5% of the 500 normal subjects mentioned previously;[63] it was confined to the right side in the majority and was bilateral in only a small percentage. The pattern has no known significance. Muscle slips originating from the lateral and posterolateral ribs can sometimes be identified as short, meniscus-shaped shadows along the lateral half of both hemidiaphragms. Although such an appearance is common in association with severe pulmonary overinflation (Fig. 10–6), as in asthma or emphysema, it may occur in normal individuals with exceptionally low descent of the diaphragm during inspiration, particularly young men; in the absence of supportive evidence, the finding should not be interpreted as a sign of air trapping.

A small eventration may occur anywhere in the diaphragm, but is seen most commonly in the anteromedial quadrant on the right. This finding also has no known functional significance. Irregularity of the contour of the left hemidiaphragm or an apparent left paracardiac mass can be caused by a dilated left inferior phrenic or pericardiacophrenic vein in patients who have inferior vena caval occlusion or narrowing.[67, 67a]

Computed Tomographic Appearance

On CT, the diaphragm can be visualized only where its upper surface interfaces with the lung and the inferior surface interfaces with intraperitoneal or retroperitoneal fat.[68] Although it is not visualized where it abuts structures of similar soft tissue attenuation, such as the liver and spleen,

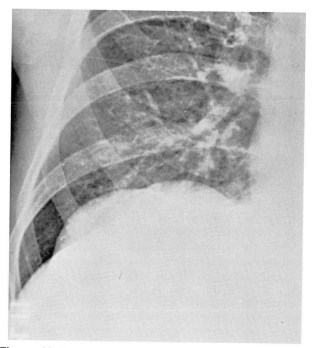

Figure 10–5. Scalloping of the Diaphragm. A radiograph of the right hemidiaphragm reveals two smooth arcuate elevations disturbing the normally smooth contour of the dome, a finding of no known significance.

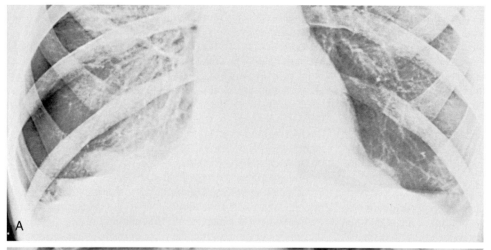

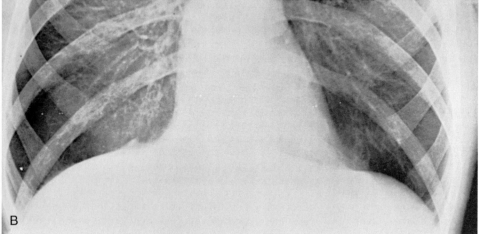

Figure 10–6. Diaphragmatic Muscle Slips. Inspiratory *(A)* and expiratory *(B)* radiographs of the lower half of the thorax of a patient with severe emphysema reveal short, meniscus-shaped shadows extending laterally from each hemidiaphragm. These muscle slips are prominent on full inspiration and disappear on expiration.

its position can be readily inferred since at all levels the lungs and pleura lie adjacent and peripheral to it whereas the abdominal viscera lie central to it (Fig. 10–7).[68]

The anterior or sternocostal portion of the diaphragm

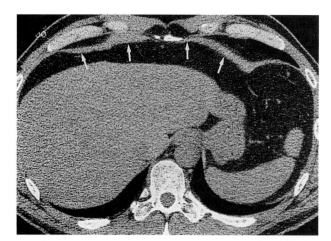

Figure 10–7. Anterior Portion of the Diaphragm. A CT scan at the level of the xiphoid demonstrates continuity between the anterior (xiphoid) and lateral (costal) diaphragmatic fibers *(arrows)*. The diaphragm is well visualized in areas where it is outlined by lung and peritoneal or retroperitoneal fat. Where it abuts structures of similar soft tissue attenuation such as the liver and spleen, it is not visualized; however, its position can be inferred because of its relation to the lungs and pleura (adjacent and peripheral to it) and the abdominal viscera (central to it).

has a variable appearance on CT that depends on the position of the central tendon relative to the xiphoid.[69, 70] Most commonly, the sternocostal portion is seen as a relatively smooth or slightly undulating soft tissue curve that is concave posteriorly, with continuity between the anterior xiphoid fibers and the lateral costal muscle (see Fig. 10–7).[69, 70] This appearance occurs when the middle leaflet of the central tendon is situated cephalad to the xiphoid; in one study, it was seen in 48% of 176 scans.[69] In the next most frequent CT appearance, the diaphragmatic line is discontinuous in the midline, the anterior diaphragmatic slips being oriented at an angle and diverging rather than converging with the lateral costal fibers (Fig. 10–8). This appearance, seen in 28% of cases in the aforementioned study,[69] occurs when the middle leaflet of the central tendon is located caudal to the level of the xiphoid. In this configuration, the transverse colon may be present anterior to the lower aspect of the heart; exclusion of a Morgagni hernia can be made by visualization of diaphragmatic fibers converging cephalad to the colon.[69, 70] Less commonly, the middle leaflet of the central tendon is located at the same level as the xiphoid, in which case the anterior portion of the diaphragm appears as a broad band with irregular, ill-defined, or angular margins.[69] In approximately 10% of people, the anterior sternal insertions of the diaphragm are either not adequately visualized or are not classifiable into one of the three patterns.[69]

The posterior or lumbar portion of the diaphragm is well visualized where the fibers arising from both the crura

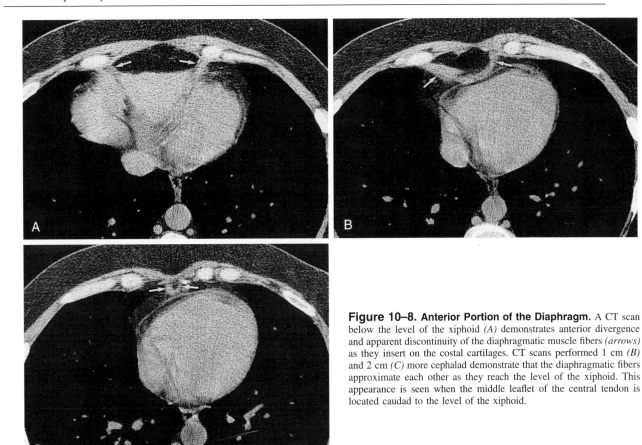

Figure 10–8. Anterior Portion of the Diaphragm. A CT scan below the level of the xiphoid *(A)* demonstrates anterior divergence and apparent discontinuity of the diaphragmatic muscle fibers *(arrows)* as they insert on the costal cartilages. CT scans performed 1 cm *(B)* and 2 cm *(C)* more cephalad demonstrate that the diaphragmatic fibers approximate each other as they reach the level of the xiphoid. This appearance is seen when the middle leaflet of the central tendon is located caudad to the level of the xiphoid.

and arcuate ligament arch forward to insert into the central tendon (Fig. 10–9). The right crus is longer than the left and arises from the anterolateral surface of the 1st, 2nd, and 3rd lumbar vertebrae;[68, 70] the left crus arises from the 1st and 2nd vertebrae. The most cephalad CT section in which the crura are visualized is at the level of the esophageal hiatus, which usually corresponds to the 10th thoracic vertebra.[68, 70] The crura are usually oval or comma shaped and have a variable thickness;[71] occasionally they have a nodular ap-

pearance (Fig. 10–10),[72] being thickest during deep inspiration.[68] The right crus is usually more prominent and thicker than the left.[68] Although the most anterior aspect of the crura can be identified in the preaortic position, laterally the crural fibers usually merge smoothly and indistinguishably with those arising from the medial arcuate ligaments.[68] The medial arcuate ligament is a tendinous arch in the fascia covering the psoas muscle, whereas the lateral arcuate ligament is a thickened band of fascia covering the anterior aspect of

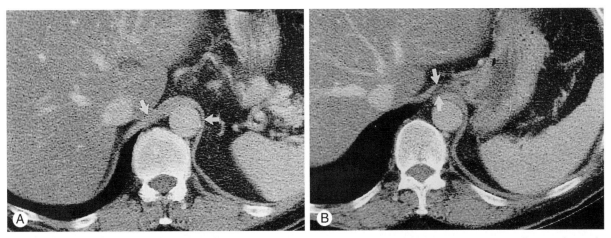

Figure 10–9. Lumbar Portion of the Diaphragm. A CT scan *(A)* demonstrates right and left crura *(arrows)* extending anterior to the aorta. Posterolaterally, the crural fibers merge smoothly and indistinguishably with fibers arising from the medial arcuate ligaments. A scan at a slightly more cephalad level *(B)* demonstrates discontinuity of the right and left crura at the level of the esophageal hiatus *(arrows)*.

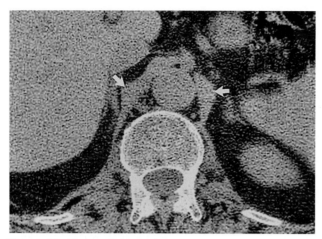

Figure 10–10. Lumbar Portion of the Diaphragm. A CT scan in a 72-year-old man demonstrates focal nodular thickening *(arrows)* of the right and left diaphragmatic crura.

the quadratus lumborum muscle.[68, 70] As with the crura, the arcuate ligaments may also have a focal nodular appearance: in one review of CT scans in 100 patients, bilateral nodularity was found in 3 and unilateral nodularity in 2;[73] the nodular areas measured approximately 9 mm in the transverse plane and 6 mm in the anteroposterior plane and extended for 4 cm in the cephalocaudal plane.

The mean thickness of the diaphragm is slightly greater in men than in women and slightly greater on the right than on the left (approximately 5 mm on the right and 4 mm on the left).[74] Although there is no significant relationship between thickness and age,[74] a generalized increase in diaphragmatic nodularity and irregularity is seen in older individuals; for example, in one study of 60 patients, focal areas of nodularity ("pseudotumors") were seen in 3% of patients between 20 and 49 years of age and in 22% between 50 and 79.[74] The authors postulated that the nodularities were due to increased laxity of the connective tissues that bind the diaphragm with age.[74] Ultrasound has also been used to measure diaphragmatic thickness and the change in diaphragmatic thickness during maximal contraction in the area of apposition. In one study of 13 healthy men, the mean value for thickness ($\pm$ SD) was 1.7 $\pm$ 0.2 mm at functional residual capacity (FRC) and 4.5 $\pm$ 0.9 mm at total lung capacity (TLC).[75]

In the aforementioned study, focal diaphragmatic defects also increased in number and severity with age, being absent in patients under 39 years of age and present in 25% of patients between 40 and 49 and 60% of patients between 70 and 79. These diaphragmatic defects occurred mainly in the posterior portion of the diaphragm and were of three types. Type 1, the most common, was a localized defect in the thickness of the diaphragm but with maintenance of diaphragm continuity. The defect typically measured approximately 5 mm in length and was not associated with protrusion of omental fat beyond the diaphragm. Type 2 represented an apparent defect in the diaphragm in which the muscle fibers appeared to separate into layers parallel to the diaphragmatic contour. This defect was also not associated with any protrusion of omental fat. Type 3 defects, present in 5% of patients between 40 and 49 years of age and in up

to 35% of patients in their eighth decade, varied from 5 mm in width to involvement of almost the entire hemidiaphragm. In this type of defect, omental fat protrudes beyond the diaphragm (Fig. 10–11).[74] Herniation of omental fat through the diaphragmatic defect, often seen in otherwise normal elderly individuals, may cause diagnostic difficulties by mimicking a lung tumor on the radiograph or a traumatic diaphragmatic hernia on CT.[74, 76, 77]

In the majority of patients, the diaphragm can be adequately visualized on conventional transverse CT sections. However, multiplanar spiral CT reformations[78] and coronal and sagittal MR images[79–81] allow better assessment of the diaphragm and its anatomic relationships with adjacent tissues. With both spiral CT[78] and fast gradient-echo MR imaging,[81] the diaphragm and peridiaphragmatic region can be scanned in a single breath-hold, thus minimizing artifacts from respiratory motion.

On CT, two thin soft tissue attenuation lines can frequently be seen adjacent to the diaphragm. One extends laterally from the esophagus below the level of the inferior pulmonary veins.[82,83] The pulmonary component of this line is formed by the intersegmental (intersublobar) septum, which separates the medial from the posterior basal segment of the lower lobe; its mediastinal component is the pulmonary ligament (Fig. 10–12).[83] In one investigation, the septum and the pulmonary ligament were seen in 58% of 80 CT examinations on the right side and in 79% on the left.[82] The other line of attenuation extends laterally from the inferior vena cava on the right side and from the posterior portion of the left ventricle on the left side.[84] Although initially believed to represent the phrenic nerve,[82] this line probably represents the inferior phrenic artery and vein (Fig. 10–13).[84] It is seen on CT in 30% to 60% of patients.[82, 84]

Diaphragmatic Excursion

A wide range of diaphragmatic excursion is seen in normal individuals. In a study of inspiratory-expiratory radiographs of 350 subjects aged 30 to 80 years without evidence of respiratory disease, Fraser found the mean excursions of the right and left hemidiaphragms to be 3.3 and 3.5 cm, respectively (unpublished data), somewhat less than the values observed by others. For example, in one study of 114 healthy young men, the range of diaphragmatic excursion was 0.8 to 8.1 cm overall, 5 to 7 cm in 57 individuals (50%), and less than 3 cm in 16 (14%);[64] there was no relationship between diaphragmatic movement and vital capacity. Unequal movement of the two hemidiaphragmatic domes was common: movement was equal in only 10 subjects, being greater on the right in 73 (never by more than 1.9 cm) and greater on the left in 31 (exceeding 1.4 cm in only 1 case). These observations are at variance with the findings in one study of older subjects[85] but agree with those obtained by others.[86, 87]

Diaphragmatic excursion can also be measured with M-mode and real-time ultrasound.[88, 89] (The intraobserver and interobserver coefficients of variation are smallest for real-time analysis.) In one investigation of 55 normal adults, the mean right and left hemidiaphragmatic excursion was 53 $\pm$ 16 (mean $\pm$ SD) and 46 $\pm$ 12 mm, respectively, and the ratio of right-to-left diaphragmatic excursion was about 1.2.[88] The shape, motion, and thickness of the diaphragm can also

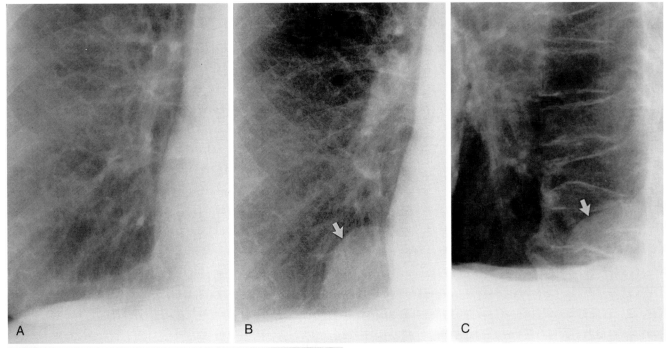

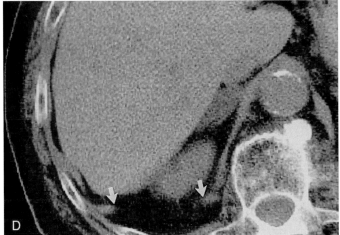

Figure 10–11. Diaphragmatic Defect with Herniation of Omental Fat. A view of the right lower aspect of the chest from a posteroanterior radiograph *(A)* in a 78-year-old woman is unremarkable. A similar view 5 years later *(B)* reveals a focal mass *(arrow)* that on the lateral radiograph *(C)* can be seen to have a posterior location *(arrow)*. The mass has a lower density than the heart and soft tissues of the abdomen, consistent with fat. A view of the right hemidiaphragm from a CT scan *(D)* reveals a focal defect *(arrows)* in its posterior aspect with herniation of omental fat. The patient had no symptoms related to the defect.

be assessed by CT and MR imaging.[90–93] For example, in one MR investigation of 10 supine normal subjects, the mean maximal excursion of the right and left hemidiaphragms was 4.4 and 4.2 cm, respectively;[92] regional motion was greater anteriorly and laterally. With CT, a large range of maximal crural diaphragmatic thickness has been reported in both men (1.8 to 18.8 mm) and women (1.8 to 21.1 mm).[90]

The Respiratory Pump

Muscle weakness and fatigue are now considered to be important determinants of ventilatory failure in almost all instances. The muscles of ventilation generally behave much as other striated muscles of the body.[94, 95] They differ in that they are under automatic as well as voluntary control; in addition, in contrast to the inertial loads facing most other skeletal muscles, the respiratory muscles must principally overcome resistive and elastic loads.[96] Unlike other muscles that are subcutaneous in position, diaphragmatic function

cannot be measured directly because of its inaccessibility, at least in humans. This disadvantage necessitates the use of a variety of indirect means of measurement, all of which have certain limitations. In the following sections we consider the components of the respiratory pump machinery under the headings of contractile mechanism and energy sources.

Contractile Mechanism

Because of rib articulation and its insertion onto the lower ribs, contraction of the diaphragm results in lifting and expansion of the chest cage. Since it also pushes down on the abdominal viscera, the increased abdominal pressure contributes to upward and outward displacement of the thorax and results in displacement of the abdominal wall outward. If the abdominal muscles are contracted during inspiration, abdominal pressure increases, descent of the diaphragm is restricted, and rib cage movement is accentuated. At the end of a quiet expiration, the diaphragm is relaxed, and pleural and abdominal pressures are equal. On

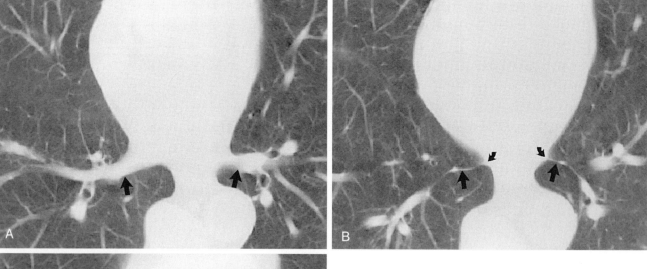

Figure 10–12. The Pulmonary Ligament. A CT scan *(A)* demonstrates the right and left inferior veins *(arrows)*. A scan at a slightly more caudad level *(B)* demonstrates right and left intersegmental septa *(straight arrows)* and the pulmonary ligaments *(curved arrows)*, which form the mediastinal attachment. A third scan at the level of the dome of the right hemidiaphragm *(C)* shows a line formed by the right inferior phrenic artery and vein *(arrow)* and the more posteriorly located pulmonary ligaments and intersegmental septa.

inspiration, intrapleural pressure becomes more negative and abdominal pressure more positive; i.e., the transdiaphragmatic pressure difference increases. When the abdominal muscles are relaxed—as they tend to be with quiet breathing

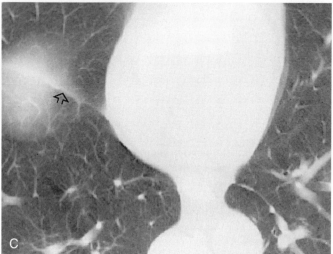

Figure 10–13. Inferior Phrenic Artery and Vein. A CT scan at the level of the dome of the diaphragm demonstrates right and left lines of attenuation *(arrows)* caused by the inferior phrenic artery and vein. The right line of attenuation extends laterally from the inferior vena cava and the left from the posterior portion of the left ventricle.

in the supine position—this increase in pressure causes protrusion of the abdominal wall. The abdominal and accessory muscles also act as fixators or positioning muscles that adjust the configuration and stiffness of the rib cage and abdomen in such a way as to optimize efficiency of the diaphragm.[96] This function is particularly evident in the upright position and especially during exercise, when abdominal muscle contraction tends to lengthen the diaphragmatic muscle fibers. Because of the length-tension relationship of skeletal muscle, the longer fibers can generate more tension for a given neuronal drive.[97]

Abdominal expiratory muscles can also aid inspiration by decreasing the end-expiratory lung volume below the relaxed volume of the rib cage and abdomen and then suddenly relaxing at the onset of inspiration. The sudden descent of the diaphragm along its passive length-tension curve represents an energy-independent inspiratory contribution. This strategy is used by normal subjects in the hyperpnea of CO_2 rebreathing and exercise[57] and in patients with bilateral diaphragmatic paralysis.[98] The maneuver is effective in the upright and lateral decubitus postures but ineffective in the supine position, thus accounting for the characteristic increase in dyspnea noted by patients with bilateral diaphragmatic paralysis when they assume the supine posture.[98]

The force generated by the contracting diaphragm is a

function of muscle fiber length and the mechanical advantage of the muscle. Like all skeletal muscles, the diaphragmatic fibers have a characteristic length-tension relationship. Thus, at a specific optimal length at which maximal overlap between actin and myosin filaments occurs, maximal force can be generated with a given stimulation. As the fibers are lengthened or shortened beyond this point, the tension generated by a given stimulus is decreased. Studies in the dog have shown that diaphragmatic muscle fibers are at nearly optimal length at FRC.[99] In contrast to the mechanical advantage given to the diaphragm by abdominal muscle contraction, hyperinflation of the lung decreases diaphragmatic efficiency by shortening muscle fiber length. This situation obviously applies chiefly to patients with obstructive lung disease,[100] but has also been shown to be true for normal individuals breathing at high lung volumes.[101, 102]

The force and transdiaphragmatic pressure generated by the diaphragm during contraction are also related to the mechanical advantage of the muscle. For a dome-shaped structure such as the diaphragm, the mechanical advantage is related to the radius of curvature: the greater the curvature (the smaller the radius of curvature), the more pressure generated for a given tension in the diaphragm (law of Laplace). It was formerly thought that this principle was an important determinant of diaphragmatic muscular function: with a decrease in lung volume and elevation of the diaphragm, the radius of curvature was thought to decrease, whereas with increasing lung volume and descent of the diaphragm, the radius of curvature was thought to increase. However, relatively recent studies suggest that changes in diaphragmatic contour may not be such an important determinant of diaphragmatic function since the radiologically determined radius of curvature of the diaphragm does not change substantially with changes in lung volume.[103, 104]

The other determinant of diaphragmatic contractility is the intensity of neural stimulation. Diaphragmatic force is maximum in humans when the phrenic nerve is stimulated at a frequency of 100 Hz; it is reduced to 94% maximum at 50 Hz, 70% maximum at 20 Hz, and 25% maximum at 10 Hz.[102] Strength of the muscle is assessed as the degree of response to maximal stimulation and varies with the length of the muscle at the time of excitation; endurance depends on the force and duration of contraction.

Energy Sources

The energy sources of respiratory muscles are oxygen, stored glycogen and protein, and nutrients extracted from the circulation; as already discussed, the abundant blood supply to the diaphragm is not a limiting factor in O_2 supply except during maximal demand.[54, 105] However, when oxygen transport to the tissues is impaired by a reduction in cardiac output or by severe hypoxemia or anemia, a critical shortage of O_2 for effective diaphragmatic activity may occur, and the body's homeostatic mechanism may be faced with the predicament of deciding which vital organs or tissues should be deprived.[100]

Experimental studies in dogs have shown that the diaphragm derives approximately half its energy requirement from oxidation of carbohydrate and the remainder from lipid substances in the blood.[105] The diaphragm is extremely resistant to anaerobic metabolism,[105] lactic acid being pro-

duced only when severely hypoxic—as may occur in severe pulmonary edema with hyperventilation, low lung compliance, arterial hypoxemia, and reduced cardiac output.[100]

Respiratory Muscle Weakness and Fatigue

Ultimately, inadequate contraction of respiratory muscles develops in all patients with ventilatory respiratory failure. The three major factors that can lead to failure of adequate inspiratory muscle function are decreased neuronal drive, weakness of the respiratory muscle, and fatigue of the muscle. In fact, the last two of these are similar in that the muscles eventually reach a point where the demand placed on them exceeds their capacity to generate force and hence pressure. However, in the case of weakness, the primary problem is a decrease in the muscles' ability to generate force against normal loads, whereas in the case of fatigue, the major problem is a failure of force generation by a normally functioning muscle against increased load.[106] Moreover, fatigue is reversible over relatively short time periods whereas weakness may be permanent or only slowly reversible.[107]

A failure of central drive with resulting ventilatory respiratory failure occurs in central neurogenic hypoventilation or drug overdosage. Failure related to weakness is seen in neuromuscular disease such as myasthenia gravis or muscular dystrophy. Muscle fatigue is the common final pathway in patients whose respiratory failure is due to the increased work of breathing that occurs in diseases such as COPD or kyphoscoliosis.

There has been much recent interest in the study of respiratory muscle fatigue.[23, 108–111] The respiratory muscles are the most fatigue-resistant muscles in the body; in addition, diaphragmatic strength has been decreased to only about 40% of normal in patients in whom intravenous curare has been administered in a dose sufficient to completely abolish hand grip and head raising.[18, 112] On the other hand, fatigue of the diaphragm can occur during hyperventilation at levels that occur during exercise in normal subjects.[112a] In humans, the critical transdiaphragmatic pressure required for fatigue is approximately 40% maximum.[113] A more rigorous determination of the force output for fatigue can be calculated as the critical tension-time index (TTI) (i.e., the TTI beyond which fatigue is inevitable).* The normal TTI for the diaphragm is 0.02, and fatigue occurs within 1 hour if it is maintained at 0.2.[114, 115] The time that it takes a muscle to fatigue depends not only on the power that it has to generate relative to its strength and the fraction of the respiratory cycle that it is active but also on the energy stores it has and the energy supplies that are delivered to it. The power output

---

*The TTI of a muscle is the product of its force as a fraction of maximal force and its duty cycle. For the repetitively contracting respiratory muscles, the duty cycle is the ratio of inspiratory time to total respiratory cycle time (T_I/T_{Tot}). For example, a TTdi value of 0.2 for the diaphragm is achieved when the transdiaphragmatic pressure generated with each breath is 40% of maximum (tension = 0.4 maximum) and the inspiratory time is half of the total respiratory cycle time (T_I/T_{Tot} = 0.5).

$$TTdi = 0.4 \times 0.5 = 0.2$$

A test to noninvasively measure global inspiratory muscle TTI has also been proposed: occluded mouth pressure 0.1 second after the start of inspiration as a fraction of maximal inspiratory mouth pressure.[116]

depends on the compliance and resistance of the respiratory system, whereas strength is related to lung volume, muscle atrophy, and overall nutritional status of the host. The factors that determine energy availability for the respiratory muscles include the oxygen content of the arterial blood supplying the muscles, respiratory muscle blood flow, substrate concentration in the blood, and the energy stores in the muscle.[108] All these factors can be altered with disease.

The resting oxygen consumption of the respiratory muscles normally ranges from 1% to 3% of total oxygen consumption and can increase markedly in the presence of cardiorespiratory disease (as high as 25% of total oxygen consumption).[117] Normal subjects breathing a hypoxic gas mixture have a significant decrease in the time to reach respiratory muscle fatigue during loaded breathing,[118, 119] and supplemental oxygen can prolong the endurance time of the respiratory and other skeletal muscles in patients who are chronically hypoxemic.[120]

The presence of weakened or fatiguing muscle before the development of hypercapnia can be suggested by physical examination and confirmed by using specific diagnostic tests of muscle strength, endurance, and fatigue.[115, 121, 122] In the relaxed and supine state, most healthy individuals have predominant abdominal rather than rib cage motion,[123] a finding that correlates with breathing with the diaphragm as opposed to the intercostal muscles.[124] By contrast, normal subjects fatigued from breathing against resistance exhibit an interesting sequence of clinical manifestations that correlates with EMG evidence of muscle fatigue and the onset of respiratory acidosis.[125] Such individuals are first noted to have very shallow and rapid breathing, followed by paradoxical movement of the abdominal wall, the exhausted and flaccid diaphragm being sucked in by the negative intrapleural pressure created by rib cage expansion. In some patients, alternation between rib cage and abdominal breathing (respiratory alternans) is observed, a presumed homeostatic maneuver that permits resting of one group of muscles while the other works.[126] These signs of diaphragmatic weakness are best detected with the patient in the supine position; the hand should be placed on the abdominal wall to exclude the possibility that the indrawing is caused by contraction of abdominal muscles. This pattern of paradoxical movement of the abdomen and rib cage is transient in patients who have respiratory muscle fatigue, but is permanent in those who have diaphragmatic paralysis. Weakness or paralysis of the chest wall musculature, such as occurs after high spinal cord section with intact diaphragmatic function, causes the opposite paradoxical movement: inward inspiratory movement of the rib cage and sternum coincident with abdominal expansion.

The various diagnostic procedures that have been developed to test respiratory muscle innervation, strength, endurance, and the presence of fatigue are described in detail in Chapter 17. Briefly, respiratory muscle strength can be measured by assessing the inspiratory and expiratory pressure at the mouth.[127, 128] This test requires patient cooperation and is open to error if the facial muscles are weakened and allow air leak; the external intercostal and accessory muscles of respiration also contribute to the results. Because of the length-tension relationship of the respiratory muscles, the pressure generated is strongly influenced by the lung volume at which it is measured.[129] Magnetometry or respiratory inductance plethysmography can be used as an objective means of determining movement of the diaphragm; the dimensions of the rib cage and abdomen are measured simultaneously and separately during the respiratory cycle.[130]

Diaphragmatic EMG, using either esophageal or surface electrodes, can be used as an index of respiratory motoneuron drive.[30, 100, 131, 132] In normal subjects, changes in inspiratory muscle pressure and ventilation have been shown to be proportionate to changes in inspiratory neural drive as assessed by diaphragmatic EMG.[132] Like random noise, the EMG is made up of a whole spectrum of frequencies. Serial measurements of patients who suffer diaphragmatic fatigue show a shift in the power spectrum, with low-frequency components increasing and those of high frequency decreasing. This shift of the high/low ratio precedes clinical evidence of fatigue and blood gas abnormalities and may therefore be an important early warning sign.[133, 134]

Perhaps the most effective means of identifying fatigue of the diaphragm is the measurement of transdiaphragmatic pressure, which is accomplished by recording the pressure in balloons placed in both the esophagus and stomach. Gastric and esophageal pressure devices and EMG have been incorporated into a single catheter.[135] If the diaphragm has become completely flaccid as a result of muscle fatigue and the patient does not contract the abdominal muscles, transdiaphragmatic pressure undergoes no change in full inspiration, the negative pleural pressure inducing a negative abdominal pressure. However, when the diaphragm is not completely flaccid, this method of assessing diaphragmatic function may not be reliable, since simultaneous contraction of the diaphragm and other inspiratory muscles results in a change in abdominal pressure that depends not only on the relative strength of contraction of the two muscle groups combined[136] but also on the degree of abdominal muscle relaxation. Studies in normal subjects have shown considerable intersubject variation during both slow and forced inspiratory maneuvers, with some individuals showing a natural tendency to low transdiaphragmatic pressure.[137, 138] Tests designed to measure respiratory muscle endurance as opposed to strength may prove to be more relevant to assessment of the eventual development of respiratory muscle fatigue and ventilatory failure.[139]

Respiratory muscle fatigue can be classified as central or peripheral fatigue. Central fatigue occurs when maximal voluntary activation of the muscle cannot be achieved, and it can be recognized by the observation of greater than voluntary contraction upon electrical stimulation of the phrenic nerve. Peripheral fatigue can be divided into high- or low-frequency fatigue. The former is a failure of force generation at high stimulation frequencies; rapid recovery from high-frequency fatigue follows cessation of an exhaustive work load (<10 minutes). Low-frequency fatigue occurs after more prolonged, lower-intensity stimulation, and recovery may take 24 hours or more.[140] High-frequency fatigue is due to failure of neuromuscular transmission, whereas low-frequency fatigue is due to impaired excitation-contraction coupling.[23, 39, 141]

Prompt recognition of inspiratory muscle weakness is important, since it clearly indicates impending ventilatory failure and death; a period of muscle rest on a ventilator and treatment of the underlying causes of the weakness or increased load may produce complete recovery. This situation is perhaps most obvious in patients in cardiogenic shock, in whom diversion of oxygen away from the respiratory muscles to other vital organs may be lifesaving.[142] Although by no means a substitute for mechanical ventilation in this situation, the demonstration that aminophylline or isoproterenol therapy improves diaphragmatic contractility[143–145] raises the possibility that still other and more powerful medications will be discovered that reduce or abolish muscle fatigue.

It is unclear whether a state of "chronic fatigue" of the inspiratory muscles contributes to ventilatory failure in patients with diseases such as COPD. Although respiratory muscle rest may be beneficial in such patients, as little as 48 hours of mechanical ventilation has been shown to induce some inspiratory muscle atrophy in experimental animals[146, 147] Like other skeletal muscles, the respiratory muscles can be trained to generate greater force, shortening, and endurance, both in normal subjects and in patients who have diseases such as COPD and chronic congestive heart failure.[148–151] In animals, training has also been shown to increase the number of slow-twitch fibers that are concerned with diaphragmatic endurance.[40, 42]

THE CHEST WALL

The structures of the thoracic wall, both soft tissue and osseous, form a complex of shadows on radiographs of the chest that may be important to radiographic analysis, and a working knowledge of their normal anatomy and variations is indispensable.

Soft Tissues

On frontal radiographs of the thorax, the soft tissues, including the skin, subcutaneous fat, and muscles, are usually distinguishable over the shoulders and along the thoracic wall. On successive examinations, a decrease or increase in their extent may constitute a valuable sign of loss or gain in weight.

The pectoral muscles form the anterior axillary fold, a structure normally visible in both men and women that curves smoothly downward and medially from the axilla to the rib cage. In men, particularly those with heavy muscular development, the inferior border of the pectoralis major muscle may be seen as a downward extension of the anterior axillary fold that passes obliquely across the middle portion of both lungs. In women, this shadow is obscured by the breasts, whose presence and size must be taken into consideration when assessing the density of the lower lung zones. Congenital absence of the pectoralis muscle is rare (Fig. 10–14).[152]

In many cases, the shadow of the sternomastoid muscle is visible as an opacity whose lateral margin parallels the spine in the medial third of the lung apices; it curves downward and laterally to blend with the companion shadow on the superior aspect of each clavicle. The latter shadow, which is 2 to 3 mm thick, parallels the superior aspect of the clavicle; it is formed by the skin and subcutaneous tissue overlying the clavicles and is rendered visible radiologically

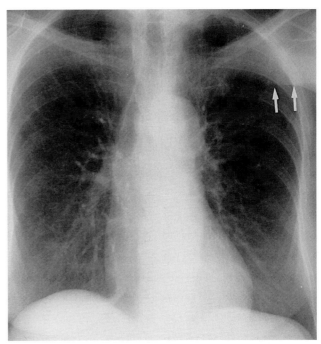

Figure 10–14. Congenital Absence of the Pectoralis Muscle. A posteroanterior chest radiograph demonstrates radiolucency of the left hemithorax and a horizontal course of the left anterior axillary fold *(arrows)* caused by absence of the left pectoralis muscle. The patient was a 67-year-old woman with congenital absence of the left pectoralis. (Note that the breast shadows are symmetric.)

by the supraclavicular fossae and the tangential direction in which the x-ray beam strikes the clavicles.

The frequency of identification of the companion shadows of the clavicles varies: in healthy subjects with no demonstrable physical abnormality, they may be bilaterally symmetric, seen more clearly on one side than the other, or invisible on both sides. Absence of a companion shadow on one side suggests enlargement of the supraclavicular lymph nodes or another pathologic process such as edema; however, one must exercise caution in interpreting such asymmetry as significant without confirmatory signs.

Sometimes the floor of the supraclavicular fossa can be identified as a saucer-shaped opacity projected behind the clavicle that runs laterally from the sternomastoid shadow.[153] In one review of frontal radiographs of 500 patients, the fossa was identified on at least one side in 145 (29%).[153] Although it can occasionally be seen as a roughly horizontal opacity suggesting a fluid level, its true nature can be readily discerned by simply following the line out laterally beyond the chest wall. The suprasternal fossa, which consists of a depression on the skin surface of the neck between the sternal heads of the sternocleidomastoid muscles, can also be infrequently identified on posteroanterior radiographs. It is roughly U or V shaped and projects immediately above the manubrium of the sternum; it is seen most frequently in cachectic or very thin individuals and in patients with severe chronic obstructive lung disease.[154] Occasionally, the suprasternal fossa simulates a fluid level in the esophagus.

Because of the fat planes separating the various muscle groups, CT and MR images allow identification of the majority of individual chest wall muscles. The outer anterior chest wall musculature is composed mainly of the pectoralis major (larger and more superficial) and the pectoralis minor (Fig. 10–15). The serratus anterior is located immediately superficial to the ribs on the lateral aspect of the thorax. The posterior chest wall musculature is more complex and includes superficial, intermediate, and deep muscles.[155] The first of these muscle groups controls arm motion and includes the trapezius, latissimus dorsi, levator scapulae, and rhomboid muscles. The intermediate muscles are inspiratory and include the superior and inferior serratus posterior muscles. The deep muscles lie adjacent to the vertebral column and regulate its motion.[155]

The external and internal intercostal muscles lie between the ribs and cannot usually be distinguished from each other on CT or MR imaging. The innermost intercostal muscles together with the parietal pleura and endothoracic fascia are visualized as a 1- to 2-mm-thick line or stripe in the interspaces along the anterior and posterior costal pleural surfaces.[156] The transversus thoracis muscle is a small muscle that arises from the lower part of the sternum and attaches to the superolateral aspect of the second to the fifth costal cartilage.[155] It is seen on CT at the level of the heart as a

thin line internal to the anterior costal cartilage (Fig. 10–16).[156] The subcostal muscles are small muscles that extend from the angle of the rib to the internal surface of the adjacent lower rib.[155] They are seen on CT in a small percentage of patients as a 1- to 2-mm-thick line covering the inner surface of a posterior rib or ribs at the level of the heart (Fig. 10–17).[156]

Bones

The Ribs

In the absence of pulmonary or pleural disease, deformity of the spine, or congenital anomalies of the ribs themselves, the rib cage should be symmetric. Both the upper and lower borders of the ribs should be sharply defined except in the middle and lower thoracic regions; here, the thin flanges created by the vascular sulci on the inferior aspects of the ribs posteriorly are viewed *en face,* which creates a less distinct inferior margin. In some individuals,

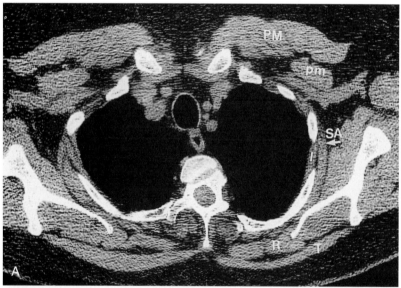

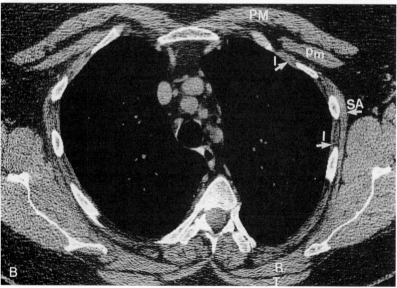

Figure 10–15. Chest Wall Muscles. CT scans (*A* and *B*) demonstrate normal chest wall muscles seen in cross section. These muscles may be divided into an anterior group (including the pectoralis major [PM] and pectoralis minor [pm]) and a posterior group (including the trapezius [T], rhomboideus [R], and the paraspinal muscles). The serratus anterior (SA) lies on the lateral aspect of the rib cage, whereas the intercostal muscles (I) lie between the ribs.

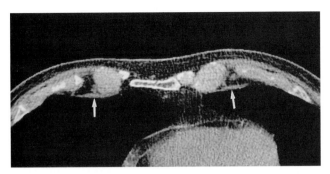

Figure 10–16. Transversus Thoracis Muscle. A magnified view of the anterior aspect of the chest from an HRCT scan demonstrates a thin line internal to the costal cartilage *(arrows)*, representing the transversus thoracis muscle. It arises from the lower part of the sternum and attaches to the superolateral aspect of the second to fifth costal cartilages.

the inferior aspects of the ribs show local superficial indentations posteriorly within 2 or 3 cm of their tubercles; these indentations should not be mistaken for pathologic rib notching, which is situated more laterally near the midclavicular line in cases of increased collateral circulation through the intercostal vessels (as in coarctation of the aorta).

Calcification* of rib cartilage is common and probably never of pathologic significance. The first rib cartilage is usually the first to calcify, often shortly after the age of 20 years. Fairly consistent differences in the pattern of costal calcification are observed in the two sexes, particularly in older individuals.[157] In one radiographic study of 100 adults, 60 of whom were male and 40 female, the upper and lower borders of cartilage were found to calcify first in men, with calcification extending in continuity with the end of the rib; calcification of the central area follows.[158] By contrast, calcification in women tends to occur first in a central location, in the form of either a solid tongue or as two

*It has been pointed out that the term *calcification* as applied to costal cartilage is a misnomer since this condition is often true ossification.[160] Despite the validity of this observation, it is difficult to overcome common usage and we shall continue to use calcification here.

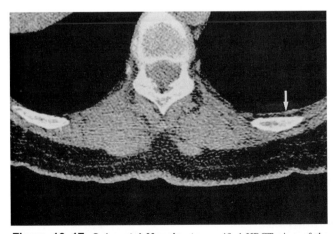

Figure 10–17. Subcostal Muscle. A magnified HRCT view of the posterior of the chest at the level of the heart demonstrates a line of soft tissue attenuation *(arrow)* internal to a left posterior rib and separated from it by a fat pad. This line is caused by the left subcostal muscle in combination with the pleura and endothoracic fascia. No soft tissue line is seen anterior to the right posterior rib.

parallel lines extending into the cartilage from the end of the rib (Fig. 10–18). These findings were confirmed in a study of the chest radiographs of 1,000 patients aged 10 to 95 years:[159] "marginal" calcification appeared in 70% of the males and 11% of the females, whereas predominantly "central" calcification was observed in 12% of the males and 76% of the females; a mixed type of calcification was observed in approximately 7% of both sexes. The relationship between age and costal cartilage calcification varied. In males, any calcification was uncommon under the age of 20, and marginal calcification increased from 3% in these young adults to 89% in men aged 60 years and over. By contrast, central calcification was observed in 45% of females under the age of 20 and increased to 88% in patients 60 years of age and older.

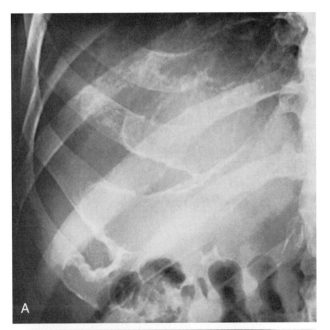

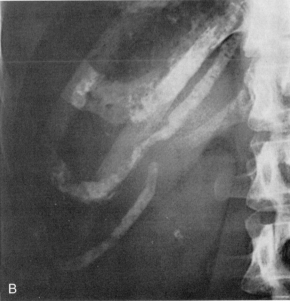

Figure 10–18. Patterns of Rib Cartilage Calcification in Men and Women. *A,* Marginal calcification in a man. *B,* Central calcification in a woman. *See* the text.

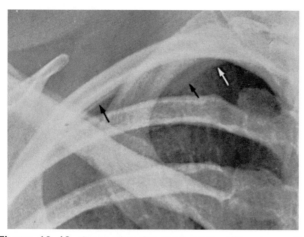

Figure 10–19. Companion Shadows of the Ribs. A magnified view of the apex of the right hemithorax reveals thin smooth shadows of water density lying roughly parallel to the inferior surfaces of the first and second ribs *(arrows).* These companion shadows are caused by perception in tangential projection of a combination of parietal and visceral pleura and the soft tissues immediately external to the pleura.

The reason for the difference in costal cartilage calcification between men and women is uncertain. In one study, all five women with a male pattern of calcification had undergone pelvic surgery, which led the authors to speculate that the process of calcification may be under hormonal control.[158] However, based on a strikingly similar pattern of costal cartilage calcification in a pair of homozygotic twins, other investigators have concluded that calcification is primarily genetically determined.[161] Whatever the pathogenesis, the sex of adult patients can be determined from the pattern of calcium deposition in the ribs in about 95% of cases.[63, 159]

Thin, smooth shadows of water density that parallel the ribs and measure 1 to 2 mm in thickness project adjacent to the inferior and inferolateral margins of the first and second ribs and to the axillary portions of the lower ribs (Fig. 10–19). In one study of 300 normal subjects in whom such companion shadows were specifically sought, they were seen adjacent to the first rib in 35% and the second rib in 31%.[63] The shadows were bilateral in approximately half the cases; when unilateral, they were more common on the right side. Companion shadows adjacent to the axillary portions of the

lower ribs were seen more often (in 75% of 700 normal subjects).

These companion shadows are caused by visualization in tangential projection of the parietal pleura and soft tissues immediately external to the pleura and should not be interpreted as local pleural thickening. They are caused by a combination of muscle, fascia, and adipose tissue between the rib and the parietal pleura,[162] the most important being fat (Fig. 10–20).[163] In one study, the thickness of soft tissue shadows accompanying the second, third, and fourth ribs was measured on the posteroanterior radiographs of 22 obese patients and 22 subjects of normal weight;[164] the mean thickness of the accompanying shadow of the second rib was 2.7 and 2.2 mm in obese males and females, respectively, as compared with 1.8 and 0.7 mm in those of normal weight. In another investigation, the thickness of the companion shadows in eight obese patients before and after weight reduction decreased from almost 3.0 mm to 1.2 mm.[163] Extrapleural fat is most abundant over the fourth to eighth ribs posterolaterally.[165]

Congenital anomalies of the ribs are relatively uncommon. Supernumerary ribs arising from the seventh cervical vertebra were identified in 1.5% of 350 normal subjects in one study (Fig. 10–21);[63] nearly all were bilateral, but many had developed asymmetrically. An extreme example has been reported of a 35-year-old man admitted to the hospital for complaints unrelated to the thorax who was found to have 15 pairs of thoracic ribs arising from 15 thoracic vertebrae;[166] he had 7 cervical and 5 lumbar vertebrae, several showing congenital anomalies. All the ribs were well developed and roughly symmetric. (The height of the patient is not recorded!) Rarely, cervical ribs articulate with the scapula (omovertebral bones) in patients who have congenital fixed elevation of the scapula (Sprengel's deformity, Fig. 10–22). Omovertebral bones occur in 30% to 40% of patients with Sprengel's deformity.[167] Other anomalies such as hypoplasia of the first rib (observed in 1.2% of 350 normal subjects in one series[63]), bifid or splayed anterior ribs, and (rarely) local fusion of ribs are usually important only in that they may give rise to an erroneous interpretation of abnormal lung density.

An intrathoracic rib is a rare congenital anomaly characterized by an accessory rib that arises within the bony thorax, more commonly on the right and from either the anterior

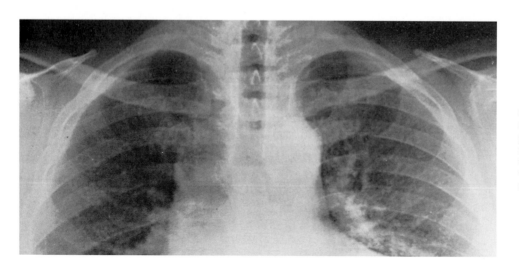

Figure 10–20. Companion Shadows of the Ribs in an Obese Subject. A view of the upper portion of the thorax from a posteroanterior radiograph of an exceptionally obese man reveals unusually wide companion shadows caused by accumulation of fat.

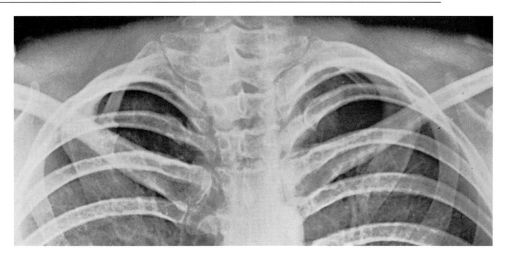

Figure 10–21. Cervical Ribs. Bilateral supernumerary ribs arise from the seventh cervical vertebra. The right rib is longer than the left and shows a synchondrosis with the medial aspect of the first rib.

surface of a rib or a contiguous vertebral body;[168–170] it usually extends downward and slightly laterally to end at or near the diaphragm. This pattern may vary; for example, in one patient the intrathoracic rib originated from the posterior portion of the left third rib and extended through lung substance to join the anterior portion of the left second rib.[168] Somewhat surprisingly, such intrathoracic ribs are unassociated with symptoms. An even rarer abnormality is an anomalous rib arising from the right side of the last sacral vertebra—a pelvic rib.[171]

Because of their oblique orientation, only a small portion of any given rib is seen on a single CT section.[155, 172] Identification of a specific rib can be made by identifying the thoracic spine level adjacent to the posterior end of the rib.[155] The first rib can be readily identified as it lies adjacent to the medial end of the clavicle at the level of the sternoclavicular joint. The second, third, and fourth ribs can usually be identified at the same level by counting posteriorly along the rib cage (Fig. 10–23).[172] By proceeding sequentially caudally, each next vertebra and corresponding rib can be identified.

Other Chest Wall Bones

Occasionally, the inferior aspect of the clavicle has an irregular notch or indentation 2 to 3 cm from the sternal

articulation; its size and shape vary from a superficial saucer-shaped defect to a deep notch 2 cm wide by 1.0 to 1.5 cm deep. These rhomboid fossae (Fig. 10–24) give rise to costoclavicular or rhomboid ligaments that radiate downward to bind the clavicles to the first rib.[152, 173] The fossae are seen in about 10% of clavicles studied anatomically,[174] but are rarely detected radiologically.[175] A tiny foramen may be seen occasionally near the superior aspect of the center of the clavicle, either unilaterally or bilaterally. This foramen permits passage of the middle supraclavicular nerve and is said to be present in 6% of dry skeletal specimens.[152]

The coracoclavicular joint is a true synovial joint between the coracoid process of the scapula and a bony process extending inferiorly from the clavicle.[176] These joints are genetically determined anatomic variants that are seen more frequently in individuals from Asia than from Europe and Africa;[176] an unusually high incidence has been noted in people from southern China. Although these joints are subject to osteophyte formation with age, they do not give rise to symptoms or disability. Another anatomic variant of no clinical significance consists of sharply circumscribed lucencies in the body of the scapula surrounded by a thin layer of cortical bone;[177] these most likely represent areas of incomplete bone formation during maturation and do not occasion symptoms.

The normal thoracic spine is straight in frontal projec-

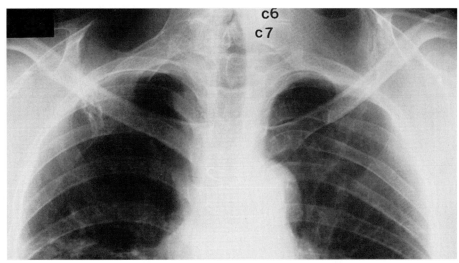

Figure 10–22. Omovertebral Bones in a Patient with Sprengel's Deformity. A view of the upper part of the chest in a 37-year-old woman demonstrates elevation of both scapulas. The left sixth (C6) and seventh (C7) cervical ribs are fused and articulate with the elevated scapula (omovertebral bones); a single right C7 omovertebral bone is present.

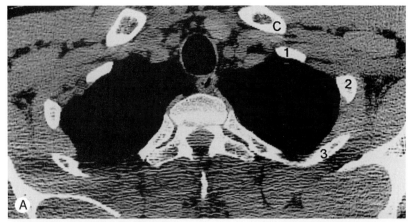

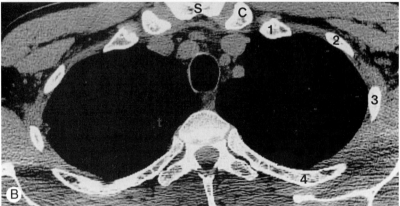

Figure 10–23. Ribs in Cross Section. An HRCT scan at the level of the thoracic inlet *(A)* demonstrates the right and left clavicles (C) and the first (1), second (2) and third (3) ribs. A second scan at the level of the sternoclavicular joint *(B)* demonstrates the upper part of the sternum (S) and the medial end of the clavicles (C). The first costal cartilage (1) and the second (2), third (3), and fourth (4) ribs can be identified by counting posteriorly along the rib cage. The fourth rib can be seen attached to the fourth thoracic vertebra.

tion and gently concave anteriorly in lateral projection. Its radiopacity in lateral projection decreases uniformly from above downward, and any deviation from this should arouse suspicion of intrathoracic disease.

The lateral and superior borders of the manubrium are the only portions of the sternum visible on frontal projections of the thorax, although the whole of the sternum should be clearly seen tangentially in lateral radiographs. The normal CT anatomy of the sternum was assessed in one study of 35

patients;[178] the body was found to be ovoid to rectangular in shape and usually possessed sharp cortical margins. In the manubrium, part of the posterior cortical margin was unsharp and irregular in 34 of 35 patients, and part of the anterior cortical margin was indistinct in 20. Interpretation of this appearance as an abnormality can be avoided by angulating the CT gantry to a position more nearly perpendicular to the manubrium, the definition of these cortical margins being rendered sharp by this maneuver.

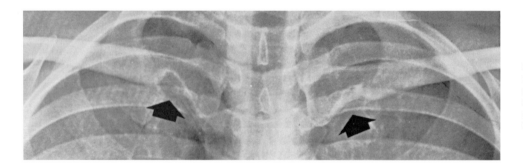

Figure 10–24. Rhomboid Fossae. An irregular notch is present in the inferior aspect of both clavicles approximately 2 cm from their sternal end *(arrows)*. These fossae give origin to the costoclavicular or rhomboid ligaments.

REFERENCES

1. Strohl KP: Upper airway muscles of respiration. Am Rev Respir Dis 124:211, 1981.
2. Derenne J-P, Macklem PT, Roussos CL: The respiratory muscles: Mechanics, control and pathophysiology. I. Am Rev Respir Dis 118:119, 1978.
3. Luce JM, Culver BH: Respiratory muscle function in health and disease. Chest 81:82, 1982.
4. Roussos C (ed): The Thorax. *In* Lenfant C (ed): Lung Biology in Health and Disease. New York, Marcel Dekker, 1995.
5. Epstein SK: An overview of respiratory muscle function. Clin Chest Med 15:619, 1994.
6. van Lunteren E, Dick TE: Intrinsic properties of pharyngeal and diaphragmatic respiratory motoneurons and muscles. J Appl Physiol 73:787, 1992.
7. Fregosi RF, Lansing RW: Neural drive to nasal dilator muscles: Influence of exercise intensity and oronasal flow partitioning. J Appl Physiol 79:1330, 1995.
8. Tangel DJ, Mezzanotte WS, White DP: Respiratory-related control of palatoglossus and levator palatini muscle activity. J Appl Physiol 78:680, 1995.
9. Korl RC, Knuth SL, Bartlett D: Selective reduction of genioglossal muscle activity by alcohol in normal human subjects. Am Rev Respir Dis 129:247, 1984.
10. Mathew OP, Abu-Osba YK, Thach BT: Influence of upper airway pressure changes on genioglossus muscle respiratory activity. J Appl Physiol 52:438, 1982.
11. Mathew OP, Abu-Osba YK, Thach BT: Genioglossus muscle responses to upper airway pressure changes: Afferent pathways. J Appl Physiol 52:445, 1982.
12. Weiner D, Mitra M, Salamone J: Effect of chemical stimuli on nerves supplying upper airway muscles. J Appl Physiol 52:530, 1982.
13. Onal E, Lopata M, O'Connor TD: Diaphragmatic and genioglossal electromyogram responses to CO_2 rebreathing in humans. J Appl Physiol 50:1052, 1981.
14. Hwang J, Bartlett D Jr, St. John WM: Characterization of respiratory-modulated activities of hypoglossal motoneurons. J Appl Physiol 55:793, 1983.
15. Gottfried SB, Strohl KP, Van De Graff W, et al: Effects of phrenic stimulation on upper airway resistance in anesthetized dogs. J Appl Physiol 55:419, 1983.
16. Hyland RH, Hutcheon MA, Perl A, et al: Upper airway occlusion induced by diaphragmatic pacing for primary alveolar hypoventilation: Implications for the pathogenesis of obstructive sleep apnea. Am Rev Respir Dis 124:180, 1981.
17. Wheatley JR, Tangel DJ, Mezzanotte WS, et al: Influence of sleep on alae nasi EMG and nasal resistance in normal men. J Appl Physiol 75:626, 1993.
18. Gal TJ, Goldberg SK: Diaphragmatic function in healthy subjects during partial curarization. J Appl Physiol 48:921, 1980.
19. De Troyer A, Loring SH: Actions of the respiratory muscles. *In* Roussos C (ed): The Thorax. *In* Lenfant C (ed): Lung Biology in Health and Disease. New York, Marcel Dekker, 1995, pp 535–563.
20. Orozco-Levi M, Gea J, Monells J, et al: Activity of latissimus dorsi muscle during inspiratory threshold loads. Eur Respir J 8:441, 1995.
21. Celli BR: Coordination and breathing retraining. *In* Roussos C (ed): The Thorax. *In* Lenfant C (ed): Lung Biology in Health and Disease. New York, Marcel Dekker, 1995, pp 2301–2319.
22. Han JN, Gayan-Ramirez G, Dekhuijzen R, et al: Rspiratory function of the rib cage muscles. Eur Respir J 6:722, 1993.
23. Edwards RHT: The diaphragm as a muscle. Mechanisms underlying fatigue. Am Rev Respir Dis 119(Suppl):81, 1979.
24. White JE, Drinnan MJ, Smithson AJ, et al: Respiratory muscle activity and oxygenation during sleep in patients with muscle weakness. Eur Respir J 8:807, 1995.
25. De Troyer A: Mechanical role of the abdominal muscles in relation to posture. Respir Physiol 53:341, 1983.
26. De Troyer A, Ninane V: Triangularis sterni: A primary muscle of breathing in the dog. J Appl Physiol 60:14, 1986.
27. De Troyer A, Ninane V, Gilmartin JJ, et al: Triangularis sterni muscle use in supine humans. J Appl Physiol 62:919, 1987.
28. Sharp JT: Respiratory muscles: A review of old and newer concepts. Lung 157:185, 1980.
29. De Troyer A, Estenne M, Ninane V, et al: Transverse abdominis muscle function in humans. J Appl Physiol 68:1010, 1990.
30. Martin JG, De Troyer A: The behaviour of the abdominal muscles during inspiratory mechanical loading. Respir Physiol 50:63, 1982.
31. Lloyd JS, Brozanski BS, Daood M, et al: Developmental transitions in the myosin heavy chain phenotype of human respiratory muscle. Biol Neonate 69:67, 1996.
32. Whitelaw WA: Topography of the diaphragm. *In* Roussos C (ed): The Thorax. *In* Lenfant C (ed): Lung Biology in Health and Disease. New York, Marcel Dekker, 1995, pp 587–616.
33. von Hayek H: The Human Lung. New York, Hafner, 1960.
34. De Troyer A, Sampson M, Sigrist S, et al: The diaphragm: Two muscles. Science 213:237, 1981.
35. Supinski G, DiMarco AF, Hussein F, et al: Analysis of the contraction of series and parallel muscles working against elastic loads. Respir Physiol 87:141, 1995.
36. Ward ME, Ward JW, Macklem PT: Analysis of human chest wall motion using a two-compartment rib cage model. J Appl Physiol 72:1338, 1992.
37. Gauthier GF, Padykula HA: Cytological studies of fiber types in skeletal muscle—a comparative study of the mammalian diaphragm. J Cell Biol 28:333, 1966.
38. Belman MJ, Sieck GS: The ventilatory muscles—fatigue, endurance and training. Chest 82:761, 1982.
39. Edwards RHT, Faulkner JA: Structure and function of the respiratory muscles. *In* Roussos C (ed): The Thorax. *In* Lenfant C (ed): Lung Biology in Health and Disease. New York, Marcel Dekker, 1995, pp 185–217.
40. Rochester D: Is diaphragmatic contractility important (editorial)? N Engl J Med 30:305, 1981.
41. Faulkner JA, Maxwell LC, Ruff GL, et al: The diaphragm as a muscle. Contractile properties. Am Rev Respir Dis 119(Suppl):89, 1979.
42. Lieberman DA, Maxwell LC, Faulkner JA: Adaptation of guinea pig diaphragm muscle to aging and endurance training. Am J Physiol 222:556, 1972.
43. Faulkner JA, Maxwell LC, Lieberman DA: Histochemical characteristics of muscle fibers from trained and detrained guinea pigs. Am J Physiol 222:836, 1972.
44. Keens TG, Bryan AC, Levison H, et al: Developmental pattern of muscle fiber types in human ventilatory muscles. J Appl Physiol 44:909, 1978.
45. Thurlbeck WM: Diaphragm and body weight in emphysema. Thorax 33:483, 1978.
46. Arora NS, Rochester DF: Effect of body weight and muscularity on human diaphragm muscle mass, thickness, and area. J Appl Physiol 52:64, 1982.
47. Butler C: Diaphragmatic changes in emphysema. Am Rev Respir Dis 114:155, 1976.
48. Hughes RL, Katz H, Sahgal V, et al: Fiber size and energy metabolites in five separate muscles from patients with chronic obstructive lung disease. Respiration 44:321, 1983.
49. Leak LV: Gross and ultrastructural morphologic features of the diaphragm. Am Rev Respir Dis 119(Suppl):3, 1979.
50. Warwick R, Williams PL (eds): Gray's Anatomy. 35th British ed. Philadelphia, WB Saunders, 1973, p 667.
51. Comtois A, Gorczyca W, Grassino A: Microscopic anatomy of the arterial diaphragmatic circulation. Clin Invest Med 7:81, 1984.
52. Comtois AS, Rochester DF: Respiratory muscle blood flow. *In* Roussos C (ed): The Thorax. *In* Lenfant C (ed): Lung Biology in Health and Disease. New York, Marcel Dekker, 1995, pp 633–661.
53. Rochester DF, Briscoe AM: Metabolism of the working diaphragm. Am Rev Respir Dis 119:101, 1979.
54. Bellmare F, Wight D, Lavigne CM, et al: Effect of tension and timing of contraction on the blood flow of the diaphragm. J Appl Physiol 54:1597, 1983.
55. Wang N-S: The preformed stomas connecting the pleural cavity and the lymphatics in the parietal pleura. Am Rev Respir Dis 111:12, 1975.
56. DeTroyer A, DeBeyl DZ, Thirion M: Function of the respiratory muscles in acute hemiplegia. Am Rev Respir Dis 123:631, 1981.
57. Derenne J-PH, Macklem PT, Roussos CH: State of the art. The respiratory muscles: Mechanics, control and pathophysiology. Part II. Am Rev Respir Dis 118:373, 1978.
58. Altose MD, DiMarco AF, Gottfried SB, et al: The sensation of respiratory muscle force. Am Rev Respir Dis 126:807, 1982.
59. Guz A: Sensory aspects of the diaphragm. Am Rev Respir Dis 119(Suppl):65, 1979.
60. Campbell EJM: The effect of muscular paralysis induced by curarization on breath holding in normal subjects. Am Rev Respir Dis 119(Suppl):67, 1979.
61. Tarver RD, Conces DJ Jr, Cory DA, et al: Imaging the diaphragm and its disorders. J Thorac Imaging 4:1, 1989.
62. Lennon EA, Simon G: The height of the diaphragm in the chest radiograph of normal adults. Br J Radiol 38:937, 1965.
63. Felson B: Chest Roentgenology. Philadelphia, WB Saunders, 1973.
64. Young DA, Simon G: Certain movements measured on inspiration-expiration chest radiographs correlated with pulmonary function studies. Clin Radiol 23:37, 1972.
65. Wittenborg MH, Aviad I: Organ influence on the normal posture of the diaphragm: A radiological study of inversions and heterotaxies. Br J Radiol 36:280, 1963.
66. Reddy V, Sharma S, Cobanoglu A: What dictates the position of the diaphragm—the heart or the liver? A review of sixty-five cases. J Thorac Cardiovasc Surg 108:687, 1994.
67. Chung JW, Im JG, Park JH, et al: Left paracardiac mass caused by dilated pericardiacophrenic vein: Report of four cases. Am J Roentgenol 160:25, 1993.
67a. Erden GA, Mavis AV, Cumhur T: Irregularity of the left hemidiaphragmatic contour caused by the dilated left inferior phrenic vein: A case report. Angiology 46:175, 1995.
68. Naidich DP, Megibow AJ, Ross CR, et al: Computed tomography of the diaphragm: Normal anatomy and variants. J Comput Assist Tomogr 7:4, 1983.
69. Gale ME: Anterior diaphragm: Variations in the CT appearance. Radiology 161:635, 1986.
70. Panicek DM, Benson CB, Gottlieb RH, et al: The diaphragm: Anatomic, pathologic, and radiologic considerations. Radiographics 8:385, 1988.
71. Williamson BRJ, Gouse JC, Rohrer DG, et al: Variation in the thickness of the diaphragmatic crura with respiration. Radiology 163:683, 1987.
72. Shin MS, Berland LL: Computed tomography of retrocrural spaces: Normal, anatomic variants, and pathologic conditions. Am J Roentgenol 145:81, 1985.
73. Silverman PM, Cooper C, Zeman RK: Lateral arcuate ligaments of the diaphragm: Anatomic variations at abdominal CT. Radiology 185:105, 1992.

74. Caskey CI, Zerhouni EA, Fishman EK, et al: Aging of the diaphragm: A CT study. Radiology 171:385, 1989.

75. Ueki J, De Bruin PF, Pride NB: In vivo assessment of diaphragm contraction by ultrasound in normal subjects. Thorax 50:1157, 1995.

76. Curley FJ, Hubmayr RD, Raptopoulos V: Bilateral diaphragmatic densities in a 72-year-old woman. Chest 86:915, 1984.

77. Worthy SA, Kang EY, Hartman TE, et al: Diaphragmatic rupture: CT findings in 11 patients. Radiology 194:885, 1995.

78. Brink JA, Heiken JP, Semenkovich J, et al: Abnormalities of the diaphragm and adjacent structures: Findings on multiplanar spiral CT scans. Am J Roentgenol 163:307, 1994.

79. Yeager BA, Guglielmi GE, Schiebler ML, et al: Magnetic resonance imaging of Morgagni hernia. Gastrointest Radiol 12:296, 1987.

80. Mirvis SE, Keramati B, Buckman R, et al: MR imaging of traumatic diaphragm rupture. J Comput Assist Tomogr 12:147, 1988.

81. Gierada DS, Curtin JJ, Erickson SJ, et al: Fast gradient-echo magnetic resonance imaging of the normal diaphragm. J Thorac Imaging 12:70, 1997.

82. Berkmen YM, Davis SD, Kazam E, et al: Right phrenic nerve: Anatomy, CT appearance, and differentiation from the pulmonary ligament. Radiology 173:43, 1989.

83. Godwin JD, Vock P, Osborn DR: CT of the pulmonary ligament. Am J Roentgenol 141:231, 1983.

84. Ujita M, Ojiri H, Ariizumi M, et al: Appearance of the inferior phrenic artery and vein on CT scans of the chest: A CT and cadaveric study. Am J Roentgenol 160:745, 1993.

85. Simon G, Bonnell J, Kazantzis G, et al: Some radiological observations on the range of movement of the diaphragm. Clin Radiol 20:231, 1969.

86. Alexander C: Diaphragm movements and the diagnosis of diaphragmatic paralysis. Clin Radiol 17:79, 1966.

87. Schmidt S: Anatomic and physiologic aspects of respiratory kymography. Acta Radiol (Diagn) 8:409, 1969.

88. Houston JG, Morris AD, Howie CA, et al: Technical report: Quantitative assessment of diaphragmatic movement—a reproducible method using ultrasound. Clin Radiol 46:705, 1992.

89. Jousela I, Tahvanainen J, Makelainen A, et al: Diaphragmatic movement studied with ultrasound during spontaneous breathing and mechanical ventilation with intermittent positive pressure ventilation (IPPV) and airway pressure release ventilation (APRV) in man. Anaesthesiol Reanim 19:43, 1994.

90. Dovgan DJ, Lenchik L, Kaye AD: Computed tomographic evaluation of maximal diaphragmatic crural thickness. Conn Med 58:203, 1994.

91. Kanematsu M, Imaeda T, Mochizuki R, et al: Dynamic MRI of the diaphragm. J Comput Assist Tomogr 19:67, 1995.

92. Gierada DS, Curtin JJ, Erickson SJ, et al: Diaphragmatic motion: Fast gradient-recalled-echo MR imaging in healthy subjects. Radiology 194:879, 1995.

93. Gauthier AP, Verbanck S, Estenne M, et al: Three-dimensional reconstruction of the in vivo human diaphragm shape at different lung volumes. J Appl Physiol 76:495, 1994.

94. Edwards RHT: Human muscle physiology and metabolism. Br Med Bull 36:159, 1980.

95. Human muscle fatigue (editorial). Lancet 2:729, 1981.

96. Sharp JT: Respiratory muscles: A review of old and newer concepts. Lung 157:185, 1980.

97. Luce JM, Culver BH: Respiratory muscle function in health and disease. Chest 81:82, 1982.

98. Loh L, Goldman M, Newsom-Davis J: The assessment of diaphragm function. Medicine (Baltimore) 56:165, 1977.

99. Newman SL, Road JD, Grassino A: Diaphragmatic contraction in postural changes. Fed Proc 42:1010, 1983.

100. Roussos C, Macklem PT: The respiratory muscles. N Engl J Med 307:786, 1982.

101. Roussos CS, Macklem PT: Diaphragmatic fatigue in man. J Appl Physiol 43:189, 1977.

102. Moxham J, Morris AJR, Spiro SG, et al: Contractile properties and fatigue of the diaphragm in man. Thorax 36:164, 1981.

103. Braun NMT, Aora NS, Rochester DF: Force-length relationship of the normal human diaphragm. J Appl Physiol 53:405, 1982.

104. Loring SH: Three-dimensional reconstruction of the in vivo human diaphragm shape at different lung volumes. J Appl Physiol 76:493, 1994.

105. Rochester DF, Briscoe AM: Metabolism of the working diaphragm. Am Rev Respir Dis 119(Suppl):101, 1979.

106. Roussos CH: The failing ventilatory pump (review). Lung 160:59, 1982.

107. Rochester DF: Respiratory muscles and ventilatory failure: 1993 perspective. Am J Med Sci 305:394, 1993.

108. Macklem PT: Respiratory muscles: The vital pump. Chest 78:753, 1980.

109. Roussos C, Macklem PT: The respiratory muscles. N Engl J Med 307:786, 1982.

110. Roussos C, Bellemare F, Moxham J: Respiratory muscle fatigue. In Roussos C (ed): The Thorax. In Lenfant C (ed): Lung Biology in Health and Disease. New York, Marcel Dekker, 1995, pp 1405–1462.

111. Roussos C, Zakynthinos S: Ventilatory failure and respiratory muscles. In Roussos C (ed): The Thorax. In Lenfant C (ed): Lung Biology in Health and Disease. New York, Marcel Dekker, 1995, pp 2071–2100.

112. Gandevia SC, McKenzie DK, Neering IR: Endurance properties of respiratory and limb muscles. Respir Physiol 53:47, 1983.

112a. Mador JM, Rodis A, Diaz J: Diaphragmatic fatigue following voluntary hyperpnea. Am J Respir Crit Care Med 154:63, 1996.

113. Derenne J-PH, Macklem PT, Roussos CH: State of the art. The respiratory

114. Bellemare F, Grassino A: Effect of pressure and timing of contraction on human diaphragmatic fatigue. J Appl Physiol 53:1190, 1982.

115. DeVito E, Grassino AE: Respiratory muscle fatigue: Rationale for diagnostic tests. In Roussos C (ed): The Thorax. In Lenfant C (ed): Lung Biology in Health and Disease. New York, Marcel Dekker, 1995, pp 1857–1879.

116. Ramonatxo M, Boulard P, Prefaut C: Validation of a noninvasive tension-time index of inspiratory muscles. J Appl Physiol 78:646, 1995.

117. Field S, Kelly SM, Macklem PT: The oxygen cost of breathing in patients with cardiorespiratory disease. Am Rev Respir Dis 126:9, 1982.

118. Jardim J, Farkas G, Prefaut C, et al: The failing inspiratory muscles under normoxic and hypoxic conditions. Am Rev Respir Dis 124:274, 1981.

119. Mannix ET, Sullivan TY, Palange P, et al: Metabolic basis for inspiratory muscle fatigue in normal humans. J Appl Physiol 75:2188, 1993.

120. Zattara-Hartmann MC, Badier M, Guillot C, et al: Maximal force and endurance to fatigue of respiratory and skeletal muscles in chronic hypoxemic patients: The effects of oxygen breathing. Muscle Nerve 18:495, 1995.

121. Macklem PT: Symptoms and signs of respiratory muscle dysfunction. In Roussos C (ed): The Thorax. In Lenfant C (ed): Lung Biology in Health and Disease. New York, Marcel Dekker, 1995, pp 1751–1762.

122. Diaz PT, Clanton TL: Clinical assessment of repiratory muscles. Phys Ther 75:983, 1995.

123. Vellody VPS, Nassery M, Balasaraswathi K, et al: Compliances of human rib cage and diaphragm-abdomen pathways in relaxed versus paralyzed states. Am Rev Respir Dis 118:479, 1978.

124. Gilbert R, Auchincloss JH, Peppi D: Relationship of rib cage and abdomen motion to diaphragm function during quiet breathing. Chest 80:607, 1981.

125. Cohen CA, Zagelbaum G, Gross D, et al: Clinical manifestations of inspiratory muscle fatigue. Am J Med 73:308, 1982.

126. Roussos C, Fixley M, Gross D, et al: Fatigue of inspiratory muscles and their synergic behaviour. J Appl Physiol 46:896, 1979.

127. Black LF, Hyatt RE: Maximal respiratory pressures; normal values and relationship to age and sex. Am Rev Respir Dis 99:696, 1969.

128. Rochester DF, Esau SA: Assessment of ventilatory function in patients with neuromuscular disease. Clin Chest Med 15:751, 1994.

129. Brancatisano A, Engel LA, Loring SH: Lung volume and effectiveness of inspiratory muscles. J Appl Physiol 74:688, 1993.

130. Konno K, Mead J: Measurement of the separate volume changes of rib cage and abdomen during breathing. J Appl Physiol 22:407, 1967.

131. Macklem PT: Respiratory muscles—the vital pump. Chest 78:753, 1980.

132. Lopata M, Zubillaga G, Evanich MJ, et al: Diaphragmatic EMG response to isocapnic hypoxic and hyperoxic hypercapnia in humans. J Lab Clin Med 91:698, 1978.

133. Gross D, Grassino A, Ross W, et al: Electromyogram pattern of diaphragmatic fatigue. J Appl Physiol 46:1, 1979.

134. Moxam J, Edwards R, Aubier M, et al: Changes in EMG power spectrum (high-to-low ratio) with force fatigue in humans. J Appl Physiol 53:1094, 1982.

135. Onal E, Lopatal M, Ginzburg AS, et al: Diaphragmatic EMG and transdiaphragmatic pressure measurements with a single catheter. Am Rev Respir Dis 124:563, 1981.

136. Macklem PT: Normal and abnormal function of the diaphragm. Thorax 36:161, 1981.

137. DeTroyer A, Estenne M: Limitations of measurement of transdiaphragmatic pressure in detecting diaphragmatic weakness. Thorax 36:169, 1981.

138. Gibson GJ, Clark E, Pride NB: Static transdiaphragmatic pressures in normal subjects and in patients with chronic hyperinflation. Am Rev Respir Dis 124:685, 1981.

139. Nickerson BH, Keens TG: Measuring ventilatory muscle endurance in humans as sustainable inspiratory pressure. J Appl Physiol 52:768, 1982.

140. Laghi F, D'Alfonso N, Tobin MJ: Pattern of recovery from diaphragmatic fatigue over 24 hours. J Appl Physiol 79:539, 1995.

141. Aubier M, Farkas G, De Troyer A, et al: Detection of diaphragmatic fatigue in man by phrenic stimulation. J Appl Physiol 50:538, 1981.

142. Field S, Kelly SM, Macklem PT: The oxygen cost of breathing in patients with cardiorespiratory disease. Am Rev Respir Dis 126:9, 1982.

143. Sigrist S, Thomas D, Howell S, et al: The effect of aminophylline on inspiratory muscle contractility. Am Rev Respir Dis 126:46, 1982.

144. Howell S, Roussos C: Isoproterenol and aminophylline improve contractility of fatigued canine diaphragm. Am Rev Respir Dis 129:118, 1984.

145. Gauthier AP, Yan S, Sliwinski P, et al: Effects of fatigue, fiber length, and aminophylline on human diaphragm contractility. Am Rev Respir Dis 152:204, 1995.

146. Aubier M: Respiratory muscles: Working or wasting. Intensive Care Med 19(Suppl):64, 1993.

147. Sieck GC: Physiological effects of diaphragm muscle denervation and disuse. Clin Chest Med 15:741, 1994.

148. Pardy RL, Rivington RN, Despas PJ, et al: The effects of inspiratory muscle training on exercise performance in chronic air flow limitation. Am Rev Respir Dis 123:426, 1981.

149. Reid WD, Dechman G: Considerations when testing and training the respiratory muscles. Phys Ther 75:971, 1995.

150. Mancini DM, Henson D, La Manca J, et al: Benefit of selective respiratory muscle training on exercise capacity in patients with chronic congestive heart failure. Circulation 91:320, 1995.

151. O'Kroy JA, Coast JR: Effects of flow and resistive training on respiratory muscle endurance and strength. Respiration 60:279, 1993.

152. Goldenberg DB, Brogdon BG: Congenital anomalies of the pectoral girdle demonstrated by chest radiography. J Can Assoc Radiol 18:472, 1967.

153. Christensen EE, Dietz GW: The supraclavicular fossa. Radiology 118:37, 1976.

154. Ominsky S, Berinson HS: The suprasternal fossa. Radiology 122:311, 1977.

155. Wechsler RJ, Steiner RM: Cross-sectional imaging of the chest wall. J Thorac Imaging 4:29, 1989.

156. Im JG, Webb WR, Rosen A, et al: Costal pleura: Appearances at high-resolution CT. Radiology 171:125, 1989.

157. Stewart JH, McCormick WF: A sex- and age-limited ossification pattern in human costal cartilages. Am J Clin Pathol 81:765, 1984.

158. Sanders CF: Sexing by costal cartilage calcification. Br J Radiol 39:233, 1966.

159. Navani S, Shah JR, Levy PS: Determination of sex by costal cartilage calcification. Am J Roentgenol 108:771, 1970.

160. King JB: Calcification of the costal cartilages. Br J Radiol 12:2, 1939.

161. Vastine JH II, Vastine MF, Arango O: Genetic influence on osseous development with particular reference to the deposition of calcium in the costal cartilages. Am J Roentgenol 59:213, 1948.

162. Zawadowski W: Über die Schattenbildunger an der Lungen-Weichteilgrenze. Fortschr Roentgenstr 53:306, 1936.

163. Gluck MC, Twigg HL, Ball MF, et al: Shadows bordering the lung on radiographs of normal and obese persons. Thorax 27:232, 1972.

164. Ominsky S, Berinson HS: The suprasternal fossa. Radiology 122:311, 1977.

165. Vix VA: Extrapleural costal fat. Radiology 112:563, 1974.

166. Foley WJ, Whitehouse WM: Supernumerary thoracic ribs. Radiology 93:1333, 1969.

167. Ogden JA, Conlogue GJ, Phillips L, et al: Sprengel's deformity: Radiology of the pathologic deformation. Skeletal Radiol 4:204, 1979.

168. Shoop JD: Transthoracic rib. Radiology 93:1335, 1969.

169. Kermond AJ: Supernumerary intrathoracic rib—an easily recognized rare anomaly. Australas Radiol 15:131, 1971.

170. Freed C: Intrathoracic rib: A case report. S Afr Med J 46:1165, 1972.

171. Sullivan D, Cornwell WS: Pelvic rib: Report of a case. Radiology 110:355, 1974.

172. Bhalla M, McCauley DI, Golimbu C, et al: Counting ribs on chest CT. J Comput Assist Tomogr 14:590, 1990.

173. Köhler A: Borderlands of the Normal and Early Pathologic in Skeletal Roentgenology. 10th ed. New York, Grune & Stratton, 1956.

174. Parsons FG: On the proportions and characteristics of the modern English clavicle. J Anat 51:71, 1917.

175. Shauffer IA, Collins WV: The deep clavicular rhomboid fossa. Clinical significance and incidence in 10,000 routine chest photofluorograms. JAMA 195:778, 1966.

176. Cockshott WP: The coracoclavicular joint. Radiology 131:313, 1979.

177. Cigtay OS, Mascatello VJ: Scapular defects: A normal variation. Am J Radiol 132:239, 1979.

178. Goodman LR, Teplick SK, Kay H: Computed tomography of the normal sternum. Am J Roentgenol 141:219, 1983.

CHAPTER *11*

The Normal Lung: Radiography

NORMAL LUNG DENSITY, 269
ALTERATION IN LUNG DENSITY, 270
  Physiologic Mechanisms, 270
  Physical (or Technical) Mechanisms, 271
  Pathologic Mechanisms, 272
PULMONARY MARKINGS, 272
PERCEPTION IN CHEST RADIOGRAPHY, 275
  Observer Error, 275
  Techniques of Radiograph Viewing, 277
  Threshold Visibility, 278
  Psychological Aspects of Radiologic
    Interpretation, 279
    Reader Fatigue, 279
    Physical Aspects, 279
    Intangible Factors, 279

As indicated in the previous chapters, the lungs are composed of a variety of tissues, each with a unique function, but together able to perform the act of respiration. Anatomists and pathologists can examine each tissue and determine its normal or abnormal characteristics. Through the application of special techniques such as computed tomography (CT), magnetic resonance (MR) imaging, and angiography, radiologists can also assess individual components of the lungs, although their methods are necessarily more gross. However, the bulk of the radiologic images that diagnosticians must interpret are plain radiographs composed for the most part of a summation of relatively low-contrast structures that form a complex group of shadows of varied definition and density. The composition of the lungs in relation to their "density"* and to their radiographic pattern has received insufficient attention in the literature, and in this section an attempt is made to clarify some of these issues.

NORMAL LUNG DENSITY

It is readily apparent that the "radiographic density" of the lung is the result of the absorptive powers of each of its component parts—gas, blood, and tissue. Although precise figures for the contributions of blood and tissue vary somewhat depending on whether the results are obtained by anatomic or physiologic methods, data have been compiled that allow a reasonable approximation.

The density of bloodless collapsed lung tissue is 1.065 gm/ml,[1] and that of blood is 1.052 gm/ml.[2] Since nonaerated lung *in vivo* consists of approximately half blood and half lung tissue,[3] the mean density of collapsed lung containing blood is approximately 1.06 gm/ml.[4] By comparison, water has a density of 1.0 gm/ml and air has a density of 0.

If we apply the *average* figures for total maximal tissue volume, derived from anatomic and physiologic estimates, and the predicted total lung capacity (TLC; 6,500 ml) of a 20-year-old man 170 cm tall,[5] the *average density* of lung is 740 gm ÷ 7,198 ml,* or 0.103 gm/ml. This figure, of course, represents the density of a structure whose composite parts are uniformly distributed, a situation that hardly pertains to the lung. Some of the radiographic density of lung is contributed by the major blood vessels, which are visible as homogeneous tapering structures with a density of 1.05 gm/ml. Since the *average* density of lung tissue is only 0.103, a considerable portion of lung tissue—logically, the air-containing parenchyma—must possess a density *less* than this to compensate for the relatively high density of the visible blood vessels.

The volumetric proportion of the three components of lung parenchyma at TLC has been measured anatomically by using a point-counting technique.[6] Air accounted for 92% and tissue and capillary blood for 8.0% (including the interstitium, endothelial and epithelial cells, vessel walls, and blood). According to these anatomic measurements, the density of lung parenchyma at TLC is estimated to be 0.08 × 1.06 gm/ml, i.e., 0.085 gm/ml. It follows that in a normal chest radiograph, all the tissue visible in the peripheral 2 cm of the lung or between vascular shadows should have a density of 0.085 gm/ml. These estimates, however, are considerably lower than those obtained by using CT[7] and MR imaging.[8]

Measurements of lung density on CT scans are based on an approximate linear relationship between attenuation of the x-ray beam and the density of materials of low atomic number such as air, blood, and lung tissue.[9] Attenuation is expressed in terms of the Hounsfield unit (HU) scale in

---

*In this context, the word "density" applies to the *weight of tissue per volume*, or specific gravity. It should not be confused with "radiographic density," which is a measure of the blackening of film caused by a reduction in silver emulsion by the incident x-ray beam. The greater the amount of radiation passing through the body, the denser the blackening of the radiograph; since the tissue density of bone is greater than that of lung, transmission of x-rays through bone is less, so bones appear relatively white in comparison to the blackness of lung. Therefore, tissue density has a connotation opposite that of radiographic density. The preferred term for a tissue more opaque to x-rays than its surrounding is an *opacity* or *radiopacity*; for example, bones have a greater opacity or radiopacity than lungs.

---

*The ratio of total weight (740 gm, with a volume of 740 ÷ 1.06 = 698 ml) to total volume (6,500 ml + 698 ml).

which water is 0 HU and air is $-1,000$ HU. Hounsfield units can be converted to tissue density by adding 1,000 to the HU value.[9] Thus, an attenuation value of -900 HU corresponds to a tissue density of 0.1 gm/ml. Estimates of lung density on CT have been shown to correspond closely to gravimetric estimates with a margin of error of approximately 4%.[9]

An early study in adult baboons demonstrated that the average lung density at TLC as assessed by CT was 0.12 gm/ml.[7] The results of similar studies in humans suggested that lung density was considerably higher, ranging from 0.16 to 0.18 gm/ml (average attenuation values ranging from -820 to -840 HU).[10–12] However, these studies were based on scans obtained at the end of a normal inspiration and not at TLC. It was subsequently shown that more accurate estimates of lung attenuation can be obtained by applying a spirometrically defined and controlled level of inspiration during CT scanning.[13, 14] Studies using spirometrically gated CT have shown that attenuation is markedly influenced by lung volume.[13, 15] Based on measurements made by using spirometrically controlled CT,[14, 15] the average lung density at TLC can be estimated to be on the order of 0.11 to 0.13 gm/ml. In a study in which 42 healthy subjects were encouraged "to make all possible efforts" to hold their breath at TLC, the mean lung density was 0.134 gm/ml.[16]

Lung density can also be estimated *in vivo* by using MR imaging. The technique is based on the assessment of lung water. In one study, a multiecho MR sequence was first validated in excised normal pig lung by comparison with gravimetric lung water content.[8] The ratio of lung water measured by MR and the gravimetric technique was 0.95 ± 0.03. The authors then used the multiecho sequence to measure lung water and estimate lung density in five normal adults. According to the MR measurements, the average lung density at TLC was 0.12 gm/ml.[8]

From estimates of lung density at TLC made on CT and MR imaging, we believe that the average lung density is approximately 0.12 gm/ml. This figure, of course, represents the average density. There is a considerable cephalocaudal gradient because of the effect of gravity.[15]

If extravascular tissue volume is assumed to be constant, overall lung density equals the ratio of its blood and gas content. The blood content can be further subdivided into a capillary component, which relates to the background density of the lung parenchyma (0.12 gm/ml), and a large vessel component, which is responsible for the visible lung markings (density, 1.05 gm/ml). Figures for total capillary blood volume vary according to the measurement technique. Physiologic techniques have yielded estimates in resting subjects of 60 to 100 ml,[17–20] whereas anatomic studies have indicated a volume of 150 to 200 ml.[6, 21]

It is important to appreciate the distinction between capillary and large vessel components of the lung with respect to their separate contributions to lung density. For example, variation in total capillary blood volume is difficult, if not impossible to appreciate subjectively on a plain radiograph of the chest. Although an increase in capillary blood volume is known to occur in both ventricular[22] and atrial septal defects[23] without a concomitant alteration in lung volume,[24] it is doubtful whether the increase in lung density that must result can be appreciated radiographically except by densitometry. In such situations, radiographic assessment

of vascular plethora (pleonemia) must be based on an increase in the size and number of visible pulmonary vessels, both arterial and venous.

These statements apply only to conditions in which perfusion is *uniformly* altered throughout the lungs—for example, in the pleonemia that accompanies an intracardiac left-to-right shunt (Fig. 11–1A) or in the oligemia of diffuse emphysema (Fig. 11–1B). When the reduction in blood flow is local, as in unilateral emphysema (Fig. 11–1C) or (occasionally) massive pulmonary embolism, alteration in density in the involved area of lung is the result of a reduction in both capillary blood volume (background density) and visible vascular shadows. Such alteration of background lung density is an exceedingly valuable radiographic sign and is referred to repeatedly throughout this book.

ALTERATION IN LUNG DENSITY

An alteration in radiographic lung density may be the result of one or more of three mechanisms.

Physiologic Mechanisms

A frequently observed physiologic variation in lung density with which every radiologist is familiar is the change that may occur from one examination to another in the same subject, depending on the depth of inspiration. Such variation is readily explained by comparing the contributions of the three components of the lung with its density. For example, again consider a 20-year-old, 170-cm-tall man and assume that pulmonary blood volume and tissue volume are reasonably constant at different degrees of lung inflation. The predicted lung volumes for such a subject are 6.5 liters (TLC), 3.4 liters (functional residual capacity [FRC]), and 1.5 liters (residual volume).[5] Assuming a total maximal tissue volume of 700 ml, average lung density at TLC is 0.12; at FRC the density is almost double (0.22), and at residual volume it is more than treble (0.40) (Fig. 11–2). Thus, assuming that total pulmonary blood volume is constant at different degrees of lung inflation, it is clear that lung density is inversely proportional to the amount of contained gas. These estimates correlate remarkably well with estimates of lung density made by MR imaging.[8] In a study of five normal volunteers, the average lung density at FRC was 0.21 gm/ml as compared with 0.12 gm/ml at TLC. Measurements of lung density on CT also show considerable variation with lung volume.[13, 15] In one study,[15] scans were obtained at lung volumes of 10%, 50%, and 90% vital capacity by using a respiratory gating device connected to the CT scanner. Differences in density were noted between the apical and basal sections of the lungs and between dependent and nondependent lung regions. On average, the lung density in the apical sections of the lung was approximately 0.17 gm/ml at 90% vital capacity, 0.25 gm/ml at 50% vital capacity, and 0.32 gm/ml at 10% vital capacity. In the basal sections, the average density was approximately 0.17 at 90% vital capacity, 0.22 at 50% vital capacity, and 0.27 at 10% vital capacity.[15]

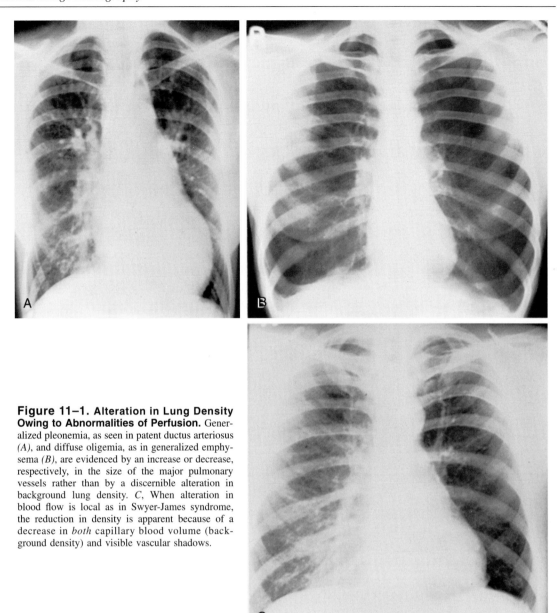

Figure 11–1. Alteration in Lung Density Owing to Abnormalities of Perfusion. Generalized pleonemia, as seen in patent ductus arteriosus *(A)*, and diffuse oligemia, as in generalized emphysema *(B)*, are evidenced by an increase or decrease, respectively, in the size of the major pulmonary vessels rather than by a discernible alteration in background lung density. *C,* When alteration in blood flow is local as in Swyer-James syndrome, the reduction in density is apparent because of a decrease in *both* capillary blood volume (background density) and visible vascular shadows.

Physical (or Technical) Mechanisms

Symmetry of radiographic density of the two lungs in a normal subject depends on proper positioning for radiography. If the patient is rotated, the lung closer to the film will be uniformly more radiopaque (whiter) than the other lung (Fig. 11–3); conversely, the lung that is farthest away from the film will be uniformly less radiopaque (more black), and a unilateral hyperlucent hemithorax will be present that can sometimes hamper interpretation. In an investigation of radiographic density using phantoms, approximately 80% of this increase in unilateral film blackening was found to be the result of asymmetric absorption of the primary x-ray beam, with the remaining 20% being due to scatter radiation.[25] Measurements of chest wall thickness showed that the x-ray beam traversed less tissue on the side of increased film blackening (or conversely, more tissue on the side of in-

creased opacity) owing chiefly to the pectoral muscles. Since rotation to the right or to the left means different things to different people (is it rotation into the right anterior oblique or left posterior oblique?), it is preferable to relate the increased opacity or increased lucency to the side that is closest to or farthest removed from the film, respectively. To reiterate, *the hemithorax closer to the film will be more radiopaque (film whiter) than the contralateral hemithorax.*

A CT study of 65 patients showed a nearly linear relationship between the degree of rotation and the change in density of the hemithoraces.[26] The change in density was almost entirely due to the anterior breast/pectoralis muscles, with little alteration being present unless these structures were present. Because of the fanlike distribution of the x-ray beam, lateral decentering of the beam also results in changes in density of the hemithoraces, although smaller than those caused by rotation.[26]

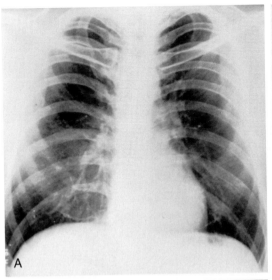
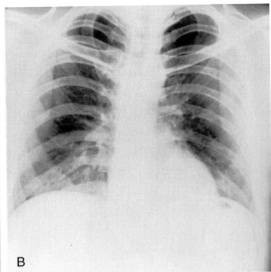
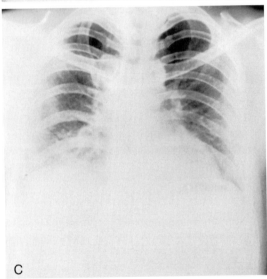

Figure 11–2. Alteration in Lung Density Owing to Changes in Lung Volume. Radiographs of the chest of a healthy 40-year-old man at total lung capacity *(A)*, functional residual capacity *(B)*, and residual volume *(C)*.

Provided that the patient is not rotated and the x-ray beam is properly centered, any discrepancy in the density of the two lungs must be interpreted as being pathologic. The etiology varies from such benign conditions as scoliosis or congenital absence of the pectoral muscles to more significant diseases such as Swyer-James syndrome; this differential diagnosis is described briefly in the following section but in considerably more detail in Chapters 18 and 19.

Pathologic Mechanisms

Excluding from consideration the contribution to radiographic density from the soft tissues of the thoracic wall and provided that physiologic and physical causes can be excluded, variation in lung density is always due to an increase or decrease in one or more of three elements—air, blood, and tissue. In the majority of clinical situations, change in density, whether increased or decreased, local or diffuse, is the result of change in all three components. Occasionally it is produced by alteration in one component

to the exclusion of the others. Examples of such "pure" alteration are the reduction in density (increased translucency) produced by pulmonary thromboembolism without infarction (in which there is a reduction in blood volume but little change in gas or tissue volume) and diffuse pulmonary inflammation (such as in sarcoidosis), in which there is an increase in extravascular tissue volume but little change in gas or blood volume.

PULMONARY MARKINGS

Correct interpretation of the chest radiograph requires a thorough knowledge of the pattern of linear markings throughout the normal lung. Such knowledge cannot be gained through didactic teaching alone; in addition, interpretation of thousands of normal chest radiographs is required to acquire the skill—perhaps the art—to be able to distinguish normal from abnormal. Discrimination of normal from abnormal radiographs requires not only familiarity with the

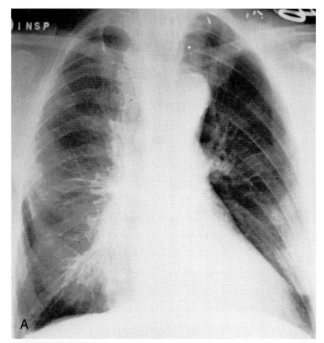

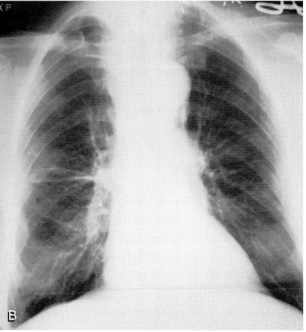

Figure 11–3. Alteration in Lung Density Owing to Improper Positioning. *A,* A radiograph of the chest in posteroanterior projection was exposed with the patient rotated slightly into the right anterior oblique position to produce an overall increase in density of the right lung as compared with the left. In *B,* positioning has been corrected and the asymmetry has disappeared.

distribution and pattern of branching of these markings but also an awareness of normal caliber, the extent of normal radiologic visibility, and changes that may occur in different phases of respiration and in various body positions. Such knowledge is necessary for two main reasons: (1) a change in the caliber of arteries and veins constitutes one of the most valuable radiologic signs of pulmonary venous and pulmonary arterial hypertension; and (2) a redistribution of

blood flow, with consequent modification of the number of radiologically visible markings, may constitute the major evidence of atelectasis or previous pulmonary resection.

The linear markings are created by the pulmonary arteries, bronchi, veins, and accompanying interstitial tissue (Figs. 11–4 and 11–5). The first two of these markings fan outward from both hila and gradually taper as they proceed distally. In the normal state they are visible up to about 1 to 2 cm from the visceral pleural surface over the convexity of the lung, at which point the lung is composed predominantly of acini.

As indicated in the section dealing with the pulmonary vasculature, the anatomic remoteness of the pulmonary veins from the arteries often renders their distinction possible on the radiograph. In the region of the pulmonary ligaments especially, these vessels should be readily distinguishable since the pulmonary veins in the lower lung zones lie almost horizontal and on a lower plane than the arteries. A horizontal line drawn across a posteroanterior radiograph of the chest at the midpoint between the apex and diaphragm separates the pulmonary artery complex in the hila (at or above this line) and the veins (below the line).[27] It is probable that in roughly 50% of individuals the upper lobe pulmonary arteries and veins cannot be distinguished on plain radiographs of the chest in posteroanterior projection.[28] When the vessels can be identified separately, the veins that drain the upper lobes always project lateral to their respective arteries—a relationship particularly valuable in the right hilar region, in which the superior pulmonary vein forms the lateral aspect of the hilum superiorly and thus produces the upper limb of its concave configuration (see Fig. 11–4). Flattening of this concavity is evidence of atelectasis of the right upper lobe or, in the presence of pulmonary venous hypertension, dilatation of the upper lobe vein.[29]

The posteroanterior chest radiograph of a normal erect subject invariably shows some discrepancy in the size of the pulmonary vessels in the upper lung zones as compared with the lower as a result of pressure-related differences in blood flow from the apex to the base (a unit volume of lung at the base of the thorax having four to eight times the blood flow of a similar volume at the apex[30]). In recumbent subjects, a decrease in the influence of gravity renders this discrepancy in vascular size minimal. In an angiographic study of the pulmonary vascular bed, the mean pulmonary vein diameter at the level of the main pulmonary artery was 7 mm in recumbent subjects and 4 mm in erect ones.[28] Since the radiographs from which these measurements were taken were exposed at a 40-inch (100-cm) target-film distance, these diameters will be considerably smaller on standard chest radiographs exposed at 6 or 10 ft (1.80 to 3 m).

Estimates of the relative blood flow to the two lungs are somewhat variable. For example, one group of investigators who used lung scanning techniques with $^{15}O_2$-labeled carbon dioxide found significantly greater blood flow through the left than the right upper zone.[31] In contrast, another group who used intravenously injected ^{131}I-MAA (macroaggregated albumin) showed a slightly greater average distribution of blood flow to the right lung than to the left—as might be expected in view of the larger size of the right lung.[32] These latter results concur with those obtained by other investigators who used ^{131}I-MAA and monitored each complete lung area by anterior and posterior scanning.[33]

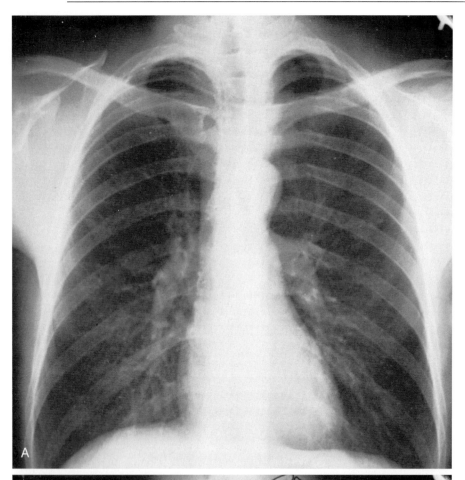

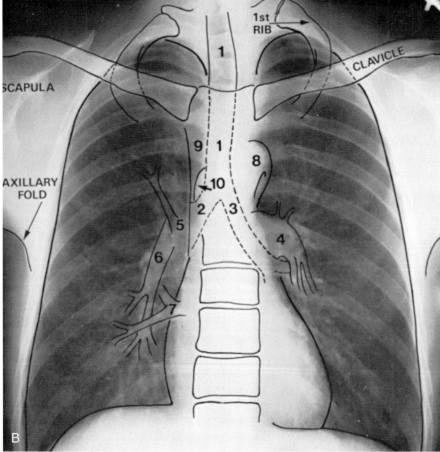

Figure 11–4. Normal Chest Radiograph, Posteroanterior Projection. *A*, Radiograph of the chest of an asymptomatic 26-year-old man in the erect position. *B*, A diagrammatic overlay shows the normal anatomic structures numbered or labeled: (1) trachea, (2) right main bronchus, (3) left main bronchus, (4) left pulmonary artery, (5) right upper lobe pulmonary vein, (6) right interlobar artery, (7) right lower and middle lobe vein, (8) aortic arch, (9) superior vena cava, and (10) azygos vein.

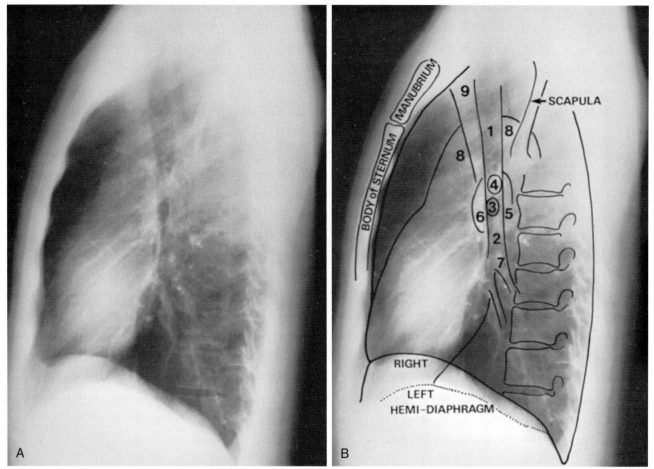

Figure 11–5. Normal Chest Radiograph, Lateral Projection. *A*, Radiograph of the chest of an asymptomatic 26-year-old man in the erect position. *B*, A diagrammatic overlay shows the normal anatomic structures numbered or labeled: (1) tracheal air column, (2) right intermediate bronchus, (3) left upper lobe bronchus, (4) right upper lobe bronchus, (5) left interlobar artery, (6) right interlobar artery, (7) confluence of pulmonary veins, (8) aortic arch, and (9) brachiocephalic vessels.

Thus, evidence favors the conclusion that blood flow in all zones of the right lung is slightly greater than that in the left.

Complex interrelationships between transthoracic pressure and pulmonary blood flow occur during inspiration and expiration and during the Valsalva and Müller maneuvers.* During inspiration, blood volume increases in the pulmonary arteries and veins and decreases in the capillaries.[34] This increase has been documented radiographically in one investigation of normal subjects in which the caliber of the right descending pulmonary artery was found to be consistently larger during inspiration than during expiration, the range of difference being 1 to 3 mm.[35]

Use of the Valsalva and Müller maneuvers to produce increases and decreases, respectively, in intra-alveolar pressure has limited application in the radiologic diagnosis of chest disease.[36] However, the Valsalva maneuver may be helpful in differentiating vascular and solid lesions, the

former being reduced in size when intra-alveolar pressure is increased whereas the latter remain unchanged (Fig. 11–6).[36, 37]

PERCEPTION IN CHEST RADIOGRAPHY

Observer Error

The radiologic diagnosis of chest disease begins with *identification* of an abnormality on a radiograph: what is not *seen* cannot be appreciated. These statements may appear self-evident, but they express an observation that deserves constant re-emphasis. The gain in confidence in the ability to *interpret* changes apparent on the radiograph must not be mistaken by radiologists for an improvement in the accuracy with which they see them in the first place. Many studies of accuracy in detecting radiographic abnormalities have revealed an astonishingly high incidence of both intraobserver and interobserver error among experienced radiologists.[38–40] For example, in one series based only on positive radiographs, interobserver error ranged from 9% to 24% and intraobserver error from 3% to 31%.[39] Since these figures are

---

*The Valsalva maneuver consists of forced expiration and the Müller maneuver of inspiration, each against a closed glottis. For proper hemodynamic effect, pressures of plus and minus 40 to 50 cm H_2O, respectively, should be maintained for 7 to 10 seconds. For radiographs to be comparable, both maneuvers should be performed at the same degree of lung inflation, preferably at the end of a quiet inspiration.

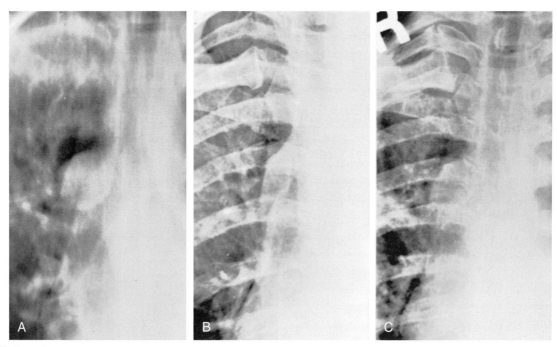

Figure 11–6. Valve of Valsalva and Müller Procedures in Distinguishing the Vascular or Solid Nature of Intrathoracic Lesions. *A*, A tomographic section of the midmediastinum reveals a well-defined circular shadow situated in the right tracheobronchial angle; the differential diagnosis includes an enlarged azygos lymph node or a markedly dilated azygos vein. *B*, A radiograph of the same area in the erect position during the Valsalva procedure reveals a marked reduction in size of the shadow. *C*, A similar projection during the Müller procedure shows a considerable increase in size of the shadow when compared with *B*. Subsequent studies proved the shadow to be a markedly dilated azygos vein associated with infradiaphragmatic interruption of the inferior vena cava.

derived from studies performed by competent, experienced observers, it is clear that radiologists should not be lulled into a false sense of security concerning their competence to "see" a lesion.

One report in which the influence of multiple readings on the detection and evaluation of radiographic abnormalities in coal workers' pneumoconiosis was described illustrates the truly astonishing level of interobserver disagreement that may occur.[41] Three groups of "readers" were used: Group A was composed of radiologists or other physicians residing in the mining areas being studied, Group B contained 24 radiologists from three departments of radiology who had considerable experience with pneumoconiosis, and Group C comprised 7 radiologists with extensive experience in the interpretation of radiographs of patients with pneumoconiosis. The A and B readers agreed in approximately 75% of their readings. However, excluding radiographs interpreted as normal by both groups of readers (leaving roughly 17,000 radiographs), 1 reader disagreed with the others in 82% of cases and agreed with only 18%! Agreement between readers in groups A and C was even worse: of 14,369 readings, there was disagreement in 75%; in fact, in only 10% did both A and C readers agree that the chest was normal. Comparison between the B and C group readings showed lower levels of disagreement than between the other two, but even here the results were rather discouraging: in 14,594 cases, there was 70% agreement and 30% disagreement between the two groups. The authors suggested four factors that were possibly responsible for the low level of observer agreement: (1) radiographs of poor technical quality; (2) a

lack of experience with the pneumoconiosis classification systems used; (3) a general lack of familiarity with the radiographic manifestations of coal workers' pneumoconiosis; and (4) inherent factors of interobserver disagreement.

Based on an analysis of eye movements, three forms of false-negative radiologic perceptual error have been defined: search, recognition, and decision-making errors.[45–47] In one study, approximately 30% of missed lung nodules were caused by failure of the radiologist to look at the area of the lesion (search error), 25% by failure of the eyes to gaze long enough at the lesion (recognition error), and 45% by the radiologist deciding after gazing at the nodule that it was not a lesion (decision-making error).[46] When gaze includes the region of the nodule, detection of the lesion is influenced by the duration of the gaze. In one study, a "dwell time" of at least 300 milliseconds led to detection of 85% of the nodules looked at directly.[47]

Error rates in the interpretation of radiographs are greater in patients with multiple abnormalities than in patients with single abnormalities.[48] The phenomenon by which detection of one abnormality interferes with the detection of other abnormalities on the same radiograph is known as "satisfaction of search."[49] It is not clear to what extent this phenomenon is due to premature termination[49] or inappropriate allocation of visual attention.[50]

The reasons for observer error are both subjective and objective and are highly complex; every physician concerned with the interpretation of chest radiographs must become thoroughly familiar with the physical and physiologic principles of perception so that errors are kept to a minimum.

Some of the more important of these principles are outlined here, but the reader is urged to review more extensive works on the subject.[49, 51–54]

Techniques of Radiograph Viewing

A radiograph can be inspected in two ways, each of which may be usefully applied to different situations. *Directed search* is a method whereby a specific pattern of inspection is carried out, commonly along such lines as thoracic and extrathoracic soft tissue, bony thorax, mediastinum, diaphragm, pleura, and finally, the lungs themselves, the latter usually by individual inspection and comparison of the zones of the two lungs from apex to base. Such a method *must* be used by radiologists in training, for it is only through the exercise of this routine during thousands of examinations that the *pattern* of the normal chest radiograph can be recognized. The alternative method of inspection is *free global search*, in which the radiograph is scanned without a preconceived orderly pattern. This technique is recommended because of objective evidence that free global search is the scanning method used by the majority of expert radiologists.[55] However, we believe that discovery of an abnormality during free-search scanning must be followed by an orderly pattern of inspection so that other, less obvious abnormalities are not overlooked.

In a study of the influence of viewing time and visual search on the interpretation of chest radiographs, a series of 10 normal and 10 abnormal radiographs were shown to 10 radiologists under two viewing conditions: (1) a 0.2- second flash; and (2) unlimited viewing time.[45] The overall accuracy of the flash viewing was surprisingly high (70% true positives) since no search was possible; as expected, performance improved with free search (97% true positives). The researchers concluded that their results supported the hypothesis that visual search begins with a global response that involves interpretation of the input from the entire retina and establishes the overall content of the visual scene, detects gross deviations from normal, and organizes subsequent foveal checking fixations.

In another study, 120 posteroanterior radiographs were shown to four observers for four different viewing times: 0.5 second, 1 second, 4 seconds, and unlimited time.[56] The cases included 40 with subtle lung cancers (lesion diameter of 1 cm or less or obscuration of the lesion by overlying structures), 40 with obvious cancers (lesion diameter of more than 1 cm and less than 4 cm), and 40 normal films. The detection of subtle and obvious lung cancers increased with incremental viewing times, but even with unlimited viewing time, on average the four radiologists missed 26% of subtle cancers. A viewing time of 0.25 second, which allows for only one visual fixation (flash viewing), allowed detection of 70% of obvious cancers. The detection rate of both subtle and obvious tumors increased considerably with viewing time up to 4 seconds; however, there was little change between a 4-second viewing time and unlimited viewing time.[56] This study thus confirms the results of a previous study in which "flash" viewing permitting only one visual fixation was shown to allow the detection of 70% of obvious abnormalities.[45] It also demonstrates that subtle and obvious tumors may be missed regardless of the length of viewing time. The observation of a false-negative rate of 13% of all lung cancers with unlimited viewing time[56] is in keeping with the findings of other studies that have shown that even experienced observers may miss 10% to 40% of relevant findings on the chest radiograph.[42–44] The value of comparing current radiographs with previous radiographs cannot be overemphasized. In a review of 27 potentially resectable lung cancers that were prospectively missed by a radiologist but were visible on the radiograph retrospectively, "the single most frequently identified cause of misdiagnosis was failure of the radiologist to evaluate the current CXRs in the context of previous CXRs."[57]

Of a somewhat different character was a study in which a number of chest films were inspected for the presence of lung nodules by five radiologists under two viewing conditions—segmented search, in which films were divided into six sections and viewed piecemeal, and global search, in which the complete film was presented and viewed in its entirety.[58] Nodules varied in edge gradient from sharp to fuzzy. As might be expected, nodules with sharper edges were identified faster, more frequently, and with higher confidence than were nodules with less sharp edges, regardless of the method of viewing. Segmented search did not increase the probability of nodule detection; rather, it led to an increase in the number of false positives and thus resulted in lower overall performance when compared with global search. We believe that the combination of initial free global search and interspersed global and checking fixations, as routinely used by expert observers,[45] provides optimal assessment of the chest radiograph.

In one study assessing the performance of observers in detecting solitary lung nodules 1.0 and 1.5 cm in diameter at viewing distances of 1.5, 3, 6, and 16 ft, no difference in observer accuracy was demonstrated for the 1.5-cm nodules at the three closest viewing distances; however, there was deterioration of about 30% at 16 ft.[59] By contrast, observer performance for the detection of 1.0-cm nodules improved as the viewing distance increased from 1.5 to 3 ft and then decreased at the two longer viewing distances. Another investigation of the visual system transfer function and optimal viewing distance for radiologists showed that viewing at a fixed distance increased the risk of failure to detect abnormalities.[60] These results support the contention that in clinical situations, multiple viewing distances are desirable. The practical application of this basic physiologic principle of viewing to everyday radiographic interpretation cannot be overstressed.[55]

Since perception of a radiographic image depends on the rate of change in illumination across the retina corresponding to the border of the x-ray shadow (the retinal illumination gradient[55]), magnification should logically reduce perception by increasing the distance across the retina over which a given change in illumination occurs. Although this observation is true for many intrapulmonary lesions whose borders are indistinct, magnification may aid in the perception of small shadows of relatively high contrast, in much the same manner as it improves the visibility of trabeculae in bone. Magnification can be helpful in the assessment of diffuse diseases of the lung in which numerous densities of relatively high contrast are crowded so closely together that they are almost indistinguishable with standard viewing; a classic example is provided by the tiny calcific shadows of alveolar microlithiasis (Fig. 11–7).

As a further means of reducing the frequency of "missing" lesions on the radiograph, the technique of *double viewing* has been advocated by several investigators.[38, 55] In one study, dual interpretation by the same observer on two occasions or by two different observers decreased by at least one third the number of positive films missed.[38] (It is important, of course, that the interpretation given on the first reading not be known at the second.) Although we cannot dispute the improvement in diagnostic accuracy to be expected from this technique, the practicality of using it routinely in large radiology departments staggers the imagination. Two compromise solutions are suggested: (1) a second reading of all films first interpreted as negative; and (2) a more universal adoption by referring physicians of personal viewing of the radiographs of their patients. Many chest physicians and surgeons become highly competent in radiologic interpretation as a result of many years of personal viewing; if this practice is carried out in consultation with the radiologist, the "second look" may reveal abnormalities missed on the first interpretation.

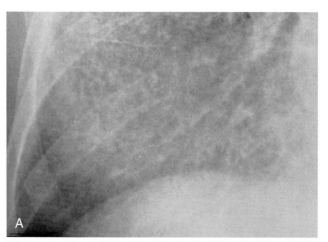

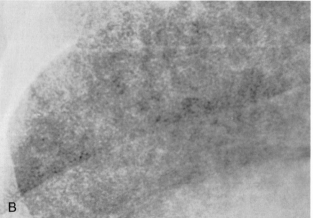

Figure 11–7. Value of Radiographic Magnification. *A*, Section of the lower portion of the right lung in a posteroanterior radiograph (photographically magnified) of a patient with pulmonary alveolar microlithiasis. The tiny calcispherytes can be visualized but tend to be confluent and thus indistinct. *B*, The same area of a radiograph made at 2:1 radiographic magnification with a 0.3-mm-focus tube. Significant improvement in visibility of the individual nodules has been obtained.

Threshold Visibility

In a study in which Lucite disks were used as test objects, it was found that a structure of unit density must be at least 3 mm in thickness to be visible on the radiograph.[61] Furthermore, it was observed that this *threshold visibility* applied only if the margins of the Lucite disks were parallel to the plane of the x-ray beam—visibility diminished progressively as the margins were increasingly beveled. A second study found that radiologists could locate the shadows of Lucite balls regularly only if the balls were at least 1 to 2 cm in diameter; balls 0.6 cm in diameter could be located only when projected over intercostal spaces, and those as small as 0.3 cm could be identified only in retrospect.[59] The difference between the 3-mm measurement in one study and the larger figures reported in the second study lies in the character of the *border* of the shadow: the 3-mm measurement applies only to lesions whose borders are sharply defined, and lesions with indistinctly defined or beveled margins (such as a sphere) must be greater than 3 mm in diameter to be visible on the radiograph. Some support is lent these observations by radiologic-pathologic studies in which it has been shown that most solitary tumors are not identifiable on the radiograph until their diameter exceeds 6 mm[59] and that a cancer less than 1.0 cm in diameter is seldom identified by standard radiographic techniques.[62]

These limits of visibility apply, of course, to individual shadows within the lung rather than to multiple diffuse nodular opacities produced, for example, by miliary tuberculosis. In the latter instance, the issue of summation of images is raised. Two opposing views have been proposed to explain the possible effect of summation. In one, it is suggested that wide distribution of a large number of small lesions throughout the lungs allows individual deposits to be visualized only when they are *not* summated and that when summation does occur, the appreciation of individual deposits is lost through blurring.[63] Another hypothesis suggests that objects of subliminal absorption may be brought above threshold by summation of their shadows.[61] Experiments based on the implantation of infraliminal spheres into inflated fixed lung specimens have shown that perfect or nearly perfect superimposition of nodules results in a visible nodular shadow whereas imperfect superimposition produces only a gray background.[64] We concur with the authors of the latter proposal that nodules as small as 1 mm in diameter may be visible by virtue of the increased x-ray absorption caused by the superimposition of individual nodules.

Certain objective reasons for missing lesions during radiologic interpretation have been clarified by studies in which postmortem radiography of the chest has been correlated with subsequent morphologic study of the lungs.[65, 66] In one such study of more than 300 cadavers, the lesions most often missed radiologically were small calcified or uncalcified nodules 3 mm or slightly more in diameter in the region of the pleura or subpleural parenchyma.[65] Many metastatic nodules measuring up to 1 cm in diameter were not identified. In addition, in 4 cases lesions measuring 2 to 5 cm in diameter that were discovered on radiography of the removed lungs were not visible even in retrospect on films taken with the lungs *in situ*. The investigators described two areas within the thorax in which it is difficult to project a lesion so that it is related to air-containing parenchyma without a superimposed confusion of overlying bones and major blood vessels: over the convexity of the lungs in close proximity to the pleura and rib cage and in the paramediastinal regions, where the shadows of the aorta, heart, and spine are quite dense. Lesions in close proximity to the diaphragm probably come within the same category. Clearly, it is important to be aware of these relatively "blind" areas in the thorax and pay particular attention to them in the development of a scanning routine.

Another area of particular importance in the interpretation of chest radiographs comprises all the structures outside the limits of the thorax. The importance to diagnosis of such abnormalities as hepatomegaly or splenomegaly, calcification in these organs, displacement or alteration in the contour of the gastric air bubble, and calcification within the thoracic soft tissues cannot be overstressed. Finally, we have been repeatedly impressed by the information to be gained from thorough inspection of the "corners and borders" of radiographs. In most departments, the name and age of the patient are inscribed on radiographs by photographic imprinting, particulars that should be noted for definite identification; similarly, an appreciation of dextrocardia or transposition of the thoracic and abdominal viscera may depend on the position of the "right" or "left" marker.

Psychological Aspects of Radiologic Interpretation

This subject is all too often neglected. Three aspects will be considered briefly, and the reader is referred to more complete discussions of this important topic.[38, 55, 67]

Reader Fatigue

The enormous increase in the use of radiologic services over the years has resulted in a significant increase in the number of examinations each radiologist may be required to make. The inevitable result is "reader fatigue." No experienced radiologist denies the diminution in visual and mental acuity that develops during the day when the workload necessitates a heavy reporting schedule. The degree of susceptibility varies, but fatigue eventually affects all to a point at which lack of efficiency accrues to the detriment of the patient. Each individual must set personal standards, but two mechanisms can be used to reduce reader fatigue to a minimum: frequent "rest periods" away from the viewbox and the establishment of a reasonable maximal number of examinations to be reported each day.

Physical Aspects

The atmosphere in which reporting is carried out deserves more attention than usually given. Quiet surroundings away from distracting influences are most desirable for necessary thought and reflection. Viewing facilities should be optimal. The illuminator is probably the least expensive and yet one of the most important pieces of apparatus in any department of radiology; all too often, however, insufficient attention is paid to such aspects as light intensity and background illumination.[38, 68] Luminance also has an important effect on the ability to visualize subtle pulmonary abnormalities on digital radiographs assessed on monitors rather than on hard copies.[69]

Intangible Factors

Intimately linked with the complex causes of observer error are several abstract phenomena that inevitably confront all radiologists but defy adequate explanation. A typical example is the variation with which the same examination may be reported from one day to another: a radiograph of the chest (often in the troublesome borderland between normal and abnormal) may be pronounced normal on Monday morning and be interpreted by the same observer as showing "diffuse reticular disease" on Friday afternoon! It is a moot point whether fatigue is the dominant influence in these intraobserver disagreements; rather, they may be more realistically ascribed to a "state of mind" that is continually fluctuating and represents an intangible influence on one's approach to a problem. Intraobserver disagreements are bound to occur, but all radiologists must constantly strive to reduce their incidence by implementing the most efficient system of radiographic perception of which they are capable.

REFERENCES

1. Hogg JC, Nepszy S: Regional lung volume and the pleural pressure gradient estimated from lung density in dogs. J Appl Physiol 27:198, 1969.
2. Altman PL, Dittmer DS: Respiration and Circulation. Bethesda MD, Federation of American Societies of Experimental Biology, 1971, p 27.
3. Staub NC: Pulmonary edema. Physiol Rev 54:678, 1974.
4. Wandtke JC, Hyde RW, Fahey PJ, et al: Measurement of lung gas volume and regional density by computed tomography in dogs. Invest Radiol 21:108, 1986.
5. Goldman HI, Becklake MR: Respiratory function tests: Normal values at median altitudes and the prediction of normal results. Am Rev Tuberc 79:457, 1959.
6. Weibel ER: Morphometrische Analyse von Zahl, Volumen and Oberfläche der Alveolen und Kapillären der menschlichen Lunge. Z Zellforsch Mikrosk Anat 57:648, 1962.
7. Hedlung L, Effmann E, Bates M, et al: Regional differences in lung density by computed tomography. Am Rev Respir Dis 125:239, 1982.
8. Mayo JR, MacKay AL, Whittall KP, et al: Measurement of lung water content and pleural pressure gradient with magnetic resonance imaging. J Thorac Imaging 10:73, 1995.
9. Hedlung LW, Vock P, Effmann EL: Evaluating lung density by computed tomography. Semin Respir Med 5:76, 1983.
10. Rosenblum LJ, Mauceri RA, Wellenstein DE, et al: Density patterns in the normal lung as determined by computed tomography. Radiology 137:409, 1980.
11. Rosenblum LJ, Mauceri RA, Wellenstein DE, et al: Density patterns in the normal lung as determined by computed tomography. Radiology 137:409, 1980.
12. Genereux GP: Computed tomography and the lung: Review of anatomic and densitometric features with their clinical application. Assoc Radiol 36:88, 1985.
13. Rienmüller RK, Behr J, Kalender WA, et al: Standardized quantitative high-resolution CT in lung disease. J Comput Assist Tomogr 15:742, 1991.
14. Kalender WA, Rienmüller R, Seissler W, et al: Measurement of pulmonary parenchymal attenuation: Use of spirometric gating with quantitative CT. Radiology 175:265, 1990.
15. Verschakelen JA, Van Fraeyenhoven L, Laureys G, et al: Differences in CT density between dependent and nondependent portions of the lung: Influence of lung volume. Am J Roentgenol 161:713, 1993.
16. Gevenois PA, Scillia P, de Maertelaer V, et al: The effects of age, sex, lung size, and hyperinflation on CT lung densitometry. Am J Roentgenol 167:1169, 1996.
17. Staub NC: The interdependence of pulmonary structure and function. Anesthesiology 24:831, 1963.
18. Roughton FJW, Forster RE: Relative importance of diffusion and chemical reaction rates in determining rate of exchange of gases in the human lung, with special reference to true diffusing capacity of pulmonary membrane and volume of blood in the lung capillaries. J Appl Physiol 11:290, 1957.
19. Bates DV, Varvis CJ, Donevan RE, et al: Variations in the pulmonary capillary blood volume and membrane diffusion component in health and disease. J Clin Invest 39:1401, 1960.
20. Newman F, Smalley BF, Thomson ML: Effect of exercise, body and lung size on CO diffusion in athletes and nonathletes. J Appl Physiol 17:649, 1962.
21. Cander L, Forster RE: Determination of pulmonary parenchymal tissue volume and pulmonary capillary blood flow in man. J Appl Physiol 14:541, 1959.
22. Flatley FJ, Constantine H, McCredie RM, et al: Pulmonary diffusing capacity and pulmonary capillary blood volume in normal subjects and in cardiac patients. Am Heart J 64:159, 1962.
23. Bucci G, Cook CD: Studies on respiratory physiology in children. VI. Lung diffusing capacity, diffusing capacity of the pulmonary membrane and pulmonary capillary blood volume in congenital heart disease. J Clin Invest 40:1431, 1961.
24. Jonsson B, Linderholm H, Pinardi G: Atrial septal defect: A study of physical working capacity and hemodynamics during exercise. Acta Med Scand 159:275, 1957.
25. Joseph AEA, Lacey GJ, Bryant THE, et al: The hypertransradiant hemithorax. The importance of lateral decentering, and the explanation for its appearance due to rotation. Clin Radiol 29:125, 1978.
26. Crass JR, Cohen AM, Wiesen E, et al: Hyperlucent thorax from rotation: Anatomic basis. Invest Radiol 28:567, 1993.
27. Simon G: Personal communication, 1965.
28. Burko H, Carwell G, Newman E: Size, location, and gravitational changes of normal upper lobe pulmonary veins. Am J Roentgenol 111:687, 1971.
29. Lavender JP, Doppman J: The hilum in pulmonary venous hypertension. Br J Radiol 35:303, 1962.
30. Glazier JB, DeNardo GL: Pulmonary function studied with the xenon[133] scanning technique. Normal values and a postural study. Am Rev Respir Dis 94:188, 1966.
31. Dollery CT, West JB, Wilcken DEL, et al: A comparison of the pulmonary blood flow between left and right lungs in normal subjects and patients with congenital heart disease. Circulation 24:617, 1961.
32. Friedman WF, Braunwald E, Morrow AG: Alterations in regional pulmonary blood flow in patients with congenital heart disease studied by radioisotope scanning. Circulation 37:747, 1968.
33. Chen JTT, Robinson AE, Goodrich JK, et al: Uneven distribution of pulmonary blood flow between left and right lungs in isolated valvular pulmonary stenosis. Am J Roentgenol 107:343, 1969.
34. Riley RL: Effect of lung inflation upon the pulmonary vascular bed. In de Reuck AVS, O'Connor M (eds): Ciba Foundation Symposium on Pulmonary Structure and Function. London, Churchill, 1962, pp 261–272.
35. Chang CH: The normal roentgenographic measurement of the right descending pulmonary artery in 1,085 cases. Am J Roentgenol 87:929, 1962.
36. Whitley JE, Martin JF: The Valsalva maneuver in roentgenologic diagnosis. Am J Roentgenol 91:297, 1964.
37. Rigler LG: Functional roentgen diagnosis: Anatomical image—physiological interpretation. Am J Roentgenol 82:1, 1959.
38. Garland LH: Studies on the accuracy of diagnostic procedures. Am J Roentgenol 82:25, 1959.
39. Garland LH: On the scientific evaluation of diagnostic procedures. Radiology 52:309, 1949.
40. Garland LH, Cochrane AL: Results of international test in chest roentgenogram interpretation. JAMA 149:631, 1952.
41. Felson B, Morgan WKC, Bristol LJ, et al: Observations on the results of multiple readings of chest films on coal miners' pneumoconiosis. Radiology 109:19, 1973.
42. Herman PG, Gerson SJ, Hessel SJ, et al: Disagreements in chest roentgen interpretation. Chest 68:278, 1975.
43. Herman PG, Hessel SJ: Accuracy and its relationship to experience in the interpretation of chest radiographs. Invest Radiol 10:62, 1975.
44. Yerushalmy J: The statistical assessment of the variability in observer perception and description of roentgenographic pulmonary shadows. Radiol Clin North Am 7:381, 1969.
45. Kundel HL, Nodine CF: Interpreting chest radiographs without visual search. Radiology 116:527, 1975.
46. Kundel HL, Nodine CF, Carmody D: Visual scanning, pattern recognition and decision-making in pulmonary nodule detection. Invest Radiol 13:175, 1978.
47. Carmody DP, Nodine CF, Kundel HL: An analysis of perceptual cognitive factors in radiographic interpretation. Perception 9:339, 1980.
48. Samuel S, Kundel HL, Nodine CF, et al: Mechanism of satisfaction of search: Eye position recordings in the reading of chest radiographs. Radiology 194:895, 1995.
49. Tuddenham WJ: Visual search, image organization, and reader error in roentgen diagnosis: Studies of the psychophysiology of roentgen image perception (Memorial Fund Lecture). Radiology 78:694, 1962.
50. Berbaum KS, Franken EA, Dorfman DD, et al: Satisfaction of search in diagnostic radiology. Invest Radiol 25:133, 1990.
51. Tuddenbaum WJ, Calvert WP: Visual search patterns in roentgen diagnosis. Radiology 76:255, 1961.
52. Kundel HL, LaFollette PS Jr: Visual search patterns and experience with radiological images. Radiology 103:523, 1972.
53. Kundel HL: Visual sampling and estimates of the location of information on chest films. Invest Radiol 9:87, 1974.
54. Kundel HL: Perception errors in chest radiography. Semin Respir Med 10:203, 1989.
55. Tuddenham WJ: Problems of perception in chest roentgenology: Facts and fallacies. Radiol Clin North Am 1:277, 1963.
56. Oestmann JW, Greene R, Kushner DC, et al: Lung lesions: Correlation between viewing time and detection. Radiology 166:451, 1988.
57. Austin JHM, Romney BM, Goldsmith LS: Missed bronchogenic carcinoma: Radiographic findings in 27 patients with a potentially resectable lesion evident in retrospect. Radiology 182:115, 1992.
58. Carmody DP, Nodine CF, Kundel HL: Global and segmented search for lung nodules of different edge gradients. Invest Radiol 15:224, 1980.
59. Spratt JS Jr, Ter-Pogossian M, Long RTL: The detection and growth of intrathoracic neoplasms: The lower limits of radiographic distinction of the antemortem size, the duration, and the pattern of growth as determined by direct mensuration of tumor diameters from random thoracic roentgenograms. Arch Surg 86:283, 1963.
60. Shea FJ, Ziskin MC: Visual system transfer function and optimal viewing distance for radiologists. Invest Radiol 7:147, 1972.
61. Newell RR, Garneau R: The threshold visibility of pulmonary shadows. Radiology 56:409, 1951.
62. Goldmeier E: Limits of visibility of bronchogenic carcinoma. Am Rev Respir Dis 91:232, 1965.
63. Resink JEJ: Is a roentgenogram of fine structures a summation image or a real picture? Acta Radiol 32:391, 1951.
64. Heitzman ER: The lung. Radiologic-Pathologic Correlations. St. Louis, CV Mosby, 1984, pp 92–98.
65. Greening RR, Pendergrass EP: Postmortem roentgenography with particular emphasis upon the lung. Radiology 62:720, 1954.
66. Beilin DS, Fink JP, Leslie LW: Correlation of postmortem pathological observations with chest roentgenograms. Radiology 57:361, 1951.
67. Riebel FA: Use of the eyes in x-ray diagnosis. Radiology 70:252, 1958.
68. Alter AJ, Kargas GA, Kargas SA, et al: The influence of ambient and viewbox light upon visual detection of low-contrast targets in a radiograph. Invest Radiol 17:402, 1982.
69. Otto D, Bernhardt TM, Rapp-Bernhardt U, et al: Subtle pulmonary abnormalities: Detection on monitors with varying spatial resolutions and maximum luminance levels compared with detection on storage phosphor radiographic hard copies. Radiology 207:237, 1998.

CHAPTER 12

The Normal Lung: Computed Tomography

ANATOMY, 281
  Bronchi and Vessels, 281
  Interlobar Fissures, 286
  Interlobular Septa, 287
  Lung Parenchyma, 287
LUNG DENSITY, 291

ANATOMY

A cross-sectional computed tomographic (CT) image of the thorax is a two-dimensional representation of a three-dimensional slice; the third dimension—slice thickness, or CT collimation—can vary from 1 to 10 mm. All structures within the three-dimensional unit (volume = voxel) of the slice are represented as a two-dimensional unit (area = pixel) on the image. Thicker sections (7- to 10-mm collimation) allow assessment of the entire lung volume, which can usually be performed during one or two single breath-holds when using the spiral CT technique. On such thick sections, vessels can be clearly identified within the lung parenchyma as they course through the slice (Fig. 12–1). However, volume averaging within the plane of section results in decreased spatial resolution, and assessment of fine parenchymal detail requires the use of 1- to 2-mm-collimation scans. The resulting thinner sections allow assessment of airways as small as 1.5 to 2 mm in diameter and vessels down to the level of the interlobular septal veins and centrilobular arteries.[1, 2] However, because of the thin section, vessels cut in cross section may be difficult to distinguish from small nodules.[3]

Because of the considerable difference between the appearance of normal lung parenchyma on thick and thin sections, it is useful to review the main CT features of each separately. To facilitate the discussion, we will refer to 7- to 10-mm-collimation scans throughout the chapter as conventional CT, regardless of whether the images have been obtained by using conventional or spiral CT technique; 1- to 2-mm-collimation CT scans are referred to as high-resolution CT (HRCT).

Bronchi and Vessels

The appearance of bronchi and vessels depends on their orientation: when imaged along their long axes, they appear as cylindrical structures that taper as they branch; when imaged at an angle to their longitudinal axes, they appear as rounded structures if perpendicular to the plane of the CT or as elliptical structures when oriented obliquely (Fig. 12–2). The outer walls of pulmonary vessels form smooth and sharply defined interfaces with the surrounding lung. Central pulmonary vessels can be readily recognized as arteries by their location adjacent to bronchi. Central pulmonary veins can be identified as they course toward the left atrium. Although it is often impossible to distinguish peripheral pulmonary arteries from veins on conventional CT, differentiation can frequently be accomplished with HRCT; with this technique, veins can be identified as structures that separate secondary pulmonary lobules, extend into interlobular septa, and (sometimes) reach the pleura (Fig. 12–3);[4] by contrast, pulmonary arteries lie near the center of the secondary pulmonary lobule and do not abut the pleura.

Conventional CT allows visualization of all lobar bronchi and about 70% of segmental bronchi.[5] The recommended protocol for assessment of these airways consists of contiguous 3- to 5-mm-thick sections obtained during a single breath-hold with either dynamic incremental or spiral CT.[6] Assessment of smaller bronchi requires the use of HRCT. The limit of CT visibility is a 1.5- to 2-mm-diameter airway;[1] smaller branches cannot be visualized because their walls are less than 0.1 mm thick and therefore below the spatial resolution of current CT scanners. In normal individuals, no airways can be visualized within 1 cm of the costal or paravertebral pleura;[7] however, they can be identified within 1 cm of the mediastinal pleura (but not abutting it) in approximately 40%.[7] The smallest pulmonary artery that can be resolved by HRCT is approximately 0.2 mm in diameter and corresponds to the artery accompanying a terminal bronchiole.[1] The distance from this artery to the border of the secondary lobule or the pleural surface ranges from 3 to 5 mm (Fig. 12–4).

The outer diameter of a bronchus is approximately equal to that of the adjacent pulmonary artery.[8] However, the *apparent* bronchial wall thickness and the diameter of bronchi and vessels are markedly influenced by the display parameters (window level and window width) used. When an incorrect parameter is used, the error in estimating the thickness or size of a structure is related to its actual thickness or size, greater fractional overestimates or underestimates being made for small structures; that is, the apparent

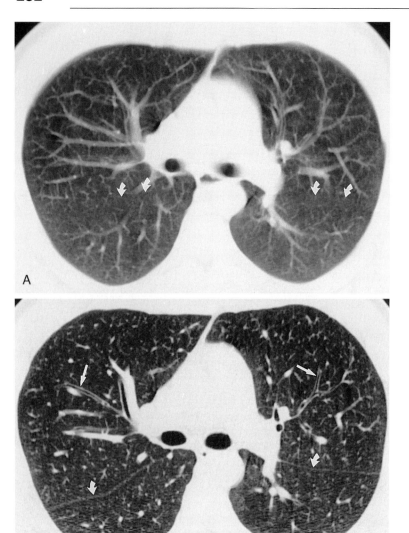

Figure 12–1. Comparison of Conventional and HRCT. A 10-mm-collimation CT scan at the level of the bronchus intermedius *(A)* demonstrates normal lung parenchyma and airways as visualized on conventional CT. Pulmonary vessels can be easily identified as they course within the 10-mm thickness of the CT section. A 1-mm-collimation HRCT scan *(B)* performed at the same level reveals sharper definition between vessels and bronchi and the adjacent lung parenchyma than seen with conventional CT. Bronchi measuring approximately 2 mm in diameter *(straight arrows)* are clearly identified on the HRCT image but not on conventional CT. Interlobar fissures *(curved arrows)* appear as sharply defined lines on the HRCT image as opposed to the broad areas of slightly increased attenuation on the corresponding conventional CT image. Both images were reconstructed with a high-resolution algorithm and photographed at a window level of −700 and window width of 1,500 HU.

Figure 12–2. Influence of Orientation of Vessels and Bronchi on CT Image. An HRCT scan illustrates vessels and bronchi running horizontally within the plane of the CT section and thus appearing as tubular structures *(straight arrows)*, bronchi and vessels running perpendicular to the plane of section and thus appearing as circular structures *(curved arrows)*, and bronchi and vessels running obliquely and thus appearing as elliptical structures *(open arrows)*.

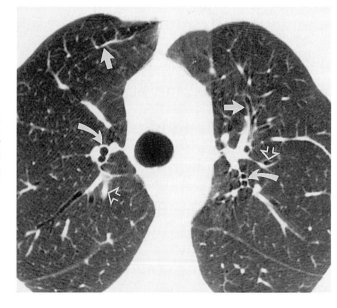

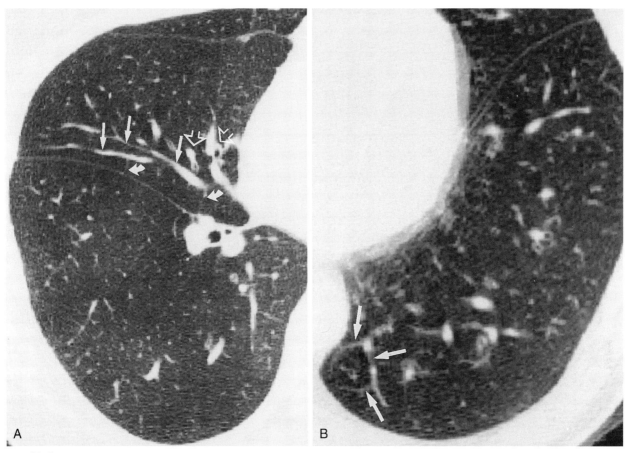

Figure 12–3. Pulmonary Veins and Interlobular Septa. A view of the right lung from an HRCT scan *(A)* reveals right middle lobe pulmonary veins *(straight arrows)* running almost horizontal to the plane of the CT section. Smaller feeding veins can be seen coming from interlobular septa near the right major fissure *(curved arrows)*. The larger veins also outline the margins of secondary pulmonary lobules. Right middle lobe pulmonary arteries and adjacent bronchi *(open arrows)* can be seen in cross section. A view of the left lower lobe from an HRCT scan *(B)* demonstrates pulmonary veins marginating a secondary pulmonary lobule *(arrows)*. An ectatic bronchiole can be seen near the center of the lobule.

change in size is inversely proportional to the size of the structure. Studies with phantoms have demonstrated that accurate assessment of the size of small parenchymal structures requires the use of a display level of −450 Hounsfield units (HU) (Fig. 12–5).[9, 10] In one investigation, hollow cylinders of sweet potato (possessing a CT attenuation value similar to that of airway wall) with diameters ranging from 1 to 5 mm and wall thickness ranging from 0.5 to 2 mm were measured with HRCT and with an optic micrometer.[10] The cylinders were placed in a sponge to simulate airways within inflated lung parenchyma. CT scans were photographed at various window levels and at window widths ranging from 100 to 750 HU. A window level of −450 HU provided measurements that were similar to those obtained with the optic micrometer; window levels of −550 to −900 HU resulted in progressive overestimation of cylinder wall thickness and underestimation of lumen diameter. No appreciable difference in measurement was obtained when using window widths between 100 and 750 HU. (The technical parameters of CT are discussed in greater detail in Chapter 13, page 311.)

The influence of window settings in the assessment of bronchial wall thickness was also evaluated in a study of inflation-fixed lungs in which measurements obtained with HRCT were compared with those obtained by using planime-

try.[11] In this study, the optimal window width was found to be 1,000 to 1,400 HU; a width narrower than 1,000 HU was associated with overestimation of bronchial wall thickness, whereas the use of widths of 1,500 to 2,000 HU led to slight underestimation of wall thickness (Fig. 12–6). For clinical practice, we recommend the use of a window level of −600 to −700 HU and a window width of 1,000 to 1,500 HU since these settings provide the best depiction of airways and lung parenchyma. However, it is important to realize that these display parameter settings result in an overestimation of the diameter of small structures and bronchial wall thickness and an underestimation of the diameter of the bronchial lumen.[9] Although a window level of −450 HU allows more accurate quantitative measurements, this setting is seldom used in clinical practice because the images are too dark and therefore do not allow adequate visualization of small parenchymal structures and focal abnormalities.[12]

Anatomically, the normal bronchial wall thickness is usually equivalent to approximately 10% to 15% of the bronchial diameter.[13, 14] This measure is slightly overestimated on CT because of inaccuracies in boundary detection, the CT measurement including the surrounding peribronchial interstitium.[14] In one study of 502 normal subsegmental bronchi in 30 patients (measurements being made by using a window level of −450 HU and a window width of 1,200

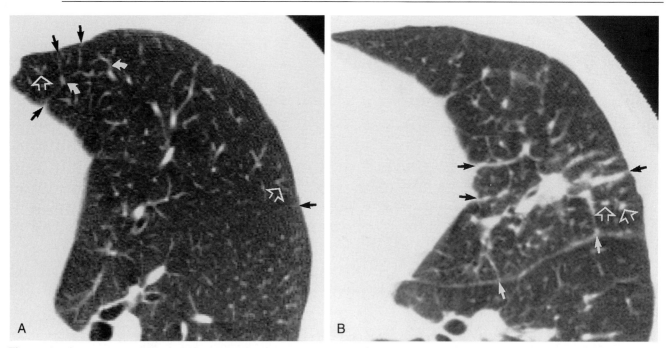

Figure 12–4. Normal and Abnormal Parenchyma. A magnified view of the left lung at the level of the lingula *(A)* from an HRCT in a 60-year-old man demonstrates normal interlobular septa *(straight arrows)* and peripheral veins *(curved arrows)* separating adjacent secondary pulmonary lobules. Small nodular and branching opacities *(open arrows)* located near the center of the secondary lobules and 3 to 5 mm from the pleura represent pulmonary arteries. An HRCT scan *(B)* in a 61-year-old man with relatively mild parenchymal abnormalities caused by sarcoidosis demonstrates thickening of the interlobular septa *(straight arrows)* and increased number and size of centrilobular opacities *(open arrows)*, findings consistent with a perilymphatic distribution of granulomas in the interlobular septal and bronchoarterial interstitium.

to 1,500 HU), the mean inner-to-outer bronchial diameter ratio was found to be 0.66 $\pm$ 0.06 (range, 0.51 to 0.86).[8] This ratio corresponds to a mean bronchial wall thickness equivalent to 17% of the luminal diameter with a range of 7% to 25%. There was no appreciable difference between measurements made by using 1.5-mm-collimation (HRCT) and 5-mm-collimation scans.[8]

In another investigation, bronchial wall area and percent wall area—i.e., wall area ÷ (wall area + luminal area)—were assessed by HRCT in six healthy men aged 25 to 50;[15] bronchial wall area was 9 mm² for airways less than 2 mm in diameter, 14 mm² for airways 2 to 4 mm in diameter, 25 mm² for airways 4 to 6 mm in diameter, and 43 mm² for airways greater than 6 mm in diameter. The relative airway wall area increased as the size of the airway decreased, the percent wall area increasing from 55% in airways greater than 6 mm in diameter to 81% in airways less than 2 mm in diameter. The apparent increase in percent wall area in smaller airways on HRCT may be due (at least in part) to increased inaccuracy in boundary detection as the airway wall becomes thinner. For example, the spatial resolution of HRCT is approximately 0.25 to 0.5 mm, whereas the thickness of the wall of a subsegmental bronchus is approximately 0.3 mm, making it difficult to obtain accurate measurements.[14]

The pulmonary artery–to–outer bronchial diameter ratio (ABR) was measured in a study of 30 patients without cardiopulmonary disease.[8] (Diameters were assessed at the level of subsegmental bronchi by using a window level of −450 HU and a window width of 1,200 to 1,500 HU.) The mean ABR was 0.98 $\pm$ 0.14 (range, 0.53 to 1.39)—a value comparable to that reported on chest radiographs in supine

normal subjects (1.04 $\pm$ 0.13).[16] Since an increased ratio of the inner bronchial diameter to the pulmonary artery diameter is one of the CT criteria for a diagnosis of bronchiectasis,[7] this ratio is another parameter that has been investigated in normal individuals. The measurement has been found to be influenced by altitude, presumably as a result of the combination of hypoxic vasoconstriction and bronchodilatation.[17–19] In one investigation of 17 normal, nonsmoking subjects living at 1,600 m and 16 living at sea level, the mean bronchoarterial ratio at a window level of −450 HU was 0.76 at altitude and 0.62 at sea level.[17] The results of this investigation are similar to those of the previous study done at sea level.[8]

Although the mean internal bronchial diameter–to–pulmonary arterial diameter and the mean outer bronchial diameter–to–pulmonary artery diameter ratios at sea level are approximately 0.65 and 1, respectively, there is considerable variation in these ratios within a given segment or lobe. In clinical practice, an inner bronchial diameter–to–pulmonary artery diameter ratio of greater than 1 is frequently considered to be indicative of bronchiectasis; however, such a ratio may be seen in normal individuals.[7, 18, 20] In one investigation of 27 healthy subjects performed in Denver (1,600-m altitude, the CT images being photographed at window levels of −700 to −800 HU and a window width of 1,400 to 1,800 HU), 15 (56%) had at least one bronchus considered subjectively to have an internal diameter greater than that of the adjacent pulmonary artery.[18] Of 142 bronchi assessed, 37 (approximately 25%) had an internal diameter greater than that of the adjacent pulmonary artery. In none of the normal subjects was the internal diameter of the bronchus more than 1.5 times greater than that of the adjacent pulmonary artery.

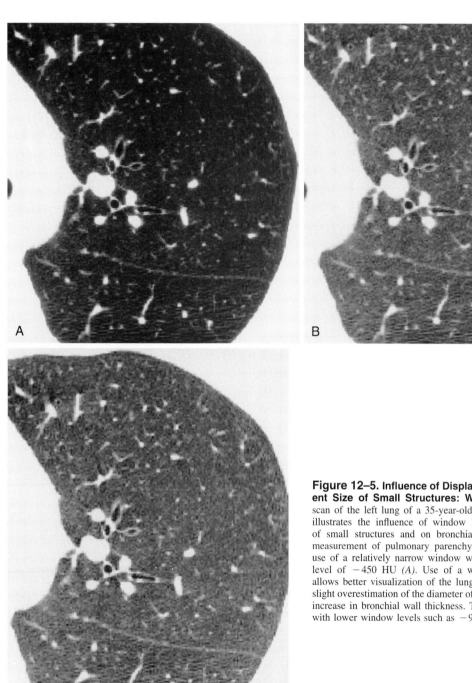

Figure 12–5. Influence of Display Parameters on Apparent Size of Small Structures: Window Level. An HRCT scan of the left lung of a 35-year-old woman with normal lungs illustrates the influence of window level on the apparent size of small structures and on bronchial wall thickness. Accurate measurement of pulmonary parenchymal structures requires the use of a relatively narrow window width (1,000) and a window level of −450 HU *(A)*. Use of a window level of −700 *(B)* allows better visualization of the lung parenchyma but results in slight overestimation of the diameter of the vessels and an apparent increase in bronchial wall thickness. This problem is accentuated with lower window levels such as −900 HU *(C)*.

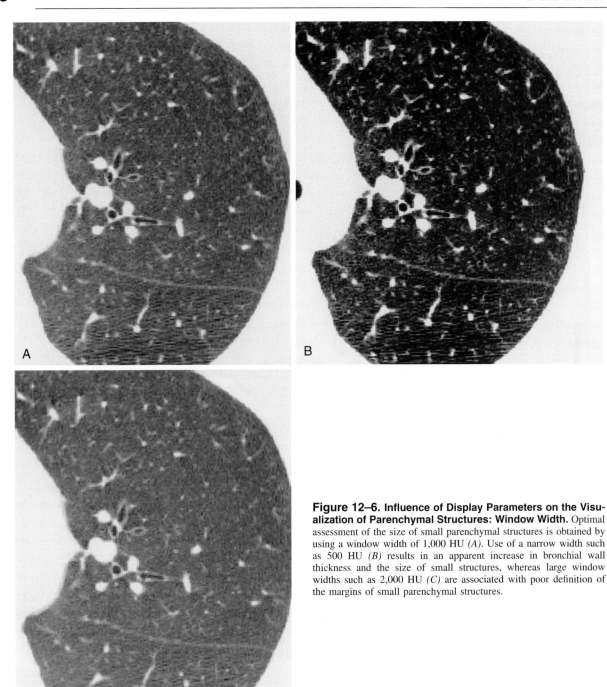

Figure 12–6. Influence of Display Parameters on the Visualization of Parenchymal Structures: Window Width. Optimal assessment of the size of small parenchymal structures is obtained by using a window width of 1,000 HU *(A)*. Use of a narrow width such as 500 HU *(B)* results in an apparent increase in bronchial wall thickness and the size of small structures, whereas large window widths such as 2,000 HU *(C)* are associated with poor definition of the margins of small parenchymal structures.

In another study performed at sea level, approximately 15% of healthy adults were considered on subjective assessment to have at least one bronchus with a bronchoarterial diameter ratio greater than 1.[7]

Interlobar Fissures

On conventional CT, the obliquely oriented major fissures can be seen as bands of either decreased or, less commonly, increased attenuation (Fig. 12–7);[21] when perpen-

dicular to the plane of section, they are visualized as lines *(see* Fig. 12–7). Whether obliquely oriented or perpendicular to the plane of section, the major fissures are characteristically seen as lines on HRCT.[21] Cardiac or respiratory motion may result in a double-fissure artefact, most frequently seen at the base of the left lung (Fig. 12–8);[22] in one review of high-resolution scans in 42 patients, this artefact was seen at one or more levels in 28 (67%).[22]

On conventional CT, the minor fissure is seen as either a broad triangular or oval area of decreased attenuation when it is horizontal (in the plane of the CT section) or as a band

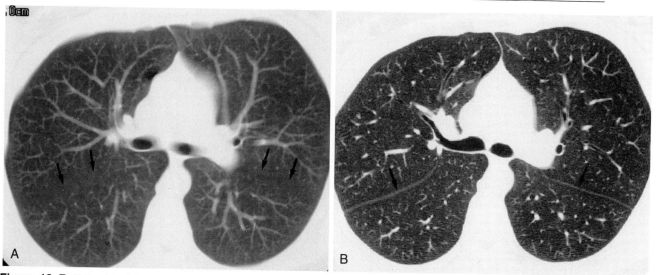

Figure 12–7. Major Interlobar Fissures on CT. A conventional CT scan *(A)* demonstrates the major right and left interlobar fissures *(arrows)* as broad bands of decreased vascularity and slightly increased attenuation. An HRCT scan at the same level *(B)* demonstrates the fissures *(arrows)* as sharply defined lines.

of decreased attenuation extending obliquely, caudally, and anteriorly (Fig. 12–9).[24] On HRCT, the fissure is usually visualized as a curvilinear line of increased attenuation that forms a quarter of a circle or a semicircle on its highest aspect just above the origin of the right middle lobe bronchus (Fig. 12–10).[24] It is most commonly located medially and occasionally laterally.[24] As it extends caudally and inferiorly, it can be visualized as a straight or slightly curved line.[24]

Interlobular Septa

Normal interlobular septa are seldom visualized on conventional CT. However, a few are normally seen on HRCT as thin, straight lines 1 to 2 cm in length and slightly more than 0.1 mm in thickness that extend to the pleural surface (Fig. 12–11; *see also* Fig. 12–3, page 283).[1, 2] They are most commonly identified in the anterior and lateral aspects of the lungs, where they are best developed;[1, 2] they are seldom seen in the central lung regions. Pulmonary veins coursing in the interlobular septa can often be identified on HRCT, particularly in the dependent lung regions. The pulmonary parenchyma between the interlobular septa and the centrilobular pulmonary arteries (lobular core) contains small vessels, bronchi, and interstitium below the resolution of CT. This area is seen as a region of homogeneous attenuation slightly greater than air.

Lung Parenchyma

Attenuation of the lung parenchyma is determined by the relative proportions of blood, gas, extravascular fluid, and pulmonary tissue.[25, 26] Normal lung parenchyma has a fairly homogeneous attenuation that is slightly greater than that of air. However, a gradient is normally present, the attenuation being greater in the dependent than in the nondependent regions (Fig. 12–12).[26–28] This gradient is attributable primarily to the influence of gravity on blood flow and lung inflation. Although the gradient is present whether the subject is supine or prone,[27] it is larger in the former position, presumably as a result of the compressive influence of mediastinal structures and the location of pulmonary veins. The gradient is also larger at the lung bases than at the lung apices.[28] The attenuation gradient is usually relatively small (on the order of 50 to 100 HU).[27, 28] In some subjects, a stripe of ground-glass attenuation measuring 2 to 30 mm in thickness is present in the most dependent lung regions.[29] This stripe—which has been referred to as subpleural dependent density or dependent opacity[14, 29]—is largely the result of passive atelectasis. Such atelectasis is reversible with a change in posture and can thus be readily distinguished from interstitial or air-space disease by repeating the scan with the patient prone (Fig. 12–13).[3, 29]

The anteroposterior increase in attenuation is not homogeneous. For example, there is typically a discontinuity at

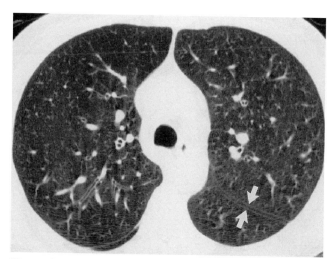

Figure 12–8. Double Fissure Artefact. An HRCT scan in a 40-year-old woman demonstrates a double fissure artefact caused by cardiac pulsation *(arrows)*. Note the blurring of the vessels in the superior segment of the left lower lobe and the normal appearance of the right major fissure.

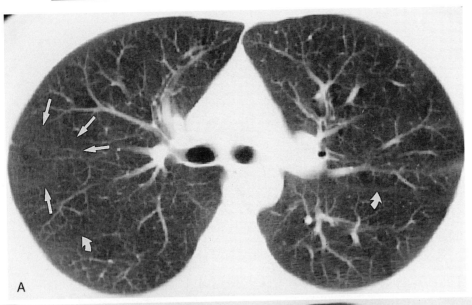

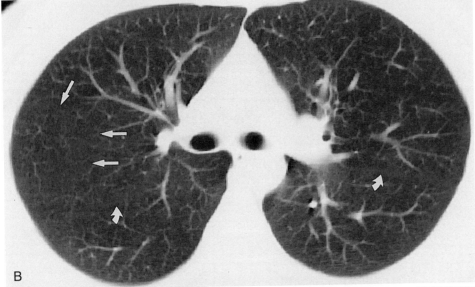

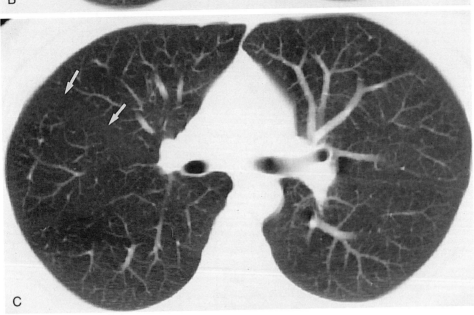

Figure 12–9. Right Minor Fissure on Conventional CT. A conventional CT scan at the level of the right upper lobe bronchus *(A)* reveals the right minor fissure as a triangular area of decreased vascularity *(straight arrows)*. The major interlobar fissures are seen as bands of slightly increased attenuation *(curved arrows)*. At the level immediately inferior to the right upper lobe bronchus *(B)*, the right minor fissure is visualized as a curvilinear area with decreased vascularity *(straight arrows)*. A section at the level of the bronchus intermedius *(C)* demonstrates the fissure as a broad band of slightly increased attenuation and decreased vascularity *(straight arrows)*.

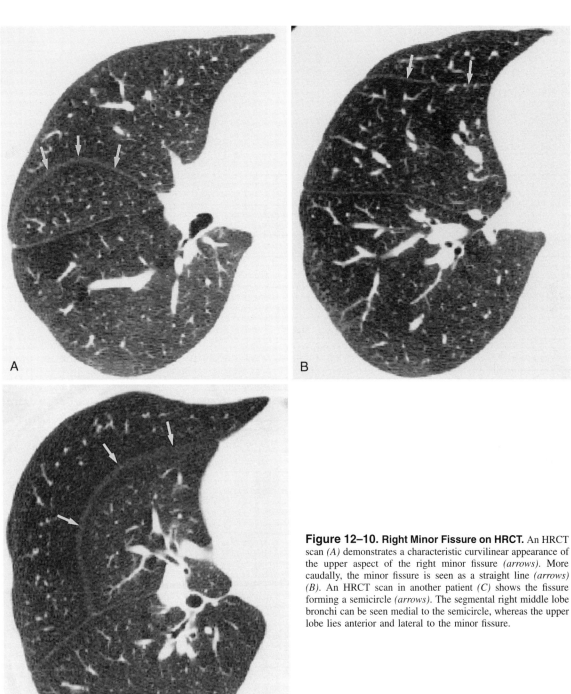

Figure 12–10. Right Minor Fissure on HRCT. An HRCT scan *(A)* demonstrates a characteristic curvilinear appearance of the upper aspect of the right minor fissure *(arrows)*. More caudally, the minor fissure is seen as a straight line *(arrows)* *(B)*. An HRCT scan in another patient *(C)* shows the fissure forming a semicircle *(arrows)*. The segmental right middle lobe bronchi can be seen medial to the semicircle, whereas the upper lobe lies anterior and lateral to the minor fissure.

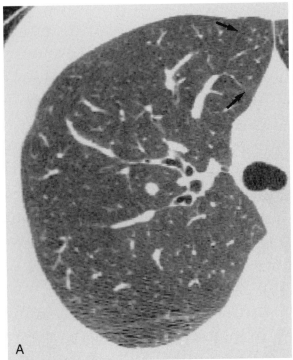

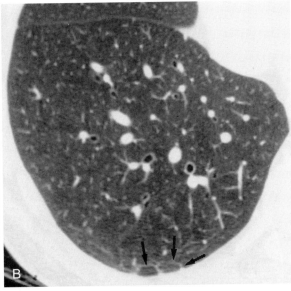

Figure 12–11. Normal Interlobular Septa. Views of the right upper *(A)* and right lower lobes *(B)* from an HRCT scan in a 35-year-old woman demonstrate normal interlobular septa *(straight arrows).*

the major fissure, with the posterior aspect of the upper lobes having greater attenuation than the anterior aspect of the lower lobes.[30] Furthermore, in some normal individuals the lingula and superior segments of the lower lobes have relatively low attenuation when compared with other lung regions;[30] although the reason for this lower attenuation is not clear, it has been attributed to a decrease in blood flow.[30] A

heterogeneous pattern of lung attenuation on HRCT, referred to as mosaic attenuation, is seen in 15% to 20% of normal adults.[20, 31]

CT scans of the chest are usually performed during suspended full inspiration. In selected cases, scans may also be performed following or during forced expiration. As lung gas volume is reduced, lung attenuation increases,[30, 32, 33]

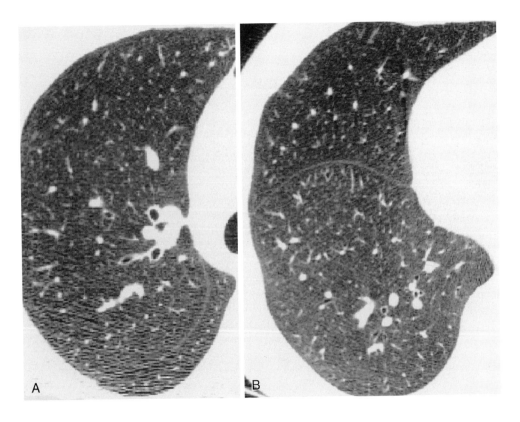

Figure 12–12. Normal Attenuation Gradient. HRCT scans through the right upper *(A)* and lower *(B)* lung zones demonstrate a normal increase in attenuation from the anterior to the posterior (dependent) lung regions. The attenuation gradient in the lower lung zones is slightly greater than in the upper.

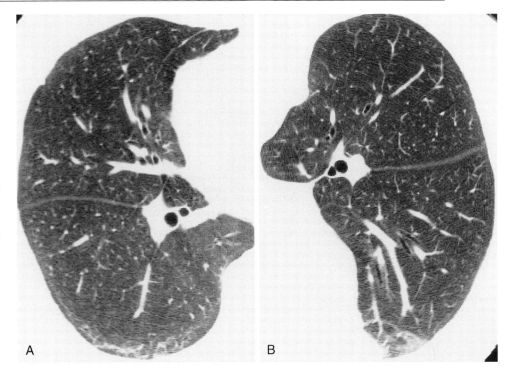

Figure 12–13. Dependent Opacity. A view of the right lung with the patient supine *(A)* demonstrates focal areas of increased opacity in the posterior dependent regions. A repeat scan with the patient prone *(B)* demonstrates the region to be normal. In the prone position, an increased opacity caused by dependent atelectasis is seen in the most anterior portion of the right middle lobe.

the increase being greater in the dependent than in the nondependent regions (Fig. 12–14).[32] However, this increase is variable in different lung regions, in one study ranging from 84 to 372 HU.[30] Furthermore, focal areas of low attenuation are frequently seen on expiratory scans, particularly in the superior segments of the lower lobes and in the anterior aspects of the right middle lobe and lingula (Fig. 12–15).[30] Such areas are presumably the result of focal air trapping.[30] The extent of air trapping in normal individuals is usually limited to small, localized areas involving a few secondary lobules; this can be seen on expiratory HRCT in up to 90% of subjects.[31] However, air trapping involving a total volume equal or greater than that of a pulmonary segment is seen in approximately 10% to 15% of normal subjects.[20, 31] Therefore, it is the extent and not simply the presence of air

trapping that is important in determining the presence of airway obstruction.

LUNG DENSITY

Measurement of lung density with CT is based on the existence of an approximately linear relationship between the attenuation of an x-ray beam of 65 keV (120 kVp) and the density of materials of low atomic number (ranging from nitrogen to water).[25, 34] Attenuation on a CT scan is expressed in terms of the Hounsfield unit scale, in which water is 0 HU and air is −1,000 HU. The relationship between the physical density—weight of tissue per unit volume—and the Hounsfield scale can be expressed by using a "scaled

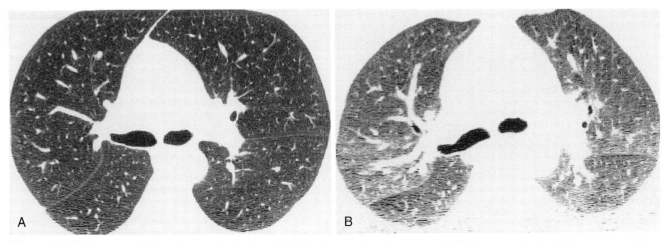

Figure 12–14. Increased Attenuation on Expiratory HRCT. Inspiratory *(A)* and expiratory *(B)* HRCT scans at the level of the main bronchi in a 35-year-old woman demonstrate the normal increase in attenuation seen at low lung volumes. The attenuation gradient from least dependent to most dependent lung regions is more readily seen on the expiratory CT scan. Note that the increase in attenuation is not homogeneous inasmuch as a discontinuity is present at the level of the major fissures, the posterior aspect of the upper lobes having greater attenuation than the superior segments of the left lower lobes.

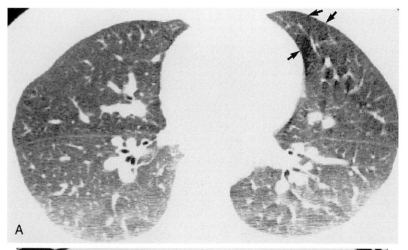

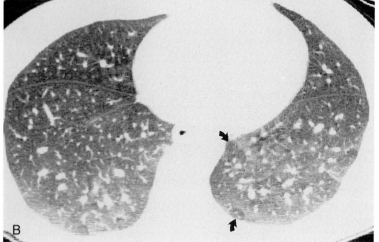

Figure 12–15. Expiratory HRCT Scans. HRCT scans (*A* and *B*) performed at the end of a maximal expiration in a 35-year-old woman with normal lungs demonstrate an attenuation gradient. Focal areas of decreased attenuation are present in the lingula *(straight arrows)* and in the lower lobes *(curved arrows)*, presumably a result of focal air trapping.

CT quotient," which is obtained by adding 1,000 to the Hounsfield value and then dividing by 1,000. With this formulation, CT quotient values that range from air to water are approximately equal to the physical density in grams per milliliter.[25, 26] For example, a CT attenuation value of −880 HU (approximately the mean value for normal lung at total lung capacity) represents a scaled CT quotient of 120 or a density equivalent of 0.12 gm/ml. The validity of this concept has been confirmed by scanning phantom materials of known density and measuring tissue density in experimental animals with CT scans and gravitometrically.[25, 26] In the latter instance, CT density has been recorded from scans of intact frozen dog thoraces and compared with the gravitometric measurement of the same volume of lung (1-cm-thick frozen slices) at the level of the scan; the CT estimate of lung density in a single slice was within 4% of the gravitometric measurement.

Normal lung attenuation is influenced by the degree of inflation and capillary blood volume and varies considerably between lung regions (Fig. 12–16) and at different times in the normal respiratory cycle. To obtain accurate measurements, it is necessary to use spirometrically gated CT. This procedure allows the selection of a specific point in the respiratory cycle at which flow can be interrupted by closing a valve in the spirometer and CT can be obtained.[33, 35] With this technique, the mean lung attenuation in a normal subject

has been shown to be approximately −760 HU at 20% vital capacity, −835 HU at 50% vital capacity, and −860 HU at 80% vital capacity.[35] By linear extrapolation it has been estimated that the mean lung attenuation away from visible vessels at 0% and 100% vital capacity would be −730 HU and −895 HU, respectively, which corresponds to a change in lung density of 0.27 to 0.105 gm/ml.[33] In a study in which HRCT was performed in 42 healthy subjects who were encouraged "to make all possible efforts to reach total lung capacity," the mean lung attenuation was found to be −866 HU, which corresponds to a mean lung density of 0.134 gm/ml.[36]

Differences in attenuation between dependent and nondependent lung regions have been assessed in an HRCT study of six healthy male volunteers.[33] Mean differences in lung attenuation between dependent and nondependent lung regions at 10%, 50%, and 90% vital capacity with the subject supine were approximately 70, 51, and 40 HU, respectively, for the apical portions of the lung and 130, 57, and 26 HU, respectively, for the basal regions. With the subject prone, the values were approximately 126, 63, and 19 HU for the upper lung zones and 112, 64, and 48 HU for the lower lung zones. This attenuation gradient was significantly greater at a lung volume of 10% vital capacity than at a volume of 90% vital capacity in both the supine and prone positions. For both positions, differences in lung attenuation for lung

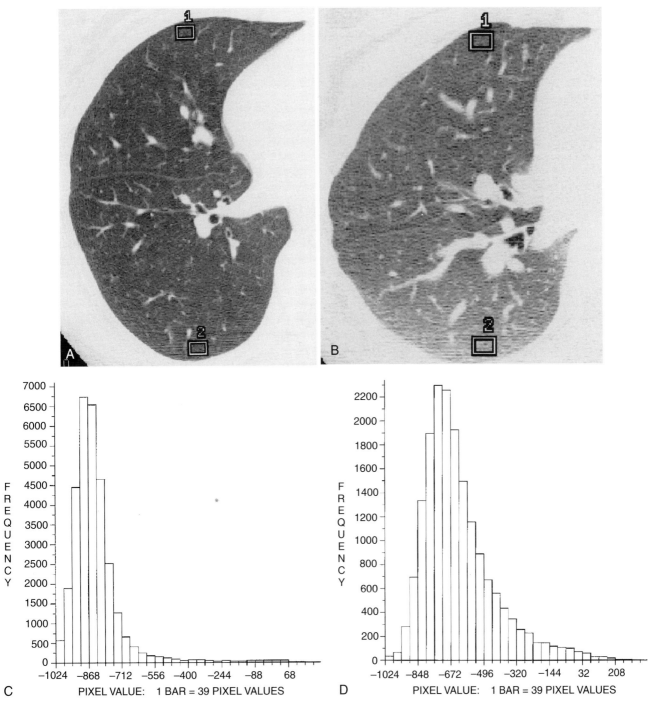

Figure 12–16. Measurements of Lung Attenuation. A view of the right lung from an HRCT scan obtained at the level of the inferior pulmonary vein at end-inspiration *(A)* reveals a slight anteroposterior gradient. Measurements of lung attenuation away from vessels in the most anterior aspect *(box 1)* showed a mean attenuation of −868 HU as compared with −823 HU in the most dependent lung region *(box 2)*. An HRCT scan performed at the same level at end-expiration *(B)* shows a diffuse increase in attenuation of the lung and an increase in the attenuation gradient. The mean attenuation in the most anterior aspect of the lung *(box 1)* was −748 HU and that in the most dependent portion *(box 2)* was −391 HU. (However, there was considerable variation in the attenuation values, the standard deviation of the four measurements ranging from 65 to 175 HU.) A plot of frequency versus pixel attenuation values *(C)* shows a wide range of attenuation values. This frequency distribution includes lung parenchyma as well as intrapulmonary vessels, except for the right inferior pulmonary vein and segmental pulmonary arteries and bronchi. Frequency distribution analysis at end-expiration *(D)* shows an overall increase in attenuation values.

volumes of 90% and 10% vital capacity were significantly greater in the dependent than in the nondependent regions. Mean differences between attenuation at lung volumes of 90% and 10% vital capacity in dependent areas were 160 HU when the subject was supine and 173 HU when the subject was prone.[33] There is also a small cephalocaudal gradient in lung density. In one investigation in which attenuation values were measured on spirometrically gated HRCT scans performed at 50% vital capacity, the mean attenuation value was -799 HU above the tracheal carina, -798 HU at the tracheal carina, and -773 HU below the carina.[37]

The regional gradient in lung expansion measured with CT has been used to estimate the pleural pressure gradient; the lung pressure-volume curve was measured and used to calculate the expected anteroposterior differences in pleural pressure that would yield the observed density gradient. The estimated value of approximately 0.25 cm H_2O per centimeter distance is virtually identical to what has been measured experimentally.[38]

Although the mean attenuation values within any given area of lung show a relatively smooth gradient from the apical to the caudal regions and from the nondependent to the most dependent regions, there is a wide range of attenuation values within any unit volume (voxel) or pixel (*see* Fig. 12–16). In one study, frequency distribution analysis demonstrated that approximately 13% of the lung had attenuation values less than -900 HU, 57% had attenuation values between -899 and -800 HU, 17% had attenuation values between -799 and -700 HU, and 13% had attenuation values greater than -699 HU.[37]

Spirometrically controlled CT has been performed in relatively few centers and has had limited application in daily clinical practice. However, since it allows accurate control of lung volume, highly reproducible measurements of lung attenuation can be obtained.[39] For example, in one study in which HRCT scans were performed twice at 50% vital capacity in 24 adult patients with pulmonary disease, the mean difference in attenuation values between the two sets of scans was only 7 HU (range, 0 to 24 HU).[39]

A number of investigators have also assessed lung attenuation values after a normal or a deep breath without the use of spirometric gating.[27, 28, 40, 41] The main disadvantage of this method is that the degree of inspiration is variable between patients and between different examinations in the same patient. Although it has been claimed that these studies were performed at total lung capacity, correlation of lung volume on CT with plethysmographic and helium dilution lung volumes in one study demonstrated that the end-inspiratory CT volumes obtained in supine patients were virtually identical to those of functional residual capacity in the sitting position.[42]

In another investigation, the normal inspiratory and dynamic expiratory attenuation values were measured in 10 healthy men by using an electron beam scanner and 3-mm collimation.[30] Considerable variation was found in the increase in lung attenuation that occurred during forced exhalation when measurements from all subjects, subject positions, lung levels, and lung regions were considered. In 3 subjects, portions of the lingula failed to show a normal increase in attenuation when compared with other segments of the lungs. In addition, 3 subjects showed air trapping in one or several secondary pulmonary lobules at various sites. Excluding those areas that appeared to trap air, the increase in lung attenuation that occurred from full inspiration to full expiration ranged from 84 to 372 HU. With the exception of a single value, in both the prone and supine positions and at all lung levels, dependent lung regions showed a greater increase in lung attenuation during rapid exhalation than did nondependent lung regions. In the supine position, the average increase in lung attenuation during exhalation was 219 HU in dependent lung regions and 171 HU in nondependent lung regions. In the prone position, the average attenuation increased by 227 HU in dependent regions and by 185 HU in nondependent regions. There was a significant correlation between the decrease in cross-sectional area and the increase in lung attenuation in each of the lung zones.

The effects of age and sex were assessed in a prospective study of 42 lifelong nonsmoking volunteers ranging in age from 23 to 71 years (mean $\pm$ SD, 42 $\pm$ 14 years).[36] Scans were performed by using 1-mm-collimation HRCT. The mean lung attenuation at total lung capacity was -866 HU (SD, 15; range, -984 to -824 HU). There was no significant difference in mean attenuation values between men and women. There was also no significant correlation between mean lung density and age, although there was slight correlation ($r = 0.39$) between age and the percentage of lung attenuation values less than -950 HU.

In summary, lung attenuation values vary considerably in different regions of the lung and are markedly influenced by lung volume. Furthermore, values are also affected by the type of CT scanner, by kilovoltage, by patient size, and by the particular region of lung being assessed.[43, 44] As a result, measurements of lung attenuation have a limited role in clinical assessment of the lung parenchyma. The one exception is the use of attenuation values to determine the presence, distribution, and extent of emphysema.

REFERENCES

1. Murata K, Itoh H, Todo G, et al: Centrilobular lesions of the lung: Demonstration by high-resolution CT and pathologic correlation. Radiology 161:641, 1986.
2. Webb WR, Stein MG, Finkbeiner WE, et al: Normal and diseased isolated lungs: High-resolution CT. Radiology 166:81, 1988.
3. Primack SL, Remy-Jardin M, Remy J, Müller NL: High-resolution CT of the lungs: Pitfalls in the diagnosis of infiltrative lung disease. Am J Roentgenol 167:413, 1996.
4. Itoh H, Murata K, Konishi J, et al: Diffuse lung disease: Pathologic basis for the high-resolution computed tomography findings. J Thorac Imaging 8:176, 1993.
5. Osborne D, Vock P, Godwin JD, et al: CT identification of broncho-pulmonary segments: 50 normal subjects. Am J Roentgenol 142:47, 1984.
6. Naidich DP, Harkin TJ: Airways and lung: Correlation of CT with fiberoptic bronchoscopy. Radiology 197:1, 1995.
7. Kim JS, Müller NL, Park CS, et al: Cylindrical bronchiectasis: Diagnostic findings at thin-section CT. Am J Roentgenol 168:751, 1997.
8. Kim SJ, Im JG, Kim IO, et al: Normal bronchial and pulmonary arterial diameters measured by thin section CT. J Comput Assist Tomogr 19:365, 1995.
9. Webb WR, Gamsu G, Wall SD, et al: CT of a bronchial phantom: Factors affecting appearance and size measurements. Invest Radiol 19:394, 1984.
10. McNamara AE, Müller NL, Okazawa M, et al: Airway narrowing in excised canine lungs measured by high-resolution computed tomography. J Appl Physiol 73:307, 1992.
11. Bankier AA, Fleischmann D, Mallek R, et al: Bronchial wall thickness: Appropriate window settings for thin-section CT and radiologic-anatomic correlation. Radiology 199:831, 1996.
12. Müller NL, Miller RR: Diseases of the bronchioles: CT and histopathologic findings. Radiology 196:3, 1995.
13. Weibel ER, Taylor CR: Design and structure of the human lung. In Pulmonary Diseases and Disorders. New York, McGraw-Hill, 1988, p 11.
14. Webb WR, Müller NL, Naidich D: High-Resolution CT of the Lung. 2nd ed. New York, Lippincott-Raven, 1996.
15. Okazawa M, Müller NL, McNamara AE, et al: Human airway narrowing measured using high resolution computed tomography. Am J Respir Crit Care Med 154:1557, 1996.
16. Woodring JH: Pulmonary artery–bronchus ratios in patients with normal lungs, pulmonary vascular plethora, and congestive heart failure. Radiology 179:115, 1991.
17. Kim JS, Müller NL, Park CS, et al: Broncho-arterial ratio on thin-section CT: Comparison between high-altitude and sea level. J Comput Assist Tomogr 21:306, 1997.
18. Lynch DA, Newell JD, Tschomper BA, et al: Uncomplicated asthma in adults: Comparison of CT appearance of the lungs in asthmatic and healthy subjects. Radiology 188:829, 1993.
19. Herold CJ, Wetzel RC, Robotham JL, et al: Acute effects of increased intravascular volume and hypoxia on the pulmonary circulation: Assessment with high-resolution CT. Radiology 183:665, 1992.
20. Worthy SA, Park CS, Kim JS, et al: Bronchiolitis obliterans after lung transplantation: High-resolution CT findings in 15 patients. Am J Roentgenol 169:673, 1997.
21. Glazer HS, Anderson DJ, DiCroce JJ, et al: Anatomy of the major fissure: Evaluation with standard and thin-section CT. Radiology 180:839, 1991.
22. Mayo JR, Müller NL, Henkelman RM: The double-fissure sign: A motion artifact on thin-section CT scans. Radiology 165:580, 1987.
23. Frija J, Schmit P, Katz M, et al: Computed tomography of the pulmonary fissures: Normal anatomy. J Comput Assist Tomogr 6:1069, 1982.
24. Berkmen YM, Auh YH, Davis SD, et al: Anatomy of the minor fissure: Evaluation with thin-section CT. Radiology 170:647, 1989.
25. Hedlund LW, Vock P, Effmann EL: Evaluating lung density by computed tomography. Semin Respir Med 5:76, 1983.
26. Hedlund LW, Vock P, Effmann EL: Computed tomography of the lung: Densitometric studies. Radiol Clin North Am 21:775, 1983.
27. Rosenblum LJ, Mauceri RA, Wellenstein DE, et al: Density patterns in the normal lung as determined by computed tomography. Radiology 137:409, 1980.
28. Genereux GP: Computed tomography and the lung: Review of anatomic and densitometric features with their clinical application. Assoc Radiol 36:88, 1985.
29. Aberle DR, Gamsu G, Ray CS: High-resolution CT of benign asbestos-related diseases: Clinical and radiographic correlation. Am J Roentgenol 151:883, 1988.
30. Webb WR, Stern EJ, Kanth N, et al: Dynamic pulmonary CT: Findings in healthy adult men. Radiology 186:117, 1993.
31. Park CS, Müller NL, Worthy SA, et al: Airway obstruction in asthmatic and healthy individuals: Inspiratory and expiratory thin-section CT findings. Radiology 203:361, 1997.
32. Robinson PJ, Kreel L: Pulmonary tissue attenuation with computed tomography: Comparison of inspiration and expiration scans. J Comput Assist Tomogr 3:740, 1979.
33. Verschakelen JA, Van Fraeyenhoven L, Laureys G, et al: Differences in CT density between dependent and nondependent portions of the lung: Influence of lung volume. Am J Roentgenol 161:713, 1993.
34. Rhodes CG, Wollmer P, Fazio F, et al: Quantitative measurement of regional extravascular lung density using positron emission and transmission tomography. Comput Assist Tomogr 5:783, 1981.
35. Kalender WA, Rienmüller R, Seissler W, et al: Measurement of pulmonary parenchymal attenuation: Use of spirometric gating with quantitative CT. Radiology 175:265, 1990.
36. Gevenois PA, Scillia P, de Maertelaer V, et al: The effects of age, sex, lung size, and hyperinflation on CT lung densitometry. Am J Roentgenol 167:1169, 1996.
37. Rienmüller RK, Behr J, Kalender WA, et al: Standardized quantitative high resolution CT in lung diseases. J Comput Assist Tomogr 15:742, 1991.
38. Coxson HO, Mayo JR, Behzad H, et al: Measurement of lung expansion with computed tomography and comparison with quantitative histology. J Appl Physiol 79:1525, 1995.
39. Kohz P, Stäbler A, Beinert T, et al: Reproducibility of quantitative, spirometrically controlled CT. Radiology 197:539, 1995.
40. Goddard PR, Nicholson EM, Laszlo G, et al: Computed tomography in pulmonary emphysema. Clin Radiol 33:379, 1982.
41. Adams H, Bernard MS, McConnochie K: An appraisal of CT pulmonary density mapping in normal subjects. Clin Radiol 43:238, 1991.
42. Kinsella M, Müller NL, Abboud RT, et al: Quantitation of emphysema by computed tomography using a "density mask" program and correlation with pulmonary function tests. Chest 97:315, 1990.
43. Müller NL, Staples CA, Miller RR, et al: "Density mask": An objective method to quantitate emphysema using computed tomography. Chest 94:782, 1988.
44. Zerhouni EA, Boukadoum M, Siddiky MA, et al: A standard phantom for quantitative CT analysis of pulmonary nodules. Radiology 149:767, 1983.

PART *II*

INVESTIGATIVE METHODS IN CHEST DISEASE

CHAPTER 13

Methods of Radiologic Investigation

CONVENTIONAL RADIOGRAPHY, 299
  Projections, 299
    Posteroanterior and Lateral Projections, 299
    Lordotic Projection, 300
    Lateral Decubitus Projection, 300
    Oblique Projection, 301
  Basic Radiographic Techniques, 301
  Special Radiographic Techniques, 303
    Inspiratory-Expiratory Radiography, 303
    Valsalva and Müller Maneuvers, 305
    Bedside Radiography, 305
    Digital Radiography, 306
      Storage Phosphor Radiography, 306
      Selenium Detector Digital Radiography, 307
      Film Digitization, 307
    Radiologic Methods for Determination of Lung Volume, 308
CONVENTIONAL TOMOGRAPHY, 309
COMPUTED TOMOGRAPHY, 309
  Technical Parameters, 311
  Radiation Dose, 313
  Indications, 314
MAGNETIC RESONANCE IMAGING, 315
  Physical Principles, 315
    Relaxation Times, 317
    Magnetic Resonance Pulse Sequences, 317
  Indications, 320
BRONCHOGRAPHY, 322
ANGIOGRAPHY, 322
  Pulmonary Angiography, 322
    Technique, 322
    Complications, 323
    Indications, 323
  Aortography, 324
    Technique, 324
    Indications, 324
  Bronchial and Intercostal Arteriography, 325
    Technique, 325
    Indications, 325
RADIONUCLIDE IMAGING, 326
  Ventilation-Perfusion Lung Scanning, 326
    Technique, 326
    Indications, 330
  Gallium 67 Lung Scanning, 331
POSITRON EMISSION TOMOGRAPHY, 332
ULTRASONOGRAPHY, 333
  Indications, 333

The approach to the diagnosis of chest disease used in this book involves two basic steps: (1) *identification* of an abnormality on the chest radiograph; and (2) *correlation* of the radiographic findings with the clinical picture to arrive at a diagnosis that takes into account the results of special radiologic procedures, laboratory tests, pulmonary function tests, scintillation scanning, and other procedures such as bronchoscopy and pathologic examination of cytology and biopsy specimens.

In this chapter we describe the radiographic methods that we use. Emphasis is placed on the techniques that have proved most valuable in our experience. Procedures that others have used to advantage but that we have found unrewarding are described briefly, together with our reasons for regarding them as less useful.

The cornerstone of radiologic diagnosis is the chest radiograph. This statement cannot be overemphasized. All other radiologic procedures, including fluoroscopy, computed tomography (CT), magnetic resonance (MR) imaging, and angiography, are strictly ancillary. With a few exceptions, to which we refer later on, establishing the *presence* of a disease process on the chest radiograph should constitute the first step in radiologic diagnosis; if this first examination does not clearly show the nature and extent of the abnormality, additional studies can be carried out to *complement* the radiograph.

CONVENTIONAL RADIOGRAPHY

Projections

Posteroanterior and Lateral Projections

The most satisfactory basic or "routine" radiographic views for evaluation of the chest are posteroanterior (PA) and lateral projections with the patient standing; such projections provide the essential requirement for proper three-dimensional assessment. In patients who are too ill to stand, anteroposterior (AP) upright or supine projections offer alternative but considerably less satisfactory views.

Situations in which the performance of routine radiography are likely to be cost effective have been the subject of considerable study.[1] In one analysis of more than 10,000 chest radiographs of hospital-based patients, investigators concluded that routine screening examinations—obtained solely because of hospital admission regulations or scheduled surgery—are not warranted in patients under 20 years of age;[2] although the authors of this study also considered that the lateral projection could be safely eliminated from routine screening examinations in patients 20 to 39 years of age, it was believed that they should be included whenever chest disease is suspected and in screening examinations of patients 40 years of age and older. In a study in which routine preoperative examinations were assessed in 905 surgical admissions, investigators carried out clinical screening for the presence of factors that would make patients more likely to have abnormal radiographs:[3] of the 368 patients who had no risk factors, only 1 had an abnormal chest radiograph; by contrast, of the 504 patients who had identifiable risk factors, 114 (23%) were found to have significant radiographic abnormalities.

In a study of routine admission chest radiographs in a Veterans Administration population known to have a high prevalence of cardiopulmonary disease, radiographic abnormalities were identified in 106 (36%) of 294 patients;[4] however, these abnormalities were new or unexpected in only 20 patients and treatment was changed because of radiographic findings in only 12 (4%). Of even greater importance was the observation that in only 1 patient might appropriate treatment have been omitted if a chest radiograph had not been obtained. From this study the investigators concluded that the impact of routine admission chest radiographs on patient care is very small, even in a population with a high prevalence of cardiopulmonary disease. Similar conclusions were drawn in a retrospective study of routine prenatal chest radiographs of 12,109 consecutive pregnant women who gave birth at the Mayo Clinic;[5] of the 48 patients who showed appreciable radiographic abnormalities, *all* had a positive history or abnormal physical findings that would have suggested the presence of disease and the requirement for chest radiography.

A study with a somewhat different slant was carried out by a Harvard group in which the contribution of chest radiography to diagnosis was assessed in 1,102 consecutive patients with chest complaints in the emergency ward and ambulatory screening clinic of a large hospital.[6] The authors found that 96% of the patients younger than 40 years of age had no radiographic abnormalities indicative of an acute process, a normal physical examination of the chest, and no hemoptysis; if radiographs in the group younger than 40 years had been limited to patients with an abnormal physical examination or hemoptysis, 58% of the patients in that group would have been spared the examination and only 2.3% of the acute radiographic abnormalities in the entire population of patients under 40 years of age would have gone undetected. It is of some interest that these researchers found that in patients older than 40 years of age, chest symptoms were a sufficient indication for chest radiography, a conclusion also reached by other investigators.[2]

In a statement promulgated by the American College of Radiology, the following criteria for screening chest x-ray examinations were recommended:[7] that all routine prenatal chest x-ray examinations be discontinued, that routine chest radiographs not be required solely because of hospital admission, that routine periodic examinations unrelated to job exposure be discontinued, and that mandated chest x-ray examinations as a condition of initial or continuing employment have not been shown to be of sufficient productivity to justify their continued use for tuberculosis detection. Table 13–1 summarizes our recommendations on the use of

Table 13–1. RECOMMENDATIONS FOR THE USE OF CHEST RADIOGRAPHS

A. Indications for Chest Radiography
  1. Signs and symptoms related to the respiratory and cardiovascular systems
  2. Follow-up of previously diagnosed thoracic disease for the evaluation of improvement, resolution, or progression
  3. Staging of intrathoracic and extrathoracic tumors
  4. Preoperative assessment of patients scheduled for intrathoracic surgery
  5. Preoperative evaluation of patients with cardiac or respiratory symptoms or patients with a significant potential for thoracic pathology that may compromise the search for the result or lead to increased perioperative morbidity or mortality
  6. Monitoring of patients with life support devices and patients who have undergone cardiac or thoracic surgery or other interventional procedures
B. Routine Chest Radiographs Are Not Indicated in the Following Situations
  1. Routine screening of unselected populations
  2. Routine prenatal chest radiographs for the detection of unsuspected disease
  3. Routine radiographs solely because of hospital admission
  4. Mandated radiographs for employment
  5. Repeated radiograph examinations on long-term facility admission

Data from American College of Radiology: ACR Standard for the Performance of Pediatric and Adult Chest Radiography. Standards: American College of Radiology, Reston, VA, 1997, p 27; and American Thoracic Society: Chest x-ray screening statements. Am Thorac News 10:14, 1984. Reprinted with permission of the American College of Radiology. No other representation of the article is authorized without express, written permission from the American College of Radiology.

chest radiographs based on a review of the literature and the recommendations of the American College of Chest Radiology[8] and the American Thoracic Society.[9]

Lordotic Projection

The lordotic projection can be made in AP or PA projection.[10] A modification of the AP view seems to possess some merit:[11] instead of assuming the rather uncomfortable lordotic pose, the patient stands erect and the x-ray tube is angled 15 degrees cephalad. The chief advantage of this modification is its reproducibility.

The lordotic projection is advocated in three situations: (1) for improving visibility of the lung apices, superior mediastinum, and thoracic inlet; (2) for locating a lesion by parallax; and (3) for identifying the minor fissure in suspected cases of atelectasis of the right middle lobe.[12, 13] Although the technique is sometimes useful in these situations, in general a direct approach by CT yields greater and more precise information and should be the procedure of choice whenever available.

Lateral Decubitus Projection

For the lateral decubitus projection, the patient lies on one side and the x-ray beam is oriented horizontally. Since the dependent hemithorax is the side being specifically examined in the majority of cases, it is desirable to elevate the thorax on a radiolucent support such as a foam cushion or mattress. The technique is particularly helpful for the identification of small pleural effusions. Less than 100 ml of fluid may be identified on well-exposed radiographs in this position, whereas radiographs taken with the patient erect seldom reveal pleural effusions of less than 300 ml.[14] Radiography in the lateral decubitus position is also useful to demonstrate a change in position of an air-fluid level in a cavity or to ascertain whether a structure that forms part of a cavity represents a freely moving intracavitary loose body (e.g., a fungus ball).

A modification of the standard lateral decubitus projection that can identify small amounts of fluid in the pleural space more precisely has been proposed.[15] In this technique, a pillow is placed under the patient's hip so that the trunk slopes downward at an angle of about 20 degrees; the lower part of the arm is extended above the head and the trunk rotated dorsally so that the scapula parallels the horizontal table (to prevent the scapula from obscuring the lower thoracic margin) (Fig. 13–1). Radiography is carried out at full expiration, when the reduced volume of the thoracic cavity raises the fluid level to its maximum. (Although the rationale is undoubtedly correct, we believe that a film taken at moderate inspiration would provide better contrast between the relatively deflated lung and adjacent pleural fluid.) This

technique allows visualization of pleural fluid collections as small as 3 to 5 ml.[15, 16]

Oblique Projection

Oblique studies are sometimes useful in locating a disease process (e.g., a pleural plaque); however, in most situations we prefer to use CT.

Basic Radiographic Techniques

It should be self-evident that diagnostic accuracy in chest disease is partly related to the quality of the radiographic images themselves. As such, it is incumbent on all radiologists to ensure that the images on which their diagnostic impressions are based are of the highest quality. Careful attention to several variables is necessary to ensure such quality.

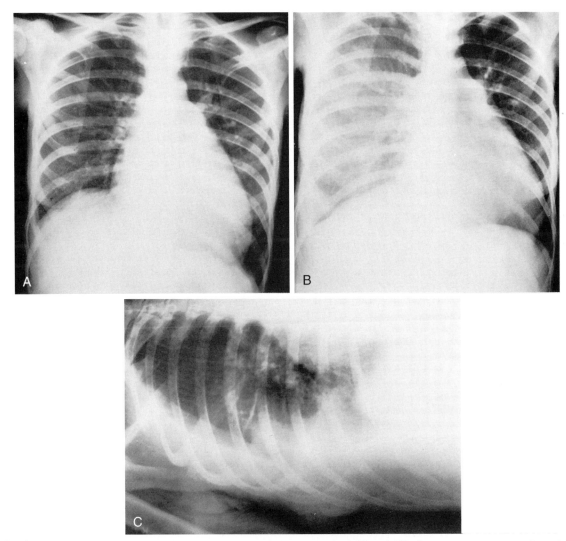

Figure 13–1. Value of Lateral Decubitus Radiography in the Assessment of Pleural Effusion. A posteroanterior radiograph in the erect position *(A)* shows apparent elevation of the right hemidiaphragm, although slight thickening of the axillary pleura in the region of the costophrenic sulcus suggests the possibility of subpulmonic effusion. A radiograph in the supine position *(B)* reveals a marked increase in opacity of the right hemithorax owing to the presence of fluid in the posterior pleural space. A lateral decubitus radiograph *(C)* shows the fluid to much better advantage along the costal margin and reveals how much fluid can be accommodated in the subpulmonic space.

Patient Positioning. Positioning must be such that the x-ray beam is properly centered, the patient's body is not rotated, and the scapulas are rotated sufficiently anteriorly so that they are projected away from the lungs. On properly centered radiographs, the medial ends of the clavicles are projected equidistant from the margins of the vertebral column.

Patient Respiration. Respiration must be fully suspended, preferably at total lung capacity (TLC). It has been shown that in erect chest radiographs, normal subjects routinely inhale to approximately 95% of TLC *without coaxing*;[17] thus, such radiographs can be of value in estimating lung volume and, by comparison with subsequent radiographs, in appreciating an increase or decrease in volume as a result of disease.

Film Exposure. Exposure factors should be such that the resultant radiograph permits faint visualization of the thoracic spine *and* the intervertebral disks on the PA radiograph so that lung markings behind the heart are clearly visible; exposure should be as short as possible, consistent with the production of adequate contrast. Unfortunately, all too frequently technical factors are such that optimal radiographic density is achieved over the lungs generally but without adequate exposure of the mediastinum or the left side of the heart (Fig. 13–2), a tendency that seriously limits radiologic interpretation. Moderate overexposure can be easily compensated for by bright illumination; underexposure, on the other hand, cannot be compensated for by any viewing technique and, since it prevents visualization of vital areas of the thorax, should not be tolerated in any circumstances. With perseverance, it is always possible to overcome problems of underexposure.

For a PA chest radiograph, the mean radiation dose at skin entrance should not exceed 0.3 mGy per exposure and the exposure time should not exceed 40 msec.[8] An optimally exposed radiograph presents the lung at a midgray level (average optical density, 1.6 to 1.9). (Optical density is a measurement of the ability of the film to stop light [film blackness], and it is equal to the logarithm of light incident on the film over light transmitted by the film [$D = \log Io/It$].) The focal-film distance should be at least 180 cm (72 inches) to minimize magnification.[8] (Focal-film distance is the distance between the focal spot of the x-ray tube and the radiograph.)

Kilovoltage. A high-kilovoltage technique appropriate to the film speed should be used;[8] for PA and lateral chest radiographs, we recommend using 115 to 150 kVp. (The abbreviation *kVp* is the peak voltage applied across the x-ray tube.) The use of high kilovoltage has several advantages over a lower range of voltage (60 to 80 kVp).[18, 19] Since the coefficients of x-ray absorption of bone and soft tissue approximate each other in the higher kilovoltage ranges, radiographic visibility of the bony thorax is reduced with only slight change in the overall visibility of lung structures. Furthermore, the mediastinum is better penetrated, thereby permitting visibility of lung behind the heart and the many mediastinal lines and interfaces whose identification is so important to the overall assessment of both the mediastinum and lungs. This technique can produce chest radiographs superior in all respects to those obtained with other techniques; in addition to better penetration of the mediastinum, films yield a clearer visibility of the pulmonary vasculature than can be obtained with lower peak kilovoltage techniques.

In a study designed to compare the detection of pulmonary nodules on chest radiographs exposed at 70 and 120 kVp, a clear improvement in observer performance was observed with the higher kilovoltage, presumably as a result of the wider latitude provided by this technique.[20] (Film latitude is the range of relative exposure [milliampere per second [mAs], expressed on a logarithmic scale, that will produce images with optical density within the accepted range for diagnostic radiology.) High kilovoltage also results in lower radiation exposure than does lower kilovoltage. The only drawback of the high-kilovoltage technique is the diminished visibility of calcium that results from the lower coefficient of x-ray absorption; however, this shortcoming has not proved troublesome in practice.

Grids and Filters. When using a grid, at least a 10:1 aluminum interspace grid with a minimum of 103 lines per inch is recommended by the American College of Radiology.[8] An alternative option uses an air gap technique in which a space of 15 cm (6 inches) is interposed between the patient and the x-ray film;[21, 22] since the air gap reduces radiation scatter by distance dispersion, no grid is required. When this technique is used, a constant focal-film distance of 10 feet is recommended.[23] In a comparative study of air gap and grid techniques, it was shown that the former can provide contrasts equal to those obtained with grids;[24] of the various combinations of distances possible, a focal-film distance of 10 feet with an air gap of 6 inches provides a good compromise. Patient exposure with an air gap technique was comparable to a no-grid, no–air gap technique and was less than that obtained with a grid.

Adequate exposure of the mediastinum while maintaining a proper level of exposure of the lung can be facilitated by the use of a tunnel wedge filter.[18, 25] Wedge filtration equalizes the densities of the thinner apical regions of the chest with those of basal regions; in addition to reducing exposure to the apices, it provides increased exposure over the width of the mediastinum. The wedge filter is constructed of various thicknesses of 0.003-inch copper foil to a maximum thickness of approximately 0.3 mm; in addition to the technical advantages of such filtration, it has been shown that a copper filter 0.32 mm thick reduces the entrance radiation exposure to the patient by 30% to 40%.[26] Despite its usefulness in equalizing exposure, the wedge filter does not necessarily improve the detectability of pulmonary parenchymal abnormalities. In a study comparing the effectiveness of the filter technique with that of the conventional (nonfilter) method, it was found that the two were not significantly different in the depiction of interstitial and airspace disease; however, the filter technique was slightly worse for the identification of nodules.[27] Another limitation of fixed filtration devices is that they are optimal only for perfectly centered radiographs in patients with the body configuration for which they are designed.[18]

Other techniques that have been developed to compensate for the large range of densities within the thorax include rapidly customized patient-specific filters[28, 29] and scanning equalization radiography.[30, 31] The latter technique incorporates a feedback system that modulates the x-ray beam intensity according to the body habitus of the individual patient. The best known of these systems is marketed as AMBER (Advanced Multiple-Beam Equalization Radiography.)[32] This system markedly improves visualization of me-

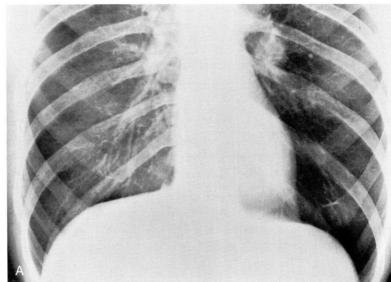

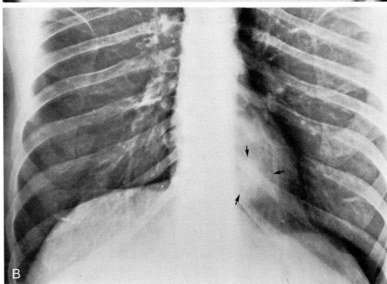

Figure 13–2. The Hazard of Radiographic Underexposure. A radiograph of the lower half of the thorax in posteroanterior projection *(A)* reveals no obvious abnormalities. The mediastinum and left side of the heart are underexposed. A more heavily exposed view (in slight lordotic projection) *(B)* demonstrates a somewhat poorly defined nodular mass situated in the lung behind the left side of the heart *(arrows)*. Even in retrospect, this lesion is not visible in *A*.

diastinal detail on PA radiographs[33] and detection of nodules overlying the mediastinum or diaphragm.[34] However, it decreases the contrast in the periphery of the lung,[35] requires a higher radiation dose,[36] has a higher cost than conventional radiography, and cannot be used for bedside examinations. It is therefore questionable whether the advantages of this system outweigh its disadvantages.

Special Radiographic Techniques

Inspiratory-Expiratory Radiography

Comparison of radiographs exposed in full inspiration (TLC) and maximal expiration (residual volume [RV]) may supply useful information in two specific situations. The main indication is the investigation of air trapping, either general or local. The former is exemplified by asthma or emphysema. In both these abnormalities, diaphragmatic excursion is reduced symmetrically and lung density changes little between expiratory and inspiratory radiographs; to demonstrate these features convincingly, expiration must be forced and preferably timed. When air trapping is local, as in bronchial obstruction or lobar emphysema, the expiratory radiograph reveals decreased ipsilateral diaphragmatic elevation, a shift of the mediastinum toward the contralateral hemithorax, and relative absence of density change in involved bronchopulmonary segments (Fig. 13–3).

The second indication for expiratory-inspiratory radiography is when pneumothorax is suspected and the visceral-pleural line is not visible on the standard inspiratory radiograph or the findings are equivocal. In these situations, a film taken in full expiration may show the line more clearly (Fig. 13–4) for two reasons: (1) at full expiration the volume of air in the pleural space is relatively greater in relation to the volume of lung, thus providing better separation of the pleural surfaces; and (2) the relationship of the pleural line to overlying ribs changes. (Despite these observations, it should be noted that the diagnosis of pneumothorax can be readily made on the inspiratory radiograph alone in the majority of cases.) In a study of 85 cases of pneumothorax and 93 without pneumothorax randomly reviewed by three independent radiologists, no statistical difference was de-

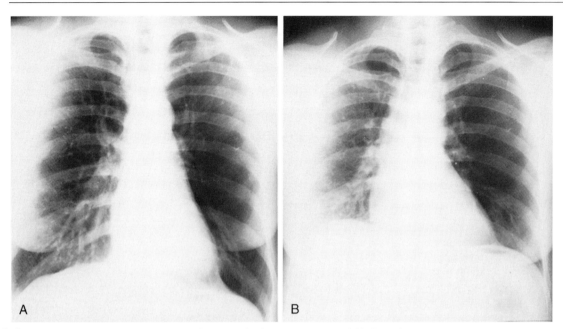

Figure 13–3. Value of Inspiratory-Expiratory Radiography in the Assessment of Air Trapping. *A,* A radiograph in full inspiration (total lung capacity) of a 31-year-old woman with unilateral obliterative bronchiolitis (Swyer-James syndrome). *B,* In full expiration (residual volume), the presence of left-sided air trapping is evidenced by a shift of the mediastinum to the right, a reduction in left hemidiaphragmatic excursion, and a marked discrepancy in overall density of the two lungs.

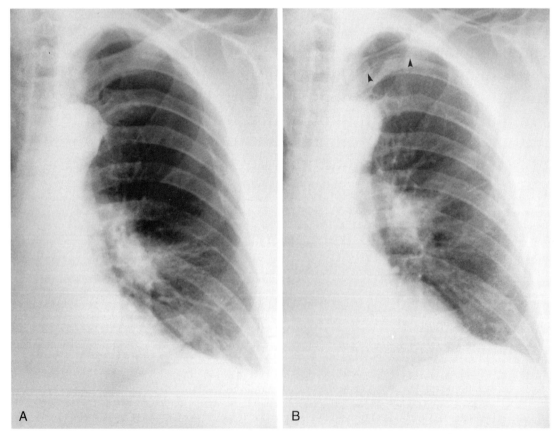

Figure 13–4. The Value of Expiration (Residual Volume) in the Demonstration of a Small Pneumothorax. Detail views of the left lung from a posteroanterior chest radiograph are shown at total lung capacity *(A)* and at residual volume *(B).* A small left apical pneumothorax is revealed. The visceral pleural line cannot be identified with conviction in *A* but can be seen clearly on the expiratory film *(arrowheads).*

tected in the sensitivity or specificity of expiratory and inspiratory radiographs for the detection of pneumothorax.[37] Four of the 85 cases were scored as definite pneumothorax on inspiration and as definitely not pneumothorax on expiration by all three readers, and 3 of the 85 cases were scored as definite pneumothorax on expiration and as definitely not pneumothorax on inspiration. As acknowledged by the authors, a limitation of this study was the method of determining whether pneumothorax was indeed present: a pneumothorax was considered present if the three observers, by consensus, agreed that it was present on either inspiratory or expiratory radiographs.

Valsalva and Müller Maneuvers

The Valsalva and Müller maneuvers—respectively consisting of forced expiration and inspiration against a closed glottis—may aid in determining the vascular or solid nature of intrathoracic masses. Lung volumes must be roughly the same on the two radiographs for accurate comparison. The end of quiet inspiration is probably the most satisfactory position from which to institute both maneuvers because it produces reasonably reproducible lung volumes and facilitates performance of the maneuvers. A change in size indicates a vascular lesion. Lack of change in size, however, is not helpful because it may occur with solid lesions or with insufficient effort. Either the erect or recumbent position can be used, depending on the information sought. Although potentially helpful, these maneuvers are seldom used in clinical practice.

Bedside Radiography

The number of requests for radiographic examination of the chest with a mobile apparatus at a patient's bedside (traditionally and almost universally called *portable*, with semantic inaccuracy) has increased enormously since its introduction owing partly to the growth of intensive care units (ICUs) and partly to the introduction of complex cardiovascular surgical procedures that require close postoperative surveillance. In many hospitals, these examinations account for 40% to 50% of all chest radiographs performed.[38]

Such radiographs are almost invariably technically inferior to those obtained in the standard manner in the radiology department itself. This inferior quality derives from multiple factors, some of which are uncontrollable (e.g., the patient's supine position, a short focal-film distance, and the restricted ability of many such patients to suspend respiration or to achieve full inspiration to TLC). Other factors, however, including the technical ones used in the exposure, are subject to control. Frequently, these radiographs are overexposed or underexposed, sometimes to a degree that limits or even precludes recognition of the subtle changes that are so important in the postoperative period. These difficulties often result in the radiologist either accepting an inferior product or arranging a repeat examination, with associated patient discomfort, increased radiation exposure, and increased cost. Some of these problems can be minimized by using a wide-latitude screen-film combination. (Film latitude is defined as the range of relative exposure [milliampere per second], expressed on a logarithmic scale, that will produce film density within the diagnostic range, i.e., between 0.25 and

2.0.) An optimally exposed bedside radiograph presents the lung at a midgray level (average optical density, approximately 1.4 to 1.7).[39] An alternative technique that is rapidly replacing the screen-film combination for bedside radiographs is digital radiography since it allows satisfactory images to be obtained over a wide range of x-ray exposures (*see* page 306).

In cooperative patients, upright radiographs at a 180-cm (72-inch) target-film distance are preferred. In uncooperative or comatose patients, semierect or supine radiographs may be performed at a 100- to 125-cm (40- to 50-inch) target-film distance.[39] It is recommended that the kilovoltage be between 80 and 100 kVp to optimize penetration and minimize scatter radiation.[38, 39] Image quality is markedly improved by using a 6:1 or an 8:1 grid;[38] however, antiscatter grids are used in only 10% to 15% of hospitals,[38] presumably because of the time and effort involved in ensuring careful alignment to avoid grid cutoff.

Since the patient is almost always postoperative or has severe illness, radiography often occurs in the supine position. Because of the shorter focal-film distance usually used and the AP direction of the x-ray beam, magnification of the heart and superior mediastinum often amounts to 15% to 20% as compared with 5% on conventional PA radiographs. Care must be taken to not misinterpret the magnification as organic enlargement. Radiography in supine patients is also liable to result in diagnostic error in relation to the pulmonary vascular shadows. As discussed previously, pulmonary blood volume is approximately 30% greater in supine than in erect subjects; as a result, pulmonary vascular shadows usually appear larger, especially in the upper lung zones. This impact of positioning is enhanced by the effect of gravity and consequent increased flow to the upper lung zones. Such a radiographic appearance must not be misinterpreted as evidence of pulmonary venous hypertension. All too frequently the degree of angulation of the thorax on bedside radiographs is not recorded, a deficiency that can lead to misinterpretation; a simple and effective device to measure patient position has been described.[40]

The diagnostic efficacy of bedside chest radiography has been the subject of several studies. In one study of the radiographs of 140 patients admitted to surgical and medical ICUs over a 2-month period (including routine morning radiographs as well as those performed after a change in clinical status), new findings or changes affecting the patient's management were found in 65% of the radiographs.[43] The findings included malpositioning of endotracheal or tracheostomy tubes (in 12% of patients in whom tubes were present), malpositioning of central venous catheters (in 9% of patients in whom catheters were present), and such interval changes as pneumothorax, atelectasis, and pulmonary edema (present in 44% of radiographs subsequent to the initial study). In another investigation, positive radiographic findings were discovered in 45% of bedside examinations;[42] the authors of this study concluded that such examinations were indicated in 94% of their cases.

The results of two studies of patients in a medical ICU indicated that 40% to 45% of routine morning radiographs had at least one clinically unsuspected finding or device malposition that influenced patient management.[43, 44] One of these studies involved a review of 1,354 examinations in a respiratory ICU;[43] the radiographs demonstrated findings that resulted in a change in the diagnostic approach or therapy in 364 (27%) and demonstrated an inadequately positioned catheter in 273 (20%). Of all bedside chest examinations, 169 (12%) resulted in the institution of a diagnostic procedure and 273 (20%) resulted in a change in therapy. Another group of investigators classified patients into four groups according to their primary diagnosis:[45] pulmonary, hemodynamically unstable cardiac, uncomplicated cardiac, and miscellaneous. Unsuspected abnormalities leading to a change in management were present in 57% of the pulmonary and unstable cardiac patients and in only 3% of the uncomplicated cardiac and miscellaneous groups suggesting that routine radiographs are indicated only in the first two groups.

In spite of these results, studies in which the role of routine morning chest radiographs has been assessed have yielded variable results, and the need for such radiographs, even for ICU patients receiving mechanical ventilation, has been questioned.[46] For example, in one study of 525 patients, the number in whom there was "major malposition" of any device was only 7 (1.3%);[47] the incidence of cardiopulmonary findings requiring immediate intervention was less than 1%. In a second study of 1,003 chest radiographs (including 480 daily routine examinations) from surgical ICU patients in which multivariate analysis was performed, the authors concluded that only the presence of a Swan-Ganz catheter or a clinically suspected abnormality justified having routine daily radiographs.[48]

From the various studies in the literature it seems reasonable to conclude that daily routine chest radiographs are indicated in ICU patients with acute cardiac or pulmonary problems, in patients receiving mechanical ventilation, and in patients with a Swan-Ganz catheter in place; they are not necessary in stable cardiac patients, patients admitted for cardiac monitoring, or ICU patients admitted because of extrathoracic disease. Chest radiographs are recommended after insertion of endotracheal tubes, central venous lines, chest tubes, and intra-aortic balloons.[47-50]

Digital Radiography

Since its inception, the discipline of diagnostic radiology has depended on photographic film as the primary vehicle for recording and interpreting the radiologic image. However, a change in this traditional approach has taken place in the form of inherently digital techniques, including diagnostic ultrasound, nuclear medicine, CT, MR imaging, and digital subtraction angiography (DSA). Although conventional radiography has lagged behind, during the past decade a number of technologic advances have enabled digital radiography to become an integral part of chest imaging. Even though its full potential has not been reached, several systems are available commercially and the clinical use of digital chest radiography is increasing at a rapid pace.

Digital radiography has a number of advantages over conventional screen-film systems.[33, 51] One of the most important is the wide exposure latitude, which is 10 to 100 times greater than the widest dynamic range of screen-film systems. During digital image processing, the systems automatically determine the range of clinically appropriate gray levels and produce an image within that range. As a result, the final image is virtually independent of absolute x-ray exposure levels. (A potential disadvantage is that patients

may receive unnecessarily high radiation doses that may not be detected because they do not result in perceptible alterations in image quality.) The wider latitude of digital systems allows them to be used in a much broader range of exposure conditions than possible with conventional systems and makes them an ideal choice in applications in which exposures are highly variable or difficult to control, such as bedside radiography. Another major advantage of digital radiography is related to the fact that it produces what are essentially electronic images; as a result, an image may be transmitted to any location, displayed at multiple sites simultaneously, and efficiently archived for later reference. The images may be displayed on video monitors (soft copy) or be printed onto film or paper (hard copy). Some of the limitations of the various digital systems include high cost, slow accessibility to stored data, and limited spatial resolution. Cost can be reduced by interpreting the images displayed on video monitors. Although several groups have demonstrated that radiologists prefer and have higher diagnostic accuracy when they use digitized hard-copy films than when they use video monitors,[52–54, 54a] others have found that image quality on monitors is comparable to that of hard copy provided the monitor has a matrix of at least 2,048 × 2,048 pixels[54b–d] and the maximum luminance is maintained at approximately 75 foot-lamberts.[54d]

Two main types of digital radiography systems are available commercially: those based on photostimulatable storage phosphor image receptors and those based on selenium-coated receptors. Also of considerable importance, particularly for teleradiology and picture archiving, is film digitization.

Storage Phosphor Radiography

Storage phosphor imaging (computed radiography) has been used mainly for bedside chest radiography because its wide dynamic range allows it to achieve consistent images over a wide range of x-ray exposures.[38, 55] Storage phosphor systems have a dynamic range of approximately 1:10,000 as compared with 1:100 for standard films;[56] that is, they are capable of producing diagnostic images over a much broader range of exposure, which results in a considerable decrease in the repeat rate for bedside chest radiographs.[57]

In the storage phosphor technology, a reusable photostimulatable phosphor rather than film is used to record the image. Plates coated with the phosphor are loaded into special cassettes that are outwardly similar to screen-film cassettes. During exposure, the receptor stores the x-ray energy and is then scanned by a laser beam, which results in the creation of visible or infrared radiation, the intensity of which corresponds to the absorbed x-ray energy. The resultant luminescence is then measured and recorded digitally.[58]

The digital image consists of a two-dimensional matrix of picture elements (pixels), each assigned a number representing the image parameter, such as the number of x-ray photons transmitted. The spatial resolution of the image is dictated by the size of the pixels relative to the size of the object to be imaged.[51] An image matrix of 2,048 × 2,048 pixels results in a spatial resolution of approximately 5 line pairs per millimeter for a pediatric chest (20 × 20 cm) and a resolution of 2.5 line pairs per millimeter for an adult chest (40 × 40 cm).[51] Spatial resolution, or resolving power, is the ability to record separate images of adjacent objects. It is determined by imaging a target made up of parallel lead strips separated by spaces equal to the width of the strips. The lead strips constitute the lines and the space between them the line pairs. A resolution of 5 line pairs per millimeter means that the system can record up to 5 lines per millimeter, each line being 0.1 mm in width and separated by a 0.1-mm gap. A pixel size of 0.2 mm or less has been shown to be necessary to achieve diagnostic accuracy equivalent to that obtained with a conventional screen-film image.[59] Larger pixel sizes limit detection of fine anatomic detail, subtle parenchymal abnormalities, and small pneumothoraces. To cover the average adult thorax, an image matrix of approximately 2,000 × 2,500 pixels is required to obtain a 0.2-mm pixel size.[33]

Another important consideration in the storage phosphor technique is the number of discrete gray levels. This parameter determines the dynamic range of the image—i.e., how well it reproduces small variations in x-ray attenuation. The number of gray levels is expressed as the number of bits. Most digital systems provide 8-bit (256 gray levels), 10-bit (1,024 gray levels), or 12-bit (4,096 gray levels) images. Optimal display is obtained with the use of 4,096 gray levels.[33]

The images obtained with storage phosphor technique can be viewed either on a high-resolution monitor or on film derived from a laser printer. The latter has been used most commonly because high-resolution monitors have lower contrast resolution.[38] Observer performance with digital radiographs displayed on a workstation is significantly lower, particularly for abnormalities associated with low-contrast information, such as interstitial lung disease.[60] Several groups have shown that films obtained by laser printing provide diagnostic information equivalent to that obtained by conventional radiography in the assessment of pulmonary, mediastinal, and pleural abnormalities (Fig. 13–5).[61, 62]

Although storage phosphor digital radiography has some advantages over conventional radiography, objective measurement of physical parameters such as spatial resolution and noise demonstrates that the overall image quality of storage phosphor radiographs is slightly inferior to that of an optimal conventional radiograph.[33] This slight loss of quality is of concern when assessing the presence of mild parenchymal abnormalities such as early interstitial disease.[33, 63] Another consideration is the relatively low quantum efficiency of storage phosphor technology, most systems requiring equal or higher radiation doses than used for conventional screen-film systems.[33] (Quantum efficiency refers to the ability of a system to absorb x-rays and to convert x-ray photons into light. The greater the quantum efficiency, the lower the exposure (milliampere-second) required to produce the same film density).

Selenium Detector Digital Radiography

Similar to the photostimulatable storage phosphor systems, selenium-based chest imaging systems use a receptor that allows a digital image to be adjusted after processing and displayed on a monitor or on film. These systems may consist of a selenium drum receptor—i.e., an aluminum drum 50 cm in diameter that is coated with a 0.5-mm-thick layer of amorphous selenium[64, 65]—or a flat plate selenium detector.[66] A grid can easily be incorporated into the system to decrease scatter.[67]

The main advantage of selenium-based detectors is considerably greater quantum efficiency than can be achieved by conventional screen-film systems and photostimulatable phosphor detectors.[67] In fact, the absorption of the selenium detector provides an effective quantum efficiency that is very close to the theoretical limit.[64] Furthermore, because of the smooth, homogeneous layer of the amorphous selenium used as the detector (as compared with the grain structure of the storage phosphor technique), the conversion process of the selenium system is relatively free of intrinsic noise sources.[64, 68] It therefore allows images to be obtained at a lower radiation dose and theoretically results in images with better diagnostic quality than can be obtained by either conventional screen-film combinations or storage phosphor techniques.[68]

In one study in which selenium detector digital chest radiography was compared with conventional PA chest radiographs, six independent observers rated the visualization obtained with the selenium detector to be better than that obtained with the conventional system in four regions (right lower lobe, upper lobes, ribs, and soft tissues), better than or equal to that obtained with the conventional system in four regions (retrocardiac, retrodiaphragmatic, hilum, and upper mediastinum), and equal to that obtained with the conventional system in four regions (right minor fissure, carina, azygoesophageal recess, and thoracic spine).[68] Some of the observers had a strong preference for the digital images, whereas others showed no preference.

Because of the advantages of the selenium system, it has been in daily routine use in some departments since 1995.[68] This system has an image matrix of 2,166 × 2,488 pixels, which results in a pixel size of 0.2 mm.[68]

Film Digitization

Film-based digital imaging systems convert standard radiographs into digital images.[69] Digitization is accomplished by measuring the transmittance of light through the film, converting the light to electronic signals with a photodetector, and quantifying the signal by using an analog-to-digital converter. A variety of methods may be used, including video cameras, scanning microdensitometers, and laser film scanners. The first of these devices produces rapid digitization but has limited spatial resolution and dynamic range.[51] Thus although the image quality is not sufficient for primary diagnosis, because of its high speed and low cost, video scanning is commonly used in teleradiology systems.[49] The best image quality is obtained with laser film scanners.[70] These devices can provide spatial resolution from 2.5 to 5 line pairs per millimeter (0.1- to 0.2-mm pixel size) and 1,026 shades of gray.[51] The quality of the image is affected not only by the digitizing technique but also by the quality of the original radiograph used for digitization.[71]

Several groups have compared the quality of digitized images with that of film; in general, the former have lower spatial resolution and result in lower diagnostic accuracy.[51, 72–74] However, in one study of 2,048-line monitors and interactive video display systems, the diagnostic accuracy associated with digitized images was found to be comparable to

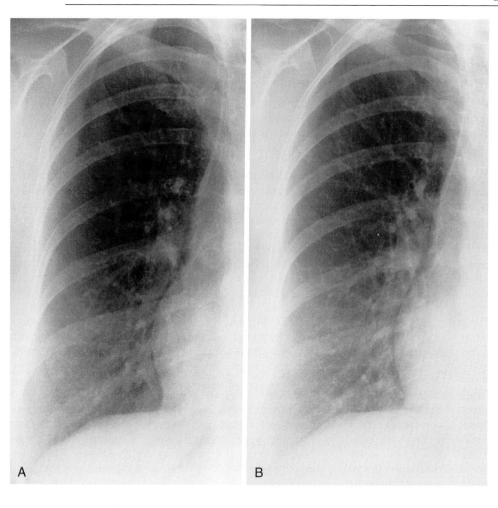

Figure 13–5. Storage Phosphor and Conventional Radiography. Views of the normal right lung of a 54-year-old woman obtained by using storage phosphor technology *(A)* and conventional radiography *(B)* demonstrate comparable visualization of parenchymal detail.

that of film.[75] Regardless of the technique used, film digitization is limited by the dynamic range of the original radiograph, involves additional expense and delay, and has lower signal-to-noise ratio than the original analog film image because of the process of digitization.[51, 76] The main applications of the procedure have been in teleradiology and storage of existing film-based examinations in picture-archiving communication systems.

Radiologic Methods for Determination of Lung Volume

Many radiographic methods have been devised for estimating lung volume; unfortunately, most are inaccurate except as a rough gauge.[77] This lack of accuracy is largely a result of the awkward shape of the thorax and difficulty in estimating the volumetric contributions of the diaphragmatic domes, heart, and pulmonary blood and tissue.

One method described in 1960 pictured the lungs as a stack of five horizontal elliptical cylindroids.[78] The volume of each of these five segments was measured and their total was the capacity of the thorax. The volumes of the heart, the right and left hemidiaphragms, the intrathoracic extracardiac blood, and the lung tissue were totaled and subtracted from the thoracic capacity to yield the total volume of gas in the lungs. Measurements thus obtained approximated those obtained by conventional means in healthy subjects and in patients with congestive heart failure, but they were significantly greater in patients with emphysema when compared

with figures obtained by gas dilution measurement of TLC. However, the results of a subsequent study showed comparable TLC values obtained with this technique and with plethysmography in patients with various chest diseases.[79]

In patients with chronic obstructive pulmonary disease (COPD), gas dilution techniques underestimate TLC whereas plethysmographic measurements using mouth pressure may overestimate it.[79a] In one study, TLC was measured by four methods: helium dilution, a volume-displacement body plethysmograph (box volume being plotted against mouth pressure), the same body plethysmograph with volume plotted against pressures measured with an esophageal balloon, and a radiologic technique.[79a] The mean TLC measurements were 6.02 ± 1.37 liters with helium dilution, 6.11 ± 1.18 liters with a radiologic technique, 6.36 ± 1.12 liters with esophageal pressure (considered to provide the closest estimate of TLC), and 6.65 ± 1.11 liters with mouth pressure.

A modification of the 1960 technique was subsequently described in light of new physiologic data on pulmonary tissue and blood volume.[80] A comparison of this modified technique with plethysmography showed comparable TLC estimates in normal subjects and in patients with pulmonary fibrosis, sarcoidosis, emphysema, or pulmonary neoplasms; however, in patients with emphysema, values obtained with the radiographic method were more accurate than those obtained by gas dilution techniques. When TLC was known, RV was readily obtained by subtracting the spirometrically obtained vital capacity. An experienced observer could make the measurements in less than 30 minutes, and the technique was highly reproducible.

A comparably accurate but faster and much simpler method for estimating TLC from chest radiographs was described in 1971.[81] According to this technique, the outlines of the lungs on PA and lateral radiographs are traced, their areas measured with a planimeter, and a regression equation applied to these measurements. Another technique was described in which the operator traces the outline of the lungs with a tracking device or cursor.[82] The operation is controlled by a programmable computer and the output is displayed on an X-Y plotter. With this technique, estimates of TLC can be obtained in less than 40 seconds. A comparison of these estimates with water displacement measurements of various phantoms revealed the former to differ from true volume by −8% to +16%.[82] However, a comparison of results derived from this technique with plethysmographically determined TLC in patients was not reported. In 1975, an additional technique was described that entails computerized graphic-to-digital conversion of tracings directly from PA and lateral radiographs.[83] The procedure can be performed in less than 60 seconds and, in a test on 53 subjects, showed good correlation with physiologic measurements ($r = 0.85$).

One group of investigators measured lung volumes on chest radiographs by using equations derived from CT.[84] The technique is based on the fact that CT reveals the true cross-sectional area of the chest, and it compares favorably with planimetric methods for estimating lung volume. A computerized planimetric method that defines the boundaries of the chest wall, heart, diaphragm, and spine on PA and lateral chest radiographs has also been described.[77] In one assessment of this method, the correlation of lung volumes measured by the planimetric method and by plethysmography in patients with and without COPD was 0.85, a value similar to that obtained by other planimetric methods.[85] Despite the relatively good correlation and similar mean values between planimetric and plethysmographic lung volumes, the poor concordance of measurements within individual subjects was such that the difference between planimetric and plethysmographic measurements of TLC had 95% confidence limits of −2.2 to 2.3 liters.[85] Similarly, although the mean inspiratory capacity obtained by planimetry was comparable to that obtained by spirometry, there were considerable discrepancies within individuals, the 95% confidence intervals between the two techniques being −1.7 to 2.5 liters.[85] In summary, radiographic methods are inferior to pulmonary function tests in the determination of lung volume.[77, 85] The one exception may be in patients with severe airway obstruction, in whom gas dilution techniques underestimate lung volume and plethysmography overestimates it.

CONVENTIONAL TOMOGRAPHY

Conventional tomography allows selective visibility of a particular layer of tissue to the exclusion of structures lying superficial or deep to it. The technique involves reciprocal movement of the x-ray tube and film at proportional velocity. This motion causes blurring of all structures not continuously "in focus" during excursions of the tube and film, so the image of only a thin "slice" is recorded in detail on the radiograph. The level of tomographic "cut" is controlled by

the ratio of the tube-object distance to the object-film distance, and therefore this level can be altered by varying the ratio. The thickness of the cut is governed by the length of the tube-film travel: the shorter the excursion, the thicker the layer recorded. Various reciprocal movements of tube and film have been developed, the most commonly used being rectilinear and pluridirectional.

In all but a few centers, conventional tomography has been completely replaced by CT, since the latter allows much better depiction of both normal anatomy and abnormal findings. Despite this advantage, a few illustrations in this book are based on conventional tomography for historical reasons and to emphasize a finding that may not be readily apparent on the chest radiograph.

COMPUTED TOMOGRAPHY

CT is based on the principle that the internal structure of an object can be reconstructed from multiple projections of it. The CT image is a two-dimensional representation of a three-dimensional cross-sectional slice, the third dimension being the section or slice thickness. The latter is also known as the collimation width and is defined by collimators between the x-ray tube and the patient. The CT image is composed of multiple picture elements (typically 512 × 512) known as pixels. A pixel is a unit area, i.e., each square on the image matrix; it reflects the attenuation of a unit volume of tissue, or voxel, that corresponds to the area of the pixel multiplied by the scan collimation. The x-ray attenuations of the structures within a given voxel are averaged to produce the image. This volume averaging results in loss of spatial resolution: the thicker the slice, the lower the ability of CT to resolve small structures. Slice thickness can be varied to provide optimal assessment. For instance, in the evaluation of fine parenchymal detail such as interlobular septa, thin sections (1- to 2-mm collimation) are superior to thicker sections (7- to 10-mm collimation). On the other hand, vessels running obliquely to the plane of section are easier to identify on thicker sections inasmuch as they course through the thickness of the slice. Moreover, as section thickness decreases, noise increases and grainier images result.

The first CT scanner was introduced into clinical practice by Godfrey Hounsfield in 1972.[86] This device consists essentially of an x-ray source, collimators, x-ray detectors, and associated electronics all mounted on a gantry that moves to produce the scan. On conventional CT, the x-ray source is rotated mechanically around the patient to produce the multiple projections required for mathematical reconstruction of the cross-sectional image. The time required to obtain the image (scan time) is determined by the time required for this rotation. In most modern CT scanners, the scan time is on the order of 1 second. A faster scanning speed can be achieved by using electron beam or spiral CT. In the former (also known as *ultrafast CT*), the x-ray beam is produced by a focused electron beam that sweeps around a tungsten ring encircling the patient. This technique allows images to be acquired in 100 msec or less and has been particularly useful in assessing dynamic changes such as tracheal configuration and cross-sectional area during forced expiration.[87]

A conventional CT scan of the chest consists of a series of individual cross-sectional slices obtained during suspended respiration. After each slice is obtained, the patient is allowed to breath while the table is moved to the next scanning position. This method of obtaining a series of individual cross-sectional images is known as incremental CT scanning. Although each image can be obtained within approximately 1 second, there is a delay of 5 to 10 seconds between images. Spiral (helical) CT is a major technical advance that allows continuous scanning while the patient is continuously moved through the CT gantry.[88] With this technique, patient translation into the gantry and x-ray source rotation occur simultaneously during data acquisition. Therefore the x-ray beam traces a helical or spiral curve in relation to the patient. Each rotation of the x-ray tube can be considered to generate data specific to an angled plane of section.[89] Cross-sectional images can be reconstructed after the data specific to each plane of section are estimated. This mathematical calculation is performed by interpolation of the spiral data above and below each plane of section. Most current spiral CT scanners reorder the projection data and perform interpolation from views separated by 180 degrees to opti-

mize resolution in the longitudinal axis.[90, 91] The position and spacing of these images can be chosen retrospectively for arbitrary table positions and at small increments.

A spiral CT scan of the entire chest may be completed during a single breath-hold or several successive short breath-holds. The continuous nature of the data acquisition allows true volumetric scanning and the production of multiple overlapping images that result in increased spatial resolution in the longitudinal axis. These overlapping reconstructions allow the production of high-quality multiplanar and three-dimensional reformations without additional radiation exposure (Figs. 13–6 and 13–7). In addition, because spiral CT allows major portions or the entire chest to be scanned during a single breath-hold, it virtually eliminates motion artefacts that otherwise degrade image quality. Spiral CT has been shown to be considerably better than conventional CT in the detection of pulmonary nodules,[92, 93] arteriovenous malformations,[94] and central airway abnormalities.[95] The shorter acquisition time allows consistent opacification of intrathoracic vessels with smaller volumes of contrast medium,[96] as well as marked improvement in the visualization of abnormalities of the superior vena cava, brachiocephalic

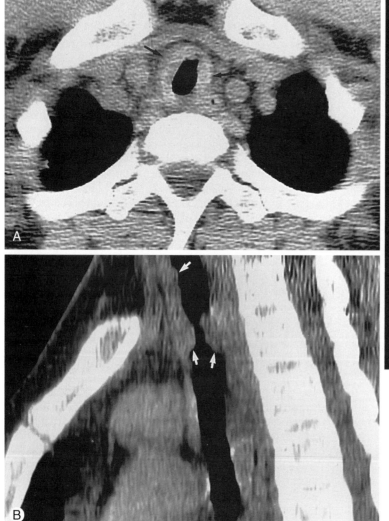

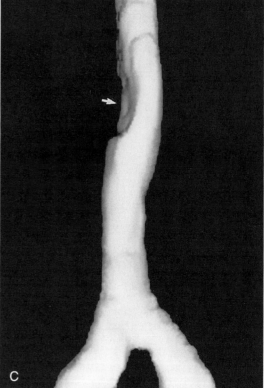

Figure 13–6. Spiral CT with Sagittal and Three-Dimensional Reconstruction. A 3-mm-collimation spiral CT scan *(A)* demonstrates circumferential thickening of the trachea *(arrows)*. The sagittal reconstruction *(B)* allows better assessment of the focal nature of the thickening as seen by narrowing of the lumen *(arrows)*. The narrowing is also well seen on the coronal three-dimensional reconstruction *(arrow in C)* of the trachea and main bronchi. The patient was a 27-year-old woman with endotracheal tuberculosis. (Case courtesy of Dr. Kyung Soo Lee, Department of Radiology, Samsung Medical Center, Seoul, Korea.)

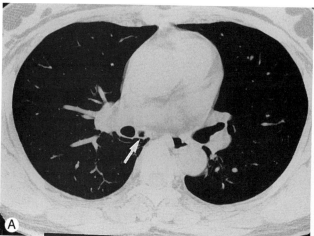

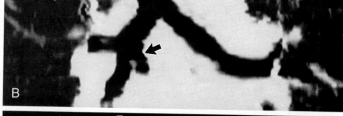

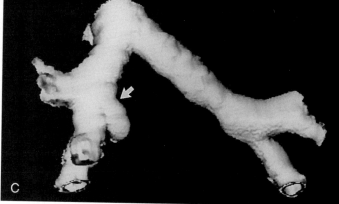

Figure 13–7. Spiral CT with Coronal and Three-Dimensional Reconstruction of an Accessory Cardiac Bronchus. A cross-sectional spiral CT image *(A)* demonstrates a localized area of air density *(arrow)* medial to the bronchus intermedius. A coronal reconstruction *(B)* demonstrates that this localized abnormality communicates with the distal right main bronchus *(arrow)*. The diagnosis of an accessory cardiac bronchus can be readily made on the coronal reconstruction. Three-dimensional reconstruction *(C)* more clearly defines the bronchial anatomy and the cardiac bronchus. The patient was a 39-year-old woman with recurrent respiratory infections. (Case courtesy of Dr. Kyung Soo Lee, Department of Radiology, Samsung Medical Center, Seoul, Korea.)

veins, aorta, and pulmonary arteries and veins (Fig. 13–8).[95–98, 98a, b] Three-dimensional image displays also allow better appreciation of the spatial relationships of various structures than a series of sections.[98c, d] Use of graphics-based software systems and volume-rendering techniques allows depiction of the luminal surface of the airways that resembles the images seen by bronchography or during bronchoscopy.[98d, e] (The technique by which luminal surface views are produced from the virtual environment of the CT database is known as *virtual bronchoscopy.*[98e])

Technical Parameters

Several operator-dependent parameters greatly influence the information provided by chest CT, the main ones being slice thickness, slice spacing, field of view, reconstruction algorithm, and image display settings (window width and level). In selected cases, intravenous contrast may be used to distinguish vessels from soft tissue lesions or detect intravascular abnormalities such as thromboemboli.

As indicated previously, all structures within the unit of

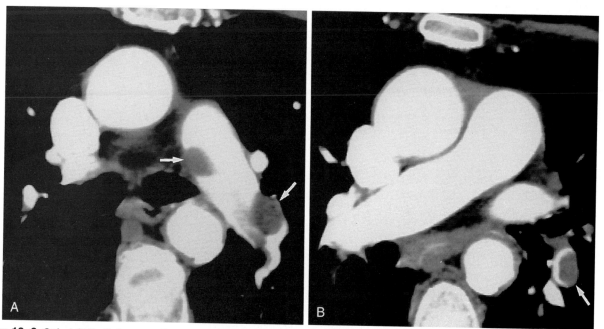

Figure 13–8. Spiral CT in Pulmonary Thromboembolism. A 3-mm-collimation spiral CT scan following the intravenous administration of contrast medium *(A and B)* demonstrates several emboli in the left main and interlobar pulmonary arteries *(arrows)*. The patient was an 84-year-old woman with acute shortness of breath.

volume represented by the slice (voxel) are averaged to produce a single CT number in the corresponding picture element (pixel). The thicker the slice, the more volume that is averaged to produce the image, thus resulting in lower spatial resolution. The optimal slice thickness is determined by the size of the structure being assessed and by the number of scans required to evaluate the patient. It has been well established that thin sections (1- to 2-mm collimation) are required for adequate assessment of the pulmonary parenchyma and peripheral bronchi (Fig. 13–9).[99–101] Adequate assessment of the patient can be obtained by performing these scans at 10-mm intervals. Although only 10% to 20% of the lung parenchyma is sampled, the improved spatial resolution allows better assessment of normal and abnormal findings than is possible with thicker sections.[102] However, this approach is not acceptable in all situations; for example, when assessing pulmonary metastases it is essential to evaluate the entire chest, preferably by using continuous spiral volumetric CT through the chest with 5- to 7-mm-thick sections. Volumetric scanning during a single breath-hold at 3- to 5-mm collimation is recommended for assessment of abnormalities involving the trachea and central bronchi.[103] Thus the optimal slice thickness is dictated by the indication for performing the CT scan.

CT scanning should be performed with a field of view large enough to encompass the patient (35 to 40 cm). In general, the largest matrix available (usually 512 × 512) should be used in image reconstruction to reduce pixel size. Using a field of view of 40 cm and a 512 × 512 matrix results in a pixel size of 0.78 mm. Targeting the image prospectively or retrospectively to a smaller field of view decreases pixel size and increases spatial resolution. For example, targeting the image to a single lung by using a field of view of 25 cm results in a pixel size of 0.49 mm. Maximal spatial resolution is usually obtained by using a field of view of 13 cm, which results in a pixel size of

0.25 mm.[104] Although small fields of view increase spatial resolution, they should be used only in selected cases as an ancillary technique since they allow assessment of only a small portion of the chest.

In the majority of cases, the CT scan data are reconstructed by using a standard or soft tissue algorithm that smooths the image and reduces visible image noise. This reconstruction algorithm is preferred in the assessment of abnormalities of the mediastinum and chest wall. However, use of a high–spatial frequency reconstruction algorithm is required for optimal assessment of the lung parenchyma.[104, 105] This algorithm reduces image smoothing and increases spatial resolution, thereby allowing better depiction of normal and abnormal parenchymal interfaces (Fig. 13–10) and thus better visualization of small vessels, bronchi, and subtle interstitial abnormalities.[105, 106] The combination of thin-section CT (1- to 2-mm collimation) and a high–spatial frequency reconstruction algorithm provides for the optimal assessment of interstitial and air-space lung disease and is referred to as high-resolution CT (HRCT) (Fig. 13–11).[100, 107]

CT numbers in the thorax range from −1,000 Hounsfield units (HU) for air in the trachea to approximately 700 HU for dense bones. The display of the CT image on the monitor (soft copy) or film (hard copy) is determined by the window level and width and is limited to 256 shades of gray. Therefore, no single window setting can adequately display all the information available on a chest CT. To display the large number of attenuation values (HU) within a limited number of shades of gray, a CT number is selected that corresponds to approximately the mean attenuation value of the tissue being examined. This center CT attenuation value is called the window level. The computer is then instructed to assign one shade of gray to a certain number of CT attenuation values above and below the window level. The range of CT numbers above and below the window level is called the window width. To adequately depict the

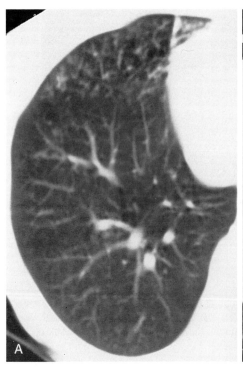
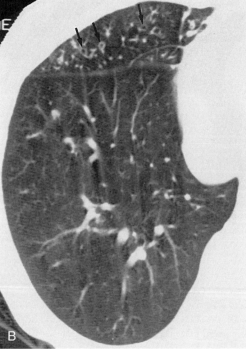

Figure 13–9. HRCT Versus Conventional CT for Bronchiectasis. A conventional 10-mm-collimation CT scan *(A)* in a 65-year-old woman demonstrates small focal areas of ground-glass attenuation and consolidation in the right middle lobe. An HRCT scan (1.5 mm collimation) *(B)* performed immediately after the conventional CT scan demonstrates right middle lobe bronchiectasis *(arrows)*. Even in retrospect the bronchiectasis cannot be seen on the conventional CT image.

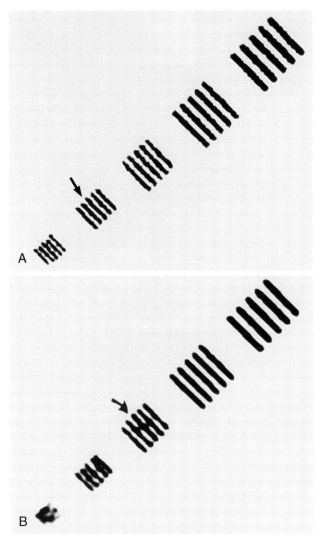

cients is negligible, provided that these structures are separated by interfaces of different attenuation properties; for example, lymph nodes in the mediastinum can usually be distinguished from each other and from other structures because of the presence of fat-containing interfaces of low attenuation. Since blood in vessels has a similar attenuation as soft tissue, differentiation of vascular structures from soft tissue abnormalities can be difficult; however, this distinction can be greatly aided by the use of intravenous injection of contrast medium, which brings about an increase in attenuation (CT numbers) proportional to the vascularity and permeability of the tissue being measured.

Radiation Dose

Comparison of radiation doses of different radiologic techniques is best assessed by the use of effective dose as defined by the International Commission on Radiological Protection.[108] The effective radiation dose allows a comparison of the radiation-related risk by taking into account not only the dose to each organ or tissue but also the amount of tissue irradiated and the relative cancer risk for each tissue. The calculated effective dose is the dose that would have to be given to the whole body to produce the same risk, and it allows comparison of nonuniform irradiation.

The mean skin dose of conventional 10-mm-collimation CT of the chest performed at 10-mm intervals is on the order of 30 to 35 mGy, which results in an effective radiation dose of approximately 8 mSv.[109, 110] As a result of the small amount of tissue irradiated, HRCT with 1- to 2-mm-thick sections at 10-mm intervals has an effective radiation dose of only 10% to 20% that of conventional CT.[110] The combined effective radiation dose of a PA and lateral chest radiograph is on the order of 0.15 mSv.[111, 112] Therefore the effective radiation dose of conventional CT of the chest is approximately equivalent to 50 PA and lateral chest radiographs, whereas an HRCT study is equivalent to 5 to 10 PA and lateral radiographs.[113] To place these exposures in perspective, it has been pointed out that the effective radiation dose of HRCT of the chest is less than 30% of the average annual effective dose received by individuals in North America from natural radiation.[113, 114]

Although conventional CT is performed at 200 to 400 mAs in most clinical settings, it has been demonstrated that acceptable diagnostic quality can be obtained in many cases with a setting as low as 20 mAs.[115] It has also been shown that acceptable HRCT images can be achieved in many cases by the use of 40 mAs.[116] In fact, by combining 1.5-mm-collimation scans at 20-mm intervals with low-dose scans (40 mAs), an acceptable quality of HRCT can be obtained with a radiation dose equivalent to that of a single AP chest radiograph.[110] It should be noted, however, that such scans have a lower signal-to-noise ratio.[116] The increased noise is due to quantum mottle and is greatly increased in large patients as compared with small or average-sized patients. (Quantum mottle refers to the lack of precision of CT attenuation numbers because of variation in the number of x-ray photons absorbed by the detector. It results in lack of uniformity of the CT image when scanning a homogeneous object such as a water bath.)

In one investigation of the relationship between diag-

Figure 13–10. High–Spatial Resolution Versus Standard Reconstruction Algorithms. Line-pair phantoms were reconstructed by using identical CT parameters and reconstruction with high–spatial resolution *(A)* and standard *(B)* algorithms. From left to right the grouped line pairs represent resolutions of 10, 8, 6.25, 5, and 3.9 line pairs per centimeter (lp/cm), respectively. Maximal resolution with the high–spatial frequency reconstruction algorithm in this example is 8 lp/cm *(straight arrow)* as compared with 6.25 lp/cm for the standard algorithm *(curved arrow)*. This represents a 28% improvement in spatial resolution.

lungs, a window level of −600 to −700 HU and a window width of 1,000 to 1,500 HU are most commonly recommended.[107] Window levels of 30 to 50 HU and window widths of 350 to 500 HU usually provide the best assessment of the mediastinum, hila, and pleura. It should be emphasized that these figures represent useful guidelines only and there are no universally accepted ideal window settings for either the lung parenchyma or the mediastinum; different windows may provide optimal assessment of particular abnormalities in individual cases.

As in most radiographic procedures, the variable forming the CT image is the difference in x-ray attenuation properties of various tissues; for example, the attenuation coefficient of fat is less than that of muscle, which is less than that of bone. Anatomic structures can often be identified by CT even though the difference in their attenuation coeffi-

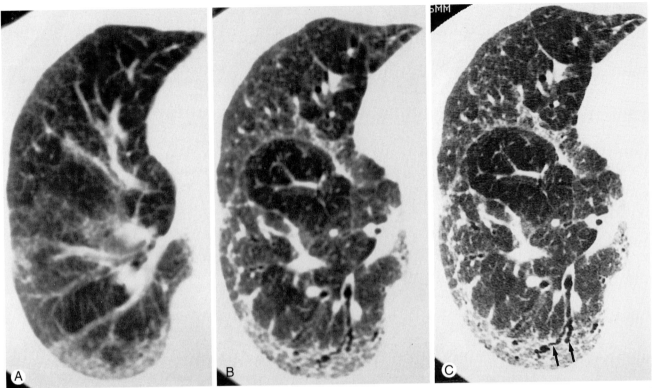

Figure 13–11. Influence of Section Thickness and Reconstruction Algorithm on Image Quality. A 10-mm-collimation CT scan *(A)* in a 71-year-old patient demonstrates poorly defined areas of increased attenuation in the right lung. The pattern and distribution of abnormalities are better visualized on the 1.5-mm-collimation CT scan *(B)*. Both *A* and *B* were reconstructed by using a standard reconstruction algorithm. An HRCT scan (1.5-mm-collimation CT scan reconstructed by using a high–spatial frequency algorithm) *(C)* allows optimal assessment of fine parenchymal detail. The edges of vessels and bronchi are more sharply defined than on the standard algorithm. The abnormalities consist of a fine reticular pattern and areas of ground-glass attenuation involving mainly the subpleural regions. Note the irregular dilatation of the posterior basal bronchi of the right lower lobe as they enter into an area of fibrosis (traction bronchiectasis *[arrows]*). The diagnosis of idiopathic pulmonary fibrosis was confirmed by open-lung biopsy.

nostic accuracy and radiation dose, chest radiographs and low-dose (80 mAs) and conventional-dose (340 mAs) HRCT scans from 50 patients with chronic infiltrative lung disease and 10 healthy control subjects were assessed by two independent observers.[117] The CT scans were obtained at only three levels—the aortic arch, the tracheal carina, and 1 cm above the right hemidiaphragm. A correct first-choice diagnosis was made more often with either CT technique than with radiography. A high confidence level in the first-choice diagnosis was reached in 42% of radiographic, 61% of low-dose CT, and 63% of conventional-dose CT interpretations, which were correct in 92%, 90%, and 96% of the studies, respectively. Use of the low-dose technique (80 mAs) at only three levels resulted in an effective radiation dose of 0.03 mSv, a value lower than the effective dose from PA and lateral chest radiographs, and was associated with significant improvement in the number of correct first-choice diagnoses made with a high degree of confidence.

Indications

Throughout this book, indications for CT examination in specific disease entities are discussed in the appropriate sections. Based on data in the literature,[107, 118, 119] the most common indications for the use of CT are presented in the following paragraphs.

Evaluation of Suspected Mediastinal Abnormalities Identified on Standard Chest Radiographs. CT can be used to differentiate the cystic or solid nature of mediastinal masses, localize such masses relative to other mediastinal structures, and to some extent determine their composition (e.g., adipose tissue). Whether mediastinal widening is pathologic or is simply an anatomic variation can also be assessed, and CT can distinguish a solid mass from a vascular anomaly or aneurysm (generally using contrast enhancement). A dilated pulmonary artery can be differentiated from a solid mass in the hilum (e.g., enlarged lymph nodes) and the presence and extent of mediastinal metastases determined in patients with pulmonary carcinoma.

Search for Occult Thymic Lesions. Thymoma or thymic hyperplasia can be detected in selected patients with myasthenia gravis when standard chest radiographs are negative or suspicious.

Determination of the Presence and Extent of Neoplastic Disease. Occult pulmonary metastases can be detected when extensive surgery is planned for a known primary neoplasm with a high propensity for lung metastases or when a solitary lung metastasis is identified on a chest radiograph; in addition, primary neoplasms can be detected in patients with positive sputum cytology and negative chest radiographs and fiberoptic bronchoscopy. Mediastinal, pleural, bone, muscle, and subcutaneous tissue involvement can be assessed and invasion into the spinal canal detected.

Search for Diffuse or Central Calcification in a Pulmonary Nodule. Figure 13–12.

Miscellaneous Indications. Additional indications include assisting in the percutaneous biopsy of lesions such as medi-

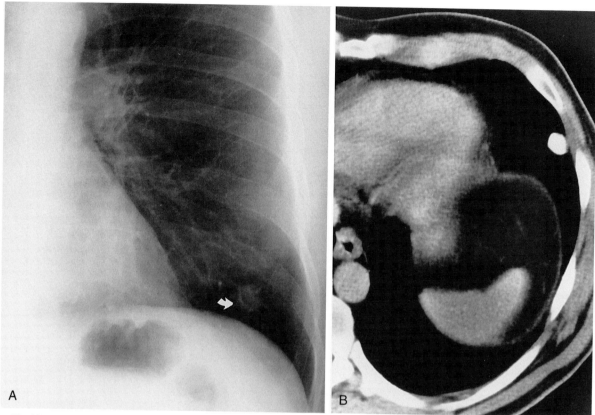

Figure 13–12. CT Demonstration of Calcified Granuloma. A magnified view of the left lung from a posteroanterior chest radiograph *(A)* in a 51-year-old man demonstrates a 1.5-cm-diameter nodule *(arrow)*. A CT scan *(B)* demonstrates that the nodule is diffusely calcified, which allows a confident diagnosis of granuloma. Even in retrospect the calcification is not evident on the chest radiograph.

astinal, pleural, or pulmonary masses when fluoroscopic guidance is inadequate; localization of loculated collections of fluid within the pleural space when standard radiographic or ultrasonic techniques prove inadequate; and assessment of the size and configuration of the thoracic aorta.

Based on data in the literature, the main indications for the use of HRCT (1- to 2-mm collimation, high–spatial frequency reconstruction algorithm) include the following:[100, 107]

Diagnosis of Bronchiectasis. *See* Figure 13–9, page 312.

Detection of Parenchymal Lung Disease. Patients with symptoms or pulmonary function abnormalities suggestive of parenchymal lung disease but normal or questionable radiographic findings can be assessed (Fig. 13–13).

Differential Diagnosis of Diffuse Lung Disease. HRCT can be used to assess patients in whom the combination of clinical and radiographic findings does not provide a confident diagnosis and further radiologic assessment is considered warranted (Fig. 13–14). This indication in particular includes patients with chronic interstitial and air-space disease and immunocompromised patients with acute parenchymal abnormalities; in such patients the differential diagnosis can be narrowed or a specific diagnosis often made on HRCT even when the radiographic findings are nonspecific.

MAGNETIC RESONANCE IMAGING

When certain atomic nuclei are placed in a magnetic field and stimulated by radio waves of a particular frequency, they will re-emit some of the absorbed energy in the form of radio signals. This phenomenon, known as nuclear magnetic resonance, has been used since shortly after World War II by organic chemists, biochemists, and physicists to identify and spectroscopically analyze intricate molecules in liquids or solids. During the early 1970s, several investigators began exploring the possibility that the technique could also produce images of sufficient resolution for medical purposes. Since then, major technologic advances have occurred, and today thoracic MR imaging plays an important role in the evaluation of abnormalities of the great vessels, mediastinum, hila, and chest wall.

Physical Principles

With the exception of the hydrogen nucleus, which consists of a single proton, atomic nuclei contain both protons and neutrons. The constituent nucleons (the generic term for a proton or neutron) each possess an intrinsic angular moment or "spin"; however, since pairs of protons or neutrons align in such a way that their spins cancel out, a *net* spin exists for a nucleus only when it contains an odd (unpaired) proton or an odd neutron. This intrinsic spin has an associated magnetic moment, so each nucleus may be considered to act as a small bar magnet. When these nuclei are exposed to a magnetic field, they experience a torque, their axis of spin rotating about the field direction as the nuclei attempt to line up parallel to the magnetic field. Any nucleus with a net spin possesses a characteristic resonant

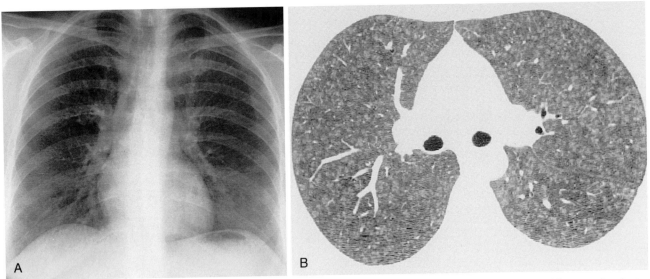

Figure 13–13. HRCT in Chronic Diffuse Lung Disease. A posteroanterior chest radiograph *(A)* in a 35-year-old woman with progressive shortness of breath demonstrates subtle bilateral areas of increased opacity. HRCT *(B)* demonstrates small rounded opacities in a centrilobular distribution. Although the radiographic findings were nonspecific, the HRCT appearance is most suggestive of extrinsic allergic alveolitis. The diagnosis was proved by open-lung biopsy.

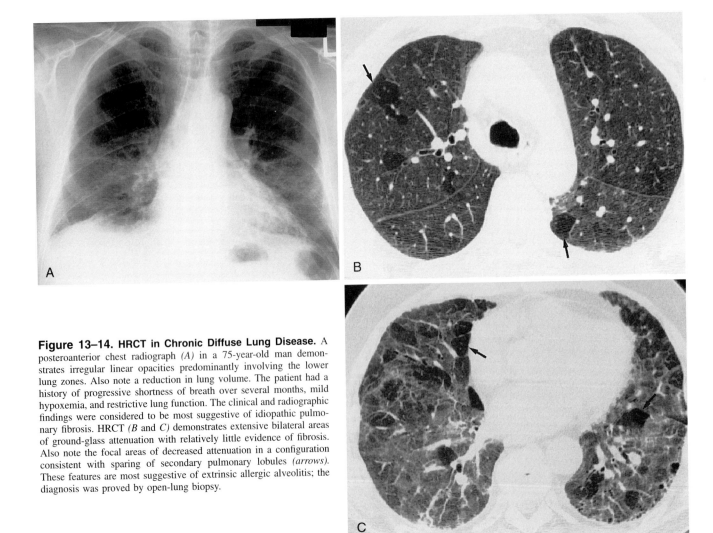

Figure 13–14. HRCT in Chronic Diffuse Lung Disease. A posteroanterior chest radiograph *(A)* in a 75-year-old man demonstrates irregular linear opacities predominantly involving the lower lung zones. Also note a reduction in lung volume. The patient had a history of progressive shortness of breath over several months, mild hypoxemia, and restrictive lung function. The clinical and radiographic findings were considered to be most suggestive of idiopathic pulmonary fibrosis. HRCT *(B and C)* demonstrates extensive bilateral areas of ground-glass attenuation with relatively little evidence of fibrosis. Also note the focal areas of decreased attenuation in a configuration consistent with sparing of secondary pulmonary lobules *(arrows)*. These features are most suggestive of extrinsic allergic alveolitis; the diagnosis was proved by open-lung biopsy.

or "precessional" frequency that is determined by the magnetic field strength and a constant (the gyromagnetic ratio, which takes into account the magnetic properties of the nuclear species in question). For a nuclear magnetic interaction to occur, the pulse of radio-frequency (RF) radiation must be at precisely the same frequency as the precessional frequency of the nucleus (also known as the Larmor frequency). The magnetic field and the net magnetization vectors are usually described by using an orthogonal coordinate system in which the z-axis is parallel to the large external magnetic field and parallel to the long axis of the patient (Fig. 13–15).

To induce the MR phenomenon, a short RF pulse is applied via a coil surrounding the patient, the RF radiation being equivalent to the application of a second, smaller magnetic field (*see* Fig. 13–15). The RF signal changes the state of the protons in the magnetic field from one of equilibrium to one of excitation. This excited state is inherently unstable and naturally decays toward the equilibrium state over a period of time. As the nuclei "relax" to their original alignment in the magnetic field, they radiate to their surroundings the absorbed energy at their characteristic or Larmor frequency. The re-emitted energy provides a signal that can be detected by a receiver coil wrapped around the patient; if there are a sufficient number of these signals and if they can be spatially resolved, an image of the distribution of the emitting nuclei can be formed.

Currently, most medical MR imaging uses hydrogen protons as the nuclei of interest because they are abundant in the body. The greater the number of hydrogen protons present, the more intense the MR signal. Several factors influence the nature of the energy emitted during MR imaging.

Relaxation Times

The signal strength during emission diminishes exponentially with a characteristic "relaxation time" that is determined in part by the general environment of the nuclei. The greater the facility to pass energy to neighboring nuclei, the more rapidly the irradiated nuclei can return to their original energy state and hence a shorter relaxation time. There are two such relaxation times, designated *T1* and *T2*.

T1. Once nuclei have been energized by an RF pulse, T1 is the time constant corresponding to exponential restoration of the magnetization *parallel* to the external field (Fig. 13–16); to put it another way, T1 represents the time required for the component of the net magnetization vector in the z direction to return to its initial value after it has been perturbed by the RF pulse (see Figs. 13–15 and 13–16). T1 is also known as the *spin-lattice* or *longitudinal relaxation time*. In a pure liquid, the return to equilibrium is exponential, and after three T1 periods have elapsed, 95% of the original magnetization will have been restored. The T1 relaxation time tends to be long for fluids (e.g., cerebrospinal fluid, hydatid cysts) and shorter in fat. Any process that increases tissue water content (e.g., edema) lengthens T1.

T2. T2 is the time constant corresponding to exponential decay of the magnetization *perpendicular* to the external field and is also known as the *spin-spin relaxation time*. After an RF pulse has tipped the nuclear magnetization vector toward the transverse plane, the components of this vector all precess together, or "in phase," and therefore appear to be stationary in the rotating reference frame. However, the precession does not remain in phase. Subtle local alterations in magnetic field strength cause some nuclei to precess at different rates from others; the RF waves from individual nuclei dephase and cancel each other out, and the sum of the nuclear magnetization vectors in the transverse plane decays to zero. The time constant for this dephasing or decay *(T2)* provides additional data about the local environment in which the hydrogen nuclei reside. During the measuring pulse, the precessing protons are brought into phase with the frequency of the radio signal (*see* Fig. 13–16).

The T2 relaxation time is due to random molecular motion that leads to signal dephasing. The latter is in turn related to the local molecular environment, T2 times being characteristically long for homogeneous environments (e.g., fluid) and short for complex tissues (e.g., muscle). An increase in tissue water secondary to congestive heart failure or pulmonary neoplasm results in lengthening of the T2 relaxation time.[120]

The MR signal is also influenced by motion of water or blood during the imaging sequence. To generate an MR signal, protons need to be excited by the RF pulse and then need to be refocused. Four interactions occur between flowing protons and the pulse sequence: (1) signal loss caused by flow through the imaging plane during the pulse sequence; (2) signal loss caused by phase-encoding misregistration; (3) signal loss caused by destructive phase interference in the voxel; and (4) signal gain caused by inflow of blood that has not yet received any RF pulses (unsaturated spins).[120] As a result of these four effects and depending on the velocity of blood flow and the image sequence used, the MR signal of flowing blood may be increased ("white blood" signal), decreased ("black blood" signal), or intermediate. A number of specialized MR pulse sequences have been devised that have special sensitivity to flow and may allow its quantification.[120, 121, 121a]

Magnetic Resonance Pulse Sequences

The RF pulse duration determines the extent to which the net magnetization rotates with respect to its original alignment. For example, a 90-degree pulse rotates the net magnetization 90 degrees; similarly, a 180-degree pulse rotates the net magnetization 180 degrees. An appropriate sequence of RF pulses may be used to emphasize either the T1 or T2 portion of the MR signal or improve the efficiency of data accumulation.[122] The more common pulse sequences include saturation recovery, inversion recovery, and spin echo.

Saturation Recovery. The saturation recovery sequence uses two 90-degree pulses separated by a time interval, TR. This interval is set to be longer than T2 but shorter than T1; thus the second pulse arrives before T1 relaxation is complete. The signal obtained depends on the extent of relaxation that has occurred during time interval TR.[122]

Inversion Recovery. If a 180-degree pulse is applied to a sample in equilibrium with a magnetic field, the net magnetization rotates so that it points in the direction opposite the external magnetic field. Following the inversion pulse, the magnetization will immediately begin to revert to its equilibrium state at a rate determined by T1. After a predetermined

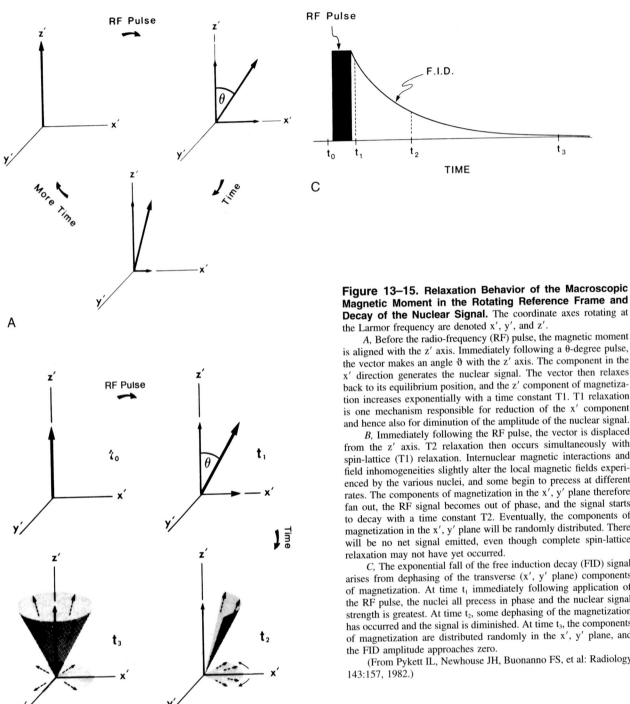

Figure 13–15. Relaxation Behavior of the Macroscopic Magnetic Moment in the Rotating Reference Frame and Decay of the Nuclear Signal. The coordinate axes rotating at the Larmor frequency are denoted x′, y′, and z′.

A, Before the radio-frequency (RF) pulse, the magnetic moment is aligned with the z′ axis. Immediately following a θ-degree pulse, the vector makes an angle ϑ with the z′ axis. The component in the x′ direction generates the nuclear signal. The vector then relaxes back to its equilibrium position, and the z′ component of magnetization increases exponentially with a time constant T1. T1 relaxation is one mechanism responsible for reduction of the x′ component and hence also for diminution of the amplitude of the nuclear signal.

B, Immediately following the RF pulse, the vector is displaced from the z′ axis. T2 relaxation then occurs simultaneously with spin-lattice (T1) relaxation. Internuclear magnetic interactions and field inhomogeneities slightly alter the local magnetic fields experienced by the various nuclei, and some begin to precess at different rates. The components of magnetization in the x′, y′ plane therefore fan out, the RF signal becomes out of phase, and the signal starts to decay with a time constant T2. Eventually, the components of magnetization in the x′, y′ plane will be randomly distributed. There will be no net signal emitted, even though complete spin-lattice relaxation may not have yet occurred.

C, The exponential fall of the free induction decay (FID) signal arises from dephasing of the transverse (x′, y′ plane) components of magnetization. At time t_1 immediately following application of the RF pulse, the nuclei all precess in phase and the nuclear signal strength is greatest. At time t_2, some dephasing of the magnetization has occurred and the signal is diminished. At time t_3, the components of magnetization are distributed randomly in the x′, y′ plane, and the FID amplitude approaches zero.

(From Pykett IL, Newhouse JH, Buonanno FS, et al: Radiology 143:157, 1982.)

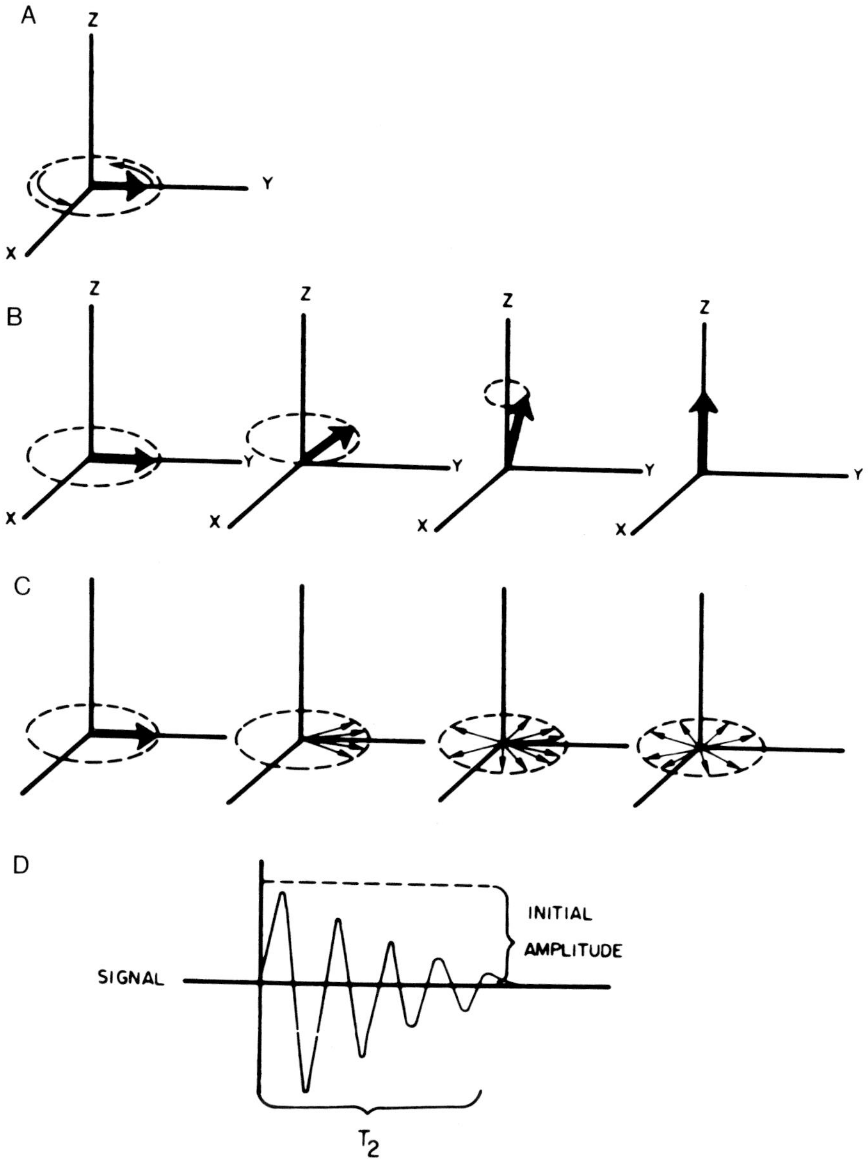

Figure 13–16. Relaxation Times T1 and T2. *A,* After a $\pi/2$ pulse, the net magnetic moment, made up of the sum of many individual dipole moments, precesses in the X-Y plane and induces a signal in the receiver coil. *B,* The signal decays in time T1 owing to spontaneous reversion of the inverted dipoles, which causes the net magnetic moment to approach the direction of Bo. *C,* Individual dipoles also drift out of phase, which disperses the net magnetic moment and causes the signal to cease in time T2. *D,* The initial amplitude of the signal is related to T1, whereas persistence of signal is a measure of T2. (From Mitchell MR, Partain LL, Price RR, et al: Appl Radiol 11:4, 1982. Brentwood Publishing Corp, a Prentice-Hall/Simon & Schuster unit of Gulf + Western, Inc.)

time, the residual net magnetization can be measured or read by rotating it 90 degrees to produce a coherent induced signal in the measuring coil. The amplitude of the resulting signal will depend both on the inversion time interval (time between the 180- and 90-degree pulses) and on tissue T1. T1 can be measured by observing the signal at several inversion time intervals.

Spin Echo. In the spin-echo sequence, a 90-degree pulse is initially applied to rotate the net magnetization into the xy plane. At the end of the pulse, nuclear magnets are initially phase coherent. They begin to rephase because of intrinsic magnetic field inhomogeneities in the tissues. At time TE/2, a 180-degree pulse is applied to cause the magnetization to refocus and form an echo at time TE (Fig. 13–17).[122] The effect of the 180-degree pulse on the precessing spins is similar to a group of runners who because they move at different speeds, spread out as they get farther from the start line; if they are suddenly told that they are running in the wrong direction, they will all turn around and, since the farthest away are the fastest, will all arrive back at the

start line together.[123] Spin-echo may be used to determine T2 without contamination from inhomogeneity effects of the magnetic field.[124]

The spin-echo sequence is the most commonly used MR technique in the chest. The separation of the successive 90-degree pulses on spin-echo MR is known as the repetition time (TR). Short repetition times are required to allow distinction between tissues with different T1 relaxation times. These short repetition times are known as *T1-weighted sequences.* In 1.5-tesla MR scanners, T1-weighted sequences have TR times ranging from 600 to 1,000 msec.[120] Because chest MR scans are cardiac (electrocardiogram) gated to decrease motion artefacts, this sequence corresponds to one RR interval.

The MR signal decays as an exponential function of the T2 relaxation time. To distinguish tissues with different T2 characteristics, a long echo time is required (≥ 80 msec). Furthermore, to maximize T2 differences and to minimize the effect of T1 relaxation, T2-weighted images require long TR intervals. Thus, T2-weighted images on cardiac-gated

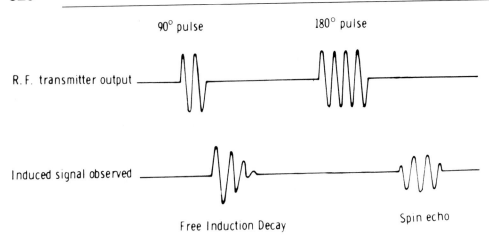

Figure 13–17. A Spin-Echo 90-τ–180-τ Pulse Sequence for Measuring T2. The 90-degree pulse produces a signal proportional to the initial magnetization induced by the static field. The signal decays partly because of spin-spin interactions but also because the static field is not perfectly homogeneous. The 180-degree pulse applied after time τ reflects the spins about a fixed axis normal to the field direction so that they refocus to give an echo signal at time 2τ. The echo amplitude, M(2τ), is given by

$$M(2\tau) = M(o)e - \frac{2\tau}{T2}$$

independent of field imperfections. (From Gore JC, Emery EW, Orr JS, et al: Invest Radiol 16:269, 1981.)

MR are obtained by using two to three RR intervals and a TE of 80 msec or more. In practice, a double-echo sequence is commonly used; that is, a TR corresponding to two or three RR intervals with both a short echo delay (TE of ≤20 msec) and a long echo delay (TE of ≥80 msec). The sequence that minimizes the T1 effect (long TR) and the T2 effect (short TE) is referred to as the *proton density sequence*. The signal on the proton density–weighted image is influenced primarily by the proton density or relative water content. Although this sequence provides the best signal-to-noise ratio, it has limited contrast (i.e., limited ability to distinguish various tissues) because it minimizes the effects of both T1 and T2 relaxation times. In summary, the intensity of the MR image depends on four parameters: nuclear density, two relaxation times called T1 and T2, and motion of the nuclei within the imaged volume.

Routine examination of the chest usually includes a T1-weighted spin-echo coronal localizer sequence. This practice allows a first impression of the normal and abnormal findings and serves as a guide for prescribing the appropriate T1-, proton density–, and T2-weighted sequences. In the majority of cases, 8- to 10-mm-thick sections are performed with 1- to 2-mm intersection gaps. Although thinner sections may provide improved spatial resolution, they result in a lower signal-to-noise ratio.

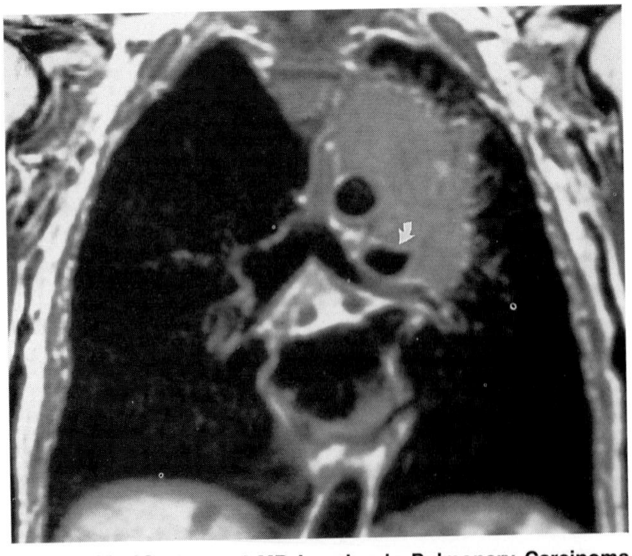

The advantages of MR imaging over CT include (1) lack of ionizing radiation; (2) direct coronal, sagittal or oblique, and transverse imaging (Fig. 13–18); (3) intrinsic contrast in blood vessels because of flow; and (4) increased soft tissue contrast because of multiple MR parameters as compared with only electron density on CT (Fig. 13–19). The main limitation of MR imaging in the chest is the presence of physiologic motion, which severely degrades image quality. Although this quality has greatly improved in recent years with the use of cardiac gating and respiratory compensation, the use of MR imaging in the assessment of lung parenchyma is still hampered by the low signal-to-noise ratio caused by the low proton density of the lungs and the loss in signal resulting from the magnetic field inhomogeneity created by the difference in diamagnetic susceptibilities between air and water. This situation creates innumerable magnetic susceptibility gradients in inflated lung that in the presence of water perfusion and diffusion lead to loss of signal at conventional (TE of 20 msec) echo delays. As a consequence, most normal lungs show little or no MR signal above background on standard MR sequences.[125] The signal in lung parenchyma can be increased by the use of specialized techniques such as ultrashort-TE, gradient-echo sequences and short-TE (≤7 msec) spin-echo sequences.[126, 127] Use of a spin-echo sequence with a short echo delay (TE of ≤7 msec) partially compensates for the very short T2 relaxation time of inflated lung parenchyma and has been shown to lead to a 3.5-fold increase in the signal-to-noise ratio from aerated lung.[127]

Indications

Evaluation of the Heart and Great Vessels. MR imaging has a well-established role in the assessment of congenital abnormalities of the heart and great vessels. It is superior to echocardiography in the assessment of adult congenital heart disease because it permits unobstructed views of all atrial, ventricular, and great vessel abnormalities.[128, 129] However, it is usually reserved for patients with nondiagnostic or equivo-

Figure 13–18. Coronal MR Imaging in Pulmonary Carcinoma. Coronal T1-weighted (TR/TE, 800/20) cardiac-gated, spin-echo MR image demonstrates a large tumor in the left upper lobe. The tumor extends into the aortopulmonary window and is associated with encasement and narrowing of the left pulmonary artery *(arrow)*. The patient had an unresectable (T4) adenocarcinoma of the lung.

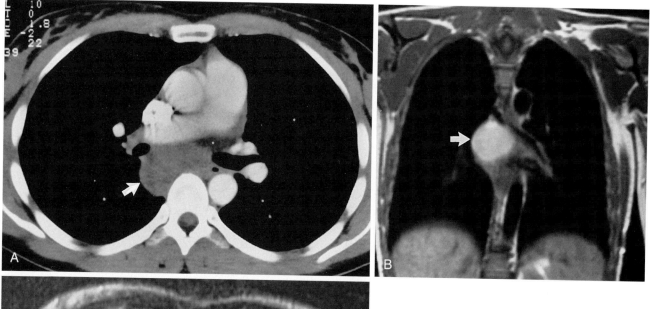

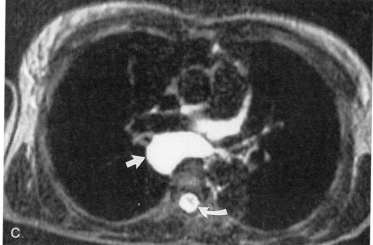

Figure 13–19. Soft Tissue and Fluid Characterization on CT and MR Imaging. A contrast-enhanced CT scan *(A)* demonstrates a large, smoothly marginated subcarinal lesion *(arrow)*. The attenuation value is consistent with either a soft tissue lesion or a cyst filled with proteinaceous material. A coronal T1-weighted (TR/TE, 923/20) spin-echo MR image *(B)* shows a subcarinal mass with high signal intensity *(arrow)*. A transverse T2-weighted (TR/TE, 2,769/100) *(C)* spin-echo MR image obtained at the same level as *A* demonstrates an area of homogeneous high signal intensity *(straight arrow)*. The high signal intensity on the T2-weighted image is diagnostic of fluid. Note that the signal in the subcarinal mass *(straight arrow)* in *C* is identical to that of cerebrospinal fluid *(curved arrow)*.

cal findings on echocardiography.[129] MR imaging also allows excellent assessment of central pulmonary artery abnormalities. Cine gradient-echo sequences allow assessment of cardiac wall motion and can detect high-velocity jets caused by ventricular septal defects, valvular regurgitation, or focal stenoses.[128, 130] Velocity-encoded cine sequences can be used to calculate blood flow.[131]

Although comparable to conventional CT in the assessment of aortic aneurysms[132] and aortic dissection,[133] MR imaging has been shown to be inferior to spiral CT.[134] In one study in which spiral CT, multiplanar transesophageal echocardiography, and MR imaging were compared, the three techniques were found to have 100% sensitivity in the detection of thoracic aortic dissection;[134] however, spiral CT had a higher specificity. Furthermore, the sensitivity in detecting aortic arch vessel involvement was 93% for spiral CT, 60% for transesophageal echocardiography, and 67% for MRI, with specificities of 97%, 85%, and 88%, respectively.

Evaluation of the Mediastinum and Hila. Currently, MR imaging is a secondary imaging modality in the mediastinum and hila that is used mainly in cases in which the CT findings are equivocal. In patients with pulmonary carcinoma, MR imaging has been shown to be superior to CT in the assess-

ment of mediastinal and vascular invasion.[135] It can also be helpful in the diagnosis of bronchogenic cysts in cases in which the CT findings are not diagnostic (see Fig. 13–19);[136] these lesions characteristically show a homogeneous high signal intensity on T2-weighted MR images because of their fluid content.

Evaluation of the Chest Wall. MR imaging allows excellent assessment of primary chest wall tumors,[137] and chest wall extension of lymphoma,[138] and pulmonary carcinoma, particularly superior sulcus tumors.[139, 140] Assessment of tumor invasion of fat and vascular involvement is most readily made with the use of T1-weighted sequences. T2-weighted sequences are optimal for differentiation of tumor and edema from surrounding muscle.[120] MR imaging is also ideally suited for the evaluation of neurogenic tumors, since it provides excellent assessment of the tissue characteristics of the mass, as well as assessment of intraspinal extension.[141, 142] MR is therefore the imaging modality of choice in the assessment of paraspinal lesions (Fig. 13–20).

Evaluation of the Lung Parenchyma. MR imaging has limited benefit in the assessment of lung parenchyma. However, several groups have demonstrated a potential role in the assessment of chronic interstitial and air-space lung dis-

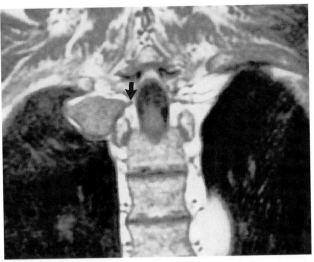

Figure 13–20. MR Imaging of Paraspinal Tumor. A coronal, spin-echo, T1-weighted MR image (TR/TE, 800/15) demonstrates a paraspinal tumor that can be seen to originate from a nerve root *(arrow)*. Surgery confirmed the diagnosis of neurofibroma.

ease[143, 144] and in the qualitative and quantitative measurement of lung water content.[145, 146] The technique can also be helpful in identifying mass lesions in a completely opacified hemithorax following pneumonectomy and in the distinction of atelectasis caused by a hilar-obstructing lesion from nonobstructive (passive) lobar atelectasis.[147]

BRONCHOGRAPHY

Until the advent of HRCT, bronchography was used to investigate the presence and extent of bronchiectasis. Because of the risks of allergic reaction to the bronchographic medium (ranging from bronchospasm through iodism to frank anaphylaxis and death) and the temporary impairment in ventilation and diffusion,[148, 149] its use was limited to patients in whom surgical resection of local disease was considered. It is now clear, however, that CT is a more valuable technique in the investigation of this disease. For example, in a 1986 study comparing HRCT (1.5-mm-thick sections) obtained every 10 mm with bronchography in 44 lungs from 36 patients, CT was found to have a sensitivity of 97% and a specificity of 93%.[150] In another investigation of 259 segmental bronchi from 70 lobes, CT was positive in 87 of 89 segmental bronchi shown to have bronchiectasis (sensitivity, 98%) and negative in 169 of 170 segmental bronchi without bronchiectasis at bronchography (specificity, 99%).[151] Similar results have been reported by other investigators.[152] Given the high diagnostic accuracy of CT and the morbidity associated with bronchography, the latter has become an outmoded imaging technique.

It has been suggested, however, that selective bronchography performed through the fiberoptic bronchoscope and using an iso-osmolar, nonionic contrast medium may be helpful in the diagnosis of bronchiectasis.[153, 154] A dimeric contrast medium is required because monomeric nonionic agents at iso-osmolar concentrations do not provide sufficient iodine concentration.[153] The technique is generally well tolerated, although headaches, nausea, and flushing may develop in some patients. It should be reserved for patients

with recurrent hemoptysis in whom the HRCT scan is normal or shows only questionable abnormalities.[155]

ANGIOGRAPHY

Angiography includes all procedures in which contrast medium is injected into vascular structures for investigating thoracic disease. These methods include pulmonary angiography, aortography, bronchial arteriography, superior vena cava angiography, and azygography. Only the general indications for their use are considered here; detailed discussion in relation to specific diseases is presented in relevant chapters.

Pulmonary Angiography

Technique

Depending on individual circumstances, pulmonary angiography can be performed by various routes: (1) by venous injection into one or both arms simultaneously through a needle or (preferably) a catheter; (2) via a catheter into the superior vena cava, right atrium, right ventricle, or main pulmonary artery; or (3) by selective injection into the right or left pulmonary artery or one of its branches. In pulmonary angiography, as in all other special angiographic procedures, individual requirements for each examination must be determined in relation to the specific circumstances. In the majority of cases, however, selective catheterization with injection of contrast into the right and left pulmonary arteries or one of their major branches is considered the method of choice. This procedure invariably produces clearer opacification of the pulmonary vascular tree than does venous or intracardiac injection,[156] a finding that relates to the fact that a diseased segment of the arterial tree causes blood to be shunted away from that segment, so a flood injection tends to opacify comparatively normal branches remote from the disease. The superior visibility following selective catheterization usually outweighs any disadvantage inherent in the catheterization procedure itself.

Pulmonary angiography may be performed by using conventional film technique or digital subtraction (DSA). The latter has several advantages, the main one being the elimination of overlapping projection of other structures so that the pulmonary vessels are visualized better (Fig. 13–21). The use of DSA also allows an approximately 25% reduction in the volume of contrast material required.[157] Besides being cost saving, this reduction also decreases the risk of acute heart failure in patients with severe chronic pulmonary arterial hypertension.[158, 159] Interobserver agreement in the interpretation of DSA images and conventional angiograms performed for the diagnosis of pulmonary embolism was assessed in one prospective study of 397 consecutive patients with nondiagnostic ventilation-perfusion lung scan results.[159] All angiograms were read immediately by the attending radiologist, by two radiologists after 6 months, and later by means of consensus of the two radiologists. Interobserver disagreement occurred in 4% to 11% of patients with DSA images as compared with 20% to 36% of patients with conventional images. Initial diagnoses were changed after the images were reviewed by consensus in 12% of patients with DSA images and 20% of patients with conventional angiograms. The authors concluded that interobserver

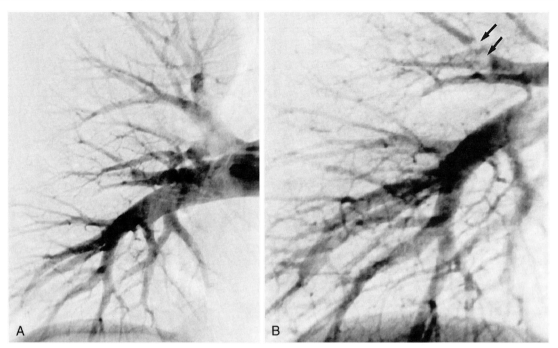

Figure 13–21. Digital Subtraction Angiography. Views from a selective right pulmonary angiogram using digital subtraction technique *(A and B)* demonstrate good visualization of the pulmonary vessels. The localized filling defects *(arrows in B)* seen in a subsegmental artery in the right middle lobe indicate the presence of pulmonary emboli.

agreement was better with intra-arterial DSA than with conventional pulmonary angiography.

The two main disadvantages of DSA are the increased breath-hold time required to obtain the image (which leads to increased motion artefacts) and the dilution of intravenous contrast material (which results in poor opacification of small pulmonary artery branches).[159] The latter can be improved considerably with the use of selective intra-arterial DSA.[159]

Complications

Although pulmonary angiography is considered to be the gold standard for the diagnosis of pulmonary thromboembolism, the procedure is only requested in a small percentage of patients with clinically suspected embolism and nondiagnostic ventilation-perfusion scans. For example, in a review of 316 consecutive cases of suspected pulmonary embolism in a large institution in the United States, only 24 of 141 patients with indeterminate ventilation-perfusion scans underwent pulmonary angiography.[160] In another survey of 360 acute care hospitals in the United Kingdom, approximately 47,000 ventilation-perfusion lung scans were obtained as opposed to only 490 pulmonary angiograms.[161]

The reluctance to request pulmonary angiograms stems to some extent from concern over the perceived risks of morbidity and mortality from the procedure.[160, 162] This reluctance is still present in spite of a considerable decrease in the number of complications over the years.[162–164] In 1980, the complications seen in 1,350 patients who underwent pulmonary angiography at Duke University were reported.[163] Three deaths (0.2%) were directly attributable to the procedure, all in patients with pulmonary arterial hypertension (systolic pressures of 75, 100, and 160 mm Hg). The most common serious complications were cardiac perforation and

endocardial and myocardial injury, which were seen in 20 patients (1.5%). In a second study from the same institution based on 1,434 patients and published in 1987, the authors found only 2 deaths directly attributable to the procedure. Other complications included reversible cardiac arrest in 5 patients and cardiac arrhythmias in 15.[164]

Since 1987, two major technical developments have occurred: the replacement of stiff end-hole catheters by multiple side-hole pigtail catheters[162] or flow-directed catheters[157] and the use of low-osmolar intravenous contrast medium.[162] In a 1996 review of 1,434 patients who underwent pulmonary angiography with nonionic contrast medium (iopamidol, 76%) and multiple side-hole pigtail catheters, major complications were found in only 4 patients (0.3%);[162] no deaths were attributed to the procedure. The major complications included respiratory arrest requiring ventilatory support (in 2 patients) and recurrent ventricular arrhythmias (in 2 more). Minor complications were seen in 11 patients (0.8%) and included arrhythmias responsive to lidocaine, catheter-induced vasovagal syncope, chest pain, and contrast-induced urticaria. In another study of 211 patients assessed with the use of selective pulmonary DSA performed with an 8-F Swan-Ganz–type flow-directed pulmonary angiography catheter and nonionic contrast material, no mortality or morbidity as a direct result of pulmonary angiography was observed.[157] In summary, with the current devices and techniques—particularly flow-directed catheters, selective pulmonary artery catheterization, and nonionic low-osmolar contrast medium—pulmonary angiography is a safe procedure even in patients with pulmonary arterial hypertension.[157, 162]

Indications

Detection of Congenital Abnormalities of the Pulmonary Vasculature. Abnormalities include agenesis or hypoplasia of a pulmonary artery, coarctation of one or more pulmonary arteries (peripheral pulmonic stenosis), and anomalous pulmonary venous drainage.

Investigation of Thromboembolic Disease. Pulmonary angiography is the gold standard in the diagnosis of acute thromboembolism (Fig. 13–22).[165–168] It is also indicated in patients with pulmonary hypertension and suspected chronic thromboembolism in whom the diagnosis cannot be confirmed with less invasive techniques such as spiral CT.

Aortography

Technique

The preferred technique for aortography is direct catheterization of the thoracic aorta percutaneously from either the femoral or brachial artery.[169, 170] An alternative method is digital subtraction aortography following injection into an arm vein or the superior vena cava;[171] although this technique provides satisfactory opacification in selected cases when direct catheterization of the aorta is contraindicated, it is seldom used in clinical practice.

Indications

Evaluation of Mediastinal Injury. Traditionally, aortography has been considered imperative in patients in whom mediastinal widening is observed radiographically following severe deceleration injuries.[172] In this situation, the procedure has been performed to distinguish purely venous hematoma from major arterial injury and to show the number and sites

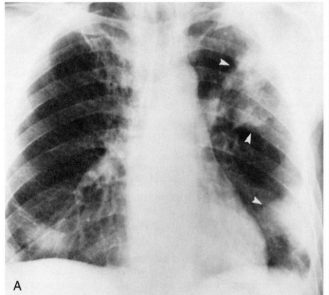

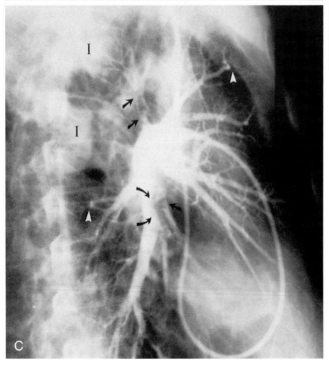

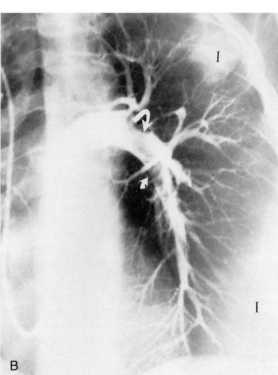

Figure 13–22. The Value of Pulmonary Angiography in the Demonstration of Thromboembolism. A conventional posteroanterior chest radiograph *(A)* discloses multiple areas of consolidation *(arrowheads)* that relate closely to a pleural surface. Selective left pulmonary angiograms in oblique *(B)* and lateral *(C)* projection (arterial phase) demonstrate multiple intraluminal filling defects *(arrows)* and amputated peripheral arteries *(arrowheads)*. Note that the vascular abnormalities subtend the infarcts identified on the conventional study *(I in B and C)*. Similar findings were present in the right pulmonary artery (not shown). The features are diagnostic of pulmonary thromboembolism and infarction.

of arterial lesions. Although chest radiography has a high sensitivity in the detection of mediastinal hemorrhage following trauma, aortography shows aortic injury in fewer than 10% of cases;[173] this overutilization is generally accepted practice because of the high mortality associated with undetected traumatic aortic disruption.[173]

The need for aortography in the evaluation of mediastinal injury can be decreased considerably with the use of CT.[174–176, 176a] In one retrospective study,[176] the findings on contrast-enhanced conventional CT scans performed to evaluate traumatic aortic injury in 677 patients were reviewed. The scans were interpreted as negative in 570 patients (84%), positive for mediastinal hematoma in 100, and technically inadequate or equivocal in 7. The 570 patients with negative CT scans had no further evaluation. Of the 100 patients with mediastinal hemorrhage on CT, abnormalities of the aorta were identified on CT in 21. The abnormalities included irregular contour of the aorta, pseudoaneurysm, intimal flap, or pseudocoarctation (Fig. 13–23). Angiography demonstrated traumatic aortic injuries in 19 (90%) of these 21 patients. In the 79 patients in whom mediastinal hemorrhage was the only finding on CT, angiography was negative for aortic injury in 77 (97%) and positive in 2.

In a prospective study of 1,518 patients with nontrivial blunt trauma who were examined with spiral CT,[176] 127 (8.4%) had abnormal CT scans of the mediastinum and underwent thoracic aortography. In 89 (70%) of the 127 patients, spiral CT demonstrated a mediastinal hematoma but a normal aorta. None of these patients had aortic tears on aortography. Spiral CT had a lower specificity (82%) than did aortography (96%). Meta-analysis of the data in the literature prior to 1996 indicates that using either mediastinal

hemorrhage or abnormalities of the aorta as an indicator for a positive CT examination provides a sensitivity of 99.3%, a specificity of 87%, a positive predictive value of 20%, and a negative predictive value of 99.9% in the diagnosis of aortic injury.[176a] Based on these results, some authors[176, 177] recommend CT in all patients with a history of blunt decelerating trauma and chest radiographic findings that are equivocal or suggestive of mediastinal hemorrhage. We and others,[178] however, prefer to use angiography in patients with radiographic findings highly suggestive of mediastinal hematoma. We also recommend CT, preferably using the spiral technique, in the screening of patients with questionable radiographic findings and in patients undergoing CT for evaluation of other injuries.[178]

Evaluation of Congenital Vascular Anomalies. Other indications for aortography include precise identification of aortic anomalies, such as patent ductus arteriosus or aortic coarctation, and the identification of anomalous vessels, such as an artery supplying a sequestered lobe.[179, 180]

Bronchial and Intercostal Arteriography

Technique

Optimal opacification of the bronchial arteries can be achieved only by selective catheterization, usually via a percutaneous transfemoral approach.[181–183] Since the arteries originate from the aorta at the level of the fifth or sixth thoracic vertebra in about 80% of patients,[184] the catheter is first advanced to this region. The catheter tip is pointed posterolaterally along the right aortic wall to locate the right bronchial artery and is pointed anterolaterally and to the left when searching for the left bronchial arteries.[185] When an artery is located, a small amount of contrast is injected to confirm its identity. Once the bronchial artery is identified, it is selectively catheterized and contrast is injected.

An important consideration in the performance of bronchial arteriography is the relationship of the bronchial arteries with the arteries supplying the spinal cord. The main blood supply to the spinal cord is via the anterior spinal artery, which originates from the intracranial branches of the vertebral arteries.[185] Another important supply is the anterior radicular artery (artery of Adamkiewicz), which most commonly originates from the aorta at the level of the lower thoracic spine (T8 to T12). This artery provides blood to the lower thoracic and lumbosacral spinal cord; in approximately 5% of cases it arises from the right intercostal-bronchial trunk.[185] In addition to these major vessels, smaller posterior spinal arteries may originate from the aorta at different levels. Extreme caution must be used when performing bronchial arteriography to avoid occlusion of any of these vessels and secondary spinal cord complications, particularly transverse myelitis.[185]

Indications

Bronchial arteriography is occasionally performed to investigate severe hemoptysis when a possible source of bleeding is not apparent from the radiograph or CT. However, more commonly it is performed as part of the assessment for therapeutic embolization of bronchial arteries in

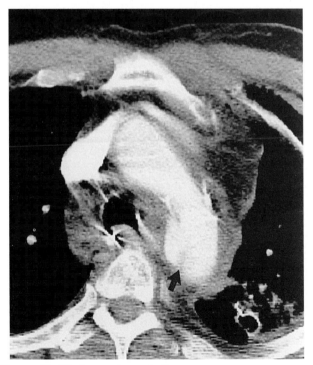

Figure 13–23. Traumatic Aortic Tear. A spiral CT scan following the intravenous administration of contrast shows focal irregularity of the contour of the aortic arch *(arrow)*. A small amount of blood is present in the mediastinum. The diagnosis of traumatic aortic tear was confirmed at surgery.

patients with life-threatening hemoptysis in whom resectional surgery is contraindicated for one reason or another (Fig. 13–24) or for stabilization of patients with massive hemoptysis prior to surgery.[185–188]

The main factors limiting long-term success of bronchial artery embolization are progression of underlying disease[189] and recruitment of systemic collaterals.[185] When patients have cataclysmic hemoptysis, it is important to recognize that the nonbronchial systemic vessels can be the source of bleeding, particularly in patients with chronic infection and pleural involvement;[190] in such cases it can be exceedingly difficult to decide what vessel or vessels to embolize.[191] A pulmonary artery source should also be considered when embolization of systemic arteries fails to control bleeding.

RADIONUCLIDE IMAGING

The number of indications for radionuclide imaging in pulmonary disorders has increased considerably over the years. The main clinical applications include diagnosis of pulmonary thromboembolism, prediction of pulmonary function after surgery, assessment of the presence of lung inflammation or infection, and assessment of lung tumors.

Lung scintigraphy involves the recording of γ-radiation produced by radiopharmaceuticals that are injected intravenously or inhaled into the air spaces. The most widely used imaging device is the scintillation or gamma camera, which records the flux of γ-radiation from the lungs in a single exposure. The most commonly used scintigraphic techniques in pulmonary nuclear medicine are ventilation-perfusion ($\dot{V}/\dot{Q}$) lung scans and gallium 67 (^{67}Ga) citrate scans. Some groups have also shown that the use of positron emission tomography (PET) with 2-[^{18}F]-fluoro-2-deoxy-D-glucose (FDG) can be helpful in distinguishing benign from malignant lung lesions and in staging pulmonary carcinoma.

Ventilation-Perfusion Lung Scanning

Technique

Currently, the radiopharmaceuticals of choice for perfusion lung scanning are either technetium 99m–labeled human albumin microspheres (^{99m}Tc-HAM) or macroaggregated albumin (^{99m}Tc-MAA) (Fig. 13–25). ^{99m}Tc-MAA particles vary in size from 10 to 150 μm, with over 90% of particles measuring between 10 and 90 μm. ^{99m}Tc-HAM particles are more uniform in size and range from 35 to 60 μm. The

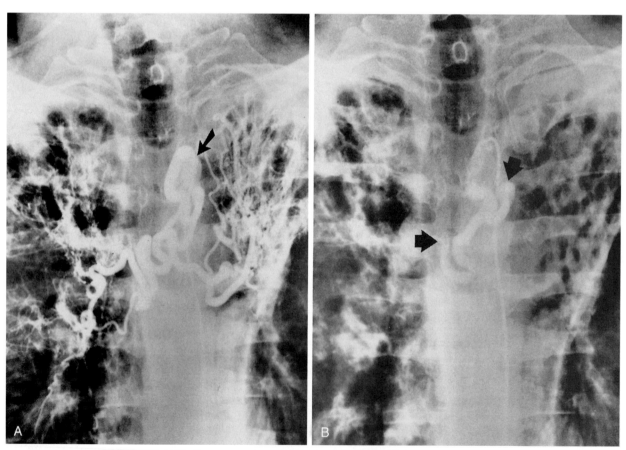

Figure 13–24. Bronchial Artery Embolization for Life-Threatening Pulmonary Hemorrhage. A bronchial artery angiogram *(A)* reveals marked dilatation of the vessel within the mediastinum and a remarkable increase in flow to a partly atelectatic left upper lobe with severe bronchiectasis; note the origin of the bronchial artery from the top of the aortic arch *(arrow)*. This 40-year-old man with cystic fibrosis had hemoptysis amounting to 600 ml during the previous 24 hours. Following the injection of polyvinyl alcohol foam (Ivalon) particles, a repeat injection of contrast medium *(B)* reveals total obstruction of both the left and right branches of the bronchial artery *(arrows)* and an absence of flow to the left upper lobe.

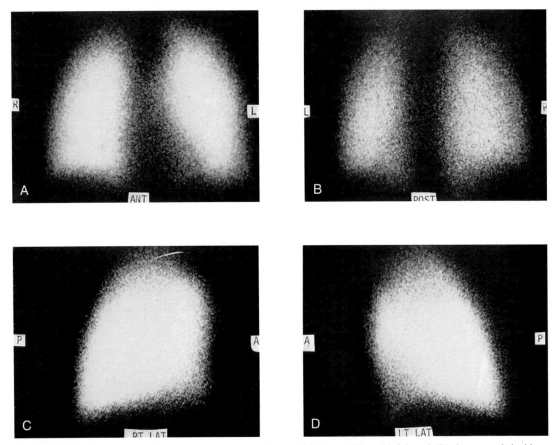

Figure 13–25. Normal Perfusion Lung Scan. Anterior *(A)*, posterior *(B)*, right lateral *(C)*, and left lateral *(D)* views recorded with a gamma camera following intravenous injection of ^{99m}Tc-labeled macroaggregated albumin show normal pulmonary perfusion.

biologic half-life of ^{99m}Tc-MAA within the lung ranges between 2 and 6 hours.

The intravenous administration of either ^{99m}Tc-HAM or ^{99m}Tc-MAA should be performed over a period of 5 to 10 respiratory cycles with the patient in the supine position, which limits the effect of gravity on regional pulmonary arterial blood flow. Following injection, particles pass through the right atrium and ventricle and lodge within precapillary arterioles in the lungs. The distribution of particles is proportional to regional pulmonary blood flow at the time of injection. The radiopharmaceutical injection is usually between 74 and 148 MBq (2 to 4 mCi) and contains 200,000 to 500,000 particles. It has been estimated that only about 0.1% of precapillary arterioles are transiently blocked in routine clinical use.[192] The number of particles injected should be reduced in patients with pulmonary hypertension, patients with right-to-left intracardiac or intrapulmonary shunts, children, and patients who have undergone pneumonectomy or single-lung transplantation. A minimum of 60,000 particles is required to obtain an even distribution of activity within the pulmonary arterial circulation and avoid potential false-positive interpretations.[192]

When scintigraphy is performed to assess pulmonary perfusion, at least six views of the lungs should be obtained, including anterior, posterior, right and left lateral, and right and left posterior oblique views. Additional right and left anterior oblique views may be helpful in selected cases. In animal studies, it has been demonstrated that perfusion imaging will detect greater than 90% of emboli that completely

occlude pulmonary arterial vessels greater than 2 mm in diameter.[193]

Perfusion scintigraphy is sensitive but nonspecific for diagnosing pulmonary disease. Virtually all parenchymal lung diseases (including neoplasms, infections, COPD, and asthma) can cause decreased pulmonary arterial blood flow within the affected lung zone. Since thromboemboli characteristically cause abnormal perfusion with preserved ventilation (mismatched defects) (Fig. 13–26) whereas parenchymal lung disease most often causes both ventilation and perfusion abnormalities in the same lung region (matched defects), combined ventilation and perfusion scintigraphy is routinely performed to improve the diagnostic specificity. Conditions in which the ventilation abnormality appears larger than the perfusion abnormality (reverse mismatch) include airway obstruction, atelectasis, and pneumonia.

The majority of the experience with ventilation imaging has been with xenon 133 (^{133}Xe). Alternative ventilation imaging techniques using ^{127}Xe, krypton 81m (^{81m}Kr), ^{99m}Tc aerosols, technegas, or pertechnegas have not been as extensively evaluated.[194] However, the available data suggest that there is no major diagnostic difference between the agents.

With ^{133}Xe, ventilation imaging is generally performed prior to perfusion imaging. An initial posterior washin or first-breath image is acquired for 100,000 counts or 10 to 15 seconds following the inhalation of 550 to 770 MBq of ^{133}Xe. Equilibrium images are then obtained while the patient rebreathes the gas within a closed system for at least 4 minutes. The washin or breath-hold images demonstrate re-

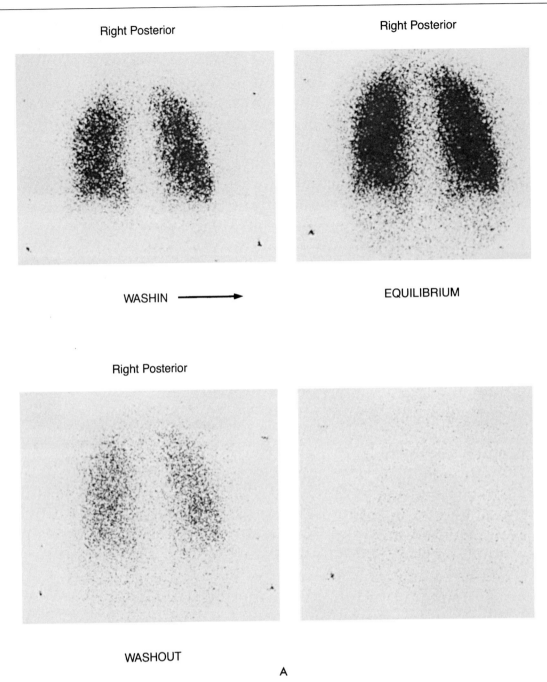

Figure 13–26. The Value of Ventilation/Perfusion Lung Scans in the Diagnosis of Thromboembolism. A xenon inhalation lung scan *(A)* discloses normal ventilation parameters during the washin, equilibrium, and washout phases. Corresponding technetium 99m–labeled macroaggregated albumin perfusion lung scans *(B, see* facing page) in anterior, posterior, and right and left posterior oblique projections identify multiple segmental filling defects throughout both lungs *(arrowheads).* These findings, in concert with the ventilation study are virtually diagnostic (high probability) of pulmonary thromboembolism. The patient was a 65-year-old man with acute dyspnea.

gional lung ventilation. Regions of the lungs that appear as defects on the washin images may normalize on the equilibrium image because of collateral ventilation. Finally, serial washout images are acquired while the patient breathes ambient air, and regional air trapping can be detected as focal areas of retained activity. Serial washout images should be initially performed in the posterior projection rather than in the left and right posterior oblique positions to maximize the number of lung segments that can be visualized. To optimize diagnostic performance of the test, patients should be imaged

in the erect position; however, if necessary, supine patients or patients receiving ventilatory assistance can also be imaged.

The imaging technique using ^{127}Xe is similar to that of ^{133}Xe; however, because ^{127}Xe has a higher energy than ^{99m}Tc, ventilation imaging with this agent may be performed following perfusion imaging. There are two advantages to performing postperfusion ventilation studies: (1) the patient can be positioned such that the lung demonstrating the greatest perfusion abnormality may be imaged optimally; and (2) ventilation imaging may be avoided in cases in which the

Anterior

Posterior

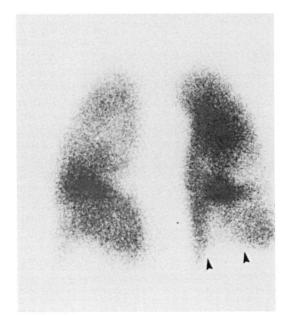

Right Posterior Oblique

Left Posterior Oblique

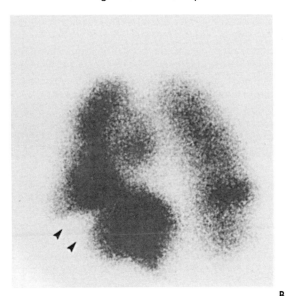 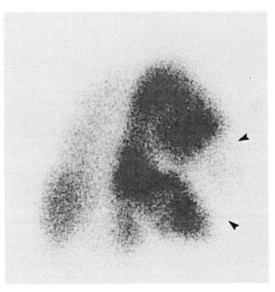

B

Figure 13–26 *Continued.*

perfusion lung scan appears normal. However, ^{127}Xe also has two major disadvantages: it is more costly than ^{133}Xe and requires medium energy collimation. When ventilation imaging is performed with either ^{133}Xe or ^{127}Xe, initial breath-hold or washin images can be obtained only in a single projection, thus limiting the comparison with perfusion images, which are obtained in multiple projections.

^{81m}Kr is another insoluble gas used to assess regional ventilation. This agent has a very short physical half-life (13 seconds), and therefore only washin or breath-hold images

can be acquired. However, the short half-life enables the acquisition of images in multiple projections, thereby allowing direct comparison with perfusion lung images. ^{81m}Kr is relatively expensive and is produced from a rubidium 81 generator. The parent radionuclide itself has a physical half-life of only 4.7 minutes; therefore the useful lifetime of the generator is only 1 day. Similar to ^{127}Xe, ventilation imaging with ^{81m}Kr is generally performed following perfusion imaging.

Ventilation imaging with ^{99m}Tc-radiolabeled aerosols

can be performed with several radiopharmaceuticals, including ^{99m}Tc-diethylenetriamine pentaacetic acid (DTPA), ^{99m}Tc-sulfur colloid, ^{99m}Tc-pyrophosphate, ^{99m}Tc-methylene diphosphonate, or ^{99m}Tc-glucoheptanate. The most commonly used agent is ^{99m}Tc-DTPA; however, it has a relatively short residence time within the lung, particularly in smokers, and for these patients ^{99m}Tc-labeled sulfur colloid or pyrophosphate may be more useful. ^{99m}Tc–labeled radioaerosols are between 0.5 and 3 μm in size and are produced by a commercially available nebulizer. For a routine ventilation study, 1.11 GBq (30 mCi) of ^{99m}Tc-DTPA in 3 ml of saline is placed within the nebulizer. High-pressure oxygen is then forced through the nebulizer and produces aerosolized droplets that are inhaled by the patient through a mask or mouthpiece. The patient generally breathes from the nebulizer for 3 to 5 minutes or until 37 MBq (1 mCi) of activity is deposited within the lungs. The distribution of activity within the lungs is proportional to regional ventilation. ^{99m}Tc–labeled radioaerosol studies are generally performed prior to perfusion imaging and multiple image projections can be obtained. Ventilation studies with ^{99m}Tc-labeled radioaerosols require minimal patient cooperation and can be performed in patients receiving ventilatory assistance. Disadvantages of ^{99m}Tc-labeled radioaerosols relate primarily to central deposition of activity in patients with airway obstruction and the amount of activity that is wasted within the nebulizer.

Because of the problem with central deposition of ^{99m}Tc-labeled radioaerosol in patients with COPD, newer agents such as ^{99m}Tc-technegas and ^{99m}Tc-pertechnegas have been developed.[194] Both of these agents are produced by burning ^{99m}Tc-pertechnetate in a carbon crucible at very high temperatures, a procedure that leads to an ultrafine radiolabeled aerosol (particle size, 0.02 to 0.2 μm). Pertechnegas is purged with 5% oxygen and 95% argon, as opposed to technegas, which is purged with 100% argon. This relatively minor difference causes profound changes in the biologic half-life. When inhaled, both agents are distributed homogeneously within the lung in proportion to the regional lung ventilation, and very little central deposition of activity is seen, even in patients with COPD. Pertechnegas readily penetrates the alveolar epithelial membrane, and its biologic half-life in the lungs is quite short (approximately 6 to 10 minutes). On the other hand, there is very little transalveolar or mucociliary clearance of technegas, and the effective half-life is essentially equal to the physical half-life. The use of both these agents requires minimal patient cooperation, and only two or three breaths are necessary to obtain sufficient activity within the lungs to perform ventilation imaging. In general, ventilation imaging with both technegas and pertechnegas is performed prior to perfusion imaging; similar to ^{99m}Tc-radiolabeled aerosols, views of the lungs can be obtained for multiple projections corresponding to the views obtained with perfusion imaging.

Indications

Diagnosis and Follow-up of Acute Pulmonary Thromboembolism.

The ventilation-perfusion (V̇/Q̇) lung scan has been shown to be a safe noninvasive technique to evaluate regional pulmonary perfusion and ventilation and has been widely used in the evaluation of patients with suspected thromboembolism (Tables 13–2 and 13–3).[195–197] Despite

Table 13–2. SENSITIVITY, SPECIFICITY, AND POSITIVE PREDICTIVE VALUE OF V̇/Q̇ LUNG SCANNING FOR DETECTING ACUTE PULMONARY THROMBOEMBOLISM USING THE ORIGINAL PIOPED INTERPRETATION CRITERIA

V̇/Q̇ SCAN INTERPRETATION	SENSITIVITY (%)	SPECIFICITY (%)	PPV (%)
High	40	98	87
High, intermediate	82	64	49
High, intermediate, low	98	12	32

V̇/Q̇, ventilation-perfusion; PIOPED, Prospective Investigation of Pulmonary Embolism Diagnosis; PPV, positive predictive value.

Data from The PIOPED Investigators: JAMA 263:2753, 1990.

these attributes and studies suggesting an underdiagnosis of thromboemboli, critics have suggested that V̇/Q̇ scanning has been overused and has minimal impact on patient management.[198–200]

The Urokinase Pulmonary Embolism Trial (UPET) was a large-scale study that used perfusion lung scanning as a screening test for the diagnosis of pulmonary thromboemboli.[201] In more than 90% of the patients enrolled in the trial, perfusion lung scanning was performed following the intravenous administration of ^{131}I-labeled MAA. Since perfusion scanning was accomplished with a rectilinear scanner, no ventilation imaging was performed. Despite using suboptimal radiopharmaceuticals and instrumentation as judged by current standards, the UPET study established perfusion lung scanning as an effective technique to diagnose pulmonary thromboembolism and to assess restoration of pulmonary blood flow following an embolic event.[201] The majority of patients who are treated for acute pulmonary thromboembolism either completely lyse their thrombus or partially recanalize their pulmonary arteries. In the UPET study, approximately 75% to 80% of perfusion defects resolved by 3 months; those defects that did not resolve by this time remained largely persistent when monitored for 1 year. (The amount of clot resolution observed in this study is probably an underestimate, since ventilation scanning was not performed and many of the unresolved perfusion defects might have been due to pre-existing chronic obstructive lung disease.) Based on data from the UPET, we would recommend

Table 13–3. EFFECT OF SELECTED RISK FACTORS ON THE PREVALENCE OF PULMONARY THROMBOEMBOLISM

V̇/Q̇ SCAN INTERPRETATION	0 RISK FACTORS*	1 RISK FACTOR*	≥2 RISK FACTORS*
High	63/77 (82%)	41/49 (84%)	56/58 (97%)
Intermediate	52/207 (25%)	40/107 (37%)	77/173 (45%)
Low/very low	14/315 (4%)	19/155 (12%)	37/179 (21%)

*Risk factors include immobilization, trauma to the lower extremities, surgery, or central venous instrumentation within 3 months of enrollment.

Results are based on the data published in Worsley DF, Alavi A, Palevsky HI: Comparison of the diagnostic performance of ventilation/perfusion lung scanning in different patient populations. Radiology 199:481, 1996.

performing a repeat perfusion lung scan approximately 3 months following the initial diagnosis of pulmonary thromboembolism to evaluate clot resolution and serve as a baseline for future comparisons.

Prediction of Pulmonary Function After Surgery. Quantitative $\dot{V}/\dot{Q}$ lung scanning has been shown to be a useful method for determining regional lung function in patients who are to undergo pulmonary resection or lung transplantation. Its major use is in the prediction of postoperative function following lobectomy or pneumonectomy. For lung carcinomas that are located in the lung periphery, ventilation and perfusion defects are usually matched and correspond to the abnormality noted on the chest radiograph. In central carcinoma, however, discrepancies between ventilation and perfusion ($\dot{V}/\dot{Q}$ mismatch) are commonly seen. In these cases, either the primary lung tumor or enlarged lymph nodes cause obstruction of the pulmonary vasculature, which in turn causes decreased perfusion to the affected lobe or segment. Thus in patients with central carcinomas, regional perfusion values correlate better with regional lung function and should be used to predict postoperative lung function.

The predicted postoperative forced expiratory volume in 1 second (FEV_1) after lobectomy or pneumonectomy is calculated by multiplying the preoperative value by the percentage of radionuclide activity in the lobes or lung that will remain after surgery.[202] An expected postoperative FEV_1 less than 0.8 liters or 35% of predicted usually precludes lung resection.

Gallium 67 Lung Scanning

The radiopharmaceutical of choice for imaging pulmonary infection and inflammation is ^{67}Ga citrate, a ferric analogue with a physical half-life of 78 hours; following intravenous administration, approximately 90% of the administered activity is bound to transferrin. The optimum time to perform thoracic imaging is 48 to 72 hours following injection. The precise mechanism of gallium localization at sites of inflammation is not completely understood but has been postulated to be related to increased vascular permeability, direct bacterial uptake of gallium (binding to siderophores), binding to lactoferrin secreted by activated leukocytes, and direct binding to circulating leukocytes.[203]

Although nonspecific, the intensity and distribution of ^{67}Ga accumulation within the lungs can be used to quantify the degree of pulmonary parenchymal inflammation.[203] According to a widely used grading scheme, 0 = activity less than soft tissue activity, 1+ = activity equal to soft tissue activity, 2+ = activity greater than soft tissue activity but less than liver activity, 3+ = activity equal to liver activity, and 4+ = activity greater than liver activity. The grade of ^{67}Ga uptake can then be multiplied by the area of the lung involved to give a gallium index. Semiquantitative indices—including the ratio of lung activity to liver activity—can also be calculated and used in serial studies of patients who have interstitial or air-space disease.

Increased gallium activity within the chest is a sensitive, but relatively nonspecific indicator of pulmonary infection or inflammation. A variety of conditions—including adult respiratory distress syndrome, pneumonia, drug reactions [busulfan, cyclophosphamide, amiodarone, contrast follow-

ing lymphangiography], pneumoconiosis, idiopathic pulmonary fibrosis, sarcoidosis, and uremic pneumonitis—may cause increased radiogallium accumulation within the lungs. Neoplastic disease such as lymphoma, leukemia, mesothelioma, or metastatic carcinoma may also cause increased radiogallium activity, although its distribution is usually more focal.

^{67}Ga scintigraphy has been used most commonly in patients with sarcoidosis, in which the typical scintigraphic appearance consists of bilateral, perihilar, or peritracheal activity (Fig. 13–27).[203] Parenchymal activity can also be seen, either with or without hilar activity; although it may be diffuse, it is usually most marked within the midlung zones with relative sparing of the upper and lower zones. This activity correlates with the presence of T lymphocytes in bronchoalveolar lavage specimens and has been shown to correlate well with response to therapy.[204–206]

Use of ^{67}Ga uptake for the assessment of disease activity, prediction of response to corticosteroids, and estimation of prognosis in idiopathic pulmonary fibrosis has been found to be disappointing.[207–210] As a result, ^{67}Ga scanning is not recommended for the assessment of patients with this condition.[211, 212]

In immunocompromised hosts, ^{67}Ga scintigraphy has a higher sensitivity than do plain chest radiographs for the detection of inflammatory disease.[213] In particular, the presence of diffuse gallium uptake within the lungs in a human immunodeficiency virus (HIV)-positive patient with a normal chest radiograph is highly suggestive of *Pneumocystis carinii* pneumonia (PCP) (Fig. 13–28). Other conditions

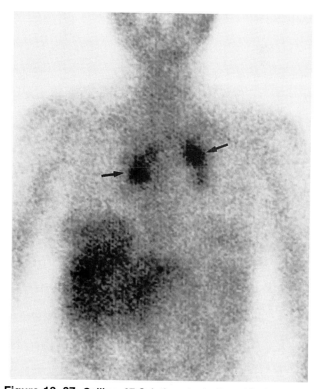

Figure 13–27. Gallium 67 Scintigraphy in Sarcoidosis. An anterior gallium 67 citrate image of the chest demonstrates bilateral symmetric perihilar increased activity *(arrows)* in a patient with active sarcoidosis. (Courtesy of Dr. Daniel Worsley, Department of Radiology, Vancouver Hospital and Health Sciences Centre, Vancouver, BC, Canada.)

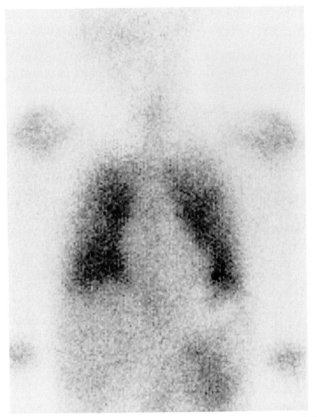

Figure 13–28. Gallium 67 Scintigraphy in *Pneumocystis carinii* Pneumonia. An anterior gallium 67 citrate image of the chest in an HIV-positive patient demonstrates intense diffuse increased accumulation of activity within both lungs, a finding characteristic of *P. carinii* pneumonia. (Courtesy of Dr. Daniel Worsley, Department of Radiology, Vancouver Hospital and Health Sciences Centre, Vancouver, BC, Canada.)

associated with diffuse lung uptake in immunocompromised patients include cytomegalovirus or cryptococcal infection and lymphoma. Although localized lung uptake may also be associated with PCP, particularly in patients treated with prophylactic aerosolized pentamidine, more often focal accumulation is related to bacterial pneumonia or lymphoma. Focal activity within the lung and corresponding regional lymph nodes is typical for *Mycobacterium avium-intracellulare* or *Mycobacterium tuberculosis* infection.[203] Kaposi's sarcoma does not accumulate ^{67}Ga, although the lesion takes up thallium 201 (^{201}Tl) chloride avidly. Sequential imaging with ^{67}Ga and ^{201}Tl chloride has been used to distinguish between Kaposi's sarcoma, PCP, and lymphoma in HIV-infected patients.[214]

High-dose ^{67}Ga scanning has also been shown to be useful in detecting mediastinal disease in both Hodgkin's and non-Hodgkin's lymphoma. (Because of the biodistribution of ^{67}Ga within the liver, spleen, and large bowel, gallium scintigraphy is less sensitive for detecting intra-abdominal or para-aortic disease.) Although Hodgkin's disease is usually gallium avid, there is some variation in the degree of uptake in the various histologic subtypes of non-Hodgkin's lymphoma: patients with intermediate- or high-grade lymphoma usually show increased accumulation of gallium, whereas uptake in low-grade lymphoma is usually less intense and sometimes absent. Currently, CT scanning is the method of

choice for the initial staging of lymphoma, ^{67}Ga imaging being most useful in detecting disease activity following therapy, when the differentiation between viable and necrotic tumor can be difficult.[215] When such post-therapy studies are performed, it is clearly important to have demonstrated that the lymphoma is gallium avid prior to therapy.

POSITRON EMISSION TOMOGRAPHY

PET is a functional imaging technique in which tomographic images are obtained following the administration of positron-emitting radiopharmaceuticals. Once emitted, positrons travel only several millimeters before losing enough energy to be susceptible to annihilation with an electron. During annihilation, the rest mass energy of the positron and electron are converted to energy, and two 511-keV γ-rays are emitted in opposite directions 180 degrees apart. The annihilation photons are simultaneously detected (coincidence detection) at opposite sides of a ring-type gantry.[216] As with CT, MR imaging, and single-photon emission computed tomography (SPECT), PET is based on the principle that a three-dimensional representation of an object can be obtained from multiple annular projections of that object. The optimum tomographic resolution of modern PET imaging systems is approximately 3 mm. The disadvantages of FDG-PET imaging relate predominantly to its inherent complexities, cost, and limited availability.

Multiheaded conventional gamma cameras, which are readily available in most nuclear medicine departments, can be equipped with ultrahigh-energy collimators to allow SPECT imaging of positron-emitting radiopharmaceuticals. The spatial resolution and sensitivity of these SPECT systems are inferior to PET systems. However, despite these limitations, diagnostic-quality images and clinically useful results have been obtained with FDG-SPECT systems.[217]

The majority of studies using PET have involved diseases of the central nervous system or heart. Several groups have shown that it may also play an important role in the chest, particularly in the assessment of neoplastic disease.[216, 216a, b] Malignant cells have increased glucose transport and metabolism related to their rapid proliferation and increased content of messenger RNA.[218–220] These biochemical alterations can be imaged by PET following administration of the glucose analogue FDG. The mechanism of uptake and initial phosphorylation of FDG is similar to that of glucose. However, once FDG is phosphorylated (FDG-6-phosphate), it is not metabolized further and remains within the cell. The amount of FDG-6-phosphate within the cell can be imaged with PET systems and is proportional to glucose uptake and metabolism. Current indications for FDG-PET imaging include distinction of benign from malignant pulmonary nodules, mediastinal staging of non–small cell pulmonary carcinoma, and differentiation between parenchymal scarring and recurrent tumor in patients who have had previous therapy for a pulmonary carcinoma.

The sensitivity and specificity of FDG-PET imaging for distinguishing malignant from benign lesions range from approximately 80% to 100% and 50% to 97%, respectively.[221–223] False-positive studies have been reported in sites of active inflammation such as aspergillosis, tuberculosis, and sarcoidosis. An additional advantage of FDG-PET in the evaluation of solitary pulmonary nodules is the ability to stage mediastinal non–small cell lung cancer.[224–226] In one study, FDG-PET imaging was compared with CT in the assessment of nodal metastases in 42 patients.[225] A total of 62 nodal stations (40 hilar/lobar, 22 mediastinal) were surgically sampled. The sensitivity and specificity for hilar/lobar lymph node station metastases when using PET imaging were 73% and 76%, respectively, as compared with 27% and 86% for CT. For mediastinal node station metastases, the sensitivity and specificity when using PET imaging were 92% and 100%, respectively, as compared with 58% and 80% for CT. In another study of 99 patients, comparison of FDG-PET imaging with CT demonstrated a sensitivity and specificity for the diagnosis of N2 disease of 83% and 94% for PET imaging versus 63% and 73% for CT, respectively.[226] These studies suggest that FDG-PET imaging is superior to CT in the detection of mediastinal lymph node metastases. The results of preliminary studies suggest that PET imaging may also have a role in the detection of extrathoracic metastases.[226a, b]

In patients with residual parenchymal abnormalities following radiotherapy for lung cancer, FDG-PET imaging can also be used to distinguish between persistent or recurrent lung cancer and radiation fibrosis. In one study of 35 patients with this diagnostic dilemma, the sensitivity and specificity for detecting recurrent tumor were 97% and 100%, respectively.[227] Only one patient—who had a very thin pleural tumor rind—had a false-negative study.

ULTRASONOGRAPHY

With respect to thoracic disease, ultrasonography has made its greatest impact in the assessment of congenital and

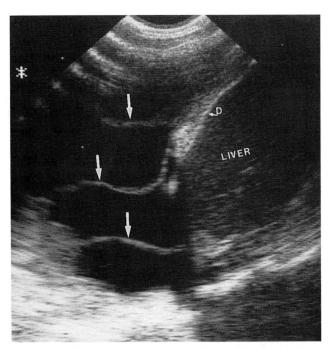

Figure 13–30. Complex Effusion on Ultrasound. Ultrasound demonstrates several septations *(arrows)* within a large right pleural effusion. Also noted are the diaphragm (D) and liver. The effusion proved to be a malignant exudate caused by mesothelioma. (Courtesy of Dr. Anne R. Buckley, Department of Radiology, Vancouver Hospital and Health Sciences Centre, Vancouver, BC, Canada.)

acquired heart disease, particularly in establishing the nature of valvular deformity, the volume of cardiac chambers, the thickness of their walls, and the effectiveness of cardiac contraction (ejection fraction). The role of ultrasound in the assessment of abnormalities of the aorta has increased considerably with the advent of transesophageal echocardiography. The procedure is also valuable for detecting pericardial effusion, assessing its size, and differentiating it from cardiomegaly and has been used to detect intravascular air bubbles in cases of pulmonary air embolism.

Because it is portable, does not use ionizing radiation, and frequently provides useful diagnostic information, ultrasound is commonly used in the diagnosis of pleural, diaphragmatic, and infradiaphragmatic abnormalities. Except for these important applications, the role of ultrasound in the diagnosis of noncardiovascular chest disease is limited by the physical composition of the intrathoracic structures: neither air nor bone transmits sound; instead, they reflect or absorb incoming sonic energy and prevent the collection of information about acoustic interfaces behind ribs or lung tissue. Sonography is therefore limited to assessment of pulmonary masses or consolidation abutting the mediastinum, chest wall, or diaphragm and to documentation of the presence and nature of pleural fluid.

Indications

Assessment of Pleural Effusions and Distinction of Effusions from Solid Pleural Lesions. Differentiation of liquid from solid pleural collections, which may be exceedingly difficult on chest radiographs, is usually easily achieved with ultrasonography.[228, 229] Although lateral decubitus chest radiographs will

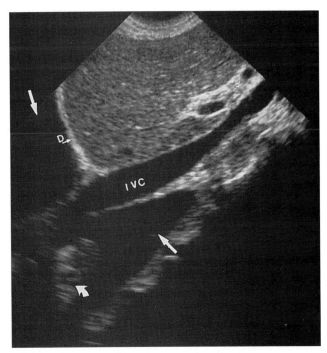

Figure 13–29. Pleural Effusion on Ultrasound. Ultrasound demonstrates a large echo-free right pleural effusion *(straight arrows)*. Also noted are an atelectatic right lung *(curved arrow)*, the diaphragm (D), the inferior vena cava (IVC), and the liver. The effusion was shown on needle aspiration to be a transudate.

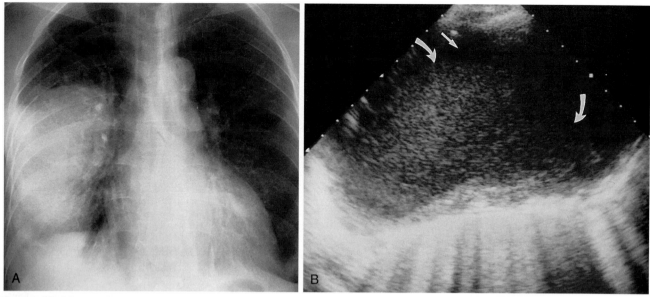

Figure 13–31. Loculated Empyema. A posteroanterior chest radiograph *(A)* demonstrates a well-defined opacity in the right hemithorax with associated pleural effusion. Ultrasound *(B)* demonstrates a small collection of echo-free fluid *(straight arrow)* and a large collection of echogenic fluid *(curved arrows)* with enhanced through transmission. Aspiration of fluid confirmed the diagnosis of empyema, which was treated by ultrasound-guided drainage.

readily demonstrate a free-flowing pleural effusion, they are not helpful in distinguishing loculated effusions from empyema or solid pleural masses. Because of its portability, bedside sonography has become a major imaging modality, not only in determining the presence of pleural fluid but also as a guide to aspiration and drainage.[230–232]

The majority of pleural fluid collections are readily identified at ultrasound as anechoic or hypoechoic collections, often delineated by echogenic aerated lung (Fig. 13–29). Although transudates and exudates have similar radiologic appearances, they may have different ultrasound characteristics.[231, 233] In one study of 50 patients, 15 of 19 (79%) effusions containing septations at ultrasound represented exudates (Fig. 13–30).[231] In another investigation of 320 patients, effusions with complex septated, complex nonseptated, or homogeneously echogenic patterns were always exudates.[233] Other findings indicative of exudative effusion include the presence of a thickened pleura or an associated pulmonary parenchymal lesion. Even though these findings are helpful, hypoechoic effusions may be either transudates or exudates.[231, 233]

Although sonography is more accurate than plain radiography in differentiating pleural fluid from solid pleural

lesions, optimal assessment requires that the performance of sonography be guided by the radiographic findings: in one analysis, combined use of the two modalities was more accurate (98%) than either radiography (68%) or sonography (92%) alone.[230]

Assessment of the Diaphragm. Ultrasonography provides excellent assessment of diaphragmatic and peridiaphragmatic masses and fluid collections and allows easy distinction of small pleural effusion from infradiaphragmatic fluid collections. The procedure has also been shown to be helpful in the diagnosis of traumatic tears of the right hemidiaphragm because the liver provides an optimal acoustic window to assess the right hemidiaphragm.[234] The presence of bowel gas usually precludes optimal sonographic assessment of the left hemidiaphragm.

Guide to Needle Biopsy and Catheter Placement. Ultrasonography allows excellent visualization of pulmonary, pleural, or mediastinal lesions in contact with the chest wall or in a juxtadiaphragmatic location, thus permitting real-time monitoring while performing fine-needle aspiration.[235] The procedure is also frequently used as a guide to the placement of catheters for pleural sclerotherapy or drainage of empyemas (Fig. 13–31).[236–238] It also allows pleural drainage to be performed at the bedside in critically ill patients.

REFERENCES

1. Robin ED, Burke CM: Routine chest x-ray examinations. Chest 90:258, 1986.
2. Sagel SS, Evens RG, Forrest JV, et al: Efficacy of routine screening and lateral chest radiographs in a hospital-based population. N Engl J Med 291:1001, 1974.
3. Rucker L, Frye EB, Staten MA: Usefulness of screening chest roentgenograms in preoperative patients. JAMA 250:3209, 1983.
4. Hubbell FA, Greenfield S, Tyler JL, et al: Special article: The impact of routine admission chest x-ray films on patient care. N Engl J Med 312:209, 1985.
5. Bonebrake CR, Noller KL, Loehnen CP, et al: Routine chest roentgenography in pregnancy. JAMA 240:2747, 1978.
6. Benacerraf BR, McLoud TC, Rea JT, et al: An assessment of the contribution of chest radiography in outpatients with acute chest complaints: A prospective study. Radiology 138:293, 1981.
7. Harris JH (Report from Chairman of the Board): Referral criteria for routine screening chest x-ray examinations. Am Coll Radiol Bull 38:17, 1982.
8. American College of Radiology: ACR Standard for the Performance of Pediatric and Adult Chest Radiography. Standards: American College of Radiology, Reston, VA, 1997, p 27.
9. American Thoracic Society: Chest x-ray screening statements. Am Thorac News 10:14, 1984.
10. Simon G: Principles of Chest X-Ray Diagnosis. 3rd ed. London, Butterworth, 1971.
11. Jacobson G, Sargent EN: Apical roentgenographic views of the chest. Am J Roentgenol 104:822, 1968.
12. Zinn B, Monroe J: The lordotic position in fluoroscopy and roentgenography of the chest. Am J Roentgenol 75:682, 1956.
13. Rundle FF, DeLambert RM, Epps RG: Cervicothoracic tumors: A technical aid to their roentgenologic localization. Am J Roentgenol 81:316, 1959.
14. Rigler LG: Roentgen diagnosis of small pleural effusion: A new roentgenographic position. JAMA 96:104, 1931.
15. Müller R, Löfstedt S: The reaction of the pleura in primary tuberculosis of the lungs. Acta Med Scand 122:105, 1945.
16. Hessén I: Roentgen examination of pleural fluid: A study of the localization of free effusion, the potentialities of diagnosing minimal quantities of fluid and its existence under physiological conditions. Acta Radiol Suppl 86:1, 1951.
17. Crapo RO, Montague T, Armstrong J: Inspiratory lung volume achieved on routine chest films. Invest Radiol 14:137, 1979.
18. Lynch PA: A different approach to chest roentgenography: Triad technique (high kilovoltage, grid, wedge filter). Am J Roentgenol 93:965, 1965.
19. Tuddenham WJ, Gibbons JF, Hale J, et al: Supervoltage and multiple simultaneous roentgenography—new technics for roentgen examination of the chest. Radiology 63:184, 1954.
20. Kelsey CA, Moseley RD, Mettler FA, et al: Comparison of nodule detection with 70-kVp and 120-kVp chest radiographs. Radiology 143:609, 1982.
21. Watson W: Gridless radiography at high voltage with air gap technique. X-Ray Focus 2:12, 1958.
22. Jackson FI: The air-gap technique, and an improvement by anteroposterior positioning for chest roentgenography. Am J Roentgenol 92:688, 1964.
23. Ailsby RL, Ghadially FN: Atypical cilia in human bronchial mucosa. J Pathol 109:75, 1973.
24. Trout ED, Kelley JP, Larson VL: A comparison of an air gap and a grid in roentgenography of the chest. Am J Roentgenol 124:404, 1975.
25. Wilkinson GA, Fraser RG: Roentgenography of the chest. Appl Radiol 4:41, 1975.
26. Rossi RP, Harnisch G, Hendee WR: Reduction of radiation exposure in radiography of the chest. Radiology 144:909, 1982.
27. Kelsey CA, Lane RG, Moseley RD, et al: Chest radiographs obtained with shaped filters: Evaluation by observer performance tests. Radiology 159:653, 1986.
28. Hasegawa BH, Naimuddin S, Dobbins JT, et al: Digital beam attenuator technique for compensated chest radiography. Radiology 159:537, 1986.
29. Peppler WW, Zink F, Naimuddin S, et al: Patient-specific beam attenuators. In Peppler WW, Alter A (eds): Proceedings of the Chest Imaging Conference 1987. Madison, WI, Medical Physics Publishing, 1987, p 6.
30. Plewes DB: A scanning system for chest radiography with regional exposure control: Theoretical considerations. Med Phys 10:646, 1984.
31. Plewes DB, Vogelstein EE: A scanning system for chest radiography with regional exposure control: Practical implementation. Med Phys 10:654, 1984.
32. Vlasbloem H, Schultze Kool LJ: AMBER: A scanning multiple-beam equalization system for chest radiography. Radiology 169:29, 1988.
33. MacMahon H, Vyborny C: Technical advances in chest radiography. Am J Roentgenol 163:1049, 1994.
34. Schultze Kool LJ, Busscher DLT, Vlasbloem H, et al: Advanced multiple-beam equalization radiography in chest radiology: A simulated nodule detection study. Radiology 169:35, 1988.
35. Chotas HG, vanMetter RL, Johnson GA, et al: Small object contrast in AMBER and conventional chest radiography. Radiology 180:853, 1991.
36. Goleijns J, Broerse JJ, Julius HW, et al: AMBER and conventional chest radiography: Comparison of radiation dose and image quality. Radiology 185:719, 1992.
37. Seow A, Kazerooni EA, Cascade PN, et al: Comparison of upright inspiratory and expiratory chest radiographs for detecting pneumothoraces. Am J Roentgenol 166:313, 1996.

38. Wandtke JC: Bedside chest radiography. Radiology 190:1, 1994.
39. American College of Radiology: ACR standard for the performance of pediatric and adult bedside (portable) chest radiography. Standards: American College of Radiology, Reston, VA, 1997, p 31.
40. Gallant TE, Dietrich PA, Shinozaki T, et al: Technical notes. Simple device to measure patient position on portable chest radiographs. Am J Roentgenol 131:169, 1978.
41. Henschke CI, Pasternack GS, Schroeder S, et al: Bedside chest radiography: Diagnostic efficacy. Radiology 149:23, 1983.
42. Janower ML, Jennas-Nocera Z, Mukai J: Utility and efficacy of portable chest radiographs. Am J Roentgenol 142:265, 1984.
43. Bakemeyer WB, Crapo RO, Calhoon S, et al: Efficacy of chest radiology in respiratory intensive care unit: A prospective study. Chest 88:691, 1985.
44. Greenbaum DM, Marschall LKE: The value of routine daily chest x-rays in intubated patients in the medical intensive care unit. Crit Care Med 10:29, 1982.
45. Strain DS, Kinasewitz GT, Vereen LE, et al: Value of routine daily chest x-rays in the medical intensive care unit. Crit Care Med 13:534, 1985.
46. Hall FM: Indications for bedside radiographs (letter). Am J Roentgenol 143:684, 1984.
47. Silverstein DS, Livingston DH, Elcavage J, et al: The utility of routine daily chest radiography in the surgical intensive care unit. J Trauma 35:643, 1993.
48. Fong Y, Whalen G, Hariri RJ, et al: Utility of routine chest radiographs in the surgical intensive care unit. Arch Surg 130:764, 1995.
49. Gray P, Sullivan G, Ostryzniuk P, et al: Value of postprocedural chest radiographs in the adult intensive care unit. Crit Care Med 20:1513, 1992.
50. Hornick PI, Harris P, Cousins C, et al: Assessment of the value of the immediate postoperative chest radiograph after cardiac operation. Ann Thorac Surg 59:1150, 1995.
51. Aberle DR, Hansell D, Huang HK: Current status of digital projectional radiography of the chest. J Thorac Imaging 5:10, 1990.
52. Kundel HL: Visual perception and image display terminals. Radiol Clin North Am 24:69, 1986.
53. Goodman LR, Foley WD, Wilson CR, et al: Pneumothorax and other lung diseases: Effect of altered resolution and edge enhancement on diagnosis with digitized radiographs. Radiology 167:83, 1988.
54. MacMahon H, Metz CE, Doi K, et al: Effect of display format on diagnostic accuracy in digital chest radiography: An ROC study. Radiology 161:203, 1986.
54a. Dawood RM, Craig JOMC, Todd-Pokrapek A, et al: Clinical diagnosis from digital displays: Results and conclusions from the St. Mary's Evaluation Project. Br J Radiol 67:1, 1994.
54b. Razavi M, Sayre JW, Taira RK, et al: Receiver-operating-characteristic study of chest radiographs in children: Digital hard-copy film versus 2K × 2K softcopy images. Am J Roentgenol 158:443, 1992.
54c. Frank MS, Jost RG, Molina PL, et al: High-resolution computer display of portable digital chest radiographs of adults: Suitability for primary interpretation. Am J Roentgenol 160:473, 1993.
54d. Otto D, Bernhardt TM, Rapp-Bernhardt U, et al: Subtle pulmonary abnormalities: Detection on monitors with varying spatial resolutions and maximum luminance levels compared with detection on storage phosphor radiographic hard copies. Radiology 207:237, 1998.
55. Goodman LR, Wilson CR, Foley WD: Digital radiography of the chest: Promises and problems. Am J Roentgenol 150:1241, 1988.
56. Schaefer CM, Greene R, Llewellyn HJ, et al: Interstitial lung disease: Impact of postprocessing in digital storage phosphor imaging. Radiology 178:733, 1991.
57. Sagel SS, Jost RG, Glazer HS, et al: Digital mobile radiography. J Thorac Imaging 5:36, 1990.
58. Sonoda M, Takano M, Miyahara J, et al: Computed radiography utilizing scanning laser stimulated luminescence. Radiology 148:833, 1983.
59. MacMahon H, Vyborny CJ, Metz CE, et al: Digital radiography of subtle pulmonary abnormalities: An ROC study of the effect of pixel size on observer performance. Radiology 158:21, 1986.
60. Thaete FL, Fuhrman CR, Oliver JH, et al: Digital radiography and conventional imaging of the chest: A comparison of observer performance. Am J Roentgenol 162:575, 1994.
61. Cox GG, Cook LT, McMillan JH, et al: Chest radiography: Comparison of high-resolution digital displays with conventional and digital film. Radiology 176:771, 1990.
62. Niklason LT, Chan HP, Cascade PN, et al: Portable chest imaging: Comparison of storage phosphor digital, asymmetric screen-film, and conventional screen-film systems. Radiology 186:387, 1993.
63. MacMahon H, Sanada S, Doi K, et al: Direct comparison of conventional and computed radiography with a dual image recording technique. Radiographics 11:259, 1991.
64. Neitzel U, Maack I, Gunther-Kohfahl S: Image quality of a digital chest radiography system based on a selenium detector. Med Phys 21:509, 1994.
65. Floyd CE, Baker JA, Chotas HG, et al: Selenium-based digital radiography of the chest: Radiologists' preference compared with film-screen radiographs. Am J Roentgenol 165:1353, 1995.
66. Papin PJ, Huang HK: A prototype amorphous selenium imaging plate system for digital radiography. Med Phys 14:322, 1987.
67. Chotas HG, Floyd CE Jr, Ravin CE: Technical evaluation of a digital chest radiography system that uses a selenium detector. Radiology 195:264, 1995.

68. van Heesewijk HPM, Neitzel U, van der Graaf Y, et al: Digital chest imaging with a selenium detector: Comparison with conventional radiography for visualization of specific anatomic regions of the chest. Am J Roentgenol 165:535, 1995.

69. Fraser RG, Sanders C, Barnes GT, et al: Digital imaging of the chest. Radiology 171:297, 1989.

70. Lo S-CB, Taira RK, Mankovich NJ, et al: Performance characteristics of a laser scanner and laser printer system for radiological imaging. Comput Radiol 10:227, 1986.

71. Kundel HL, Mezrich JL, Brickman I, et al: Ditigal chest imaging: Comparison of two film image digitizers with a classification task. Radiology 165:747, 1987.

72. Goodman LR, Foley WD, Wilson CR, et al: Digital and conventional chest images: Observer performance with film digital radiography system. Radiology 158:27, 1986.

73. Goodman LR, Foley WD, Wilson CR, et al: Pneumothorax and other lung diseases: Effect of altered resolution and edge enhancement on diagnosis with digitized radiographs. Radiology 167:83, 1988.

74. MacMahon H, Metz CE, Doi K, et al: Digital chest radiography: Effect on diagnostic accuracy of hard copy, conventional video, and reversed gray scale video display formats. Radiology 168:669, 1988.

75. Hayrapetian A, Aberle DR, Huang HK, et al: Comparison of 2048-line digital display formats and conventional radiographs: an ROC study. Am J Roentgenol 152:1113, 1989.

76. Glazer HS, Muka E, Sagel SS, et al: New techniques in chest radiography. Radiol Clin North Am 32:711, 1994.

77. Spence DPS, Kelly YJ, Ahmed J, et al: Critical evaluation of computerised x-ray planimetry for the measurement of lung volumes. Thorax 50:383, 1995.

78. Barnhard HG, Pierce JA, Joyce JW, et al: Roentgenographic determination of total lung capacity. A new method evaluated in health, emphysema and congestive heart failure. Am J Med 28:51, 1960.

79. O'Shea J, Lapp NL, Russakoff AD, et al: Determination of lung volumes from chest films. Thorax 25:544, 1970.

79a. Paré PD, Wiggs BJR, Coppin CA: Errors in the measurement of total lung capacity in chronic obstructive lung disease. Thorax 38:468, 1983.

80. Loyd HM, String ST, DuBois AB: Radiographic and plethysmographic determination of total lung capacity. Radiology 86:7, 1966.

81. Harris TR, Pratt PC, Kilburn KH: Total lung capacity measured by roentgenograms. Am J Med 50:756, 1971.

82. Jaffe CC: A new technique for rapid determination of quantitative data from radiographs. Radiology 103:451, 1972.

83. Herman PG, Sandor T, Mann BE, et al: Rapid computerized lung volume determination from chest roentgenograms. Am J Roentgenol 124:477, 1975.

84. Friedman PJ, Brimm JE, Botkin MC, et al: Measuring lung volumes from chest films using equations derived from computed tomography. Invest Radiol 19:263, 1984.

85. Pierce RJ, Brown DJ, Holmes M, et al: Estimation of lung volumes from chest radiographs using shape information. Thorax 34:725, 1979.

86. Hounsfield GN: Computerized transverse axial scanning (tomography). I. Description of system. Br J Radiol 46:1016, 1973.

87. Stern EJ, Graham CM, Webb WR, et al: Normal trachea during forced expiration: Dynamic CT measurements. Radiology 187:27, 1993.

88. Kalender WA, Seissler W, Klotz E, et al: Spiral volumetric CT with single-breath-hold technique, continuous transport, and continuous scanner rotation. Radiology 176:181, 1990.

89. Bressler Y, Skrabacz CZ: Optimal interpolation in helical scan computed tomography. Proc ICASSP 3:1472, 1989.

90. Polacin A, Kalender WA, Marchal G: Evaluation of section sensitivity profiles and image noise in spiral CT. Radiology 185:29, 1992.

91. Crawford CR, King K: Computed tomography scanning with simultaneous patient translation. Med Phys 17:967, 1990.

92. Costelo P, Anderson W, Blume DL: Pulmonary nodules: Evaluation with spiral volumetric CT. Radiology 179:875, 1991.

93. Remy-Jardin M, Remy J, Giraud F, et al: Pulmonary nodules: Detection with thick-section spiral CT versus conventional CT. Radiology 187:513, 1993.

94. Remy J, Remy-Jardin M, Wattinne L, et al: Pulmonary arteriovenous malformations: Evaluation with CT of the chest before and after treatment. Radiology 182:809, 1992.

95. Naidich DP: Helical computed tomography of the thorax. Radiol Clin North Am 32:759, 1994.

96. Costello P, Dupuy DE, Ecker CP, et al: Spiral CT of the thorax with reduced volume of contrast material: A comparative study. Radiology 183:663, 1992.

97. Costello P, Ecker CP, Tello R, et al: Assessment of the thoracic aorta by spiral CT: Pictorial essay. Am J Roentgenol 158:1127, 1992.

98. Remy-Jardin M, Remy J, Wattinne L, et al: Central pulmonary thromboembolism: Diagnosis with spiral volumetric CT with the single–breath-hold technique—comparison with pulmonary angiography. Radiology 185:381, 1992.

98a. Rubin GD: Helical CT angiography of the thoracic aorta. J Thorac Imaging 12:128, 1997.

98b. Mayo JR, Remy-Jardin M, Müller NL, et al: Pulmonary embolism: Prospective comparison of spiral CT with ventilation-perfusion scintigraphy. Radiology 205:447, 1997.

98c. Fram EK, Godwin JD, Putman CE: Three-dimensional display of the heart, aorta, lungs and airway using CT. Am J Roentgenol 139:1171, 1982.

98d. Remy-Jardin M, Remy J, Artaud D, et al: Volume rendering of the tracheobronchial tree: Clinical evaluation of bronchographic images. Radiology 208:761, 1998.

98e. Higgins WE, Ramaswamy K, Swift RD, et al: Virtual bronchoscopy for three-dimensional pulmonary image assessment: State of the art and future needs. RadioGraphics 18:761, 1998.

99. Müller NL, Miller RR: State-of-the-art: Computed tomography of chronic diffuse infiltrative lung disease. Am Rev Respir Dis 142:1206, 1990.

100. Müller NL: Clinical value of high resolution CT in chronic diffuse lung disease. Am J Roentgenol 157:1163, 1991.

101. McGuinness G, Naidich DP: Bronchiectasis: CT/clinical correlations. Semin Ultrasound CT MR 16:395, 1995.

102. Leung AN, Staples CA, Müller NL: Chronic diffuse infiltrative lung disease: Comparison of diagnostic accuracy of high-resolution and conventional CT. Am J Roentgenol 157:693, 1991.

103. Naidich DP, Harkin TJ: Airways and lung: Correlation of CT with fiberoptic bronchoscopy. Radiology 197:1, 1995.

104. Mayo JR, Webb WR, Gold R, et al: High resolution CT of the lungs: An optimal approach. Radiology 163:507, 1987.

105. Zwirewich CV, Terrif B, Müller NL: High-spatial-frequency (bone) algorithm improves quality of standard CT of the thorax. Am J Roentgenol 153:1169, 1989.

106. Mayo JR: The high resolution CT technique. Semin Roentgenol 26:104, 1991.

107. Webb WR, Müller NL, Naidich DP (eds): High Resolution CT of the Lung. New York, Lippincott-Raven, 1996.

108. International Commission on Radiological Protection: Report 60: The recommendations of the International Commission on Radiological Protection, 1990. Ann ICRP 21:1, 1991.

109. Nishizawa K, Maruyama T, Takayama M, et al: Determinations of organ doses and effective dose equivalents from computed tomographic examination. Br J Radiol 64:20, 1991.

110. Mayo JR, Jackson SA, Müller NL: High-resolution CT of the chest: Radiation dose. Am J Roentgenol 160:479, 1993.

111. United Nations Scientific Committee on the Effects of Atomic Radiation: Sources, Effects and Risks of Ionizing Radiation: Report of the Scientific Committee on the Effects of Atomic Radiation. New York, United Nations, 1988.

112. Geleigns J, Broerse JJ, Julius HW, et al: AMBER and conventional chest radiography: Comparison of radiation dose and image quality. Radiology 185:719, 1992.

113. Naidich DP, Pizzarello D, Garay SM, Müller NL: Is thoracic CT performed often enough? Chest 106:331, 1994.

114. National Research Council Committee on the Biological Effects of Ionizing Radiations: Health Effects of Exposure to Low Levels of Ionizing Radiations (BEIR V). Washington, DC, National Academy Press, 1990.

115. Naidich DP, Marshall CH, Gribbin C, et al: Low-dose CT of the lungs: Preliminary observations. Radiology 175:729, 1990.

116. Zwirewich CV, Mayo JR, Müller NL: Low-dose high-resolution CT of lung parenchyma. Radiology 180:413, 1991.

117. Lee KS, Primack SL, Staples CA, et al: Chronic infiltrative lung disease: Comparison of diagnostic accuracies of radiography and low- and conventional-dose thin-section CT. Radiology 191:669, 1994.

118. Society for Computed Body Tomography: Special report. New indications for computed body tomography. Am J Roentgenol 133:115, 1979.

119. Naidich DP, Zerhouni EA, Siegelman SS (eds): Computed Tomography and Magnetic Resonance of the Thorax. New York, Raven Press, 1991.

120. Mayo JR: Magnetic resonance imaging of the chest: Where we stand. Radiol Clinc North Am 32:795, 1994.

121. Firmin DN, Nayler GL, Kilner PJ, et al: Application of phase shifts in NMR for flow measurement. Magn Reson Med 14:230, 1990.

121a. Boxerman JL, Mosher TJ, McVeigh ER, et al: Advanced MR imaging techniques for evaluation of the heart and great vessels. RadioGraphics 18:543, 1998.

122. Harms SE, Morgan TJ, Yamanashi WS, et al: Principles of nuclear magnetic resonance imaging. RadioGraphics 4(Suppl):26, 1984.

123. Pavlicek W, Modic M, Weinstein M: Pulse sequence and significance. Radiographics 4(Suppl):49, 1984.

124. Pykett IL, Newhouse JH, Buonanno FS, et al: Nuclear magnetic resonance. Principles of nuclear magnetic resonance imaging. Radiology 143:157, 1982.

125. Gamsu G, Sostman D: Magnetic resonance imaging of the thorax. Am Rev Respir Dis 139:254, 1989.

126. Bergin CJ, Glover GH, Pauly JM: Lung parenchyma: Magnetic susceptibility in MR imaging. Radiology 180:845, 1991.

127. Mayo JR, McKay A, Müller NL: MR imaging of the lungs: Value of short TE spin-echo pulse sequences. Am J Roentgenol 159:951, 1992.

128. Higgins CB, Sakuma H: Heart disease: Functional evaluation with MR imaging. Radiology 199:307, 1996.

129. Higgins CB, Caputo GR: Role of MR imaging in acquired and congenital cardiovascular disease. Am J Roentgenol 161:13, 1993.

130. Sechtem U, Pflugfelder PW, White RD, et al: Cine MR imaging: Potential for the evaluation of cardiovascular function. Am J Roentgenol 148:239, 1987.

131. Kondo C, Caputo GR, Semelka R, et al: Right and left ventricular stroke volume measurements with velocity-encoded cine MR imaging: In vitro and in vivo validation. Am J Roentgenol 157:9, 1991.

132. Glazer HS, Gutierrez FR, Levitt RG, et al: The thoracic aorta studied by MR imaging. Radiology 157:149, 1985.

133. Kersting-Sommerhoff BA, Higgins CB, White RD, et al: Aortic dissection: Sensitivity and specificity of MR imaging. Radiology 166:651, 1988.

134. Sommer T, Fehske W, Holzknecht N, et al: Aortic dissection: A comparative study of diagnosis with spiral CT, multiplanar transesophageal echocardiography, and MR imaging. Radiology 199:347, 1996.

135. Webb WR, Gatsonis C, Zerhouni EA, et al: CT and MR imaging in staging non–small cell bronchogenic carcinoma: Report of the radiologic diagnostic oncology group. Radiology 178:705, 1991.

136. Nakata H, Egashira K, Watanabe H, et al: MRI of bronchogenic cysts. J Comput Assist Tomogr 17:267, 1993.

137. Fortier MV, Mayo JR, Swensen SJ, Müller NL: MR imaging of chest wall lesions. RadioGraphics 14:597, 1994.

138. Bergin CJ, Healy MV, Zincone GE, et al: MR evaluation of chest wall involvement in malignant lymphoma. J Comput Assist Tomogr 14:928, 1990.

139. Heelan RT, Demas BE, Caravelli JF, et al: Superior sulcus tumors: CT and MR imaging. Radiology 170:637, 1989.

140. McLoud TC, Filion RB, Edelman RR, et al: MR imaging of superior sulcus carcinoma. J Comput Assist Tomogr 13:233, 1989.

141. Flickinger FW, Yuh WT, Behrendt DM: Magnetic resonance imaging of mediastinal paraganglioma. Chest 94:652, 1988.

142. Siegel MJ, Jamroz GA, Glazer HS, et al: MR imaging of intraspinal extension of neuroblastoma. J Comput Assist Tomogr 10:593, 1986.

143. Müller NL, Mayo JR, Zwirewich CV: Value of MR imaging in the evaluation of chronic infiltrative lung disease: Comparison with CT. Am J Roentgenol 158:1205, 1992.

144. Primack SL, Mayo JR, Hartman TE, et al: MR imaging of infiltrative lung disease: Comparison with pathologic findings in 22 patients. J Comput Assist Tomogr 18:233, 1994.

145. Cutillo AG, Morris AH, Ailion DC, et al: Determination of lung water content and distribution by nuclear magnetic resonance imaging. J Thorac Imaging 1:39, 1986.

146. Mayo JR, MacKay A, Whittall K, et al: Measurement of lung water content and pleural pressure gradient with magnetic resonance imaging. J Thorac Imaging 10:73, 1995.

147. Herold CJ, Kuhlman JE, Zerhouni EA: Pulmonary atelectasis: Signal patterns with MR imaging. Radiology 178:715, 1991.

148. Christoforidis AJ, Nelson SW, Tomashefski JF: Effects of bronchography on pulmonary function. Am Rev Respir Dis 85:127, 1962.

149. Suprenant E, Wilson A, Bennett L, et al: Changes in regional pulmonary function following bronchography. Radiology 91:736, 1968.

150. Grenier P, Maurice F, Musset D, et al: Bronchiectasis: Assessment by thin-section CT. Radiology 161:95, 1986.

151. Young K, Aspestrand F, Kolbenstvedt A: High resolution CT and bronchography in the assessment of bronchiectasis. Acta Radiol 32:439, 1991.

152. Giron J, Skaff F, Maubon A, et al: The value of thin-section CT scans in the diagnosis and staging of bronchiectasis: Comparison with bronchography in a series of fifty-four patients. Ann Radiol 31:25, 1988.

153. Morcos SK, Baudouin SV, Anderson PB, et al: Iotrolan in selective bronchography via the fiberoptic bronchoscope. Br J Radiol 62:383, 1989.

154. Morcos SK, Anderson PB: Airways and the lung: Bronchography through the fiberoptic bronchoscope [comment]. Radiology 200:612, 1996.

155. Naidich DP, Harkin TJ: Airways and lung: CT versus bronchography through the fiberoptic bronchoscope. Radiology 200:613, 1996.

156. Cicero R, del Castillo H: Lobar and segmental angiopneumography in pulmonary disease. Acta Radiol 45:42, 1956.

157. van Rooij WJ, den Heeten GJ, Sluzewski M: Pulmonary embolism: Diagnosis in 211 patients with use of selective pulmonary digital subtraction angiography with a flow-directed catheter. Radiology 195:793, 1995.

158. Nicod P, Peterson K, Levine M, et al: Pulmonary angiography in severe chronic pulmonary hypertension. Ann Intern Med 107:565, 1987.

159. van Beek EJR, Bakker AJ, Reekers JA: Pulmonary embolism: Interobserver agreement in the interpretation of conventional angiographic and DSA images in patients with nondiagnostic lung scan results. Radiology 198:721, 1996.

160. Schluger N, Henschke C, King T, et al: Diagnosis of pulmonary embolism at a large teaching hospital. J Thorac Imaging 9:180, 1994.

161. Cooper TJ, Hayward MWJ, Hartog M: Survey on the use of pulmonary scintigraphy and angiography for suspected pulmonary thromboembolism in the UK. Clin Radiol 43:243, 1991.

162. Hudson ER, Smith TP, McDermott VG, et al: Pulmonary angiography performed with iopamidol: Complications in 1,434 patients. Radiology 198:61, 1996.

163. Mills SR, Jackson DC, Older RA, et al: The incidence, etiologies, and avoidance of complications of pulmonary angiography in a large series. Radiology 136:295, 1980.

164. Perlmutt LM, Braun SD, Newman GE, et al: Pulmonary arteriography in the high-risk patient. Radiology 162:187, 1987.

165. Stein PD, Hull RD, Saltzman HA, et al: Strategy for diagnosis of patients with suspected acute pulmonary embolism. Chest 103:1553, 1993.

166. Kelley MA, Carson JL, Palevsky HI, et al: Diagnosing pulmonary embolism: New facts and strategies. Ann Intern Med 114:300, 1991.

167. Oudkerk M, van Beek EJR, van Putten WLJ, et al: Cost-effectiveness analysis of various strategies in the diagnostic management of pulmonary embolism. Arch Intern Med 153:947, 1993.

168. Oser RF, Zuckerman DA, Gutierrez FR, et al: Anatomic distribution of pulmonary emboli at pulmonary angiography: Implications for cross-sectional imaging. Radiology 199:31, 1996.

169. Seldinger SI: Catheter replacement of the needle in percutaneous arteriography: A new technique. Acta Radiol 39:368, 1953.

170. Petasnick JP: Radiologic evaluation of aortic dissection. Radiology 180:297, 1991.

171. Guthaner DF, Miller DC: Digital subtraction angiography of aortic dissection. Am J Roentgenol 141:157, 1983.

172. Davies ER, Roylance J: Aortography in the investigation of traumatic mediastinal haematoma. Clin Radiol 21:297, 1970.

173. Raptopoulos V: Chest CT for aortic injury: Maybe not for everyone. Am J Roentgenol 162:1053, 1994.

174. Richardson P, Mirvis SE, Scorpio R, et al: Value of CT in determining the need for angiography when findings of mediastinal hemorrhage on chest radiographs are equivocal. Am J Roentgenol 156:272, 1991.

175. Madayag MA, Kirshenbaum KJ, Nadimpalli SR, et al: Thoracic aortic trauma: Role of dynamic CT. Radiology 179:853, 1991.

176. Gavant ML, Menke PG, Fabian T, et al: Blunt traumatic aortic rupture: Detection with helical CT of the chest. Radiology 197:125, 1995.

176a. Mirvis SE, Shanmuganathan K, Miller BH, et al: Traumatic aortic injury—diagnosis with contrast-enhanced thoracic CT: Five-year experience at a major center. Radiology 200:413, 1996.

177. Fisher RG, Chasen MH, Lamki N: Diagnosis of injuries of the aorta and brachiocephalic arteries caused by blunt chest trauma: CT vs aortography. Am J Roentgenol 162:1047, 1994.

178. Hunink MGM, Bos JJ: Triage of patients to angiography for detection of aortic rupture after blunt chest trauma: Cost-effectiveness analysis of using CT. Am J Roentgenol 165:27, 1995.

179. Sutton D, Samuel RH: Thoracic aortography in intralobar lung sequestration. Clin Radiol 14:317, 1963.

180. Turk LN III, Lindskog GE: The importance of angiographic diagnosis in intralobar pulmonary sequestration. J Thorac Cardiovasc Surg 41:299, 1961.

181. Nordenström B: Selective catheterization and angiography of bronchial and mediastinal arteries in man. Acta Radiol 6:13, 1967.

182. Darke CS, Lewtas NA: Selective bronchial arteriography in the demonstration of abnormal systemic circulation in the lung. Clin Radiol 19:357, 1968.

183. Miyazawa K, Katori R, Ishikawa K, et al: Selective bronchial arteriography and bronchial blood flow: Correlative study. Chest 57:416, 1970.

184. Cauldwell EW, Siekert RG, Lininger RE, et al: The bronchial arteries: An anatomic study of 150 human cadavers. Surg Gynecol Obstet 86:395, 1948.

185. Roberts AC: Bronchial artery embolization therapy. J Thorac Imaging 5:60, 1990.

186. Remy J, Smith M, Lemaitre L, et al: Treatment of massive hemoptysis by occlusion of a Rasmussen aneurysm. Am J Roentgenol 135:605, 1980.

187. Remy J, Arnaud A, Fardou H, et al: Treatment of hemoptysis by embolization of bronchial arteries. Radiology 122:33, 1977.

188. Cohen AM, Doershuk CF, Stern RC: Bronchial artery embolization to control hemoptysis in cystic fibrosis. Radiology 175:401, 1990.

189. Uflacker R, Kaemmerer A, Neves C, et al: Management of massive hemoptysis by bronchial artery embolization. Radiology 146:627, 1983.

190. North LB, Boushy SF, Houk VN: Bronchial and intercostal arteriography in non-neoplastic pulmonary disease. Am J Roentgenol 107:328, 1969.

191. Vujic I, Pyle R, Hungerford GD, et al: Angiography and therapeutic blockade in the control of hemoptysis. The importance of nonbronchial systemic arteries. Radiology 143:19, 1982.

192. Heck LL, Duley JW: Statistical considerations in lung scanning with Tc-99m albumin particles. Radiology 113:675, 1975.

193. Alderson PO, Doppman JL, Diamond SS, et al: Ventilation-perfusion lung imaging and selective pulmonary angiography in dogs with experimental pulmonary emboli. J Nucl Med 19:164, 1978.

194. James JM, Herman KJ, Lloyd JJ, et al: Evaluation of 99Tcm Technegas ventilation scintigraphy in the diagnosis of pulmonary embolism. Br J Radiol 64:711, 1991.

195. Hull RD, Raskob GE, Coates G, et al: A new noninvasive management strategy for patients with suspected pulmonary embolism. Arch Intern Med 149:2549, 1989.

196. Hull RD, Raskob GE, Ginsberg JS, et al: A noninvasive strategy for the treatment of patients with suspected pulmonary embolism. Arch Intern Med 154:289, 1994.

197. The PIOPED Investigators: Value of the ventilation/perfusion scan in acute pulmonary embolism. JAMA 263:2753, 1990.

198. Hull RD, Raskob GE: Low-probability lung scan findings: A need for a change. Ann Intern Med 114:142, 1991.

199. Robin ED: Overdiagnosis and overtreatment of pulmonary embolism: The emperor may have no clothes. Ann Intern Med 87:775, 1977.

200. Robinson PJ: Lung scintigraphy—doubt and certainty in the diagnosis of pulmonary embolism. Clin Radiol 40:557, 1989.

201. UPET Investigators: The Urokinase Pulmonary Embolism trial: A national cooperative. Circulation 47(Suppl 2):46, 1973.

202. Ali MK, Mountain CF, Ewer MS, et al: Predicting loss of pulmonary function after pulmonary resection for bronchogenic carcinoma. Chest 77:337, 1980.

203. Line BR: Scintigraphic studies of inflammation in diffuse lung disease. Radiol Clin North Am 29:1095, 1991.

204. Rizzato G, Blasi A: A European survey on the usefulness of 67Ga lung scans in assessing sarcoidosis. Experience in 14 research centers in seven different countries. Ann N Y Acad Sci 465:463, 1986.

205. Lawrence EC, Teague RB, Gottlieb MS, et al: Serial changes in markers of disease activity with corticosteroid treatment in sarcoidosis. Am J Med 74:747, 1983.

206. Baughman RP, Fernandez M, Bosken CH, et al: Comparison of gallium 67 scanning, bronchoalveolar lavage, and serum angiotensin-converting enzyme levels in pulmonary sarcoidosis. Predicting response to therapy. Am Rev Respir Dis 129:676, 1984.

207. Schwarz MI: Idiopathic pulmonary fibrosis (medical staff conference). West J Med 149:199, 1988.

208. Scott-Miller K, Smith EA, Kinsella M, et al: Lung disease associated with progressive systemic sclerosis: Assessment of interlobar variations by bronchoalveolar lavage and comparison with noninvasive evaluation of disease activity. Am Rev Respir Dis 141:301, 1990.

209. Gelb AF, Dreisen RB, Epstein JD, et al: Immune complexes, gallium lung scans, and bronchoalveolar lavage in idiopathic interstitial pneumonitis-fibrosis. Chest 84:148, 1983.

210. Pantin CF, Valind SO, Sweatman M, et al: Measures of the inflammatory response in cryptogenic fibrosing alveolitis. Am Rev Respir Dis 138:1234, 1988.

211. Raghu G: Idiopathic pulmonary fibrosis: A rational clinical approach. Chest 92:148, 1987.

212. Whitcomb ME, Dixon GF: Gallium scanning, bronchoalveolar lavage, and the national debt. Chest 85:719, 1984.

213. Miller RF: Nuclear medicine and AIDS. Eur J Nucl Med 16:103, 1990.

214. Lee VW, Fuller JD, O'Brien MJ, et al: Pulmonary Kaposi sarcoma in patients with AIDS: Scintigraphic diagnosis with sequential thallium and gallium scanning. Radiology 180:409, 1991.

215. Front D, Israel O: The role of Ga-67 scintigraphy in evaluating the results of therapy of lymphoma patients. Semin Nucl Med 25:60, 1995.

216. Patz EF, Goodman PC: Positron emission tomography imaging of the thorax. Radiol Clin North Am 32:811, 1994.

216a. Rege SD, Hoh CK, Glaspy JA, et al: Imaging of pulmonary mass lesions with whole-body positron emission tomography and fluorodeoxyglucose. Cancer 72:82, 1993.

216b. Chinn R, Ward R, Keyes JW, et al: Mediastinal staging of non-small-cell cancer with positron emission tomography. Am J Respir Crit Care Med 152:2090, 1995.

217. Margin WH, Delbeke D, Patton JA, et al: Detection of malignancies with SPECT versus PET, with 2-[fluorine-18]fluoro-2-deoxy-D-glucose. Radiology 198:225, 1996.

218. Warburg O: On the origin of cancer cells. Science 123:309, 1956.

219. Weber G: Enzymology of cancer cells part 1. N Engl J Med 296:486, 1977.

220. Weber G: Enzymology of cancer cells part 2. N Engl J Med 296:541, 1977.

221. Gupta NC, Frank AR, Dewan NA: Solitary pulmonary nodules: Detection of malignancy with PET with 2-[F-18]-fluoro-2-deoxy-D-glucose. Radiology 184:441, 1992.

222. Patz EF, Lowe VJ, Hoffman J, et al: Focal pulmonary abnormalities: Evaluation with F-18 fluorodeoxyglucose PET scanning. Radiology 88:487, 1993.

223. Sazon DAD, Santiago SM, Hoo GWS, et al: Fluorodeoxyglucose-positron emission tomography in the detection and staging of lung cancer. Am J Respir Crit Care Med 153:417, 1996.

224. Wahl RL, Quint LE, Greenough RL, et al: Staging of mediastinal non–small cell lung cancer with FDG PET, CT and fusion images: Preliminary prospective evaluation. Radiology 191:371, 1994.

225. Patz EF, Lowe VJ, Goodman PC, et al: Thoracic nodal staging with PET imaging with 18FDG in patients with bronchogenic carcinoma. Chest 108:1617, 1995.

226. Valk PE, Pounds TR, Hopkins DM, et al: Staging non–small cell lung cancer by whole-body positron emission tomographic imaging. Ann Thorac Surg 60:1573, 1995.

226a. Bury T, Dowlati A, Paulus P, et al: Evaluation of the solitary pulmonary nodule by positron emission tomography imaging. Eur Resp J 9:410, 1996.

226b. Erasmus JJ, Patz EF Jr, McAdams HP, et al: Evaluation of adrenal masses in patients with bronchogenic carcinoma using 18F-fluorodeoxy-glucose positron emission tomography. Am J Roentgenol 168:1357, 1997.

227. Patz EF Jr, Lowe VJ, Hoffman JM, et al: Persistent or recurrent bronchogenic carcinoma: Detection with PET and 2-[F-18]-2-deoxy-D-glucose. Radiology 191:379, 1994.

228. Müller NL: Imaging of the pleura. Radiology 186:297, 1993.

229. McLoud TC, Flower CDR: Imaging the pleura: Sonography, CT, and MR Imaging. Am J Roentgenol 156:1145, 1991.

230. Lipscomb DJ, Flower CDR, Hadfield JW: Ultrasound of the pleura: An assessment of its clinical value. Clin Radiol 32:289, 1981.

231. Hirsch JH, Rogers JV, Mack LA: Real-time sonography of the pleural opacities. Am J Roentgenol 136:297, 1981.

232. O'Moore PV, Mueller PR, Simeone JF, et al: Sonographic guidance in diagnostic and therapeutic interventions in the pleural space. Am J Roentgenol 149:1, 1987.

233. Yang PC, Luh KT, Chang DB, et al: Value of sonography in determining the nature of pleural effusion: Analysis of 320 cases. Am J Roentgenol 159:29, 1992.

234. Somers JM, Gleeson FV, Flower CD: Rupture of the right hemidiaphragm following blunt trauma: The use of ultrasound in diagnosis. Clin Radiol 42:97, 1990.

235. Ikezoe J, Morimoto S, Arisawa J, et al: Percutaneous biopsy of thoracic lesions: Value of sonography for needle guidance. Am J Roentgenol 154:1181, 1990.

236. Morrison MC, Mueller PR, Lee MJ, et al: Sclerotherapy of malignant pleural effusion through sonographically placed small-bore catheters. Am J Roentgenol 158:41, 1992.

237. O'Moore PV, Mueller PR, Simeone FJ, et al: Sonographic guidance in diagnostic and therapeutic interventions in the pleural space. Am J Roentgenol 159:1, 1987.

238. Klein JS, Schultz S, Heffner JE: Interventional radiology of the chest: Image-guided percutaneous drainage of pleural effusions, lung abscess, and pneumothorax. Am J Roentgenol 164:581, 1995.

CHAPTER 14

Methods of Pathologic Investigation

CYTOLOGY, 339
  Sputum and Bronchial Washings and Brushings, 339
    Technical Considerations, 339
    Diagnostic Features and Yield, 340
  Bronchoalveolar Lavage, 343
  Pleural Fluid, 343
    Benign Cells, 344
    Malignant Cells, 344
    Miscellaneous Cytologic Findings, 345
  Fine-Needle Aspiration, 345
    Transthoracic Needle Aspiration, 345
    Transmucosal Needle Aspiration, 347
    Intraoperative Needle Aspiration, 348
  Aspiration from Intravascular Catheters, 348
EXAMINATION OF EXCISED LOBES AND WHOLE
LUNGS, 348
SPECIAL PATHOLOGIC TECHNIQUES, 351
  Examination of the Pulmonary Vasculature and
    Airways, 351
  Lung Culture, 351
  Electron Microscopy, 351
    Transmission Electron Microscopy, 351
    Scanning Electron Microscopy, 354
  Immunochemistry, 355
  Morphometry, 356
  Cytogenetics, 356
  Flow Cytometry, 356
  Molecular Biology, 358

In many pulmonary diseases, diagnosis is not possible despite consideration of the results of radiologic and clinical investigations and of routine laboratory tests and function studies. In this situation it is often necessary to obtain cells or tissue for pathologic examination, on the basis of which a definitive diagnosis is possible in many instances. The techniques used to obtain cytologic specimens, as well as a summary of the principles involved in the examination of tissue and cellular material, are discussed in this chapter; the techniques and indications for tissue biopsy are discussed in Chapter 15 (*see* page 341).

CYTOLOGY

The practice of cytology is concerned primarily with the morphologic features of individual cells or small clusters of cells. Although most useful in the diagnosis of malignancy, cytologic studies can also detect acellular material or cellular changes suggestive of specific benign diseases. Interpretation of the findings in specimens submitted for cytologic analysis varies somewhat with the origin of the material and the technique by which it is obtained. Thus, the following discussion can be divided into four sections: (1) sputum, bronchial washings, and bronchial brushings (sampling the airway surface and, to a lesser extent, the lung parenchyma); (2) bronchoalveolar lavage (BAL) fluid (sampling primarily the lung parenchyma); (3) pleural fluid; and (4) pulmonary or mediastinal material aspirated via a thin needle.

Sputum and Bronchial Washings and Brushings

Cells and other material suitable for cytologic examination are most often obtained from the lungs by spontaneous or induced expectoration of sputum, by bronchial washing or brushing performed during endoscopy, and by BAL (*see* farther on).[1] It has also been suggested that in some anesthetized patients, analysis of secretions suctioned from the endotracheal tube might be useful as a screening procedure for carcinoma.[2]

Technical Considerations

Sputum is best collected by having patients rinse their mouth with water and then expectorate a deep cough specimen into a wide-mouthed collecting jar; the optimal time is generally considered to be early morning just after rising. Inadequate samples are fairly common and account for as many as 25% to 30% of specimens in some series[3, 4] and approximately 15% in the literature as a whole;[5] the most common causes are insufficient material or lack of sputum altogether (indicated by the absence of alveolar macrophages).[4] Careful explanation to the patient of the necessity for a deep cough should help reduce the incidence of such inadequate specimens. When sputum production is truly minimal and specimens are repeatedly inadequate, it may be helpful to induce deep expectoration by having the patient inhale an aerosolized heated solution of saline (or, less commonly other substances such as propylene glycol or sulfur dioxide).[6–10] Since bronchoscopy may be followed by repeated deep coughing, some physicians obtain postbronchoscopic specimens for cytologic analysis; however, it has been argued that the procedure is not cost effective for this purpose.[11]

Once collected, sputum may be processed in several ways. In one widely used method ("pick and smear"), the freshly expectorated sample is brought to the laboratory where it is examined for tissue fragments or for areas of discolored, blood-tinged mucus. Specimens from these areas, as well as from randomly chosen mucus, are then smeared evenly over glass slides and immediately fixed in 95% ethyl alcohol or by cytospray without air drying. Since the number of unsatisfactory specimens decreases as the number of smears increases,[12] at least two slides should be prepared. The slides are then stained, usually by the Papanicolaou method, and examined by a cytotechnologist and/or a cytopathologist.

Although widely used, this direct smear technique has two disadvantages: first, the lack of fixative in the collecting jar makes it difficult to obtain either multiple specimens over an extended period or a single specimen at a site remote from the laboratory; second, and more important, since only a small portion of the expectorated mucus is usually sampled, malignant cells could be missed. A variety of prefixation and concentration techniques have been proposed to overcome these drawbacks. One method has been to dissolve the mucus to yield a less viscous fluid that can either be passed through a Millipore filter[13, 14] or centrifuged to provide a cell-rich residue that can be smeared on a slide.[15] Many mucolytic substances have been used for this purpose, including urea, hydrogen peroxide, detergents, enzymes (including hyaluronidase, papain, ficin, pancreatin, trypsin, and chymotrypsin[13, 16]), acetylcysteine,[17] hydrochloric acid,[18] dithiothreitol,[19, 20] and several commercial agents.[14, 15] Although most of these agents are not widely used because of the relatively tedious nature of the procedure and less than optimal cell morphology, some investigators have found cell preservation to be adequate and the number of positive cases to be increased.[19, 21]

In a second method, proposed by Saccomanno and associates in 1963,[22] sputum is expectorated into a jar containing 50% ethyl or isopropyl alcohol (which itself contains 2% polyethylene glycol); the alcohol acts as a fixative that permits the collection of sputum specimens over a period of several days. In the laboratory, the sputum-alcohol mixture is placed in a household-type food blender and blended at the highest speed for a short period, effectively emulsifying the mucus and resulting in a fluid that can be centrifuged. When the supernatant is discarded, the residual concentrated cellular material is smeared on glass slides, dried, and stained.

This procedure results in a substantial increase in the number of cells, both benign and malignant, available for examination. For example, Saccomanno and colleagues found that it increased the number of satisfactory smears (containing at least a few alveolar macrophages) from about 70% in the direct smear method to 92%.[22] In one study in which a known number of malignant cells were added to sputum specimens, investigators identified malignant cells in 14 of 39 slides prepared by the direct smear method from samples containing approximately 50 malignant cells per milliliter of sputum; the discovery rate dropped to only 2 of 40 slides when the concentration was decreased to 24 cells per milliliter.[23] By contrast, in specimens prepared by the

Saccomanno method, all 42 slides prepared from sputum containing 6 cells per milliliter were positive. The researchers concluded that efficiency of detection was increased 24-fold by using the Saccomanno method.

Despite these apparent benefits, the procedure is not endorsed by all cytopathologists.[1] Because it entails the use of a blender, it has been criticized as a potential mechanism for aerosol spread of infection.[1] In addition, the Saccomanno method has been found by some investigators to result in relatively poor cell preservation (particularly for small cell carcinoma[24]) and to have a diagnostic sensitivity inferior to that of the pick-and-smear method.[24–26]

Sputum samples have also been formalin-fixed and embedded in paraffin to yield blocks from which multiple sections can be cut and stained in the same manner as tissue fragments obtained by biopsy.[5, 27] In the hands of some investigators, this procedure has yielded good results; for example, in one study of 4,297 sputum specimens from 1,889 patients (219 of whom were shown to have carcinoma by radiologic or pathologic means), the sensitivity for a positive diagnosis was approximately 85% with examination of three specimens.[5] However, since the technique is time consuming (in the study just cited, nine slides with 27 sections were examined for each patient) and the details of cellular morphology are often suboptimal (at least in the experience of some investigators[29]), it is not commonly used.

The technical problems associated with sputum processing are less likely to be encountered in samples obtained by endoscopic bronchial washing or brushing since the amount of mucus is usually relatively small (although mucolytic agents have also been used in these specimens to optimize cell visualization, in some instances with good results[21]). Specimens derived by direct brushing of a bronchial abnormality should be taken before biopsy to diminish the degree of blood contamination. They can be smeared directly onto glass slides and rapidly fixed in the endoscopy room; it has also been suggested that the cell-rich fluid obtained by agitating the brush in saline should be filtered in an attempt to increase the yield of diagnostic cells.[30]

Bronchial washings (typically consisting of about 5 ml of fluid instilled and aspirated through the bronchoscope) can be passed through a membrane filter or, preferably, centrifuged and the resulting cell-rich button smeared on slides and, if sufficient in amount, prepared into a cell block for histologic examination;[31] the latter procedure has been shown by some investigators to increase the likelihood of a positive diagnosis by approximately 5% to 10%.[32, 33] It also enables the performance of immunocytochemistry, which may be useful in the diagnosis of lymphoma.[34] If the cell button is scanty in material, it can be processed in a cytospin apparatus.

Diagnostic Features and Yield

The principal purpose of cytologic examination of sputum and specimens obtained by bronchial washing and brushing is the detection of malignancy. It has been repeatedly shown that such examination is worthwhile: in large series of patients with confirmed lung cancer, positive diagnoses range from 50% to 90%;[35–39] in a 1992 literature review of the diagnostic accuracy of sputum specimens, the overall sensitivity was found to be approximately 65% and the specificity, 98%.[5] Although the yield from sputum specimens has been reported to be approximately equal to that from bronchial washings,[36] the latter will be available for cytologic examination in most cases since bronchoscopy is almost always performed in patients with suspected pulmonary carcinoma. In most cases, malignant cells derived by one technique will also be identified in cytologic specimens from the other two; in a small number, however, use of the three modes of investigation is complementary. For example, in one study of 57 patients subsequently proved to have carcinoma, brush specimens were positive in 52 (91%) and washings in 50 (88%);[41] the combined positive yield was 96%. Correlation between the number of positive diagnoses obtained from washings and brushings and from biopsy specimens is also high, although the two procedures are again complementary in a small number of cases.[11, 42, 43]

Because bronchoscopy is usually indicated in patients who have suspected pulmonary carcinoma and because the diagnostic yield of the procedure is greater than that of sputum cytology, it has been argued that sputum analysis should be limited to those individuals in whom surgery is not contemplated or bronchoscopy has been unsuccessful.[25, 25a] In fact, largely because of the easy availability and high yield of bronchoscopy and TTNA, sputum cytology has been less used in recent years and is now a relatively uncommon means of establishing a diagnosis of pulmonary carcinoma.[28, 40, 40a] Nevertheless, some have argued that it is still a cost-effective first procedure in patients who have central lesions.[28]

Although most often used to establish a diagnosis of carcinoma in a patient with a radiologically evident lesion, brushing of specific bronchial branches has been found by some investigators also to be valuable in confirming the presence and identifying the location of carcinoma in sputum-positive, radiologically negative patients.[44]

False-positive results (the reporting of malignant cells in the absence of true neoplasm) in specimens of sputum and in bronchial washings and brushings are uncommon, such results being reported in 1% to 3% of cases in most series.[39, 45, 46] Reasons include specimen mix-up, "floaters" (i.e., clusters of malignant cells derived from a patient other than the one in question as a result of specimen handling in the laboratory), inexperience of the cytopathologist, evaluation of poorly preserved or inadequately prepared specimens, and misinterpretation of reactive epithelial atypia as neoplastic.[47–50] The last reason is most common in the presence of pneumonia[51] or pulmonary infarction.[52, 53] Cytologic features suggestive of radiotherapy or chemotherapeutic drug effect are often evident in the cells of patients undergoing such therapy;[54] nevertheless, differentiation of these cells from malignant ones may also be difficult in some cases.[55] Although malignant cells may be found in sputum specimens in the absence of radiologic abnormality (e.g., in carcinoma *in situ*), this situation should always be viewed with suspicion; the diagnostic slides should be reviewed in consultation with the reporting cytopathologist and, if the material is still believed to indicate malignancy, the possibility of specimen mix-up should be considered. The cytologic features of sputum obtained from individuals who have never smoked have been described;[56] as might be expected, metaplastic or dysplastic epithelial changes are rare.

As with false-positive diagnoses, there are a variety of reasons for false-negative results. As might be expected, one of the most important is an insufficient amount of material for analysis; it has been repeatedly shown that the yield of malignant cells increases with the number of specimens examined, regardless of whether they are sputum, washings, brushings, or a combination of these.[4, 5, 35, 39, 57] The increase in yield can be substantial; for example, in one study of 449 cases of proven lung carcinoma, positive diagnoses obtained by sputum cytology increased from 40% on the first sample to 80% after examination of five specimens.[4] Positive cytologic diagnoses are made more often with central than with peripheral neoplasms and with large tumors more frequently than with small ones;[4, 36, 57, 58] for example, in one series the true-positive rate for tumors less than 2 cm in diameter was only 15%, whereas for those greater than 2 cm, it was 82%.[4] Histopathologic type has also been shown to correlate with positive diagnosis, squamous cell carcinoma generally having a higher frequency than adenocarcinoma or large cell carcinoma;[4, 58, 59] this finding is probably explained by the much more frequent central location and intrabronchial growth of the squamous cell variety. Some investigators have found that lesions in the upper lobes are associated with a smaller yield than those in the lower lobes.[58, 59]

Metastatic neoplasms are less commonly detected than are primary lung carcinomas, probably because they tend to invade pulmonary parenchyma rather than the proximal airways;[60] nevertheless, discovery rates of 30% to 55% have been reported.[9, 39, 61, 62] Rare cases of metastatic sarcoma have also been identified by sputum analysis.[62a] We are not aware of precise figures concerning the yield of positive diagnoses in patients who have pulmonary lymphoma; however, there is no doubt that the diagnosis can be made confidently in some.[34]

The reliability of cytologic examination in typing specific forms of pulmonary carcinoma is somewhat difficult to assess given the problems associated with histologic classification (*see* page 1084); nevertheless, as a generalization, it is probably reasonable to say that there is a relatively high degree of accuracy for the better-differentiated tumors (Fig. 14–1). Typing accuracy is also somewhat related to specific tumors; in general, the cytologic diagnosis has been found to agree with the histologic diagnosis in about 40% to 80% of large cell carcinomas, 75% to 85% of adenocarcinomas, 85% to 95% of squamous cell carcinomas, and 90% to 95% of small cell carcinomas.[4, 38, 39, 63] From a practical point of view, the distinction between small cell and non–small cell carcinoma can be made with confidence in the vast majority of cases.

In benign disease, examination of sputum and bronchial washings and brushings is most useful for the detection and characterization of infectious organisms. Bacteria are most commonly identified by Gram or Ziehl-Neelsen stains (procedures that are often carried out in the microbiology laboratory); however, more sensitive and specific immunochemical and molecular techniques are being increasingly used and, in some instances (e.g., legionellosis and some forms of mycobacterial infection), have been shown to be of value in definitive and rapid diagnosis. Virus-induced cytopathologic changes may be suggestive of a specific organism[64] and provide supportive evidence of the etiology of a pneumonia before the results of serologic or cultural investigations are available. Many fungi and parasites can also be seen on

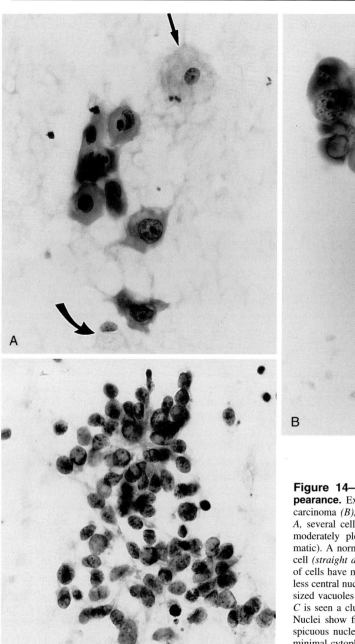

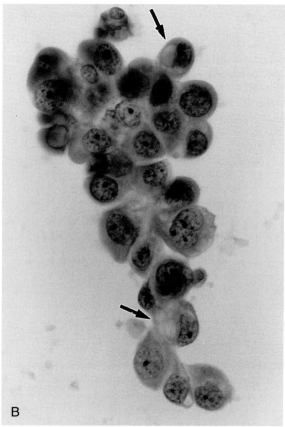

Figure 14–1. Pulmonary Carcinoma—Cytologic Appearance. Examples of squamous cell carcinoma *(A),* adenocarcinoma *(B),* and small cell carcinoma *(C)* are illustrated. In *A,* several cells have abundant, dense cytoplasm and enlarged, moderately pleomorphic nuclei, some very dark (hyperchromatic). A normal goblet cell *(curved arrow)* and oral squamous cell *(straight arrow)* are present for comparison. In *B,* a cluster of cells have moderately pleomorphic nuclei containing more or less central nucleoli. The cytoplasm of some cells shows variably sized vacuoles *(arrows),* suggesting glandular differentiation. In *C* is seen a cluster of cells smaller than those in either *A* or *B.* Nuclei show finely granular (dispersed) chromatin with inconspicuous nucleoli. They are also closely opposed, indicative of minimal cytoplasm. (A, ×300; B, ×500; C, ×400.)

Papanicolaou stain, thus allowing the cytopathologist to suggest or confirm such conditions as invasive or allergic bronchopulmonary aspergillosis,[65] cryptococcosis, or filariasis.[66] In some situations, identification of a specific organism is fairly common: for example, one group of investigators reported finding structures diagnostic of *Echinococcus granulosus* in 8 (33%) of 24 cases of hydatid disease;[67] similarly, a definitive diagnosis of *Pneumocystis carinii* pneumonia can be made in many patients with the acquired immunodeficiency syndrome (AIDS) by identifying silver-positive organisms in specimens of induced or expectorated sputum.[68, 68a]

Cytologic examinations in noninfectious, non-neoplas-

tic diseases are less likely to be productive, although there are a few exceptions. For example, in the appropriate clinical setting, the presence of macrophages containing lipid supports a diagnosis of lipid pneumonia or fat embolism.[69, 70] Similarly, the finding of hemosiderin-laden macrophages indicates previous intrapulmonary hemorrhage and is consistent with conditions such as Goodpasture's syndrome or idiopathic pulmonary hemorrhage. The identification of asbestos bodies virtually assures a history of occupational exposure to the mineral[70a] and the documentation of elastin fibers in potassium hydroxide preparations has been said to be supportive evidence for the presence of necrotizing pneumonia.[71]

Bronchoalveolar Lavage

BAL is a relatively noninvasive means of sampling both cellular and acellular components of the lung parenchyma.[72] The procedure involves the instillation of saline into the peripheral lung parenchyma via a wedged fiberoptic bronchoscope.[73] For clinical purposes, 20- to 50-ml aliquots are injected and recovered by gentle suction to avoid airway trauma and collapse. A total of 100 to 300 ml of normal saline can be instilled; about 40% to 60% of the injected volume is usually recovered.[73] When disease is focal, lavage should be directed to the site of greatest abnormality; when diffuse, lavage of the middle lobe, lingula, or lower lobes allows for better fluid recovery than does lavage of the upper lung zones.[74] A portion of the lavage fluid can be processed in the same manner as bronchial washings for routine cytologic evaluation; in addition, specific types of inflammatory cells can be counted and substances within the fluid analyzed. Since the initial aliquot recovered may contain artefactually high numbers of neutrophils and respiratory epithelial cells, it has been proposed that this sample be analyzed separately or discarded.[75, 76] Criteria for identifying unsatisfactory specimens have been proposed and include a paucity of alveolar macrophages, an excessive number of airway epithelial cells, the presence of a mucopurulent exudate, and excessive degenerative cellular changes.[77]

The procedure is generally well tolerated, even in patients who have asthma[78] or are critically ill and mechanically ventilated.[79–81] Nevertheless, it can cause significant decreases in FEV_1 and A–a oxygen gradient in asthmatic patients,[82a] and careful monitoring of such individuals is warranted. In one series of 119 patients with pulmonary interstitial disease (many of whom underwent more than one procedure), complications included fever (2.5%), pneumonitis (0.4%), hemorrhage (0.7%), and bronchospasm (0.7%);[82] none of these complications required therapy. Interestingly, fever following the procedure is probably related to the release of proinflammatory cytokines from alveolar macrophages activated by the instillation of fluid into the airways rather than infection.[83] Pneumothorax has been documented rarely.[84] A moderate impairment in gas exchange may be seen in sicker patients.[79, 80] Focal areas of consolidation corresponding to the region undergoing lavage are common on chest radiographs;[85] clearing usually occurs within 24 hours.

BAL has been used for diagnosis and in the experimental investigation of numerous pulmonary diseases. Its most important clinical use is in the diagnosis of infection in immunocompromised hosts, especially patients with AIDS;[86–92, 92a] in the latter situation, the procedure is particularly valuable in the diagnosis of *P. carinii* pneumonia. Culture of BAL fluid is clearly an important diagnostic procedure in this setting; quantitative techniques may be used to help differentiate colonization from true infection (the presence of 10^3 colony-forming units per milliliter generally being used as the threshold for a clinically significant result[93–95] [*see* page 719]). In addition to culture, the diagnosis of a specific infection is sometimes made by the cytopathologist on the basis of the morphologic, histochemical, or immunohistochemical characteristics of a particular organism;[96–100] it has also been accomplished by analyzing BAL fluid by polymerase chain reaction (PCR) for the presence of organism-specific DNA.[101–103] Measurement of various substances in BAL fluid may also be diagnostically useful in some cases; for example, levels of adenosine deaminase have been found to be increased in patients with tuberculosis and sarcoidosis,[104] and it has been proposed that ventilator-associated pneumonia may be identified by assay for BAL fluid endotoxin[105] and pneumococcal pneumonia by the detection of pneumococcal antigen on countercurrent immunoelectrophoresis and latex agglutination.[106]

BAL can also be useful in the diagnosis of neoplasia, particularly peripheral tumors that are not visualized endoscopically; in this situation, it yields a positive diagnosis in approximately 65% to 70% of patients.[107, 108] The procedure has also been found to yield a large number of positive diagnoses in patients with Hodgkin's and non-Hodgkin's lymphoma[109, 110, 110a] and metastatic carcinoma (appearing as either multiple nodules or lymphangitic carcinomatosis).[109, 111] With respect to the latter situation, it should be remembered that reactive Type II epithelial cells are common in interstitial pneumonitis and the organizing phase of diffuse alveolar damage (adult respiratory distress syndrome) and their atypia may be severe enough to mimic carcinoma.[112, 113]

A variety of other less common pulmonary abnormalities have also been investigated for the diagnostic utility of BAL. Those in which the procedure has proved to be diagnostically helpful in some cases include drug-induced pneumonitis,[114] lipidoses,[115, 116] diffuse pulmonary hemorrhage,[117] asbestosis,[118, 119] lipid pneumonia, alveolar proteinosis, fat embolism,[70] and Langerhans' cell histiocytosis.[120]

In addition to diagnosis, BAL has been an important technique in treating alveolar proteinosis[120a] and in enhancing the understanding of mechanisms of lung injury, inflammation, repair, and fibrosis in many pulmonary diseases,[121, 122] including pneumoconiosis,[123, 124, 124a] idiopathic pulmonary fibrosis,[125] immunologically mediated connective tissue disease,[126] sarcoidosis,[127, 127a] extrinsic allergic alveolitis,[128] Langerhans' cell histiocytosis,[129] eosinophilic lung disease,[130] drug-induced disease,[131] asthma,[132, 133] AIDS,[134] and chronic obstructive pulmonary disease.[135] Much of this research has been related to the investigation of inflammatory and immune-mediator cells and their secretions. Approximately 95% of normal individuals have fewer than 25×10^4 cells per milliliter of lavage fluid (the mean in one study of 111 subjects being $12.7 \pm 9.1 \times 10^4$);[136] of these cells, the great majority (about 85% to 100%) are macrophages. Most of the remaining cells are lymphocytes, neutrophils, and eosinophils; generally they represent fewer than 1% of all cells when present and are totally absent in most healthy individuals.[136]

Pleural Fluid

For cytologic examination, pleural fluid should be collected in a clean jar. If rapid transportation to the laboratory is not feasible, cellular morphology will usually be reasonably well preserved without fixative for at least 24 hours at refrigerator temperature.[137] Once in the laboratory, the fluid may be treated in the same fashion as bronchial wash specimens, i.e., passed through a membrane filter or centrifuged; in the latter situation, the resulting cell-rich button is smeared on glass slides or, if minimal in amount, processed by cytospin technique. When sufficient material is obtained, a portion of the button should be fixed in formalin and processed for histologic examination; as with transthoracic needle aspiration, the latter procedure frequently yields small tissue fragments on which standard stains as well as histochemical and immunohistochemical investigations can be performed, sometimes greatly facilitating diagnosis.[138] Bloody effusions can be difficult to evaluate, not only because of problems in making smears but also because of the large number of red cells that obscure cellular morphology; several techniques have been proposed to obviate these problems, including density-gradient centrifugation, sedimentation, filtration, and microhematocrit procedures.[139, 140]

As with cytologic examination of pulmonary secretions, the primary feature of diagnostic importance in pleural fluid is the exclusion or confirmation of malignancy. In addition, the number and nature of inflammatory and other cells within the effusion may provide valuable clues concerning etiology. Finally, in a number of uncommon conditions, acellular material or unusual cellular alterations are suggestive of a specific benign diagnosis. In addition to histochemical and immunohistochemical studies, ancillary techniques such as flow cytometry, cytogenetic analysis, and electron microscopy are sometimes useful or indispensable in making a definitive diagnosis.[141] Additional details concerning the composition of pleural effusions, including biochemical features, are given in Chapter 69 (*see* page 2741).

Benign Cells

Erythrocytes. Red blood cell (RBC) counts greater than 10,000/mm³ are common to all types of effusion and therefore of no discriminatory value.[142] A grossly bloody effusion in which the RBC count is high only in the first part of the aspirate should suggest traumatic hemorrhage ("bloody tap"). Apart from this situation, a grossly bloody effusion or one containing 100,000 RBCs per cubic millimeter is much more likely to be of neoplastic than tuberculous origin; other causes include trauma, pulmonary infarction, and (rarely) benign asbestos effusion.

Neutrophils. A large number of neutrophils in pleural fluid usually indicates the presence of bacterial pneumonia; however, this situation can also occur with primary pleural bacterial infection, pancreatitis, pulmonary infarction, and (occasionally) malignant neoplasms and tuberculosis.[142] Although polymorphonuclear leukocytosis predominates in the early stages of tuberculous effusion, it is rapidly superseded by lymphocytosis;[143] thus, an effusion that has been present for longer than a few days and contains more than 50% neutrophils is unlikely to be caused by tuberculosis.

Lymphocytes. An effusion containing 50% or more lymphocytes is almost certainly either tuberculous or neoplastic;[142, 144] for example, in one series of 31 patients with an exudative effusion having a predominance of small lymphocytes, 30 were proved to be caused by either tuberculosis or cancer.[142] Although lymphocyte predominance may be seen in either disease, most effusions caused by neoplasms contain an admixture of other cell types, thus resulting in a polymorphous cellular population. By contrast, the lymphocyte-rich effusion of tuberculosis typically contains a paucity of mesothelial or other mononuclear or polymorphonuclear inflammatory cells;[137, 142] in fact, the cellular uniformity may be so marked as to suggest the possibility of small lympho-

cytic lymphoma.[145] There is also evidence that the specific type of lymphocyte that predominates in pleural fluid may have diagnostic significance. For example, in one investigation of 70 fluid samples (42 pleural and 28 peritoneal), numbers of natural killer cells were found to be markedly elevated in 14 of 15 patients with carcinoma and only 1 of 55 without.[146]

Eosinophils. Eosinophilic pleural effusion may or may not be associated with blood eosinophilia and occurs in a variety of conditions. One of the more common associations is pleural trauma: in one series of 127 effusions with greater than 20% eosinophils, a history of recent surgery, trauma, spontaneous pneumothorax, or transthoracic aspiration was found in 81 (64%).[137] The pathogenesis of eosinophilia in these situations is not clear. The presence of air within the pleural space has been proposed as the common denominator;[147, 148] however, the experimental production of eosinophilia by the intraperitoneal injection of blood suggests that other factors, either alone or in combination, may also be involved.[149] There is experimental evidence that eosinophil colony-stimulating factor and interleukins-3 and -5 released from macrophages within the fluid may be involved in both proliferation and survival of the eosinophils.[150]

A variety of other clinical conditions have been implicated in pleural fluid eosinophilia.[148, 151, 152] Pulmonary infections, including histoplasmosis, coccidioidomycosis, and actinomycosis, are occasional causes,[142, 152, 154, 154a] as are parasitic infestations such as amebiasis, ascariasis, and ruptured hydatid cyst. An especially high incidence has been noted in patients with paragonimiasis, presumably related to the transpleural migration of this organism. Effusions that accompany immunologic abnormalities such as rheumatoid disease[137, 152] and drug-induced hypersensitivity[151, 155] are only occasionally associated with increased eosinophils. A high proportion of benign asbestos-related effusions have been found to show eosinophilia,[148] and pulmonary infarction is also said to be a relatively frequent cause.[137]

Despite this rather extensive list of etiologies, quite frequently there is no clinical correlation at all,[148, 151, 154a] and perhaps the most important diagnostic point is that tuberculous and neoplastic effusions only occasionally contain a substantial number of eosinophils.[137, 142, 152, 156] (However, the converse is not true: up to 20% of eosinophilic effusions have been associated with a malignant neoplasm.[154a])

Malignant Cells

The proportion of positive cytologic diagnoses from pleural effusions of malignant origin ranges from 33% to 87%;[142] most authors report a sensitivity of about 50%.[142, 157–159] Definitive diagnosis may be difficult, chiefly as a result of the cytologically atypical changes that can occur in reactive mesothelial cells. As with sputum and bronchial washing specimens, repeated examinations are likely to increase the yield of positive diagnoses.[142] In one investigation, the use of more than one staining/fixative technique was also found to be associated with a higher number of positive diagnoses.[160] In one review of the literature, an overall false-positive rate of about 0.5% was found for several combined series.[161] In patients with cancer in whom no malignant cells are identified in the effusion, it is possible that the effusion is secondary to pneumonia distal to an obstructing pulmonary carcinoma or to a lymphatic obstruction.[162]

As mentioned previously, the use of one or more special techniques can sometimes aid in the diagnosis or exclusion of malignancy.[146] For example, combining cytogenetic analysis with cytologic examination is said to increase the true-positive yield to over 80%[159] and has been found by some investigators to specifically help in the diagnosis of mesothelioma.[163] Electron microscopy is of value in selected cases,[164, 165] particularly in confirming mesothelial differentiation in malignant cells. Tissue culture of aspirated cells has also been shown to be diagnostic in some cases;[166] however, the procedure is time consuming and relatively expensive and yields results that are not substantially better than those with conventional cytologic techniques.

Analysis of cell DNA content or proliferative index by flow cytometry or image analysis has been assessed by several investigators.[167–169] Although the specificity for malignancy has been reported to be between 95% and 100% (in one review of nine reports, the false-positive rate was found to be 2.5%[170]), the sensitivity is only about 55% to 65% (i.e., approximately 35% to 45% of malignant effusions are composed of diploid cells).[171] Nevertheless, some malignancies that appear benign by cytologic evaluation have been identified by the presence of an aneuploid population. As a result, it has been suggested that the presence of aneuploidy should prompt a careful review of cytologic material and the examination of additional specimens.[169] There is evidence that the combined use of image analysis and assessment of immunoreactivity to specific antigens (such as Ber-EP4[172] or cytokeratin[173]) may improve the diagnostic accuracy.

Numerous immunocytochemical studies have been performed in an attempt to identify antibodies that can aid in the distinction between reactive mesothelial cells and malignant cells and between malignant mesothelial cells and metastatic carcinoma.[153] The use of a panel of antibodies to such substances as keratins, vimentin, carcinoembryonic antigen, leu-M1, Ber-EPA, and epithelial membrane antigen is generally thought to be most helpful for the latter task;[174–178] a positive reaction to various substances such as bcl-2, p53 gene product, and P-170 glycoprotein has been found to be highly specific and moderately sensitive in the former.[179, 180] These issues are discussed more fully in Chapter 72 (*see* page 2816).

Miscellaneous Cytologic Findings

Although various benign diseases may be diagnosed or suggested from the examination of material or altered cells within a pleural effusion, this situation is very uncommon. Examples include endometriosis,[181] infectious diseases such as echinococcosis[182] and aspergillosis,[183] rheumatoid disease,[184] ruptured mediastinal teratoma,[185] lymphangioleiomyomatosis,[186] and systemic lupus erythematosus.[187, 188]

Fine-Needle Aspiration

Unlike other procedures such as transthoracic (core) needle biopsy and mediastinoscopy, which produce true tissue fragments, fine-needle aspiration results in a specimen that consists predominantly of individual cells or small clusters of cells. It is a technique with high reliability and minimal patient discomfort and complications and has thus become an important method in the diagnosis of lung disease, particularly cancer and, to a lesser extent, infection. Aspirates can be taken across the chest wall (transthoracic needle aspiration), across the bronchial wall (transbronchial needle aspiration), or directly during mediastinoscopy or thoracotomy (intraoperative needle aspiration). The relative merits of needle biopsy versus needle aspiration are considered on page 370.

Transthoracic Needle Aspiration

Transthoracic needle aspiration (TTNA) was first described in the late nineteenth century as a technique to obtain the microorganisms responsible for acute pneumonia; subsequent investigators documented its use in the diagnosis of lung cancer.[189, 190] In the 1930s a cutting needle for lung biopsy was introduced;[191] along with several technical modifications, this method allowed the removal of an actual core of tissue and resulted in rapid replacement of the fine-needle aspiration technique. With the recognition of considerably greater morbidity and mortality associated with cutting needles without the advantage of greater diagnostic yield in the diagnosis of malignancy in most settings, TTNA has experienced a resurgence. This preference has been positively influenced by the increased expertise of cytopathologists and operators performing the procedure.[192]

Technical Considerations. The procedure consists of sucking fluid and cells into a syringe through a long, narrow-gauge needle inserted percutaneously into a parenchymal lesion. Most clinicians use needles of 20 to 22 gauge (equivalent to an external diameter of about 1 mm) because of the relatively low incidence of complications and a good yield.[193–195] The use of an ultrathin needle (24 to 25 gauge) has been advocated by some who claim a similar yield with fewer complications.[196]

The many different needles that are available may be classified into two general types: single-pass needles and multiple-pass coaxial needles.[197] The former are inserted directly into the lesion and removed immediately after aspiration. The coaxial system consists of an outer guiding needle and an inner aspiration needle; after the guide needle has been positioned adjacent to the lesion, the inner aspiration needle is advanced through it into the lesion itself. Following aspiration, the inner needle is withdrawn and the outer needle is left in place to facilitate further sampling.[197] Both systems have advantages and disadvantages. The single-pass system creates a smaller hole and minimizes the time that the needle is in place across the pleura; however, if the sample is inadequate, the whole procedure needs to be repeated. The coaxial system allows repeated sampling of the lesion but has the disadvantage of requiring a larger-bore outer needle (e.g., a 19-gauge outer needle for a 22-gauge aspiration needle).[194]

TTNA may be performed under fluoroscopic,[198–200] computed tomographic (CT),[195, 201, 202] or in cases that have an adequate acoustic window, ultrasound guidance.[203, 204] The choice between fluoroscopic and CT guidance is influenced by size and location of the lesion, as well as by personal preference of the radiologist and the availability of fluoroscopic and CT facilities.[197] CT guidance is recommended for biopsy of lesions adjacent to the mediastinum or hilum, for small nodules, or for situations in which an oblique or angled biopsy approach is required.[197, 202] The patient is positioned on the biopsy table or CT scanner in such a way as to allow the shortest needle route and the fewest pleural surfaces to be traversed.[205] When the needle is judged to be inserted properly, it is rotated while applying vigorous suction. To increase the diagnostic yield, it is important to make multiple aspirations.[207] Ideally, a portion of the aspirate should be stained and examined at the time of the procedure (in a manner analogous to performing frozen sections on tissue);[208–210] this practice enables rapid assessment of the adequacy of the specimen so that repeat aspirations or cutting needle biopsy can be performed immediately in an attempt to increase the diagnostic yield.[211, 220]

Aspirated material may be evacuated directly onto glass slides, smeared, and immediately fixed by cytospray technique or in 95% alcohol (some cytopathologists prefer to air-dry a portion of the sample). The needle contents may also be expelled into saline or 50% alcohol and transported to the laboratory, the fluid then being processed in the same manner as bronchial wash or pleural fluid specimens (*see* page 343.) As with the latter material, processing of a portion of the sample as a cell block frequently provides tissue fragments for histologic examination and for histochemical and immunohistochemical analysis and has been shown to increase the sensitivity of the procedure;[212, 213] the determination of a specific type of malignancy may also be greatly facilitated. If indicated, a portion of the aspirated sample can be processed for electron microscopic examination.[214–216]

The two main indications for fine-needle aspiration in chest disease are the diagnosis of pulmonary malignancy and determination of the etiology of serious pneumonia when noninvasive diagnostic methods have failed. (Although TTNA can also yield material sufficient for the diagnosis of mediastinal tumors such as lymphoma, thymoma, and neurilemmoma,[219] the use of cutting needle biopsy has been advocated for this situation to obtain more tissue for histologic examination [*see* page 369].[217]) Since the negative predictive value of TTNA is as low as 70% in the diagnosis of pulmonary malignancy,[218] we believe that it is not generally indicated if there is an intention to proceed with resection of a lesion regardless of the result of the test. Although some physicians argue that it should still be performed to identify cases of small cell carcinoma (which would then be treated nonsurgically), most would recommend resection of peripheral small cell carcinomas in otherwise operable patients (particularly since several cases initially diagnosed as small cell carcinoma on fine-needle aspiration have been proved at resection to be atypical carcinoid tumors).[202, 205] Thus, we believe that biopsy of a peripheral lesion strongly suspected of being a carcinoma merely to establish the diagnosis or cell type preoperatively is not warranted. (An exception to this "rule" may apply in geographic regions in which TTNA yields a relatively high proportion of specific benign diagnoses, such as in areas where coccidioidomycosis is endemic.)

In patients with suspected pulmonary carcinoma, there are thus two major indications for TTNA: (1) when a cytologic diagnosis must be established in a patient judged to be unresectable on clinical or radiologic grounds; and (2) to determine the cell type in a lesion suspected of being either a metastasis or a second primary pulmonary carcinoma. Although some believe that the procedure is also indicated to establish a diagnosis in a patient who is a poor surgical risk and in whom a positive biopsy would permit acceptance of the risk, the poor negative predictive power of a test result in this clinical situation makes such reasoning doubtful (*see* page 347).

Contraindications to TTNA include a suspicion that the lesion may be an echinococcal cyst; the presence of severe pulmonary arterial hypertension, a bleeding disorder, anticoagulant therapy or uncontrollable cough; and inability of the patient to tolerate a complicating pneumothorax.[221] Serious complications are rare and can usually (although not always[222]) be avoided by the use of ultrathin needles.[223, 224] In one review of the literature in 1982, only 12 deaths were identified, most of which were caused by hemorrhage;[225] air embolism[226, 227] and massive pneumothorax[225] are occasional causes.

Pneumothorax is the most common complication; however, it is not usually severe, with fewer than a third of affected patients requiring aspiration of the pleural space through either a malleable sigmoid needle or an intercostal drainage tube.[228–231] The risk of pneumothorax increases with larger needle diameter,[232, 233] procedures that cross more than one visceral pleural surface,[234] an increased number of passes,[235] and the presence of underlying chronic obstructive lung disease;[236, 237] it is minimized with the use of ultrathin (24 to 25 gauge) needles.[232] The majority of operators have used 20- to 23-gauge needles and have reported pneumothorax rates of 20% to 30%.[238–241]

Significant bleeding into the lung or pleural space is uncommon when the needle used is more than 20 gauge;[242, 243] in one investigation of 50 patients in whom aspiration was performed with an ultrathin needle of 24 or 25 gauge, the incidence of pneumothorax and hemorrhage was 8% and 4%, respectively;[232] these low figures compare with an incidence of 30% and 10%, respectively, in 2,062 patients culled from the literature who underwent biopsies with 16- to 20-gauge needles. The procedure itself usually results in little discomfort for the patient; it is interesting that pain upon puncture of the lesion, although rare in most tumors, appears to be relatively common in neurogenic tumors of the mediastinum.[244] One important, albeit rare complication of TTNA is spread of disease from the primary site along the needle track. As might be expected, this complication has been documented most commonly for neoplasms;[245, 246] however, infections such as cutaneous blastomycosis[247] and tuberculous pleurisy[248] have also been reported.

Several investigators have assessed the intraobserver and interobserver reproducibility of cytologic diagnosis in TTNA specimens.[249, 250] In one review of 100 cases, the concordance in the diagnosis of malignancy was 90% between two observers and 94% by the same observers at different times;[249] agreement on the specific histologic type of tumor was 80% between observers and 85% by the same cytopathologist. In a second study, also of 100 cases, interobserver agreement in the diagnosis of malignancy was 85%;[250] intraobserver reproducibility was 100% for the cytologist experienced with TTNA and 90% for the relatively inexperienced observer.

Diagnostic Features and Yield. As with other cytologic techniques, the most important use of TTNA is in the establishment of a diagnosis of pulmonary carcinoma. The overall sensitivity in reported series varies from about 70% to 95% (5% to 30% false negatives);[193, 195, 199, 220, 251–254] most reports are in the 85% to 95% range. The diagnostic yield is higher in peripheral pulmonary lesions than in central ones,[251] although it is still appreciable in the latter site; for example, in one study in which the diagnostic yield of TTNA was compared with that of sputum cytology, the former was superior irrespective of the location of the tumor.[255] Diagnostic yield is also closely related to size of the aspirated nodule;[251] nodules less than 1 cm in diameter have been found by some investigators to be associated with a sensitivity for diagnosis of about 60%.[251, 256] Since the most common cause of false-negative diagnoses is sampling error,[257, 258] the number of such cases can be decreased by assessing specimen adequacy during the procedure.

False-positive diagnoses have been documented in 0.5% to 2% of cases in most series;[255] with experienced cytopathologists, the lower figure can probably be expected. As with other cytologic specimens, a variety of underlying pulmonary conditions have been associated with an incorrect diagnosis of malignancy;[259] the most common is probably tuberculosis.[225] Diagnostic errors have also been documented in aspirates of mediastinal tumors,[260] although precise incidence figures are unavailable. In a large study of performance parameters conducted by the American College of Pathologists that involved 436 institutions and almost 12,000 TTNA specimens (approximately 40% of which had histologic material for review), the overall results were as follows: sensitivity, 89%; specificity, 96%; positive predictive value, 99%; and negative predictive value, 70%.[218]

As with sputum and bronchial washing/brushing specimens, the correlation between cytologic and histologic diagnoses of specific tumors types is generally good for the better-differentiated tumors; for example, in one investigation of 109 specimens for which there was adequate clinical and histologic follow-up, the accuracy of cytologic diagnoses was as follows: squamous cell carcinoma, 70%; adenocarcinoma, 86%; small cell carcinoma, 95%; and large cell carcinoma, 57%.[261]

Metastatic neoplasms may be differentiated from primary lung carcinoma in a substantial number of cases. In many instances, comparison of tissue fragments within a cell block with slides of a known extrathoracic primary will provide the diagnosis. In addition, the cytologic features of some neoplasms (such as renal cell carcinoma or colonic adenocarcinoma[262]) are occasionally sufficiently characteristic to suggest an extrathoracic origin without examining actual tissue fragments. Electron microscopic[263, 264] and/or immunohistochemical[265–267, 267a] examination is also useful in selected cases in identifying a specific type of tumor.

Although the principal application of TTNA is in the determination of malignancy and its cell type, a specific diagnosis of a benign condition is occasionally possible. Since small tissue fragments are often included in the aspirate, especially when larger-bore needles are used, virtually any pulmonary disease that has characteristic histopathologic changes may be identified.[225, 269] Nevertheless, the majority of studies using fine-needle aspiration have been associated with a sensitivity of only 40% to 50% for the diagnosis of specific benign lesions.[195, 199, 252] (The diagnostic yield can be increased with the use of transthoracic cutting needles;[201, 270, 271, 271a] for example, in one study of 122 patients in which coaxially placed, 20-gauge, automated transthoracic needle biopsy was compared with fine-needle aspiration biopsy under CT guidance, the former allowed a specific diagnostic rate of 100% for benign lesions as compared with 44% when fine-needle aspiration was used.[201] The advantages and disadvantages of this technique are discussed farther on [*see* page 370].)

The most common benign diseases to be diagnosed by TTNA are infections. Obviously, culture of aspirated material is the most important aspect of tissue analysis in these cases, and material for this purpose should always be submitted to the microbiology laboratory when there is a suspicion that a lesion might be of infectious etiology. Some investigators have also found that analysis of aspirated fluid for the presence of bacterial antigen by latex agglutination or PCR increases the diagnostic yield.[272, 272a] Cytologic examination itself occasionally provides the initial or only etiologic diagnosis of the pneumonia.[306] A variety of bacteria, fungi (including *P. carinii*),[306] and parasites (such as *Dirofilaria*[273] and *Echinococcus*[274]) may be identified by either routine or special stains, immunochemical techniques, or PCR.[274a] Tissue fragments consistent with active granulomatous inflammation can also be detected in TTNA specimens; the presence of finely granular or calcified necrotic material, corresponding to areas of caseous necrosis, is also suggestive of a granulomatous process. The most common underlying lesion in these cases is tuberculosis;[275, 276] occasionally, other infections or noninfectious disease such as Wegener's granulomatosis can be suggested.[277]

In one series of 108 immunocompromised patients in whom biplane fluoroscopy was used for needle placement, one or more etiologic organisms were identified in 79 presumed infectious episodes.[278] In another study of nonventilated patients with nosocomial pneumonia, TTNA with an ultrathin needle led to modification of the initial antibiotic therapy in 29 of 97 patients, including 12 in whom the initially chosen empiric regimen was ineffective.[224] TTNA is also useful in the diagnosis of some infections in patients with organ transplants[222] and in patients with AIDS (although its sensitivity has not been compared with that of induced sputum in this setting).[279]

Many benign neoplastic and non-neoplastic lesions can also be definitely diagnosed by TTNA, including hamartoma,[280] nodular amyloidosis,[281] solitary fibrous tumor,[282] splenosis,[283] thymoma, posterior mediastinal neurogenic tumors, and lipoma.[225] The diagnosis of other non-neoplastic conditions may also be suggested by the cellular background of the smear: for example, the presence of fragments of vegetable material implies aspiration pneumonia[284] and the finding of numerous blood cells and hemosiderin-laden macrophages suggests the diagnosis of pulmonary infarction.[285]

Transmucosal Needle Aspiration

Although needle aspiration of mediastinal lesions may be carried out percutaneously,[229, 286] a transbronchial or transtracheal approach has also been used.[287–293] Such transmucosal needle aspiration may be accomplished through either a rigid or a flexible fiberoptic bronchoscope. When the latter instrument is used, lesions that are peripherally situated in the lung can be aspirated, even when they are not visible through the bronchoscope, provided that the aspiration is performed with fluoroscopic guidance.[294] It is important that aspiration be carried out before other procedures such as bronchial brushing or biopsy to minimize contamination of the aspirate by mechanically displaced material from the airway wall. Aspirated material is handled in the laboratory in the same fashion as that derived by TTNA.

The technique has been used most often for establishing a diagnosis of primary malignancy and in the staging of known lung carcinoma; it has also been used occasionally to confirm a diagnosis of sarcoidosis and to establish the presence of nodal mycobacterial disease in patients infected with HIV.[206] With respect to cancer staging, negative findings do not preclude the need for further staging;[293] however, confirmation of metastatic carcinoma or the identification of small cell carcinoma may obviate the need for additional staging procedures and provide a guide to appropriate nonsurgical therapy.[291] The procedure has been particularly advocated for the diagnosis of necrotic bronchial carcinoma, vascular bronchial tumors (such as carcinoid tumor), peribronchial or submucosal carcinoma (such as in lymphangitic carcinomatosis), superior sulcus tumors (via the trachea), and subcarinal or hilar lymph node enlargement.[289] Satisfactory sampling of subcarinal lymph nodes can be obtained in about 90% of cases;[295] as is true of most procedures, the yield improves with experience and training.[296] Complications are few and generally not serious and include minimal, usually transient hemoptysis and low-grade fever (occasionally associated with bacteremia);[297, 298] pneumothorax or significant hemorrhage caused by puncture of a large pulmonary artery or the aorta is rare.[289, 291]

Material adequate for interpretation is procured by experienced aspirators in approximately 80% of centrally located tumors;[289] the sensitivity of subcarinal sampling for malignancy has ranged from 50%[299] to almost 90%.[300] As might be expected, the yield is significantly less for peripheral tumors (particularly those associated with a normal carina at bronchoscopy[301]) and for tumors in other peribronchial lymph nodes, the sensitivity in the latter situation generally being about 30%.[289, 302, 303] As with TTNA, the yield is much greater when specimen adequacy is assessed during the procedure.[290, 304, 305] Some investigators have found the use of 18- or 19-gauge needles as opposed to 22 gauge to be associated with a greater diagnostic yield without an increase in complications.[300, 307] The addition of ultrasound guidance may be useful for sampling smaller lymph nodes or for more precise identification of nodes in institutions in which immediate evaluation of the adequacy of the sample is not available.[308, 308a]

Intraoperative Needle Aspiration

Fine-needle aspiration is used by some surgeons to make a definitive diagnosis of malignancy during thoracotomy or mediastinoscopy in patients in whom the diagnosis of cancer has not been established preoperatively. Diagnostic accuracy ranges from 95% to 100%, and smears prepared at the operating table can be stained and interpreted within 10 minutes.[309–312] Some investigators have also used touch

imprints of mediastinal lymph nodes sampled at the time of thoracotomy.[313]

Aspiration from Intravascular Catheters

Cells and tissue fragments can also be aspirated from blood obtained via a wedged Swan-Ganz catheter ("microvascular pulmonary cytology").[314] Although the reliability of the technique has been questioned,[315] it has been used in the diagnosis of pulmonary fat, tumor and amniotic fluid embolism, and lymphangitic carcinoma.[314, 316, 317]

EXAMINATION OF EXCISED LOBES AND WHOLE LUNGS

Pulmonary lobes that have been surgically excised or whole lungs that have been removed either surgically or at autopsy can be examined by a variety of techniques. To some extent, the method of examination depends on the suspected nature of the underlying disease: for example, injection of the pulmonary artery with contrast medium might be the procedure of choice in a case of suspected arteriovenous fistula, and incineration of lung tissue and analysis of the residue may be desirable in the presence of pneumoconiosis. However, these special techniques are impractical and unnecessary as a routine, and in the great majority of cases the most appropriate method of investigation is inflation and fixation of the lung with formalin, followed by serial slicing.

The easiest and most widely used method of fixation is to distend the lung to apparent full inflation by introducing formalin into the bronchi under positive pressure. This fixation method is conveniently performed by elevating a container above the lung, the most suitable maximal pressure head ranging from 25 to 50 cm of formalin; a smaller pressure head can be obtained by raising the lung in relation to the fluid level in the reservoir. A full head of pressure may be required to inflate the lungs of patients who died in status asthmaticus, with lower pressures used for lungs of older patients and those suspected of having emphysema.

After inflation, the most proximal airways are clamped and the lung or lobe left for a period of time in a large vat of formalin. Although the tissue may be firm enough to be adequately cut after only 2 to 3 hours, specimens are best left overnight and examined the following day. After examination of the pleural surface, the specimen should be cut with a sharp knife in even sections 1 to 1.5 cm thick. Sectioning may be performed in any plane, but we find the sagittal orientation most convenient for general use since it exposes a relatively large area of tissue per cut; however, in some circumstances, transverse cuts are desirable for correlation with CT images. The cut slices can be rinsed in running water to remove formalin and then laid out on a board for detailed examination. In addition to systematic inspection of the parenchyma, airways, vessels, and lymph nodes, palpation of grossly unremarkable areas should be performed to identify the occasional abnormality that is not apparent visually.

Examination of a slice under the dissecting microscope may reveal abnormalities in greater detail than can be achieved with the naked eye; although uncommonly performed, this practice can be helpful in the assessment of emphysema, particularly following impregnation of the slices with barium and immersion in water.[318] In exceptional cases, ultrathin, whole-lung sections may be cut and mounted on paper to better observe the extent and severity of disease and to preserve specimens (Fig. 14–2);[319] this procedure is most useful in emphysema and pneumoconiosis. A rapid method of preparing these sections has been described,[320] as well as a modified technique for the study of normal and diseased pulmonary arteries.[321]

Although we believe slicing after formalin instillation and fixation is the most valuable method for examining lungs or lobes, the technique can be criticized on several points.

1. Overinflation may lead to artefactual distortion of lung architecture. After removal from the body, the lung's expansion is no longer limited by the chest wall, so *in vitro* inflation to maximal capacity can theoretically produce volumes larger than existed *in vivo*. However, it has been established that lung volumes at apparent full inflation are similar to predicted total lung capacity,[322] which implies that lung size is limited to some extent by the pleura. Thus the potential deleterious effects of overinflation do not appear to pose a significant problem.

2. When a lung is distended and left without a constant head of pressure, it diminishes 20% to 30% in volume, even when the bronchus is clamped. The greater part of this decrease in volume occurs in the first few hours after inflation, and it is largely complete within 12 hours. Some of it

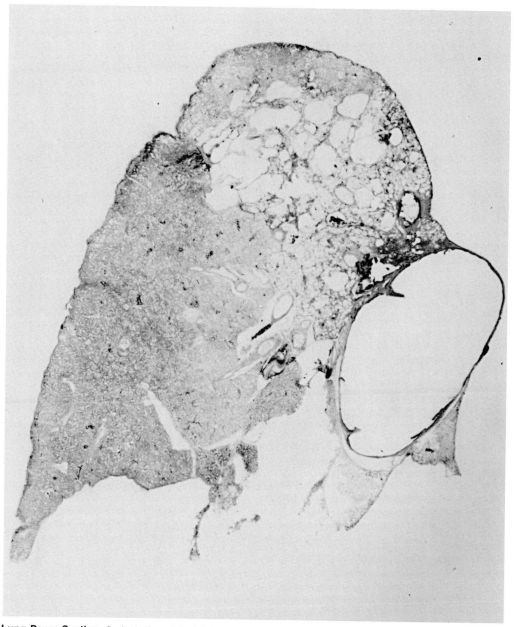

Figure 14–2. Lung Paper Section. Sagittal slice of the left lung taken near the hilum and reproduced at actual size. The slice measures about 100 μm in thickness and was obtained by cutting a whole lung on a specially designed giant microtome (commercial bacon slicers have also been used for the same purpose). The ultrathin slice was floated on a water bath and mounted on paper. Centrilobular emphysema is easily seen in the upper lobe and a large bulla is evident in the lingula.

is the result of leakage through pleural tears, but decreased volume also occurs in "airtight" lungs, presumably from tissue shrinkage and through diffusion of gas and fixative. Although not a significant factor for routine diagnosis, this volume loss can be minimized if necessary by the use of constant pressure during fixation.[323]

3. It is not possible to take fresh lung tissue for special studies once the lung has been fixed. One of the more obvious circumstances in which fresh lung tissue may be important is pulmonary infection, in which culture may be the definitive diagnostic method. Thus in surgically excised specimens in which a preoperative diagnosis has not been made, it is mandatory that appropriate swabs and/or portions of abnormal tissue be taken for culture before fixation. The same applies to lungs removed at postmortem examination from patients with suspected pneumonia, especially when the host is immunocompromised or may have an unusual pulmonary disease. Similar provisos hold in some situations for the procurement of fresh tissue for immunohistochemical analysis (e.g., in cases of pulmonary lymphoma), electron microscopy, flow cytometry, and molecular biologic procedures. In most cases in which fresh tissue is taken, the pleural incision used to obtain the appropriate tissue can be sutured or clamped and the lung subsequently inflated and fixed sufficiently for proper examination.

4. It is more difficult to examine pulmonary arteries and bronchi in fixed, sliced specimens than in fresh lungs in which these structures have been opened continuously along their walls. The latter technique has its own deficiencies related to transection of the airways and vessels themselves; however, a technique has been described by which artefacts associated with such cutting can be limited.[323a] Nevertheless, appropriate examination of the vasculature and bronchi in fixed lungs can usually be performed by careful inspection and comparison of each slice with its neighbor.

5. Pulmonary edema may be difficult to recognize histologically in fixed inflated specimens as a result of the flooding of air spaces by formalin. However, the diagnosis can also be made with a reasonable degree of confidence in whole lungs by documenting an increase in lung weight unassociated with significant air-space disease (other than edema) histologically. When the diagnosis is suspected, a small portion of lung can also be excised and the incision clamped before inflation of the entire specimen.

6. Postmortem radiographs for radiologic-pathologic correlation are not possible or are of poor quality once the lung is filled with fixative.

Despite these potential disadvantages, we believe that the identification and anatomic localization of many abnormalities can be much better appreciated in distended, fixed lung slices than in the distorted, limp tissue of uninflated, unfixed lung. In addition, appreciation of the nature and extent of disease microscopically is usually superior in the former situation (Fig. 14–3). Thus we believe that the advantages of this technique far outweigh the disadvantages and recommend that simple distention by liquid formalin be the routine procedure for examination of all lungs, whether of autopsy or surgical origin.

Several additional techniques have been proposed to obtain specimens suitable for special investigations such as morphometric analysis and radiologic-pathologic correlation.

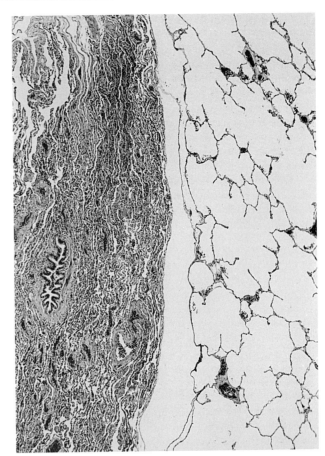

Figure 14–3. Effect of Formalin Inflation on Appreciation of Lung Structure. The pulmonary tissue on one side of an interlobular septum was not fixed by formalin inflation and is thus almost totally atelectatic, making interpretation of any disease that might be present very difficult. By contrast, the structure of the adjacent parenchyma, which had been adequately inflated with formalin, is clearly evident. (×40.)

Some researchers have advocated inflation and fixation by formaldehyde gas rather than fluid.[324–327] This technique results in specimens that are said to be ideal for demonstration purposes and for the study of three-dimensional morphology;[324] in addition, excellent radiologic-pathologic correlation can be achieved.[325, 326] However, depending to some extent on the temperature of the formaldehyde vapor as well as the severity of parenchymal disease, the tissue may be inadequately fixed and the histology poor.[327] Inflation by formalin steam does not dehydrate the lungs as rapidly as gas alone, and preservation for histologic studies is said to be much better.[327, 328]

Some workers have also suggested using a combination of liquid inflation-fixation and air-drying.[329–331] In this technique, a mixture of formalin, polyethylene glycol, and alcohol is insufflated into the bronchi; after fixation (about 48 hours), the lung is dried by blowing air through the bronchus at a constant pressure of about 20 mm Hg. Use of these techniques results in adequately preserved specimens from which excellent gross and histologic correlation with radiologic abnormalities can be obtained (Fig. 14–4).[332–336] (A modified method in which the lung is first fixed by formalin and then insufflated with polyethylene glycol has been said to result in even better histologic detail.[331])

Radiologic-pathologic correlation has also been attempted by postmortem radiography. The appearance of the chest radiograph when using this technique is similar to that taken antemortem during quiet breathing or at expiration.[337] However, since it is desirable to use special halters to suspend the body in a vertical position, the procedure has seldom been used.

SPECIAL PATHOLOGIC TECHNIQUES

Examination of the Pulmonary Vasculature and Airways

Several substances have been used for morphologic investigation of the pulmonary vasculature. One of the most satisfactory is the Schlesinger mass,[338] the basic ingredient of which is gelatin, which is kept liquid at room temperature by potassium iodide and solidifies upon the addition of formalin. Barium sulfate or other radiopaque material can be added to obtain radiographic visibility (Fig. 14–5), and dyes can be used to enable identification of different components of the vasculature both grossly and microscopically. A technique enabling radiographic visualization of the bronchial arteries of lungs post mortem has also been described.[339]

Specimen bronchography can be performed by using either the Schlesinger mass or fine-particle barium or lead insufflated into the bronchial tree. Casts of the pulmonary vasculature or bronchial tree have been made with several materials, including wax, celluloid,[340] vinyl, polyester and styrene polymer resins,[340–342] and silicone rubber.[343] An especially effective representation of the pulmonary and bronchial vascular systems and the airways can be accomplished by injection of Batson's solution of varying colors;[344] after the selected material has hardened, the surrounding lung is digested in acid to leave permanent casts of the injected structure. In addition to gross visual inspection, the casts can be examined by scanning electron microscopy to reveal the fine structure of the airways or vessels. A method of preparing a hollow cast of the bronchial tree has also been described.[345]

Lung Culture

Although many microorganisms can be appreciated in tissue sections or cytologic preparations through the use of routine histochemical stains, immunochemical techniques, or PCR, it is clear that culture is desirable and often essential for definitive identification and typing. Thus samples should be taken for culture under sterile conditions at the time that tissue fragments, respiratory tract secretions, or pleural fluid specimens are acquired in any patient who might have an infection.

Although postmortem lung cultures should also be taken in the appropriate circumstances, their results must be assessed with caution. There are two major problems in the interpretation of such results: (1) the high incidence of positive cultures in the absence of clinical or pathologic evidence of true infection;[346–348] and (2) the poor correlation in some studies between antemortem and postmortem culture results[349] and between pulmonary histology and culture re-

sults.[349] Reasons for the high percentage of positive cultures obtained in the absence of apparent infection include inadequacy of sterile technique during procurement of the culture, the presence of commensal organisms in patients with chronic diseases such as cystic fibrosis, and perimortem aspiration of oropharyngeal secretions.

The most meaningful postmortem culture results are obtained with the following procedures:[350] (1) cultures should be taken under sterile conditions immediately after the thorax has been entered and before the large vessels and the gastrointestinal tract have been incised; (2) the pleural surface of a palpably or visibly abnormal area of lung should be seared with a hot spatula or soldering iron; the seared area should then be incised with a scalpel and the underlying parenchyma either swabbed or cut into a small tissue fragment with sterile instruments; and (3) the lung parenchyma adjacent to the cultured area should be sectioned and fixed for histologic examination.

Confidence in the clinicopathologic significance of a positive culture requires the presence of at least some of the following: (1) absence of organisms normally considered skin or oropharyngeal commensals such as *Staphylococcus epidermidis*; (2) the presence of a pure culture of one organism in more than one site, either in lung and blood or in two different foci in the same or both lungs; (3) the presence of histologic evidence of infection in the tissue adjacent to that yielding the positive culture (inflammation, with or without the presence of organisms demonstrated with Gram or other stains); and (4) a heavy growth of organisms. To the extent that these features are not present, the relevance of a positive culture must be questioned.

There is evidence that quantitative determination of bacterial growth may be helpful in determining which postmortem cultures are significant. In one study of 50 lungs, histologic evidence of pneumonia or bronchitis was felt to be present in 18.[351] Of these 18 lungs, culture of the adjacent lung parenchyma grew greater than 10^5 organisms per milliliter of tissue in all but 1 instance; although 21 of the lungs without histologic evidence of infection also had positive cultures, in only 3 were the counts greater than 10^5 per milliliter. A technique involving culture from imprints derived from fresh[352] or microtome sections of frozen lung[353] has also been said to yield reliable results.

Electron Microscopy

It is usually unnecessary to examine pulmonary, pleural, or mediastinal tissue by electron microscopy for diagnostic purposes, the application of this technique in lung disease being primarily in research. Nevertheless, it is helpful in some instances and indispensable in others in establishing a precise diagnosis.[216, 354, 355, 355a]

Transmission Electron Microscopy

In transmission electron microscopy (TEM), an electron beam is focused on an ultrathin section of tissue and an image produced by collecting the transmitted electrons on a screen or photographic plate. Because of the necessity for a small tissue specimen (usually on the order of 0.25 × 0.25 mm in the final prepared state), one of the major limitations

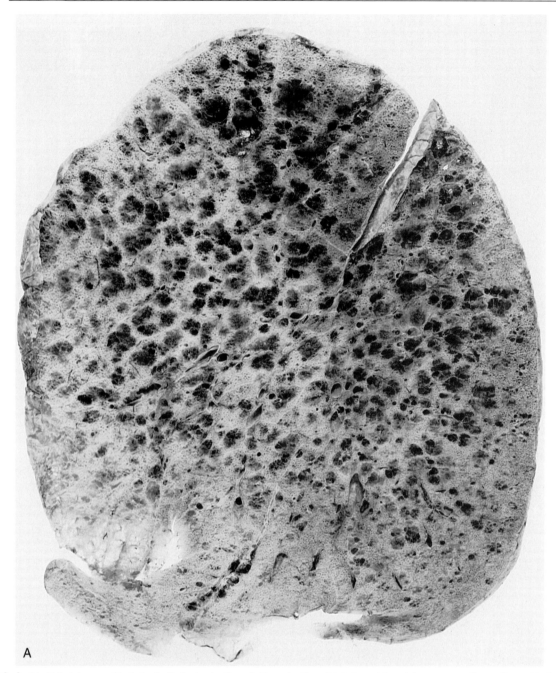

Figure 14–4. Air-Dried Lung—Radiologic-Pathologic Correlation. A slice of left lung *(A)* and its corresponding radiographic image *(B)* are illustrated. A moderate degree of centrilobular emphysema is evident as patchy, relatively well demarcated parenchymal spaces (highlighted by black [anthracotic] pigment on the gross specimen). The lung was fixed for 48 hours with a mixture of formalin, polyethylene glycol, and alcohol. It was then dried by air insufflation at a constant pressure of about 20 mm Hg for 48 hours.

of the technique is related to sampling, diagnostic conclusions being considered reliable only when the tissue examined is clearly representative of the disease process. Careful handling and fixation of tissue are also essential since autolysis rapidly results in ultrastructural changes that can obscure proper interpretation, especially in diseased lungs.[356] A convenient and adequate fixative is a cold-buffered mixture of 4% formaldehyde and 1% glutaraldehyde, although a buffered solution of either alone may be adequate for initial fixation. Tissue fragments should be small (about 1 mm³) to allow for adequate fixative penetration. Specimens obtained

via bronchoscopy, thoracoscopy, or TTNA can be placed directly in fixative by the endoscopist or aspirator; open-lung biopsy specimens should be referred immediately to a pathologist who can appropriately sample and mince the tissue. Fluid aspirated from the pleural space can be centrifuged and the resulting pellet fixed and processed for TEM; preservation of ultrastructural detail in this instance has been reported to be adequate even after a delay in fixation.[357]

Although generally not as adequate for interpretation as biopsy material, tissue obtained at autopsy can also be used, and several techniques have been advocated to obviate post-

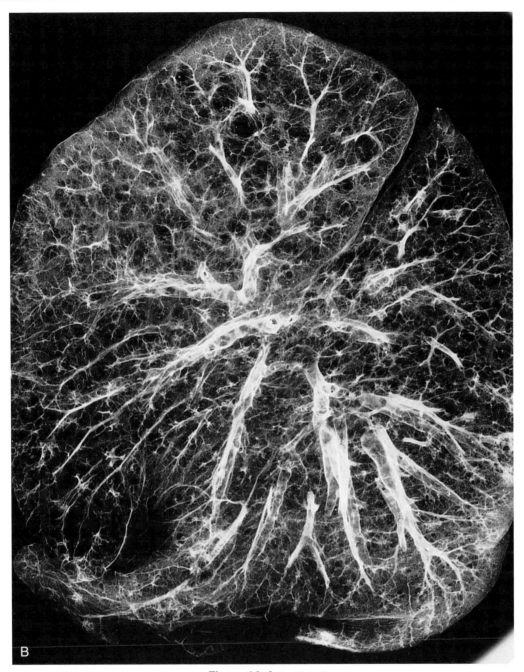

Figure 14–4 *Continued*

mortem autolysis. Some pathologists have performed "immediate autopsies" within 3 to 5 minutes of death; however, although the procedure results in adequate tissue preservation, this practice is impractical in most situations.[358] One group of investigators injected glutaraldehyde into the lung percutaneously within 30 minutes of death, the glutaraldehyde being mixed with a dye to localize the injected region upon evisceration;[356] although useful for examining normal lungs or diffuse lung disease, this technique is less helpful for focal abnormalities, in which precise localization of the areas to inject may be difficult. Tracheobronchial tissue obtained up to 5 hours post mortem and placed in Krebs-Henseleit solution perfused with oxygen and carbon dioxide may be remarkably well preserved.[359] Samples for TEM can

also be retrieved from paraffin-embedded tissue or from cut and stained sections on glass slides. Although in these circumstances cellular details are usually obscured, structures such as neurosecretory granules or viral particles may be sufficiently well preserved to help establish a diagnosis.[360]

Only a brief review of some of the diagnostic applications of TEM will be given here. Although the identity of the etiologic agent in pneumonia is determined most reliably by culture or immunohistochemical analysis and less often by light microscopy, ultrastructural examination will occasionally establish the presence of an organism and may indicate the specific type, particularly in the case of viral infections, in which the characteristics of size and morphology enable precise characterization of some species. Preser-

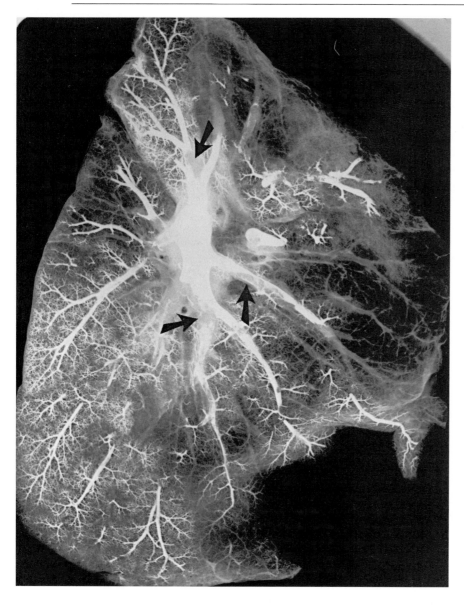

Figure 14–5. Postmortem Pulmonary Angiogram. A radiograph of a 1-cm-thick slice of the left lung shows multiple filling defects *(arrows)* in the proximal vessels corresponding to thromboemboli; the small vessels are normal (although some have failed to opacify). The specimen was injected via the pulmonary artery with a barium gelatin mixture, fixed with an ethylene glycol-alcohol solution, and air-dried.

vation of viral particles is usually good, and tissue or cells obtained from blocks or even slides years after fixation have been found to harbor recognizable virions.[360, 361] TEM is essential for diagnosis and characterization of the dyskinetic cilia syndrome,[362] since the basic abnormality cannot be accurately determined by other means.

Although not usually essential, electron microscopic findings are sufficiently characteristic to help confirm the diagnosis of a variety of metabolic abnormalities, including amyloidosis, alveolar proteinosis, and some storage diseases.[363] Intracytoplasmic Birbeck granules are characteristic of the Langerhans' cells of Langerhans' cell histiocytosis, and their identification may help confirm the diagnosis (Fig. 14–6); although identification of these granules is not usually necessary in specimens obtained by open or transbronchial biopsy, analysis of cells obtained by BAL may obviate the need for such an invasive procedure.[364, 365] TEM examination of the lungs, unlike that of the kidneys, is usually unrewarding in immunologic disease of presumed immune complex origin; only rarely have basement membrane–dense deposits consistent with such complexes been identified.[366]

Of more widespread use is the application of TEM to the diagnosis of pulmonary neoplasms in both biopsy and cytologic specimens.[367] Occasionally, it is the definitive diagnostic technique in tracheobronchial gland carcinomas[368, 369] and other uncommon neoplasms.[370, 371] Although largely supplanted by immunohistochemical analysis, the identification of neurosecretory granules may aid in the diagnosis of small cell carcinoma and carcinoid tumor in selected cases, especially when only small amounts of tissue are available from transbronchial biopsy or TTNA. Classification of pulmonary sarcoma is often aided by ultrastructural findings, and most neoplasms with a sarcomatous appearance should be examined in this fashion (in conjunction with immunohistochemical techniques) before a specific diagnosis is applied. In pleural effusions, TEM is useful in differentiating mesothelioma from metastatic carcinoma[164, 372] and, occasionally, in distinguishing primary from metastatic lung carcinoma.[165]

Scanning Electron Microscopy

In scanning electron microscopy (SEM), an electron beam sweeps over and interacts with the surface of the

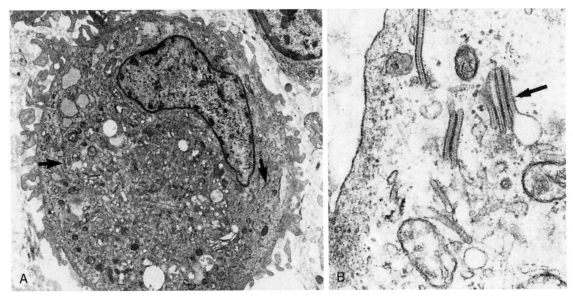

Figure 14–6. Langerhans' Cell Histiocytosis—Transmission Electron Microscopy. *A,* This TEM section shows a cell with numerous microvilli and cytoplasmic granules suggestive of a macrophage. Higher magnification of regions indicated by *arrows (B)* showed tubular structures composed of thin parallel membranes surrounding finely granular material (Birbeck granules). The presence of these structures identifies the cell as a Langerhans' cell; the finding of a large number of such cells in bronchoalveolar lavage fluid supports a diagnosis of Langerhans' cell histiocytosis. (A, ×1000; B, ×50,650.)

specimen, thereby resulting in several forms of secondary radiation;[373–376] depending on the nature of the radiation and the means used to image it, important characteristics of a specimen can be revealed. SEM is not encumbered by the two major problems encountered with tissue used for TEM. Tissue preservation is not as critical since fine ultrastructural detail is not observed, so formalin-fixed, paraffin-embedded material is adequate. In addition, substantially larger tissue sections can be examined, which makes the problem of sampling considerably less important. Techniques have been described for examining cells obtained from bronchial secretions and pleural fluid by both light microscopy and SEM.[377–380]

SEM images are produced when secondary electrons are collected and amplified to obtain a detailed three-dimensional representation of the surface morphology of an object (Fig. 14–7). Although undoubtedly beautiful and of value in understanding the pathogenesis and morphology of pulmonary disease, such images are not usually helpful in establishing a diagnosis. However, some investigators have suggested that they can be of value in differentiating benign, atypical, and malignant cells in pleural effusions.[381–383]

Of far greater importance in diagnosis are other forms of emitted radiation. Backscattered electrons are emitted in numbers proportional to the atomic number of the material from which they emanate. Since most foreign substances have an atomic number greater than that of carbon, they cause a brighter image than does surrounding tissue, and the technique is thus useful in identifying such substances in very small amounts (up to 50 nm in diameter).[373, 384] In addition, x-rays emitted from an object can be examined by wavelength or energy dispersion spectrometry to provide a precise analysis of the elemental composition of the portion of the sample examined. The primary use of SEM is thus in the study of pneumoconiosis, in which particulate material can be identified and its composition analyzed precisely. Since the different images can be correlated, the technique

can provide accurate information about the location of specific particulates within cells or tissue. Although other techniques are available to identify the type and quantity of retained dust within the lung in cases of pneumoconiosis—including high-temperature ashing, microincineration, plasma ashing and etching, and wet-chemical or enzyme digestion[376, 385]—these techniques cannot provide information about the anatomic location of the dust.

Immunochemistry

The development of techniques for the immunochemical demonstration of tissue antigens has been one of the major advances in diagnostic pathology, and these techniques

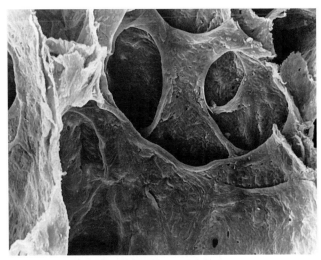

Figure 14–7. Scanning Electron Micrograph of Pulmonary Emphysema. The illustration shows lung parenchyma with a decreased number of alveolar septa and relatively large discontinuities in their walls.

are now indispensable in confirming or establishing a diagnosis in many situations. In pulmonary disease, immunochemical studies are usually performed on fresh or fixed tissue sections or on cytologic preparations obtained by needle aspiration.[386]

Immunofluorescence tests are performed by applying an antibody conjugated with fluorescein dye to a tissue section or cytologic preparation.[387] After washing, the material is examined with a fluorescent microscope to enable appreciation of the fluorescent antibody-antigen complex. In the lung, the technique is particularly useful in confirming a diagnosis of Goodpasture's syndrome;[388] it has also been used for identifying infectious organisms such as *Legionella* species[389] and subtypes of *Streptococcus pneumoniae*.[390] The potential for other uses is limited predominantly by the ingenuity of pulmonary researchers and by the development of specific antibodies;[387] for example, one group of investigators has reported high sensitivity and specificity of anti–angiotensin-converting enzyme antibody for the granulomas of sarcoidosis.[391]

Immunofluorescence tests have three major problems: (1) the necessity in most cases for using frozen tissue (ideally snap-frozen at $-70°$ C or less at the time of excision); (2) the difficulty in some instances of localizing the foci of positive immunofluorescence histologically; and (3) the natural fading of fluorescence in many cases, thereby resulting in the lack of a permanent tissue record. To overcome these difficulties, a variety of immunoenzymatic techniques have been developed that can be used on formalin-fixed paraffin-embedded tissue on which the application of an appropriate counterstain results in histologic details that are of sufficient clarity to locate regions of positive reactivity precisely. Methods have also been developed for use on cells exfoliated from the airways or aspirated from pleural fluid or parenchymal tumors.[386, 392–394]

Basically, immunoenzymatic techniques involve the conjugation of a diagnostic antibody with an enzyme (most frequently peroxidase), the application of this combination to a tissue section, and the addition of a substrate (such as diaminobenzidine in the case of peroxidase) that reacts with the enzyme to produce a visible compound. These techniques have been used in the study of immunologic lung disease, for the identification of microorganisms, and in the diagnosis of pulmonary, pleural, and mediastinal neoplasms.[395] A variety of antibodies have been developed in an attempt to characterize subtypes of pulmonary carcinoma more precisely and to distinguish neoplasms such as mesothelioma from metastatic adenocarcinoma or mediastinal lymphoma from thymoma. Other applications include distinguishing metastatic from primary pulmonary neoplasms, identifying bronchioloalveolar carcinoma, and precisely classifying pulmonary sarcomas.

Morphometry

Morphometry is concerned with the estimation of quantity or measurements such as diameter, volume, and thickness by counting points and line segments superimposed on a two-dimensional image.[396] In the lung, the latter is usually a standard hematoxylin and eosin–stained tissue section or a TEM photomicrograph. Although its application in the study

of normal lung was pioneered in 1963[397] and it has since been used extensively for this purpose and for the study of disease processes,[398, 399] the use of morphometry as a *diagnostic* procedure in pulmonary disease has been minimal. Its greatest application has been in developmental anomalies, in which it is of value in characterizing such conditions as pulmonary hypoplasia[400, 401] and neonatal lobar emphysema.[402, 403] Computer-generated morphometric analysis has also been investigated in the diagnosis of pleural effusions.[404]

Cytogenetics

The principal use of cytogenetic investigation in the diagnosis of chest disease is in relation to malignant pleural effusions;[159, 405] when combined with routine cytologic examination, diagnostic accuracy has been reported to be almost 85%.[406] In one investigation of 61 pleural effusions, numerical or structural chromosomal abnormalities were identified in 29 (85%) of the 34 malignant cases and none of those that were benign.[407] In another study of 10 effusions associated with mesothelioma, cytogenetic abnormalities, including deletions involving 1p, 3p, and 22q, were found in all samples;[408] standard cytologic examination was considered to be diagnostic of mesothelioma in 5 cases, suggestive of the disease in 4, and benign in 1.

Flow Cytometry

Flow cytometry is a technique that enables rapid and reliable quantification of various cellular characteristics, including cell size and shape. With respect to thoracic disease, it is used most often in the analysis of cell DNA content and proliferative activity; it can also be used for specific typing and quantification of lymphocyte subsets in the investigation of lymphoproliferative disorders and non-neoplastic immunologic disease. (Estimates of cellular DNA can also be made by using image analysis techniques in which an operator can select the cells to be quantitated by observing them on a monitor; since samples undergoing flow cytometry generally contain benign as well as malignant cells [e.g., inflammatory and connective tissue cells], this technique theoretically yields a more uniform cell population for analysis.)

The substrate material may be tissue fragments, free cells in fluid (such as pleural effusion) or pulmonary secretions (such as bronchial washings), or TTNA specimens. Fresh (unfixed or fast-frozen) tissue is necessary for lymphocyte subset analysis and is preferable for DNA determination; however, formalin-fixed, paraffin-embedded material may also be used for the latter purpose. Areas of hemorrhage, necrosis, and fibrosis should be minimized to reduce background noise. In the laboratory, the tissue fragment is mechanically or enzymatically dissociated to form a cell suspension. The cells are incubated with various substances to remove cell membranes and cytoplasm, and the free nuclei are incubated with a fluorescent dye such as propidium iodide, which attaches to DNA; other substances such as the tumor markers p53 and c-myc can also be labeled with specific antibodies.[409] The cells are then forced under pressure through a flow chamber into a single file that is exposed to a monochromatic light source such as produced by an argon laser. Lenses collect the light emitted from the passing cells on a photomultiplier tube; the resulting electrical signals are converted to digital form, which can be displayed in a variety of ways, most often as a histogram (Fig. 14–8).

Since the amount of DNA in the nucleus varies with the normal cell cycle, flow cytometric measurements can give an idea of the proliferative activity of the cells within a specific sample. The normal cell cycle can be divided into resting (G_0) and presynthetic (G_1) phases characterized by a diploid (2N) amount of DNA, into postsynthetic (G_2) and mitotic (M) phases with a tetraploid (4N) value, and into an intermediate synthetic (S) phase. Since malignant neoplasms are often composed of aneuploid cells (i.e., cells that are not diploid), determination of the type and degree of aneuploidy can theoretically aid in the distinction between a benign and a malignant process. For example, in one study of bronchial washings from 73 patients, flow cytometric analysis had a sensitivity and specificity for the detection of carcinoma similar to that of routine cytology.[409a] Others have found the combination of flow cytometry and cytology to increase diagnostic sensitivity.[409b]

Ploidy determination has also been used in an effort to predict prognosis and response to therapy. The proliferative index is related to the proportion of cells in the synthetic phase; it can be calculated from the data represented on the histogram and has also been used in assessing tumor prognosis. Many flow cytometric investigations have been performed on pulmonary, pleural, and mediastinal neoplasms in an attempt to document the usefulness of flow cytometry in predicting tumor behavior. Most pulmonary carcinomas are aneuploid, the reported incidence ranging from about 45% to 95%;[410–413] overall, the best estimate is probably about 70%. Multiple aneuploid populations are not uncommon,[411, 412] perhaps corresponding to the heterogeneity that is frequently observed histologically. Although some investigators have documented a significant association between the presence of aneuploidy and regional lymph node metastases,[414, 415]

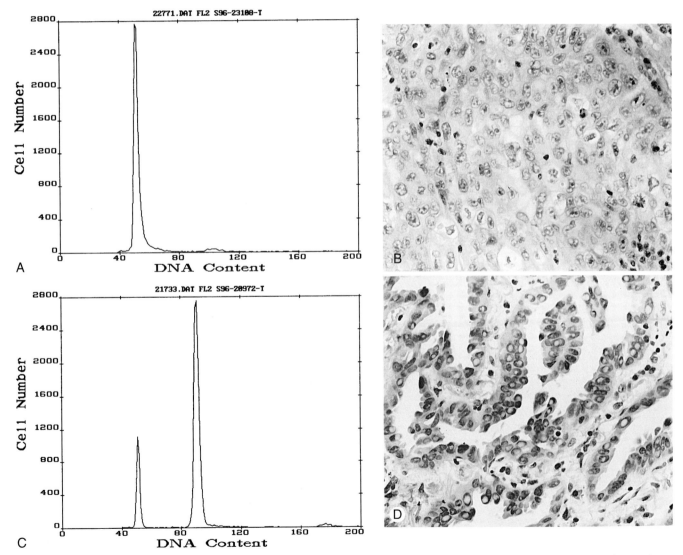

Figure 14–8. Pulmonary Carcinoma—Flow Cytometric Analysis. Plots of DNA content versus cell number for two pulmonary carcinomas show an essentially diploid population in *A* (corresponding to the large cell carcinoma illustrated in *C*) and a clearly aneuploid population in *B* (corresponding to the bronchioloalveolar carcinoma in *D*). Note that the histologically better differentiated tumor in these two examples is associated with the poorer cytometric data.

most have found no consistent association between aneuploidy and tumor stage.[410, 411, 416–419] The majority (albeit not all[413, 420]) have also found a significantly better prognosis for diploid than for aneuploid non–small cell carcinomas (approximately 65% versus 40% survival rates over follow-up periods of 1 to more than 5 years);[410–412, 417–419, 421–423] although this survival advantage appears to be independent of stage (at least for Stages I to III), there is evidence that it is most closely associated with a squamous cell histologic subtype.[410, 421, 424, 425] Similar prognostic results have been documented by some investigators for the proliferative index, those with a relatively low index surviving longer.[423]

As might be expected, aneuploidy has generally been found to be more common in small cell carcinoma than in atypical or typical carcinoid tumors (the numbers for the three tumors being approximately 90%, 60%, and 30%, respectively).[416, 426–428] Some (albeit not all[424]) investigators have demonstrated better survival with diploid than with aneuploid tumors.[428] (The use and results of flow cytometry in the diagnosis of cancer in pleural fluid specimens are discussed on page 2816.)

As indicated previously, quantification of lymphocyte and macrophage subsets also has important applications in pulmonary disease. For this purpose, cells are identified and sorted according to the presence of various antibodies conjugated to a fluorescent dye such as fluorescein isothiocyanate. The procedure is somewhat different from DNA assessment, since viable cells need to be examined (dead cells take up antibodies nonspecifically). As a result, the technique is particularly useful in the analysis of BAL fluid;[429, 430] however, appropriately handled lung biopsy and TTNA specimens can also be analyzed.[430a] The technique has been employed most often in the evaluation of lymphoproliferative disorders. For example, the finding of BAL lymphocytosis characterized by a high percentage of B cells that show light chain restriction (i.e., a predominance of either κ or λ surface light chain) is highly suggestive of low-grade B-cell lymphoma.[431] Other potential applications of flow cytometric analysis of BAL fluid include the assessment of Ia-positive T lymphocytes as a prognostic indicator in sarcoidosis,[432] asbestosis,[432a] and idiopathic pulmonary fibrosis; assessment of CD4/CD8 ratios in the investigation of acute rejection, infection, and obliterative bronchiolitis in patients with lung transplants;[433, 434] and investigation of macrophage subtypes in patients with AIDS,[435] tuberculosis,[436] or pulmonary carcinoma.[437]

Assessment of blood lymphocyte types is also of proven or potential value in some forms of pulmonary disease. The best example is probably the determination of CD4/CD8 (helper/suppressor) T-cell ratios in patients with AIDS. However, there is also evidence that the helper/suppressor ratio

may be related to prognosis in patients with small cell carcinoma.[438]

Molecular Biology

The field of molecular biology is undergoing rapid development, and its use is likely to be invaluable in diagnosis and the assessment of prognosis of some forms of pleural, pulmonary, and mediastinal disease. Three areas of current application are immunohistochemical identification of genetic markers of carcinoma, establishment of a diagnosis of lymphoma by gene rearrangement studies, and identification of pathogenic organisms or neoplastic cells by PCR.

Several genes, including K-*ras*, *p53*, *her2/neu*, and *myc*, are involved in the control of growth and differentiation of both normal and malignant cells. Identification of these genes in cells from BAL or sputum specimens or tissue sections by immunohistochemical or other techniques may be useful in detecting early pulmonary carcinoma or in predicting the prognosis of low-stage tumors.[439, 440] A variety of recombinant DNA techniques can be used to identify rearrangements of genes that encode for B-cell immunoglobulins or T-cell surface antigens. In this fashion, the clonality of a lymphoid population can be established, monoclonality being considered a strong indicator of malignancy. The procedure has been used on pulmonary tissue fragments, pleural fluid, and BAL fluid.[441–443]

PCR is a process that enables the identification of minute amounts of a specific DNA or RNA sequence through enzymatic amplification by DNA polymerase. The procedure uses two oligonucleotide primers complementary to a portion of a DNA or RNA sequence that is characteristic of the target to be identified (the template). (For RNA, the sample is first subjected to reverse transcription so that complementary DNA is obtained.) The DNA in the sample is denatured by heating, and the sample is then incubated with the primers, which anneal to the template during cooling. DNA polymerase (which is included in the reaction mixture) acts to extend the complementary areas; repeated cycles of denaturation, annealing, and extension lead to massive amplification of the number of complementary copies, which can then be detected on an agarose gel.

The procedure can be applied to fluids (e.g., pleural effusion, BAL, or gastric aspirate), sputum, bronchial brushings, and fresh or paraffin-embedded tissue fragments. In pulmonary disease, it has been most widely used in the identification of infectious organisms, principally *Mycobacterium tuberculosis* (*see* page 845),[444–446] but also organisms such as *Mycoplasma pneumoniae*,[447] *P. carinii*,[448] cytomegalovirus,[449] and *Aspergillus* species.[102] Because some tumors have fairly consistent genetic abnormalities, the possibility of identifying minute amounts in fluid or fine-needle aspiration specimens is also theoretically possible.[450]

REFERENCES

1. Young JA: Techniques in pulmonary cytopathology. J Clin Pathol 46:589, 1993.
2. Chalon J, Tang CK, Klein GS, et al: Routine cytodiagnosis of pulmonary malignancies. Arch Pathol Lab Med 105:11, 1981.
3. Ahlbom G, Winslov J: Outpatient sputum cytology in the diagnosis of lung cancer. Scand J Respir Dis 58:227, 1977.
4. Ng ABP, Horak GC: Factors significant in the diagnostic accuracy of lung cytology in bronchial washing and sputum samples. II. Sputum samples. Acta Cytol 27:397, 1983.
5. Böcking A, Biesterfeld S, Chatelain R, et al: Diagnosis of bronchial carcinoma on sections of paraffin-embedded sputum. Sensitivity and specificity of an alternative to routine cytology. Acta Cytol 36:37, 1992.
6. Olsen CR, Froeb HF, Palmer LA: Sputum cytology after inhalation of heated propylene glycol: A clinical correlation. JAMA 178:668, 1961.
7. Kim BM, Froeb HF, Palmer L, et al: Clinical experience with cytologic examination of sputum obtained by heated aerosols. Am Rev Respir Dis 87:836, 1963.
8. Umiker WO: A new vista in pulmonary cytology: Aerosol induction of sputum. Dis Chest 39:512, 1961.
9. Fontana RS, Carr DT, Woolner LB, et al: An evaluation of methods of inducing sputum production in patients with suspected cancer of the lung. Proc Mayo Clin 37:113, 1962.
10. Allan WB, Whittlesey P: The results of the experimental use of sulfur dioxide in the production of material for cell studies in lung cancer. Ann Intern Med 52:326, 1980.
11. Bender BL, Cherock M-A, Sotos SN: Effective use of bronchoscopy and sputa in the diagnosis of lung cancer. Diagn Cytopathol 1:183, 1985.
12. Russell WO, Neidhardt HW, Mountain CF, et al: Cytodiagnosis of lung cancer. A report of a four-year laboratory, clinical, and statistical study with a review of the literature on lung cancer and pulmonary cytology. Acta Cytol 7:1, 1963.
13. Chang JP, Anken M, Russell WO: Liquefaction and membrane filtration of sputum for the diagnosis of cancer. Am J Clin Pathol 37:584, 1962.
14. McCarty SA: Solving the cytopreparation problem of mucoid specimens with a mucoliquefying agent (Mucolexx) and nucleopore filters. Acta Cytol 16:221, 1972.
15. Liu W: Concentration and fractionation of cytologic elements in sputum. Acta Cytol 10:368, 1966.
16. Pharr SL, Farber SM: Cellular concentration of sputum and bronchial aspirations by tryptic digestion. Acta Cytol 6:447, 1962.
17. Bonime RG: Improved procedure for the preparation of pulmonary cytology smears. Acta Cytol 16:543, 1972.
18. Taplin DJ: Malignant cells in sputum: A simple method of liquefying sputum. J Med Lab Technol 23:252, 1966.
19. Tang C-S, Kung ITM: Homogenization of sputum with dithiothreitol for early diagnosis of pulmonary malignancies. Acta Cytol 37:689, 1993.
20. Tang C-S, Tang CMC, Kung ITM: Dithiothreitol homogenization of prefixed sputum for lung cancer detection. Diagn Cytopathol 10:76, 1994.
21. Hees K, Lebeau PB: Comparison of conventional and thinprep preparations of mucoid cytology samples. Diagn Cytopathol 12:181, 1995.
22. Saccomanno G, Saunders RP, Ellis H, et al: Concentration of carcinoma or atypical cells in sputum. Acta Cytol 7:305, 1963.
23. Ellis HD, Kernosky JJ: Efficiency of concentrating malignant cells in sputum. Acta Cytol 7:372, 1963.
24. Perlman EJ, Erozan YS, Howdon A: The role of the Saccomanno technique in sputum cytopathologic diagnosis of lung cancer. Am J Clin Pathol 91:57, 1989.
25. Gledhill A, Bates C, Henderson D, et al: Sputum cytology: A limited role. J Clin Pathol 50:566, 1997.
25a. Goldberg-Kahn B, Healy JC, Bishop JW: The cost of diagnosis: A comparison of four different strategies in the workup of solitary radiographic lung lesions. Chest 111:870, 1997.
26. Rizzo T, Schumann GB, Riding JM: Comparison of the pick and smear and Saccomanno methods for sputum cytologic analysis. Acta Cytol 34:875, 1990.
27. Abramson W, Dzenis V, Hicks S: Cytologic study of sputa and exudates using paraffin tubes. Acta Cytol 8:306, 1964.
28. Raab SS, Hornberger J, Raffin T: The importance of sputum cytology in the diagnosis of lung cancer: A cost-effectiveness analysis. Chest 112:937, 1997.
29. Johnston WW, Frable WJ: Diagnostic Respiratory Cytopathology. New York, Masson Publishing, 1979.
30. Smith MJ, Kini SR, Watson E: Fine needle aspiration and endoscopic brush cytology. Comparison of direct smears and rinsings. Acta Cytol 24:456, 1980.
31. Ahlqvist J: Fine needle aspiration and brush specimens. Simultaneous embedding in paraffin and enrichment. Acta Cytol 37:503, 1993.
32. Calabretto ML, Giol L, Sulfaro S: Diagnostic utility of cell-block from bronchial washing in pulmonary neoplasms. Diagn Cytopathol 15:191, 1996.
33. Flint A: Detection of pulmonary neoplasms by bronchial washings. Are cell blocks a diagnostic aid? Acta Cytol 37:21, 1993.
34. Bardales RH, Powers CN, Frierson HF Jr, et al: Exfoliative respiratory cytology in the diagnosis of leukemias and lymphomas in the lung. Diagn Cytopathol 14:108, 1996.
35. Johnston WW, Bossen EH: Ten years of respiratory cytopathology at Duke University Medical Center. 1. The cytopathologic diagnosis of lung cancer during the years 1970 to 1974, noting the significance of specimen number and type. Acta Cytol 24:103, 1980.
36. Rosa UW, Prolla JC, da Silva Gastal E: Cytology in diagnosis of cancer affecting the lung. Results in 1,000 consecutive patients. Chest 63:203, 1973.
37. Hartveit F: Time and place of sputum cytology in the diagnosis of lung cancer. Thorax 36:299, 1981.
38. Ng ABP, Horak GC: Factors significant in the diagnostic accuracy of lung cytology in bronchial washing and sputum samples. 1. Bronchial washings. Acta Cytol 27:391, 1983.
39. Risse EKJ, van't Hof MA, Laurini RN, et al: Sputum cytology by the Saccomanno method in diagnosing lung malignancy. Diagn Cytopathol 1:286, 1985.
40. Steffee CH, Segletes LA, Geisinger KR: Changing cytologic and histologic utilization patterns in the diagnosis of 515 primary lung malignancies. Cancer 81:105, 1997.
40a. Blumenfeld W, Singer M, Glanz S, et al: Fine-needle aspiration as the initial diagnostic modality in malignant lung disease. Diagn Cytopathol 14:268, 1996.
41. Muers MF, Boddington MM, Cole M, et al: Cytological sampling at fiberoptic bronchoscopy: Comparison of catheter aspirates and brush biopsies. Thorax 37:457, 1982.
42. Naryshkin S, Daniels J, Young NA: Diagnostic correlation of fiberoptic bronchoscopic biopsy and bronchoscopic cytology performed simultaneously. Diagn Cytopathol 8:119, 1992.
43. Matsuda M, Horai T, Nakamura S, et al: Bronchial brushing and bronchial biopsy: Comparison of diagnostic accuracy and cell typing reliability in lung cancer. Thorax 41:475, 1986.
44. Sato M, Saito Y, Nagamoto N, et al: Diagnostic value of differential brushing of all branches of the bronchi in patients with sputum positive or suspected positive for lung cancer. Acta Cytol 37:879, 1993.
45. Hinson KFW, Kuper SWA: The diagnosis of lung cancer by examination of sputum. Thorax 18:350, 1963.
46. Laurie W: Sputum cytology in the diagnosis of bronchial carcinoma. Med J Aust 1:205, 1966.
47. Naryshkin S, Young NA: Respiratory cytology: A review of non-neoplastic mimics of malignancy. Diagn Cytopathol 9:89, 1993.
48. Naryshkin S, Bedrossian CWM: Selected mimics of malignancy in sputum and bronchoscopic cytology specimens. Diagn Cytopathol 13:443, 1995.
49. Johnston WW: Type II pneumocytes in cytologic specimens. A diagnostic dilemma. Am J Clin Pathol 97:608, 1992.
50. Ritter JH, Wick MR, Reyes A, et al: False-positive interpretations of carcinoma in exfoliative respiratory cytology. Report of two cases and a review of underlying disorders. Am J Clin Pathol 104:133, 1995.
51. Johnston WW: Ten years of respiratory cytopathology at Duke University Medical Center. III. The significance of inconclusive cytopathologic diagnoses during the years 1970 to 1974. Acta Cytol 26:759, 1982.
52. Bewtra C, Dewan N, O'Donahue WJ Jr: Exfoliative sputum cytology in pulmonary embolism. Acta Cytol 27:489, 1983.
53. Scoggins WG, Smith RH, Frable WJ, et al: False-positive cytological diagnosis of lung carcinoma in patients with pulmonary infarcts. Ann Thorac Surg 24:474, 1977.
54. Öztek I, Baloglu H, Üskent N, et al: Chemotherapy- and radiotherapy-induced cytologic alterations in the sputum of patients with inoperable lung carcinoma. Role in follow-up. Acta Cytol 40:1265, 1996.
55. Koss LG, Melamed MR, Mayer K: The effect of busulfan on human epithelia. Am J Clin Pathol 44:385, 1965.
56. Schumann GB, Roby TJ, Swan GE, et al: Quantitive sputum cytologic findings in 109 nonsmokers. Am Rev Respir Dis 139:601, 1989.
57. Ng ABP, Horak GC: Factors significant in the diagnostic accuracy of lung cytology in bronchial washing and sputum samples. 1. Bronchial washings. Acta Cytol 27:391, 1983.
58. Clee MD, Sinclair DJM: Assessment of factors influencing the result of sputum cytology in bronchial carcinoma. Thorax 36:143, 1981.
59. Umiker WO: False-negative reports in the cytologic diagnosis of cancer of the lung. Am J Clin Pathol 28:37, 1957.
60. Broghamer WL, Richardson ME, Faurest S, et al: Cytologic negativity in the diagnosis of secondary pulmonary neoplasms. Diagn Cytopathol 1:85, 1985.
61. Rosenberg BF, Spjut HJ, Gedney MM: Exfoliative cytology in metastatic cancer of the lung. N Engl J Med 261:226, 1959.
62. Kern WH, Schweizer CW: Sputum cytology of metastatic carcinoma of the lung. Acta Cytol 20:514, 1976.
62a. Ali SZ, Kronz JD, Plowden KM, et al: Metastatic pulmonary leiomyosarcoma: Cytopathologic diagnosis on sputum examination. Diagn Cytopathol 18:280, 1998.
63. Johnston WW, Frable WJ: Cytopathology of the respiratory tract: A review. Am J Pathol 84:371, 1976.
64. Naib ZM, Stewart JA, Dowdle WR, et al: Cytological features of viral respiratory tract infections. Acta Cytol 12:162, 1968.
65. Chen KTK: Cytology of allergic bronchopulmonary aspergillosis. Diagn Cytopathol 9:82, 1993.
66. Anupindi L, Sahoo R, Rao RV, et al: Microfilariae in bronchial brushing cytology of symptomatic pulmonary lesions. A report of two cases. Acta Cytol 37:397, 1993.
67. Vercelli-Retta J, Mānana G, Reissenweber NJ: The cytologic diagnosis of hydatid disease. Acta Cytol 26:159, 1982.

68. Pitchenik AE, Ganjei P, Torres A, et al: Sputum examination for the diagnosis of *Pneumocystis carinii* pneumonia in the acquired immunodeficiency syndrome. Am Rev Respir Dis 133:226, 1986.

68a. Metersky ML, Aslenzadeh J, Stelmach P: A comparison of induced sputum and expectorated sputum for the diagnosis of *Pneumocystis carinii* pneumonia. Chest 113:1555, 1998.

69. Corwin RW, Irwin RS: The lipid-laden macrophage as a marker of aspiration in parenchymal lung disease. Am Rev Respir Dis 132:576, 1985.

70. Mimoz O, Edouard A, Beydon L, et al: Contribution of bronchoalveolar lavage to the diagnosis of posttraumatic pulmonary fat embolism. Intensive Care Med 21:973, 1995.

70a. Wheeler TM, Johnson EH, Coughlin D, et al: The sensitivity of detection of asbestos bodies in sputa and bronchial washings. Acta Cytol 32:647, 1988.

71. Shlaes DM, Lederman M, Chmielewski R, et al: Elastin fibers in the sputum of patients with necrotizing pneumonia. Chest 83:885, 1983.

72. Taskinen EI, Tukiainen PS, Alitalo RL, et al: Bronchoalveolar lavage. Cytological techniques and interpretation of the cellular profiles. *In* Rosen PP, Fechner RE (eds): Pathology Annual. Part 2. Vol 29. E Norwalk, CT, Appleton & Lange, 1994, pp 121–155.

73. Kvale PA: Bronchoscopic biopsies and bronchoalveolar lavage. Chest Surg Clin North Am 6:205, 1996.

74. Costabel U: Bronchoalveolar lavage: A standardized procedure or a technical dilemma? Eur Respir J 4:776, 1991.

75. Klech H, Pohl W: Technical recommendations and guidelines for bronchoalveolar lavage (BAL). Eur Respir J 2:561, 1989.

76. Reynolds HY: Bronchoalveolar lavage. Am Rev Respir Dis 135:250, 1987.

77. Chamberlain DW, Braude AC, Rebuck AS: A critical evaluation of bronchoalveolar lavage. Criteria for identifying unsatisfactory specimens. Acta Cytol 31:599, 1987.

78. Smith DL, Deshazo RD: Bronchoalveolar lavage in asthma. Am Rev Respir Dis 148:523, 1993.

79. Montravers P, Gauzit R, Dombret MC, et al. Cardiopulmonary effects of bronchoalveolar lavage in critically ill patients. Chest 104:1541, 1993.

80. Papazian L, Colt HG, Scemama F, et al: Effects of consecutive protected specimen brushing and bronchoalveolar lavage on gas exchange and hemodynamics in ventilated patients. Chest 104:1548, 1993.

81. Steinberg KP, Mitchell DR, Maunder RJ, et al: Safety of bronchoalveolar lavage in patients with adult respiratory distress syndrome. Am Rev Respir Dis 148:556, 1993.

82. Strumpf IJ, Feld MK, Cornelius MJ, et al: Safety of fiberoptic bronchoalveolar lavage in evaluation of interstitial lung disease. Chest 80:268, 1981.

82a. Spanevello A, Migliori GB, Satta A: Bronchoalveolar lavage causes decrease in Pao₂, increase in (A–a) gradient value, and bronchoconstriction in asthmatics. Respir Med 92:191, 1998.

83. Krause A, Hohberg B, Heine F, et al: Cytokines derived from alveolar macrophages induce fever after bronchoscopy and bronchoalveolar lavage. Am J Respir Crit Care Med 155:1793, 1997.

84. Krueger JJ, Sayre VA, Karetzky MS: Bronchoalveolar lavage–induced pneumothorax. Chest 94:440, 1988.

85. Gurney JW, Harrison WC, Sears K, et al: Bronchoalveolar lavage: Radiographic manifestations. Radiology 163:71, 1987.

86. Stover DE: Diagnosis of pulmonary disease in the immunocompromised host. Semin Respir Med 10:89, 1989.

87. Meduri GU, Stover DE, Greeno RA, et al: Bilateral bronchoalveolar lavage in the diagnosis of opportunistic pulmonary infections. Chest 100:1272, 1991.

88. Sternberg RI, Baughman RP, Dohn MN, et al: Utility of bronchoalveolar lavage in assessing pneumonia in immunosuppressed renal transplant recipients. Am J Med 95:358, 1993.

89. Xaubet A, Torres A, Marco F, et al: Pulmonary infiltrates in immunocompromised patients. Chest 95:130, 1989.

90. Breuer R, Lossos IS, Lafair JS, et al: Utility of bronchoalveolar lavage in the assessment of diffuse pulmonary infiltrates in non-AIDS immunocompromised patients. Respir Med 84:313, 1990.

91. Rust M Albera C, Carratu L, et al: The clinical use of BAL in patients with pulmonary infections. Eur Respir J 3:954, 1990.

92. Abati A, Cajigas A, Holland SM, et al: Chronic granulomatous disease of childhood: Respiratory cytology. Diag Cytopathol 15:98, 1996.

92a. Pagano L, Pagliari G, Basso A, et al: The role of bronchoalveolar lavage in the microbiological diagnosis of pneumonia in patients with haematological malignancies. Ann Med 29:535, 1997.

93. Speich R, Wust J, Hess T, et al: Prospective evaluation of a semiquantitative dip slide method compared with quantitative bacterial cultures of BAL fluid. Chest 109:1423, 1996.

94. Kollef MH, Bock KR, Richards RD, et al: The safety and diagnostic accuracy of minibronchoalveolar lavage in patients with suspected ventilator-associated pneumonia. Ann Intern Med 122:743, 1995.

95. Cantral DE, Tape TG, Reed EC: Quantitative culture of bronchoalveolar lavage fluid for the diagnosis of bacterial pneumonia. Am J Med 95:601, 1993.

96. Linder J, Vaughan WP, Armitage JO, et al: Cytopathology of opportunistic infection in bronchoalveolar lavage. Am J Clin Pathol 88:421, 1987.

97. Zaman SS, Seykora JT, Hodinka RL, et al: Cytologic manifestations of respiratory syncytial virus pneumonia in bronchoalveolar lavage fluid. A case report. Acta Cytol 40:546, 1996.

98. Wheeler RR, Bardales RH, North PE, et al: Toxoplasma pneumonia: Cytologic diagnosis by bronchoalveolar lavage. Diagn Cytopathol 11:52, 1994.

99. Newsome AL, Curtis FT, Culbertson CG, et al: Identification of acanthamoeba in bronchoalveolar lavage specimens. Diagn Cytopathol 8:231, 1992.

100. Solans EP, Yong S, Husain AN: Bronchioloalveolar lavage in the diagnosis of CMV pneumonitis in lung transplant recipients: An immunocytochemical study. Diagn Cytopathol 16:350, 1997.

101. Cagle PT, Buffone G, Holland VA, et al: Semiquantitative measurement of cytomegalovirus DNA in lung and heart-lung transplant patients by in vitro DNA amplification. Chest 101:93, 1992.

102. Tang CM, Holden DW, Aufauvre-Brown A, et al: The detection of *Aspergillus* spp. by the polymerase chain reaction and its evaluation in bronchoalveolar lavage fluid. Am Rev Respir Dis 148:1313, 1993.

103. Brugiere O, Vokurka M, Lecossier D, et al: Diagnosis of smear-negative pulmonary tuberculosis using sequence capture polymerase chain reaction. Am J Respir Crit Care Med 155:1478, 1997.

104. Albera C, Mabritto I, Ghio P, et al: Adenosine deaminase activity and fibronectin levels in bronchoalveolar lavage fluid in sarcoidosis and tuberculosis. Sarcoidosis 10:18, 1993.

105. Pugin J, Auckenthaler R, Delaspre O, et al: Rapid diagnosis of Gram negative pneumonia by assay of endotoxin in bronchoalveolar lavage fluid. Thorax 47:547, 1992.

106. Jimenez P, Meneses M, Saldias F, et al: Pneumococcal antigen detection in bronchoalveolar lavage fluid from patients with pneumonia. Thorax 49:872, 1994.

107. Pirozynski M: Bronchoalveolar lavage in the diagnosis of peripheral, primary lung cancer. Chest 102:372, 1992.

108. Linder J, Radio SJ, Robbins RA, et al: Bronchoalveolar lavage in the cytologic diagnosis of carcinoma of the lung. Acta Cytol 31:796, 1987.

109. Poletti V, Romagna M, Allen KA, et al: Bronchoalveolar lavage in the diagnosis of disseminated lung tumors. Acta Cytol 39:472, 1995.

110. Wisecarver J, Ness MJ, Rennard SI, et al: Bronchoalveolar lavage in the assessment of pulmonary Hodgkin's disease. Acta Cytol 33:527, 1989.

111. Levy H, Horak DA, Lewis MI: The value of bronchial washings and bronchoalveolar lavage in the diagnosis of lymphangitic carcinomatosis. Chest 94:1028, 1988.

112. Stanley MW, Henry-Stanley MJ, Gajl-Peczalska KJ, et al: Hyperplasia of type II pneumocytes in acute lung injury. Cytologic findings of sequential bronchoalveolar lavage. Am J Clin Pathol 97:669, 1992.

113. Biyoudi-Vouenze R, Tazi A, Hance AJ, et al: Abnormal epithelial cells recovered by bronchoalveolar lavage: Are they malignant? Am Rev Respir Dis 142:686, 1990.

114. Huang M-S, Colby TV, Goellner JR, et al: Utility of bronchoalveolar lavage in the diagnosis of drug-induced pulmonary toxicity. Acta Cytol 33:533, 1989.

115. Tabak L, Yilmazbayhan D, Kilicaslan Z, et al: Value of bronchoalveolar lavage in lipidoses with pulmonary involvement. Eur Respir J 7:409, 1994.

116. Carson KF, Williams CA, Rosenthal DL, et al: Bronchoalveolar lavage in a girl with Gaucher's disease. A case report. Acta Cytol 38:597, 1994.

117. Pérez-Arellano JL, Garcia J-EL, Macias MCG, et al: Hemosiderin-laden macrophages in bronchoalveolar lavage fluid. Acta Cytol 36:26, 1992.

118. De Vuyst P, Dumortier P, Moulin E, et al: Diagnostic value of asbestos bodies in bronchoalveolar lavage fluid. Am Rev Respir Dis 136:1219, 1987.

119. Roggli VL, Coin PG, MacIntyre NR, et al: Asbestos content of bronchoalveolar lavage fluid. A comparison of light and scanning electron microscopic analysis. Acta Cytol 38:502, 1994.

120. Auerswald U, Barth J, Magnussen H: Value of CD-1–positive cells in bronchoalveolar lavage fluid for the diagnosis of pulmonary histiocytosis X. Lung 169:305, 1991.

120a. Bingisser R, Kaplan V, Zollinger A, et al: Whole-lung lavage in alveolar proteinosis by a modified lavage technique. Chest 113:1718, 1998.

121. Goldstein RA, Rohatgi PK, Bergofsky EH, et al: Clinical role of bronchoalveolar lavage in adults with pulmonary disease. Am Rev Respir Dis 142:481, 1990

122. Helmers RA, Hunninghake GW: Bronchoalveolar lavage in the nonimmunocompromised patients. Chest 96:1184, 1989.

123. Costabel U, Teschler H: Inflammation and immune reactions in interstitial lung disease (ILD) associated with inorganic dust exposure. Eur Respir J 3:363, 1990.

124. Costabel U, Donner CF, Haslam PL, et al: Occupational lung disease due to inhalation of inorganic dust. Eur Respir J 3:946, 1990.

124a. Fontenot AP, Kotzin BL, Comment CE, et al: Expansions of T-cell subsets expressing particular T-cell receptor variable regions in chronic beryllium disease. Am J Respir Cell Mol Biol 18:581, 1998.

125. Haslam PL, Poulter LW, Rossi GA, et al: The clinical role of BAL in idiopathic pulmonary fibrosis. Eur Respir J 3:940, 1990.

126. Wallaert B, Rossi GA, Sibille Y: Collagen-vascular diseases. Eur Respir J 3:942, 1990.

127. Poulter LW, Rossi GA, Bjermer L, et al: The value of bronchoalveolar lavage in the diagnosis and prognosis of sarcoidosis. Eur Respir J 3:943, 1990.

127a. Kodama N, Yamaguchi E, Hizawa N, et al: Expression of RANTES by bronchoalveolar lavage cells in nonsmoking patients with interstitial lung diseases. Am J Respir Cell Mol Biol 18:526, 1998.

128. Semenzato G, Bjermer L, Costabel U, et al: Extrinsic allergic alveolitis. Eur Respir J 3:945, 1990.

129. Danel C, Israel-Biet D, Costabel U, et al: The clinical role of BAL in pulmonary histiocytosis X. Eur Respir J 3:949, 1990.

130. Danel C, Israel-Biet D, Costabel U, et al: The clinical role of BAL in eosinophilic lung diseases. Eur Respir J 3:950, 1990.

131. Danel C, Israel-Biet D, Costabel U, et al: Drug induced pneumonitis. Eur Respir J 3:952, 1990.

132. Fabbri LM, De Rose V, Godard PH, et al: Bronchial asthma. Eur Respir J 3:958, 1990.

133. Smith DL, Deshazo RD: Bronchoalveolar lavage in asthma. Am Rev Respir Dis 148:523, 1993.

134. Willsie SK, Herndon BL, Miller L, et al: Soluble versus cell-bound CD4, CD8 from bronchoalveolar lavage: Correlation with pulmonary diagnoses in human immunodeficiency virus–infected individuals. J Leukoc Biol 59:813, 1996.

135. Pozzi E, De Rose V, Rennard SI, et al: Chronic bronchitis and emphysema. Eur Respir J 3:959, 1990.

136. Merchant RK, Schwartz DA, Helmers RA, et al: Bronchoalveolar lavage cellularity. The distribution in normal volunteers. Am Rev Respir Dis 146:448, 1992.

137. Spriggs AI, Boddington MM: The Cytology of Effusions. New York, Grune & Stratton, 1968, pp 1–39.

138. Dekker A, Bupp PA: Cytology of serous effusions. An investigation into the usefulness of cell blocks versus smears. Am J Clin Pathol 70:855, 1978.

139. Yam LT, Janckila AJ: A simple method of preparing smears from bloody effusions for cytodiagnosis. Acta Cytol 27:114, 1983.

140. Nagasawa T, Nagasawa S: Enrichment of malignant cells from pleural effusions by Percoll density gradients. Acta Cytol 27:119, 1983.

141. Nance KV, Silverman JF: The utility of ancillary techniques in effusion cytology. Diagn Cytopathol 8:185, 1992.

142. Light RW, Erozan YS, Ball WC Jr: Cells in pleural fluid. Their value in differential diagnosis. Arch Intern Med 132:854, 1973.

143. Antony VB, Repine JE, Harada RN, et al: Inflammatory responses in experimental tuberculosis pleurisy. Acta Cytol 27:355, 1983.

144. Mestitz P, Pollard AC: The diagnosis of tuberculous pleural effusion. Br J Dis Chest 53:86, 1959.

145. Spieler P: The cytologic diagnosis of tuberculosis in pleural effusions. Acta Cytol 23:374, 1979.

146. Green LK, Griffin J: Increased natural killer cells in fluids. A new, sensitive means of detecting carcinoma. Acta Cytol 40:1240, 1996.

147. Spriggs AI: Pleural eosinophilia due to pneumothorax (letter). Acta Cytol 23:425, 1979.

148. Adleman M, Albelda SM, Gottlieb J, et al: Diagnostic utility of pleural fluid eosinophilia. Am J Med 77:915, 1984.

149. Chapman JS, Reynolds RC: Eosinophilic response to intraperitoneal blood. J Lab Clin Med 51:516, 1958.

150. Nakamura Y, Ozaki T, Kamei T, et al: Factors that stimulate the proliferation and survival of eosinophils in eosinophilic pleural effusion: Relationship to granulocyte/macrophage colony-stimulating factor, interleukin-5, and interleukin-3. Am J Respir Cell Mol Biol 8:605, 1993.

151. Veress JF, Koss LG, Schreiber K: Eosinophilic pleural effusions. Acta Cytol 23:40, 1979.

152. Campbell GD, Webb WR: Eosinophilic pleural effusion: A review with the presentation of seven new cases. Am Rev Respir Dis 90:194, 1964.

153. Bedrossian CWM: Special stains, the old and the new: The impact of immunocytochemistry in effusion cytology. Diagn Cytopathol 18:141, 1998.

154. Curran WS, Williams AW: Eosinophilic pleural effusion: A clue in differential diagnosis. Arch Intern Med 111:809, 1963.

154a. Rubins JB, Rubins HB: Etiology and prognostic significance of eosinophilic pleural effusions. Chest 110:1271, 1996.

155. Petusevsky ML, Faling J, Rocklin RE, et al: Pleuropericardial reaction to treatment with dantrolene. JAMA 242:2772, 1979.

156. Järvinen KAJ, Kahanpää A: Prognosis in cases with eosinophilic pleural effusion: 17 cases followed for five to twelve years. Acta Med Scand 164:245, 1959.

157. Naylor B, Schmidt RW: The case for exfoliative cytology of serous effusions. Lancet 1:711, 1964.

158. Chrétien J: Needle biopsy of the pleura: A simple procedure often more efficient than the classical methods. Abbottempo 1:25, 1963.

159. Dewald GW, Hicks GA, Dines DE, et al: Cytogenetic diagnosis of malignant pleural effusions: Culture methods to supplement direct preparations in diagnosis. Mayo Clin Proc 57:488, 1982.

160. Venrick MG, Sidawy MK: Cytologic evaluation of serous effusions. Processing techniques and optimal number of smears for routine preparation. Am J Clin Pathol 99:182, 1993.

161. Kutty CPK, Remeniuk E, Varkey B: Malignant-appearing cells in pleural effusion due to pancreatitis. Case report and literature review. Acta Cytol 24:412, 1980.

162. Decker DA, Dines DE, Payne WS, et al: The significance of a cytologically negative pleural effusion in bronchogenic carcinoma. Chest 74:640, 1978.

163. Granados R, Cibas ES, Fletcher JA: Cytogenetic analysis of effusions from malignant mesothelioma. A diagnostic adjunct to cytology. Acta Cytol 38:711, 1994.

164. Gondos B, McIntosh KM, Renston RH, et al: Application of electron microscopy in the definitive diagnosis of effusions. Acta Cytol 22:297, 1978.

165. Posalaky Z, McGinley D, Posalaky IP: Electron microscopic identification of the colorectal origins of tumor cells in pleural fluid. Acta Cytol 25:45, 1981.

166. Monif GRG, Stewart BN, Block AJ: Living cytology. A new diagnostic technique for malignant pleural effusions. Chest 69:626, 1976.

167. Banks ER, Jennings CD, Jacobs S: Comparative assessment of DNA analysis in effusions by image analysis and flow cytometry. Diagn Cytopathol 10:62, 1994.

168. Fuhr JE, Kattine AA, Sullivan TA, et al: Flow cytometric analysis of pulmonary fluids and cells for the detection of malignancies. Am J Pathol 141:211, 1992.

169. Rijken A, Dekker A, Taylor S, et al: Diagnostic value of DNA analysis in effusions by flow cytometry and image analysis. A prospective study on 102 patients as compared with cytologic examination. Am J Clin Pathol 95:6, 1991.

170. Zarbo RJ: Flow cytometric DNA analysis of effusions: A new test seeking validation. Am J Clin Pathol 95:2, 1991.

171. Huang MS, Tsai MS, Hwang JJ, et al: Comparison of nucleolar organiser regions and DNA flow cytometry in the evaluation of pleural effusion. Thorax 49:1152, 1994.

172. Matter-Walstra KW, Kraft R: Atypical cells in effusions: Diagnostic value of cell image analysis combined with immunocytochemistry. Diagn Cytopathol 15:263, 1996.

173. Guber A, Cohen R, Ronah R, et al: Flow cytometric analysis and cytokeratin typing of human lung tumors. A preliminary study. Chest 105:138, 1994.

174. Lee JS, Nam JH, Lee MC, et al: Immunohistochemical panel for distinguishing between carcinoma and reactive mesothelial cells in serous effusions. Acta Cytol 40:631, 1996.

175. Daste G, Serre G, Mauduyt MA, et al: Immunophenotyping of mesothelial cells and carcinoma cells with monoclonal antibodies to cytokeratins, vimentin, CEA, and EMA improves the cytodiagnosis of serous effusions. Cytopathology 2:19, 1991.

176. Estaeban JM, Yokota S, Husain S, et al: Immunocytochemical profile of benign and carcinomatous effusions: A practical approach to difficult diagnosis. Am J Clin Pathol 94:698, 1990.

177. Maguire B, Whitaker D, Carrello S, et al: Monoclonal antibody Ber-EPA: Its use in the differential diagnosis of malignant mesothelioma and carcinoma in cell blocks of malignant effusions and FNA specimens. Diagn Cytopathol 10:130, 1994.

178. Mezger J, Stotzer O, Schilli G, et al: Identification of carcinoma cells in ascitic and pleural fluid: Comparison of four panepithelial antigens with carcinoembryonic antigen. Acta Cytol 36:75, 1992.

179. Mullick SS, Green LK, Ramzy I, et al: p53 gene product in pleural effusions. Practical use in distinguishing benign from malignant cells. Acta Cytol 40:855, 1996.

180. Tiniakos DG, Healicon RM, Hair T, et al: p53 immunostaining as a marker of malignancy in cytologic preparations of body fluids. Acta Cytol 39:171, 1995.

181. Zaatari GS, Gupta PK, Bhagavan BS, et al: Cytopathology of pleural endometriosis. Acta Cytol 26:227, 1982.

182. Jacobson ES: A case of secondary echinococcosis diagnosed by cytologic examination of pleural fluid and needle biopsy of pleura. Acta Cytol 17:76, 1973.

183. Reyes CV, Kathuria S, MacGlashan A: Diagnostic value of calcium oxalate crystals in respiratory and pleural fluid cytology. A case report. Acta Cytol 23:65, 1979.

184. Nosanchuk JS, Naylor B: A unique cytologic picture in pleural fluid from patients with rheumatoid arthritis. Am J Clin Pathol 50:330, 1968.

185. Cobb CJ, Synn J, Cobb SR, et al: Cytologic findings in an effusion caused by rupture of a benign cystic teratoma of the mediastinum into a serous cavity. Acta Cytol 29:1015, 1985.

186. Itami M, Teshima S, Asakuma Y: Pulmonary lymphangiomyomatosis diagnosed by effusion cytology. A case report. Acta Cytol 41:522, 1997.

187. Kelley S, McGarry P, Hutson Y: Atypical cells in pleural fluid characteristic of systemic lupus erythematosus. Acta Cytol 15:357, 1971.

188. Osamura RY, Shioya S, Handa K, et al: Lupus erythematosus cells in pleural fluid; cytologic diagnosis in two patients. Acta Cytol 21:215, 1977.

189. Horder TJ: Lung puncture: A new application of clinical pathology. Lancet 2:1345, 1909.

190. Dudgeon LS, Patrick CV: A new method for the rapid microscopical diagnosis of tumors: With an account of 200 cases so examined. Br J Surg 15:250, 1927.

191. Silverman I: A new biopsy needle. Am J Surg 40:671, 1938.

192. Sterrett G, Whitaker D, Glancy J: Fine-needle aspiration of lung, mediastinum and chest wall. A clinicopathologic exercise. In Sommers SC, Rosen PP (eds): Pathology Annual. Part 2. Vol 17. E Norwalk, CT, Appleton & Lange, 1982, p 197.

193. Stanley JH, Fish GD, Andriole JG, et al: Lung lesions: Cytologic diagnosis by fine-needle biopsy. Radiology 162:389, 1987.

194. Li H, Boiselle PM, Shepard JAO, et al: Diagnostic accuracy and safety of CT-guided percutaneous needle aspiration biopsy of the lung: Comparison of small and large pulmonary nodules. Am J Roentgenol 167:105, 1996.

195. Westcott JL, Rao N, Colley DP: Transthoracic needle biopsy of small pulmonary nodules. Radiology 202:97, 1997.

196. Zavala DC, Schoell JE: Ultra-thin needle aspiration of the lung in infectious and malignant disease. Am Rev Respir Dis 123:125, 1981.

197. Tarver RD, Conces DJ Jr: Interventional chest radiology. Radiol Clin North Am 32:689, 1994.

198. Todd TRJ, Weisbrod G, Tao LC, et al: Aspiration needle biopsy of thoracic lesions. Ann Thorac Surg 32:154, 1981.

199. Greene R, Szyfelbein WM, Isler RJ, et al: Supplementary tissue-core histology from fine-needle transthoracic aspiration biopsy. Am J Roentgenol 144:787, 1985.

200. Westcott JL: Direct percutaneous needle aspiration of localized pulmonary lesions: Results in 422 patients. Radiology 137:31, 1980.

201. Klein JS, Salomon G, Stewart EA: Transthoracic needle biopsy with a coaxially placed 20-gauge automated cutting needle: Results in 122 patients. Radiology 198:715, 1996.

202. vanSonnenberg E, Casola G, Ho M, et al: Difficult thoracic lesions: CT-guided biopsy experienced in 150 cases. Radiology 167:457, 1988.

203. Lee L-N, Yang P-C, Kuo S-H, et al: Diagnosis of pulmonary cryptococcosis by ultrasound guided percutaneous aspiration. Thorax 48:75, 1993.

204. Pedersen OM, Aasen TB, Gulsvik A: Fine needle aspiration biopsy of mediasti-

nal and peripheral pulmonary masses guided by real-time sonography. Chest 89:504, 1986.

205. Perlmutt LM, Johnston WW, Dunnick NR: Percutaneous transthoracic needle aspiration: A review. Am J Roentgenol 152:451, 1989.

206. Harkin TJ, Ciotoli C, Addrizzo-Harris DJ, et al: Transbronchial needle aspiration (TBNA) in patients infected with HIV. Am J Respir Crit Care Med 157:1913, 1998.

207. Jereb M, Us-Krasovec M: Thin needle biopsy of chest lesions: Time-saving potential. Chest 78:288, 1980.

208. Yam LT, Levine H: Rapid cytologic diagnosis of percutaneous needle aspirates of peripheral pulmonary lesions. Am J Clin Pathol 59:648, 1973.

209. Pak HY, Yokota SB, Teplitz RL: Rapid staining techniques employed in fine needle aspiration (letter). Acta Cytol 27:81, 1983.

210. Yang GCH, Alvarez II: Ultrafast Papanicolaou stain. An alternative preparation for fine needle aspiration cytology. Acta Cytol 39:55, 1995.

211. Santambrogio L, Nosotti M, Bellaviti N, et al: CT-guided fine-needle aspiration cytology of solitary pulmonary nodules—a prospective randomized study of immediate cytologic evaluation. Chest 112:423, 1997.

212. Smith MJ, Kini SR, Watson E: Fine needle aspiration and endoscopic brush cytology. Comparison of direct smears and rinsings. Acta Cytol 24:456, 1980.

213. Kern WH, Haber H: Fine needle aspiration minibiopsies. Acta Cytol 30:403, 1986.

214. Akhtar M, Bakry M, Al-Jeaid AS, et al: Electron microscopy of fine-needle aspiration biopsy specimens: A brief review. Diagn Cytopathol 8:278, 1992.

215. Kurtz SM: Rapid ultrastructural examination of FNAs in the diagnosis of intra-thoracic tumors. Diagn Cytopathol 8:289, 1992.

216. Neill JSA, Silverman JF: Electron microscopy of fine-needle aspiration biopsies of the mediastinum. Diagn Cytopathol 8:272, 1992.

217. Morrissey B, Adams H, Gibbs AR, et al: Percutaneous needle biopsy of the mediastinum: Review of 94 procedures. Thorax 48:632, 1993.

218. Zarbo RJ, Fenoglio-Preiser CM: Interinstitutional database for comparison of performance in lung fine-needle aspiration cytology. A College of American Pathologists Q-probe study of 5264 cases with histologic correlation. Arch Pathol Lab Med 116:463, 1992.

219. Powers CN, Silverman JF, Geisinger KR, et al: Fine-needle aspiration biopsy of the mediastinum: A multi-institutional analysis. Am J Clin Pathol 105:168, 1996.

220. Logrono R, Kurtycz DFI, Sproat IA, et al: Multidisciplinary approach to deep-seated lesions requiring radiologically guided fine-needle aspiration. Diagn Cytopathol 18:338, 1998.

221. Flower CDR, Verney GI: Percutaneous needle biopsy of thoracic lesions: An evaluation of 300 biopsies. Clin Radiol 30:215, 1979.

222. de Vivo F, Pond GD, Rhenman B, et al: Transtracheal aspiration and fine needle aspiration biopsy for the diagnosis of pulmonary infection in heart transplant patients. J Thorac Cardiovasc Surg 96:696, 1988.

223. Zavala DC, Schoell JE: Ultra-thin needle aspiration of the lung in infectious and malignant disease. Am Rev Respir Dis 123:125, 1981.

224. Dorca J, Manresa F, Esteban L, et al: Efficacy, safety and therapeutic relevance of transthoracic aspiration with ultrathin needle in nonventilated nosocomial pneumonia. Am J Respir Crit Care Med 151:1491, 1995.

225. Sterrett G, Whitaker D, Glancy J: Fine-needle aspiration of lung, mediastinum and chest wall. A clinicopathologic exercise. *In* Sommers SC, Rosen PP (eds): Pathology Annual. Part 2. Vol 17. E Norwalk, CT, Appleton & Lange, 1982, p 197.

226. Westcott JL: Air embolism complicating percutaneous needle biopsy of the lung. Chest 63:108, 1973.

227. Omenaas E, Moerkve O, Thomassen L, et al: Cerebral air embolism after transthoracic aspiration with a 0.6 mm (23 gauge) needle. Eur Respir J 2:908, 1989.

228. Gibney RTN, Man GCW, King EG, et al: Aspiration biopsy in the diagnosis of pulmonary disease. Chest 80:300, 1981.

229. Jereb M, Us-Krasovec M: Transthoracic needle biopsy of mediastinal and hilar lesions. Cancer 40:1354, 1977.

230. Sagel SS, Ferguson TB, Forrest JV, et al: Percutaneous transthoracic aspiration needle biopsy. Ann Thorac Surg 26:399, 1978.

231. Allison DJ, Hemingway AP: Percutaneous needle biopsy of the lung. BMJ 282:875, 1981.

232. Zavala DC, Schoell JE: Ultra-thin needle aspiration of the lung in infectious and malignant disease. Am Rev Respir Dis 123:125, 1981.

233. Perlmutt LM, Johnston WW, Dunnick NR: Percutaneous transthoracic needle aspiration: A review. Am J Roentgenol 152:451, 1989.

234. Greene RE: Transthoracic needle aspiration biopsy. *In* Athanasoulis CA (ed): Interventional Radiology. Philadelphia, WB Saunders, 1982, pp 587–634.

235. Moore EH, Shepard JO, McLoud TC, et al: Positional precautions in needle aspiration lung biopsy. Radiology 175:733, 1990.

236. Fish GD, Stanley JH, Miller KS, et al: Postbiopsy pneumothorax: Estimating the risk by chest radiography and pulmonary function tests. Am J Roentgenol 150:71, 1988.

237. Miller KS, Fish GD, Stanley JH, et al: Prediction of pneumothorax rate in percutaneous needle aspiration of the lung. Chest 93:872, 1988.

238. Perlmutt LM, Braun SD, Newman GE, et al: Timing of chest film follow-up after transthoracic needle aspiration. Am J Roentgenol 146:1049, 1986.

239. Stanley JH, Fish GD, Andriole JG, et al: Lung lesions: Cytologic diagnosis by fine-needle biopsy. Radiology 162:389, 1987.

240. Li H, Boiselle PM, Shepard JO, et al: Diagnostic accuracy and safety of CT-guided percutaneous needle aspiration biopsy of the lung: Comparison of small and large pulmonary nodules. Am J Roentgenol 167:105, 1996.

241. Westcott JL, Rao N, Colley DP: Transthoracic needle biopsy of small pulmonary nodules. Radiology 202:97, 1997.

242. Fontana RS, Miller WE, Beabout JW, et al: Transthoracic needle aspiration of discrete pulmonary lesions: Experience in 100 cases. Med Clin North Am 54:961, 1970.

243. Sanders DE, Thompson DW, Pudden BJE: Percutaneous aspiration lung biopsy. Can Med Assoc J 104:139, 1971.

244. Dahlgren SE, Ovenfors C-O: Aspiration biopsy diagnosis of neurogenous mediastinal tumours. Acta Radiol Diagn 10:289, 1970.

245. Muller NL, Bergin CJ, Miller RR, et al: Seeding of malignant cells into the needle track after lung and pleural biopsy. J Can Assoc Radiol 37:192, 1986.

246. Nagasaka T, Nakashima N, Nunome H: Needle tract implantation of thymoma after transthoracic needle biopsy. J Clin Pathol 46:278, 1993.

247. Carter RR III, Wilson JP, Turner HR, et al: Cutaneous blastomycosis as a complication of transthoracic needle aspiration. Chest 91:917, 1987.

248. Cazzadori A, Di Perri G, Marocco S, et al: Tuberculous pleurisy after percutaneous needle biopsy of a pulmonary nodule. Respir Med 88:477, 1994.

249. Taft PD, Szyzfelbein WM, Greene R: A study of variability in cytologic diagnoses based on pulmonary aspiration specimens. Am J Clin Pathol 73:36, 1980.

250. Francis D, Hojgaard K: Transthoracic aspiration biopsy. A study on diagnostic reproducibility. Acta Pathol Microbiol Scand 85:889, 1977.

251. Layfield LJ, Coogan A, Johnston WW, et al: Transthoracic fine needle aspiration biopsy. Sensitivity in relation to guidance technique and lesion size and location. Acta Cytol 40:687, 1996.

252. Moulton JS, Moore PT. Coaxial percutaneous biopsy technique with automated biopsy devices: Value in improving accuracy and negative predictive value. Radiology 186:515, 1993.

253. Tao LC, Pearson FG, Delarue NC, et al: Percutaneous fine-needle aspiration biopsy: 1. Its value to clinical practice. Cancer 45:1480, 1980.

254. Poe RH, Tobin RE: Sensitivity and specificity of needle biopsy in lung malignancy. Am Rev Respir Dis 122:725, 1980.

255. Dahlgren SE, Lind B: Comparison between diagnostic results obtained by transthoracic needle biopsy and by sputum cytology. Acta Cytol 16:53, 1972.

256. Berquist TH, Bailey PB, Cortese DA, et al: Transthoracic needle biopsy: Accuracy and complications in relation to location and type of lesion. Mayo Clin Proc 55:475, 1980.

257. Zakowski MF, Gatscha RM, Zaman MB: Negative predictive value of pulmonary fine needle aspiration cytology. Acta Cytol 36:283, 1992.

258. Cagle PT, Kovach M, Ramzy I: Causes of false results in transthoracic fine needle lung aspirates. Acta Cytol 37:16, 1993.

259. Silverman JF: Inflammatory and neoplastic processes of the lung: Differential diagnosis and pitfalls in FNA biopsies. Diagn Cytopathol 13:448, 1995.

260. Geisinger KR: Differential diagnostic considerations and potential pitfalls in fine-needle aspiration biopsies of the mediastinum. Diagn Cytopathol 13:436, 1995.

261. Mitchell ML, King DE, Bonfiglio TA, et al: Pulmonary fine-needle aspiration cytopathology: A five-year correlation study. Acta Cytol 28:72, 1984.

262. Michel RP, Lushpihan A, Ahmed MN: Pathologic findings of transthoracic needle aspiration in the diagnosis of localized pulmonary lesions. Cancer 51:1663, 1983.

263. Davies DC, Russell AJ, Tayar R, et al: Transmission electron microscopy of percutaneous fine needle aspirates from lung: A study of 70 cases. Thorax 42:296, 1987.

264. Taccagni G, Cantaboni A, Dell'Antonio G, et al: Electron microscopy of fine needle aspiration biopsies of mediastinal and paramediastinal lesions. Acta Cytol 32:868, 1988.

265. Mottolese M, Venturo I, Rinaldi M, et al: Combinations of monoclonal antibodies can distinguish primary lung tumors from metastatic lung tumors sampled by fine needle aspiration biopsy. Cancer 64:2493, 1989.

266. Kung ITM, Chan S-K, Lo ESF: Application of the immunoperoxidase technique to cell block preparations from fine needle aspirates. Acta Cytol 34:297, 1990.

267. Domagala WM, Markiewski M, Tuziak T, et al: Immunocytochemistry on fine needle aspirates in paraffin miniblocks. Acta Cytol 34:291, 1990.

267a. Raab SS, Slagel DD, Hughes JH, et al: Sensitivity and cost-effectiveness of fine-needle aspiration with immunocytochemistry in the evaluation of patients with a pulmonary malignancy and a history of cancer. Arch Pathol Lab Med 121:695, 1997.

268. O'Reilly PE, Brueckner J, Silverman JF: Value of ancillary studies in fine needle aspiration cytology of the lung. Acta Cytol 38:144, 1994.

269. Fraser RS: Transthoracic needle aspiration. The benign diagnosis. Arch Pathol Lab Med 115:751, 1991.

270. Goralnik CH, O'Connell DM, El Yousef SJ, et al: CT-guided cutting-needle biopsies of selected chest lesions. Am J Roentgenol 151:903, 1988.

271. Clore F, Virapongse C, Saterfiel J: Low-risk large-bore biopsy of chest lesions. Chest 96:538, 1989.

271a. Boiselle PM, Shepard JA, Mark EJ, et al: Routine addition of an automated biopsy device to fine-needle aspiration of the lung: A prospective assessment. Am J Roentgenol 169:661, 1997.

272. Bella F, Tort J, Morera M-A, et al: Value of bacterial antigen detection in the diagnostic yield of transthoracic needle aspiration in severe community acquired pneumonia. Thorax 48:1227, 1993.

272a. Ruiz-Gonzalez A, Nogues A, Falguera M, et al: Rapid detection of pneumococcal antigen in lung aspirates: Comparison with culture and PCR. Respir Med 91:201, 1997.

273. Hawkins AG, Hsiu J-G, Smith RM, et al: Pulmonary dirofilariasis diagnosed by fine needle aspiration biopsy: A case report. Acta Cytol 29:19, 1985.

274. Saenz-Santamaria J, Moreno-Casado J, Nunez C: Role of fine-needle biopsy in the diagnosis of hydatid cyst. Diagn Cytopathol 13:229, 1995.

274a. Shim JJ, Cheong HJ, Kang E-Y, et al: Nested polymerase chain reaction for detection of *Mycobacterium tuberculosis* in solitary pulmonary nodules. Chest 113:20, 1998.

275. Dahlgren SE, Ekstrom P: Aspiration cytology in the diagnosis of pulmonary tuberculosis. Scand J Respir Dis 53:196, 1972.

276. Das DK, Bhambhani S, Pant JN, et al: Superficial and deep-seated tuberculous lesions: Fine-needle aspiration cytology diagnosis of 574 cases. Diagn Cytopathol 8:211, 1992.

277. Pitman MB, Szyfelbein WM, Niles J, et al: Clinical utility of fine needle aspiration biopsy in the diagnosis of Wegener's granulomatosis. A report of two cases. Acta Cytol 36:222, 1992.

278. Castellino RA, Blank N: Etiologic diagnosis of focal pulmonary infection in immunocompromised patients by fluoroscopically guided percutaneous needle aspiration. Radiology 132:563, 1979.

279. Falguera M, Nogues A, Ruiz-Gonzales A, et al: Transthoracic needle aspiration in the study of pulmonary infections in patients with HIV. Chest 106:697, 1994.

280. Dahlgren S: Needle biopsy of intrapulmonary hamartoma. Scand J Respir Dis 47:187, 1966.

281. Tomashefski JF Jr, Cramer SF, Abramowsky C, et al: Needle biopsy diagnosis of solitary amyloid nodule of the lung. Acta Cytol 24:224, 1980.

282. Dusenbery D, Grimes MM, Frable WJ: Fine-needle aspiration cytology of localized fibrous tumor of pleura. Diagn Cytopathol 8:444, 1992.

283. Carlson BR, McQueen S, Kimbrell F, et al: Thoracic splenosis. Diagnosis of a case by fine needle aspiration cytology. Acta Cytol 32:91, 1988.

284. Covell JL, Feldman PS: Fine needle aspiration diagnosis of aspiration pneumonia (phytopneumonitis). Acta Cytol 28:77, 1984.

285. Silverman JF, Weaver MD, Shaw R, et al: Fine needle aspiration cytology of pulmonary infarct. Acta Cytol 29:162, 1985.

286. Adler OB, Resenberger A, Peleg H: Fine-needle aspiration biopsy of mediastinal masses: Evaluation of 136 experiences. Am J Roentgenol 140:893, 1983.

287. Wang KP, Terry P, Marsh B: Bronchoscopic needle aspiration biopsy of paratracheal tumors. Am Rev Respir Dis 118:17, 1978.

288. Wang KP, Marsh BR, Summer WR, et al: Transbronchial needle aspiration for diagnosis of lung cancer. Chest 80:48, 1981.

289. Nguyen G, York EL, Jones RL, et al: Transmucosal needle aspiration biopsy via the fibreoptic bronchoscope. Value and limitations in the cytodiagnosis of tumours and tumour-like lesions of the lung. *In* Rosen PP, Fechner RE (eds): Pathology Annual. Part 1. Vol 26. E Norwalk, CT, Appleton & Lange, 1992, p 105.

290. Roche DH, Wilsher ML, Gurley AM: Transtracheal needle aspiration. Diagn Cytopathol 12:106, 1995.

291. Harrow EM, Wang K-P: The staging of lung cancer by bronchoscopic transbronchial needle aspiration. Chest Surg Clin North Am 6:223, 1996.

292. Wang KP: Flexible transbronchial needle aspiration biopsy for histologic specimens. Chest 88:860, 1995.

293. Utz JP, Patel AM, Edell ES: The role of transcarinal needle aspiration in the staging of bronchogenic carcinoma. Chest 104:1012, 1993.

294. Wang KP, Haponik EF, Britt EJ, et al: Transbronchial needle aspiration of peripheral pulmonary nodules. Chest 6:819, 1984.

295. Vansteenkiste J, Lacquet LM, Demedts M, et al: Transcarinal needle aspiration biopsy in the staging of lung cancer. Eur Respir J 7:265, 1994.

296. de Castro FR, Lopez FD, Serda GJ: Relevance of training in transbronchial fine-needle aspiration technique. Chest 111:103, 1997.

297. Witte MC, Opal SM, Gilbert JG, et al: Incidence of fever and bacteremia following transbronchial needle aspiration. Chest 89:85, 1986.

298. Watts WJ, Green RA: Bacteremia following transbronchial fine needle aspiration. Chest 85:295, 1984.

299. Schenk DA, Bower JH, Bryan CL, et al: Transbronchial needle aspiration staging of bronchogenic carcinoma. Am Rev Respir Dis 134:146, 1986.

300. Schenk DA, Chambers SL, Derdak S, et al: Comparison of the Wang 10-gauge and 22-gauge needles in the mediastinal staging of lung cancer. Am Rev Respir Dis 147:1251, 1993.

301. Shure D: Bronchoscopy: Transbronchial biopsy and needle aspiration. Chest 95:1130, 1989.

302. Salathe M, Soler M, Bolliger CT, et al: Transbronchial needle aspiration in routine fibreoptic bronchoscopy. Respiration 59:5, 1992.

303. Harrow E, Halber M, Hardy S, et al: Bronchoscopic and roentgenographic correlates of a positive transbronchial needle aspiration in the staging of lung cancer. Chest 100:1592, 1991.

304. Wilsher ML, Gurley AM: Transtracheal aspiration using rigid bronchoscopy and a rigid needle for investigating mediastinal masses. Thorax 51:197, 1996.

305. Shannon JJ, Bude RO, Orens JB, et al: Endobronchial ultrasound-guided needle aspiration of mediastinal adenopathy. Am J Respir Crit Care Med 153:1424, 1996.

306. Krane JF, Renshaw AA: Relative value and cost-effectiveness of culture and special stains in fine-needle aspirates of the lung. Acta Cytol 42:305, 1998.

307. Mehta AC, Kavuru MS, Meeker DP, et al: Transbronchial needle aspiration for histology specimens. Chest 96:1228, 1989.

308. Shannon JJ, Bude RO, Orens JB, et al: Endobronchial ultrasound-guided aspiration of mediastinal adenopathy. Am J Respir Crit Care Med 153:1424, 1996.

308a. Gress FG, Savides TJ, Sandler A, et al: Endoscopic ultrasonography, fine-needle aspiration biopsy guided by endoscopic ultrasonography, and computed tomography in the preoperative staging of non-small-cell lung cancer: A comparison study. Ann Intern Med 127:604, 1997.

309. DeCaro LF, Pak HY, Yokota S, et al: Intraoperative cytodiagnosis of lung tumors by needle aspiration. J Thorac Cardiovasc Surg 85:404, 1983.

310. Pantzar P, Meurala H, Koivuniemi A, et al: Preoperative fine needle aspiration biopsy of lung tumors. Scand J Thorac Cardiovasc Surg 17:51, 1983.

311. Cappellari JO, Thompson EN, Wallenhaupt SL: Utility of intraoperative fine needle aspiration biopsy in the surgical management of patients with pulmonary masses. Acta Cytol 38:707, 1994.

312. Cartwright DM, Howell LP: Intraoperative cytology as an elective surgical procedure. Analysis of 57 cases. Acta Cytol 37:280, 1993.

313. Clarke MR, Landreneau RJ, Borochovitz D: Intraoperative imprint cytology for evaluation of mediastinal lymphadenopathy. Ann Thorac Surg 57:1206, 1994.

314. Masson RG, Ruggieri J: Pulmonary microvascular cytology: A new diagnostic application of the pulmonary artery catheter. Chest 88:908, 1985.

315. Giampaolo C, Schneider V, Kowalski BH, et al: The cytologic diagnosis of amniotic fluid embolism: A critical reappraisal. Diagn Cytopathol 3:126, 1987.

316. Castella X, Valles J, Cabezuelo MA, et al: Fat embolism syndrome and pulmonary microvascular cytology. Chest 101:1710, 1992.

317. Bhuvaneswaran JS, Venkitachalam CG, Sandhyamani S: Pulmonary wedge aspiration cytology in the diagnosis of recurrent tumour embolism causing pulmonary arterial hypertension. Int J Cardiol 39:209, 1993

318. Heard BE: A pathological study of emphysema of the lungs with chronic bronchitis. Thorax 13:136, 1958.

319. Gough J, Wentworth JE: The use of thin sections of entire organs in morbid anatomical studies. J R Microbiol Soc 69:231, 1949.

320. Whimster WF: Rapid giant paper sections of lungs. Thorax 24:737, 1969.

321. Ferencz C, Greco J: A method for the three-dimensional study of pulmonary arteries. Chest 57:428, 1970.

322. Thurlbeck WM: The geographic pathology of pulmonary emphysema and chronic bronchitis. I. Review. Arch Environ Health 14:16, 1967.

323. Heard BE, Esterly JR, Wootliff JS: A modified apparatus for fixing lungs to study the pathology of emphysema. Am Rev Respir Dis 95:311, 1967.

323a. McCulloch TA, Rutty GN: Postmortem examination of the lungs: A preservation technique for opening the bronchi and pulmonary arteries individually without transection problems. J Clin Pathol 51:163, 1998.

324. Blumenthal BJ, Boren HG: Lung structure in three dimensions after inflation and fume fixation. Am Rev Respir Dis 79:764, 1959.

325. Wright BM, Slavin G, Kreel L, et al: Postmortem inflation and fixation of human lungs. A technique for pathological and radiological correlations. Thorax 29:189, 1974.

326. Mittermayer C, Wybitul K, Rau WS, et al: Standardized fixation of human lung for radiology and morphometry; description of a "two chamber" system with formaldehyde vapor inflation. Pathol Res Pract 162:115, 1978.

327. Silverton RE: Gross fixation methods used in the study of pulmonary emphysema. Thorax 20:289, 1965.

328. Weibel ER, Vidone RA: Fixation of the lung by formalin steam in the controlled state of air inflation. Am Rev Respir Dis 84:856, 1961.

329. Markarian B: A simple method of inflation-fixation and air drying of lungs. Am J Clin Pathol 63:20, 1975.

330. Sutinen S, Pääkkö P, Lahti R: Post-mortem inflation, radiography and fixation of human lungs. A method for radiological and pathological correlations and morphometric studies. Scand J Respir Dis 60:29, 1979.

331. Satoh K, Sato A, Nagahara Y, et al: Improved method of preparation of inflated-fixed lung for radiologic-pathologic correlation. J Thorac Imaging 9:112, 1994.

332. Pääkkö P, Sutinen S, Lahti R: Pattern recognition in radiographs of excised air-inflated human lungs. I. Circulatory disorders in non-emphysematous lungs. Eur J Respir Dis 62:21, 1981.

333. Pääkkö P, Sutinen S, Lahti R: Pattern recognition in radiographs of excised air-inflated human lungs. II. Acute inflammation in non-emphysematous lungs. Eur J Respir Dis 62:33, 1981.

334. Pääkkö P: Pattern recognition in radiographs of excised air-inflated human lungs. III. Chronic interstitial and granulomatous inflammation, scars, and lymphangitis carcinomatosa in non-emphysematous lungs. Eur J Respir Dis 62:289, 1981.

335. Sutinen S, Pääkkö P, Lohela P, et al: Pattern recognition in radiographs of excised air-inflated human lungs. IV. Emphysema alone and with other common lesions. Eur J Respir Dis 62:297, 1981.

336. Hruban RH, Meziane MA, Zerhouni EA, et al: High resolution computed tomography of inflation-fixed lungs. Pathologic-radiologic correlation of centrilobular emphysema. Am Rev Respir Dis 136:935, 1987.

337. Hampton AO, Castleman B: Correlation of postmortem chest teleroentgenograms with autopsy findings. With special reference to pulmonary embolism and infarction. Am J Roentgenol 43:305, 1940.

338. Schlesinger MJ: New radiopaque mass for vascular injection. Lab Invest 6:1, 1957.

339. Cudkowicz L, Armstrong JB: Observations on the normal anatomy of the bronchial arteries. Thorax 6:343, 1951.

340. Tompsett DH: Anatomical Techniques. London, E & S Livingstone, 1970.

341. Liebow AA, Hales MR, Lindskog GE, et al: Plastic demonstrations of pulmonary pathology. J Bull Int Assoc Med Museums 27:116, 1947.

342. Hojo T: Scanning electron microscopy of styrene-methylethylketone casts of the airway and the arterial system of the lung. Scanning Microsc 7:287, 1993.

343. Phalen RF, Oldham MJ: Airway structures. Tracheobronchial airway structure as revealed by casting techniques. Am Rev Respir Dis 128(Suppl):1, 1983.

344. Charan NB, Turk GM, Dhand R: The role of bronchial circulation in lung abscess. Am Rev Respir Dis 131:121, 1985.

345. Timbrell V, Bovan NE, Davies AS, et al: Hollow casts of lungs for experimental purposes. Nature 225:97, 1970.

346. Dolan CT, Brown AL Jr, Ritts RE Jr: Microbiological examination of postmortem tissues. Arch Pathol 92:206, 1971.

347. Koneman EW, Davis MA: Postmortem bacteriology. III. Clinical significance of microorganisms recovered at autopsy. Am J Clin Pathol 61:28, 1974.

348. Koneman EW, Minckler TM, Shires DG, et al: Postmortem bacteriology: II. Selection of cases for culture. Am J Clin Pathol 55:17, 1971.

349. Fabregas N, Torres A, El-Ebiary M, et al: Histopathologic and microbiologic aspects of ventilator-associated pneumonia. Anesthesiology 84:760, 1996.

350. de Jongh DS, Loftis JW, Green GS, et al: Postmortem bacteriology. A practical method for routine use. Am J Clin Pathol 49:424, 1968.

351. Knapp BE, Kent TH: Postmortem lung cultures. Arch Pathol 85:200, 1968.

352. Fung JC, Sun T, Kilius I, et al: Printcultures for postmortem microbiology. Ann Clin Lab Sci 13:83, 1983.

353. Zanen-Lim OG, Zanen HC: Postmortem bacteriology of the lung by printculture of frozen tissue. A technique for in situ culture of microorganisms in whole frozen organs. J Clin Pathol 33:474, 1980.

354. Wang N-S: Applications of electron microscopy to diagnostic pulmonary pathology. Hum Pathol 14:888, 1983.

355. Ravinsky E, Qinonez GE, Paraskevas M, et al: Processing fine needle aspiration biopsies for electron microscopic examination. Experience implementing a procedure. Acta Cytol 37:661, 1993.

355a. Panchal A, Koss MN: Role of electron microscopy in interstitial lung disease. Curr Opinion Pulmon Med 3:341, 1997.

356. Bachofen M, Weibel ER, Roos B: Postmortem fixation of human lungs for electron microscopy. Am Rev Respir Dis 111:247, 1975.

357. Gondos B, McIntosh KM, Renston RH, et al: Application of electron microscopy in the definitive diagnosis of effusions. Acta Cytol 22:297, 1978.

358. Trump BF, Valigorsky JM, Jones RT, et al: The application of electron microscopy and cellular biochemistry to the autopsy. Observations on cellular changes in human shock. Hum Pathol 6:499, 1975.

359. Ferguson CC, Richardson JB: A simple technique for the utilization of postmortem tracheal and bronchial tissues for ultrastructural studies. Hum Pathol 9:463, 1978.

360. Pinkerton H, Carroll S: Fatal adenovirus pneumonia in infants. Correlation of histologic and electron microscopic observations. Am J Pathol 65:543, 1971.

361. Smith J, Coleman DV: Electron microscopy of cells showing viral cytopathic effects in Papanicolaou smears. Acta Cytol 27:605, 1983.

362. Editorial: "Immotile-cilia" syndrome and ciliary abnormalities induced by infection and injury. Am Rev Respir Dis 124:107, 1981.

363. Skikne MI, Prinsloo I, Webster I: Electron microscopy of lung in Niemann-Pick disease. J Pathol 106:119, 1972.

364. Basset F, Soler P, Jaurand MC, et al: Ultrastructural examination of bronchoalveolar lavage for diagnosis of pulmonary histiocytosis X: Preliminary report on four cases. Thorax 32:303, 1977.

365. Kullberg FC, Funahashi A, Siegesmund KA: Pulmonary eosinophilic granuloma: Electron microscopic detection of X-bodies on lung lavage cells and transbronchoscopic lung biopsy in one patient. Ann Intern Med 96:188, 1982.

366. Kuhn C: Systemic lupus erythematosus in a patient with ultrastructural lesions of the pulmonary capillaries previously reported in the Review as due to idiopathic pulmonary hemosiderosis. Am Rev Respir Dis 106:931, 1972.

367. Quinonez GE, Ravinsky E, Paraskevas M, et al: Contribution of transmission electron microscopy to fine-needle aspiration biopsy diagnosis: Comparison of cytology and combined cytology and transmission electron microscopy with final histological diagnosis. Diagn Cytopathol 15:282, 1996.

368. Heard BE, Dewar A, Firmin RK, et al: One very rare and one new tracheal tumour found by electron microscopy: Glomus tumour and acinic cell tumour resembling carcinoid tumours by light microscopy. Thorax 37:97, 1982.

369. Heilman E, Feiner H: The role of electron microscopy in the diagnosis of unusual peripheral lung tumours. Hum Pathol 9:589, 1978.

370. Chumas JC, Lorelle CA: Pulmonary meningioma. A light- and electron-microscopic study. Am J Surg Pathol 6:795, 1982.

371. Katzenstein A-LA, Maurer JJ: Benign histiocytic tumor of lung. A light- and electron-microscopic study. Am J Surg Pathol 3:61, 1979.

372. Domagala W, Woyke S: Transmission and scanning electron microscopic studies of cells in effusions. Acta Cytol 19:214, 1975.

373. Abraham JL: Recent advances in pneumoconiosis: The pathologist's role in etiologic diagnosis. In Thurlback WM, Abell MR (eds): The Lung: Structure, Function, and Disease. Baltimore, Williams & Wilkins, 1978.

374. Lapenas DJ, Davis GS, Gale PN, et al: Mineral dusts as etiologic agents in pulmonary fibrosis: The diagnostic role of analytical scanning electron microscopy. Am J Clin Pathol 78:701, 1982.

375. Ghadially FN: Invited review. The technique and scope of electron-probe x-ray analysis in pathology. Pathology 11:95, 1979.

376. Vallyathan NV, Green FHY, Craighead JE: Recent advances in the study of mineral pneumoconiosis. In Sommers SC, Rosen PP (eds): Pathology Annual. Part 2. Vol 15. New York, Appleton-Century-Crofts, 1980.

377. Domagala W, Kahan AV, Koss LG: A simple method of preparation and identification of cells for scanning electron microscopy. Acta Cytol 23:140, 1979.

378. Mikel UV, Johnson FB: A simple method for the study of the same cells by light and scanning electron microscopy. Acta Cytol 24:252, 1980.

379. Becker SN, Wong JY, Marchiondo AA, et al: Scanning electron microscopy of alcohol-fixed cytopathology specimens. Acta Cytol 25:578, 1980.

380. Ito E, Kudo R, Miyoshi M, et al: Transmission and scanning electron microscopic study of the same cytologic material. Acta Cytol 32:588, 1988.

381. Takenaga A, Matsuda M, Horai T, et al: Scanning electron microscopy in the study of lung cancer. New technique of comparative studies on the same lung cancer cells by light microscopy and scanning electron microscopy. Acta Cytol 21:90, 1977.

382. Kaneshima S, Kiyasu Y, Kudo H, et al: An application of scanning electron microscopy to cytodiagnosis of pleural and peritoneal fluids. Comparative observation of the same cells by light microscopy and scanning electron microscopy. Acta Cytol 22:490, 1978.

383. Gondos B, Lai CE, King EB: Distinction between atypical mesothelial cells and malignant cells by scanning electron microscopy. Acta Cytol 23:321, 1979.

384. McMahon JT: Analytical electron microscopy in pneumoconiosis. Cleveland Clin Q 52:503, 1985.

385. Davis JMG, Gylseth B, Morgan A: Assessment of mineral fibres from human lung tissue. Thorax 41:167, 1986.

386. Suthipintawong C, Leong AS-Y, Vinyuvat S: Immunostaining of cell preparations: A comparative evaluation of common fixatives and protocols. Diagn Cytopathol 15:167, 1996.

387. Pertschuk LP, Kim DS, Brigati DJ: Nonrenal practical applications of immunofluorescence in diagnostic pathology. In Sommers SC, Rosen PP (eds): Pathology Annual. Part 1, Vol 14. New York, Appleton-Century-Crofts, 1979.

388. Beechler CR, Enquist RW, Hunt KK, et al: Immunofluorescence of transbronchial biopsies in Goodpasture's syndrome. Am Rev Respir Dis 121:869, 1980.

389. Lowry BS, Vega FG Jr, Hedlund KW: Localization of Legionella pneumophila in tissue using FITC-conjugated specific antibody and a background stain. Am J Clin Pathol 77:601, 1982.

390. Wicher K, Kalinka C, Mlodozeniec P, et al: Fluorescent antibody technic used for identification and typing of Streptococcus pneumoniae. Am J Clin Pathol 77:72, 1982.

391. Pertschuk LP, Silverstein E, Friedland J: Immunohistologic diagnosis of sarcoidosis; detection of angiotensin-converting enzyme in sarcoid granulomas. Am J Clin Pathol 75:350, 1981.

392. Walts AE, Said JW: Specific tumor markers in diagnostic cytology. Immunoperoxidase studies of carcinoembryonic antigen, lysozyme, and other tissue antigens in effusions, washes, and aspirates. Acta Cytol 27:408, 1983.

393. To A, Dearnaley DP, Ormerod MG, et al: Indirect immunoalkaline phosphatase staining of cytologic smears of serous effusions for tumor marker studies. Acta Cytol 27:109, 1983.

394. Dalquen P, Bittel D, Gudat F, et al: Combined immunoreaction and Papanicolaou's stain on cytological smears. Pathol Res Pract 181:50, 1986.

395. Tubbs RR: Pulmonary immunohistology. Cleve Clin Q 52:473, 1985.

396. Loud AV, Anversa P: Biology of disease. Morphometric analysis of biologic processes. Lab Invest 50:250, 1984.

397. Weibel ER: Morphometry of the Human Lung. New York, Academic Press, 1963.

398. Chang L-Y, Mercer RR, Pinkerton KE, et al: Quantifying lung structure. Experimental design and biologic variation in various models of lung injury. Am Rev Respir Dis 143:625, 1991.

399. Pesce CM: Biology of disease. Defining and interpreting diseases through morphometry. Lab Invest 56:568, 1987.

400. Cooney TP, Thurlbeck WM: Pulmonary hypoplasia in Down's syndrome. N Engl J Med 307:1170, 1982.

401. Williams AJ, Vawter G, Reid LM: Lung structure in asphyxiating thoracic dystrophy. Arch Pathol Lab Med 108:658, 1984.

402. Hislop A, Reid L: New pathological findings in emphysema of childhood: 2. Overinflation of a normal lobe. Thorax 26:190, 1971.

403. Henderson R, Hislop A, Reid L: New pathological findings in emphysema of childhood: 3. Unilateral congenital emphysema with hypoplasia—and compensatory emphysema of contralateral lung. Thorax 26:195, 1971.

404. Walts AE, Morimoto R, Marchevsky AM: Computerized interactive morphometry and the diagnosis of lymphoid-rich effusions. Am J Clin Pathol 99:570, 1993.

405. Bousfield LR, Greenberg ML, Pacey F: Cytogenetic diagnosis of cancer from body fluids. Acta Cytol 29:768, 1985.

406. DeWald G, Dines DE, Weiland LH, et al: Usefulness of chromosome examination in the diagnosis of malignant pleural effusions. N Engl J Med 295:1494, 1976.

407. Metintas M, Ozdemir N, Solak M, et al: Chromosome analysis in pleural effusions. Efficiency of this method in the differential diagnosis of pleural effusions. Respiration 61:330, 1994.

408. Granados R, Cibas ES, Fletcher JA: Cytogenetic analysis of effusions from malignant mesothelioma. A diagnostic adjunct to cytology. Acta Cytol 38:711, 1994.

409. Morkve O, Halvorsen OJ, Stangeland L, et al: Quantitation of biological tumor markers (p53, c-myc, Ki-67 and DNA ploidy) by multiparameter flow cytometry in non–small-cell lung cancer. Int J Cancer 52:851, 1992.

409a. Deinlein E, Sander U, Greiner C, et al: Diagnostic significance of flow cytometric analysis applied to the detection of cancer cells in bronchial washing fluid. Anal Quant Cytol Histol 10:360, 1988.

409b. Fuhr JE, Kattine AA, Sullivan TA, et al: Flow cytometric analysis of pulmonary fluids and cells for the detection of malignancies. Am J Pathol 141:211, 1992.

410. Volm M, Drings P, Mattern J, et al: Prognostic significance of DNA patterns and resistance-predictive tests in non–small cell lung carcinoma. Cancer 56:1396, 1985.

411. Tirindelli-Danesi D, Teordori L, Mauro F, et al: Prognostic significance of flow cytometry in lung cancer. A 5-year study. Cancer 60:844, 1987.

412. Salvati F, Teodori L, Trinca ML, et al: The relevance of flow-cytometric DNA content in the evaluation of lung cancer. J Cancer Res Clin Oncol 120:233, 1994.

413. Granone P, Cardillo G, Rumi E, et al: DNA flow cytometric analysis in patients with operable non–small cell lung carcinoma. Eur J Cardiothorac Surg 7:351, 1993.

414. Volm M, Bak M, Hahn EW, et al: DNA and S-phase distribution and incidence of metastasis in human primary lung carcinoma. Cytometry 9:183, 1988.
415. Ayabe H, Tomita M, Kawahara K, et al: DNA stemline heterogeneity of non–small cell lung carcinomas and differences in DNA ploidy between carcinomas and metastatic nodes. Lung Cancer 11:201, 1994.
416. Bunn PA Jr, Carney DN, Gazdar AF, et al: Diagnostic and biological implications of flow cytometric DNA content analysis in lung cancer. Cancer Res 43:5026, 1983.
417. Volm M, Drings P, Mattern J, et al: Prognostic significance of DNA patterns and resistance-predictive tests in non–small cell lung carcinoma. Cancer 56:1396, 1985.
418. Cibas ES, Melamed MR, Zaman MB, et al: The effect of tumor size and tumor cell DNA content on the survival of patients with stage I adenocarcinoma of the lung. Cancer 63:1552, 1989.
419. Carey FA, Prasad US, Walker WS, et al: Prognostic significance of tumor deoxyribonucleic acid content in surgically resected small-cell carcinoma of lung. J Thorac Cardiovasc Surg 103:1214, 1992.
420. Morkve O, Halvorsen OJ, Skjaerven R, et al: Prognostic significance of p53 protein expression and DNA ploidy in surgically treated non–small cell lung carcinomas. Anticancer Res 13:571, 1993.
421. Sahin AA, Ro JY, El-Naggar AK, et al: Flow cytometric analysis of the DNA content of non–small cell lung cancer. Ploidy as a significant prognostic indicator in squamous cell carcinoma of the lung. Cancer 65:530, 1990.
422. Salvati F, Teodori L, Trinca ML, et al: The relevance of flow-cytometric DNA content in the evaluation of lung cancer. J Cancer Res Clin Oncol 120:233, 1994.
423. Filderman AE, Silvestri GA, Gatsonis C, et al: Prognostic significance of tumor proliferative fraction and DNA content in stage I non–small cell lung cancer. Am Rev Respir Dis 146:707, 1992.
424. Visakorpi T, Holli K, Hakama M: High cell proliferation activity determined by DNA flow cytometry and prognosis in epidermoid lung carcinoma. Acta Oncol 34:605, 1995.
425. Rice TW, Bauer TW, Gephardt GN, et al: Prognostic significance of flow cytometry in non–small-cell lung cancer. J Thorac Cardiovasc Surg 106:210, 1993.
426. Vindelov LL, Hansen HH, Christensen IJ, et al: Clonal heterogeneity of small-cell anaplastic carcinoma of the lung demonstrated by flow-cytometric DNA analysis. Cancer Res 40:4295, 1980.
427. Larsimont D, Kiss R, de Launoit Y, et al: Characterization of the morphonuclear features and DNA ploidy of typical and atypical carcinoids and small cell carcinomas of the lung. Am J Clin Pathol 94:378, 1990.
428. Jones DJ, Haseleton PS, Moore M: DNA ploidy in bronchopulmonary carcinoid tumours. Thorax 43:195, 1988.
429. Thomas M, von Eiff M, Brandt B, et al: Immunophenotyping of lymphocytes in bronchoalveolar lavage fluid. A new flow cytometric method vs standard immunoperoxidase technique. Chest 108:464, 1995.
430. Dauber JH, Wagner M, Brunsvold S, et al: Flow cytometric analysis of lymphocyte phenotypes in bronchoalveolar lavage fluid: Comparison of a two-color technique with a standard immunoperoxidase assay. Am J Respir Cell Mol Biol 7:531, 1992.
430a. Zaer FS, Braylan RC, Zander DS, et al: Multiparametric flow cytometry in the diagnosis and characterization of low-grade pulmonary mucosa-associated lymphoid tissue lymphomas. Mod Pathol 11:525, 1998.
431. Poletti V, Romagna M, Gasponi A, et al: Bronchoalveolar lavage in the diagnosis of low-grade, MALT type, B-cell lymphoma in the lung. Monaldi Arch Chest Dis 50:191, 1995.
432. Suzuki K, Tamura N, Iwase A, et al: Prognostic value of Ia + T lymphocytes in bronchoalveolar lavage fluid in pulmonary sarcoidosis. Am J Respir Crit Care Med 154:707, 1996.
432a. Sprince NL, Oliver LC, McLoud TC, et al: T-cell alveolitis in lung lavage of asbestos-exposed subjects. Am J Ind Med 21:311, 1992.
433. Crim C, Keller CA, Dunphy CH, et al: Flow cytometric analysis of lung lymphocytes in lung transplant recipients. Am J Respir Crit Care Med 153:1041, 1996.
434. Whitehead BF, Stoehr C, Finkle C, et al: Analysis of bronchoalveolar lavage from human lung transplant recipients by flow cytometry. Respir Med 89:27, 1995.
435. Wasserman K, Subklewe M, Pothoff G, et al: Expression of surface markers on alveolar macrophages from symptomatic patients with HIV infection as detected by flow cytometry. Chest 105:1324, 1994.
436. Kuo HP, Yu CT: Alveolar macrophage subpopulations in patients with active pulmonary tuberculosis. Chest 104:1773, 1993.
437. McDonald CF, Hutchinson P, Atkins RC: Delineation of pulmonary alveolar macrophage subpopulations by flow cytometry in normal subjects and in patients with lung cancer. Clin Exp Immunol 91:126, 1993.
438. Studnicka M, Wirnsberger R, Neumann M, et al: Peripheral blood lymphocyte subsets and survival in small-cell lung cancer. Chest 105:1673, 1994.
439. Jacobson DR, Fishman CL, Mills NE: Molecular genetic tumor markers in the early diagnosis and screening of non–small-cell lung cancer. Ann Oncol 3:S3, 1995.
440. Cagle PT: Molecular pathology of lung cancer and its clinical relevance. Monogr Pathol 36:134, 1993.
441. Betsuyaku T, Munakata M, Yamaguchi E, et al: Establishing diagnosis of pulmonary malignant lymphoma by gene rearrangement analysis of lymphocytes in bronchoalveolar lavage fluid. Am J Respir Crit Care Med 149:526, 1994.
442. Keicho N, Oka T, Takeuchi K, et al: Detection of lymphomatous involvement of the lung by bronchoalveolar lavage. Application of immunophenotypic and gene rearrangement analysis. Chest 105:458, 1994.
443. Kavuru MS, Tubbs R, Miller ML, et al: Immunocytometry and gene rearrangement analysis in the diagnosis of lymphoma in an idiopathic pleural effusion. Am Rev Respir Dis 145:209, 1992.
444. de Lassence A, Lecossier D, Pierre C, et al: Detection of mycobacterial DNA in pleural fluid from patients with tuberculous pleurisy by means of the polymerase chain reaction: Comparison of two protocols. Thorax 47:265, 1992.
445. Pierre C, Olivier C, Lecossier D, et al: Diagnosis of primary tuberculosis in children by amplification and detection of mycobacterial DNA. Am Rev Respir Dis 147:420, 1993.
446. Yuen KY, Chan KS, Chan CM, et al: Use of PCR in routine diagnosis of treated and untreated pulmonary tuberculosis. J Clin Pathol 46:318, 1993.
447. Tjhie JH, van Kuppeveld FJ, Roosendaal R, et al: Direct PCR enables detection of *Mycoplasma pneumoniae* in patients with respiratory tract infections. J Clin Microbiol 32:11, 1994.
448. Honda J, Hoshino T, Natori H, et al: Rapid and sensitive diagnosis of cytomegalovirus and *Pneumocystis carinii* pneumonia in patients with haematological neoplasia by using capillary polymerase chain reaction. Br J Haematol 86:138, 1994.
449. Chehab FF, Xiao X, Kan YW, et al: Detection of cytomegalovirus infection in paraffin-embedded tissue specimens with the polymerase chain reaction. Mod Pathol 2:75, 1989.
450. Shibata D, Almoguera C, Forrester K, et al: Detection of c-K-ras mutations in fine-needle aspirates from human pancreatic adenocarcinomas. Cancer Res 50:1279, 1990.

CHAPTER 15

Endoscopy and Diagnostic Biopsy Procedures

ENDOSCOPIC PROCEDURES, 366
    Laryngoscopy, 366
    Esophagoscopy and Upper Gastrointestinal Endoscopy, 367
    Bronchoscopy, 367
        Technical Considerations, 367
        Indications and Yield, 367
BIOPSY PROCEDURES, 369
    Bronchial Biopsy, 369
    Transbronchial Biopsy, 369
    Transthoracic Needle Biopsy, 370
    Thoracoscopy and Video-Assisted Thoracoscopic Surgery, 371
    Open Lung Biopsy by Thoracotomy, 372
    Closed Pleural Biopsy, 372
    Mediastinoscopy and Anterior Mediastinoscopy, 373
    Scalene Lymph Node Biopsy, 374

In some cases of pulmonary disease, tissue biopsy is necessary to confirm or establish a diagnosis. As with material acquired for cytologic assessment (*see* page 339), biopsy can be accomplished by a number of techniques, each of which has its own type and rate of complications and diagnostic yield. It is unrealistic to make hard-and-fast rules regarding what type of lesion requires a biopsy and which procedure should be used; each case must be considered individually, with both the patient and the clinical situation taken into account. Before discussing specific techniques, it is appropriate to emphasize several features that are common to all.

1. Despite the fact that reported instances of mortality are rare and morbidity is seldom serious, it must be remembered that *every* method of obtaining tissue can result in complications. Thus, biopsy is only indicated if there is at least some reasonable chance that it will provide information guiding specific and useful therapy.

2. When considering the merits of a particular technique, it is necessary to take into account both the experience of its proponents—who will generally obtain results superior to those of less experienced investigators—and the specific expertise available in the local milieu. In fact, the various techniques have been infrequently compared by the same observer. In an extensive review of the literature in which the results of biopsies in chronic diffuse lung disease were compared, the combined results of a number of investigators

gave total yields of 63% for cutting needle biopsy, 72% for transbronchial biopsy, and 94% for open-lung biopsy.[1]

3. In most circumstances, the procedure chosen should be influenced by the particular diagnosis suspected clinically. For example, a lymph node in the supraclavicular fossa might simply be aspirated if the clinical situation suggests a diagnosis of metastatic pulmonary carcinoma; however, it might be excised completely if lymphoma is suspected.

4. Although biopsy is usually performed to obtain material for histologic study, in many cases it is essential that some tissue be sent to the microbiology laboratory for culture.

5. It is important to remember that a biopsy often samples only a portion of a particular disease process. Thus because of possible variation in distribution and severity, especially in diffuse pulmonary disease, the findings in one biopsy specimen cannot necessarily be extrapolated to all regions.

6. Correlation of clinical, radiologic, and pathologic findings frequently provides a more precise diagnosis than is possible with each alone, and close cooperation between specialists should be encouraged.

ENDOSCOPIC PROCEDURES

Fiberoptic bronchoscopy is the endoscopic procedure of most use to chest physicians. However, laryngoscopy and upper gastrointestinal endoscopy sometimes play important roles in the evaluation of patients who have pulmonary disease.

Laryngoscopy

The larynx can be examined indirectly by the use of a mirror or directly; the latter may be combined with bronchoscopy. Laryngoscopy should be performed in any patient who complains of a persistent, dry, hacking or brassy cough, particularly when the cough is associated with hoarseness. The vocal cords should be well seen, not only to exclude a local lesion but also to detect paralysis that would account for the hoarseness. In the latter instance, chest radiography or CT may reveal a mediastinal lesion.

Esophagoscopy and Upper Gastrointestinal Endoscopy

Pulmonary disease may occur in association with several esophageal abnormalities, and the diagnosis may be facilitated by direct endoscopic examination of the esophagus. Aspiration pneumonia may be secondary to esophageal diverticula, achalasia, or stenosis from peptic ulceration or neoplasia. When the origin of expectorated blood is not known, direct view of the upper gastrointestinal tract may detect bleeding esophageal varices or peptic ulceration. Diffuse pulmonary disease can also occur in association with dysphagia in patients with progressive systemic sclerosis, in which case esophagoscopy and esophageal motility studies may be required to confirm the diagnosis.

Bronchoscopy

Flexible fiberoptic bronchoscopy is a safe and relatively easy procedure that has proved extremely useful in the diagnosis and management of many pulmonary diseases; the ease of access to the lung parenchyma by lavage and biopsy has also made it a valuable research tool for the investigation of disease pathogenesis. Guidelines for use of the procedure have been published by the American Thoracic Society (Table 15–1).[2]

Technical Considerations

Satisfactory bronchoscopy requires the patient's confidence in the bronchoscopist; explanation of the procedure and reassurance take only a few minutes and may greatly facilitate examination. Differences of opinion exist regarding the need for prebronchoscopic sedation, the type of anesthesia, the indications for rigid versus flexible fiberoptic bronchoscopy, and the method of insertion of the instrument.[3, 4] There appears to be general agreement that atropine sulfate is indicated prior to the procedure,[5] since it not only reduces bronchial secretions but also may prevent bradycardia and reflex bronchoconstriction produced by the stimulation of vagal nerve endings.[6] However, it should be remembered that the drug tends to dry secretions, and removal of tenacious secretions may be more difficult after its use. In addition, some investigators have been unable to confirm its theoretical benefits by objective assessment.[6a] Ideally, the drug should be administered about 1½ hours prior to the procedure to allow for the elimination of accumulated secretions and to block further secretions from forming.[3] Although some form of sedation is commonly advocated and is almost certainly necessary in children who are going to be examined under local anesthesia, it is not an absolute requirement in adults.[7, 8] It is our usual practice to administer intravenous midazolam prior to bronchoscopy; however, we omit such sedation under some circumstances (for example, an ambulatory patient who is unaccompanied).

Lidocaine is currently the topical anesthetic of choice for bronchoscopy.[3, 9] It can be applied directly to the upper airways[9] and can be injected through the bronchoscopic channel or nebulized for anesthesia of the lower airways.[3, 10] Although the drug can be safely administered in high doses to patients without liver or cardiovascular disease,[11] central nervous system toxicity can occur in small patients or in those in whom the drug is metabolized slowly;[12] methemoglobinemia has also been reported in a susceptible individual.[13] In one trial, intratracheal cocaine in combination with lidocaine nasal jelly, benzocaine lozenges, and the application of 10% lidocaine spray to the posterior pharynx furnished better results than those obtained by the same preparatory regimen in combination with nebulized lidocaine.[14] It should be borne in mind that some local anesthetics have antibacterial action; for example, tetracaine inhibits the growth of *Mycobacterium tuberculosis* in culture,[15, 16] and lidocaine (even without preservative) is said to inhibit the growth of fungi and nontuberculous bacteria.[3] Fortunately, the concentration of lidocaine found in specimens is usually well below the maximum inhibitory concentration of these organisms.[3]

On the rare occasion when general rather than local anesthesia is used, the patient should be closely monitored in the postbronchoscopic period for hypoventilation occasioned by the anesthetic or by neuromuscular blocking agents.[17] Resuscitative facilities should be available for even routine endoscopic procedures. Fiberoptic bronchoscopy has a role to play in emergency situations at the bedside as well, notably in the intensive care unit.[18] It is our practice to administer supplemental oxygen to all patients during this procedure. Routine chest radiography following bronchoscopy is not justified.[19, 20]

As indicated previously, diagnostic bronchoscopy is a relatively safe procedure in experienced hands, the mortality in several large series ranging from 0% to 0.1%.[21–26] Major complications include pneumonia,[4, 21, 27, 28] aspiration of gastric contents,[29] septic shock with acute pulmonary edema,[30] pneumothorax, and hemorrhage (the last two almost always associated with transbronchial biopsy).[21, 22, 24, 25, 31] In a large mail survey of randomly selected members of the American College of Chest Physicians, more than three quarters of the 871 respondents reported a major complication (bleeding of more than 50 ml, respiratory distress, pneumothorax, or death) rate of less than 2.5% and more than 80% reported a minor complication (hypoxemia, arrhythmia, bleeding of less than 50 ml) rate of less than 10%.[4] The incidence of complications is probably related to the experience of those performing the procedure and the presence of conditions increasing the risk of the intervention, such as recent myocardial infarction, bleeding disorders, refractory hypoxemia, and unstable arrhythmias. Bronchoscopy has been performed safely in the elderly,[32] in acutely ill mechanically ventilated patients,[33] and in patients who have asthma[34, 35] or significant thrombocytopenia.[36]

Indications and Yield

A major indication for bronchoscopy is the acquisition of material for the diagnosis of suspected pulmonary infection. Use of protected specimen brushing or quantitative bronchoalveolar lavage appears to be helpful in differentiating true pathogens from colonizing organisms in the airway,[37–40] a distinction of particular importance in patients with adult respiratory distress syndrome who are mechanically ventilated. Bronchoscopy with lavage is also a valuable tool in the diagnosis of infection in an immunocompromised host,[41, 42] especially patients with the acquired immunodeficiency syndrome (AIDS).[43, 44]

Table 15–1. GUIDELINES FOR FIBEROPTIC BRONCHOSCOPY IN ADULTS

A. Diagnostic Uses
1. To evaluate lung lesions of unknown etiology that appear on the chest roentgenogram as a density, infiltrate, atelectasis, or localized hyperlucency.
2. To assess airway patency.
3. To investigate unexplained hemoptysis, unexplained cough (or change in the nature of a cough), localized wheeze, or stridor.
4. To search for the origin of suspicious or positive sputum cytology.
5. To investigate the etiology of unexplained paralysis of a vocal cord or hemidiaphragm, superior vena cava syndrome, chylothorax, or unexplained pleural effusion.
6. To evaluate problems associated with endotracheal tubes such as tracheal damage, airway obstruction, or tube placement.
7. To stage lung cancer preoperatively and subsequently to evaluate, when appropriate, the response to therapy.
8. To obtain material for microbiologic studies in suspected pulmonary infections.
9. To evaluate the airways for suspected bronchial tear or other injury after thoracic trauma.
10. To evaluate a suspected tracheoesophageal fistula.
11. To determine the location and extent of respiratory tract injury after acute inhalation of noxious fumes or aspiration of gastric contents.
12. To obtain material for study from the lungs of patients with diffuse or focal lung diseases.

B. Therapeutic Uses
1. To remove retained secretions or mucous plugs not mobilized by conventional noninvasive techniques.
2. To remove foreign bodies.
3. To remove abnormal endobronchial tissue or foreign material by use of forceps or laser techniques.
4. To perform difficult intubations, e.g., in patients with cervical spondylitis, dental problems, myasthenia gravis, acromegaly, achalasia, full stomach, small bowel obstruction, and trauma to the head, neck, larynx, or trachea.

C. Research Applications
Multiple and varied applications include but are not limited to the study of tracheal mucous velocity, regional gas exchange, cilial structure and function, and the chemical and cellular nature of material obtained by bronchoalveolar lavage.

D. Conditions Involving Increased Risk
As in all clinical situations, the risk of bronchoscopy must be weighed against the potential benefit for the patient. Sound clinical judgment and careful assessment of each patient must predominate, especially in decisions regarding the need for hospitalization. Increased risk situations include
1. Lack of patient cooperation.
2. Recent myocardial infarction or unstable angina.
3. Partial tracheal obstruction.
4. Unstable bronchial asthma.
5. Respiratory insufficiency associated with moderate to severe hypoxemia or any degree of hypercarbia.
6. Uremia and pulmonary hypertension (possibility of serious hemorrhage after biopsy).
7. Lung abscess (danger of flooding the airway with purulent material).
8. Immunosuppression (danger of postbronchoscopy infection).
9. Obstruction of the superior vena cava (possibility of bleeding and laryngeal edema).
10. Debility, advanced age, and malnutrition.
11. Unstable cardiac arrhythmia.
12. Respiratory failure requiring mechanical ventilation.
13. Disorders requiring laser therapy, biopsy of lesions obstructing large airways, or multiple transbronchial lung biopsies.

The danger of a serious complication from bronchoscopy is especially high in patients with the following conditions:
1. Malignant arrhythmia.
2. Profound refractory hypoxemia.
3. Severe bleeding diathesis that cannot be corrected when biopsy is anticipated.

In most situations involving increased risk, patient safety requires hospitalization and overnight observation after the procedure.

E. Contraindications
1. Absence of consent from the patient or the patient's representative.
2. Bronchoscopy by an inexperienced person without direct supervision.
3. Bronchoscopy without adequate facilities and personnel to care for such emergencies as cardiopulmonary arrest, pneumothorax, or bleeding.
4. Inability to adequately oxygenate the patient during the procedure.

F. Additional Comments
1. In most patients with undiagnosed pulmonary disorders and in those requiring therapeutic intervention, bronchoscopy is but one component of their overall evaluation or treatment.
2. The fiberoptic bronchoscope is the instrument of choice when bronchoscopy is needed for patients on mechanical ventilators or in those with disease or trauma involving the skull, jaws, or cervical spine.
3. The rigid open-tube bronchoscope is the instrument of choice during massive hemoptysis.
4. Outpatients may be bronchoscoped in the hospital in a day-care setting.
5. When out-of-hospital bronchoscopy is performed, there should be adequate facilities and personnel to care for emergencies and to properly handle specimens.
6. Bronchoscopy should not be used routinely as a substitute for conventional noninvasive techniques for mobilizing pulmonary secretions.
7. Bronchoscopy is not a routine initial procedure in the evaluation of unexplained cough.
8. Bronchoscopy is not routinely necessary to obtain sputum for diagnostic study in cases of pneumonia or acute bronchitis.

From Burgher LW, Jones FL, Patterson JR, et al: Am Rev Respir Dis 136:1066, 1987. Official Statement of the American Thoracic Society. © American Lung Association.

Bronchoscopy is the primary diagnostic tool in patients with suspected pulmonary carcinoma; in addition, it is essential in the assessment of resectability and staging of patients with central tumors.[44a] Clinical symptoms of unexplained hemoptysis, prolonged cough, or change in the character of the cough, as well as findings of a focal wheeze or stridorous breathing, all suggest the possibility of underlying malignancy. The etiology of unexplained vocal cord or hemidiaphragm paralysis, superior vena cava syndrome, chylothorax, or pleural or pericardial effusion might well be determined by bronchoscopic examination of the airways; the source of malignant cells detected on cytologic examination of airway secretions may also be determined at bronchoscopy.[45] Radiographic findings of atelectasis, focal hyperinflation, and recurrent or poorly resolving pneumonia strongly suggest the presence of occult endobronchial obstruction, whereas the utility of bronchoscopy in the evaluation and diagnosis of radiographic central masses is self-evident.[46] Although commonly performed in patients with solitary pulmonary nodules, the usefulness of the procedure in this setting has been questioned (*see* page 1193).[47]

The importance of careful and appropriate case selection to the enhancement of diagnostic yield cannot be overly stressed. For example, bronchoscopy is useful for the diagnosis of neoplasia in patients with pleural effusion if there is associated hemoptysis or radiographic abnormalities suggesting a tumor; however, the yield is poor if these features are lacking.[48, 49] Similarly, in patients with hemoptysis and a normal or nonspecific chest radiograph, bronchoscopy is much more likely to yield a diagnosis of cancer in patients who are older or who have recurrent hemoptysis or a history of smoking.[52] Bronchoscopy has little role in the initial investigation of most patients with chronic refractory cough; however, it may be useful in the diagnosis of this symptom in patients in whom the history, physical examination, pulmonary function testing, and empiric therapy have failed to determine its etiology or lead to its resolution.[52]

Other diagnostic uses of bronchoscopy include the evaluation of airway patency, endotracheal or endobronchial tube placement, airway damage associated with prolonged endotracheal intubation or other trauma,[53] tracheal-esophageal fistula, and inhalational airway injury.[2] Proponents of bronchoscopy using tissue autofluorescence have reported improved sensitivity for the detection of early carcinoma and dysplasia of the bronchial mucosa in comparison to standard bronchoscopy.[54–56] Some bronchoscopists have used endoscopic ultrasound to determine the depth of tumor infiltration into the bronchial wall or adjacent structures; such examination may also provide information complementary to that of conventional radiography and CT in the assessment of mediastinal and hilar lymph node involvement by carcinoma so that the optimal site for transbronchial lymph node biopsy can be chosen.[57, 58] Bronchoscopy allows bronchoalveolar lavage and transbronchial biopsy; as discussed farther on (*see* page 370), material from these procedures is important in the diagnosis of a variety of infections and other causes of diffuse infiltrative lung disease.[59]

Bronchoscopy also serves a number of therapeutic functions. It is commonly used in the treatment of alveolar proteinosis, in which it may be lifesaving. The techniques of endobronchial laser and other resectional surgery, brachytherapy, and stent placement are helpful in re-establishing airway patency in a variety of clinical situations.[60–67] Bronchoscopic visualization of the airway is invaluable to the anesthetist and intensivist in the performance of difficult intubation[2, 68, 69] and in the placement of double-lumen tubes for thoracic surgery.[68] It has been used for the placement of sealants to close bronchopleural fistulas[70, 71] and in the removal of foreign bodies,[72, 73] inspissated secretions, or mucous plugs[5, 74] not cleared from the airway by less invasive means. Bronchoscopic biopsy has been credited with the cure of a patient with carcinoma *in situ*,[75] and we have seen other examples of this serendipitous outcome.

Although the fiberoptic bronchoscope is suitable for most procedures, rigid bronchoscopy is preferable for the management of massive hemoptysis,[2] stent placement, and laser resection of endobronchial tissue.[64, 76]

BIOPSY PROCEDURES

The bronchial approach for obtaining histologic or cytologic material for diagnosis is used not only because of its high yield but also because of the low incidence of complications. Tissue can be obtained directly from endoscopically visible lesions (bronchial biopsy) and by transbronchial biopsy of the lung parenchyma. Lavage is useful for obtaining samples from the lung periphery for microbiologic or cytologic analysis (*see* page 343).

Bronchial Biopsy

The principal value of proximal airway bronchoscopic biopsy is in the diagnosis of malignancy and the establishment of tumor cell type. A diagnosis of sarcoidosis can also often be confirmed; other abnormalities, such as benign endobronchial neoplasms and endobronchial tuberculosis, are detected less commonly. Endoscopically visible lesions in the proximal bronchial tree can be brushed, washed, aspirated with a needle, or biopsied with forceps. The first three of these procedures have already been discussed; with respect to total yield, they are complementary to tissue biopsy (*see* page 342).[77, 78]

The overall diagnostic yield of biopsies of tumors that are bronchoscopically visible ranges from about 90% to 95%.[79–81] Multiple biopsies are useful; for example, in one investigation the diagnostic yield was 92% with brushings and a single forceps biopsy and 96% with multiple biopsies.[81] Because of the small amount of tissue sampled, agreement between tumor histologic type on biopsy and excised specimens is not always present; for example, in one investigation of 107 non–small cell tumors, a discrepancy between the two was found in 41 (38%).[82] However, the distinction between small cell and non-small cell carcinoma is very dependable.

Transbronchial Biopsy

Anderson is given credit for the first description of transbronchial biopsy (TBB) following his observation that bronchial biopsy specimens of small airways harvested during the course of rigid bronchoscopy often contained lung parenchyma.[83] The techniques used to perform TBB have been well described.[84] Although there is some debate concerning appropriate instrumentation,[84, 85] large forceps obtain significantly more alveolar tissue than do small ones.[86] In the setting of infection, larger tissue samples are associated with an increased diagnostic yield.[87] The procedure can be performed safely in outpatients[88, 89] and without fluoroscopy in patients with diffuse parenchymal radiographic abnormalities.[90–92] Complications of "significant" bleeding and pneumothorax occur in fewer than 2% of patients in skilled hands.[88, 89] Temperature greater than 38° C occurred in 5 of 50 (10%) patients in one series;[93] no bacteremia was detected. Uncorrected coagulopathy, uremia, a platelet count of less than $50,000/\mu l$, and pulmonary hypertension are strong relative contraindications.[94]

The most fruitful and widespread application of TBB is in the diagnosis of diffuse lung disease. It yields diagnostic material in a high proportion of patients who have sarcoidosis and lymphangitic carcinomatosis[84, 95–97] and has an important role in the diagnosis of rejection and the exclusion of opportunistic infection in lung transplant recipients.[94] The procedure can also yield specific diagnoses of more uncommon diseases such as Langerhans' cell histiocytosis, pulmonary alveolar proteinosis, Goodpasture's syndrome, eosinophilic pneumonia, and Wegener's granulomatosis.[84, 84a] It is generally not helpful in the diagnosis and management of idiopathic pulmonary fibrosis.[84] Although largely supplanted by bronchoalveolar lavage, TTB also has a high diagnostic yield in patients with AIDS and *Pneumocystis carinii* pneumonia or in those with sputum smear–negative tuberculosis.[84]

TTB has also been used in the diagnosis of peripheral tumors. For example, in one study of 46 peripheral carcinomas less than 2 cm in diameter, the experienced bronchoscopists were able to obtain a diagnosis of malignancy in 45 cases by using localizing bronchography, a curet, and fluoroscopy.[98] When fluoroscopy is used without bronchography, the diagnostic yield in malignant lesions ranges from 70% to 90%;[99–102] as might be expected, the yield for benign lesions is considerably lower.[100, 103]

Transthoracic Needle Biopsy

Transthoracic needle biopsy (TTNB) is a procedure whereby a core of lung, lymph node, or tumor tissue is obtained by the use of a cutting needle. The optimal technique for performing the procedure as well as range of instruments available with their purported advantages and disadvantages have been reviewed.[104, 104a, b] Although several passes may be required in some cases,[105, 106] only two aspirations are necessary in the majority.[107]

TTNB offers no advantage over fine-needle aspiration (transthoracic needle aspiration [TTNA]) in the diagnosis of pulmonary carcinoma[108–112] and has substantially higher complication rates. However, the larger samples provided by cutting needle biopsies are more likely to be diagnostic in benign lesions,[113–117] including those characterized by more diffuse disease such as vasculitis and infection.[118–122] There is also substantial evidence that TTNB under CT guidance is useful in the examination of hilar and mediastinal masses for the staging of lung cancer;[123–126] however, it is not appropriate for the examination of normal-sized nodes and may not enable precise histologic classification of lymphoma.[127] It is safer, less costly, and better tolerated than thoracotomy or mediastinoscopy.[104]

Most TTNB procedures can be done under fluoroscopic guidance, an approach that is suitable when the lesion is visible in two 90-degree planes.[126] When this approach is not possible, CT is useful for determining the optimal approach; it offers superb resolution of anatomic structures (thereby lessening the risk of vascular complications), permits documentation of needle position within the lesion, helps avoid biopsy of necrotic areas in larger lesions, and is useful in planning the simplest and safest route for needle placement.[104] Ultrasound guidance is also helpful in avoiding the necrotic centers of some lung masses[128] and may be used when a lesion abuts the pleura.

The most common complication of TTNB is pneumothorax. In one series of 122 patients who underwent biopsy with a 20-gauge automated cutting needle, it developed in 54%;[129] 15% required catheter drainage. Although it has been suggested that CT-guided biopsy may result in an increased frequency of pneumothorax, following the documentation of a 37% rate in one review,[130] most studies have been associated with a rate of about 20% to 25% (values similar to those of TTNA under fluoroscopic guidance).[106, 131] The most important risk factor for pneumothorax is the presence of obstructive lung disease; in one study, patients who had normal spirometric test results and radiographs that did not demonstrate any findings suggestive of air-flow obstruction had a 7% pneumothorax rate;[132] by contrast, pneumothorax developed in approximately 45% of patients with radiographic and spirometric findings of obstructive lung disease, many requiring chest tube placement.

Although severe hemorrhage is more likely to occur with the use of larger biopsy needles,[104, 133, 134] even small needles have been associated with fatal hemorrhage in patients with coagulopathy.[135] Overall, hemoptysis occurs in 10% to 15% of patients.[136–138] Other rarer complications of TTNB include cerebral air embolism[138a, b] (which some have estimated to be the most common cause of death from this procedure[139]) lobar or lung torsion,[139a, b] and seeding of the needle tract by malignant cells.[140] In one study of 502 carefully selected patients who underwent biopsy with a Hausser needle (a 14-gauge cutting needle), pneumothorax developed in 43 (9%) (only 12 necessitating chest tube drainage), 3 experienced hemothorax requiring chest tube drainage, 27 (5%) had hemoptysis of less than 30 ml, and 5 had an intrapulmonary hematoma;[141] no fatalities were reported.

Some have attributed their high diagnostic yield and low complication rate when performing TTNB in patients with both consolidation[119] and lung nodules[142] to the use of ultrasound guidance; 3 of the 60 patients examined had minor complications. Exclusion of higher-risk patients, such as those who are uncooperative or who have significant chronic obstructive pulmonary disease or bleeding diathesis, can also diminish complication rates. In one study of 228 patients with diffuse lung disease in whom such selection was undertaken, serious complications were few;[122] although pneumothorax developed in 25% of the patients, only 2 (1%) required chest tube placement.

In conclusion, the diagnostic accuracy of TTNB is high,[120, 143, 144] and careful attention to patient selection will minimize the risk of complications and maximize the number of patients who will benefit from the procedure.[122]

Thoracoscopy and Video-Assisted Thoracoscopic Surgery

Thoracoscopy is a procedure in which the visceral and parietal pleura can be directly examined by insertion of an instrument through a small incision in the chest wall.[145] Although first described as a diagnostic tool by the Swedish internist H.C. Jacobaeus,[146] it found its most widespread early use in the lysis of pleural adhesions to maintain "therapeutic" pneumothoraces in patients with tuberculosis.[147] The advent of video technology and development of appropriate instrumentation has allowed video-assisted thoracoscopic surgery (VATS) to extend this minimally invasive approach to the performance of a wide variety of diagnostic and therapeutic maneuvers in the chest.[148–151]

The primary use of "medical" thoracoscopy is for the diagnosis of pleural disease.[152, 152a] After pneumothorax induction, an endoscope (thoracoscope, fiberoptic bronchoscope, or mediastinoscope) is inserted through an incision in an intercostal space and the pleura is examined; biopsy of the pleura or underlying lung can be performed through the same or a second opening in the thoracic cage. Anesthesia can be local,[153] regional,[154] or general.[155] The procedure appears to be well tolerated by both children and adults,[151, 156, 157] including patients who demonstrate some degree of hypoxemia prior to its initiation.[158] In addition to diagnosis, thoracoscopy has also been useful in the management of recurrent pneumothorax associated with apical "blebs," the lesions having been successfully resected via the thoracoscope under local anaesthesia.[159]

There is good evidence that thoracoscopic biopsy is the diagnostic method of choice in the investigation of patients with persistent pleural effusion in whom a diagnosis has not been established by closed pleural biopsy and/or fluid aspiration. For example, in one series of 150 patients with malignant effusion, the diagnosis was established in 131 (87%), whereas the combined yield of needle biopsy and pleural fluid cytology was only 41%.[160] In a second series of 102 patients with pleural effusion (91 patients) or pleural masses (11 patients) in whom there was no diagnosis after the examination of pleural fluid and closed biopsy specimens, thoracoscopy established a diagnosis in 95;[157] the procedure had a sensitivity of 96% and a negative predictive value of 93% for the diagnosis of pleural malignancy. In this series, 2 patients had major complications without mortality (vascular collapse with ventricular tachycardia in 1 patient and massive subcutaneous emphysema in another); minor complications such as air leak, fever, or minor bleeding at the biopsy site occurred in 5.5%. These results were similar to those found in a retrospective review of 182 patients at the Cleveland Clinic, in which the diagnostic sensitivity for malignancy was found to be 95%.[161] Fifteen per cent of patients in this series had a major complication such as bleeding requiring transfusion, prolonged air leak, empyema, pneumonia, wound infection, entry into the peritoneum, congestive heart failure, pneumothorax, myocardial infarction, pulmonary laceration, or seizure; 1 death was directly attributed to the thoracoscopy itself. Thoracoscopy is of particular

value in the diagnosis of mesothelioma;[162] in one study of 153 patients with this tumor, it confirmed the diagnosis in 150,[162] results that are comparable to those of thoracotomy.[163]

The development of VATS technology has added both complexity to and opportunity for the diagnosis and treatment of lung disease. In contrast to "medical" thoracoscopy, VATS is usually performed under general anesthesia in the operating room with selective lung ventilation.[150] Trocars and cannulas are used to establish ports for viewing, whereas a variety of sophisticated instruments are used for surgery. Although direct comparisons to open thoracotomy are scanty, purported advantages of the procedure include reduced pain with faster recovery and the ability to operate with greater safety on sicker patients.[164–167] Disadvantages include increased cost and invasiveness in comparison to thoracentesis and closed pleural biopsy; in addition, the opportunity for bimanual palpation and binocular inspection of the lung is lost, and there is a decreased ability to control hemorrhage in comparison to open thoracotomy.[150]

Thoracoscopy has also been used to provide biopsy material in patients with diffuse interstitial lung disease, the diagnostic yield ranging from 90% to 100%.[168–170] In one retrospective investigation, 22 patients undergoing VATS for biopsy of diffuse interstitial disease were compared with 21 patients who had undergone open-lung biopsy in the preceding 6-month period;[171] although the operative time and amount of tissue obtained were similar for the two procedures, VATS was associated with significant reductions in the length of pleural drainage, hospital stay, and complications. In similar studies, VATS provided better visualization of the lung, shorter hospitalization, and fewer complications than did open-lung biopsy.[166, 172] Another group of investigators compared patients undergoing VATS with patients undergoing conventional posterolateral thoracotomy for a variety of indications, including diffuse lung disease;[173] the VATS patients had a shorter length of stay and less analgesia requirement than did the thoracotomy patients. Although other workers have found that the VATS approach to the diagnosis of interstitial lung disease increased cost with no counterbalancing advantages,[174] most have found it to be the procedure of choice when transbronchial biopsies have yielded inconclusive results or are not considered appropriate. Open-lung biopsy is indicated when the patient is mechanically ventilated, unstable, or suffering from a coagulopathy.[150]

VATS may also be used to assess the mediastinum for the staging of lung cancer. The procedure allows biopsy of lymph nodes that are difficult to reach or inaccessible by cervical mediastinoscopy or anterior mediastinotomy,[175] including the posterior subcarinal nodes, paraesophageal nodes, inferior pulmonary ligament nodes, and (at times) the hilar nodes.[150] Despite these advantages, the procedure does not replace the need for staging mediastinoscopy, which enables better assessment of superior mediastinal disease and is associated with lower complication rates and a shorter duration of hospital stay.[176, 177] In addition, hilar lymph nodes are not always accessible by VATS; for example, in one study of 11 patients with malignant N1 nodes and lung cancer, only 6 were successfully identified.[178] Based on this preliminary information, it seems reasonable to conclude that VATS exploration of the mediastinum may confirm unresectability in some patients with cancer and enlarged mediastinal nodes on CT scan in whom cervical mediastinoscopy is negative, thereby avoiding a full thoracotomy. If the nodes prove to be benign and no other contraindications (such as parietal pleural involvement by tumor) are detected, curative resection can immediately follow the VATS biopsy. Some authors have suggested that VATS should precede thoracotomy for cancer;[179] however, the cost-benefit ratio of this strategy remains to be determined. VATS can also be used to obtain tissue for diagnosis in patients with mediastinal masses when TTNB has failed to provide a diagnosis or is inappropriate.[180, 181]

When the etiology of a solitary peripheral pulmonary nodule is unclear after less invasive investigation, thoracoscopy offers a means of excisional biopsy. If the nodule proves to be pulmonary carcinoma on frozen section examination, thoracotomy can be performed at the same time for more appropriate staging and for assurance of adequacy of the resection; on the other hand, if it is shown to be benign or a metastasis, the patient can be spared full thoracotomy.[181a] Patients who have limited lung reserve precluding lobectomy can also be offered resection of a carcinoma with minimal excision of lung tissue.[182, 183] A number of techniques have been described to aid in localization of the nodule at the time of VATS.[184–186] When compared with wedge resection via thoracotomy, there is no cost advantage to a VATS resection;[183–187] however, pain and duration of the hospital stay are less.[183, 187] VATS can also be used in the management of chest trauma, allowing the identification and control of bleeding sites and the repair of diaphragmatic injuries.[187a, b]

Complications of VATS are similar to those of medical thoracoscopy and include bleeding, air leak, tumor seeding at the entry site, fever, wound infection, and death.[150, 151, 188, 189] In one study of 266 VATS procedures over a 1-year period, complications were identified in 10%;[190] there were no deaths. Prolonged air leak occurred in approximately 4% of the cases, wound infection in 2%, and significant bleeding in 2%; in 11 patients (4%), thoracotomy was required after the VATS approach failed to achieve its intended goal. It was the authors' impression that patients had less pain and resumed normal activity more quickly. The VATS study group reported 38 deaths (2.1%) among 1,820 cases performed at over 40 institutions; no patients died intraoperatively and many of the deaths were not directly attributable to the procedure.[191] An analysis of 307 VATS procedures in the elderly (including segmental and lobar resection) revealed a mortality rate of less than 1%, major morbidity extending the length of stay in 7% and minor complications occurring in 9%.[192] The median length of stay was 4 days for patients aged 65 to 79 years, and 5 days for those aged 80 to 90; the authors concluded that these results compared favorably with those reported in the literature for thoracotomy.

Open Lung Biopsy by Thoracotomy

In this technique, the chest is opened through a standard thoracotomy incision or through a limited incision large enough to allow removal of a fragment of tissue measuring 2 to 3 cm in diameter. Some have preferred a modified Chamberlain approach, in which the thorax is entered in the second interspace, for easy access to all pulmonary lobes

and the mediastinum.[193] When a small incision is used, pulmonary parenchyma is ballooned out by exerting positive pressure on the lung, a clamp is applied, and the tissue is removed. This technique is particularly applicable when the disease is so diffuse that any portion of the lung is likely to be abnormal. When disease is more confined, a full thoracotomy incision is recommended so that the surgeon can examine the lung and choose the best site for biopsy; although the larger incision is not associated with higher morbidity or mortality, it usually necessitates a longer hospital stay.

Selection of the appropriate site for biopsy is clearly important. Areas of discrete disease should be removed *en bloc* if small enough to be included in the specimen; if more extensive disease is present, the biopsy should include an area of transition between abnormal and apparently normal lung. It is probably unwise to biopsy only very abnormal areas since these areas may show end-stage disease in which the etiology may be difficult to determine.[193] Our own recommendation is that samples from more than one site should be taken if surgically feasible to have a better appreciation of the spectrum of pulmonary disease; however, some investigators have found that when appropriate samples are taken from areas of radiologic abnormality, biopsies from additional sites are unnecessary.[194] The tip of the lingula not uncommonly shows nonspecific chronic vascular changes and fibrosis, and it has been argued that this region should be avoided for biopsy;[195] however, in one investigation of 20 patients with diffuse lung disease, biopsies of the lingula and a separate region of lung yielded similar results.[196]

In general, the biopsy specimens should be submitted to a pathologist as soon as possible after excision. Portions may then be selected for ancillary investigations (such as electron microscopy, immunofluorescence, and flow cytometry), and frozen sections can be performed to provide a preliminary diagnosis or to assess adequacy of the biopsy material. When appropriate, material should be sent for culture. The remaining tissue can then be fixed and used for permanent histologic sections. Techniques have been described for inflating biopsy specimens to help eliminate difficulties in interpretation associated with alveolar collapse.[197, 198]

When performed by an experienced surgeon, open-lung biopsy may have a mortality rate roughly equivalent to that of needle biopsy. In one review of 502 patients who underwent the procedure for the diagnosis of chronic interstitial lung disease, a mortality rate of only 0.3% and a complication rate of 2.5% were identified.[193] However, based on a review of 2,290 cases reported in the literature, mortality and complication rates have been calculated to be 1.8% and 7.0%, respectively.[1] These latter figures are probably more realistic estimates given the tendency for open biopsy to be performed in sicker patients.

Closed Pleural Biopsy

The most common method of obtaining fragments of pleural tissue for histologic examination is TTNB, a procedure that can be performed at the same time as thoracentesis.[199] The two needles most commonly used are the Cope and Abrams. Others have reported equivalent or better efficacy with more recently developed instruments such as the Raja[200] or Tru-cut needle.[201, 202] The latter (and similar instruments) is particularly valuable in the diagnosis of diffuse pleural thickening when guided by ultrasound or by CT.[203, 203a] Success with these needles depends largely on the skill of the operator,[204] the selection of patients, and the number of specimens taken. Evidence that the last of these is important was provided by one study of 55 patients with pleural effusion, 33 of which were malignant or granulomatous;[205] up to 10 specimens were obtained from individual patients at one site only, and in 32 of the 33 patients the pathologic abnormality was present in only some of the specimens.

We prefer the Abrams needle for pleural biopsy. When the anesthetic has been infiltrated and the 22-gauge needle is in the effusion, a clamp is applied to the needle, flush with the skin; 20 ml of pleural fluid is drawn into the syringe, the syringe and needle are withdrawn, and the fluid is sent for appropriate analysis. A clamp is applied to the biopsy needle at the same distance from the sharp trocar tip as from the point of the needle to its clamp. A small incision is made with a scalpel through anesthetized skin and subcutaneous tissue, and the biopsy needle, with its inner (cutting) cylinder in the closed position and with a three-way stopcock and 50-ml syringe attached to its adapter, is introduced through the anesthetized muscle and pleura until the clamp reaches the thoracic wall. The inner cutting cylinder is then rotated to allow fluid to pass through the side opening in the needle and into the syringe. Often the fluid is slightly blood tinged from trauma inflicted by the trocar, which is why specimens for diagnostic purposes should be taken before the pleural biopsy needle is introduced. The biopsy needle is withdrawn slowly, with some pressure on the needle toward the side containing the biopsy notch; the notch is placed laterally or inferiorly to avoid intercostal vessels, and when the parietal pleura slips into the notch, withdrawal of the needle is suddenly interrupted. At this point, the cutting cylinder is rotated while maintaining pressure, thereby closing the hole and cutting a biopsy specimen from the pleura. The biopsy port is then opened, the specimen aspirated into the syringe, and the process repeated without withdrawing the needle from the chest cavity.

Inability to obtain fluid during attempted thoracentesis may indicate empyema, the material being too thick to pass through a 22-gauge needle. When the clinical circumstances suggest empyema, a 16-gauge needle should be inserted after production of a satisfactory degree of anesthesia. Empyema can be diagnosed on gross examination of aspirated fluid. In cases of loculated effusion, the exploring needle should be withdrawn and reinserted at different angles (a situation in which adequate infiltration of anesthetic in the parietal pleura is particularly important). When no fluid is withdrawn at the first attempt despite strong evidence of its presence, thoracentesis should be repeated in higher or lower interspaces, after further anesthesia.

Although complications are rare and usually mild, severe hemorrhage into the chest wall and pleural cavity may occur. Mediastinal and subcutaneous emphysema have also been reported,[205, 206] and there have been cases of pulmonary neoplasm developing along needle tracks;[207–209] the latter complication is more common in patients who have mesothelioma.

The chief value of TTNB of the pleura is in the diagnosis of cancer and tuberculosis. Since granulomatous disease other than tuberculosis seldom involves the pleura, the finding of necrotizing or non-necrotizing granulomas is usually accepted as an indication of tuberculous infection, even when microorganisms are not identified. The sensitivity for the diagnosis ranges from about 70% to 90%.[210–214] Rarely, histologic findings in patients with rheumatoid disease suggest that an effusion is a manifestation of this condition;[215] pleural granulomatous inflammation consistent with sarcoidosis and associated with an effusion is even less common.[216, 217] The diagnostic yield in patients with neoplastic involvement of the pleura, when combined with cytology, ranges from about 65% to 85%.[211, 212, 214, 218] One group has combined TTNB with percutaneous pleural brushing; in their hands, a diagnosis of malignancy was confirmed in 31 (91%) of 34 patients.[281a]

In patients in whom the nature of a pleural effusion has not been established following thoracentesis, needle biopsy of the pleura should be performed. Biopsy may also be combined with the initial examination of pleural fluid when the diagnosis of tuberculosis is suspected, inasmuch as the yield of thoracentesis alone is poor in this situation. If such closed pleural biopsy fails to yield a diagnosis, we recommend direct biopsy by thoracoscopy.

Mediastinoscopy and Anterior Mediastinotomy

The main indications for mediastinal biopsy are the staging and (less often) the diagnosis of pulmonary carcinoma. Primary mediastinal neoplasms can also be diagnosed, as can certain benign conditions such as sarcoidosis.[218b]

The mediastinum can be evaluated surgically by a variety of techniques other than thoracotomy. The first described—cervical mediastinoscopy—is carried out through an incision in the suprasternal notch;[219] the soft tissue adjacent to the trachea is dissected, and biopsy material is removed under direct vision through a rigid mediastinoscope. The space explored consists of the upper half of the mediastinum, including tissues around the intrathoracic portion of the trachea, the tracheal bifurcation, and the proximal part of the main bronchi. Complications are uncommon and usually not serious; in one review of 20,000 procedures, complications were found in fewer than 2.5% (mortality was less than 0.5%).[220] Major bleeding can be the result of inadvertent biopsy of the aorta or innominate artery. The left recurrent laryngeal nerve may be damaged by biopsy in the area of the left tracheobronchial angle. Pneumothorax may occur on either side, but is more common on the right. Accidental tear of the tracheobronchial wall can also cause an air leak, and the esophagus has occasionally been perforated in the subcarinal area. Rarely, stroke has followed compression of the innominate artery by the mediastinoscope against the manubrium. As with most surgical interventions, the rate of complications diminishes with experience.[221]

When the subaortic and anterior mediastinal lymph nodes need to be assessed, techniques other than cervical mediastinoscopy must be used.[222, 223] Extended cervical mediastinoscopy has been employed by some surgeons in conjunction with the standard method.[222] In this procedure, tissue is examined from the anterolateral surface of the anterior aortic arch to the lateral portion of the pericardium in front of the left superior pulmonary vein. This practice allows biopsy of lymph nodes to which left upper lobe carcinomas preferentially metastasize.[222] The more familiar anterior (parasternal) mediastinotomy is used by most thoracic surgeons to sample lymph nodes (both hilar and mediastinal), lung parenchyma, and masses on the left side and in the anterosuperior mediastinum.[223] Right anterior mediastinotomy allows biopsy of mediastinal masses and lung parenchyma, as well as hilar and mediastinal lymph nodes on the right side.

Anterior mediastinotomy has the advantage of permitting more extensive exploration of the mediastinum and more accurate assessment of neoplastic extension to the hila than is permitted by cervical mediastinotomy.[225–227] The examination is performed via a 6-cm incision in the second intercostal space lateral to the sternal border.[223] Complications are infrequent and include superficial wound infection (in approximately 2.5% of cases), pneumothorax (in 2%), hemorrhage controlled by direct pressure (in 1.8%), and recurrent laryngeal nerve palsy (in fewer than 1%).[223] Anterior mediastinotomy can be performed safely in the outpatient setting and, when necessary, in conjunction with cervical mediastinoscopy and bronchoscopy.[223] The procedure is a good means of assessing resectability of left upper lobe carcinomas; unresectability at thoracotomy because of mediastinal lymph node involvement that was not previously appreciated at anterior mediastinotomy has been found in fewer than 8% of patients.[223, 228]

Scalene Node Biopsy

Scalene lymph node biopsy consists of the removal of tissue lying on the scalene group of muscles in the supraclavicular fossa, including the medial fat pad.[229] The advent of sophisticated imaging techniques and the ease of other procedures such as fine-needle aspiration have markedly reduced the role of the procedure in the staging of pulmonary carcinoma and in the diagnosis of nonmalignant disease. In experienced hands, it is a relatively minor procedure; however, major complications include local large vessel injury, lymphatic fistulas, Horner's syndrome, and infection extending into the mediastinum.[230] A review of 186 scalene lymph node biopsies at the Massachusetts General Hospital showed a 6% incidence of such complications, fatal in 2 cases.[231]

Scalene lymph nodes that are palpable almost always contain pathologic tissue;[232, 233] in a review of the literature it was noted that palpable nodes were involved by neoplasm in 475 (83%) of 576 cases of pulmonary carcinoma.[232] When nodes are not palpable, the diagnostic yield of biopsy is low;[232, 234, 235] in this circumstance, the role of biopsy is limited to the staging of some N2 or N3 patients for the purpose of entry into aggressive treatment protocols.[236] In general, fine-needle biopsy of palpable nodes is the procedure of choice to confirm metastasis in the setting of pulmonary carcinoma; however, excisional biopsy is preferable for adequate tumor classification in patients with known or suspected lymphoma.

REFERENCES

1. Wall CP, Gaensler EA, Carrington CB, et al: Comparison of transbronchial and open biopsies in chronic infiltrative lung diseases. Am Rev Respir Dis 123:280, 1981.
2. Burgher LW, Jones FL, Patterson JR, et al: Guidelines for fiberoptic bronchoscopy in adults. Am Rev Respir Dis 136:1066, 1987.
3. Reed AP: Preparation of the patient for awake flexible fiberoptic bronchoscopy. Chest 101:244, 1992.
4. Prakash UB, Offord KP, Stubbs SE: Bronchoscopy in North America: The ACCP survey. Chest 100:1668, 1991.
5. Henke CA, Hertz M, Gustafson P: Combined bronchoscopy and mucolytic therapy for patients with severe refractory status asthmaticus on mechanical ventilation: A case report and review of the literature. Crit Care Med 22:1880, 1994.
6. Belen J, Neuhaus A, Markowitz D, et al: Modification of the effect of fiberoptic bronchoscopy on pulmonary mechanics. Chest 79:516, 1981.
6a. Williams T, Brooks T, Ward C: The role of atropine premedication in fiberoptic bronchoscopy using intravenous midazolam sedation. Chest 113:1394, 1998.
7. Pearce SJ: Fibreoptic bronchoscopy: Is sedation necessary? BMJ 281:779, 1980.
8. Colt HG, Morris JF: Fiberoptic bronchoscopy without premedication. Chest 98:1327, 1990.
9. Kirkpatrick MB: Lidocaine topical anesthesia for flexible bronchoscopy. Chest 96:965, 1989.
10. Foster WM, Hurewitz AN: Aerosolized lidocaine reduces dose of topical anesthetic for bronchoscopy. Am Rev Respir Dis 146:520, 1992.
11. Berger R, McConnell JW, Phillips B, et al: Safety and efficacy of using high dose topical and nebulized anesthesia to obtain endobronchial cultures. Chest 95:299, 1989.
12. Wu FL, Razzaghi A, Souney PF: Seizure after lidocaine for bronchoscopy: Case report and review of the use of lidocaine in airway anesthesia. Pharmacotherapy 13:72, 1993.
13. Kotler RL, Hansen-Flaschen J, Casey MP: Severe methaemoglobinaemia after flexible fiberoptic bronchoscopy. Thorax 44:234, 1989.
14. Graham DR, Hay JG, Clague J, et al: Comparison of three different methods used to achieve local anaesthesia for fiberoptic bronchoscopy. Chest 102:704, 1992.
15. Erlich H: Bacteriologic studies and effects of anesthetic solutions on bronchial secretions during bronchoscopy. Am Rev Respir Dis 84:414, 1961.
16. Conte BA, Laforet EG: The role of the topical anesthetic agent in modifying bacteriologic data obtained by bronchoscopy. N Engl J Med 267:957, 1962.
17. Godden DJ, Willey RF, Fergusson RJ, et al: Rigid bronchoscopy under intravenous general anaesthesia with oxygen Venturi ventilation. Thorax 37:532, 1982.
18. Barrett CR Jr: Flexible fiberoptic bronchoscopy in the critically ill patient. Methodology and indications. Chest 73(Suppl):746, 1978.
19. Milam MG, Evins E, Sahn SA: Immediate chest roentgenography following fiberoptic bronchoscopy. Chest 96:477, 1989
20. Frazier WD, Pope TL Jr, Findley LJ: Pneumothorax following transbronchial biopsy. Chest 97:539, 1990.
21. Pereira W Jr, Kovnat DM, Snider GL: A prospective cooperative study of complications following flexible fiberoptic bronchoscopy. Chest 73:813, 1978.
22. Lukomsky GI, Ovchinnikov AA, Bilal A: Complications of bronchoscopy: Comparison of rigid bronchoscopy under general anesthesia and flexible fiberoptic bronchoscopy under topical anesthesia. Chest 79:316, 1981.
23. Credle WF Jr, Smiddy JF, Elliott RC: Complications of fiberoptic bronchoscopy. Am Rev Respir Dis 109:67, 1974.
24. Mitchell DM, Emerson CJ, Collyer J, et al: Fibreoptic bronchoscopy: Ten years on. BMJ 281:360, 1980.
25. Pue CA, Pacht ER: Complications in fiberoptic bronchoscopy at a university hospital. Chest 107:430, 1995.
26. Sen RP, Walsh TE: Serious complications of fiberoptic bronchoscopy. Chest 94:22, 1988.
27. Timms RM, Harrell JH: Bacteremia related to fiberoptic bronchoscopy. A case report. Am Rev Respir Dis 111:555, 1975.
28. Beyt BE Jr, King DK, Glew RH: Fatal pneumonitis and septicemia after fiberoptic bronchoscopy. Chest 72:105, 1977.
29. Hammer DL, Aranda CP, Galati V, et al: Massive intrabronchial aspiration of contents of pulmonary abscess after fiberoptic bronchoscopy. Chest 74:306, 1978.
30. de Fijter JW, van der Hoeven JG, Eggelmeijer F, et al: Sepsis syndrome and death after bronchoalveolar lavage. Chest 104:1296, 1993.
31. Cordasco EM, Mehta AC, Ahmad M: Bronchoscopically induced bleeding. Chest 100:1141, 1991.
32. Knox AJ, Mascie-Taylor BH, Page RL: Fibreoptic bronchoscopy in the elderly: Four years' experience. Br J Dis Chest 82:290, 1988.
33. Trouillet JL, Guiguet M, Gibert C, et al: Fiberoptic bronchoscopy in ventilated patients. Chest 97:927, 1990.
34. Djukanovic R, Wilson JW, Lai CKW, et al: The safety aspects of fiberoptic bronchoscopy, bronchoalveolar lavage, and endobronchial biopsy in asthma. Am Rev Respir Dis 143:772, 1991.
35. Bleecher ER, McFadden ER Jr, Hurd SS, et al: Investigative bronchoscopy in subjects with asthma and other obstructive pulmonary disease. Chest 101:297, 1992.
36. Weiss SM, Hert RC, Gianola FJ, et al: Complications of fiberoptic bronchoscopy in thrombocytopenia patients. Chest 104:1025, 1993.
37. Chastre J, Trouillet JL, Fagon JY: Diagnosis of pulmonary infections in mechanically ventilated patients. Semin Respir Infect 11:65, 1996.
38. Chastre J, Fagon JY, Trouillet JL: Diagnosis and treatment of nosocomial pneumonia in patients in intensive care units. Clin Infect Dis 21:226, 1996.
39. Allen RM, Dunn WF, Limper AH: Diagnosing ventilator-associated pneumonia: The role of bronchoscopy. Mayo Clin Proc 69:962, 1994.
40. Örtqvist A, Kalin M, Lejdeborn L, et al: Diagnostic fiberoptic bronchoscopy protected brush culture in patients with community-acquired pneumonia. Chest 97:576, 1990.
41. Schulman LL, Smith CR, Drusin R, et al: Utility of airway endoscopy in the diagnosis of respiratory complications of cardiac transplantation. Chest 93:960, 1988.
42. Willcox PA, Bateman ED, Potgieter PD, et al: Experience with fiberoptic bronchoscopy in the diagnosis of pulmonary shadows in renal transplant recipients over a 12-year period. Respir Med 84:297, 1990.
43. Ekdahl K, Eriksson L, Rollof J, et al: Bronchoscopic diagnosis of pulmonary infections in a heterogeneous nonselected group of patients. Chest 103:1743, 1993.
44. Coker RJ, Mitchell DM: The role of bronchoscopy in patients with HIV disease. Int J STD AIDS 5:172, 1994.
44a. Gasparini S: Bronchoscopic biopsy techniques in the diagnosis and staging of lung cancer. Monaldi Arch Chest Dis 52:392, 1997.
45. Edell ES, Cortese DA: Bronchoscopic localization and treatment of occult lung cancer. Chest 96:919, 1989.
46. Su WJ, Lee PY, Perng RP: Chest roentgenographic guidelines in the selection of patients for fiberoptic bronchoscopy. Chest 103:1198, 1993.
47. Torrington KG, Kern JD: The utility of fiberoptic bronchoscopy in the evaluation of the solitary pulmonary nodule. Chest 104:1021, 1993.
48. Chang SC, Perng RP: The role of fiberoptic bronchoscopy in evaluation of the causes of pleural effusions. Arch Intern Med 149:855, 1989.
49. Kelly P, Falouh M, O'Brien A, et al: Fiberoptic bronchoscopy in the management of lone pleural effusion: A negative study. Eur Respir J 3:397, 1990.
50. Poe RH, Israel RH, Marin MG, et al: Utility of fiberoptic bronchoscopy in patients with hemoptysis and a nonlocalizing chest roentgenogram. Chest 92:70, 1988.
51. O'Neill KM, Lazarus AA: Hemoptysis—indications for bronchoscopy. Arch Intern Med 151:171, 1991.
52. Sen RP, Walsh TE: Fiberoptic bronchoscopy for refractory cough. Chest 99:33, 1991.
53. Hara KS, Prakash UBS: Fiberoptic bronchoscopy in the evaluation of acute chest and upper airway trauma. Chest 96:627, 1989.
54. Lam S, MacAulay C, Hung J, et al: Detection of dysplasia and carcinoma in situ with a lung imaging fluorescence endoscope device. J Thorac Cardiovasc Surg 105:1035, 1993.
55. Lam S, MacAulay C, Palcic B: Detection and localization of early lung cancer by imaging techniques [review]. Chest 103(Suppl):12, 1993.
56. Lam S, Kennedy T, Unger M, et al: Localization of bronchial intraepithelial neoplastic lesions by fluorescence bronchoscopy. Chest 113:696, 1998.
57. Lam S, Becker HD: Future diagnostic procedures (review). Chest Surg Clin North Am 6:363, 1996.
58. Golderg BB, Steiner RM, Liu JB, et al: US-assisted bronchoscopy with use of miniature transducer-containing catheters. Radiology 190:233, 1994.
59. Feinnsilver SH, Fein AM, Niederman MS, et al: Utility of fiberoptic bronchoscopy in nonresolving pneumonia. Chest 98:1322, 1990.
60. Edell ES: Future therapeutic procedures. Chest Surg Clin North Am 6:381, 1996.
61. Spratling L, Speiser BL: Endoscopic brachytherapy. Chest Surg Clin North Am 6:293, 1996.
62. Colt HG: Laser bronchoscopy. Chest Surg Clin North Am 6:277, 1996.
63. Freitag L, Firusian N, Stamatis G, et al: Bronchoscopy—the role of bronchoscopy in pulmonary complications due to mustard gas inhalation. Chest 100:1436, 1991.
64. Pierce RJ: Lasers, brachytherapy and stents—keeping the airways open. Respir Med 85:263, 1991.
65. Maiwand MO, Homasson J-P: Cryotherapy for tracheobronchial disorders. Clin Chest Med 16:427, 1995.
66. Colt HG, Dumon J-F: Airway stents: Present and future. Clin Chest Med 16:465, 1995.
67. Helmers RA, Sanderson DR: Rigid bronchoscopy: The forgotten art. Clin Chest Med 16:393, 1995.
68. Lee AC, Wu CL, Feins RH, et al: The use of fiberoptic endoscopy in anesthesia. Chest Surg Clin North Am 6:329, 1996.
69. Ovassapian A, Randel GI: The role of the fiberscope in the critically ill patient. Crit Care Clin 11:29, 1995.
70. York EL, Lewall DB, Hirji M, et al: Endoscopic diagnosis and treatment of postoperative bronchopleural fistula. Chest 97:1390, 1990.
71. McManigle JE, Fletcher GL, Tenholder MF: Bronchoscopy in the management of bronchopleural fistula. Chest 97:1235, 1990.
72. Lan RS, Lee CH, Chiang YC, et al: Use of fiberoptic bronchoscopy to retrieve bronchial foreign bodies in adults. Am Rev Respir Dis 140:1734, 1989.
73. Kelly SM, Marsh BR: Airway foreign bodies. Chest Surg Clin North Am 6:253, 1996.

74. Tsao TCY, Tsai YH, Lan RS, et al: Treatment for collapsed lung in critically ill patients. Chest 97:435, 1990.
75. Infeld M, Gerblich A, Subramanyan S, et al: Focus of bronchial carcinoma in situ eradicated by endobronchial biopsy. Chest 94:1107, 1988.
76. Brutinel WM, Cortese DA, Edell ES, et al: Complications of Nd:YAG laser therapy. Chest 94:902, 1988.
77. Muers MF, Boddington MM, Cole M, et al: Cytological sampling at fiberoptic bronchoscopy: Comparison of catheter aspirates and brush biopsies. Thorax 37:457, 1982
78. Arroliga AC, Matthay RA: The role of bronchoscopy in lung cancer. Clin Chest Med 14:87, 1993.
79. Dreisin RB, Albert RK, Talley PA, et al: Flexible fiberoptic bronchoscopy in the teaching hospital: Yield and complications. Chest 74:144, 1978.
80. Rudd RM, Gellert AR, Boldy DAR, et al: Bronchoscopic and percutaneous aspiration biopsy in the diagnosis of bronchial carcinoma cell type. Thorax 37:462, 1982.
81. Popovich J Jr, Kvale PA, Eichenhorn MS, et al: Diagnostic accuracy of multiple biopsies from flexible fiberoptic bronchoscopy—a comparison of central versus peripheral carcinoma. Am Rev Respir Dis 125:521, 1982.
82. Chuang MT, Marchevsky A, Teirstein AS, et al: Diagnosis of lung cancer by fibreoptic bronchoscopy: Problems in the histological classification of non–small cell carcinomas. Thorax 39:175, 1984.
83. Andersen HA, Fontana RS, Harrison EG Jr: Transbronchoscopic lung biopsy in diffuse pulmonary disease. Dis Chest 48:187, 1965.
84. Shure D: Bronchoscopy: Transbronchial biopsy and needle aspiration. Chest 95:1130, 1989.
84a. Schnabel A, Holl-Ulrich K, Dalhoff K, et al: Efficacy of transbronchial biopsy in pulmonary vaculitides. Eur Respir J 10:2738, 1997.
85. Smith LS, Seaquist M, Schillaci RF: Comparison of forceps used for transbronchial lung biopsy. Chest 87:574, 1985.
86. Loube DI, Johnson JE, Wiener D, et al: The effect of forceps size on the adequacy of specimens obtained by transbronchial biopsy. Am Rev Respir Dis 148:1411, 1993.
87. Fraire AE, Cooper SP, Greenberg SD, et al: Transbronchial lung biopsy. Chest 102:748, 1992.
88. Blasco LH, Hernandez IMS, Garrido VV, et al: Safety of the transbronchial biopsy in outpatients. Chest 99:562, 1991.
89. Ahmad M, Livingston DR, Golish JA, et al: The safety of outpatient transbronchial biopsy. Chest 90:403, 1986.
90. Milligan SA, Luce JM, Golden J, et al: Transbronchial biopsy without fluoroscopy in patients with diffuse roentgenographic infiltrates and the acquired immunodeficiency syndrome. Am Rev Respir Dis 137:486, 1988.
91. De Fenoyl O, Capron F, Lebeau B, et al: Transbronchial biopsy without fluoroscopy: A five year experience in outpatients. Thorax 44:956, 1989.
92. Anders GT, Johnson JE, Bush BA, et al: Transbronchial biopsy without fluoroscopy. Chest 94:557, 1988.
93. Witte MC, Opal SM, Gilbert JG, et al: Incidence of fever and bacteremia following transbronchial needle aspiration. Chest 89:85, 1986.
94. Kvale PA: Bronchoscopic biopsies and bronchoalveolar lavage. Chest Surg Clin North Am 6:205, 1996.
95. Haponik EF, Summer WR, Terry PB, et al: Clinical decision making with transbronchial lung biopsies: The value of nonspecific histologic examination. Am Rev Respir Dis 125:524, 1982.
96. Puksa S, Hutcheon MA, Hyland RH: Usefulness of transbronchial biopsy in immunosuppressed patients with pulmonary infiltrates. Thorax 38:146, 1983.
97. Zellweger J-P, Leuenberger PJ: Cytologic and histologic examination of transbronchial lung biopsy. Eur J Respir Dis 63:94, 1982.
98. Ono R, Loke J, Ikeda S: Bronchofiberoscopy with curette biopsy and bronchography in the evaluation of peripheral lung lesions. Chest 79:162, 1981.
99. Popovich J Jr, Kvale PA, Eichenhorn MS, et al: Diagnostic accuracy of multiple biopsies from flexible fiberoptic bronchoscopy—a comparison of central versus peripheral carcinoma. Am Rev Respir Dis 125:521, 1982.
100. Radke JR, Conway WA, Eyler WR, et al: Diagnostic accuracy in peripheral lung lesions: Factors predicting success with flexible fiberoptic bronchoscopy. Chest 76:176, 1979.
101. Zavala DC, Rossi NP, Rodman NF, et al: A new mobile catheter for obtaining bronchial brush biopsies. Diagnostic results in 50 patients with suspicious pulmonary lesions and negative bronchoscopies. Am Rev Respir Dis 106:541, 1972.
102. Katis K, Inglesos E, Zachariadis E, et al: The role of transbronchial needle aspiration in the diagnosis of peripheral lung masses or nodules. Eur Respir J 8:963, 1995.
103. Wallace JM, Deutsch AL: Flexible fiberoptic bronchoscopy and percutaneous needle lung aspiration for evaluating the solitary pulmonary nodule. Chest 81:665, 1982.
104. Salazar AM, Westcott JL: The role of transthoracic needle biopsy for the diagnosis and staging of lung cancer. Clin Chest Med 14:99, 1993.
104a. Klein JS, Zarka MA: Transthoracic needle biopsy: An overview. J Thorac Imaging 12:232, 1997.
104b. Moore EH: Needle-aspiration lung biopsy: A comprehensive approach to complication reduction. J Thorac Imaging 12:259, 1997.
105. Perlmutt LM, Johnston WW, Dunnick NR: Percutaneous transthoracic needle aspiration: A review. Am J Roentgenol 152:451, 1989.
106. Westcott JL, Rao N, Colley DP: Transthoracic needle biopsy of small pulmonary nodules. Radiology 202:97, 1997.
107. Williams AJ, Santiago S, Lehrman S, et al: Transcutaneous needle aspiration of solitary pulmonary masses: How many passes? Am Rev Respir Dis 136:452, 1987.
108. Dull WL: Needle aspiration biopsy in suspected pulmonary carcinoma. Respiration 39:291, 1980.
109. Tao LC, Pearson FG, Delarue NC, et al: Percutaneous fine-needle aspiration biopsy: 1. Its value to clinical practice. Cancer 45:1480, 1980.
110. Zavala DC, Schoell JE: Ultra-thin needle aspiration of the lung in infectious and malignant disease. Am Rev Respir Dis 123:125, 1981.
111. Todd TRJ, Weisbrod G, Tao LC, et al: Aspiration needle biopsy of thoracic lesions. Ann Thorac Surg 32:154, 1981.
112. Poe RH, Tobin RE: Sensitivity and specificity of needle biopsy in lung malignancy. Am Rev Respir Dis 122:725, 1980.
113. Morgenroth A, Pfeuffer HP, Austgen M, et al: Six years' experience with perithoracic core needle biopsy in pulmonary lesions. Thorax 44:177, 1989.
114. Arakawa H, Nakajima Y, Kurihara Y, et al: CT-guided transthoracic needle biopsy: A comparison between automated biopsy gun and fine needle aspiration. Clin Radiol 51:503, 1996.
115. Klein JS, Salomon G, Stewart EA: Transthoracic needle biopsy with a coaxially placed 20-gauge automated cutting needle: Results in 122 patients. Radiology 198:715, 1996.
116. Milman N: Percutaneous lung biopsy with a fine bore cutting needle (Vacu-Cut): Improved results using drill technique. Thorax 50:560, 1995.
117. Yuan A, Yang PC, Chang DB, et al: Ultrasound guided aspiration biopsy for pulmonary tuberculosis with unusual radiographic appearances. Thorax 48:167, 1993.
118. Yang PC, Chang DB, Yu C, et al: Ultrasound guided percutaneous cutting biopsy for the diagnosis of pulmonary consolidations of unknown aetiology. Thorax 47:457, 1992.
119. Haramati LB: CT-guided automated needle biopsy of the chest. Am J Roentgenol 165:53, 1995.
120. Gruden JF, Klein JS, Webb WR: Percutaneous transthoracic needle biopsy in AIDS: Analysis in 32 patients. Radiology 189:567, 1993.
121. Staroselsky AN, Schwarz Y, Man A, et al: Additional information from percutaneous cutting needle biopsy following fine-needle aspiration in the diagnosis of chest lesions. Chest 113:1522, 1998.
122. Niden AH, Salem F: A safe high-yield technique for cutting needle biopsy of the lung in patients with diffuse lung disease. Chest 111:1615, 1997.
123. Rosenberger A, Adler O: Fine needle aspiration biopsy in the diagnosis of mediastinal lesions. Am J Roentgenol 131:239, 1978.
124. Adler OB, Resenberger A, Peleg H: Fine-needle aspiration biopsy of mediastinal masses: Evaluation of 136 experiences. Am J Roentgenol 140:893, 1983.
125. Gardner D, vanSonnenberg E, D'Agostino HB, et al: CT-guided transthoracic needle biopsy. Cardiovasc Intervent Radiol 14:17, 1991.
126. vanSonnenberg E, Casola G, D'Agostino HB, et al: Interventional radiology in the chest. Chest 102:608, 1992.
127. Welch TJ, Sheedy PF 2d, Johnson CD, et al: Radiology 171:493, 1989.
128. Pan JF, Yang PC, Chang DB, et al: Needle aspiration biopsy of malignant lung masses with necrotic centers. Chest 103:452, 1993.
129. Klein JS, Salomon G, Stewart EA: Transthoracic needle biopsy with a coaxially placed 20-gauge automated cutting needle: Results in 122 patients. Radiology 198:715, 1996.
130. Salazar AM, Westcott JL: The role of transthoracic needle biopsy for the diagnosis and staging of lung cancer. Clin Chest Med 14:99, 1993.
131. Li H, Boiselle PM, Shepard JO, et al: Diagnostic accuracy and safety of CT-guided percutaneous needle aspiration biopsy of the lung: Comparison of small and large pulmonary nodules. Am J Roentgenol 167:105, 1996.
132. Fish GD, Stanley JH, Miller KS, et al: Postbiopsy pneumothorax: Estimating the risk by chest radiography and pulmonary function tests. Am J Roentgenol 150:71, 1988.
133. Berquist TH, Bailey PB, Cortese DA, et al: Transthoracic needle biopsy: Accuracy and complications in relation to location and type of lesion. Mayo Clin Proc 55:475, 1980.
134. Perlmutt LM, Johnston WW, Dunnick NR: Percutaneous transthoracic needle aspiration: A review. Am J Roentgenol 152:451, 1989.
135. Milner LB, Ryan K, Gullo J: Fatal intrathoracic hemorrhage after percutaneous aspiration lung biopsy. Am J Roentgenol 132:280, 1979.
136. Ballard GL, Boyd WR: A specially designed cutting aspiration needle for lung biopsy. Am J Roentgenol 130:899, 1978.
137. Mehnert JH, Brown MJ: Percutaneous needle core biopsy of peripheral pulmonary masses. Am J Surg 136:151, 1978.
138. McEvoy RD, Begley MD, Antic R: Percutaneous biopsy of intrapulmonary mass lesions: Experience with a disposable cutting needle. Cancer 51:2321, 1983.
138a. Aberle DR, Gamsu G, Golden JA: Fatal systemic arterial air embolism following lung needle aspiration. Radiology 165:351, 1987.
138b. Baker BK, Awwad EE: Computed tomography of fatal cerebral air embolism following percutaneous aspiration biopsy of the lung. J Comput Assist Tomogr 12:1082, 1988.
139. Lillington GA: Hazards of transthoracic needle biopsy of the lung. Ann Thorac Surg 48:163, 1989.
139a. Graham RJ, Heyd RL, Raval VA, et al: Lung torsion after percutaneous needle biopsy of lung. Am J Roentgenol 159:35, 1992.
139b. Fogarty JP, Dudek G: An unusual case of lung torsion. Chest 108:575, 1995.
140. Müller NL, Bergin CJ, Miller RR, et al: Seeding of malignant cells into the needle track after lung and pleural biopsy. Can Assoc Radiol J 37:192, 1986.
141. Morgenroth A, Pfeuffer HP, Austgen M, et al: Six years' experience with perithoracic core needle biopsy in pulmonary lesions. Thorax 44:177, 1989.

142. Yuan A, Yang PC, Chang DB, et al: Ultrasound-guided aspiration biopsy of small peripheral pulmonary nodules. Chest 101:926, 1992.

143. Arakawa H, Nakajima Y, Kurihara Y, et al: CT-guided transthoracic needle biopsy: A comparison between automated biopsy gun and fine needle aspiration. Clin Radiol 51:503, 1996.

144. Klein JS, Salomon G, Stewart EA: Transthoracic needle biopsy with a coaxially placed 20-gauge automated cutting needle: Results in 122 patients. Radiology 198:715, 1996.

145. Mathur PN, Astoul P, Boutin C: Medical thoracoscopy. Technical details. Clin Chest Med 16:479, 1995.

146. Jacobaeus HC: Über die Möglichkeit, die Zystoskopie bei Untersuchung Seröser Höhlungen anzuwenden. Munch Med Wochenschr 57:2090, 1910.

147. Braimbridge MV: The history of thoracoscopic surgery. Ann Thorac Surg 56:610, 1993.

148. Walker WS, Craig SR: Video-assisted thoracoscopic pulmonary surgery—current status and potential evolution. Eur J Cardiothorac Surg 10:161, 1996.

149. Salo JA: The role of video-thoracoscopy in the diagnosis and treatment of chest disease. Ann Med 26:401, 1994.

150. Harris RJ, Kavuru MS, Rice TW, et al: The diagnostic and therapeutic utility of thoracoscopy. Chest 108:828, 1995.

151. Colt HG: Thoracoscopy. Chest 108:324, 1995.

152. Mathur PN, Loddenkemper R: Medical thoracoscopy. Clin Chest Med 16:487, 1995.

152a. Loddenkemper R: Thoracoscopy—state of the art. Eur Respir J 11:213, 1998.

153. Weissberg D, Kaufman M, Zurkowski Z: Pleuroscopy in patients with pleural effusion and pleural masses. Ann Thorac Surg 29:205, 1980.

154. Rodgers BM, Ryckman FC, Moazam F, et al: Thoracoscopy for intrathoracic tumors. Ann Thorac Surg 31:414, 1981.

155. Boutin C, Viallat JR, Cargnino P, et al: Thoracoscopic lung biopsy: Experimental and clinical preliminary study. Chest 82:44, 1982.

156. Janik JS, Nagaraj HS, Groff DB: Thoracoscopic evaluation of intrathoracic lesions in children. J Thorac Cardiovasc Surg 83:408, 1982.

157. Menzies R, Charbonneau M: Thoracoscopy for the diagnosis of pleural disease. Ann Intern Med 114:271, 1991.

158. Faurschou P, Madsen F, Viskum K: Thoracoscopy: Influence of the procedure on some respiratory and cardiac values. Thorax 38:341, 1983.

159. Nezu K, Keiji K, Tojo T, et al: Thoracoscopic wedge resection of blebs under local anesthesia with sedation for treatment of a spontaneous pneumothorax. Chest 111:230, 1997.

160. Boutin C, Viallat JR, Cargnino P, et al: Thoracoscopy in malignant pleural effusions. Am Rev Respir Dis 124:588, 1981.

161. Harris RJ, Kavuru MS, Mehta AC, et al: The impact of thoracoscopy on the management of pleural disease. Chest 107:845, 1995.

162. Boutin C, Loddenkemper R, Astoul P: Diagnostic and therapeutic thoracoscopy: Techniques and indications in pulmonary medicine. Tuber Lung Dis 74:225, 1993.

163. Loddenkemper R, Boutin C: Thoracoscopy: Present diagnostic and therapeutic indications. Eur Respir J 6:1544, 1993.

164. Mack MJ, Aronoff RJ, Acuff TE, et al: Present role of thoracoscopy in the diagnosis and treatment of diseases of the chest. Ann Thorac Surg 54:403, 1992.

165. Landreneau RJ, Hazelrigg SR, Ferson PF, et al: Thoracoscopic resection of 85 pulmonary lesions. Ann Thorac Surg 54:415, 1992.

166. Ferson PF, Landreneau RJ, Dowling RD, et al: Comparison of open versus thoracoscopic lung biopsy for diffuse infiltrative pulmonary disease. J Thorac Cardiovasc Surg 106:194, 1993.

167. Lewis RJ, Caccavale RJ, Sisler GE, et al: One hundred consecutive patients undergoing video-assisted thoracic operations. Ann Thorac Surg 54:421, 1992.

168. Boutin C, Viallat JR, Cargnino P, et al: Thoracoscopic lung biopsy: Experimental and clinical preliminary study. Chest 82:44, 1982.

169. Dijkman JH, van der Meer JWM, Bakker W, et al: Transpleural lung biopsy by the thoracoscopic route in patients with diffuse interstitial pulmonary disease. Chest 82:76, 1982.

170. Marchandise FX, Vandenplas O, Wallon J, et al: Thoracoscopic lung biopsy in interstitial lung disease. Acta Clin Belg 47:165, 1992.

171. Bensard DD, McIntyre RC Jr, Waring BJ, et al: Comparison of video thoracoscopic lung biopsy to open lung biopsy in the diagnosis of interstitial lung disease. Chest 103:765, 1993.

172. Carnochan FM, Walker WS, Cameron EW: Efficacy of video assisted thoracoscopic lung biopsy: An historical comparison with open lung biopsy. Thorax 49:361, 1994.

173. Rubin JW: Video-assisted thoracic surgery: The approach of choice for selected diagnosis and therapy. Eur J Cardiothorac Surg 8:431, 1994.

174. Molin LJ, Steinberg JB, Lanza LA: VATS increases costs in patients undergoing lung biopsy for interstitial lung disease. Ann Thorac Surg 58:1598, 1994.

175. Landreneau RJ, Hazelrigg SR, Mack MJ, et al: Thoracoscopic mediastinal lymph node sampling: Useful for mediastinal lymph node stations inaccessible by cervical mediastinoscopy. J Thorac Cardiovasc Surg 106:554, 1993.

176. Ginsberg RJ: Thoracoscopy: A cautionary note. Ann Thorac Surg 56:801, 1993.

177. Gossot D, Toledo L, Fritsch S, et al: Mediastinoscopy vs thoracoscopy for mediastinal biopsy—results of a prospective nonrandomized study. Chest 110:1328, 1996.

178. Wain JC: Video-assisted thoracoscopy and the staging of lung cancer. Ann Thorac Surg 56:776, 1993.

179. Yim AP: Routine video-assisted thoracoscopy prior to thoracotomy. Chest 109:1099, 1996.

180. Kern JA, Daniel TM, Tribble CG, et al: Thoracoscopic diagnosis and treatment of mediastinal masses. Ann Thorac Surg 56:92, 1993.

181. Gossot D, Fritsch S, Halimi B, et al: The diagnostic value of thoracoscopy in solid masses of the mediastinum. Rev Mal Respir 12:29, 1995.

181a. Ferson PF, Keenan RJ, Luketich JD: The role of video-assisted thoracic surgery in pulmonary metastases. Chest Surg Clin North Am 8:59, 1998.

182. Mack MJ, Hazelrigg SR, Landreneau RJ, et al: Thoracoscopy for the diagnosis of the indeterminate solitary pulmonary nodule. Ann Thorac Surg 56:825, 1993.

183. Allen MS, Deschamps C, Lee RE, et al: Video-assisted thoracoscopic stapled wedge excision for indeterminate pulmonary nodules. J Thorac Cardiovasc Surg 106:1048, 1993.

184. Shennib H: Intraoperative localization techniques for pulmonary nodules. Ann Thorac Surg 56:745, 1993.

185. Shennib H, Bret P: Intraoperative transthoracic ultrasonographic localization of occult lung lesions. Ann Thorac Surg 55:767, 1993.

186. Mack MJ, Shennib H, Landreneau RJ, et al: Techniques for localization of pulmonary nodules for thoracoscopic resection. J Thorac Cardiovasc Surg 106:550, 1993.

187. Hazelrigg SR, Nunchuck SK, Landreneau RJ, et al: Cost analysis for thoracoscopy: Thoracoscopic wedge resection. Ann Thorac Surg 56:633, 1993.

187a. Frame SB: Thoracoscopy for trauma. Int Surg 82:223, 1997.

187b. Liu DW, Liu HP, Lin PJ, et al: Video-assisted thoracic surgery in treatment of chest trauma. J Trauma 42:670, 1997.

188. Johnstone PA, Rohde DC, Swartz SE, et al: Port site recurrences after laparoscopic and thoracoscopic procedures in malignancy. J Clin Oncol 14:1950, 1996.

189. Chen YM, Wu MF, Lee PY, et al: Necrotizing fasciitis: Is it a fatal complication of tube thoracostomy?—report of three cases. Respir Med 86:249, 1992.

190. Kaiser LR, Bavaria JE: Complications of thoracoscopy. Ann Thorac Surg 56:796, 1993.

191. Hazelrigg SR, Nunchuck SK, LoCicero J 3d: Video assisted thoracic surgery study group data. Ann Thorac Surg 56:1039, 1993.

192. Jaklitsch MT, DeCamp MM Jr, Liptay MJ, et al: Video-assisted thoracic surgery in the elderly. Chest 110:751, 1996.

193. Gaensler EA, Carrington CB: Open biopsy for chronic diffuse infiltrative lung disease: Clinical, roentgenographic and physiological correlations in 502 patients. Ann Thorac Surg 30:411, 1980.

194. Chechani V, Landreneau RJ, Shaikh SS: Open lung biopsy for diffuse infiltrative disease. Ann Thorac Surg 54:296, 1992.

195. Newman SL, Michel RP, Wang N-S: Lingular lung biopsy: Is it representative? Am Rev Respir Dis 132:1084, 1985.

196. Wetstein L: Sensitivity and specificity of lingular segmental biopsies of the lung. Chest 90:383, 1986.

197. Churg A: An inflation procedure for open lung biopsies. Am J Surg Pathol 7:69, 1983.

198. Brody AR, Craighead JE: Preparation of human lung biopsy specimens by perfusion-fixation. Am Rev Respir Dis 112:645, 1975.

199. DeFrancis N, Klosk E, Albano E: Needle biopsy of the parietal pleura: A preliminary report. N Engl J Med 252:948, 1955.

200. Ogirala RG, Agarwal V, Vizioli LD, et al: Comparison of the Raja and the Abrams pleural biopsy needles in patients with pleural effusion. Am Rev Respir Dis 147:1291, 1993.

201. Chang DB, Yang PC, Luh KT, et al: Ultrasound-guided pleural biopsy with Tru-cut needle. Chest 100:1328, 1991.

202. McLeod DT, Ternouth I, Nkanza N: Comparison of the Tru-cut biopsy needle with the Abrams punch for pleural biopsy. Thorax 44:794, 1989.

203. Scott EM, Marshall TJ, Flower CD, et al: Diffuse pleural thickening: Percutaneous CT-guided cutting needle biopsy. Radiology 194:867, 1995.

203a. Hsu WH, Chiang CD, Hsu JY, et al: Value of ultrasonically guided needle biopsy of pleural masses: An underutilized technique. J Clin Ultrasound 25:119, 1997.

204. Walsh LJ, MacFarlane JT, Manhire AR, et al: Audit of pleural biopsies: An argument for a pleural biopsy service. Respir Med 88:503, 1994.

205. Mungall IPF, Cowen PN, Cooke NT, et al: Multiple pleural biopsy with the Abrams needle. Thorax 35:600, 1980.

206. Scerbo J, Keltz H, Stone DJ: A prospective study of closed pleural biopsies. JAMA 218:377, 1971.

207. Mestitz P, Purves MJ, Pollard AC: Pleural biopsy in the diagnosis of pleural effusion: A report of 200 cases. Lancet 2:1349, 1958.

208. Schachter EN, Basta W: Subcutaneous metastasis of an adenocarcinoma following a percutaneous pleural biopsy. Am Rev Respir Dis 107:283, 1973.

209. Jones FL Jr: Subcutaneous implantation of cancer: A rare complication of pleural biopsy. Chest 57:189, 1970.

210. Kirsch CM, Kroe DM, Jensen WA, et al: A modified Abrams needle biopsy technique. Chest 108:982, 1995.

211. Poe RH, Israel RH, Utell MJ, et al: Sensitivity, specificity, and predictive values of closed pleural biopsy. Arch Intern Med 144:325, 1984.

212. Prakash UB, Reiman HM: Comparison of needle biopsy with cytologic analysis for the evaluation of pleural effusion: Analysis of 414 cases. Mayo Clin Proc 60:158, 1985.

213. Yew WW, Chan CY, Kwan SY, et al: Diagnosis of tuberculous pleural effusion by the detection of tuberculostearic acid in pleural aspirates. Chest 100:1261, 1991.

214. Bueno EC, Clemente GM, Castro CB, et al: Cytologic and bacteriologic analysis of fluid and pleural biopsy specimens with Cope's needle: Study of 414 patients. Arch Intern Med 150:1190, 1990.

215. Tserkézoglou A, Metakidis S, Papastamatiou-Tsimara H, et al: Solitary rheumatoid nodule of the pleura and rheumatoid pleural effusion. Thorax 33:769, 1978.

216. Gardiner IT, Uff JS: Acute pleurisy in sarcoidosis. Thorax 33:124, 1978.
217. Nelson DG, Loudon RG: Sarcoidosis with pleural involvement. Am Rev Respir Dis 108:647, 1973.
218. Sison BS, Weiss Z: Needle biopsy of the parietal pleura in patients with pleural effusions. BMJ 2:298, 1962.
218a. Emad A, Rezaian GR: Closed percutaneous pleural brushing: A new method for diagnosis of malignant pleural effusions. Respir Med 92:659, 1998.
218b. Mentzer SJ, Swanson SJ, Scott J, et al: Mediastinoscopy, thoracoscopy, and video-assisted thoracic surgery in the diagnosis and staging of lung cancer. Chest 112:239S, 1997.
219. Carlens E: Mediastinoscopy: A method for inspection and tissue biopsy in the superior mediastinum. Dis Chest 36:343, 1959.
220. Kirschner PA: Cervical mediastinoscopy. Chest Surg Clin North Am 6:1, 1996.
221. Sarin CL, Nohl-Oser HC: Mediastinoscopy: A clinical evaluation of 400 consecutive cases. Thorax 24:585, 1969.
222. Ginsberg RJ: Extended cervical mediastinoscopy. Chest Surg Clin North Am 6:21, 1996.
223. Olak J: Parasternal mediastinoscopy (Chamberlain procedure). Chest Surg Clin North Am 6:31, 1996.
224. Lopez L, Varela A, Freixinet J, et al: Extended cervical mediastinoscopy: Prospective study of fifty cases. Ann Thorac Surg 57:555, 1994.
225. Chandler SB, Stemmer EA, Calvin JW, et al: Mediastinal biopsy for indeterminate chest lesions. Thorax 21:533, 1966.

226. McNeill TM, Chamberlain JM: Diagnostic anterior mediastinotomy. Ann Thorac Surg 2:532, 1966.
227. Evans DS, Hall JH, Harrison GK: Anterior mediastinotomy. Thorax 28:444, 1973.
228. Deneffe G, Lacquet LM, Gyselen A: Cervical mediastinoscopy and anterior mediastinotomy in patients with lung cancer and radiologically normal mediastinum. Eur J Respir Dis 64:613, 1983.
229. Daniels AC: A method of biopsy useful in diagnosing certain intrathoracic diseases. Dis Chest 16:360, 1949.
230. Thomas HS, Bloomer WE, Orloff MJ: Scalene lymph node biopsy. Dis Chest 53:316, 1968.
231. Skinner DB: Scalene-lymph-node biopsy: Reappraisal of risks and indications. N Engl J Med 268:1324, 1963.
232. Brantigan JW, Brantigan CO, Brantigan OC: Biopsy of nonpalpable scalene lymph nodes in carcinoma of the lung. Am Rev Respir Dis 107:962, 1973.
233. Lal S, Poole GW: Scalene-node biopsies. Lancet 2:112, 1963.
234. Schatzlein MH, McAuliffe S, Orringer MB, et al: Scalene node biopsy in pulmonary carcinoma: When is it indicated? Ann Thorac Surg 31:322, 1981.
235. Bernstein MP, Ferrara JJ, Brown L: Effectiveness of scalene node biopsy for the staging of lung cancer in the absence of palpable adenopathy. J Surg Oncol 29:46, 1985.
236. Lee JD, Ginsberg RJ: Lung cancer staging: The value of ipsilateral scalene lymph node biopsy performed at mediastinoscopy. Ann Thorac Surg 62:338, 1996.

CHAPTER 16

The Clinical History and Physical Examination

CLINICAL HISTORY, 379
  Symptoms of Respiratory Disease, 380
    Cough and Expectoration, 380
      Clinical Features, 380
      Etiology, 380
      Complications, 382
    Hemoptysis, 382
    Chest Pain, 385
      Pleural Pain, 385
      Mediastinal Pain, 386
      Chest Wall Pain, 386
    Dyspnea, 387
    Miscellaneous Symptoms, 389
  Past Medical and Personal History, 389
CLINICAL HISTORY, 379
PHYSICAL EXAMINATION, 391
  Examination of the Chest, 391
    Inspection, 391
    Palpation, 392
    Percussion, 392
    Auscultation, 392
      Normal Breath Sounds, 393
      Adventitious Breath Sounds, 394
  Examination of the Heart and Systemic
    Vasculature, 395
  Extrathoracic Manifestations of Pulmonary
    Disease, 396
    Clubbing and Hypertrophic Osteoarthropathy, 396
    Cyanosis, 397

CLINICAL HISTORY

In the first edition of this book, the authors clearly stated that their aim was to define "an approach to the diagnosis of diseases of the chest based on the abnormal roentgenogram." Although we still agree with this approach and with the fundamental significance of the chest radiograph in the diagnosis of pulmonary disease, we believe that it is also important to emphasize the clinical history as the other cornerstone of pulmonary diagnosis. The significance of this aspect of investigation is illustrated by the observation that most chest radiographs are taken because the history directs the attention of the physician to the chest. Of equal or even greater importance is the fact that the key to the diagnostic solution of an abnormal radiographic pattern most often lies in an awareness of the patient's complaints.

Good history taking is an art. It requires that the patient be at ease, confident in the physician's ability, and prepared to divulge all pertinent details that will enable him or her to identify the cause of the malady. Of particular importance is the avoidance of an atmosphere of haste, although often the physician must patiently return a digressing patient to a discussion of pertinent information. After the initial description of respiratory complaints by the patient, the physician should elicit further details. For example, arriving at the significance of dyspnea requires more information regarding its onset: was it sudden or gradual? Concerning its severity, does it occur when the patient is walking slowly in the street or only when running upstairs? Does it require exertion to develop or does it occur even at rest? At what time of day is it particularly obvious? Is it made worse by lying flat? The patient's answers to these questions and to others intended to clarify additional symptoms frequently give the physician a good idea of the diagnosis by the time the history has been taken.

In addition to questions related specifically to current chest symptomatology, any pertinent information concerning past illnesses and personal habits should be elicited. Of prime importance in lung disease is information concerning the patient's tobacco consumption, particularly with respect to quantity and mechanism (e.g., primary cigarette smoking as opposed to secondhand exposure to the smoke from a spouse). Areas of current and previous residence and travel should be ascertained; even a brief exposure elsewhere can result in an infection or infestation that might otherwise be overlooked. A history of exposure in the home to allergens or organic dust known to cause extrinsic allergic alveolitis should be sought when appropriate. Similarly, a complete and chronologic work history may suggest that the patient's complaints are the result of exposure to a specific substance known to be an occupational hazard or may identify nonspecific dust or fumes responsible for chronic cough and expectoration. Since drug reactions can imitate virtually any pulmonary syndrome, a complete drug history is mandatory in all patients. Because of the common and sometimes atypical involvement of the lungs in patients with the acquired immunodeficiency syndrome, risk factors for human immunodeficiency virus (HIV) infection should also be determined. Finally, since lung disease is frequently only one manifestation of a more general process or is secondary to a disease involving other organs, an account of the function of other body systems is essential.

The principal symptoms of respiratory disease are cough, expectoration, hemoptysis, dyspnea, and pain. These symptoms are considered in greater detail, after which further consideration is given to the pertinence of personal, occupational, and residential history and to disease of other organ systems commonly associated with respiratory disorders.

Symptoms of Respiratory Disease

Cough and Expectoration

Cough is a defense mechanism designed to protect against the inhalation of noxious substances and rid the conducting airways of aspirated foreign material and excessive respiratory tract secretions. The prevalence of chronic cough is high, particularly in cigarette smokers, in whom more than 30% of men and 25% of women have the symptom.[1-4] Despite these figures, there is evidence that women have a more sensitive cough reflex than men.[4a] Although smokers may not seek attention for chronic cough and sputum production, the presence of these symptoms may predict future decline in lung function[1] and may be associated with the more ominous symptom of breathlessness.[3, 5] Chronic cough is also surprisingly frequent in people who do not smoke, approximately 5% of individuals in the general non-smoking population complaining of the symptom.[6] Epidemiologic surveys have linked the likelihood of cough in some of these people to indoor[7-10] or outdoor[10-12] air pollution. Cough is also a symptom of more than 100 diseases,[13] ranging from the trivial to the most serious; as such, it always signals the need for further evaluation. However, clinically stable patients subjected to obvious irritant exposure such as tobacco smoke should avoid exposure (e.g., quit smoking) before costly and unnecessary investigation of the nature of their cough is undertaken.

Clinical Features

The etiology of a patient's cough can often be deduced from the history alone. Questions should be asked concerning its time course (is it acute or chronic?), its character (is it productive or dry, and if the former, what is the nature of the expectorated sputum?), its provoking features, and the presence of additional clinical features.

Although the character of a cough rarely indicates the disease process responsible, it may suggest its site of origin. Patients with chronic postnasal drip frequently describe a cough that originates from a need to "clear the throat," and both the physician and patient recognize it as originating in the upper respiratory tract. The cough is often described as "hacking"—a short, dry, frequently repeated cough, different from the deep, "loose" cough of patients with disease in the bronchi or lung parenchyma. Patients with tracheal lesions sometimes have a "brassy" cough, whereas a "bovine" sound has been described in association with laryngeal paralysis. When patients have narrowing in the upper airways significant enough to cause cough, the breath sounds may have a stridorous or "Darth Vader" quality. A prolonged change in the character of a cough in a current or previous smoker should alert the clinician to the possibility of an underlying endobronchial neoplasm; such a change can also be caused by endobronchial suture material in a patient who has undergone resection for pulmonary carcinoma.[14, 15]

The character and quantity of expectorated material may also suggest a specific etiology. Patients who have chronic bronchitis typically expectorate small quantities of mucoid material; with acute bronchitis, the expectorated material may become more abundant, yellow or green in color, and (sometimes) blood streaked. Saccular bronchiectasis typically gives rise to copious, purulent, and often blood-streaked expectoration every day. The gelatinous, "rusty" expectoration formerly associated with pneumococcal pneumonia has rarely been seen since the advent of antibiotics, and bacterial pneumonia is now more commonly associated with thick yellow or greenish sputum. A foul or fetid odor should suggest infection from fusospirochetal or anaerobic organisms, usually in cases of lung abscess. Casts of the bronchial tree consisting of strands of inspissated mucus can be seen in cases of bronchitis, asthma, or mucoid impaction, the last often in association with allergic bronchopulmonary aspergillosis. Occasionally, expectorated material greatly exceeds the amount generally seen in bronchitis; although the etiology of such "bronchorrhea" is obscure in many cases,[16] in some it is associated with bronchioloalveolar carcinoma.[17] Rarely, expectoration of hair (tricoptysis) or bile (biliptysis) is a clue to the presence of an intrapulmonary teratoma or bronchobiliary fistula.[18] Sometimes it is difficult to differentiate sputum from saliva; in such circumstances, demonstration of alveolar macrophages in material submitted for cytologic analysis will establish its pulmonary origin.

The time of occurrence of the cough may also be useful in determining its etiology. Most people with chronic cough complain that it is worse when they lie down at night; this nocturnal change is particularly evident in those who have bronchiectasis or a postnasal drip from chronic sinusitis. Patients with chronic bronchitis or bronchiectasis also expectorate on arising in the morning. Episodes of coughing caused by asthma or left-sided heart failure frequently occur at night and may awaken the patient. A cough in association with or shortly after the ingestion of food should suggest aspiration.

Etiology

The etiology of cough is best considered in two groups—acute and chronic. The cause of the former is usually apparent from the clinical context. By far the most frequent is the common cold, which is accompanied by cough in approximately 85% of cases.[19] This cough may be related to lower respiratory tract infection by the virus, to postnasal drip resulting from rhinitis and/or sinusitis (which may be occult),[20] or to throat clearing secondary to pharyngitis or laryngitis. The diagnosis of acute cough in association with more serious disease such as pneumonia, aspiration, congestive heart failure, pulmonary hemorrhage, or pulmonary thromboembolism is usually suggested by other symptoms and/or the associated clinical setting. For example, cough associated with breathlessness, peripheral edema, orthopnea, and paroxysmal nocturnal dyspnea clearly suggests a diagnosis of biventricular heart failure, whereas in a debilitated, elderly hospitalized patient with new onset of cough, the possibility of pneumonia and/or aspiration should be considered.

Patients with chronic cough defying easy diagnosis are commonly referred to chest physicians for consultation. It is likely that these patients are not representative of "chronic coughers" in the population at large. Smokers, who frequently have chronic cough, seldom complain of it and may even be surprised to learn that cough is not a normal phenomenon. Such individuals have generally been excluded[21, 22] or under-represented[23] in series concerned with chronic cough. When the cause of cough remains obscure after obtaining a history, physical examination, chest radiograph, and lung function studies, the application of a systematic "anatomic, diagnostic protocol" has proved useful in diagnosis.[21–24] Investigations focused on tissues rich in cough receptors have led to the appreciation that most cough in this clinical context can be explained by postnasal drip, asthma, or gastroesophageal reflux. In some investigations, about 20% of patients have been considered to have "postinfectious" cough;[21] although this etiology is clearly valid in some patients, the number of such cases may have been overestimated because of a failure to fully investigate other specific causes. It is important to remember that up to 25% of patients may have more than one cause of cough;[21] for example, patients with allergic rhinitis may also have asthma.

The most common cause of cough in patients whose diagnosis is unclear after initial evaluation (including spirometry) is postnasal drip secondary to rhinitis and/or sinusitis of a variety of causes, including allergic and perennial rhinitis, vasomotor rhinitis, and rhinitis medicamentosa. The importance of postnasal drip as a cause of chronic cough is illustrated by one report of 45 patients, 39 (87%) of whom experienced at least initial resolution of cough with the use of antihistamine/decongestant medication.[25] Diagnosis of this condition is usually based on a history of chronic nasal discharge, a sensation of something dripping down the back of the throat, or frequent clearing of the throat. Physical examination of the nasopharynx and oropharynx reveals mucoid or mucopurulent secretions and a cobblestone appearance of the pharyngeal mucosa. Occasionally, cough is the only clinical manifestation of "postnasal drip," in which case radiologic studies may be required to confirm a diagnosis of sinusitis.[26] Despite the prolonged duration of cough in many of these patients, it typically resolves with appropriate therapy.[21–24, 27]

Chronic cough may also be the principal clinical manifestation of patients with asthma.[25, 28, 29] A history of intercurrent wheezing, family or personal atopy, or worsening of cough following exposure to allergens or irritants should reinforce the clinician's suspicion of this relationship. The presence of these features increases the post-test probability that occult asthma is important in explaining the cough when nonspecific bronchial provocation tests are performed.[30, 31] In fact, this diagnosis has been documented in about one quarter of all patients with cough in several series.[21–24] An intriguing report of seven patients with chronic cough and eosinophilic bronchitis in the absence of asthma or airway hyper-responsiveness adds to the complexity of the diagnosis of chronic cough;[32] fortunately, such patients seem to be rare.

Gastroesophageal reflux is also a common cause of chronic cough; in fact, cough is frequently the only manifestation of this disorder.[33–36] Although there is a paucity of placebo-controlled trials of antireflux therapy in patients with chronic cough and proven reflux, the evidence associating the two is compelling and includes a number of clinical and experimental observations.

1. Studies using esophageal pH monitoring have shown a significant correlation of cough frequency with the severity of reflux.[33, 35, 36]

2. Experiments in which acid or saline has been applied to the lower part of the esophagus of patients with cough and gastroesophageal reflux have shown a striking association of acid infusion with cough.[34] Although some investigators have not been able to confirm the induction of cough by direct instillation of acid in the esophagus,[35] this does not by itself negate the association since specific episodes of reflux do not necessarily cause an immediate cough;[35–38] in fact, patients cough much more frequently than they have reflux events, an observation more in keeping with the conclusion that reflux has caused the cough instead of cough causing the reflux.

3. Clearance of esophageal acid following reflux is impaired in patients with cough when compared with control subjects.[39]

4. Finally, although treatment might need to be prolonged, therapy for reflux leads to resolution of the cough.[21–24, 35]

The pathogenesis of reflux-associated cough is not entirely clear. Aspiration of acid into the lungs is likely to be responsible in only a small minority of patients.[35, 40] Instead, there is considerable evidence implicating a vagally mediated reflex, including (1) the demonstration that cough induced by exposure of the lower part of the esophagus to acid can be prevented by the prior inhalation of an anticholinergic bronchodilator or by prior installation of a local anesthetic into the esophagus;[34] (2) the observation that there is a decrease in lung function in patients with asthma following installation of acid in the lower portion of the esophagus;[41, 42] and (3) the demonstration that patients who have reflux without cough or endoscopically demonstrable esophagitis have a reduced cough threshold as assessed by capsaicin provocation testing.[43]

Capsaicin testing evaluates the role of cough sensitivity or susceptibility in the pathogenesis of cough.[44] An increased cough response to this agent is independent of changes in airway reactivity as measured by histamine provocation;[45, 46] an abnormal test result may be seen in patients with cough of both known and unknown causes. The finding that patients with chronic cough related to reflux and other nonasthmatic etiologies have mononuclear cell infiltration and epithelial damage in the airway mucosa supports the idea that more than esophageal irritation is necessary to cause cough.[47] The etiology of the airway inflammation in this context is unknown.

Bordetella pertussis infection may be a more common cause of chronic cough in adults than is generally appreciated,[48] particularly in those who have contact with infected children.[49] In one study of 79 such adults, the mean duration of cough was 54 days;[49] 80% suffered from cough longer than 3 weeks. Although frank whooping was uncommon (8%), cough followed by vomiting or choking and cough disturbing sleep were each seen in about 50% of patients. In another review of 75 unselected adults with cough of 2 weeks' or more duration, serologic evidence for pertussis was found in 16 (21%);[50] no patient had a positive culture for *B. pertussis*.

With the increasing use of angiotensin-converting enzyme inhibitors in the management of hypertension and heart failure, these agents have become an important cause of chronic cough in the population of patients at risk, the latter occurring in at least 10% of users (*see* page 2570).[51-55] The complication is more common in women than men.[56] Cough typically diminishes promptly after withdrawal of treatment with the drug; however, patients with mild cough may also improve despite continuation of the offending agent.[57]

Whether stress or anxiety can be a cause of chronic cough has not been carefully examined. Certainly, some patients with chronic cough become quite anxious about their condition. For example, in one study of 30 adults with chronic cough who were evaluated by a validated psychological symptom questionnaire, somatization scores were in the clinically significant range in 10.[58] However, these patients had other recognized causes of chronic cough, and it is unclear whether their anxiety was an additional causative influence or simply a secondary effect. In a random sample of 800 subjects chosen from a larger cohort of participants in the European Community Respiratory Health Survey in Uppsala, Sweden, there was a significant correlation between chronic nonproductive cough and female gender (odds ratio, 1.8) and anxiety (odds ratio, 1.7).[59]

Complications

The complications of cough are numerous and range from minor irritation to incapacitation (such as stress incontinence or interference with speech and sleep) to death (e.g., when cough syncope occurs while driving a vehicle).[13, 60] The stresses placed on the body during coughing may injure a number of organs and tissues, including the back;[61] ribs;[62, 63] esophagus (with perforation and mediastinitis[64]); larynx;[65] surgical or accidental wounds (causing disruption); subconjunctival, nasal, anal, and dermal veins (disruption of the latter causing petechiae and purpura);[60] pelvic floor (causing stress incontinence);[65] abdominal muscles;[66, 67] pleura (resulting in pneumothorax and/or pneumomediastinum);[68] bronchi;[69] and lung (causing interstitial emphysema).[70]

Neurologic complications of cough include "benign" cough headache,[71] cerebral air embolism (as reported in a patient maintained on positive-pressure ventilation[71a]), vertebral artery dissection,[72] seizure,[73] and cough syncope. "Benign" cough headache has been described as the initial symptom in a patient with a cerebral aneurysm;[74] "cough" toothache has also been described.[75] Patients with cough syncope are usually of stocky build and smoke and drink heavily. Although commonly attributed to cerebral ischemia from decreased cardiac output secondary to the abrupt rise in intrathoracic pressure, syncope can occur before a decline in peripheral blood pressure and after a single cough.[76] Cough syncope has also been reported to occur as a complication of whooping cough in both children[71] and adults[78] and in association with intracerebral neoplastic or vascular disease.[79, 80]

In addition to its effects on blood pressure, cough may produce several other cardiovascular complications. If severe

enough, it may result in dislodgment of venous or cardiac mural thrombi with pulmonary or systemic embolization. It may also cause the displacement of right heart or central venous catheters and may even kink or knot ventriculoatrial shunts placed for the management of hydrocephalus.[13] Rarely, cough has been associated with ventricular tachycardia.[81]

Hemoptysis

Hemoptysis (expectoration of blood) is an alarming symptom to the patient and physician alike and often indicates serious underlying pathology. It always warrants the taking of a careful history and obtaining chest radiographs; many patients also require more extensive investigation.

Irrespective of the amount of blood produced, it is important as a first consideration to distinguish a pulmonary source of bleeding from one outside the lung. The latter may include the nose, nasopharynx, esophagus, or upper gastrointestinal tract. Difficulty in diagnosis is particularly likely when vomited blood is aspirated into the airways or when expectorated blood is swallowed. In our experience and that of others,[82] this confusion is especially apt to occur when there is major bleeding from the upper airway above the larynx.

The patient may have a nosebleed, with some blood trickling into the pharynx and causing cough and expectoration. The pharynx itself may bleed because of its involvement in an ulcerative process. Bleeding from these sites or from the gums can usually be distinguished clinically from hemoptysis originating in the lower respiratory tract: in the former situation, the patient is more likely to be able to localize the source of bleeding; in addition, the patient often describes "spitting" or "hawking" of blood rather than expectoration and cough. When there is doubt about the source of bleeding, the patient should be assumed to have lung disease and should be examined accordingly.

There may also be confusion about whether blood is arising from the lung or gastrointestinal tract. Blood originating from the former site is usually bright red, often frothy, and usually provokes cough. It may be mixed with sputum or purulent secretions and often occurs in the context of a history of known lung disease. By contrast, blood originating in the esophagus or gastrointestinal tract is usually dark red or black and never frothy. It may be associated with nausea and vomiting and may be mixed with food particles. A history of upper gastrointestinal tract or hepatic disease, such as duodenal ulcer or cirrhosis, should increase the suspicion of such nonpulmonary bleeding.

Published series of causes of hemoptysis generally include patients who have undergone fiberoptic bronchoscopy and do not reflect the profile of patients seen in the office setting; for example, young patients who have a single episode of blood streaking during an attack of acute bronchitis are often not represented in such reviews. Thus, it is somewhat difficult to generalize reported figures of the frequency of the various causes of hemoptysis to the entire population. Incidence figures are also related to specific geographic areas or social groups. For example, in one investigation of elderly males from Los Angeles, 29% suffered from pulmonary carcinoma and 23% had bronchitis; in 22%, the cause of the hemoptysis was "idiopathic."[83] In another review of 208 patients seen at Hadassah Hospital in Jerusalem between 1980 and 1995, bronchiectasis (20%), bronchitis (18%), lung cancer (19%), and pneumonia (16%) accounted for most of the cases;[84] active tuberculosis was seen in only 1.4% of these patients. In other regions, different proportions of disease might be expected; for example, paragonimiasis is likely to be important in patients from parts of Southeast Asia[85] as is tuberculosis in patients from areas in which the background prevalence is high.[86]

The differential diagnosis of hemoptysis divorced from any clinical and radiographic context is extensive (Table 16–1).[87] The character of expectorated blood may sometimes suggest the underlying disease process. As already mentioned, simple streaking of mucoid material can occur in bronchitis; however, it may also denote a more serious condition such as tuberculosis or carcinoma. When sputum is frankly bloody and does not contain mucoid or purulent

material, it is more likely to be the result of pulmonary infarction than pneumonia, particularly if it persists unchanged for several days. Bloody material mixed with pus should suggest pneumonia or lung abscess in acute illness and bronchiectasis in chronic disease. When the blood is diluted so that it has a pink and sometimes frothy appearance, pulmonary edema secondary to left-sided heart failure should be suspected.

An approach to the diagnosis and management of hemoptysis can be conveniently discussed according to the amount of expectorated blood.

Minor Hemoptysis. There is considerable difference of opinion regarding the definition of minor versus major hemoptysis. For the purposes of this discussion, however, we regard the former as small amounts of blood streaking of sputum or the infrequent expectoration of less than 5 ml of pure blood at any time.

Table 16–1. CAUSES OF HEMOPTYSIS*

Infectious
  Bacterial
    Lung abscess[290]
    Bronchitis[291]
    Tuberculosis
    Bronchiectasis (including cystic fibrosis)
    "Chronic pneumonia"[292]
  Viral[293]
  Fungal[294–297]
    Mycetoma
  Parasitic[298]
    Paragonimiasis (in endemic areas)

Cardiovascular
  Left ventricular failure
  Pulmonary thromboembolism with infarction[299]
  Mitral stenosis
  Tricuspid endocarditis with septic embolism[300]
  Pulmonary hypertension
  Aneurysms
    Aortic aneurysm[301, 302]
    Subclavian artery aneurysm[303]
    Left ventricular pseudoaneurysm[304]
  Vascular prostheses[305]
  Arteriovenous malformation[306]
  Portal hypertension with tracheobronchial varices[307]
  Absence of the inferior vena cava[308]
  Pulmonary artery agenesis with lung systemic vascularization[309]

Neoplastic
  Pulmonary carcinoma
    Squamous cell carcinoma
    Small cell carcinoma
  Carcinoid tumor
  Tracheobronchial gland tumors
  Metastatic carcinoma/sarcoma

Traumatic
  Aortic tear
  Lung contusion
  Lithotripsy[310]
  Ruptured bronchus
  Tracheocarotid fistula[311]
  Bronchoscopy[312]
  Swan-Ganz catheterization[313]
  Lung biopsy
  Transtracheal aspirate
  Lymphangiography
  Hickman catheter–induced cavabronchial fistula[314]

Immunologic
  Vasculitides[315, 316]
    Wegener's granulomatosis
    Systemic lupus erythematosus
  Goodpasture's syndrome
  Idiopathic pulmonary hemosiderosis
  Other lung-renal syndromes

Drugs and toxins
  Anticoagulants[317, 317a]
  Cocaine[318]
  Penicillamine[319]
  Trimellitic anhydride[318]
  Solvents[318]
  Amiodarone[320]

Miscellaneous
  Increased bleeding tendency
    Coagulopathy
    Thrombocytopenia
  Amyloidosis[321, 322]
  Broncholithiasis[323]
  Endometriosis[324–326]
  Thoracic splenosis[327]
  Aspirated foreign body
  Intralobar sequestration[328, 329]
  Radiation[330]
  Lymphangiomyomatosis[331]
  Factitious[332]
  Bronchiolitis obliterans organizing pneumonia (BOOP)[333]
  Lipid pneumonia[333a]

*Most common causes indicated in bold type.

In any circumstance, minor hemoptysis is an indication for a chest radiograph; in most cases, culture of expectorated sputum for mycobacteria is also appropriate. Although bronchoscopy is also indicated in many patients, in some it is reasonable to forgo this procedure in others.[88] Such patients include (1) those with a strong clinical history of a nonneoplastic disease process that can explain the bleeding (e.g., bronchiectasis); (2) those with a demonstrated site of extrapulmonary bleeding; (3) those whose clinical status is so poor that no action would be taken regardless of the bronchoscopic findings; and (4) those who are nonsmokers and who have no findings on chest radiography suggesting a neoplasm. However, if hemoptysis recurs despite antibiotic therapy for presumed endobronchial infection, direct visualization of the airways is indicated.

When the chest radiograph is normal or does not demonstrate any findings suggestive of malignancy, certain clinical features indicate a higher risk of undetected pulmonary carcinoma. These include a history of smoking, age greater than 40 years, male sex, and recurrent bleeding.[89–91] HRCT and bronchoscopy are indicated in such patients and are complementary in establishing the etiology of hemoptysis. CT scanning may demonstrate carcinomas not apparent on the radiograph (Fig. 16–1) or beyond the reach of the bronchoscope[92, 93] and can aid in determining the stage and extent of central tumors.[94] In addition, HRCT scans may reveal foci of bronchiectasis inapparent or ill defined on plain radiographs (Fig. 16–2).[93, 94] On the other hand, bronchoscopy may reveal mucosal abnormalities that are inapparent on CT scanning, including squamous metaplasia and carcinoma *in situ*, bronchitis, and other mucosal lesions such as Kaposi's sarcoma.[92, 94] Although the prognosis of patients with hemoptysis who have normal chest radiographs and nondiagnostic bronchoscopic findings is generally good,[95, 96] clinically evident carcinoma will ultimately develop in a sig-

nificant number of those who have the aforementioned risk factors (e.g., 6 [5.6%] of 106 such patients in one series[90]).

Massive Hemoptysis. Definitions of massive hemoptysis quoted in the literature vary widely, and it is not surprising that statements concerning the prognosis of the condition and its suggested management are varied. Thus, amounts of expectorated blood ranging from 100 ml/day[97] to 150 ml/hr[98] to more than 1,000 ml/day[99] have been considered "massive" by different investigators.

Massive hemoptysis is most commonly seen with tuberculosis (both active and bacteriologically inactive), bronchiectasis, carcinoma, abscess, and fungus balls.[100] Increasing amounts of expectorated blood and an increasing rate of blood loss are associated with higher mortality;[99, 101, 102] other features that are associated with higher mortality rates include aspiration of blood in the contralateral lung,[103] the presence of hypotension at the initial examination,[99] underlying poor lung function precluding surgical intervention,[97, 99, 102, 103] and the presence of specific underlying conditions such as pulmonary carcinoma.[99, 104] For example, the mortality in two series of patients managed medically was 22% and 29% overall;[97, 99] however, when only potentially operable patients managed medically were considered, the mortality rate was 1.6% and 11%, respectively.

Although bronchial artery embolization has not been the subject of a randomized controlled trial, almost all patients undergoing the procedure will cease bleeding.[105–109] Failure to control bleeding with a first procedure may indicate a source in the pulmonary artery.[110] Control of bleeding in lesions that have associated pleural thickening may be particularly difficult.[111] Despite initial success, recurrent hemoptysis occurs in the following months in up to one third of patients; some of these recurrences may be fulminant and result in a fatal outcome.[112] Fatal hemoptysis has also occurred in apparently stable patients awaiting continuing in-

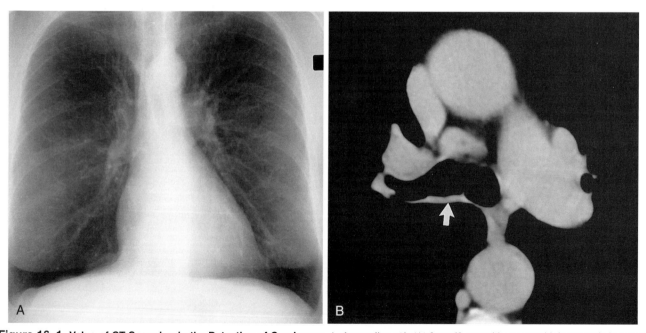

Figure 16–1. Value of CT Scanning in the Detection of Carcinoma. A chest radiograph *(A)* from 63-year-old woman with hemoptysis is normal. A CT scan (5-mm-collimation spiral CT) *(B)* demonstrates focal thickening of the posterior wall of the right main bronchus *(arrow)*. Bronchoscopic biopsy confirmed the presence of squamous cell carcinoma. (Although an enlarged paratracheal lymph node is also seen on the CT scan, mediastinoscopy was negative.)

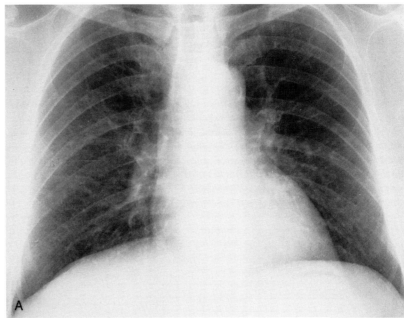

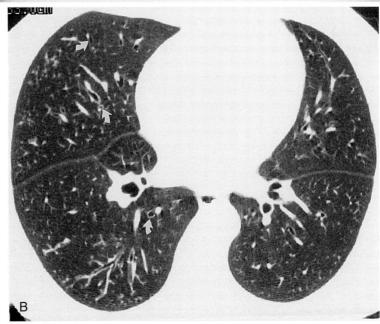

Figure 16–2. Value of CT Scanning in Detection of Bronchiectasis. A chest radiograph *(A)* from a 52-year-old man is normal. HRCT *(B)* demonstrates bronchiectasis in the right middle and lower lobes *(arrows).*

vestigation in the hospital for massive hemoptysis after initial stabilization (as in 8 of 123 such patients in one series).[113]

Chest Pain

The great majority of cases of chest pain that require evaluation are acute in nature. Chronic pain is less common but may be a difficult and sometimes unsolvable diagnostic problem. Thoracic pain can be considered in three categories according to its origin: the pleura, the mediastinum, and the chest wall. The many and varied causes of acute chest pain have been the subject of an extensive review.[114]

Pleural Pain

Since the lung and visceral pleura lack sensory pain innervation, disease of these structures alone may progress to an advanced stage, including death, without producing even minor pain. The parietal pleura, on the other hand, has a rich sensory network derived from the intercostal and diaphragmatic nerves. The nerve endings are stimulated by inflammation and stretching of the pleura and not, as was believed in the past, by the friction of visceral against parietal pleura.

Pleural pain may vary in degree from lancinating discomfort during slight inspiratory effort to a less severe but still sharp pain that may "catch" the patient at the end of a maximal inspiration. It often disappears or is reduced to a dull ache during expiration or breath-holding. Pressure over the intercostal muscles in the area of pain may or may not elicit discomfort; when it does, the pain is mild when compared with that produced by deep breathing. This situation contrasts with chest wall pain, which is associated with a palpable zone of tenderness, sometimes severe and often localized to a small area.

Except when it involves the diaphragm, the diseased area of pleura typically underlies the area in which pain is perceived. The central part of the diaphragm is innervated by the phrenic nerve, and the sensory afferent fibers enter the cervical cord mainly in the third and fourth cervical posterior nerve roots; hence irritation of the central portion of the diaphragmatic pleura is referred to the neck and the upper part of the shoulder. The outer parts of the diaphragmatic pleura are supplied by lower intercostal nerves that enter the thoracic cord in the 7th to 12th dorsal posterior nerve roots; irritation of this portion of the pleura thus causes referred pain in the lower part of the thorax or upper portion of the abdomen.

Pleural pain usually signifies inflammatory or malignant disease, either of the pleura itself or of the lung parenchyma immediately adjacent to the region of affected pleura. Chest pain is also commonly experienced by patients in areas adjacent to bronchiectatic lung, even without apparent current infection.[115] Pneumothorax is another condition that is frequently manifested by pleural pain; although the mechanism of pleura irritation is not known, the pain is generally made worse by deep inspiration and may have an aching quality or be felt simply as a tightness in the chest.

Mediastinal Pain

Pain originating in the mediastinum varies considerably in quality as a result of the several organs it contains. The trachea, esophagus, pericardium, aorta, heart, thymus, and many lymph nodes are situated in the mediastinum, and disease involving any of these organs may cause pain in that region. It should also be borne in mind that inflammation or neoplastic infiltration of the mediastinal soft tissue itself may cause discomfort.

The quality, intensity, and radiation of the pain, as well as its precipitating factors, are important in determining its origin. Pain in the retrosternal or precordial area is particularly frequent, the most common cause clearly being myocardial ischemia. It is typically described as "squeezing," "pressing," or "choking" and may extend to the neck or down the left or both arms. Although most commonly related to the myocardium, retrosternal pain typical of this tissue may in fact originate elsewhere. For example, the severe pain caused by myocardial infarction may be closely simulated by massive pulmonary thromboembolism; in this case the mechanism is thought to be related to acute pulmonary hypertension. A "squeezing" pain identical to that of angina pectoris may be also experienced by patients with severe chronic pulmonary hypertension. Acute pericarditis may also cause pain confusingly similar to that produced by myocardial disease; the pain often has a precordial distribution but may be made worse by breathing or swallowing and be relieved by bending forward.[116] Dissecting aneurysm of the aorta may give rise to a similar retrosternal pain and should be suspected when it radiates to the back and down the abdomen into the lower limbs. Its onset is typically abrupt and may be associated with circulatory collapse.

Other forms of retrosternal pain are less likely to be confused with that originating in the myocardium. A local aneurysm of the aorta may cause "boring" retrosternal or back pain when it erodes the sternum, ribs, or vertebrae. Esophageal disease may give rise to "burning" pain and is usually associated with the ingestion of food. Patients who have regurgitation of acid gastric juice complain that the pain is worse when they lie down or bend over; it may be relieved when they stand. (However, as discussed farther on, symptoms of reflux may be absent in some patients whose chest pain is the result of esophageal disease.) A common retrosternal sensation, which presumably originates in sensory nerve endings of the tracheal mucosa, is the painful rawness experienced by patients with infection of the upper respiratory tract and a dry, hacking cough.

In some instances, the etiology of acute chest pain that resembles angina pectoris is not established despite admission to an intensive care unit and subsequent exclusion of ischemic heart disease by testing. In one series of 89 such patients, only 2 were subsequently readmitted with myocardial infarction;[117] after 1 year of follow-up, 75% of the remainder were in their original employment as compared with only 36% of a group of patients considered to have heart disease. In another review of 100 patients with chest pain and normal coronary angiography undertaken because of a suspicion of ischemic heart disease, 69 were felt to have some type of chest wall tenderness; however, in only 16 could the pain of which they complained be reproduced by direct palpation.[118] Conversely, although atypical, the presence of chest wall tenderness cannot be used to exclude the diagnosis of an acute myocardial infarct.[119]

Patients with panic disorder may also have chest pain. In one series of 441 patients seen at an emergency room complaining of chest pain, panic disorder was diagnosed in 108 (24%);[120] the condition was unrecognized by the attending cardiologist in 98% of cases, and most patients were discharged from the emergency room with a diagnosis of noncardiac chest pain. The criteria for the diagnosis have been reviewed.[121]

Some patients who complain of angina-like chest pain but whose evaluation fails to reveal coronary artery disease have a disorder of esophageal function.[40] For example, in one study of 28 consecutive patients newly referred to a cardiologist for chest pain, 10 (36%) were found to have esophageal reflux.[122] However, other investigators have found no relationship between chest pain and abnormal esophageal function and have questioned whether routine measurement of esophageal motility and pH is useful in the evaluation of patients with chest pain in the absence of coronary artery disease.[123] It is possible that other tests of esophageal dysfunction may be more appropriate in this setting;[123a] for example, balloon distention of the esophagus ("impedance planimetry") in 24 consecutive patients with angina-like chest pain and negative cardiac evaluation revealed an abnormal threshold for pain perception and reproduction of the chest pain in 20.[124] No subjects in a control group had this response.

Chest Wall Pain

Pain originating in or referred to the chest wall that is not the result of parietal pleural irritation is common. Each year, approximately 10% to 20% of the 200,000 patients who have normal angiograms undertaken for investigation of presumed cardiac disease are thought in the end to suffer from this affliction.[125] Patients with chest wall pain also constitute a significant minority of patients seen in the emergency room for noncardiac chest pain.[125]

Pain in this region may originate in the muscles, intercostal nerves, vertebrae, or ribs. When chest wall pain appears to originate in the intercostal muscles, there may be a history of trauma that produced strain or even tearing; however, more often no obvious precipitating cause can be found, and the pain is considered to reflect myositis or fibrositis. In our experience, local pain and tenderness in this tissue are frequently associated with acute infection of the tracheobronchial tree accompanied by dry, often paroxysmal cough. In such cases, tenderness may be elicited by pressure over the painful area, usually in the anterolateral lower intercostal muscles. This form of pain can be differentiated from true "pleural pain" by its limited or lack of increase during deep inspiration, its aggravation by coughing or trunk movement, and its persistence between paroxysms of coughing. Muscle pain not associated with the dry cough of an acute respiratory infection or with direct trauma to the intercostal muscles requires careful investigation to exclude other conditions that may cause referred pain.

Another type of chest wall pain is that due to pressure on or inflammation of a posterior nerve root (radicular pain). This form occurs in the specific intercostal nerve distribution and typically radiates around the chest from behind; in some cases, it is localized to one area. Usually the pain is described as dull and aching and is made worse by movement, particularly during coughing. It may be caused by degenerative joint disease, a protruded intervertebral disk, rheumatoid spondylitis, malignant disease involving the vertebrae, or inflammatory or malignant disease within the spinal canal. A variety of intercostal nerve root pain whose origin may be difficult to identify before appearance of the typical rash is that due to herpes zoster. The pain is usually described as "burning," most often over a wide area unilaterally along the pathway of one or more intercostal nerves.

Pain confined to the vertebral and paravertebral regions is usually caused by inflammatory or neoplastic disease of the vertebrae. Percussion over the vertebral spines may elicit local tenderness. Costovertebral joint pain may be pleuritic in nature, but is reproduced by palpation over the affected joint.[125] An unusual form of pain that usually occurs in bone and lasts for an hour or more after the ingestion of even small amounts of alcohol may be experienced by patients with Hodgkin's disease or other neoplasms.[126]

Disease of the ribs, particularly fracture, is a relatively common cause of chest wall pain. In addition to obvious trauma, fractures may result from prolonged episodes of severe coughing. Rib pain may also be caused by metastatic carcinoma, multiple myeloma or, rarely, a primary sarcoma. The pain is usually appreciated before a mass develops; at first it is poorly localized, but later it is manifested as a dull, boring ache over the area of bone destruction. The costochondral or costosternal junctions of the ribs, as well as the sternoclavicular junction, may be the site of perichondritis; when associated with tenderness and swelling, the condition is known as *Tietze's syndrome*. Usually the pain is persistent and described as "gnawing" or "aching." This condition is generally idiopathic, but care must be taken to exclude bacterial infection. The syndrome is also seen in association with spondyloarthropathy and the sternocos-

toclavicular hyperostosis seen in connection with a variety of skin disorders.[125]

A common transitory chest wall pain of undetermined origin has been described by the name "precordial catch."[127] Typically it is a severe, sharp pain that comes on suddenly during inspiration, either at rest or during mild activity. It usually occurs on the left side of the chest in the region of the cardiac apex and lasts from 30 seconds to 5 minutes.[116] The invariable reaction to the pain is a brief suspension of respiration, followed by shallow breathing while the pain disappears gradually. Its onset is often associated with poor posture, improvement of which sometimes relieves the pain. The importance of the affliction lies solely in its differentiation from other chest pain of more serious consequence.

Dyspnea

Dyspnea—shortness of breath or literally "difficult" breathing—is a common respiratory symptom that should be distinguished from tachypnea (a rapid respiratory rate that may or may not be associated with a sensation of impaired breathing) and hyperpnea (breathing more deeply and perhaps more rapidly than normal). A dictionary definition of dyspnea as "the subjective difficulty or distress in breathing, frequently rapid breathing, usually associated with serious disease of the heart or lungs"[128] does little to illuminate the wide variety of sensations experienced by patients with this symptom. Attempts have been made to quantify the language of breathlessness and correlate patients' descriptions with specific diagnoses.[129–131] Such work suggests that the quality of respiratory sensations varies with different diseases; however, no particular sensation or set of sensations has sufficient sensitivity or specificity to have diagnostic value *in isolation*. A discussion of the physiologic basis of dyspnea is given on page 242.

Clinical evaluation—of which history is a major part—is important in assessing dyspnea; in one study, its etiology was correctly anticipated on the basis of clinical assessment alone in approximately two thirds of patients seen at a pulmonary clinic for the evaluation of chronic dyspnea.[132] A detailed description by the patient of the specific features of the dyspnea is most useful in differentiating organic causes of shortness of breath from functional dyspnea. The latter is related to tension or anxiety and is a common cause of shortness of breath; in one series, functional dyspnea was believed to be responsible for approximately 20% of cases of chronic dyspnea unexplained by history, physical examination, chest radiography, and spirometry.[133] Functional dyspnea is often associated with other symptoms but can occur independently. Usually it is described as an inability to take a deep breath or get air "down to the bottom of the lungs." Patients often spontaneously demonstrate dyspnea by taking a deep breath; if not, it is helpful to ask them to breathe as they do when short of breath. They will respond by taking a deep breath and, as history taking continues, may unconsciously repeat the sighing respirations from time to time. In dyspnea of organic cause, on the other hand, the sensation is more difficult to describe; patients may say that they are "short-winded" or "puff" and on request will demonstrate hyperpnea.

The circumstances in which dyspnea occurs are also helpful in differentiating functional from "organic" dyspnea.

Shortness of breath only during exertion is the hallmark of organic disease. By contrast, patients who are short of breath at rest and not during exercise almost invariably have functional dyspnea; they may say that shortness of breath occurs when they are at home after a busy day or while they are "sitting around doing nothing." "Even now, talking to you, doctor," they might add as they take a deep inspiration. (An exception to this observation is a patient with spasmodic asthma, who may be able to indulge in strenuous exercise without shortness of breath in the intervals between periodic attacks of extreme dyspnea.) On direct questioning, a patient with functional dyspnea may give a history of chronic tension or episodes of acute anxiety precipitating the dyspnea; however, such an association is often not present.

Dyspnea of functional origin may be associated with a variety of symptoms. Some patients complain of weakness and fatigue, symptoms that they confuse with dyspnea. When associated with hyperventilation, a sensation of "pins and needles" in the fingertips, chest pain or tightness, muscle spasm, dizziness, palpitations, and panic may be experienced, especially in situations that induce anxiety such as a visit to a crowded supermarket.[134, 135] Normal subjects rendered hypocapnic and alkalotic through hyperventilation experience a feeling of unreality and lightheadedness, alteration in awareness, and tingling and numbness of the hands, feet, and circumoral area, sensations presumably caused by hypocapnia.[136, 137] However, they are not usually bothered by precordial discomfort or sweating, symptoms that probably relate to associated anxiety in patients with hyperventilation syndrome.

Identification of panic disorder in a patient does not exclude coexistent pulmonary pathology. In fact, there is every reason to believe that patients with pulmonary disease, especially those with COPD, have a high rate of panic disorder.[121] The symptoms of panic disorder and pulmonary disease overlap, and panic anxiety can reflect underlying cardiopulmonary disease and dyspnea can reflect an underlying anxiety disorder.[121] Moreover, successful treatment of panic in patients with both disorders can improve their functional status and quality of life by relieving anxiety and dyspnea.[121]

Quantification of the severity of dyspnea and elucidation of the circumstances that provoke it may be helpful in arriving at a correct etiologic diagnosis. A number of formal scales have been devised to express this quantification in a precise manner,[138] including the Medical Research Council of Great Britain scale, the Oxygen Cost Diagram, the Baseline Dyspnea Index, the Chronic Respiratory Questionnaire,[139] and the Modified Dyspnea Index.[140] These scales attempt to describe the severity of dyspnea provoked by a defined activity and are a refinement of the key components of history taking.

In patients who have chronic obstructive pulmonary disease (COPD), careful prodding reveals a history of slowly progressive dyspnea; that is, with time the severity of dyspnea increases when performing the same activity, and activities requiring less effort come to provoke dyspnea. Both aspects are important and often require elucidation by the clinician. A careful history should include evaluation of the patient's baseline level of activity, activities that commonly provoke dyspnea, and the severity of dyspnea provoked. The time course of deteriorating symptoms usually matches that of deteriorating pulmonary function and occurs gradually over many years. However, patients may also report relatively discreet episodes of worsening of dyspnea, often in association with upper respiratory tract infection or with certain climactic conditions, a reflection of variation in severity of the underlying air-flow obstruction.

The acute onset of dyspnea also may stem from several disease processes. A patient who has been in good health and in whom such dyspnea develops suddenly usually has pneumothorax. Uncommonly, such dyspnea is the initial episode of asthma or the first indication of mitral stenosis or myocardial infarction. Acute dyspnea may also occur with pneumonia or diffuse bronchiolitis; however, in these conditions there are usually premonitory symptoms of fever and cough, with or without infection of the upper respiratory tract, which readily differentiates them. The sudden onset of dyspnea, often with obvious hyperpnea and tachycardia, in an ill or a postoperative patient may denote pulmonary thromboembolism.

The inability to lie flat because of a feeling of suffocation or shortness of breath (*orthopnea*) or a history of waking during the night with shortness of breath (*paroxysmal nocturnal dyspnea*) strongly suggest organic disease. These symptoms are usually associated with left ventricular failure, but they may also occur in patients with asthma, COPD, or bilateral diaphragmatic paralysis[141] in the absence of heart disease. *Platypnea* (shortness of breath relieved by recumbency) is a much rarer symptom than orthopnea or paroxysmal nocturnal dyspnea that also indicates organic disease. It has been associated with pneumonectomy,[142, 143] upper airway malignancy,[144] constrictive pericarditis,[145] intestinal ileus in the context of a COPD exacerbation,[146] right-to-left shunt through a patent foramen ovale[146a] (in some cases associated with "aortic elongation"[146b]), and cirrhosis with pulmonary arteriovenous shunting.[147]

Dyspnea is physiologic during pregnancy.[148, 149] Approximately 15% of women experience shortness of breath during the first trimester, 50% by 20 weeks' gestation, and 75% by 30 weeks; however, this symptom rarely increases in severity during the final weeks before delivery.[148] It is likely that the pathogenesis of dyspnea in this circumstance results from a combination of the hyperventilation produced by increased circulating progesterone[150] and the physiologic effects of an elevated diaphragm. Dyspnea that is acute, severe, and progressive; occurs at rest; or is associated with other signs and symptoms of lung or heart disease is abnormal and warrants further careful evaluation.[151]

The evaluation of symptoms that may accompany dyspnea is also important in establishing a correct diagnosis. In COPD, dyspnea that develops during exertion is frequently preceded by a long history of cough and expectoration. In patients with angina pectoris, dyspnea may be so closely linked to "tightness" in the chest that they may have difficulty determining which symptom limits their activity and may even be unable to differentiate one sensation from another. In such patients, this combination of symptoms is usually associated with exertion and characteristically requires immediate and complete cessation of activity. This situation contrasts with the dyspnea during exertion experienced by patients with emphysema, who may be able to continue activity at a slower pace. Patients with heart disease who cannot increase their cardiac output to meet the tissues' demand for extra oxygen during exercise may experience not only shortness of breath but also weakness.[152] In patients with asthma, dyspnea is often accompanied by chest tightness, wheezing, and cough and is characteristically worse at night or in the early morning hours.

Miscellaneous Symptoms

Hoarseness occurs whenever one vocal cord fails to come into firm apposition with its fellow. It is usually the direct result of laryngeal disease; occasionally, a primary pulmonary or mediastinal abnormality is the cause, invariably as a result of damage to the recurrent laryngeal nerve as it courses between the left main bronchus and pulmonary artery (*see* farther on).

In neonates, hoarseness is usually caused by laryngomalacia or laryngeal paralysis. In children, an acute onset of hoarseness is most often attributable to infection or to aspiration of a corrosive agent or foreign body. Infectious causes include croup (acute laryngotracheitis, usually caused by parainfluenza virus), laryngotracheobronchitis (following measles, parainfluenza, or respiratory syncytial virus infection), and acute epiglottitis (caused most commonly by *Haemophilus influenzae*, type B).

In adults, sudden onset of hoarseness indicates infection, trauma, allergic edema, or inhalation of noxious fumes.[153] As in children, acute infectious laryngitis is caused by one of a variety of viruses; patients who talk a lot, either from habit or in their occupation, may regain their normal voice only with difficulty. If the symptom persists for more than 3 weeks, the vocal cords should be examined for evidence of another etiology such as a "singer's nodule," contact ulcer, granulomatous inflammatory process such as tuberculosis, or epithelial proliferation (leukoplakia or carcinoma).[153] Hoarseness is also common in patients who use high-dose inhaled corticosteroids for the management of asthma.

The most common pulmonary cause of persistent hoarseness is unilateral abductor paralysis as a result of recurrent laryngeal nerve dysfunction, usually from extension of pulmonary carcinoma into the aortopulmonary window. The nerve may be similarly impaired by dilatation of the pulmonary artery in cases of pulmonary hypertension or by an aortic aneurysm in the same area (Ortner's syndrome).[154]

Fever should suggest infection, particularly when the chest radiograph reveals an air-space opacity; if the fever is accompanied by a teeth-chattering chill, the pneumonia is probably pneumococcal in origin. Fever can also occur with malignancy (especially lymphoma), pulmonary infarction, atelectasis, aspiration of noxious chemicals,[155] obliterative bronchiolitis (with or without organizing pneumonia), drug reactions, and a variety of immunologic diseases such as allergic alveolitis, eosinophilic pneumonia, allergic bronchopulmonary aspergillosis and pulmonary vasculitis.

Confusion, irrationality, and even *coma* can occur as a result of underlying pulmonary disease, particularly in the elderly; these signs are usually associated with hypoxemia or hypercapnia and often with impairment of the cerebral circulation. When they develop abruptly, a number of precipitating disease processes should be considered, including pneumonia, thromboembolism or fat embolism, and hypercalcemia secondary to squamous cell carcinoma. In the appropriate clinical setting, it is also important to rule out secondary infection or metastatic carcinoma to the brain.

Halitosis (foul-smelling breath) is multifactorial in origin[156] and is most commonly related to a disorder of the oral cavity; however, it is sometimes a manifestation of anaerobic lung infection.

Past Medical and Personal History

Although the information gleaned from a patient's respiratory symptoms and chest radiographs will often be sufficient to enable a confident diagnosis, in many cases additional knowledge of past respiratory or current nonrespiratory disease, personal habits, travel to or residence in other regions, and occupational history is useful (and sometimes essential) in establishing a correct diagnosis.

Past Medical History. Knowledge of the past history may influence interpretation of the current illness in several ways. For example, a patient's respiratory symptoms or an abnormal chest radiograph may represent no more than residua of previous active disease. In addition, some diseases such as tuberculosis or carcinoma tend to recur, whereas other conditions represent complications of previous disease, either of the lungs themselves or of extrapulmonary organs. Examples of the former include the development of aspergilloma in an inactive tuberculous cavity, pneumothorax in a patient who has idiopathic pulmonary fibrosis, or empyema in a patient with bronchiectasis. Perhaps the most common example of the latter is the development of metastatic carcinoma to the lungs. In addition to careful questioning of the patient about prior illness, it is mandatory that previous chest radiographs be obtained for comparison with current studies, a task that should always be assumed by the treating physician.

Patients should also be thoroughly questioned about their use of medications. It is important to remember that almost any clinical syndrome can be secondary to the effects of a drug (*see* page 2537). For example, a variety of acute and chronic pulmonary infections occur in patients who are receiving immunosuppressive therapy, lipoid pneumonia may follow the use of nose drops or laxatives containing mineral oil, and respiratory failure may be wholly or partly attributable to recent sedation.

Personal Habits. The presence and degree of a patient's cigarette consumption are clearly of significance in assessing suspected cases of pulmonary carcinoma or COPD. The current and previous smoking history should be obtained and an attempt made to quantify it in terms of the number of pack-years smoked (by tradition using a standardized "pack" size of 20 cigarettes). It is important to remember that a history of smoking cessation does not always hold up to objective confirmation.[157] Because of the potential importance of "secondhand" smoking, knowledge of the personal tobacco use of people with whom the patient lives and has lived is also relevant.

Heavy alcohol intake may result in decreased resistance to infection and an increased risk of aspiration. All patients should be questioned about risk factors for infection with HIV, including sexual practices, intravenous drug use, and history of blood transfusion or the use of blood products.

Inquiry about contact with animals, both domestic and wild, may be very helpful in diagnosis, as exemplified by bronchospasm related to a household pet, ornithosis from a sick bird in the home, Hantavirus pneumonia following exposure to mouse droppings, or Q fever from the inhalation of dust contaminated by sheep or cattle.

Residence and Travel History. A history of residence in or travel through an area in which specific infectious organisms are known to be endemic may be an important clue in diagnosis. Because of the multifarious manifestations of pulmonary infections, this information is potentially important in almost every case of pleuropulmonary disease. For example, a patient who has recently resided in India and who has bronchospasm, leukocytosis, and eosinophilia very likely has tropical eosinophilia, a pulmonary mass in a young farmer from Greece or Italy may well be a hydatid cyst, chronic cor pulmonale in an Egyptian may represent schistosomiasis, and a patient from Vietnam who has chronic hemoptysis may have paragonimiasis.

Although less common than infectious organisms, exposure to other environmental agents in specific sites may also be important in the pathogenesis of pleuropulmonary disease and should be questioned in the appropriate circumstances. For example, cases of mesothelioma have been associated with the presence of asbestos in the soil in certain parts of Greece[158] and Cyprus.[159]

Family History. In pulmonary disease, this aspect is most important with respect to a potential source of infection. Tuberculosis is the most serious of the pulmonary diseases that spread in the home; however, *Mycoplasma pneumoniae*, pertussis, and many viral infections may also be disseminated throughout a household, and knowledge of a recent family illness may be significant in the investigation of a patient who has an acute pneumonia.

Some pulmonary diseases have a familial incidence and a clearly defined dominant or recessive pattern of inheritance. These include cystic fibrosis; some forms of emphysema,[160] interstitial pulmonary fibrosis[161] and pulmonary hypertension; hereditary telangiectasia; ciliary dyskinesia (immotile ciliary syndrome); and alveolar microlithiasis. Most of these conditions are rare, and they may be recognized only when a family history of one of them is revealed.

A variety of other pulmonary diseases are also influenced by heredity, although their expression is strongly affected by environmental factors. Asthma and allergic rhinitis are the most important of these diseases. These conditions, which have been termed "complex genetic disorders," are not inherited in a simple mendelian fashion and are probably related to a variety of gene variants with variable penetrance. Several groups have also reported an association between pulmonary carcinoma and a family history of lung cancer (*see* page 1082).[162–167]

Occupational History. An occupational history should be part of every clinical history of patients with chest disease inasmuch as virtually any pulmonary syndrome may be related to exposure to noxious agents in the workplace. In addition to aiding in the identification of a specific disease, recognition of the relationship of the work environment to the patient's illness prevents further potentially damaging exposure of the worker to the harmful agent, allows for suitable compensation to be considered, may identify other workers at risk for illness, and may lead to the application

of suitable preventive public health measures. Knowledge of the occupational history is particularly important in the evaluation of patients with interstitial lung disease, asthma, malignancy, and chronic air-flow obstruction.

All work experiences should be determined in descending chronologic order, with particular attention paid to the nature of the work and the type of potential exposure. The physician should appreciate that different jobs may be associated with exposure to a specific agent (for example, miners, millers, insulators, pipe fitters, plumbers, ship builders, electricians, and painters may all be exposed to asbestos) and that an individual in a specific occupation may come in contact with many potentially harmful substances (for example, a welder may be exposed to metal fumes, iron, silica, various silicates [including asbestos], and carbon monoxide[168]). It should also be remembered that people can be exposed to dust and fumes from areas adjacent to those in which they normally work, and enquiry concerning these sites of potential exposure is also warranted.

The duration and intensity of exposure to a suspected noxious agent should be ascertained. The worker should be asked whether other workers with similar jobs have become ill or are receiving compensation for a work-related disorder. For acute illnesses, an appreciation that symptoms worsen at work and improve on vacation or during weekends supports the hypothesis that some substance in the workplace is the cause of the disease; however, in a patient who has asthma, this observation does not help to distinguish between the nonspecific effect of irritant exposure and asthma caused by a specific occupational sensitizing agent.

When considering the possibility of an association between occupation and pulmonary disease, it should be remembered that exposure to potentially harmful agents can also occur in the home. Examples include a person who engages in pottery making as a hobby (in whom silicosis may develop), an individual who keeps pet birds (in whom ornithosis or extrinsic allergic alveolitis may develop), and a woman handling the clothing of her husband who works in an asbestos mine (in whom mesothelioma may develop as a result of "secondhand" asbestos exposure).

Systemic Inquiry. A description of the association between pulmonary disease and diseases of other organs would be a description of most of the field of internal medicine. Reviews of the neurologic,[169] ocular,[170] and skin[171] manifestations of lung disease exemplify the complexity of these associations.

Knowledge of systemic disease can be of great help in diagnosis. The mere fact that certain other organs or tissues are involved may suggest a specific condition; for example, a patient with diffuse lung disease who has Raynaud's phenomenon and difficulty swallowing almost certainly has progressive systemic sclerosis, and the combination of lung cavities, sinusitis, and hematuria is highly suggestive of Wegener's granulomatosis. In some instances the pulmonary disease is secondary to disease of another organ; for example, inquiry may reveal symptoms indicating a primary site for multiple nodules of metastatic carcinoma in the lung. In other cases, systemic symptoms are secondary to the pulmonary disease itself. For example, small cell carcinoma of the lung may be associated with several forms of neuromuscular disease, symptoms of which may suggest the diagnosis of this specific form of cancer. Similarly, a diagnosis of chronic pulmonary insufficiency and respiratory failure may be suspected after eliciting a history of headache, confusion, tremor, twitching, or somnolence.[172, 173]

PHYSICAL EXAMINATION

Examination of the Chest

Although there appears to be an increasing reliance on radiographic and physiologic tests in the diagnosis of known or suspected lung disease, we believe that physical examination remains an integral part of clinical assessment. Nevertheless, the reliability of physical examination can also be seriously questioned. In our experience and that of others,[174–178] there is important disagreement between physicians in the eliciting of physical signs. For example, in one study of a group of patients with pulmonary findings, 28% of the diagnoses made on the basis of physical examination alone were incorrect.[178] Although agreement on physical findings exceeded that predicted by chance, four experienced examiners who assessed the same patient agreed on the physical findings only 55% of the time.[178] The more reliable of the physical findings—such as reduced percussion note, pleural friction rub, and wheeze—were associated with agreement among physicians only 50% more often than predicted by chance.[178]

Despite its inherent limitations, we believe that skills in physical examination are important and that the information obtained may be complementary to that derived from chest radiography and physiologic and laboratory testing. A few examples will suffice to show the value of this sometimes neglected procedure. In the office, home, and sometimes even the hospital bed, examination may be the only immediate tool available for assessment of the patient; for example, appreciation of tension pneumothorax in a mechanically ventilated patient may be necessary long before a chest radiograph can be obtained. A breathless patient with a normal chest radiograph may be pale or may have findings on physical examination of pulmonary hypertension or thyrotoxicosis; in these circumstances, the physical examination provides the direction for further investigation. The finding of an enlarged lymph node in the right supraclavicular fossa of a patient with lung cancer may affect the staging and diagnostic approach. When physical examination of the chest and the history are normal, moderate chronic air-flow obstruction is very unlikely to be present.[179] Perhaps more telling than all these specific examples is the observation that the more skilled physicians are in physical examination of the chest, the less likely they are to arrive at an incorrect diagnosis. For example, in one study in which a group of 24 physicians examined four patients for the presence or absence of 18 physical signs, the 8 participants who made no errors in diagnosis in any patient disagreed with their colleagues in the interpretation of any single finding only 3.9 times;[178] by contrast, of the 9 physicians who made diagnostic errors 2 to 4 times, there was disagreement in the reporting of any given clinical sign 7 to 19 times. To some extent then, the problems of observer inconsistency in physical examination maneuvers might be simply a lack of skill.

The front of the thorax is best examined when the patient is supine, and the back should be examined in the sitting or standing position. Patients who are too weak to sit upright unaided should be supported by someone standing at the foot of the bed holding their hands; when sitting upright is impossible because of extreme weakness or serious illness, the patient should lie on the right side and then roll over on the left side, the uppermost hemithorax being examined in turn. Examination of the chest is a comparative exercise: each region of one side should be compared with the same area on the other side, a rule that applies equally for inspection, palpation, percussion, and auscultation.

Inspection

Inspection is typically well under way by the time the physical examination has begun. Throughout history taking, the physician has ample opportunity to learn much about the patient. Does the patient appear sick or well, oriented or disoriented, thin or fat, blue or yellow, sober or drunk? Does he or she smell of tobacco smoke? Are the fingers clubbed or yellow with nicotine or are there the characteristic harlequin nails of one who has recently quit smoking (yellow discoloration of the distal portion of the nail and normal color at the base as a result of new nail growth following smoking cessation)?[180] Is cough present, and if so, what is its character? What are the rate and pattern of breathing? Are accessory respiratory muscles being used? Are Cheyne-Stokes respirations present? What is the character of speech (the severity of illness altering the pattern of speech in some cases[181])? Are there abnormalities such as hoarseness, stridor, and wheezing?

In the examining room, the skin should be inspected for its color and evidence of collateral venous circulation. A local lag in inspiratory movement of the chest wall may not be obvious during quiet breathing, and for this reason the patient should be asked to take a deep breath and the movements of the thoracic cage on the two sides compared. The respiratory rate can be a valuable early indicator of respiratory dysfunction; its usefulness as a screening method for detecting lower respiratory tract infection has been demonstrated in the postoperative period[182] and in geriatric patients.[183]

The thoracic cage should be inspected for evidence of deformity and symmetry of movement. Asymmetrical expansion may be the only physical sign indicating disease of the lung or pleura. It involves loss of elasticity of the underlying tissues or compensatory spasm of the intercostal and diaphragmatic musculature in the vicinity to avoid pain on movement. This sign may be present in acute disease such as atelectasis, pneumonia, or pleuritis or may indicate a chronic or inactive fibrotic process of the lung or pleura; in the latter case, it is often associated with scoliosis of the dorsal aspect of the spine with convexity toward the diseased side.

When loss of volume is considerable, whether caused by an acute or chronic process, there is often a shift of the mediastinum; this shift is detectable as displacement of the apical cardiac impulse and the trachea toward the involved side. With fibrosis and particularly with atelectasis, the lower intercostal spaces may demonstrate abnormal indrawing during inspiration. Intercostal and subcostal indrawing during inspiration (Hoover's sign) is commonly seen in patients who have severe COPD.

Of even greater importance than assessment of the asynchrony of expansion of the two hemithoraces is the assessment of respiratory muscle function (abdominal motion and its pertinence to diaphragmatic contraction are described on page 419). Observation of the patient in the supine position helps determine the relative contribution to inspiration of diaphragmatic and intercostal muscle function. Indrawing of the abdominal wall on inspiration, or alternating predominance of abdominal and thoracic movement, suggests paralysis or fatigue of the diaphragm and may be a marker of impending ventilatory failure.

Palpation

A suspected lag detected on inspection of the chest may be confirmed when a hand is placed on each hemithorax while the patient breathes deeply. The relative contribution of the respiratory muscles can also be assessed by palpation of the abdominal, intercostal, and accessory muscles during inspiration. The apical cardiac impulse and the trachea should be palpated, a shift from normal position indicating loss of volume or a relative increase in the volume of one hemithorax in comparison to the other. The left parasternal region may be palpated to determine whether a heave denoting right ventricular hypertrophy is present. When clinically indicated, the intercostal spaces and ribs should be palpated to identify tumor masses and elicit any tenderness to pressure. The axillae and the cervical region should also be explored carefully to detect enlarged lymph nodes, particularly in patients with suspected malignancy or infection.

Tactile or vocal fremitus is the feeling of a vibration on the chest wall with the spoken voice. The palm or side of the hand is placed on alternate sides of the chest in a symmetric manner as the patient says "ninety-nine," and asymmetry in vibration is noted. Increased vibration is felt in conditions in which sound transmission is increased such as pneumonia; decreased vibration is felt when sound transmission is reduced, such as with pleural effusion, lobar atelectasis, or fibrothorax.

In common practice, signs such as altered fremitus and regional chest wall lag are looked for only when pathology is strongly suspected or in an attempt to distinguish one abnormality (such as consolidation) from another (such as effusion). They should not be part of the routine examination of a healthy individual who has normal chest auscultation.

Percussion

Except in a ceremonial sense, percussion is also generally not part of the routine physical examination of a healthy patient. Nevertheless, it may provide valuable clues to the presence of disease; for example, percussion may indicate the presence of small amounts of subpulmonic fluid in situations in which the chest radiograph is equivocal. It should be stressed that the percussing finger only assesses the superficial 5 cm of lung tissue; no matter how much force is used in this method of examination, the central portion of the lung remains "silent." Also, the differences in percussion note are perceived not only by the ears but also by touch; over solid tissue, the examining fingers appreciate a difference in vibration as well as a sensation of resistance that

can be distinguished from the elasticity felt over air-containing areas.

As with inspection, the chest wall should be percussed in an orderly fashion, with identical areas compared on each side. Since the degree of resonance is influenced by the thickness of the chest wall and the volume of lung underlying the percussing finger, "normal" percussion differs both from patient to patient and from area to area in the same patient. The percussion note in disease and in health may vary from tympanitic (over the stomach gas bubble) to flat (over the liver), sounds readily detectable by even the inexperienced. Between these extremes are degrees of hyper-resonance and dullness whose significance can be evaluated only with experience.

The percussion note is produced by vibration of the percussed finger and sympathetic vibrations of the chest wall and underlying tissues and organs. The quality of the note is determined by its loudness, pitch, and timbre. The amplitude of vibrations (loudness) is much less over solid organs such as the heart and liver than over healthy lung, which because of its elasticity vibrates more. Loudness also depends on the force of the stroke and the thickness of the chest wall. An accumulation of fluid between the percussed finger and underlying lung will also reduce loudness. Resonance elicited by percussion over normal lung is distinguishable from the dull note obtained over a solid organ by the rapidity of vibrations (pitch) and by overtones superimposed on the basic note (timbre); a resonant note has a lower pitch and more overtones. The difference between a normal, resonant note and a tympanitic note—as is heard on percussion over gas in the stomach—is due largely to the difference in timbre.

In the presence of lung disease, the percussion note varies from the impaired resonance heard over an area of pneumonia that is partially consolidated, to the dullness over a completely consolidated or collapsed segment or lobe, to the extreme dullness or flatness associated with a large accumulation of pleural fluid. At the other end of the scale, the note is hyper-resonant in cases of emphysema and pneumothorax and is sometimes tympanitic over large superficial cavities or a particularly large pneumothorax. An unusual form of resonance known as *skodaic resonance* is sometimes heard over a partly compressed upper lung region when the lower portion is collapsed by pleural effusion; the note has a "boxy" quality and the mechanism of its production is unknown.

A relatively new technique termed *auscultatory percussion* is performed by auscultating the chest posteriorly while gently percussing the manubrium and comparing one side with the other.[184, 185] A high degree of accuracy in determining the presence of lung masses has been demonstrated in some studies.[185] In addition, strikingly high sensitivity and specificity for detecting pleural effusion and distinguishing effusion from elevation of the hemidiaphragm have been documented with the use of "auscultatory percussion" in one blinded, controlled evaluation.[185] Although this technique does not appear to be in common use, these descriptions of its diagnostic accuracy suggest that it should be.

Auscultation

Auscultation of the lungs is best performed with a stethoscope with small internal volume and small end piece–

skin contact.[186] The quality and intensity of the breath sounds, as well as the presence or absence of adventitious noises, are ascertained by listening with the bell or diaphragm held firmly against the chest while the patient breathes quietly and then deeply. The design of the stethoscope has been criticized because it can amplify or attenuate sounds within the spectrum of clinical interest.[187] The use of computer technology has provided new information concerning the mechanisms of sound production and new measurements of possible clinical relevance.[187]

Normal Breath Sounds

The quality of normal breath sounds varies from region to region depending on the proximity of larger bronchi to the chest wall. In the axillae or at the lung bases, a vesicular sound that has been likened to the rustle of wind in the trees is heard during inspiration and often early in expiration. The sound of air flow has a somewhat different quality over the trachea and upper retrosternal area; the pitch is higher, and expiration is clearly audible and lasts longer than inspiration. Between the scapulae and anteriorly under the clavicles, particularly on the right side, the breath sounds assume the characteristics of both vesicular and bronchial air flow and are described as bronchovesicular.

The intensity of breath sounds should be appraised. When a subject sitting erect inspires from residual volume, air first enters the uppermost part of the lungs so that in the apical zones the maximal intensity of breath sounds occurs at low lung volumes and is synchronous with maximal air flow. By contrast, over the lung bases the intensity is maximal somewhat later in the inspiratory cycle, at approximately 30% to 50% of vital capacity, again associated with maximal air flow. Inspiration is louder than expiration, which is short and may not even be heard.[188] Use of the term *air entry* to describe regional pulmonary ventilation makes some sense since lung sound amplitude varies primarily with the square of the air flow.[187] In patients with emphysema, a good correlation has been found between weak and absent breath sounds heard through a stethoscope and poor ventilation of the lungs estimated by radioactive xenon.[189, 190] This relationship is the result of diminished air flow and not alterations in the lung parenchyma per se.[191] Phonopneumography has also confirmed some clinical assumptions concerning the intensity of breath sounds.[160, 188, 192–196] This technique uses magnetic tape to record breath sounds while the phase of respiration and air-flow velocity are correlated by a pneumotachograph signal. Using phonopneumography to analyze breath sounds in normal subjects with controlled lung volume and air flow, gravity-related unevenness of regional pulmonary ventilation has been noted[160] and confirmed with radioactive xenon.[197, 198]

Many factors may contribute to a reduction or abolition of vesicular breathing. Intensity depends on the thickness of the chest wall and the region of the lung examined, as well as on the depth of respiration and air flow.[199] It may be difficult to hear breath sounds during shallow breathing caused by weakness or neuromuscular disease. Diminished breath sounds may result from complete obstruction of a lobar or segmental bronchus or a reduction in lung compliance secondary to edema or fibrosis of interstitial tissue. Diminished flow under conditions of severe air-flow obstruc-

tion also may result in very faint breath sounds. Finally, the transmission of breath sounds may be interrupted by an excess of subcutaneous fat or may be completely suppressed by fluid or air in the pleural cavity.

The mechanism of production of normal breath sounds is not completely understood; however, it is widely accepted that the inspiratory portion of the normal lung sound is generated primarily within the lobar and segmental airways, whereas the expiratory component is generated more proximally.[187] Acoustic measurements have confirmed the dependence of sound frequency on body height, with children having a higher frequency of sound than adults.[200] Sounds also differ considerably between the central and peripheral portions of the respiratory tract. Measurement of the intensity of breath sounds at the mouth while eliminating such adventitious sounds as wheezing and stridor shows that the sound of breathing in this location is generated by turbulent flow in the upper respiratory tract;[201, 202] when turbulent flow is reduced by the inspiration of helium, breath sounds at the mouth are attenuated. Attenuation of breath sounds by breathing a helium-oxygen mixture is especially pronounced at higher frequencies, which suggests that flow turbulence is the major determinant of lung sounds at these frequencies.[203] This in turn suggests that the bulk of low-frequency sound propagation to the chest wall occurs in the lung parenchyma, whose acoustic properties are only weakly determined by its gas content.[187] A reduction in bronchial caliber, as in asthma, also increases turbulence by increasing flow velocity, thus augmenting the intensity of the inspiratory sound heard at the mouth in this condition.[201, 202]

At the relatively low frequencies and long wavelengths associated with lung sounds, the large airway walls vibrate in response to intraluminal sound, which allows significant sound energy to be transmitted directly into the surrounding lung parenchyma;[187] at the same time, the entire branching network of airways behaves much like a single nonrigid tube open at its distal end to the relatively large air volumes in the smaller airways and alveoli. At higher audible frequencies, the airway walls become effectively rigid because of their inherent mass, which allows more sound energy to remain within their lumens. Estimates of the mechanical/acoustic impedance mismatch between the lung parenchyma and the chest wall suggest that the latter can account for an order of magnitude decrease in the amplitude of sound propagation and significant alterations in the timing and waveform shape of adventitious lung sounds. However, how the airways, lung parenchyma, and chest wall interact to produce the measurable acoustic properties of the thorax remains a matter of debate.[187]

Auscultation over the glottis normally reveals a high-pitched noise during inspiration, followed by a pause and then by a higher-pitched, louder and longer sound during expiration. This expiratory sound, which is also heard very well over the trachea, is modified slightly in the bronchi, in which it becomes even more high pitched. Tracheal sounds are produced by turbulence and therefore, at a given flow, depend on the dimensions of the trachea. It is believed that the difference between these sounds and those heard at the periphery is related to both a dampening effect of the "spongy" lung tissue and the entry of air from thousands of relatively narrow terminal bronchioles into their acini.[160] The observation that voluntary laryngeal sounds are not heard at the periphery of the lung[204] suggests that the vesicular inspiratory sound is produced by turbulence in airways larger than 2 mm but distal to the main bronchi. Expiratory sounds, heard poorly in the lung periphery, originate from the main bronchi and the trachea, but not the glottis.

When the underlying parenchyma partly or completely loses its air content, such as in pneumonia or adhesive atelectasis, the quality of breath sounds may change from vesicular to bronchovesicular or bronchial. Consolidated or airless lung tissue is an excellent conductor of high-pitched, prolonged expiratory sounds that emanate from adjacent bronchi. Occasionally, when the lung is consolidated, a cavity serves as a resonating chamber, breath sounds having a hollow, reverberating, low-pitched quality known as *cavernous*. Another modification of the noise of bronchial air flow is *amphoric* breathing, a high pitched, metallic sound that occurs when there is a tension pneumothorax over a collapsed lung, usually with an open bronchopleural fistula. Given the rarity of these conditions and diminishing skills in physical examination, these alterations from the usual and easily recognized sound of bronchial breathing heard in consolidation are unlikely to be appreciated by most physicians.

Voice sounds may also provide clues to pathologic abnormalities. During quiet speech, a soft, confused, barely audible sound is normally heard over lung tissue distant from large bronchi. In the presence of consolidation or adhesive atelectasis, voice sounds become more distinct and produce a noise known as *bronchophony*. In many such cases, words are distinctly audible over the involved area when the patient whispers "one, two, three"; this "whispering pectoriloquy" does not occur in the absence of bronchial breath sounds and is a useful confirmatory sign of pneumonic consolidation. Consolidation of lung tissue or its compression by a massive pleural effusion may also result in *egophony* (defined as a change in timbre of the spoken voice [e.g., *ee* as in bee to an *a*-like sound resembling a bleating goat] but not in pitch or volume).[205] When a large accumulation of fluid compresses the lower portion of the lung, the voice sounds sometimes have a nasal quality over the upper part of the lung (analogous to skodaic resonance on percussion). When voice sounds are loud in comparison to the opposite side and breath sounds in the same region are reduced, bronchial stenosis is probably present on that side.[206]

Adventitious Lung Sounds

Several attempts have been made to standardize the terminology of abnormal (adventitious) lung sounds.[207, 208] Discontinuous sounds are known as *crackles* and may be coarse or fine. Continuous sounds that are high pitched are called *wheezes*; when of lower pitch, they are known as *rhonchi*. The use of this terminology in practice is inconsistent and variable,[209, 210] a deficiency that confounds the inherent inaccuracy in physical examination that is the result of expected interobserver variability in the description of subtle events. To avoid these problems, we stress the necessity of using this terminology in a consistent fashion. Adventitious sounds may be divided into those having their origin in the airways and lung parenchyma, those related to the pulmonary vasculature, and those originating in the pleura.

Airways and Lung Parenchyma. Crackles are discontinuous noises that may be fine (relatively high-pitched sounds usually heard at the end of inspiration as air enters the acinar unit) or coarse (the low-pitched, bubbling sounds that result from the accumulation of secretions in larger bronchi and the trachea).[207, 211, 212]

Crackles are present more often during inspiration, when air flow is faster. They may be elicited during a rapid, deep breath, or—particularly when they are fine—during a deep breath after maximal expiration ended by a cough ("post-tussive rales"). Coarse crackles are heard as edema fluid or exudate moves up the bronchial tree and may be audible in patients with bronchopneumonia, bronchiectasis, or chronic granulomatous diseases such as tuberculosis or the mycoses. Fine crackles are sometimes detected at the lung bases at the end of a deep inspiration in individuals without clinically significant pulmonary disease; such individuals are likely to be obese and the crackles may diminish in intensity or even disappear after several deep inspirations. In healthy individuals, these crackles can be heard and recorded anteriorly at the lung bases near the end of a slow inspiration from residual volume;[213–215] they are believed to represent the inflation of atelectatic acini[213] or the opening of collapsed basilar bronchioles.[215]

More frequently, fine crackles are indicative of significant pulmonary disease, in which case they are usually persistent and often occur in showers. Such crackles may be present in several conditions, most commonly pulmonary edema, pneumonia, and interstitial fibrosis. When heard during late inspiration in dependent lung regions in the lateral decubitus position only, they may be an early sign of pneumonia in an acutely ill, coughing patient.[216] During the course of pneumonia, initially coarse crackles may become finer and occur later during inspiration.[217] They are not present in patients with upper airway infection or bronchitis. In patients who have diffuse interstitial disease associated with general loss of lung volume, crackles have a high-pitched superficial quality; they do not disappear on coughing and may represent the passage of air into atelectatic units as small airways previously held closed by surface forces explosively open.[187] The reproduction of breath sounds and adventitious sounds visually has clearly shown different patterns of crackles in cases of pulmonary fibrosis and pneumonia, those in the former being shorter in duration and period than the coarse crackles of pneumonia.[187]

Waveform and spectral analysis separates the waveform of crackles into two segments: a starting segment, in which the sound is determined by the pressure ratio at the site of the airway opening, and a decay segment, which may be modified by the resonant frequency of the lung.[218] Such analysis can confirm and quantify the character of coarse and fine crackles and the differences between them[219–221] and may have diagnostic importance.[221–223] For example, time-expanded waveform analysis of crackles in asbestos-exposed subjects has shown that this technique is more sensitive than auscultation and has a sensitivity for the diagnosis of asbestosis that equals that of HRCT.[224] However, these techniques are not widely available or widely studied, and whether they will have practical importance remains to be determined.

In contrast with crackles, other adventitious sounds that originate in the bronchopulmonary tree are continuous. The presence of wheezes or rhonchi indicates partial obstruction of a bronchial lumen; therefore, they are louder during expiration when the airways are narrower, although they may also be heard in inspiration. Wheezes may be heard at a distance without the aid of a stethoscope. Sounds produced by turbulent flow in the large airways may also be audible without the aid of a stethoscope and produce the characteristic noisy breathing of patients with partial obstruction of the lower part of the trachea or main bronchus. Rhonchi or wheezes not appreciated during quiet breathing may become audible when the rate of air flow is increased during fast, deep breathing or when the airways are narrowed during maximal expiration; however, this finding has little diagnostic importance.[225] A particular form of continuous sound is known as *stridor*, which is an especially loud "musical" sound of constant pitch that is caused by obstruction of the larynx or trachea;[202] it may be heard during either inspiration or expiration or throughout the entire respiratory cycle.

Because of their pathogenesis, the finding of a wheeze or rhonchus is an important clue to the presence of airway disease. If they disappear or change character with time or during coughing, a partly obstructing mucous plug should be suspected. Local wheezes or rhonchi that do not disappear with coughing should suggest the possibility of an endobronchial neoplasm. The term *wheezing respirations* is used sometimes to denote the persistent inspiratory and expiratory sounds heard all over the chest during bronchospasm. That wheezing in patients with chronic air-flow obstruction indicates bronchospasm has been shown in a comparative bronchodilator study of such individuals with and without wheezing,[226] only the former showing a positive response. In patients with asthma, there is an association between the proportion of the respiratory cycle occupied by wheeze, the intensity and pitch of the wheeze, and the severity of airway obstruction.[227, 228]

Pulmonary Vasculature. A continuous murmur heard on auscultation over the lung in a location inconsistent with a cardiac or aortic origin may be related to a pulmonary arteriovenous fistula. A search for this abnormality may be initiated by the discovery on a chest radiograph of a solitary nodule whose characteristics suggest arteriovenous communication, with or without clinically evident mucocutaneous lesions of multiple hereditary telangiectasia (Osler-Weber-Rendu disease).[229, 230] More frequently, a continuous murmur is a chance finding in severe bronchiectasis, particularly of the upper lobes;[231] in this circumstance, the murmur originates from bronchial artery–pulmonary artery anastomoses, the pressure gradient causing an audible murmur and sometimes a palpable thrill. The anastomoses may be of such magnitude that flow in the main pulmonary artery is reversed.[231] A systolic murmur or a murmur that extends beyond the second heart sound may be audible over the lung in patients who have partly obstructing emboli in the proximal pulmonary arteries.[232]

Pleura. A third group of adventitious sounds represents manifestations of pleural disease. The most common of these sounds is related to inflammation of the pleura with the formation of a sticky, fibrinous exudate on their surfaces. Because of this exudate, a rubbing, rasping, or leathery sound (known as a *friction rub*) may be heard as the visceral lining moves against the parietal lining. The sound may be heard during both inspiration and expiration, particularly in

areas in which excursion of the thoracic cage is greatest; it disappears when fluid forms and separates the two membranes. The noise is usually associated with pain. Its disappearance during breath-holding but not during coughing renders it unlike rhonchi caused by partial bronchial obstruction by mucus, which it can closely resemble. The sound is indicative of primary pleural disease caused by trauma, neoplasm, or inflammation or secondary disease related to underlying pulmonary neoplasia, infarction, or pneumonia.

Several sounds relate to the presence of air, with or without fluid, in the pleural cavity. Some of these sounds, such as the Hippocratic succussion splash and the bell sound[233] (the latter produced by tapping one coin against another placed on the chest wall), are of historic interest only. Hamman[234] described a crunching or clicking sound over the lower retrosternal area that is synchronous with the heartbeat. This sound is often audible with a stethoscope and may be noticed by the patient when lying on the left side. Although Hamman thought that the sound was pathognomonic of air in the mediastinum, it is in fact more commonly associated with a left pneumothorax.[235, 236] The sound is of diagnostic importance in that it may be present with small (radiographically undetectable) collections of air.[236]

Examination of the Heart and Systemic Vasculature

Clinical examination of the heart is essential in every case of suspected pulmonary disease since certain abnormalities may provide important clues to its etiology. For example, disease affecting either the pulmonary parenchyma or vasculature may cause pulmonary arterial hypertension, which may be manifested by right ventricular heave, accentuated pulmonic component of the second sound, or pulmonic or tricuspid regurgitant murmurs. In some cases of pulmonary edema secondary to mitral stenosis or acute left ventricular failure, convincing radiologic evidence of cardiac enlargement is absent; in such cases, a mitral valve murmur, severe arterial hypertension, or clinical signs of left ventricular strain such as gallops or heaves may suggest the cause of the edema.

Measurement of systemic arterial blood pressure may also yield clues to the nature of the pulmonary disease. Normally, systolic arterial pressure falls 5 mm Hg or less during inspiration. Pulsus paradoxus consists of an exaggerated inspiratory fall in systemic blood pressure, usually when venous return to the right side of the heart is impaired during inspiration (as in shock, right ventricular failure, cardiac tamponade, and massive pulmonary thromboembolism). Paradoxical pulse also may be found when the intrathoracic pressure swing is excessive, as may occur with obstruction of either the upper or lower airways (particularly severe asthma), in which case it appears to be the result of a reduction in pulmonary venous return[237] or an increase in left ventricular afterload (as a result of large negative intrathoracic pressure reducing cardiac output during inspiration).[238] When interpreting the significance of a pulsus paradoxus, it should be remembered that the "abnormality" is occasionally present in some normal young subjects.

Reversed pulsus paradoxus—a *rise* in arterial systolic and diastolic pressure during inspiration—has been described in patients with congenital subaortic stenosis and in those receiving intermittent inspiratory positive-pressure breathing for left ventricular failure;[78] the finding apparently results from the increased stroke output of the left ventricle.

Measurement of blood pressure during a Valsalva maneuver may be useful in identifying left ventricular failure in patients with severe chronic air-flow obstruction.[239] Patients with air-flow obstruction and left ventricular failure may not show the usual "sine wave" pattern of blood pressure change when normal breathing resumes. In healthy individuals performing a Valsalva maneuver, an initial transient rise in pressure is followed by a fall in pressure as the maneuver is maintained; this in turn is followed by recovery to a pressure higher than the original.

Extrathoracic Manifestations of Pulmonary Disease

The potential for diseases of the chest to have manifestations outside the lungs has been mentioned earlier. Specific findings are discussed in the sections dealing with the relevant diseases. The following section deals with clubbing and cyanosis, abnormalities that should be sought in all patients with disease of the lungs or pleura.

Clubbing and Hypertrophic Osteoarthropathy

These abnormalities are well known historically: in French, clubbing is still referred to as "hippocratism digital" (after Hippocrates) and skeletal changes characteristic of hypertrophic osteoarthropathy (HOA) have been seen in specimens dating from 4,000 years ago.[240]

The term *clubbing* refers to swelling of the soft tissue of the distal portions of the fingers and toes. By contrast, HOA is localized principally to the periosteum of the phalanges and distal portions of the arms and legs. Since not all cases of osteoarthropathy are pulmonary in origin, HOA has replaced the older term *hypertrophic pulmonary osteoarthropathy.*[241, 242] The terms are not synonymous: clubbing frequently occurs in the absence of full-blown osteoarthropathy, and the latter occasionally occurs without clubbing. When the two do coexist, there is no relationship between the severity of clubbing and HOA. Confusion of simple clubbing with HOA is probably responsible for the great variation in reported incidence of these two conditions in patients with pulmonary carcinoma (ranging from 2% to almost 50%).

Although the disorders are usually secondary (most often to cardiac or pulmonary disease), they may be idiopathic, in which case they are known as *pachydermoperiostosis.*[242] Thyroid acropachy, a rare disorder that occurs in association with various diseases of the thyroid gland, should probably be regarded as a distinct entity; it consists of clubbing of the fingers and toes and periosteal new bone formation that involves the hands and feet predominantly rather than the long bones.[243]

Four criteria are generally accepted for a diagnosis of clubbing: (1) increased bulk of the terminal digital tuft; (2) change in the angle between the nail and the proximal skin to greater than 180 degrees; (3) sponginess of the nail bed and periungual erythema; and (4) increased nail curvature. When all these changes are present or when at least one is severe, clubbing is readily recognizable. Unfortunately, its

detection at an early stage is highly subjective and subject to considerable interobserver variation. In an attempt to overcome this shortcoming, methods of objectively assessing the presence and degree of clubbing have been devised and are of particular use in epidemiologic studies.[244, 245, 245a]

Clubbing itself is typically asymptomatic, and it must be borne in mind that most patients do not recognize the change in their terminal phalanges when it is first brought to their attention. This failure to recognize such a subtle, insidious change may be costly, since it may be a marker of a potentially treatable disease. It is thus important not to accept without question patients' statements that their fingers have looked the same all their lives; further investigation is essential before the primary or familial nature of the abnormality can be established.

Although typically bilateral and symmetric, clubbing is occasionally unilateral in patients with vascular abnormalities of a limb (such as aneurysm or infective arteritis[245b]) or in patients with brachial plexus compression; it has also been reported on the affected side in patients with severe hemiplegia and in the toes (with or without involvement of the left hand) in those with patent ductus arteriosus associated with reversal of blood flow.[243]

The pathogenesis of clubbing is not completely understood. In some patients, blood flow to the digits is clearly increased.[246, 247] Although the precise mechanism of this phenomenon is not known, it is probable that the opening of arteriovenous anastomoses (Sucquet-Hoyer canals) in the fingers is involved. Postmortem angiography of clubbed and normal hands has not revealed any quantitative difference in the larger vessels;[248] however, capillaroscopy has shown an increase in small vessel vasculature in the former.[249] Although various markers of inflammation, including ferritin,[250] bradykinin, adenine nucleotides, 5-hydroxytryptamine, and the prostaglandins E and $F_{2\alpha}$[251] may be involved in this proliferation, there is no convincing evidence to incriminate any one of them. However, there is evidence from a number of studies that release of vasoactive compounds and platelet-derived growth factor from large platelets and platelet clumps trapped in the peripheral circulation may be important.[252-257] It is also possible that other growth factors,[258, 259] including tumor-related growth hormone,[260, 260a] may be involved in some cases (although the significance of the latter has been disputed).[261]

In cyanotic congenital heart disease, idiopathic pulmonary fibrosis, and subacute bacterial endocarditis, clubbing is common but HOA is rare.[243] Clubbing can also be seen in patients with far-advanced tuberculosis,[262] but only rarely in association with HOA;[263] of 309 patients admitted consecutively to a tuberculosis sanatorium, only 3 had the latter complication (2 with cancer and the other with a pyogenic abscess).[264]

The clinical diagnosis of HOA requires the presence of deep-seated pain and/or joint symptoms, including arthralgia with swelling and stiffness, affecting mainly the fingers, wrists, ankles, and knees. Radiographs usually show subperiosteal new bone formation in the long bones of the lower extremities, and some consider this finding essential to the diagnosis.[265] Changes may be apparent on bone scan prior to radiographic change.

Except in the rare idiopathic form, clubbing or osteoarthropathy is virtually pathognomonic of visceral disease, the primary organ of involvement having either vagal or glossopharyngeal innervation (Table 16–2).[243, 266] Malignant neoplasms account for 90% of the typical cases of HOA associated with lung disease, the majority being primary but a few metastatic.[267] The most common metastatic neoplasm is soft tissue sarcoma associated with a pleura-based mass.[268] Osteoarthropathy is usually detected before or at the time of diagnosis of the underlying disease, but occasionally is manifested years later.[269]

As with clubbing, the pathogenesis of HOA is not fully understood. It is generally agreed that the earliest morphologic change in the limbs is an overgrowth of highly vascular connective tissue, followed by subperiosteal new bone formation. As in simple clubbing, blood flow to the extremities is increased; in HOA, however, most of this augmented flow appears to be shunted through arteriovenous communications in the areas of osteoarthropathy.[272] In the great majority of cases, the increase in blood flow to the extremities appears to be secondary to a reflex mechanism, the vagus nerve serving as the afferent pathway; the efferent pathway is unknown, but is considered to be hormonal (neuropeptide) rather than neuronal.[243] Since HOA often disappears after removal of an associated intrathoracic tumor, the stimulus to this reflex arc presumably comes directly from the tumor itself or indirectly as a result of tissue damage distal to it.[271]

The hormones responsible are not entirely evident. Increased estrogen production has been reported in some cases of HOA of variable etiology;[272] there is also evidence that increased levels of circulating estrogens may at least exacerbate symptoms, as in the rare cases of HOA that develop in

Table 16–2. CAUSES OF HYPERTROPHIC OSTEOARTHROPATHY*

Pulmonary disease
  Primary carcinoma
  Metastatic carcinoma/sarcoma[334–337]
  Pulmonary artery sarcoma[337a]
  Lymphoma[338, 339]
  Leukemia[340]
  Pneumocystis carinii pneumonia[341, 342]
  Tuberculosis[343]
  Sarcoidosis[344, 345]
  Alveolar microlithiasis[346]
  Adult respiratory distress syndrome[347]
  Cystic fibrosis[348]
  Idiopathic pulmonary fibrosis[349]
  Interstitial pneumonitis and fibrosin associated with
    polymyositis[349a]
  Behçet's disease[349b]

Disease of extrapulmonary organs
  Laryngeal carcinoma[350]
  Diaphragmatic disease[356]
  Thymic carcinoma[352]
  Esophageal carcinoma[353]
  Gastrointestinal polyposis[354]
  Heart disease[355, 356]
  Palmoplantar keratoderma[356a]

Underlying syndrome or condition
  Antiphospholipid antibody syndrome[357]
  Pregnancy[358, 359]
  Purgative abuse[360]
  POEMS[351]

*Most common causes indicated in bold type.

pregnant women, in whom symptoms promptly abate after delivery.[273] Growth hormone produced by a pulmonary tumor has also been implicated occasionally.[274] Hypoxia has also been hypothesized to be a possible mechanism; however, the absence of arterial hypoxemia in many cases of bilateral upper and lower limb HOA suggests that it is relatively unimportant.

As indicated previously, some cases of HOA are not associated with demonstrable disease elsewhere in the body. This unusual condition, known as pachydermoperiostosis, is recognized as having an autosomal form of inheritance with marked variability in expressivity, males being more severely affected than females.[275] A family pedigree has been described in which the abnormality was associated with Crohn's disease and antineutrophil cytoplasmic antibodies.[275a] The disease has its onset around puberty and is associated with a distinctive thickening and furrowing of the skin of the forehead, face, and scalp (cutis verticis gyrata), severe facial acne, clubbing, and periosteal new bone formation.[275–277] Pachydermoperiostosis should not be confused with primary or hereditary digital clubbing, which is present at birth and not usually accompanied by the symptoms or radiographic findings of HOA. Although to the best of our knowledge there have been no studies directed at elucidating the early pathogenesis of pachydermoperiostosis, physiologic and radiologic investigation of this condition in its established state has clearly shown a decrease in circulation to the extremities,[275, 278] which presumably accounts for the excessive resorption of the distal phalanges of the hands and feet (acrolysis).[276]

As indicated earlier, HOA usually resolves with removal of a "causal" tumor. It has regressed following chemotherapy without objective response in the primary lesion,[279] and radiotherapy of a metastatic lesion without treatment of the primary lung tumor.[280] It has also been shown to resolve following reversal of causal liver[281] and lung[282] conditions after transplantation, and to undergo spontaneous resolution.[283]

Cyanosis

Cyanosis is a blue or bluish gray discoloration of the skin and mucous membranes caused by an excessive blood concentration of reduced hemoglobin. It is most obvious in the nail beds or buccal mucosa and is best appreciated in adequate daylight; it is virtually unrecognizable under a fluorescent lamp.[284] It is estimated that 5 gm of hemoglobin per deciliter of blood in the capillaries of the area observed have to be reduced before cyanosis is visible; as a result, this sign is never present in patients with severe anemia.[285] Conversely, it is more readily apparent in patients with polycythemia.

Cyanosis may be classified as *central*, when it is the result of inadequate saturation of arterial blood leaving the left side of the heart, or *peripheral*, when the mechanism is related to sluggish blood flow in the peripheral (systemic) vessels and excessive removal of oxygen in the adjacent tissue. In patients with normal hemoglobin concentrations and normal perfusion, central cyanosis can be appreciated by most observers under appropriate lighting conditions when the arterial oxygen saturation is about 75%.[286]

The pathogenesis of central cyanosis is related to the

development of hypoxemia, which may have several mechanisms. As discussed elsewhere (*see* page 108), ventilation-perfusion abnormalities are responsible for most of the gas exchange defects in parenchymal lung disease. In patients with severe chronic air-flow obstruction, hypoventilation can also contribute to hypoxemia. In other lung diseases such as severe acute air-space pneumonia with circulatory collapse, both central and peripheral factors undoubtedly contribute to cyanosis: the venous blood in pulmonary capillaries encounters airless acini, and the same blood stagnates in systemic capillaries, thus allowing for excessive removal of oxygen by the tissues.

Cardiac conditions with a right-to-left shunt may engender a central form of cyanosis but are differentiated from pulmonary conditions by the clinical findings and the results of pulmonary function tests. Previously inapparent right-to-left cardiac shunts may also become evident as a result of pulmonary disease when pulmonary vascular resistance increases and allows blood to flow from the right to the left atrium through a patent foramen ovale; we have seen this condition in pulmonary thromboembolic disease, where it may be associated with systemic arterial emboli, and it has been reported to occur following pneumonectomy in a patient with COPD.[287] Arterial oxygen desaturation as a result of shunting also occurs in association with cirrhosis of the liver, but the desaturation is rarely severe enough to cause cyanosis.

Peripheral cyanosis may be either paroxysmal and precipitated by cold, as in Raynaud's disease, or general and prolonged, in which case it is often associated with systemic hypotension and physical signs of circulatory collapse. The former type occurs in progressive systemic sclerosis, which commonly involves the lung. Such acrocyanosis may also be idiopathic[288] and has been seen in association with severe anorexia nervosa.[289] Prolonged peripheral cyanosis is more common in primary heart disease than in pulmonary disease; when it does occur in association with cor pulmonale and hypoxemia, it indicates a poor prognosis.

When the cyanosis is central in origin, the nail beds are usually deep blue or blue-gray and the skin is warm, whereas peripheral cyanosis is usually associated with cold, clammy skin and dusky, livid nail beds. Frequently, it is not possible on appearance alone to differentiate with certainty between central and peripheral cyanosis, and other clinical findings may not indicate the cause. However, the degree of oxygen saturation of arterial blood will provide the distinction.

When the pathogenesis of cyanosis is obscure, methemoglobinemia or sulfhemoglobinemia should be considered (*see* page 3068). The former is rarely primary and congenital; more commonly, it results from the ingestion of drugs, including nitrates, chlorates, quinones, aniline dyes, sulfonamide derivatives, acetanilid, and phenacetin. Sulfhemoglobinemia and methemoglobinemia may occur simultaneously, usually from ingestion of the same drugs, in which case the cyanosis is lead colored. When either of these conditions is present, the venous blood is brownish even after being shaken in air for 15 minutes. The diagnosis can be confirmed by spectroscopic analysis to identify the absorption bands.

REFERENCES

1. Sherman CB, Xu X, Speizer FE, et al: Longitudinal lung function decline in subjects with respiratory symptoms. Am Rev Respir Dis 146:855, 1992.
2. Dow L, Coggon D, Osmond C, et al: A population survey of respiratory symptoms in the elderly. Eur Respir J 4:267, 1991.
3. Lundback B, Stjernberg N, Nystrom L, et al: Epidemiology of respiratory symptoms, lung function and important determinants. Report from the Obstructive Lung Disease in Northern Sweden Project. Tuber Lung Dis 75:116, 1994.
4. Krzyzanowski M, Robbins DR, Lebowitz MD: Smoking cessation and changes in respiratory symptoms in two populations followed for 13 years. Int J Epidemiol 22:666, 1993.
4a. Dicpinigaitis PV, Rauf K: The influence of gender on cough reflex sensitivity. Chest 113:1319, 1998.
5. Cullinan P: Persistent cough and sputum: Prevalence and clinical characteristics in south east England. Respir Med 86:143, 1992.
6. Brown CA, Crombie IK, Smith WC, et al: The impact of quitting smoking on symptoms of chronic bronchitis: Results of the Scottish Heart Health Study. Thorax 46:112, 1991.
7. Viegi G, Paoletti P, Carrozzi L, et al: Effects of home environment on respiratory symptoms and lung function in a general population sample in north Italy. Eur Respir J 4:580, 1991.
8. Behera D, Jindal SK: Respiratory symptoms in Indian women using domestic cooking fuels. Chest 100:385, 1991.
9. Ng TP, Hui KP, Tan WC: Respiratory symptoms and lung function effects of domestic exposure to tobacco smoke and cooking by gas in non-smoking women in Singapore. J Epidemiol Community Health 47:454, 1993.
10. Xu X, Wang L: Association of indoor and outdoor particulate level with chronic respiratory illness. Am Rev Respir Dis 148:1516, 1993.
11. Schwartz J, Dockery DW, Neas LM, et al: Acute effects of summer air pollution on respiratory symptoms reporting in children. Am J Respir Crit Care Med 150:1234, 1994.
12. Krzyzanowski M, Lebowitz MD: Changes in chronic respiratory symptoms in two populations of adults studied longitudinally over 13 years. Eur Respir J 5:12, 1992.
13. Leith DE, Butler JP, Sneddon SZ, et al: Cough. In Fishman AP, Macklem PT, Meade J (eds): Handbook of Physiology. Section 3. The Respiratory System. Vol 3. Mechanics of Breathing, Part 1. Bethesda, MD, American Physiological Society 1986, p 315.
14. Shure D: Endobronchial suture. Chest 100:1193, 1991.
15. Albertini RE: Cough caused by exposed endobronchial sutures. Ann Intern Med 94:205, 1981.
16. Calin A: Bronchorrhoea. BMJ 4:274, 1972.
17. Storey CF, Knudtson KP, Lawrence BJ: Bronchiolar ("alveolar cell") carcinoma of the lung. J Thorac Surg 26:331, 1953.
18. Koch KA, Crump JM, Monteiro CB: A case of biliptysis. J Clin Gastroenterol 20:49, 1995.
19. Curley FJ, Irwin RS, Pratter MR, et al: Cough and the common cold. Am Rev Respir Dis 138:305, 1988.
20. van Duijn NP, Brouwer HJ, Lamberts H: Use of symptoms and signs to diagnose maxillary sinusitis in general practice: Comparison with ultrasonography. BMJ 305:684, 1992.
21. Irwin RS, Curley FJ, French CL: Chronic cough. Am Rev Respir Dis 141:640, 1990.
22. Hoffstein V: Persistent cough in nonsmokers. Can Respir J 1:40, 1994.
23. Poe RH, Harder RV, Israel RH, et al: Chronic persistent cough. Chest 95:723, 1989.
24. Irwin RS, Corrao, Pratter MR: Chronic persistent cough in the adult: The spectrum and frequency of causes and successful outcome of specific therapy. Am Rev Respir Dis 123:413, 1981.
25. Pratter MR, Bartter T, Akers S, et al: An algorithmic approach to chronic cough. Ann Intern Med 119:977, 1993.
26. Baker HL: The many faces of atypical sinusitis. J Natl Med Assoc 85:773, 1993.
27. Irwin RS, Pratter MR, Holland PS, et al: Postnasal drip causes cough and is associated with reversible upper airway obstruction. Chest 85:346, 1984.
28. Corrao WM, Braman SS, Irwin RS: Chronic cough as the sole presenting manifestation of bronchial asthma. N Engl J Med 300:633, 1979.
29. O'Connell EJ, Rojas AR, Sachs MI: Cough-type asthma: A review. Ann Allergy 66:278, 1991.
30. Gilbert R, Auchincloss JH: Post-test probability of asthma following methacholine challenge. Chest 97:562, 1990.
31. Palmeiro EM, Hopp RJ, Biven RE, et al: Probability of asthma based on methacholine challenge. Chest 101:630, 1992.
32. Gibson PG, Dolovich J, Denburg J, et al: Chronic cough: Eosinophilic bronchitis without asthma. Lancet 1:1346, 1989.
33. Irwin RS, Zawacki JK, Curley FJ, et al: Chronic cough as the sole presenting manifestation of gastroesophageal reflux. Am Rev Respir Dis 140:1294, 1989.
34. Ing AJ, Ngu MC, Breslin AB: Pathogenesis of chronic persistent cough associated with gastroesophageal reflux. Am J Respir Crit Care Med 149:160, 1994.
35. Irwin RS, French CL, Curley FJ, et al: Chronic cough due to gastroesophageal reflux. Chest 104:1511, 1993.
36. Ing AJ, Ngu MC, Breslin AB: Chronic persistent cough and gastro-oesophageal reflux. Thorax 46:479, 1991.
37. Paterson WG, Murat BW: Combined ambulatory esophageal manometry and dual-probe pH-metry in evaluation of patients with chronic unexplained cough. Dig Dis Sci 39:1117, 1994.
38. Laukka MA, Cameron AJ, Schei AJ: Gastroesophageal reflux and chronic cough: Which comes first? J Clin Gastroenterol 19:100, 1994.
39. Ing AJ, Ngu MC, Breslin AB: Chronic persistent cough and clearance of esophageal acid. Chest 102:1668, 1992.
40. Gastal OL, Castell JA, Castell DO: Frequency and site of gastroesophageal reflux in patients with chest symptoms. Chest 106:1793, 1994.
41. Schan CA, Harding SM, Haile JM, et al: Gastroesophageal reflux–induced bronchoconstriction. Chest 106:731, 1994.
42. Ducoloné A, Vandevenne A, Jouin H, et al: Gastroesophageal reflux in patients with asthma bronchitis. Am Rev Respir Dis 135:327, 1987.
43. Ferrari A, Olivieri M, Sembenini C, et al: Tussive effect of capsaicin in patients with gastroesophageal reflux without cough. Am J Respir Crit Care Med 151:557, 1995.
44. Midgren B, Hansson L, Karlsson JA, et al: Capsaicin-induced cough in humans. Am Rev Respir Dis 146:347, 1992.
45. O'Connell F, Thomas VE, Pride NB, et al: Capsaicin cough sensitivity decreased with successful treatment of chronic cough. Am J Respir Crit Care Med 150:374, 1994.
46. Karlsson JA: A role for capsaicin sensitive, tachykinin containing nerves in chronic coughing and sneezing but not in asthma: A hypothesis. Thorax 48:396, 1993.
47. Boulet LP, Milot J, Boutet M, et al: Airway inflammation in non-asthmatic subjects with chronic cough. Am J Respir Crit Care Med 149:482, 1994.
48. Keitel WA, Edwards KM: Pertussis in adolescents and adults: Time to reimmunize? Semin Respir Infect 10:51, 1995.
49. Postels-Multani S, Schmitt HJ, Wirsing von Konig CH, et al: Symptoms and complications of pertussis in adults. Infection 23:139, 1995.
50. Wright SW, Edwards KM, Decker MD, et al: Pertussis infection in adults with persistent cough. JAMA 273:1044, 1995.
51. Fletcher AE, Palmer AJ, Bulpitt CJ: Cough with angiotensin-converting enzyme inhibitors: How much more of a problem? J Hypertens Suppl 12:43, 1994.
52. Yesil S, Yesil M, Bayata S, et al: ACE inhibitors and cough. Angiology 45:805, 1994.
53. Karlberg BE: Cough and inhibition of the renin-angiotensin system. J Hypertens Suppl 11:49, 1993.
54. Simon SR, Black HR, Moser M, et al: Cough and ACE inhibitors. Arch Intern Med 22:153, 1993.
55. Choudry NB, Fuller RW: Sensitivity of the cough reflex in patients with chronic cough. Eur Respir J 5:296, 1992.
56. Blackie SP, Hilliam C, Porter R, et al: Captopril associated cough is not due to increased airway responsiveness. Can Respir J 1:235, 1994.
57. Reisin L, Schneeweiss A: Complete spontaneous remission of cough induced by ACE inhibitors during chronic therapy in hypertensive patients. J Hum Hypertens 6:333, 1992.
58. Carney IK, Gibson PG, Murree-Allen K, et al: A systematic evaluation of mechanisms in chronic cough. Am J Respir Crit Care Med 156:211, 1997.
59. Ludviksdottir D, Bjornsson E, Janson C, et al: Habitual coughing and its associations with asthma, anxiety, and gastroesophageal reflux. Chest 109:1262, 1996.
60. Irwin RS, Widdecombe J: Cough. In Murray JF, Nadel JA (ed): Textbook of Respiratory Medicine. 2nd ed. Philadelphia, WB Saunders, 1994, pp 529–544.
61. Torrington KG, Adornato BT: Cough radiculopathy—another cause of pain in the neck. West J Med 141:379, 1984.
62. Roberge RJ, Morgenstern MJ, Osborn H: Cough fracture of the ribs. Am J Emerg Med 2:513, 1984.
63. Sternfeld M, Hay E, Eliraz A: Postnasal drip causing multiple cough fractures. Ann Emerg Med 21:587, 1992.
64. Banks JG, Bancewicz J: Perforation of the oesophagus: Experience in a general hospital. Br J Surg 68:580, 1981
65. Banyai AL, Joannides M: Cough hazard. Chest 29:52, 1956.
66. Horsburgh AG: Medical memoranda. Rupture of the rectus abdominis muscle. BMJ 2:898, 1962.
67. Brotzman GL: Rectus sheath hematoma: A case report. J Fam Pract 33:194, 1991.
68. Birrer RB, Calderon J: Pneumothorax, pneumomediastinum, and pneumopericardium following Valsalva's maneuver during marijuana smoking. N Y State J Med 84:619, 1984.
69. Benedict EB: Rupture of the bronchus from bronchoscopy during a paroxysm of coughing. JAMA 178:509, 1961.
70. Macklin MT, Macklin CC: Malignant interstitial emphysema of the lungs and mediastinum as an important occult complication in many respiratory diseases and other conditions: An interpretation of the clinical literature in the light of laboratory experiment. Medicine (Baltimore) 23:281, 1944.
71. Sands GH, Newman L, Lipton R: Cough, exertional, and other miscellaneous headaches. Med Clin North Am 75:733, 1991.
71a. Ulyatt DB, Judson JA, Trubuhovich, et al: Cerebral arterial air embolism associated with coughing on a continuous positive airway pressure circuit. Crit Care Med 19:985, 1991.
72. Herr RD, Call G, Banks D: Vertebral artery dissection from neck flexion during paroxysmal coughing. Ann Emerg Med 21:88, 1992.

73. Tanaka T, Inoue H, Aizawa H, et al: Case of cough syncope with seizure. Respiration 61:48, 1994.
74. Smith WS, Messing RO: Cerebral aneurysm presenting as cough headache. Headache 33:203, 1993.
75. Moncada E, Graff-Radfor SB: Cough headache presenting as a toothache: A case report. Headache 33:240, 1993.
76. Kerr A Jr, Eich RH: Cerebral concussion as a cause of cough syncope. Arch Intern Med 108:248, 1961.
77. Haslam RH, Freigang B: Cough syncope mimicking epilepsy in asthmatic children. Can J Neurol Sci 12:45, 1985.
78. Jenkins P, Clarke SW: Cough syncope: A complication of adult whooping cough. Br J Dis Chest 75:311, 1981.
79. Morgan-Hughes JA: Cough seizures in patients with cerebral lesions. BMJ 2:494, 1966.
80. Linzer M, McFarland TA, Belkin M, et al: Critical carotid and vertebral arterial occlusive disease and cough syncope. Stroke 23:1017, 1992.
81. Reisin L, Blaer Y, Jafari J, et al: Cough-induced nonsustained ventricular tachycardia. Chest 105:1583, 1994.
82. Premachandra DJ, Prinsley PR, McRae D: Massive haemorrhage from the vallecula: A diagnostic difficulty. Case report. Eur J Surg 157:297, 1991.
83. Santiago S, Tobias J, Williams AJ: A reappraisal of the causes of hemoptysis. Arch Intern Med 151:2449, 1991.
84. Hirshberg B, Biran I, Glazer M, et al: Hemoptysis: Etiology, evaluation, and outcome in a tertiary referral hospital. Chest 112:440, 1997.
85. Razaque MA, Mutum SS, Singh TS: Recurrent haemoptysis? Think of paragonimiasis. Trop Doctor 21:153, 1991.
86. Yaacob I, Harun Z, Ahmad Z: Fiberoptic bronchoscopy—a Malaysian experience. Singapore Med J 32:26, 1991.
87. Cahill BC, Ingbar DH: Massive hemoptysis: Assessment and management. Clin Chest Med 15:147, 1994.
88. Weaver LJ, Solliday N, Cugell DW: Selection of patients with hemoptysis for fiberoptic bronchoscopy. Chest 76:7, 1979.
89. Poe RH, Israel RH, Martin MG, et al: Utility of fiberoptic bronchoscopy in patients with hemoptysis and a nonlocalizing chest roentgenogram. Chest 93:68, 1988.
90. Lederle FA, Nichol KL, Parenti CM: Bronchoscopy to evaluate hemoptysis in older men with nonsuspicious chest roentgenograms. Chest 95:1043, 1989.
91. O'Neil KM, Lazarus AA: Hemoptysis: Indications for bronchoscopy. Arch Intern Med 151:171, 1991.
92. Set PA, Flower CD, Smith IE, et al: Hemoptysis: Comparative study of the role of CT and fiberoptic bronchoscopy. Radiology 189:677, 1993.
93. Millar AB, Boothroyd AE, Edwards D, et al: The role of computed tomography (CT) in the investigation of unexplained haemoptysis. Respir Med 86:39, 1992.
94. McGuinness G, Beacher JR, Harkin TJ, et al: Hemoptysis: Prospective high-resolution CT/bronchoscopic correlation. Chest 105:1155, 1994.
95. Adelman M, Haponik EF, Bleecker ER, et al: Cryptogenic hemoptysis: Clinical features, bronchoscopic findings, and natural history in 67 patients. Ann Intern Med 102:829, 1985.
96. Heimer D, Bar-Ziv J, Scharf SM: Fiberoptic bronchoscopy in patients with hemoptysis and nonlocalizing chest roentgenograms. Arch Intern Med 145:1427, 1985.
97. Bobrowitz ID, Ramakrishna S, Shim Y-S: Comparison of medical versus surgical treatment of major hemoptysis. Arch Intern Med 143:1343, 1983.
98. Garzon AA, Cerruti MM, Golding ME: Exsanguinating hemoptysis. J Thorac Cardiovasc Surg 84:829, 1982.
99. Corey R, Hla KM: Major and massive hemoptysis: Reassessment of conservative management. Am J Med Sci 294:301, 1987.
100. Stoller JK: Diagnosis and management of massive hemoptysis: A review. Respir Care 37:564, 1992.
101. Garzon AA, Cerruti MM, Golding ME: Exsanguinating hemoptysis. Thor Cardiovasc Surg 84:829, 1982.
102. Crocco JA, Rooney JJ, Fankushen DS, et al: Massive hemoptysis. Arch Intern Med 121:495, 1968.
103. Garzon AA, Gourin A: Surgical management of massive hemoptysis: A ten-year experience. Ann Surg 187:267, 1978.
104. Ferris EJ: Pulmonary hemorrhage: Vascular evaluation and interventional therapy. Chest 80:710, 1981.
105. Remy J, Arnaud A, Fardou H, et al: Treatment of hemoptysis by embolization of bronchial arteries. Radiology 122:33, 1977.
106. Uflacker R, Kaemmerer, Picon PD, et al: Bronchial artery embolization in the management of hemoptysis: Technical aspects of long-term results. Radiology 157:637, 1985.
107. Lampmann LE, Tjan TG: Embolization therapy in haemoptysis. Eur J Radiol 18:15, 1994.
108. Hayakawa K, Tanaka F, Torizuka T, et al: Bronchial artery embolization for hemoptysis: Immediate and long-term results. Cardiovasc Intervent Radiol 15:154, 1992.
109. Cremaschi P, Nascimbene C, Vitulo P, et al: Therapeutic embolization of bronchial artery: A successful treatment in 209 cases of relapse hemoptysis. Angiology 44:295, 1993.
110. Rabkin JE, Astafjev VI, Gothman LN, et al: Transcatheter embolization in the management of pulmonary hemorrhage. Radiology 163:361, 1987.
111. Tamura S, Kodoma T, Otsuka N, et al: Embolotherapy for persistent hemoptysis: The significance of pleural thickening. Cardiovasc Intervent Radiol 16:85, 1993.
112. Knott-Craig CJ, Oostuizen JG, Rossouw G, et al: Management and prognosis of

113. massive hemoptysis. Recent experience with 120 patients. J Thorac Cardiovasc Surg 105:394, 1993.
113. Conlan AA, Hurwitz SS, Krige L, et al: Massive hemoptysis: Review of 123 cases. J Thorac Cardiovasc Surg 85:120, 1983.
114. Schneider RR, Seckler SG: Evaluation of acute chest pain. Med Clin North Am 65:53, 1981.
115. Munro NC, Currie DC, Garbett ND, et al: Chest pain in chronic sputum production: A neglected symptom. Respir Med 83:339, 1989.
116. Lichstein E, Seckler SG: Evaluation of acute chest pain. Med Clin North Am 57:1481, 1973.
117. Wilcox RG, Roland JM, Hampton JR: Prognosis of patients with "chest pain? cause." BMJ 282:431, 1981.
118. Wise CM, Semble EL, Dalton CB: Musculoskeletal chest wall syndromes in patients with noncardiac chest pain: A study of 100 patients. Arch Phys Med Rehabil 73:147, 1992.
119. Herr CH: The diagnosis of acute myocardial infarction in the emergency department; Part 1. J Emerg Med 10:455, 1992.
120. Fleet RP, Dupuis G, Marchand A, et al: Panic disorder in emergency departmental chest pain patients: Prevalence, comorbidity, suicidal ideation, and physician recognition. Am J Med 101:371, 1996.
121. Smoller JW, Pollack MH, Otto MW, et al: Panic anxiety, dyspnea and respiratory disease. Am J Respir Crit Care Med 154:6, 1996.
122. Voskuil J-H, Cramer MJ, Breumelhof R, et al: Prevalence of esophageal disorders in patients with chest pain newly referred to a cardiologist. Chest 109:1210, 1996.
123. Frobert O, Funch-Jensen P, Bagger JP: Diagnostic value of esophageal studies in patients with angina-like chest pain and normal coronary angiograms. Ann Intern Med 124:959, 1996.
123a. Lemire S. Assessment of clinical severity and investigation of uncomplicated gastroesophageal reflux disease and noncardiac angina-like chest pain. Canadian Journal of Gastroenterology 11:37B, 1997.
124. Rao SS, Gregersen H, Hayek B, et al: Unexplained chest pain: The hypersensitive, hyperreactive, and poorly compliant esophagus. Ann Intern Med 124:950, 1996.
125. Wise CM: Chest wall syndromes. Curr Opin Rheumatol 6:197, 1994.
126. Brewin TB: Alcohol intolerance in neoplastic disease. BMJ 2:437, 1966.
127. Miller AJ, Texidor TA: The "precordial catch," a syndrome of anterior chest pain. Ann Intern Med 51:461, 1959.
128. Stedman's Medical Dictionary. Baltimore, Williams & Wilkins, 1966.
129. Elliott MW, Adams L, Cockcroft A, et al: The language of breathlessness. Am Rev Respir Dis 144:826, 1991.
130. Simon PM, Schwartzstein RM, Weiss JW, et al: Distinguishable types of dyspnea in patients with shortness of breath. Am Rev Respir Dis 142:1009, 1990.
131. Mahler DA, Harver A, Lentine T, et al: Descriptors of breathlessness in cardiorespiratory disease. Am J Respir Crit Care Med 154:1357, 1996.
132. Pratter MR, Curley FJ, Dubois J, et al: Cause and evaluation of chronic dyspnea in a pulmonary disease clinic. Arch Intern Med 149:2277, 1989.
133. DePaso WJ, Winterbauer RH, Lusk JA, et al: Chronic dyspnea unexplained by history, physical examination, chest roentgenogram and spirometry. Chest 100:1293, 1991.
134. Patten JP: Pins and needles. Br J Hosp Med 20:334, 1978.
135. Saisch SG, Wessely S, Gardner WN: Patients with acute hyperventilation presenting to an inner-city emergency department. Chest 110:952, 1996.
136. Saltzman HA, Heyman A, Sieker HO: Correlation of clinical and physiological manifestations of sustained hyperventilation. N Engl J Med 268:1431, 1963.
137. Gardner WN: The pathophysiology of hyperventilation disorders. Chest 109:516, 1996.
138. Mahler DA, Wells CK: Evaluation of clinical methods for rating dyspnea. Chest 93:580, 1988.
139. Guyatt GH, Townsend M, Keller J, et al: Measuring functional status in chronic lung disease: Conclusions from a randomized control trial. Respir Med 85:33, 1991.
140. Stoller JK, Ferranti R, Feinstein AR: Further specification and evaluation of a new clinical index for dyspnea. Am Rev Respir Dis 134:1129, 1986.
141. Mier-Jedrzejowicz A, Brophy C, Moxham J, et al: Assessment of diaphragm weakness. Am Rev Respir Dis 137:877, 1988.
142. Timmermans C, Frans E, Herregods C, et al: Platypnea-orthodeoxia syndrome: A report of two cases. Acta Cardiol 49:217, 1994.
143. Mercho N, Stoller JK, White RD, et al: Right-to-left interatrial shunt causing platypnea after pneumonectomy: A recent experience and diagnostic value of dynamic magnetic resonance imaging. Chest 105:931, 1994.
144. Schwenk NR, Schapira RM, and Byrd JC, Laryngeal carcinoma presenting as platypnea. Chest 106:1609, 1994.
145. Mashman WE, Silverman ME: Platypnea related to constrictive pericarditis. Chest 105:636, 1994.
146. DesJardin JA, Martin RJ: Platypnea in the intensive care unit: A newly described cause. Chest 104:1308, 1993.
146a. Al Khouzaie T, Busser JR. A rare cause of dyspnea and arterial hypoxemia. Chest 112:1681, 1997.
146b. Popp G, Melek H, Garnett AR Jr. Platypnea-orthodeoxia related to aortic elongation. Chest 112:1682, 1997.
147. Byrd RP Jr, Lopez PR, Joyce BW, et al: Platypnea, orthodeoxia, and cirrhosis. J Ky Med Assoc 90:189, 1992.
148. Milne JA, Howie AD, Pack AI: Dyspnoea during normal pregnancy. Br J Obstet Gynaecol 85:260, 1978.
149. Weinberger SE, Weiss ST, Cohen WR, et al: Pregnancy and the lung. Am Rev Respir Dis 121:559, 1980.

150. Field SK, Bell SG, Cenaiko DF, et al: Relationship between inspiratory effort and breathlessness in pregnancy. J Appl Physiol 71:1897, 1991.

151. Zeldis SM: Dyspnea during pregnancy. Distinguishing cardiac from pulmonary causes. Clin Chest Med 13:567, 1992.

152. Lipscomb DJ, Edwards RHT: Computer simulation of physiological factors contributing to hyperventilation and breathlessness in cardiac patients. Br J Dis Chest 74:47, 1980.

153. Ludman H: ABC of ENT: Hoarseness and stridor. BMJ 282:715, 1981.

154. Chan P, Lee CP, Ko JT, et al: Cardiovocal (Ortner's) syndrome: Left recurrent laryngeal nerve palsy associated with cardiovascular disease. Eur J Med 1:492, 1992.

155. Meduri GU, Mauldin GL, Wunderink RG, et al: Causes of fever and pulmonary densities in patients with clinical manifestations of ventilator-associated pneumonia. Chest 106:221, 1994.

156. Attia EL, Marshall KG: Halitosis. Can Med Assoc J 126:1281, 1982.

157. Harber P, Tashkin D, Shimozaki S, et al: Veracity of disability claimants self-reports of current smoking status. Chest 93:561, 1988.

158. Constantopoulos SH, Malamou-Mitsi VD, Goudevenos JA, et al: High incidence of malignant pleural mesothelioma in neighbouring villages of northwestern Greece. Respiration 51:266, 1987.

159. McConnochie K, Simonato L, Mavrides P, et al: Mesothelioma in Cyprus: The role of tremolite. Thorax 42:342, 1987.

160. Eriksson S: Pulmonary emphysema and alpha₁-antitrypsin deficiency. Acta Med Scand 175:197, 1964.

161. Sharief N, Crawford OF, Dinwiddie R: Fibrosing alveolitis and desquamative interstitial pneumonitis. Pediatr Pulmonol 17:359, 1994.

162. Shaw GL, Falk RT, Pickle LW, et al: Lung cancer risk associated with cancer in relatives. J Clin Epidemiol 44:429, 1991.

163. McDuffie HH: Clustering of cancer in families of patients with primary lung cancer. J Clin Epidemiol 44:69, 1991.

164. He XZ, Chen W, Liu ZY, et al: An epidemiological study of lung cancer in Xuan Wei County, China: Current progress. Case-control study on lung cancer and cooking fuel. Environ Health Perspect 94:9, 1991.

165. Liu ZY, HE XZ, Chapman RS: Smoking and other risk factors for lung cancer in Xuanwei, China. Int J Epidemiol 20:26, 1991.

166. Osann KE: Lung cancer in women: The importance of smoking, family history of cancer, and medical history of respiratory disease. Cancer Res 51:4893, 1991.

167. Ambrosone CB, Rao U, Michalek AM, et al: Lung cancer histologic types and family history of cancer. Analysis of histologic subtypes of 872 patients with primary lung cancer. Cancer 72:1192, 1993.

168. Sferlazza SJ, Beckett WS: The respiratory health of welders. Am Rev Respir Dis 143:1134, 1991.

169. Chitkara RK, and Khan FA: Neurologic manifestations of lung disease. Sem in Respir Med 9:395, 1988.

170. James DG, Graham E: Oculopulmonary syndromes. Semin Respir Med 9:380, 1988.

171. Sharma OP, Nam H: Cutaneous manifestations of pulmonary disease. Semin Respir Med 9:385, 1988.

172. Austen FK, Carmichael MW, Adams RD: Neurologic manifestations of chronic pulmonary insufficiency. N Engl J Med 257:579, 1957.

173. Alexander JK, Amad KH, Cole VW: Observations on some clinical features of extreme obesity, with particular reference to cardiorespiratory effects. Am J Med 32:512, 1962.

174. Smylie HC, Blendis LM, Armitage P: Observer disagreement in physical signs of the respiratory system. Lancet 2:412, 1965.

175. Comroe JH, Botelho S: The unreality of cyanosis in the recognition of arterial anoxemia. Am J Med Sci 214:1, 1947.

176. Regan GM, Tagg B, Thomson ML: Subjective assessment and objective measurement of finger clubbing. Lancet 1:530, 1967.

177. Pyke DA: Finger clubbing: Validity as a physical sign. Lancet 2:352, 1954.

178. Spiteri MA, Cook DG, Clarke SW: Reliability of eliciting physical signs in examination of the chest. Lancet 1:873, 1988.

179. Badgett RG, Tanaka DJ, Hunt DK, et al: Can moderate chronic obstructive pulmonary disease be diagnosed by historical and physical findings alone? Am J Med 94:188, 1993.

180. Verghese A, Krish G, Howe D, et al: The harlequin nail. Chest 97:236, 1990.

181. Lee L, Loudon RG, Jacobson BH, et al: Speech breathing in patients with lung disease. Am Rev Respir Dis 147:1199, 1993.

182. Gravelyn TR, Weg JG: Respiratory rate as an indicator of acute respiratory dysfunction. JAMA 244:1123, 1980.

183. McFadden JP, Price RC, Eastwood HD, et al: Raised respiratory rate in elderly patients: A valuable physical sign. BMJ 284:626, 1982.

184. Guarino JR, Guarnin JC: Auscultatory percussion: A simple method to detect pleural effusion. J Gen Intern Med 9:71, 1994.

185. Guarino JR: Auscultatory percussion of the chest. Lancet 1:1332, 1980.

186. Hampton CS, Chaloner A: Which stethoscope? BMJ 4:388, 1967.

187. Pasterkamp H, Kraman SS, Wodicka GR: State of the art: Respiratory sounds: Advances beyond the stethoscope. Am J Respir Crit Care Med 156:974, 1997.

188. Banaszak EF, Kory RC, Snider GL: Phonopneumography. Am Rev Respir Dis 107:449, 1973.

189. Nairn JR, Turner-Warwick M: Breath sounds in emphysema. Br J Dis Chest 63:29, 1969.

190. Ploysongsang Y, Paré JAP, Macklem PT: Correlation of regional breath sounds with regional ventilation in emphysema. Am Rev Respir Dis 126:526, 1982.

191. Schreur HJW, Sterk PJ, Vanderschoot J, et al: Lung sound intensity in patients with emphysema and in normal subjects at standardised airflows. Thorax 47:674, 1992.

192. Cugell DW: Use of tape recordings of respiratory sound and breathing pattern for instruction in pulmonary auscultation. Am Rev Respir Dis 104:948, 1971.

193. Weiss EB, Carlson CJ: Recording of breath sounds. Am Rev Respir Dis 105:835, 1972.

194. Charbonneau G, Racineux JL, Sudraud M, et al: An accurate recording system and its use in breath sounds: Spectral analysis. J Appl Physiol 55:1120, 1983.

195. Ploysongsang Y: The lung sounds phase angle test for detection of small airway disease. Respir Physiol 53:203, 1983.

196. Loudon RG: Auscultation of the lung. Clin Notes Respir Dis 21:3, 1982.

197. Milic-Emili J, Henderson JAM, Dolovich MB, et al: Regional distribution of inspired gas in the lung. J Appl Physiol 21:749, 1966.

198. Dollfuss RE, Milic-Emili J, Bates D: Regional ventilation of the lung, studied with boluses of ¹³³Xe. Respir Physiol 2:234, 1967.

199. Shykoff BE, Ploysongsand Y, Chang HK: Airflow and normal lung sounds. Am Rev Respir Dis 137:872, 1988.

200. Sanchez I, Pasterkamp H: Tracheal sound spectra depend on body height. Am Rev Respir Dis 148:1083, 1993.

201. Forgacs P, Nathoo AR, Richardson HD: Breath sounds. Thorax 26:288, 1971.

202. Forgacs P: The functional basis of pulmonary sounds. Chest 73:399, 1978.

203. Pasterkamp H, Sanchez I: Effect of gas density on respirator sounds. Am J Respir Crit Care Med 153:1087, 1996.

204. Kraman SS: Does laryngeal noise contribute to the vesicular lung sound? Am Rev Respir Dis 124:292, 1981.

205. Sapira JD. About egophony. Chest 108:865, 1995.

206. Jones FL: Poor breath sounds with good voice sounds. Chest 93:312, 1988.

207. Mikami R, Murao M, Cugell DW, et al: International Symposium on Lung Sounds: Synopsis of Proceedings. Chest 92:343, 1987.

208. Pulmonary Terms and Symbols—a report of the ACCP-ATS Joint Committee on Pulmonary Nomenclature. Chest 67:583, 1975.

209. Pasterkamp H, Montogomery M, Wiebicke W: Nomenclature used by health care professionals to describe breath sounds in asthma. Chest 92:347, 1987.

210. Wilkins RL, Dexter JR, Murphy RLH, et al: Lung sound nomenclature survey. Chest 98:886, 1990.

211. Loudon R, Murphy RLH: Lung sounds. Am Rev Respir Dis 130:663, 1984.

212. Murphy RLH, Holford SK, Knowler WC: Visual lung-sound characterization by time-expanded waveform analysis. N Engl J Med 296:968, 1977.

213. Ploysongsang Y, Schonfield SA: Mechanics of production of crackles after atelectasis during low-volume breathing. Am Rev Respir Dis 126:413, 1982.

214. Thacker RE, Kraman SS: The prevalence of auscultatory crackles in subjects without lung disease. Chest 81:672, 1982.

215. Workum P, Holford SK, Delbano EA, et al: The prevalence and character of crackles (rales) in young women without significant lung disease. Am Rev Respir Dis 126:921, 1982.

216. Gilbert VE: Detection of pneumonia by auscultation of the lungs in the lateral decubitus positions. Am Rev Respir Dis 140:1012, 1989.

217. Piirlä P: Changes in crackle characteristics during the clinical course of pneumonia. Chest 102:176, 1992.

218. Mori M, Kinoshita K, Morinari H, et al: Waveform and spectral analysis of crackles. Thorax 35:843, 1980.

219. Munakata M, Ukita H, Doi I, et al: Spectral and waveform characteristics of fine and coarse crackles. Thorax 46:651, 1991.

220. Hoevers J, Loudon RG: Measuring crackles. Chest 98:1240, 1990.

221. Piirilä P, Sovijärvi ARA, Kaisla T, et al: Crackles in patients with fibrosing alveolitis, bronchiectasis, COPD, and heart failure. Chest 99:1076, 1991.

222. Al Jarad N, Davies SW, Logan-Sinclair R, et al: Lung crackle characteristics in patients with asbestosis, asbestos-related pleural disease and left ventricular failure using a time-expanded waveform analysis—a comparative study. Respir Med 88:37, 1994.

223. Bettencourt PE, Del Bono EA, Spiegelman D, et al: Clinical utility of chest auscultation in common pulmonary diseases. Am J Respir Crit Care Med 150:1291, 1994.

224. Jarad NA, Strickland B, Bothamley G, et al: Diagnosis of asbestosis by a time-expanded waveform analysis, auscultation, and high-resolution computed tomography: A comparative study. Thorax 48:347, 1993.

225. King DK, Thompson BT, Johnson DC: Wheezing on maximal forced exhalation in the diagnosis of atypical asthma. Ann Intern Med 110:451, 1989.

226. Marini JJ, Pierson DJ, Hudson LD, et al: The significance of wheezing in chronic airflow obstruction. Am Rev Respir Dis 120:1069, 1979.

227. Shim CS, Williams MH Jr: Relationship of wheezing to the severity of obstruction in asthma. Arch Intern Med 143:890, 1983.

228. Baughman RP, Loudon RG: Quantitation of wheezing in acute asthma. Chest 86:718, 1984.

229. Moyer JH, Glantz G, Brest AN: Pulmonary arteriovenous fistulas: Physiologic and clinical considerations. Am J Med 32:417, 1962.

230. Annamalai A, Ranganathan C, Radhakrishan MA: Pulmonary arteriovenous aneurysm with a major systemic component. Indian J Radiol 13:172, 1959.

231. Victor S, Lakshmikanthan C, Shankar G, et al: Continuous murmur as a sequel of augmented collateral circulation in suppurative lung disease: Report of three cases. Chest 62:504, 1972.

232. Colman NC: Pathophysiology of pulmonary embolism. In Leclerc JR (eds): Venous Thromboembolic Disorders. Philadelphia, Lea & Febiger, 1991, pp 65.

233. Fagge CH: In Pye-Smith (ed): The Principles and Practice of Medicine. 2nd ed. London, Churchill, 1888.

234. Hamman L: Spontaneous mediastinal emphysema. Bull Johns Hopkins Hosp 64:1, 1939.
235. Scadding JG, Wood P: Systolic clicks due to left-sided pneumothorax. Lancet 2:1208, 1939.
236. Semple T, Lancaster WM: Noisy pneumothorax: Observations based on 24 cases. BMJ 1:1342, 1961.
237. Squara P, Dhainaut JF, Schremmer B, et al: Decreased paradoxic pulse from increased venous return in severe asthma. Chest 97:377, 1990.
238. Scharf SM: Cardiovascular effects of airways obstruction (review). Lung 169:1, 1991.
238a. Massumi RA, Mason DT, Vera Z, et al: Reversed pulsas paradoxus. N Engl J Med 289:1272, 1973.
239. Zema MJ, Masters AP, Margouleff D: Dyspnea: The heart or the lungs? Chest 85:59, 1984.
240. Martinez-Lavin M, Mansilla J, Pineda C, et al: Evidence of hypertrophic osteoarthropathy in human skeletal remains from pre-Hispanic Mesoamerica. Ann Intern Med 120:238, 1994.
241. Martinez-Lavin M, Matucci-Cerinic M, Jajic I, et al: Hypertrophic osteoarthropathy: Consensus on its definition, classification, assessment and diagnostic criteria. J Rheumatol 20:1386, 1993.
242. Carcassi U: History of hypertrophic osteoarthropathy. Clin Exp Rheumatol 7:3, 1992.
243. Shneerson JM: Digital clubbing and hypertrophic osteoarthropathy: The underlying mechanisms. Br J Dis Chest 75:113, 1981.
244. Waring WW, Wilkinson RW, Wiebe RA, et al: Quantitation of digital clubbing in children: Measurements of casts of the index finger. Am Rev Respir Dis 104:166, 1971.
245. Sly RM, Ghazanshahi S, Buranakul B, et al: Objective assessment for digital clubbing in Caucasian, Negro, and Oriental subjects. Chest 64:687, 1973.
245a. Baughman RP, Gunther KL, Buchsbaum JA, et al: Prevalence of digital clubbing in bronchogenic carcinoma by a new digital index. Clin Exp Rheumatol 16:21, 1998.
245b. Martinez-Leon JI, Sanchez-Guzman AR, Bohorquez-Sierra JC, et al: Subperiosteal new bone formation in association with vascular graft sepsis. J Vasc Surg 26:895, 1997.
246. Mendlowitz M: Measurements of blood flow and blood pressure in clubbed fingers. J Clin Invest 20:113, 1941.
247. Racoceanu SN, Mendlowitz M, Suck AF, et al: Digital capillary blood flow in clubbing: 85 Kr studies in hereditary and acquired cases. Ann Intern Med 75:933, 1971.
248. Currie AE, Gallagher PJ: The pathology of clubbing: Vascular changes in the nail bed. Br J Dis Chest 82:382, 1988.
249. Fara EF, Baughman RP: A study of capillary morphology in the digits of patients with acquired clubbing. Am Rev Respir Dis 140:1063, 1989.
250. Shneerson JM, Jones BM: Ferritin, finger clubbing and lung diseases. Thorax 36:688, 1981.
251. Lemen RJ, Gates AJ, Mathé AA, et al: Relationships among digital clubbing, disease severity, and serum prostaglandins $F_{2\alpha}$ and E concentrations in cystic fibrosis patients. Am Rev Respir Dis 117:639, 1978.
252. Larkin J: Miscellaneous neurologic, cardiac, pulmonary, and metabolic disorders with rheumatic manifestations. Curr Opin Rheumatol 6:111, 1994.
253. Silveri F, Carlino G, Cervini C: The "endothelium/platelet unit" in hypertrophic osteoarthropathy. Clin Exp Rheumatol 7:61, 1992.
254. Martinez-Lavin M: Pathogenesis of hypertrophic osteoarthropathy. Clin Exp Rheumatol 7:49, 1992.
255. Vazquez-Abad D, Martinez-Lavin M: Macrothrombocytes in the peripheral circulation of patients with cardiogenic hypertrophic osteoarthropathy. Clin Exp Rheumatol 9:59, 1991.
256. Dickinson CJ: The aetiology of clubbing and hypertrophic osteoarthropathy. Eur J Clin Invest 23:330, 1993.
257. Matucci-Cerinic M, Martinez-Lavin M, Rojo F, et al: Von Willebrand factor antigen in hypertrophic osteoarthropathy. J Rheumatol 19:765, 1992.
258. Hojo S, Fujita J, Yamadori I, et al: Hepatocyte growth factor and digital clubbing. Intern Med 36:44, 1997.
259. Hirakata Y, Kitamura S: Elevated serum transforming growth factor-beta 1 level in primary lung cancer patients with finger clubbing. Eur J Clin Invest 26:820, 1996.
260. Gosney MA, Gosney JR, Lye M: Plasma growth hormone and digital clubbing in carcinoma of the bronchus. Thorax 45:545, 1990.
260a. El-Salhy M, Simonsson M, Stenling R, et al: Recovery from Marie-Bamberger's syndrome and diabetes insipidus after removal of a lung adenocarcinoma with neuroendocrine features. J Intern Med 243:171, 1998.
261. Yorgancioglu A, Akin A, Demtray M, et al: The relationship between digital clubbing and serum growth hormone level in patients with lung cancer. Monaldi Arch Chest Dis 51:185, 1996.
262. Macfarlane JT, Ibrahim M, Tor-Agbidye S: The importance of finger clubbing in pulmonary tuberculosis. Tubercle 60:45, 1979.
263. Kelly P, Manning P, Corcoran P, et al: Hypertrophic osteoarthropathy in association with pulmonary tuberculosis. Chest 99:769, 1991.
264. Skorneck AB, Ginsburg LB: Pulmonary hypertrophic osteoarthropathy (periostitis): Its absence in pulmonary tuberculosis. N Engl J Med 258:1079, 1958.
265. Yacoub MH: Relation between the histology of bronchial carcinoma and hypertrophic pulmonary osteoarthropathy. Thorax 20:537, 1965.
266. Doyle L: Some considerations of hypertrophic osteoarthropathy. Br J Dis Chest 74:314, 1980.
267. Coury C: Hippocratic fingers and hypertrophic osteoarthropathy: A study of 350 cases. Br J Dis Chest 54:202, 1960.
268. Lokich JJ: Pulmonary osteoarthropathy: Association with mesenchymal tumor metastases to the lungs. JAMA 238:37, 1977.
269. Perkins PJ: Delayed onset of secondary hypertrophic osteoarthropathy. Am J Roentgenol 130:561, 1978.
270. Rutherford RB, Rhodes BA, Wagner HN Jr: The distribution of extremity blood flow before and after vagectomy in a patient with hypertrophic pulmonary osteoarthropathy. Dis Chest 56:19, 1969.
271. Huckstep RL, Bodkin PE: Vagotomy in hypertrophic pulmonary osteoarthropathy associated with bronchial carcinoma. Lancet 2:343, 1958.
272. Ginsburg J, Brown JB: Increased oestrogen excretion in hypertrophic pulmonary osteoarthropathy. Lancet 2:1274, 1961.
273. Borden EC, Holling HE: Hypertrophic osteoarthropathy and pregnancy. Ann Intern Med 71:577, 1969.
274. Greenberg PB, Beck C, Martin TJ, et al: Synthesis and release of human growth hormone from lung carcinoma in cell culture. Lancet 1:350, 1972.
275. Rimoin DL: Pachydermoperiostosis (idiopathic clubbing and periostosis): Genetic and physiologic considerations. N Engl J Med 272:923, 1965.
275a. Compton RF, Sandborn WJ, Yang H, et al: A new syndrome of Crohn's disease and pachydermoperiostosis in a family. Gastroenterology 112:241, 1997.
276. Hedayati H, Barmada R, Skosey JL: Acrolysis in pachydermoperiostosis: Primary or idiopathic hypertrophic osteoarthropathy. Arch Intern Med 140:1087, 1980.
277. Matucci-Cerinic M, Lotti T, Calviere S, et al: The spectrum of dermatological symptoms of pachydermoperiostosis (primary hypertrophic osteoarthropathy): A genetic, cytogenic, and ultrastructural study. Clin Exp Rheumatol 7:45, 1992.
278. Kerber RE, Vogl A: Pachydermoperiostosis. Arch Intern Med 132:245, 1973.
279. Dalgleish AG: Hypertrophic pulmonary osteoarthropathy: Response to chemotherapy without documented tumour response. Aust N Z J Med 13:513, 1983.
280. Rao GM, Guruprakash GH, Poulose KP, et al: Improvement in hypertrophic pulmonary osteoarthropathy after radiotherapy to metastasis. Am J Roentgenol 133:944, 1979.
281. Pitt P, Mowat A, Williams R, et al: Hepatic hypertrophic osteoarthropathy and liver transplantation. Ann Rheum Dis 53:338, 1993.
282. Sansores RH, Villalba-Caloca J, Ramirez-Venegas A, et al: Reversal of digital clubbing after lung transplantation. Chest 107:283, 1995.
283. Sagar VV, Mecklenburg RL, Piccone JM: Resolution of bone scan changes in hypertrophic pulmonary osteoarthropathy in untreated carcinoma of the lung. Clin Nucl Med 3:427, 1978.
284. Kelman GR, Nunn JF: Clinical recognition of hypoxaemia under fluorescent lamps. Lancet 1:1400, 1966.
285. Lundsgaard C, Van Slyke DD: Cyanosis. Medicine (Baltimore) 2:1, 1923.
286. Martin L, Khalil H: How much reduced hemoglobin is necessary to generate central cyanosis? Chest 97:182, 1990.
287. Dlabal PW, Stutts BS, Jenkins DW, et al: Cyanosis following right pneumonectomy: Importance of patent foramen ovale. Chest 81:370, 1982.
288. Martinez R, Saponaro A, Russo R, et al: Effects of sympathetic stimulation on microcirculatory dynamics in patients with essential acrocyanosis: A study using mental stress. Panminerva Med 35:9, 1993.
289. Bhanji S, Mattingly D: Acrocyanosis in anorexia nervosa. Postgrad Med J 67:33, 1991.
290. Philpott NJ, Woodhead MA, Wilson AG, et al: Lung abscess: A neglected cause of life threatening haemoptysis. Thorax 48:674, 1993.
291. Spark RP, Sobonya RE, Armbruster RJ, et al: Pathologic bronchial vasculature in a case of massive hemoptysis due to chronic bronchitis. Chest 99:504, 1991.
292. Nakazawa H, Tsuburaya T, Watanabe H, et al: Chronic bronchopneumonia with recurrent hemoptysis and resultant severe anemia. Respiration 58:332, 1991.
293. Liam CK, Yap BH, Lam SK: Dengue fever complicated by pulmonary haemorrhage manifesting as haemoptysis. J Trop Med Hygiene 96:197, 1993.
294. Athayde J, Shore ET: Invasive pulmonary aspergillosis presenting as massive hemoptysis in a nonimmunocompromised host. Chest 103:960, 1993.
295. Groll A, Renz S, Gerein V, et al: Fatal haemoptysis associated with invasive pulmonary aspergillosis treated with high-dose amphotericin B and granulocyte-macrophage colony-stimulating factor (GM-CSF). Mycoses 35:67, 1992.
296. Harada M, Manabe T, Yamashita K, et al: Pulmonary mucormycosis with fatal massive hemoptysis. Acta Pathol Jpn 42:49, 1992.
297. Panos RJ, Barr LF, Walsh TJ, et al: Factors associated with fatal hemoptysis in cancer patients. Chest 94:1008, 1988.
298. Razauqe MA, Mutum SS, Singh TS: Recurrent haemoptysis? Think of paragonimiasis. Trop Doct 21:153, 1991.
299. Chang JC, Cregler LL: Hemoptysis in a patient with congestive heart failure and pulmonary emboli. J Natl Med Assoc 86:383, 1994.
300. Webb DW, Thadepalli H: Hemoptysis in patients with septic pulmonary infarcts from tricuspid endocarditis. Chest 76:99, 1979.
301. Casadevall J, Alvarez-Sala R, Prados C, et al: Dissection of ascending aorta. A new cause of alveolar hemorrhage? J Cardiovasc Surg 35:327, 1994.
302. Urschel JD: The diagnostic importance of computed tomography in aortobronchial fistula—a case report. Angiology 44:817, 1993.
303. Wu MH, Lai WW, Lin MY, et al: Massive hemoptysis caused by a ruptured subclavian artery aneurysm. Chest 104:612, 1993.
304. Jain A, Strickman NE, Hall RJ, et al: An unusual complication of left ventricular pseudoaneurysm: Hemoptysis. Chest 93:429, 1988.
305. Michelon G, Mullany CJ, Viggiano RW, et al: Massive pulmonary hemorrhage complicating mitral prosthetic valve obstruction. Chest 103:1903, 1993.

306. Ference BA, Shannon TM, White RI Jr, et al: Life-threatening pulmonary hemorrhage with pulmonary arteriovenous malformation and hereditary hemorrhagic telangiectasia. Chest 106:1387, 1994.

307. Youssef AI, Escalante-Glorsky S, Bonnet RB, et al: Hemoptysis secondary to bronchial varices associated with alcoholic liver cirrhosis and portal hypertension. Am J Gastroenterol 89:1562, 1994.

308. Ashour MH, Jain SK, Kattan KM, et al: Massive haemoptysis by congenital absence of a segment of inferior vena cava. Thorax 48:1044, 1993.

309. Lip GY, Dunn FG: Unilateral pulmonary artery agenesis: A rare cause of haemoptysis and pleuritic chest pain. Int J Cardiol 40:121, 1993.

310. Malhotra V, Rosen RJ, Slepian RL: Life-threatening hypoxemia after lithotripsy in an adult due to shock-wave–induced pulmonary contusion. Anesthesiology 75:529, 1991.

311. Billy ML, Snow NJ, Haug RH: Tracheocarotid fistula with life-threatening hemorrhage: Report of case. J Oral Maxillofac Surg 52:1331, 1994.

312. Cordasco EM Jr, Mehta AC, Ahmad M: Bronchoscopically induced bleeding. A summary of nine years' Cleveland clinic experience and review of the literature. Chest 100:1141, 1991.

313. DeLima LG, Wynands JE, Bourke ME, et al: Catheter-induced pulmonary artery false aneurysm and rupture: Case report and review. J Cardiothorac Vasc Anesth 8:70, 1994.

314. Winkler TR, Hanlin RJ, Hinke TD, et al: Unusual cause of hemoptysis. Hickman-induced cava-bronchial fistula. Chest 102:1285, 1992.

315. Rocha MP, Guntupalli KK, Moise KJ Jr, et al: Massive hemoptysis in Takayasu's arteritis during pregnancy. Chest 106:1619, 1994.

316. Lakhkar BN, Nagaraj MV, Shenoy DP, et al: Bilateral pulmonary aneurysm in Behçet's disease (a case report). J Postgrad Med 38:47, 1992.

317. Nathan PE, Torres AV, Smith AJ, et al: Spontaneous pulmonary hemorrhage following coronary thrombolysis. Chest 101:1150, 1992.

317a. Chang Y-C, Patz EF Jr, Goodman PC: Significance of hemoptysis following thrombolytic therapy for acute myocardial infarction. Chest 109:727, 1996.

318. Cahill BC, Ingbar DH: Massive hemoptysis. Assessment and management. Clin Chest Med 15:147, 1994.

319. Macarron P, Garcia Diaz JE, Azofra JA, et al: D-Penicillamine therapy associated with rapidly progressive glomerulonephritis. Meph Dialysis Transplant 7:161, 1992.

320. Vizioli LD, Cho S: Amiodarone-associated hemoptysis. Chest 105:305, 1994.

321. Chow LT, Chow WH, Shum BS: Fatal massive upper respiratory tract haemorrhage: An unusual complication of localized amyloidosis of the larynx. J Laryngol Otol 107:51, 1993.

322. Hoffman R: Hemoptysis during sexual arousal. An unusual manifestation of amyloidosis. Chest 104:980, 1993.

323. McLean TR, Beall AC Jr, Jones JW: Massive hemoptysis due to broncholithiasis. Ann Thorac Surg 52:1173, 1991.

324. Wood DJ, Krishnan K, Stocks P, et al: Catamenial haemoptysis: A rare cause. Thorax 48:1048, 1993.

325. Bateman ED, Morrison SC: Catamenial haemoptysis from endobronchial endometriosis—a case report and review of previously reported cases. Respir Med 84:157, 1994.

326. Elliot DL, Barker AF, Dixon LM: Catamenial hemoptysis—new methods of diagnosis and therapy. Chest 87:687, 1985.

327. Cordier JF, Gamondes JP, Marx P, et al: Thoracic splenosis presenting with hemoptysis. Chest 102:626, 1992.

328. Rubin EM, Garcia H, Horowitz MD, et al: Fatal massive hemoptysis secondary to intralobar sequestration. Chest 106:954, 1994.

329. Koyama A, Sasou K, Nakao H, et al: Pulmonary intralobar sequestration accompanied by aneurysm of an anomalous arterial supply. Intern Med 31:946, 1992.

330. Makker HK, Barnes PC: Fatal haemoptysis from the pulmonary artery as a late complication of pulmonary irradiation. Thorax 46:609, 1991.

331. Fliegel E, Chitkara RK, Azueta V, et al: Fatal hemoptysis in lymphangiomyomatosis. NY State J Med 91:66, 1991.

332. Baktari JB, Tashkin DP, Small GW: Factitious hemoptysis—adding to the differential diagnosis. Chest 105:943, 1994.

333. Mroz BJ, Sexauer WP, Meade A, et al: Hemoptysis as the presenting symptom in bronchiolitis obliterans organizing pneumonia. Chest 111:1775, 1997.

333a. Haro M, Murcia I. Nunez A, et al: Massive haemoptysis complicating exogenous lipid pneumonia. European Respiratory Journal 11:507, 1998.

334. Banerjee AK, Carvalho P: Hypertrophic pulmonary osteoarthropathy due to a pulmonary metastasis from a soft tissue sarcoma. Clin Nucl Med 16:270, 1991.

335. Vico P, Delcorde A, Rahier I, et al: Hypertrophic osteoarthropathy and thyroid cancer. J Rheumatol 19:1153, 1992.

336. Davies RA, Darby M, Richards MA: Hypertrophic pulmonary osteoarthropathy in pulmonary metastatic disease. A case report and review of the literature. Clin Radiol 43:268, 1991.

337. Golimbu C, Marchetta P, Firooznia H, et al: Hypertrophic osteoarthropathy in metastatic renal cell carcinoma. Urology 22:669, 1983.

337a. Loredo JS, Fedullo PF, Piovella F, et al: Digital clubbing associated with pulmonary artery sarcoma. Chest 109:1651, 1996.

338. Benfield GFA: Primary lymphosarcoma of lung associated with hypertrophic pulmonary osteoarthropathy. Thorax 34:279, 1979.

339. Lofters WS, Walker TM: Hodgkin's disease and hypertrophic pulmonary osteoarthropathy. Complete clearing following radiotherapy. West Indian Med J 27:227, 1978.

340. Bhandari S, Wodzinski MA, Reilly JT: Reversible digital clubbing in acute myeloid leukaemia. Postgrad Med J 70:457, 1994.

341. May T, Rabaud C, Amiel C, et al: Hypertrophic pulmonary osteoarthropathy associated with granulomatous *Pneumocystis carinii* pneumonia in AIDS. Scand J Infect Dis 25:771, 1993.

342. Bhat S, Heurich AE, Vaquer RA, et al: Hypertrophic osteoarthropathy associated with *Pneumocystis carinii* pneumonia in AIDS. Chest 96:1208, 1989.

343. Kelly P, Manning P, Corcoran P, et al: Hypertrophic osteoarthropathy in association with pulmonary tuberculosis. Chest 99:769, 1991.

344. Shah A, Bhagat R: Digital clubbing in sarcoidosis. Indian J Chest Dis Allied Sci 34:217, 1992.

345. Hashmi S, Kaplan D: Asymmetric clubbing as a manifestation of sarcoid bone disease. Am J Med 93:471, 1992.

346. Emri S, Coplu L, Selcuk ZT, et al: Hypertrophic pulmonary osteoarthropathy in a patient with pulmonary alveolar microlithiasis. Thorax 46:145, 1991.

347. Wadhwa N, Balsam D, Ciminera P: Hypertrophic osteoarthropathy in a young child with adult respiratory distress syndrome (ARDS) secondary to burns. Pediatr Radiol 22:539, 1993.

348. Braude S, Kennedy H, Hodson M, et al: Hypertrophic osteoarthropathy in cystic fibrosis. BMJ 288:822, 1984.

349. Galko B, Grossman RF, Day A, et al: Hypertrophic pulmonary osteoarthropathy in four patients with interstitial pulmonary disease. Chest 88:94, 1985.

349a. Grathwohl KW, Thompson JW, Riordan KK, et al: Digital clubbing associated with polymyositis and interstitial lung disease. Chest 108:1751, 1995.

349b. Benekli M, Gullu IH: Hippocratic fingers in Behçet's disease. Postgraduate Medical Journal 73:575, 1997.

350. Cohen PR: Hypertrophic pulmonary osteoarthropathy and tripe palms in a man with squamous cell carcinoma of the larynx and lung. Report of a case and review of cutaneous paraneoplastic syndromes associated with laryngeal and lung malignancies. Am J Clin Oncol 16:268, 1993.

351. Martinez-Lavin M: Hypertrophic osteoarthropathy. Current Opinion in Rheumatology 9:83, 1997.

352. Ilhan I, Kutluk T, Gogus S, et al: Hypertrophic pulmonary osteoarthropathy in a child with thymic carcinoma: An unusual presentation in childhood. Med Pediatr Oncol 23:140, 1994.

353. Polkey MI, Cook GR, Thomson AD, et al: Clubbing associated with oesophageal adenocarcinoma. Postgrad Med J 67:1015, 1991.

354. Erkul PE, Ariyurek OM, Altinok D, et al: Colonic hamartomatous polyposis associated with hypertrophic osteoarthropathy. Pediatr Radiol 24:145, 1994.

355. Martinez-Lavin M: Cardiogenic hypertrophic osteoarthropathy. Clin Exp Rheumatol 7:19, 1992.

356. Doyle L: Some considerations of hypertrophic osteoarthropathy. Br J Dis Chest 74:314, 1980.

356a. Barraud-Klenovsek MM, Lubbe J, Burg G: Primary digital clubbing associated with palmoplantar keratoderma. Dermatology 194:302, 1997.

357. Harris AW, Harding TA, Gaitonde MD, et al: Is clubbing a feature of the antiphospholipid antibody syndrome? Postgrad Med J 69:748, 1993.

358. Editorial: Finger clubbing and hypertrophic pulmonary osteoarthropathy. BMJ 2:785, 1977.

359. Borden EC, Holling HE: Hypertrophic osteoarthropathy and pregnancy. Ann Intern Med 71:577, 1969.

360. Armstrong RD, Crisp AJ, Grahame R, et al: Hypertrophic osteoarthropathy and purgative abuse. BMJ 282:1836, 1981.

CHAPTER 17

Methods of Functional Investigation

PREDICTED NORMAL VALUES OF PULMONARY
FUNCTION, 405
   Lung Volumes, 406
      Vital Capacity, 406
      Functional Residual Capacity, Residual Volume, and Total
        Lung Capacity, 407
RESPIRATORY INDUCTIVE PLETHYSMOGRAPHY, 408
MEASUREMENT OF FORCED EXPIRATORY VOLUME
AND FLOW, 408
   Bronchodilator Response, 409
   Density Dependence of Maximal Expiratory Flow, 409
   Additional Tests of Forced Expiration, 410
MAXIMAL VOLUNTARY VENTILATION, 410
PRESSURE-VOLUME CHARACTERISTICS OF THE
LUNG, 410
DYNAMIC COMPLIANCE, 411
RESISTANCE, 412
THE SINGLE-BREATH NITROGEN WASHOUT, 413
TESTS OF SMALL AIRWAY FUNCTION, 414
TESTS OF DIFFUSING CAPACITY, 414
MEASUREMENT OF INEQUALITY OF VENTILATION-
PERFUSION RATIOS, 416
MEASUREMENT OF RESPIRATORY CONTROL, 416
   Ventilatory Response Curves, 417
   Mouth Occlusion Pressures, 418
   Breathing Pattern Analysis, 419
   Electromyography and Electroneurography, 419
TESTS OF RESPIRATORY MUSCLE
PERFORMANCE, 419
INHALATION CHALLENGE TESTS, 420
   Nonspecific Bronchial Reactivity, 420
   Specific Inhalation Challenge, 423
   Exercise-Induced Bronchoconstriction and Isocapnic
      Hyperventilation, 423

Pulmonary function tests can have a useful role in several aspects of respiratory disease. Indications for respiratory function tests can be broadly categorized as follows: (1) to resolve whether symptoms and signs such as dyspnea, cough, or cyanosis are of respiratory origin; (2) to manage and monitor the progression of disease or response to therapy in patients with recognized pulmonary disorders; (3) to assess the risk for the development of pulmonary dysfunction and complications resulting from therapeutic interventions such as operative procedures and drugs; (4) to quantify the degree of disability in environmental or occupational lung disease; (5) to carry out epidemiologic surveys of population groups suspected of having acquired pulmonary disease as a result of exposure to dust or fumes; and (6) to screen health status as part of a regular clinical assessment or on behalf of a third party (e.g., insurance company). Methods used for assessing pulmonary function range from simple, standardized techniques that can be performed rapidly and accurately on large groups of subjects to detailed methods for measuring disturbed respiratory physiology that are time consuming and require sophisticated instrumentation. At one end of this spectrum, spirometry or measurement of peak expiratory flow can be performed by personnel with relatively little training in the office, at the bedside, or in the emergency department; at the other end, assessment of diaphragmatic muscle function may require the insertion of gastric and esophageal catheters, measurement of respiratory muscle electromyograms (EMGs), and even phrenic nerve stimulation, procedures that require sophisticated recording devices and considerable technical skill. The more detailed methods that elucidate respiratory pathophysiologic abnormalities are less readily available and often represent some of the "fringe" benefits in pulmonary research centers. The choice of which tests should be performed in a given setting depends on the purpose of the study.

Assessment of pulmonary function can be conveniently divided into three levels of increasing sophistication. The *first* includes the measurement of vital capacity (VC) and maximal expiratory flow rates and an assessment of the gas-exchanging ability of the lungs by measurement of arterial blood gas tensions. Spirometry is a measure of forced expiratory volume in one second (FEV_1), forced vital capacity (FVC), the ratio of FEV_1/FVC, and peak expiratory flow. These parameters can be readily measured with recently developed simple, inexpensive, and portable devices.[1] Their use has been advocated as an integral part of the physical examination of adult patients and has been suggested as a means of "preventive medicine."[2] In fact, spirometry can now be considered as integral a part of the assessment of a patient with suspected lung disease as measurement of blood pressure in patients with cardiovascular disease. Measurement of arterial blood gas tensions can also be considered a first-line investigation in the assessment of respiratory dysfunction, properly performed and interpreted tests yielding valuable information regarding both pulmonary and metabolic status. The use of pulse oxymetry is rapidly becoming a first-line pulmonary function test in some settings and can be especially valuable when serial measurements of the adequacy of gas exchange are required.

The *second level* of investigation of altered lung function includes measurement of the subdivisions of lung volume and estimation of the diffusing capacity of the lung. Measurements of functional residual capacity, total lung capacity, and residual volume by the helium dilution technique or whole-body plethysmography can be performed using a number of devices, as can steady-state or single-breath diffusing capacity; when coupled with spirometry and blood gas determination, these investigations serve as the basic "screening tests" of lung function in most major hospitals.[3]

Following these tests, if doubt still exists about the nature and severity of a pulmonary disorder, a variety of *third-level* procedures may be used. More detailed description of altered lung mechanics can be obtained using measurement of airway and pulmonary resistance and the pressure-volume relationship of the lung. Respiratory control can be assessed by measuring the ventilatory responses to O_2 and CO_2 and inspiratory and expiratory muscle strength. Quantitative and qualitative descriptions of the distribution of ventilation and perfusion can be made using radioactive gases and aerosols. The clinical usefulness of measuring nonspecific bronchial reactivity has been amply demonstrated, and this measurement serves as a means of both diagnosing "reactive airway disease" and quantifying its severity and progression. Since dyspnea on exertion is a major complaint of patients with respiratory disease, it is appropriate to study the physiology of such patients while they are exercising; circuits are commercially available that allow measurement of workload, ventilation, O_2 uptake, CO_2 production, and the cardiovascular response to exercise. Such measurements of exercise performance also serve as an excellent objective measurement of disability.

Whatever their degree of complexity, lung function tests must be interpreted and correlated with clinical and radiologic data to be valid. Without the added information from these sources, interpretation of pulmonary function tests shows wide variability among individual readers.[4]

PREDICTED NORMAL VALUES OF PULMONARY FUNCTION

Interpretation of the results of pulmonary function tests is based on the degree of deviation from predicted normal values calculated from regression equations that take into account attributes such as age, sex, height, weight, and race that are known to contribute to variations in lung function. A wide range of scatter among "normal" individuals is related to genetic and environmental factors, the contribution of which has been investigated by comparing measurements of lung function in monozygotic and dizygotic twins.[5, 6] The results of these studies suggest that both heredity and the prenatal and postnatal environment influence baseline lung function.

Deciding whether a measurement of lung function in an individual is abnormal is often difficult; the decision depends not only on the variability of the parameter measured in a normal population but also on the variability of the test itself. Although it is often advocated that lung function tests be considered abnormal only when the value deviates by 20% or more from the mean normal value, this approach is simplistic and can be misleading.[7] The normal

range for a test may be defined by calculating 95% confidence limits (2 × standard error of the estimate); alternatively one can define the lower 5% of a reference population as below the lower limit of normal. Although the latter approach results in a 5% false-positive rate, this is generally considered acceptable.[8] The commonly used ±20% approach assumes that the variation increases as the value increases, thus overestimating the actual variation between subjects with large lung volumes or flow rates and underestimating the variation in subjects with small volumes or flow rates.[9, 10] Ninety-five per cent confidence intervals and lower 5% cutoffs are now available for many parameters of lung function and, with computer-derived report forms, can provide individualized normal ranges. Interindividual variation in lung function differs greatly between tests: for example, in a normal population the FEV_1/FVC ratio has a narrow 95% confidence limit, whereas forced expiratory flow over the middle of forced vital capacity (FEF_{25-75}) and highly effort-dependent measurements such as maximal inspiratory and expiratory pressure have much larger limits.

Prediction equations for lung function are often inaccurate at the extremes of age—for older individuals because smaller samples of normal subjects have been examined and for younger individuals as a result of the complex changes in lung function that occur during maturation. Although most lung function variables reach their optimal value in early adult life and then decline, the age-related decline does not begin at the same age for all parameters, which makes calculation of predicted normal values by backward or forward extrapolation inaccurate.[11]

The influence of weight can also be a confounding variable when included in prediction equations: in young, growing individuals, increased body weight is associated with large volumes and flow as a result of increasing respiratory muscle strength; however, in later life, increased weight may be associated with decreasing lung function owing to "obesity effects" such as decreased functional residual capacity.[12] For the same reasons, the influence of weight may be different in tall versus short people.[13] Ethnic variations in static and dynamic lung function must also be taken into account, and normal standards for each measurement must be obtained on the population concerned.[8, 12, 14–20] Many of the earlier prediction formulas were derived from populations that included a substantial number of smokers; more recent studies have recognized the subtle alterations in lung function that occur in smokers, and prediction equations and 95% confidence limits are now available for most measurements of lung function based on data from nonsmokers. These alterations will be referred to in the individual sections dealing with specific function tests. Prediction equations for lung function are generally based on cross-sectional data. Longitudinal analysis of lung function in large cohorts has also been used in some studies and offers the advantage that individual variation in the rate of change (growth or decline) of a lung function measurement can be defined.

Although one use of pulmonary function testing is to compare the values obtained in an individual with those of a normal population, monitoring the progress of a patient over time or assessing the response to acute or chronic therapy has the advantage of using the patient's own values as a control, thus permitting greater accuracy in detecting changes in lung function. Detection of a significant change or lack of change in any test over time or in response to an intervention is again dependent on the intrinsic variability of the test. This variability can be measured as the coefficient of variation of repeated tests, which is defined as a standard deviation of repeated tests divided by the mean. The coefficient of variation varies widely among lung function tests, but in general is much narrower than the 95% confidence limits observed in the population.[21] Coefficients of variation for many pulmonary function tests have been determined and will be referenced in the individual sections that follow. A number of comprehensive reviews of standardization of techniques, reference values, and analysis of lung function are useful reference sources.[8, 22–26]

Lung Volumes

Lung volumes and capacities can be appreciated by studying the diagram in Figure 17–1. Four volumes can be identified: (1) *tidal volume* (VT), the amount of gas moved in and out of the lung with each respiratory cycle; (2) *residual volume (RV),* the amount remaining in the lung after maximal expiration and the only volume that cannot be measured directly by spirometry; (3) *inspiratory reserve volume* (IRV), the additional gas that can be inspired from the end of a quiet inspiration; and (4) *expiratory reserve volume* (ERV), the additional amount of gas that can be expired from the resting or end-expiratory level. There are also four capacities, each of which contains two or more volumes: (1) *total lung capacity* (TLC), the gas contained in the lung at the end of maximal inspiration; (2) *vital capacity* (VC), the amount that can be expired after maximal inspiration or inspired after maximal expiration; (3) *inspiratory capacity* (IC), the amount of gas that can be inspired from the end of quiet expiration; and (4) *functional residual capacity* (FRC), the volume of gas remaining in the lung at the end of quiet expiration.

Vital Capacity

Although this volume of gas can be measured from the end of maximal expiration to full inspiration (inspiratory VC), it is usually expressed as the amount of air expelled from the lungs after maximal inspiration (expiratory VC). In fact, the most reported measurement is FVC, which is the amount of air that can be exhaled forcefully from the lung after maximal inspiration. In patients with obstructive pulmonary disease, FVC can be as much as 1 liter less than inspired VC as a result of dynamic compression of airways with gas trapping on expiration and failure to detect expired volume at low flow rates.[27, 28]

VC and FVC are usually measured using spirometers of various design, and predicted normal values with 95% confidence limits based on age, sex, height, and (in some instances) weight and age are readily available.[9, 13, 29, 30] VC varies with the position of the patient, being less in the supine than in the erect posture. Although VC and FVC serve little purpose as *independent* measures of pulmonary function, they can be of much value when considered in conjunction with the results of other tests; for example, their measurement is simple and the results are a useful index of day-to-day changes in the clinical status of patients with neuromuscular disease (although in these patients measurements of inspiratory pressure are more sensitive in detecting improvement or deterioration). The FEV$_1$/FVC ratio is a much more useful index than FVC alone and allows separation of patients with ventilatory abnormalities into those with "restrictive" or "obstructive" patterns. In obstructive pulmonary disease the ratio of FEV$_1$ to FVC is generally reduced, whereas in restrictive lung disease, FVC is reduced with preservation or an increase in FEV$_1$/FVC.

The subdivisions of VC, particularly IC and IRV, are rarely used in assessing pulmonary function. ERV may be markedly reduced in patients who are obese. VT varies greatly in normal subjects, and this measurement by itself is seldom of much value; however, multiplication of VT by the respiratory rate per minute gives the minute volume, and in

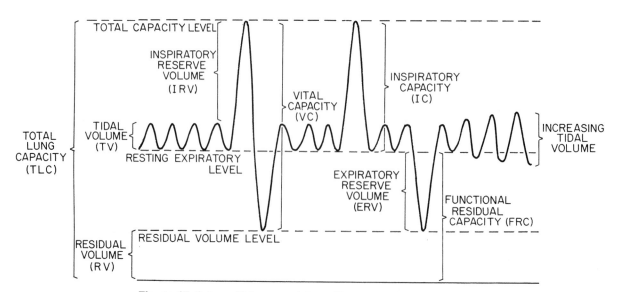

Figure 17–1. Lung Volumes and Capacities. *See* the text for descriptions.

some patients the level of alveolar hypoventilation can be suggested by these two indices alone. In addition, analysis of the pattern of generation of V_T can be useful as an indicator of respiratory drive.

Functional Residual Capacity, Residual Volume, and Total Lung Capacity

FRC is determined chiefly by the balance between the outward recoil of the chest wall and the inward recoil of the lung, although both active inspiratory muscle activity during expiration and flow limitation during tidal breathing can increase FRC above the static value. When flow limitation occurs during tidal breathing, dynamic hyperinflation results and alveolar pressure remains positive even at end expiration. This phenomenon has been termed *intrinsic positive end-expiratory pressure (auto-PEEP)*. FRC, RV, and TLC can be determined by either inert gas inhalation techniques or body plethysmography. The former includes single- and multiple-breath tests, using a closed circuit and helium or an open circuit and nitrogen used as the inert gases. (Helium and nitrogen are used because they do not participate in gas exchange.) In the open-circuit technique, the patient breathes 100% oxygen for 7 minutes and all expired gas is collected; FRC is calculated by multiplying the amount of gas expired during this period by the percentage of nitrogen in the expired gas. RV is then determined by subtracting ERV measured with a spirometer from the calculated FRC, and TLC is determined by adding IC to FRC. With the closed-circuit method, the patient breathes from a spirometer of known volume containing helium of known concentration. At the beginning of the study, the helium concentration in the lungs is zero; as the patient breathes in and out of the spirometer, the gas mixes between the spirometer and lungs until the concentration of helium is the same in both. FRC is calculated from the concentration of helium before and at the end of study and the known volume of the spirometer.

$$FRC = \frac{Spirometer\ volume \times Initial\ He\ concentration}{Final\ He\ concentration}$$

Again, RV and TLC are calculated by subtracting ERV and adding IC, respectively. Both the closed-circuit helium and open-circuit nitrogen techniques are subject to error because they do not detect trapped gas, which does not communicate with the tracheobronchial tree; as a result, they can seriously underestimate FRC, particularly in patients with obstructive lung disease, bullae, or other intrathoracic noncommunicating accumulations of gas. In addition, they are time consuming and repeated measurements are difficult to perform.[31] The techniques have the advantage that they can be performed on anesthetized or ventilated patients.[32] A modification of the N_2 washout method entailing forced rebreathing has been reported to offer advantages over the helium dilution technique in obstructed patients but is not in widespread clinical use.[33] The inert gas methods can be modified for use as a single-breath measurement by using either helium or nitrogen; however, although this adaptation may be useful for screening purposes in normal subjects, it seriously underestimates FRC in patients with airway obstruction.[9, 34, 35] The helium dilution technique has been used to independently estimate the FRC of each lung by

temporarily occluding one main bronchus with an inflatable balloon, but this technique is also not in widespread clinical use.[36]

The other major method of measuring FRC is based on Boyle's law and uses a body plethysmograph (body box). Boyle's law states that the product of the volume and pressure of gas is constant at constant temperature ($V_1 \times P_1 = V_2 \times P_2$). To measure FRC plethysmographically, the airway is closed at FRC and the subject pants against the closed airway, thus generating changes in mouth and pleural pressure and small increases and decreases in lung volume caused by compression and decompression of thoracic gas. The relationship between changes in thoracic gas volume and mouth or pleural pressure ($\Delta V/\Delta P$) can be calibrated so that intrathoracic volume can be derived and RV and TLC obtained by having the subject perform a VC maneuver immediately after measurement of FRC. The method has the theoretical advantage that all gas subjected to swings in intrathoracic pressure is measured, whether or not the gas communicates with the tracheobronchial tree.

Two types of body box are commonly used: in the first (termed a pressure box), changes in thoracic volume during panting are measured by corresponding changes in pressure within the box; in the second (constant-pressure or volume displacement body plethysmograph), changes in thoracic volume are measured using a highly sensitive spirometer. Although plethysmographic measurements of FRC have long been considered "the gold standard," there is evidence that their accuracy is affected both by the pattern of panting and (especially) by the severity of any accompanying air-flow obstruction.[37, 38] One assumption of the plethysmographic technique is that only intrathoracic and not intra-abdominal gas is subjected to swings in pressure; this assumption has been shown to be untrue since variable abdominal gas compression occurs when panting is accomplished by diaphragmatic or intercostal muscle action.[39, 40] A second erroneous assumption implicit in the plethysmographic method for the determination of FRC is that swings in mouth pressure accurately reflect swings in alveolar pressure, which compresses and decompresses intrathoracic gas. Although this assumption may be true in normal subjects, phase and amplitude differences in alveolar and mouth pressure swings can occur as a result of a combination of intrathoracic airway narrowing and an extrathoracic compliant trachea or oral cavity; this artefact can lead to an overestimation of the true intrathoracic gas volume,[41, 42] an error that can be diminished by using intraesophageal instead of mouth pressure to measure FRC.[43–46]

In patients with asthma and other obstructive pulmonary diseases, measurements of FRC and TLC made with esophageal rather than mouth pressure yield values that are closer to measurements obtained radiographically, which suggests that in this setting the standard plethysmographic technique can overestimate thoracic gas volume.[47, 48] The phase and amplitude differences between mouth pressure and changes in thoracic gas volume increase with increasing air-flow obstruction[43] and with increasing panting frequency.[48–51] These artefacts account for a significant proportion of the apparent acute increases in TLC seen in asthmatics in whom bronchoconstriction is induced.[44, 45, 52] The most accurate measurement of FRC and TLC in severely obstructed patients is obtained by the plethysmographic method with esophageal rather than mouth pressure, especially when manual support of the compliant cheeks is used during panting at low frequency (less than 1 Hz). Despite these problems, measurement of thoracic gas volume by plethysmography is very reproducible, the coefficient of variation in normal subjects being approximately 4%; however, this figure increases slightly in obstructed patients.[53]

TLC may also be determined from posteroanterior and lateral chest radiographs, a procedure that can be accomplished by experienced workers in less than 5 minutes. Measurement of TLC with radiographic methods is discussed in more detail in Chapter 13.[54, 55] Prediction equations for TLC are available.[9, 37, 56] RV increases with age, as does the RV/TLC ratio, but there is little change in FRC or TLC.

RESPIRATORY INDUCTIVE PLETHYSMOGRAPHY

Respiratory inductive plethysmography (RIP) is a technique to measure lung volumes noninvasively.[57, 58] The apparatus used consists of coils of wire that are insulated and positioned around the rib cage and abdomen; the coils are oscillated with a high-frequency signal and emit a frequency-modulated signal that is related to the changes in enclosed volume of the rib cage and abdomen. The coils therefore give a signal that is proportional to the cross-sectional area enclosed within them, and using various calibration techniques the electrical output from the rib cage and abdominal coils can be summed and equated to volume change measured using a spirometer. The major advantage of RIP is that it can measure volume without the behavioral changes in breathing pattern that may occur with the use of a mouthpiece.

A number of studies have shown that RIP is reasonably accurate, although it may be affected by changes in body position.[59–64] The technique can be used for measurements of VC and expiratory flow rates, although its accuracy in dynamic maneuvers is somewhat less than that of the spirometer.[65, 66] Even though it has been used to monitor ventilation during exercise, it has found its main uses in studying the pattern of breathing,[67] measuring lung volume changes during mechanical ventilation,[68] monitoring inhalation patterns during smoking, and characterizing apneic periods during sleep.[69]

MEASUREMENT OF FORCED EXPIRATORY VOLUME AND FLOW

The forced expiratory maneuver is the most widely used and standardized test of lung function.[22, 70] Expired volume can be plotted against time (Fig. 17–2) to yield a spirogram from which FEV_1, FVC, and FEF_{25-75} (formerly termed *the maximal midexpiratory flow rate,* or MMFR) can be derived. Expired volume can also be plotted against the instantaneous expiratory flow rate to yield a flow-volume curve. Flow at specific percentages of the forced expired VC, such as $\dot{V}max_{50}$ and $\dot{V}max_{25}$, can in turn be determined from the flow-volume curve. Standards for performance and interpretation of spirometry and flow-volume curves have been adopted by the European Respiratory Society and the American Thoracic Society.[26, 71] Although performance of

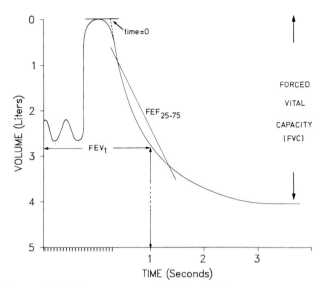

Figure 17–2. Measurement of Ventilatory Volumes. Measurements derived from a maximal forced expiration provide the most readily obtained and useful assessment of lung function. Volume in liters is plotted against time in seconds while the subject forcibly exhales from total lung capacity. The volume-versus-time slope is back-extrapolated to determine 0 time, and the expired volume in 1 second (FEV_1) is measured and compared with predicted values, as well as with the measured forced vital capacity (FVC). The FEV_1/FVC ratio serves as a volume-independent measure of expiratory air-flow obstruction. The average flow over the middle half of the forced expiratory volume (FEF_{25-75}) is obtained as the slope of the volume-time plot between 25% and 75% of FVC.

the maximal expiratory flow maneuver is a relatively simple and standardized procedure, interpretation of the abnormalities is more complicated. The determinants of maximal expiratory flow include the elastic recoil properties of the lung, the resistance of the airways, and the collapsibility of the larger airways where flow limitation occurs.

The interest in forced expiration as a measurement of dynamic lung function stems largely from the fact that it is a relatively effort-independent measurement and is highly reproducible; three to five measurements of forced expiration are usually obtained. A number of methods have been suggested for selecting the best values for FVC, FEV_1, and FEF_{25-75}: (1) choose the forced expiration with the largest sum of FEV_1 and FVC[72] (recommended for selection of the best FEF_{25-75} and flow-volume curve[26, 73]), (2) from three curves select the largest FEV_1 and FVC even if they are not on the same curve[10] (recommended for selection of FEV_1 and FVC[26]), (3) define FEV_1 and FVC as the mean of the three best of five curves,[74] and (4) construct a composite curve matched at TLC or on the descending slope of the flow-volume curve.[72, 75]

Although the forced expiratory maneuver is effort independent up to a point, submaximal efforts can result in paradoxically high values of FVC, FEV_1, and FEF_{25-75}, especially in patients with obstructive pulmonary disease.[76, 77] The significance of these differences is unclear. In normal subjects, FEV_1 and FVC are very reproducible (95% confidence limits, ±5%), but in obstructed patients this variability increases to approximately 12% when measured on the same day.[21] There is more short-term variability in the measurements in subjects who have a wheeze, a significant bronchodilator response, or documented airway hyper-responsiveness.[78] The variability also increases with longer time periods between measurements, presumably as a result of variability in both the flow-measuring device and the subject.[79] The development of portable handheld electronic spirometers that rely on the conversion of a flow signal to a volume signal has allowed the practical application of spirometry in a variety of settings, but the validity and reproducibility of some of these devices are less than with volume displacement spirometers.[1, 80, 81]

When compared with FVC and FEV_1, there is a much higher coefficient of variation for repeated measurements of FEF_{25-75}, $\dot{V}max_{50}$, and $\dot{V}max_{25}$,[21, 82–84] a variability that increases with the degree of pulmonary dysfunction.[85] The coefficient of variation for FEF_{25-75} and $\dot{V}max_{50}$ for repeated measurements in a normal subject is about 20% but increases to as high as 30% in patients with airway obstruction. There is also more variation between individuals for FEF_{25-75} and $\dot{V}max_{50}$ than for FEV_1 and FVC. The 95% confidence limits for FEV_1 and FVC in a population are 20%; for FEF_{25-75} and $\dot{V}max_{50}$ to be judged abnormal, values should be more than 40% below predicted.[21, 84, 86] Excellent prediction equations based on large groups of normal nonsmokers are available for FEV_1, FVC, $\dot{V}max_{50}$, $\dot{V}max_{25}$, and FEF_{25-75}.[8, 13, 30] Separate prediction equations have been developed for African Americans[87] and Asians,[88] as well as for the elderly.[89] There has been a recent surge of interest and activity in the measurement of lung function in infants and children.[90–92]

Another valuable test of lung function is the peak expiratory flow (PEF) (defined as the largest expiratory flow achieved during a maximally forced effort from a position of maximal inspiration expressed in liters per minute.)[26] Since the measurement of PEF is much more effort dependent than are other measures of FEF, subjects must be encouraged to perform the maneuver as vigorously as possible. In addition, measurement of PEF requires the use of an instrument with a very high frequency response since it is such a dynamic measurement.[93, 94] These factors combine to make PEF a more variable measurement than either FEV_1 or FVC.

Although the forced expiratory maneuver is the standard test of lung function, additional valuable information can be derived from a forced inspiratory maneuver and comparison of forced inspiratory and expiratory flow at equal volumes.[95] The use of inspiratory and expiratory flow-volume curves in the diagnosis of upper airway obstruction is discussed in detail in Chapter 52 (*see* page 2047).

Bronchodilator Response

Measurements of maximal expiratory flow and volume are frequently used to quantify the reversibility of air-flow obstruction. The purposes of assessing bronchodilator response are to test the potential therapeutic benefit that can be derived by bronchodilator therapy and to aid in distinguishing reversible forms of air-flow obstruction such as asthma from relatively irreversible forms of obstruction (chronic obstructive pulmonary disease [COPD], bronchiectasis, etc). To decide whether a significant improvement has occurred, it is necessary to know the reproducibility of the individual measurements:[21, 96] the 95% confidence limits for acute changes in spirometric variables are 71% for the PEF

rate, 15% for FVC, 12% for FEV_1, 17% for FEV_1/FVC, and 45% for FEF_{25-75}.[96] A beneficial effect of bronchodilators should not be reported unless improvement beyond these limits is observed.

The FEV_1 is probably the best single test for assessing bronchodilator response;[8, 97] although specific airway conductance or forced oscillation measures of respiratory impedance can be used, these tests are probably less reproducible and impractical.[98, 99] The change in FEV_1 following the administration of a bronchodilator can be expressed as per cent initial FEV_1, as per cent predicted FEV_1, or in absolute units. Expressing the results as per cent predicted FEV_1 is the most accurate in separating those who have asthma from those who have COPD.[100] It is of interest that some patients who have reversible bronchoconstriction respond to bronchodilators by showing a predominant increase in their flow rates (ΔFEV_1) whereas others primarily increase their expired volume (ΔFVC); it is useful to combine the changes in these variables when assessing bronchodilator response.[101] In fact, some patients obtain considerable symptomatic relief from inhaled bronchodilators despite a decrease in the FEV_1/FVC ratio, which makes this value a poor estimate of bronchodilator response.[102, 103] Although one group has shown a decrease in the bronchodilating effectiveness of a β-adrenergic agonist in older subjects,[104] others have shown preserved bronchodilator responsiveness as a function of age.[105, 106]

Density Dependence of Maximal Expiratory Flow

In contrast to FVC, maximal expiratory flow increases after patients are equilibrated with a low-density gas mixture such as 80% helium/20% oxygen. In normal subjects, the flows increase over most of the VC range, but at a point low in the VC range, flow of the two gases becomes equal (volume of isoflow [$Viso\dot{V}$]). It has been suggested that the increase in flow with the low-density He/O_2 mixture and $Viso\dot{V}$ are influenced by the predominant site of airway narrowing:[107, 108] gas density has an important influence on resistance in airways where flow is turbulent but does not affect resistance where flow is laminar. Although flow in the larger central airways is turbulent, gas flow in small airways is laminar because of their enormous cross-sectional area and low linear flow velocity. The theory predicts that if the major site of air-flow limitation is in large airways (where a turbulent flow pattern exists), breathing the low-density He/O_2 will substantially increase expiratory flow rates; by contrast, if the major site of flow limitation is in more peripheral airways (where a laminar flow pattern exists), He/O_2 will have no effect. The magnitude of the He/O_2 effect can be quantified by calculating the density dependence of maximum expiratory flow ($\dot{V}max$):

$$\Delta \dot{V} max = \frac{\begin{array}{c}\textit{Maximal expiratory flow breathing}\\ \textit{He/O}_2 - \textit{Maximal expiratory}\\ \textit{flow breathing air}\end{array}}{\begin{array}{c}\textit{Maximal expiratory flow}\\ \textit{breathing air}\end{array}}$$

$Viso\dot{V}$ is determined by matching the air and He/O_2 flow-volume curve at TLC or RV. Although $\Delta\dot{V}max$ and $Viso\dot{V}$

have been advocated as potentially sensitive tests of early small airway obstruction, a number of clinical studies have questioned their usefulness.[109-111] Part of this disenchantment stems from their marked variability and poor reproducibility.[112-118] One way to determine the reproducibility and therefore the potential sensitivity of a test is to calculate the signal-to-noise ratio, which is the standard deviation of the measurement between individuals divided by the standard deviation of the measurement within an individual on repeated testing: the higher the ratio, the better the test in separating groups or measuring changes in an individual. In one investigation of various functional parameters, the signal-to-noise ratio for FVC was 49; for FEV_1, 26; for PEF, 15; for $\dot{V}max_{50}$, 6.5; for $\Delta\dot{V}max_{50}$, 0.42; for $\Delta\dot{V}max_{25}$, 0.29; and for $Viso\dot{V}$, 0.7.[119] Despite these limitations, measurements of the density dependence of maximal expiratory flow have been used in the diagnosis of upper airway obstruction. However, it does not add to the information derived from inspiratory and expiratory flow-volume curves (*see also* page 2047).[120]

Additional Tests of Forced Expiration

With the advent of practical on-line computers, flow, volume, and time signals during forced expiration can be analyzed digitally in an attempt to provide additional information about the mechanisms limiting maximal expiratory flow. Such analysis includes computer averaging of a number of flow-volume curves, measurement of the slope ratio on the descending slope of the curve (tangent slope/chord slope at any volume), calculation of the total expiratory time, and measurement of the area under the maximal expiratory flow-volume curve.[120-124] In addition, partial flow-volume curves consisting of maximal expirations initiated from the end of a normal tidal breath have been used to bypass the normal bronchodilator effect of a TLC inspiration.[125] Applying negative pressure at the mouth during tidal exhalation to see whether this maneuver increases expiratory flow has been suggested as a technique to determine whether patients who have COPD are flow-limited during tidal breathing.[126] Tussometry—a noninvasive technique that involves analyzing the air-flow waveform produced by a voluntary cough—has also been advocated to assess laryngeal function.[127]

An interesting approach to the separation of factors limiting maximal expiratory flow is measurement of the maximal expiratory flow–elastic recoil curve.[128] As shown in Figure 17–3, analysis of such a curve can theoretically establish the major contributor to flow limitation. Although prediction equations for normal upstream resistance have been derived, systematic comparison of the results of this technique with those of pathologic examination has not been performed.[128]

MAXIMAL VOLUNTARY VENTILATION

Maximal voluntary ventilation is the volume of air exhaled in a specified period of time during repetitive maximal respiratory effort expressed in liters per minute. The duration of the test should be between 12 and 15 seconds.[26]

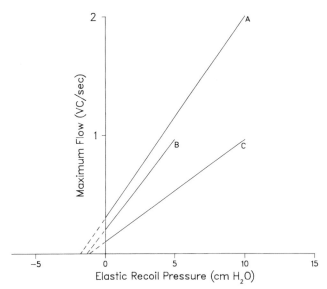

Figure 17–3. Maximal Expiratory Flow/Elastic Recoil Curve. Maximal expiratory flow can be decreased because of decreases in elastic recoil of the lung and/or increases in the resistance upstream from the flow-limiting site: upstream resistance. Theoretically, the importance of these factors can be quantified by construction of a maximal flow–elastic recoil plot. Maximal flow at different lung volumes is plotted against the measured recoil pressure at that lung volume. *Curve A* in the figure represents a normal relationship. Peak flow reaches approximately 2 vital capacities per second, and flow diminishes as recoil decreases. The slope of the line $\Delta\dot{V}max/\Delta P$ is upstream conductance. *Curve B* represents the relationship in a patient in whom loss of recoil is the *sole* cause of decreased flow. Maximal flow is decreased to less than half of normal because of decreased recoil pressures, but the conductance ($\Delta\dot{V}max/\Delta P$) is normal. *Curve C* represents a patient in whom the decrease in flow is *solely* related to a narrowing of the airways and a decrease in upstream conductance. The recoil pressures achieved are normal but the flow at any recoil pressure is decreased and the slope $\Delta\dot{V}max/\Delta P$ is decreased. While this is theoretically useful, we have found that the majority of patients who have chronic obstructive pulmonary disease show decreased flow as a result of a combination of decreased recoil and decreased upstream conductance. Patients who have pure emphysema, such as occurs in association with α_1-antitrypsin deficiency, show a curve like *B*.

The results are influenced by the properties of the lung and airways and correlate with FEV_1; however, they are also influenced by inspiratory muscle performance: the expiratory phase of such forced ventilation is determined by the mechanical properties of the airways and lung parenchyma, whereas the inspiratory portion is determined by the speed of shortening of the inspiratory muscles and is closely linked with maximal inspiratory pressure.[129-131]

PRESSURE-VOLUME CHARACTERISTICS OF THE LUNG

As discussed in Chapter 1 (*see* page 53), compliance is the relationship between the volume of air inhaled and the pressure necessary to overcome the elastic recoil of the lung. To avoid the effect of resistance and the pressure necessary to overcome it, measurements of lung compliance and recoil are done during "static maneuvers." A complete pressure-volume curve of the lung is obtained by plotting lung volume in liters against the transpulmonary pressure over a range of volumes from TLC to FRC or lower. Transpulmonary pressure (PL) is measured by a transducer that compares mouth pressure with esophageal pressure measured with a thin-walled balloon positioned in the midportion of the esophagus. Volume is measured by electrical integration of a pneumotachograph flow signal, by a spirometer, or (ideally) by a volume displacement body plethysmograph. The pressure-volume curve is a measure of lung tissue elasticity, which is related to elastin and collagen fibers as well as to surface forces. Pressure-volume data are collected during quasistatic deflation from TLC or with stepwise interruption of expiratory flow from TLC (Fig. 17–4). The curves tend to be sigmoid in shape,[132] although above FRC the pressure-volume data approximate an exponential function.[133–135]

A number of parameters derived from the pressure-volume curve reflect the elastic recoil properties of the lung (Fig. 17–5). The maximal elastic recoil pressure that the patient can generate at TLC (PLmax) reflects the elastic recoil properties of the lung as well as the inspiratory muscle strength. Elastic recoil pressures at various percentages of TLC (PL90, PL80, PL70, and so on) can also be examined in addition to the more standard measurement of compliance. Compliance is calculated as the volume change in liters divided by the transpulmonary pressure change over the relatively linear portion of the pressure-volume curve near FRC. Compliance has the disadvantage of being dependent on lung size, thus making comparison between individuals difficult; to circumvent this problem, a number of investigators have suggested fitting the pressure-volume data to an exponential equation:[133–135]

$$V = A - Be^{-K/P}$$

where A is the theoretical maximal lung volume achievable at infinite transpulmonary pressure, B is the lung volume at a transpulmonary pressure of zero, k is the shape constant that reflects the overall compliance of the lung irrespective of lung size, and P is the transpulmonary pressure. Prediction equations for normal values of k, PLmax, and elastic recoil

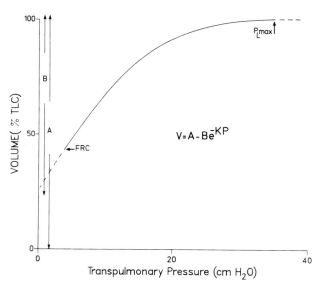

Figure 17–5. Elastic Recoil Properties of the Lung. A schematic pressure-volume curve of the lung is presented in which lung volume as a percentage of total lung capacity (TLC) (predicted or actual) is plotted against transpulmonary pressure obtained by comparing mouth and esophageal pressures. The pressure-volume behavior may be described by using various measurements from the P-V curve, including maximal elastic recoil (P$_L$ max), elastic recoil pressure at various percentages of TLC (i.e., P$_{L90}$, P$_{L60}$, and so on), and compliance—the slope of the $\Delta V/\Delta P$ plot in the relatively linear range near FRC. These all have the disadvantage of describing only a portion of the curve. The whole curve can be fitted to an exponential function such as the equation described by Colebatch and associates,[133] in which V = volume, A = the theoretical maximal lung volume at infinite transpulmonary pressure, B = the volume difference between A and the 0 transpulmonary pressure intercept, P = transpulmonary pressure, and k = the exponent that describes the shape of the P-V curve. The ratio B/A defines the position of the curve, whereas the exponential constant k describes the shape of the whole P-V curve.

pressures at various percentages of TLC have been derived from the study of large groups of normal, nonsmoking subjects.[136] The variability in these measurements has also been assessed in normal subjects: the elastic recoil pressure at 90% of TLC (PL90) and the natural logarithm of the exponential constant k have been found to be the most reproducible, with coefficients of variation of 9% and 6%, respectively.[137, 138] An increased k correlates with the severity of emphysema measured morphologically, and a decreased k has been reported in some patients with interstitial fibrosis.[134, 139] However, the curve-fitting analysis has not been found useful in distinguishing emphysematous from nonemphysematous excised human lungs.[140] In a study in which various-sized mammalian lungs were compared, k was found to increase with mean alveolar size;[141] it is possible that it reflects an overall loss of elastic recoil and enlargement of air-space size rather than the gross morphologic changes of emphysema. It has been suggested that since k is a reflection of the mean alveolar size, it can be used to estimate alveolar surface area during life.[142]

DYNAMIC COMPLIANCE

Although the compliance of the lung is normally measured during static maneuvers, dynamic compliance (Cdyn) can be measured during breathing as volume change divided

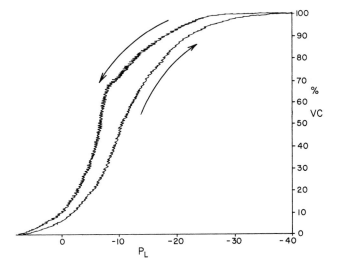

Figure 17–4. Pressure-Volume Curve. A pressure-volume tracing of a young male adult is measured in both inspiration and expiration from residual volume to total lung capacity and back to residual volume. The upper curve represents the expiratory tracing. Notice the more horizontal appearance (decrease in compliance) as total lung capacity is reached.

by the changes in transpulmonary pressure at points of zero flow. In most normal subjects, Cdyn is very similar to static compliance over the range of V_T and does not vary with respiratory frequencies up to 100 breaths per minute. Maintenance of the relationship between nonresistive pressure drop and volume change with increasing respiratory frequency reflects the remarkably synchronous action of acinar units throughout the lung. If there is any patchy obstruction of small airways or patchy alteration in regional lung compliance, regional time constant variations increase.*

With increased frequency of breathing, when the respiratory cycle time becomes shorter than the time constant of some units, Cdyn decreases as breathing frequency increases (frequency dependence of compliance). This decrease in compliance with increasing breathing frequencies is therefore a measure of the inequalities of time constants in the lung and is indirectly a reflection of heterogeneity in small airway resistance and acinar compliance. The test has been shown to correlate with measurements of unevenness of ventilation[143] and has been advocated as a test of small airway obstruction.[144, 145] However, although it may be one of the most specific and sensitive tests of small airway dysfunction, it has not gained wide acceptance clinically because it requires expensive equipment, technical expertise, and the placement of an esophageal pressure catheter.[146]

RESISTANCE

Resistance is pressure divided by flow ($R = P/\dot{V}$). In the lung, either airway resistance (Raw) or pulmonary resistance (RL) is generally measured. The former is the difference between mouth and alveolar pressure divided by flow and is measured in a constant-volume body plethysmograph or by a flow interruption technique. Enclosed within the body box, the subject pants through a pneumotachograph: the flow signal is plotted against alveolar pressure swings, estimated by changes in box pressure. With a closed system, box pressure varies only because alveolar gas is compressed and decompressed during panting, and variation in box pressure therefore reflects variations in alveolar pressure. Box pressure swings can be calibrated for alveolar pressure by comparing mouth and box pressure swings during obstructed breaths. The flow interruption technique to measure airway resistance is noninvasive and requires minimal patient cooperation, which makes it ideal for infants and ventilated subjects.[147] The method is based on the transient interruption of air flow at the mouth for a brief period, during which alveolar pressure equilibrates with mouth pressure. Measurement of mouth pressure is used to estimate alveolar pressure immediately prior to the interruption, and the ratio of this pressure to flow prior to interruption gives airway resistance.[148]

Raw can also be expressed as its reciprocal, conduc-

tance (Gaw); since resistance varies with lung volume in a hyperbolic fashion and conductance varies in a linear fashion, both should be corrected for the effects of lung volume. Specific airway conductance (SGaw) is airway conductance per unit lung volume and can be obtained by dividing Gaw by the lung volume at which it is measured; specific airway resistance (SRaw) is the product of airway resistance and the thoracic gas volume at which the measurement is made.[149]

Pulmonary resistance (RL) is obtained by dividing the difference between mouth and esophageal pressure (PL) by flow. An esophageal balloon is introduced in the manner described earlier for measurement of the pressure-volume curve of the lung, and a differential pressure transducer compares mouth and pleural pressure during breathing at varying frequencies. Since the pressure difference between the mouth and the pleural space during breathing reflects both the resistive and elastic properties of the lung, the portion of the transpulmonary pressure swing caused by elastic recoil must be subtracted to measure the true pressure-flow relationship. This calculation can be done electronically,[150] by breathing at resonant frequency (the frequency at which inertial and elastic forces cancel each other), or by measuring pressure changes at points of isovolume on inspiration and expiration.[151] Cardiac motion can result in esophageal pressure artefacts, thus influencing the accuracy of the technique; however, this problem can be overcome by a circuit that averages the pressure-flow relationship over a number of breaths.[152] No standardized prediction formulas or normal values are available for either airway or pulmonary resistance.

A simple noninvasive method of measuring the resistance of the total respiratory system (Rrs) uses forced oscillations at varying frequencies during tidal breathing. Small pulses of flow are generated at the mouth by a loudspeaker, and the relationship between the output of the loudspeaker and the resultant flow can be analyzed to give values for total respiratory system resistance and reactance.[146] Respiratory system resistance can be measured over a wide range of frequencies; the frequency dependency of resistance and reactance has been suggested as a sensitive test of early small airway dysfunction.[153–156] The forced oscillation technique has the advantages of being easy to perform, noninvasive, and not requiring cooperation of the patient. Normal values and an estimate of reproducibility are available.[154, 157] The four methods of measuring resistance have been compared in normal subjects before and after methacholine-induced bronchoconstriction; although they gave very similar values at baseline, the flow interruption technique and Rrs were less sensitive in detecting bronchoconstriction.[158]

The measurement of airway or pulmonary resistance by whatever method represents the sum of the resistance of each generation of airways arranged in series and the airways within such generation arranged in parallel. In normal subjects, the bulk of the resistance to air flow is across the larynx and large central airways, where the total cross-sectional area is least and where the flow pattern is most turbulent and therefore most costly in terms of pressure loss. Although no noninvasive technique has been devised to accurately measure the contribution to total pulmonary resistance of various sizes and generations of airways, a bronchoscopic method has been used to show that there is uniform

---

*The time constant of a lung unit is the product of its resistance and compliance. Since the units of resistance are centimeters of water per liter per second and those of compliance are liters per centimeter of water, the units of their product are seconds. The time constant of a lung unit gives an estimate of the time that it takes for the unit to completely fill with gas when a step change of pressure is applied to it. A long time constant, reflecting slow filling and emptying, can occur because of high resistance and/or high compliance.

narrowing of central and peripheral airways in asthmatic subjects following the inhalation of methacholine.[159]

THE SINGLE-BREATH NITROGEN WASHOUT

The single-breath nitrogen washout test can be used as a measure of the distribution of inspired gas. The test is carried out by having the patient inhale a VC breath of pure oxygen, beginning the inhalation from RV and maintaining the inspiratory flow rate at less than 0.5 liter per second. During the subsequent slow exhalation (flow, 0.5 liter per second) from TLC back to RV, the expired nitrogen concentration measured at the mouth is plotted against the expired volume on an XY recorder or oscilloscope. Changes in volume and nitrogen concentration during progressive exhalation can be described by five phases (Fig. 17–6): *Phase 1* represents the emptying of dead space, which contains pure oxygen and no nitrogen; *Phase 2* represents the rapid increase in nitrogen that occurs with the arrival of alveolar gas at the mouth; *Phase 3* is the slow, slight rise in nitrogen concentration that occurs during the alveolar plateau; *Phase 4* is the abrupt increase in nitrogen concentration that occurs in most normal subjects as RV is approached; and *Phase 5* is an irregular, abrupt decrease in nitrogen concentration that occurs immediately before RV is reached.

Anatomic dead space and an inert gas dilution measurement of TLC can be calculated from the single-breath nitrogen washout test.[160] Closing volume is the volume above RV at which Phase 4 begins and reflects closure of dependent airways. The addition of RV and closing volume gives closing capacity, which can be expressed as a percentage of TLC. The slope of the alveolar plateau (Phase 3) reflects the uniformity of alveolar ventilation and is calculated for the linear portion of the alveolar plateau, expressed as per cent change per liter. The upward-sloping plateau normally found is related to the asynchronous emptying of lung units that have different starting nitrogen concentrations; however, recent studies suggest that because of diffusive pendelluft at branch points subtending lung units of varying pathway length, an upward-sloping alveolar plateau can exist despite synchronous and homogeneous volume changes throughout the lung. (Diffusive pendelluft occurs when gas diffuses "backward" against the direction of bulk flow at a branch point when the concentration of that gas coming from one unit is different from that of the other.[161])

The use of N_2 per liter as a measurement of the unevenness of alveolar ventilation was suggested by Comroe and Fowler in 1951.[162] By concentrating nitrogen within the alveolar space, continuing gas exchange during slow expiration also contributes to the upward-sloping Phase 3 and the height of Phase 4.[162, 163] The beginning of Phase 4 coincides with the onset of airway closure, initially in the gravity-dependent portions of the lung. Closing volume can also be measured by monitoring expired N_2 without prior inhalation of O_2; the apical-to-base differences in resident N_2 concentration are sufficient to detect the onset of Phase 4.[163a] In disease, premature airway closure produces an elevated closing volume and closing capacity; the upward slope of Phase 3 is exaggerated owing to regional differences in distribution of the inhaled oxygen and asynchronous emptying of lung units. An increased closing capacity and slope of Phase 3 can relate to changes in small airways or alterations in elastic recoil of the lung secondary to elastic tissue disruption, diminished surface forces, or both. The downward-sloping Phase 5 is thought to be related to the onset of flow limitation in the uppermost regions of the lung that results in an increased contribution from the already flow-limited lower regions.[164]

Closing volume can also be measured by using a bolus technique that involves inhalation at RV of a small amount of xenon,[165, 166] argon,[167] or helium.[168] Since airways supplying gravity-dependent lung zones are closed at RV, the inert gas is preferentially distributed to the upper lung zones, the lower zones being filled with room air or oxygen, depending on which is used to complete the inspiration. During the next expiration from TLC, the inert gas is measured at the mouth and its concentration recorded against expired vol-

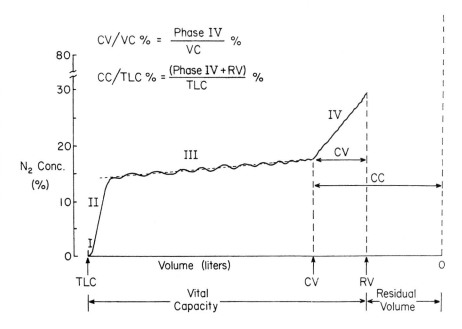

Figure 17–6. The Single-Breath Nitrogen Washout. In this test, the expired nitrogen concentration (vertical axis) is plotted against expired volume starting at total lung capacity (TLC) and ending at residual volume (RV). Phase I represents dead space gas with 0 nitrogen; Phase III represents alveolar nitrogen concentration; the slope of Phase III is increased with unevenness of distribution of ventilation. Phase IV begins at closing volume (CV) and represents the increasing contribution of gas from nitrogen-rich nondependent lung regions after the basilar regions have closed. In this diagram, Phase V is not depicted. VC, vital capacity; CC, closing capacity.

$$CV/VC\,\% = \frac{Phase\ IV}{VC}\,\%$$

$$CC/TLC\,\% = \frac{(Phase\ IV + RV)}{TLC}\,\%$$

ume. Values for closing volume and closing capacity are similar with the bolus and single-breath nitrogen washout techniques.[169] The latter can also be performed on excised postmortem lungs, in which case closing capacity has been shown to correlate with peripheral airway inflammation.[170] Prediction equations based on age and sex for definition of normal values and 95% confidence limits are described for closing volume, closing capacity, and the slope of Phase 3 of the single-breath nitrogen washout test;[171, 172] the intertest variability of parameters derived from the single-breath test have also been calculated.[173]

The distribution of inspired gas can also be measured by a multiple-breath technique in which the patient breathes 100% O_2 for 7 minutes.[174] When the distribution of inspired air is uniform, the nitrogen content of an "alveolar" sample at the end of 7 minutes should be 2.5% or less. In patients with impaired distribution, 10 to 20 minutes may elapse before the nitrogen content of poorly ventilated areas has been replaced by oxygen, so the nitrogen content of the alveolar sample at 7 minutes may greatly exceed 2.5%.

A third method for determining the distribution of inspired gas uses a helium closed-circuit apparatus, the result being expressed as the mixing efficiency.[175, 176]

TESTS OF SMALL AIRWAY FUNCTION

After the study of Hogg and his colleagues,[177] which showed that the major site of increased resistance in COPD is the small airways, and that of Macklem and Mead,[178] which indicated that small airways normally represent a small fraction of total airway resistance, there was considerable research interest in the development of screening tests to detect early abnormalities in small airway function. The basic hypothesis behind these efforts was that mild small airway abnormalities undetected by conventional measurements may be the harbinger of eventual symptomatic airflow limitation.[179] The single-breath nitrogen washout curve, the density dependence of maximal expiratory flow measured by using a helium-oxygen mixture, and measurements of air flow at low lung volumes have all been evaluated as potential tests to detect such preclinical small airway pathology.

Epidemiologic studies have shown that the results of these tests are in fact abnormal in an appreciable number of asymptomatic smokers,[180, 181] and it was the hope that these abnormalities might allow detection of early lung dysfunction and the institution of appropriate measures to prevent progression to advanced disease.[182] However, although there has been controversy regarding the value of such screening,[183, 184] it appears that the tests may not offer advantages over simple spirometry in detecting the progression of airflow obstruction.[185, 186] One reason that small airway tests have been less discriminating than was originally hoped in identifying smokers at risk for the development of progressive disease is the marked intersubject and intrasubject variability in test results.[187–189] In addition, it has not been convincingly shown that the rate of decrease in forced expiratory flow in smokers correlates with abnormalities in small airway function. In summary, at present the status of "small airway tests" does not warrant their institution as routine

screening procedures for the identification of patients at risk for the development of COPD.

TESTS OF DIFFUSING CAPACITY

Although diffusing capacity was formerly calculated for the diffusion of oxygen, carbon monoxide has replaced this gas for technical reasons. The diffusing capacity (DLCO) or transfer factor (TLCO) for carbon monoxide is computed as follows:

$$DLCO = \frac{\textit{Millimeters of CO taken up by}}{\textit{Mean alveolar Pco}} \atop - \textit{mean capillary Pco}$$

The amount of CO taken up by capillary blood is calculated by subtracting expired volume times the CO concentration of expired gas from inspired volume times the CO concentration of inspired gas. Determination of the denominator of the equation is subject to error, especially in the presence of pulmonary disease. In normal subjects, once the dead space has been emptied, a sample of expired gas accurately reflects mean alveolar Pco; since the normal mean capillary CO is so small that it can be ignored, the diffusing capacity can be calculated reliably. However, in diseased lungs that have relatively underventilated areas that empty late, the normal sharp division between dead space and alveolar gas is lost, and the expired gas sample might not reflect the mean alveolar Pco.

Several techniques for measuring diffusing capacity with CO have been devised, the main differences among them being the length of time that the gas is kept in the lungs and the methods of determining mean alveolar Pco.[190–196] The three major methods are the single-breath, the rebreathing, and the steady-state methods. The single-breath method was originally devised in an attempt to prove that oxygen was not secreted from alveolar gas into capillary blood as had been suggested by Haldane.[191] The test was reintroduced in the early 1950s, and initial technical difficulties were rectified by a number of modifications. Using standardized methodology, the single-breath method is the most widely used test for estimating diffusing capacity.[83, 192, 193, 197–202] The test is carried out by having the subject exhale to RV and then take a greater than 90% VC breath of a gas containing 0.3% CO, 10% He, 21% or 17% O_2, and the balance nitrogen (the European standard is to use 17% rather than 21% oxygen[201]). After rapid inspiration of the gas, breath is held for 9 to 11 seconds near TLC, the first 0.75 to 1.0 liter of expired gas is discarded, and the next liter, representative of alveolar gas, is collected and analyzed for helium and CO. The helium dilution is used to calculate the alveolar volume (VA), as well as the initial concentration of CO in the alveolar space. The test can be repeated at brief intervals ($\geq$4 minutes); two tests that agree within 5% are required.[199] In patients who have a small VC, a washout volume of 0.5 liter and a sample volume of 0.5 liter are recommended; alternatively, the steady-state method can be used.[199] A modified test using a 3-second breath-hold can be used during exercise.[203]

One limitation of the single-breath method is that uptake of CO from the lungs is actually occurring during the inspiratory and expiratory phases of the single breath, although the calculations assume that all CO uptake occurs during breath-holding. This assumption can lead to significant error, especially with prolonged inspiration and expiration in patients with obstructive pulmonary disease. A modification of the technique uses a rapid-response CO analyzer and three separate equations to calculate CO uptake during the inhalation, exhalation, and breath-holding periods;[204–206] this modification gives values for DLCO that are more accurate and are unaffected by prolonged expiration. An additional modification made feasible with the rapid-response analyzer is measurement of the diffusing capacity and pulmonary capillary blood flow continuously during expiration at 10% lung volume decrements from 80% to 20% of VC. DLCO is not related to lung volume in normal subjects but decreases at low lung volumes in patients with obstructive lung disease.[207] This technique has the advantage that breath-holding is not required, which makes it potentially useful during exercise. Abnormalities in diffusion at low lung volumes represent a potentially sensitive index of early lung disease.[196, 207–210] Although these modifications of the standardized single-breath diffusing capacity technique have provided valuable data, they are not recommended at present for the routine clinical assessment of patients;[200] however, measurement during constant exhalation may be useful in subjects who have impaired lung function and difficulty holding their breath for 10 seconds.[211]

Single-breath and steady-state DLCO is dependent on the lung volume at which breath-holding or tidal breathing occurs. For example, following pneumonectomy or with the chest wall restriction that occurs in conditions such as kyphoscoliosis, a patient may have a reduced DLCO without an intrinsic gas exchange abnormality in the remaining or restricted lung.[212] This observation led to the suggestion that specific diffusing capacity (the diffusing capacity divided by the alveolar volume at which it was measured [DL/VA]) would be a more accurate measurement; this relationship is abbreviated to TL/VA or KCO in Europe.[201, 213–215] However DLCO does not decrease linearly with lung volume, so DL/VA increases as lung volume decreases in normal subjects; therefore a submaximal inspiratory effort can cause spuriously high values of DL/VA.[216] Another method that avoids the effect of alveolar volume is measurement of the time constant of disappearance of alveolar CO during the breath-holding period.[217]

The rebreathing method of measuring gas diffusion involves 10 seconds of rebreathing from a small bag containing CO and helium. The technique can also be used to provide an estimate of thoracic gas volume, pulmonary capillary blood volume, and capillary blood flow.[218–220] Advantages of the technique are that it can be used during mechanical ventilation[218, 221] and in patients who are unable to breath-hold. It is also possible to perform the test at the bedside for the detection of alveolar hemorrhage through demonstration of an elevated DLCO.[194]

The steady-state techniques require the inhalation of carbon monoxide gas mixtures for several breaths until alveolar PCO remains constant. With knowledge of the expired volume and mixed expired CO concentration, the uptake of carbon monoxide is easily determined; however, accurate determination of the mean alveolar PCO is again a source of

error. A number of techniques have been used to calculate mean alveolar PCO, including end-tidal sampling, use of the Bohr equation with an assumed dead space (VD)/VT ratio, and use of the Bohr equation with a measured VD/VT (which requires arterial puncture for measurement of arterial PCO2.[149]) In addition to measurement of diffusing capacity, the fractional removal of carbon monoxide (FCO) can be calculated during a steady-state test; this measurement can help confirm the accuracy of the diffusing capacity value since both decrease simultaneously in most cases.[222] The fractional uptake of carbon monoxide is the amount removed divided by the amount inspired:

$$CO\ uptake\ per\ cent = \frac{CO\ inspired\ -\ CO\ expired}{CO\ inspired}$$

The diffusing capacity can be influenced by factors that alter the alveolar capillary membrane or pulmonary capillary blood volume. Table 17–1 summarizes the various factors that can affect the measurement of diffusing capacity[223] (*see* also Fig. 2–29, page 108).

Since the transfer of carbon monoxide is limited by diffusion and not perfusion, pulmonary blood volume (Vc) rather than pulmonary blood flow is important. Pulmonary capillary blood volume is multiplied by the kinetic constant theta (θ), which is the rate of combination of carbon monoxide and red blood cells. Theta is affected by the oxygen saturation of hemoglobin. Thus Vc × θ = the blood volume component of diffusing capacity. The membrane (DM) and Vc × θ contributions to diffusing capacity can be calculated separately by measuring the diffusing capacity using different inspired PO2 values. In normal subjects, the two components contribute approximately equally to the measured DLCO, although morphometric techniques suggest that the Vc × θ component is the more important.[224, 225]

The extent to which the measurement of diffusing capacity is affected by the distribution of ventilation and perfusion depends on the method used. Steady-state methods are most sensitive to mismatching and are affected by the distribution of ventilation with respect to lung volume, perfusion, and diffusing capacity. The fractional uptake of carbon

Table 17–1. PHYSIOLOGIC DETERMINANTS OF DIFFUSING CAPACITY

Alveolar capillary membrane
  Lung volume
  Surface area
  Thickness
  Gravity
Pulmonary capillary blood volume
  Position: increased DLCO going from standing to sitting to lying
  Müller or Valsalva maneuvers during breath-hold
  Hemoglobin concentration (increased carboxyhemoglobin-anemia effect)
  Hemoglobin affinity for oxygen (θ)
  Gravity
Distribution of ventilation relative to perfusion
  Affects steady-state method especially
  Affects fractional uptake of CO (FCO) least
Backpressure of carbon monoxide
  Cigarette smoking
  Environmental or industrial exposure

monoxide (FCO) is least affected by the distribution of ventilation; however, it is very sensitive to VD/VT and thus to respiratory frequency and VT.[226] With control of frequency, reliable prediction equations for FCO have been described in normal subjects.[227]

All methods of measurement of DLCO assume that the blood carboxyhemoglobin concentration and therefore the backpressure for carbon monoxide are virtually zero. However, an elevated carboxyhemoglobin concentration associated with smoking or industrial exposure can influence the measurement. Smokers can have levels of carboxyhemoglobin as high as 10%, which results in an approximate 1% decrease in measured DLCO for every 1% increase in carboxyhemoglobin.[228] Correction for this error does not completely return the diffusing capacity of most smokers back to normal values, however, and even asymptomatic smokers with otherwise normal pulmonary function have values of diffusing capacity that are approximately 80% of predicted normal.[199] The presence of carboxyhemoglobin has an "anemia-like" effect in addition to the backpressure increase; in addition, some components of cigarette smoke may vasoconstrict the pulmonary vasculature and reduce pulmonary capillary blood volume.[229] Most of the smoking effect is rapidly reversed following smoking cessation.[230]

Since diffusing capacity is dependent on pulmonary capillary blood volume or, more correctly, on the product of blood volume and hemoglobin concentration, factors that increase or decrease pulmonary blood volume or hemoglobin concentration also affect DLCO. The effects of anemia and polycythemia have been investigated in a number of studies.[231–235] In one study of 50 patients free of cardiopulmonary disease whose hemoglobin values ranged from 6.7 to 16.8 gm/dl, the calculated correction factor was 7% for each gram of hemoglobin.[235] In another study of 90 nonsmokers whose hematocrits ranged from 28% to 64%, it was suggested that a 1.4% adjustment (plus or minus) be made in per cent DLCO predicted for each per cent change in hematocrit above or below 44%.[232] Factors that acutely affect pulmonary capillary blood volume can also affect measured DLCO: for example, the recruitment of pulmonary vascular bed during exercise results in a substantial increase in DLCO within seconds.[236] DLCO also increases when one breathes through an inspiratory resistance, presumably as a result of negative intrathoracic pressure and recruitment of blood volume, an effect that correlates with the DLCO increase during exercise. Asthmatic subjects frequently have an increased single-breath DLCO, possibly as a result of recruitment of capillary blood volume secondary to their more negative pleural pressure swings.[237, 238] Drugs such as nitroglycerin, which can shift blood volume from the pulmonary capillary bed to the systemic capillary bed, result in a decrease in diffusing capacity.[239] An increase in DLCO in the supine position is largely related to an increase in pulmonary capillary blood volume;[240] the more substantial increase during weightlessness is caused by an increase in both the membrane component (DM) and Vc × θ.[241] Changes in pulmonary capillary blood volume may be responsible for the fluctuations in DLCO that occur during the normal menstrual cycle[242] and during the cold pressor test.[243] A decreased DM appears to be responsible for the decrease in DLCO that occurs in chronic congestive heart failure.[244] A decrease in DM is also responsible for the transient decrease in DLCO that occurs

after maximal exercise;[245, 246] the decrease is accompanied by an increase in lung density on computed tomography, which suggests that it is related to mild interstitial edema.[247]

The effect of increased blood volume on diffusing capacity does not distinguish increased blood volume in the vascular space of the lung from intra-alveolar blood; the diffusing capacity may be markedly increased in patients with pulmonary hemorrhage, and its measurement has been recommended for the diagnosis of this condition.[248, 249] Decreased DLCO has been reported in alcoholic patients, but values may be normal when corrected for anemia and smoking.[249] An isolated, lower than normal DLCO is not an uncommon finding during routine pulmonary function testing. In one study of 60 patients who had dyspnea but otherwise normal pulmonary function tests, an abnormal DLCO at rest was sensitive, but not specific for abnormal gas exchange during an exercise test.[250] An isolated reduction in DLCO has also been shown to be predictive of subsequent symptomatic pulmonary hypertension in systemic sclerosis.[251]

Early studies that calculated prediction equations for single-breath DLCO were "contaminated" by smokers; more recent studies of large numbers of nonsmokers with calculated 95% confidence limits are available.[214, 236, 248] Racial and gender differences in DLCO and DLCO/VA have been reported, with lower values in Asian and African American populations.[252, 253] Separate prediction equations have been developed for healthy children.[254] Reference normal values have also been reported for the rebreathing technique for estimating diffusing capacity.[219] Reference values from numerous studies and an approach to selecting appropriate reference values for individual laboratories are well described in a comprehensive review.[8]

MEASUREMENT OF INEQUALITY OF VENTILATION-PERFUSION RATIOS

Methods for the assessment of ventilation-perfusion ratios are described in detail in Chapter 2 (*see* page 111). The most commonly used technique to detect a disturbance in V̇/Q̇ ratios involves calculation of the alveolar-arterial gradient for oxygen by using the simplified alveolar air equation. An increase in "physiologic" dead space can be measured by using the Bohr equation, and venous admixture or true intrapulmonary shunt can be calculated. Radionuclides are now commonly used in the study of regional ventilation-perfusion inequality;[255–257] the multiple–inert gas technique provides the most accurate description of the distribution of ventilation-perfusion ratios, although it does not provide regional information.

MEASUREMENT OF RESPIRATORY CONTROL

Alveolar hypoventilation accompanied by an elevated arterial PCO₂ and decreased arterial PO₂ is the final common pathway of many pulmonary disorders. The clinical challenge is to determine why hypoventilation has occurred: is the hypoventilation occurring because the patient *will not* breathe sufficiently or *cannot* breathe sufficiently?[258] Hypoventilation can have its origin in impaired central or peripheral chemoreceptor responsiveness, defective transmission of central inspiratory activity to the respiratory muscles, failure of respiratory muscle action because of muscle fatigue or weakness, or an inability of the muscular activity to generate sufficient ventilation because of increased impedance of the respiratory system. Although it is customary to think of alveolar hypoventilation as primarily a lung problem, it is evident that metabolic, neurologic, and muscular disorders can lead to or at least contribute to the process. The list of disorders associated with depressed central ventilatory drive is ever lengthening and includes encephalitis, cerebrovascular disease affecting the medulla, Parkinson's syndrome, myxedema, obesity-hypoventilation syndrome, narcotic addiction, bilateral spinothalamic lesions, metabolic alkalosis, bulbar poliomyelitis, carotid endarterectomy, cyanotic congenital heart disease, familial dysautonomia, and chronic exposure to high altitude.[259]

The first step in the investigation of "can't versus won't" is measurement of lung volumes and flow rates, since hypoventilation caused by increased impedance alone does not occur unless the FEV_1 is less than about 1.2 liters. If hypoventilation is present with adequate ventilatory reserve, more detailed investigation of respiratory control is warranted.

It is difficult to quantify respiratory center output. The measurement closest to central neutral drive is the electrical neurogram of the phrenic nerve, but this test is difficult and invasive and is rarely used. The output can also be measured by a recording of the EMG of the diaphragm or another inspiratory muscle, but this is already one step removed from the electrical output of the respiratory center; the EMG is also invasive and can be applied only to some of the respiratory muscles (diaphragm and intercostals). Mouth pressure measured 100 msec after obstruction of the airway gives an estimate of respiratory center output unaffected by the impedance of the respiratory system,[277] but influenced by the length-tension relationship and strength of the respiratory muscles. Measurements of the work of breathing or of ventilation itself are frequently used as indicators of respiratory drive but are influenced by the resistance and compliance of the lung and by neuromuscular function. One method for clinical assessment of respiratory control involves separation of the respiratory cycle into its components: tidal volume/inspiratory time (V_T/T_I), a measure of mean inspiratory flow, and the ratio of inspiratory time over total respiratory cycle time, or T_I/T_{tot}. It has been suggested that V_T/T_I is a measure of central inspiratory activity and T_I/T_{tot} reflects respiratory center timing.[260, 261]

Ventilatory Response Curves

The ventilatory response to carbon dioxide can be measured using a steady-state or rebreathing technique.[261, 262] With the former, at least two concentrations of CO_2 are used, and relative hyperoxia is ensured during the procedure by adding a high concentration of inspired oxygen to the circuit. The difficulty with this technique is that arterial and brain tissue PCO_2 are dependent to some extent on the ventilatory response, and thus CO_2 is not a true independent variable; in addition, the technique is cumbersome to perform and requires measurement of arterial PCO_2 for accuracy.

The most widely used method of assessing CO_2 respon-

siveness entails rebreathing of CO_2, the subject breathing from a bag containing CO_2 at approximately the level of mixed venous PCO_2 (7%);[263, 264] the bag size is approximately 1 liter greater than VC and contains an enriched oxygen mixture to prevent hypoxemia during the test. The mixed venous, arterial, and alveolar PCO_2 concentrations come into equilibrium within 30 to 60 seconds; this phase is followed by a linear increase in CO_2 concentration of between 3 and 6 mm Hg per minute as a result of the endogenous production of carbon dioxide. A single ventilatory response curve requires approximately 4 minutes to obtain, and reproducible tests of the ventilatory response can be obtained at intervals as short as 10 minutes.[265] The results are expressed as the slope of the ventilatory response, $\Delta V/\Delta PCO_2$, the relationship being linear with an intercept on the CO_2 axis, which reflects the starting arterial PCO_2 (Fig. 17–7). The range of ventilatory response to CO_2 is remarkably wide among healthy subjects, in whom an approximate 16-fold variation of 0.57 to 8.17 liters per minute per millimeter Hg rise in CO_2 has been measured.[262, 266] Although this variation can be explained partly by genetic factors (as demonstrated in studies of twins) and partly by differences in lung size, considerable residual variation exists.[267] The ventilatory response to hypercapnia is decreased if nasal rather than mouth breathing is used, which suggests that upper airway receptors can modify the ventilatory response.[268, 269] On the other hand, the ventilatory response to added resistive loads is also decreased during nasal breathing, so the decreased ventilation in both instances may be secondary to the increased resistance that accompanies nasal breathing.[270] Normal values for ventilatory responses to CO_2 have been derived.[271] A method

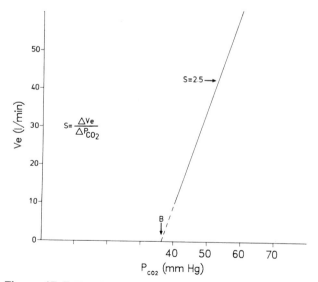

Figure 17–7. The CO_2 Ventilatory Response Curve. The ventilatory response curve to increasing levels of CO_2 serves as a measure of respiratory chemosensitivity. A linear relationship between ventilation and end-tidal CO_2 is observed using the rebreathing method, and chemosensitivity is quantified as the slope of the curve

$$\frac{\Delta Ve}{\Delta PCO_2}.$$

A normal curve in which the $\Delta Ve/\Delta PCO_2$ is 2.5 liters per minute per mm Hg is depicted. There is a wide range of normal for this slope, and the relationship can be changed by alterations in central drive, neuromuscular function, or respiratory system impedance.

to examine "dynamic chemoresponsiveness" has been proposed in which the ventilatory response to a variety of concentrations of CO_2 is assessed;[272] however, the clinical usefulness of this modification has not been determined.

The hypoxic ventilatory response can be measured with single-breath tests using 100% oxygen or 100% nitrogen or with steady-state or rebreathing methods. Measurements derived from the steady-state method typically reveal a curvilinear, hyperbolic relationship between ventilation and end-tidal or arterial PO_2 (Fig. 17–8). Ventilation changes little until arterial PO_2 reaches values of approximately 50 or 60 mm Hg, after which it increases sharply. The curvilinearity makes it difficult to fit a curve to the ventilation-versus-PO_2

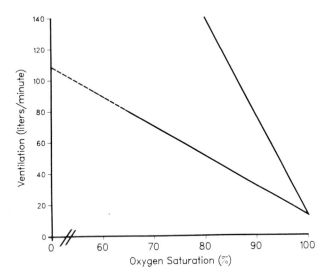

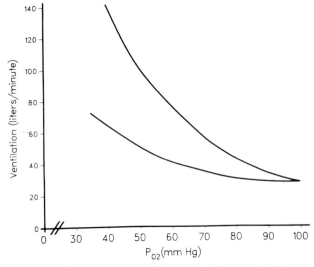

Figure 17–8. The Ventilatory Response to Hypoxemia. The ventilatory response to hypoxemia is tested by plotting ventilation versus changes in oxygen saturation *(upper panel)* or PO_2 *(lower panel)*. A wide range of normal responses is shown by these two representative curves, which are at the upper and lower limits of normal responses. The advantage of using O_2 saturation as the independent variable is that linear relationships are produced that allow easier comparison within or between subjects. The linear relationship does not mean that the peripheral chemoreceptors sense saturation but rather is the result of combining two curvilinear relationships: that between PO_2 and O_2 saturation and that between PO_2 and ventilation.

relationship to obtain a meaningful quantification of the response. The most commonly used function is a hyperbolic equation in which a shape constant (A) is used to quantify the response.[262] It is important to maintain end-tidal PCO_2 constant throughout the hypoxemic ventilatory response, which is accomplished by adding CO_2 to the inspiration circuitry.

A rebreathing technique similar to that used for CO_2 in which ventilation is plotted against arterial oxygen saturation measured with an ear oximeter (Fig. 17–8) has also been developed to assess the hypoxic ventilatory response.[273] This technique has two advantages: (1) the saturation directly reflects arterial PO_2 and is unaffected by any A-a O_2 gradient that may be present, unlike measurements of end-tidal PO_2, and (2) the relationship between ventilation and PO_2 is linear, thus allowing the response to be more easily quantified. The fact that there is a linear relationship between saturation and ventilation does not mean that arterial saturation is the pertinent signal that stimulates the peripheral chemoreceptors. A reduction in oxygen content produced by carbon monoxide poisoning or anemia has no effect on the ventilatory response curve. The linear relationship is a fortuitous occurrence that reflects a combination of two curvilinear relationships, one between PO_2 and ventilation and the other between PO_2 and arterial saturation.[259] As with CO_2, the range of normal ventilatory response to hypoxemia is extremely wide, with a mean value of 1.47 liters per minute per per cent fall in arterial saturation; 80% of healthy normal subjects have a slope between 0.6 and 2.75.[262] Studies have shown that the acute ventilatory response to hypoxemia, as customarily measured, overestimates the sustained hypoxemic response in normal subjects and obstructed patients.[274, 274a, b] A relationship exists between the ventilatory response to CO_2 and O_2 in individuals.

Additional tests to measure chemoreceptor responsiveness have been suggested, including measurement of the ventilatory response during transient exposure (four to seven breaths) to hypoxic or hyperoxic gas mixtures and measurement of breath-holding time;[275, 276] however, neither of these tests has proved as useful or as reproducible as the ventilatory response curves.

Mouth Occlusion Pressures

The ventilatory response to CO_2 and O_2 depends heavily on the impedance of the respiratory system. Thus a patient might have a normal neural output from a normally functioning respiratory center but the translation of that neural output to ventilation might be impaired purely on a mechanical basis. In an attempt to get one step closer to the true output of the respiratory center, a technique has been developed to measure mouth occlusion pressure following the first 0.1 sec of an occluded breath.[277] This technique is accomplished while the patient is breathing tidally at rest or during various stages of a ventilatory response curve to O_2 or CO_2. Periodically and unknown to the subject, the mouthpiece is temporarily occluded for at least 100 msec at the onset of inspiration; the pressure generated by the inspiratory muscles at this time is termed the *P0.1*[277, 278] An occlusion this brief is undetected by the subject, so behavioral alterations in the breathing pattern do not interfere with the measurement.[279] P0.1 can be measured during sleep by using a face mask.[280]

Measurement of occlusion pressure is not without its problems: recruitment of abdominal muscles during expiration can result in a decrease in FRC below the static equilibration point between the lung and the chest wall so that the initial inspiratory pressure generated at the mouth will be contributed to by the sudden relaxation of the abdominal muscles and the elastic recoil of the respiratory system.[281] In one investigation of patients with obstructive lung disease—in whom pleural pressure swings may be nonuniform—P0.1 measured at the mouth was significantly less than esophageal pressure at 0.1 second, presumably reflecting the same artefact that interferes with measurement of plethysmographic thoracic gas volume in these patients.[282] Despite these problems, measurement of occlusion pressure has distinct advantages over measurements of the work of breathing or ventilation in the assessment of neural drive to the inspiratory muscles since it is unaffected by the flow resistance or compliance properties of the respiratory system. P0.1 is a useful index of the neuromuscular component of the respiratory output in that it indicates the pressure potential available for inspiration in any given condition.[283] Using the occlusion pressure technique, studies have shown that patients with ventilatory impairment may have normal or even supranormal drive, the decreased ventilation being attributable solely to the increased impedance of the respiratory system.[284] Mouth occlusion pressure can be used as an indicator of respiratory drive in intubated patients and may assist in weaning decisions.[285]

Breathing Pattern Analysis

Analysis of the breathing pattern as a method of assessing the control of ventilation has also been suggested.[286] Ventilation at rest or during stimulated breathing can be divided into a flow component and a timing component.

$$V_E = V_T/T_I \times T_I/T_{tot}$$

where V_T/T_I is the mean inspiratory flow (tidal volume divided by inspiratory time) and T_I/T_{tot} is the duty cycle (ratio of inspiratory time to total respiratory cycle time). An increase in ventilation can be achieved by increasing V_T/T_I and keeping T_I/T_{tot} constant or by increasing T_I/T_{tot} and keeping V_T/T_I constant. The V_T/T_I component is thought to reflect neural output from the respiratory center, whereas the T_I/T_{tot} relationship reflects the timing element.[283] The value of separating the inspiratory flow and duty cycle components in the investigation of various disease states is not clearly defined. It is likely, however, that continued clinical investigation will reveal specific alterations in breathing patterns in certain conditions.[275]

Electromyography and Electroneurography

Direct measurement of the electrical activity in respiratory muscles is one step closer to the respiratory center output. An EMG of the diaphragm can be recorded using surface electrodes placed on the fifth, sixth, and seventh intercostal spaces close to the costochondral junctions or using an esophageal electrode.[283, 287] Inspiratory intercostal muscle activity can be measured using surface electrodes in the second and third anterior intercostal spaces but can be contaminated by electrical activity from other muscles. Finally, electrodes can be inserted directly into inspiratory or expiratory respiratory muscles. Short of placing intracranial electrodes, direct recording of phrenic nerve electrical activity is the closest one can come to measuring respiratory center output; however, this procedure is rarely performed in a clinical setting.[283]

TESTS OF RESPIRATORY MUSCLE PERFORMANCE

The final step in the assessment of respiratory control involves measurement of the output of neurologic activity as reflected in respiratory muscle performance. Respiratory muscle weakness may be suspected on routine lung function testing when there is lung restriction (decreased VC and TLC) with relatively preserved RV and lung diffusing capacity corrected for alveolar volume (DL/VA).[288] The simplest means to test inspiratory and expiratory muscle strength is to measure maximal inspiratory and expiratory pressures (MIP and MEP or PImax and PEmax) at the mouth. The arithmetic mean of these values can be used to represent an index of respiratory muscle strength.[289] Simple, portable devices that can be used on a ward or in the intensive care unit have been developed for this purpose.[290, 291]

The technique involves having a subject make maximal inspiratory and expiratory efforts against a closed mouthpiece in which a small leak has been constructed to avoid glottic closure and generation of pressure using the buccal and oropharyngeal muscles. The pressures generated depend on the lung volume at which the test is performed[292] since this volume influences the length-tension relationship and the mechanical advantage of various respiratory muscles. Thus, MIP is generated near RV and MEP near TLC when expiratory muscles are lengthened.[293] MIP and MEP are highly variable between subjects and depend on motivation and learning;[294, 294a, b] they also depend on age and, to some extent, on weight and the ratio of height to weight.[295–297] However, these variables explain little of the variance, and most of the predicted values take into account only age and sex.[290, 293, 298–301, 301a] In practice, values of MIP greater than 80 cm H_2O and values of MEP greater than 100 cm H_2O exclude clinically significant inspiratory or expiratory muscle weakness.[289] Some patients find the performance of MIPs painful or awkward, and a more natural maneuver for estimating inspiratory muscle strength—the sniff nasal inspiratory pressure—has been suggested and validated as an alternate method,[302, 303] although the tests may not be strictly comparable.[303a] Inspiratory muscle strength can also be assessed by measuring maximal mouth pressure generated during bilateral supramaximal phrenic nerve stimulation in the neck.[303b, c]

Measurement of MIP and MEP gives an overall estimate of respiratory muscle performance; measurement of maximal transdiaphragmatic pressure (Pdi max) gives a specific estimate of diaphragmatic strength. This latter measurement is obtained by comparing pleural with gastric pressure during maximal inspiratory effort against a closed mouthpiece[304–306] or with an open airway during a voluntary sniff (sniff Pdi).[307] Although no normal predicted values are available for Pdi max, they are similar to MIP in subjects in whom both have been measured. Transdiaphragmatic pressure measurement has proved useful in the detection of bilateral or unilateral diaphragmatic paralysis.[304, 308] An additional approach to the assessment of diaphragmatic strength is the measurement of transdiaphragmatic pressure during a single stimulation of the phrenic nerves in the neck;[309, 310] "twitch tension" produced by the stimulation is enhanced after vigorous voluntary contraction of the inspiratory muscles (twitch potentiation).[310a] A recent modification of this technique uses stimulation with a magnet, which circumvents the use of inaccurate surface electrodes or painful needle electrodes[311, 382] (although the results may not be strictly comparable[383]). Stimulation of the phrenic nerve can also be accompanied by measurement of the diaphragmatic electromyogram (EMG) using surface, intradiaphragmatic, or intraesophageal electrodes.[384, 385, 385a] The conduction velocity along the phrenic nerve, which is measured as the latency between phrenic stimulation and the appearance of the EMG signal, can be used as a measure of phrenic nerve integrity. The conduction pathway from the cerebral cortex or cervical spinal cord to the respiratory muscles can also be assessed using magnetic stimulation of the cortex and simultaneous measurement of respiratory muscle EMG.[386–388]

A new and potentially useful test for assessing diaphragmatic contractile function is the phonomyogram. This technique uses small microphones that are applied to the skin over the diaphragm; the acoustic signal produced during contraction is linearly related to the transdiaphragmatic pressure and to the size of the action potential.[389] Ultrasound can also be used to assess diaphramatic contraction.[309, 391] In addition to measurements of maximal pressures that estimate strength, respiratory muscle endurance can be measured by progressively loading the inspiratory muscles with increasing resistances until maximal sustainable pressure is achieved.[312–315]

The respiratory muscles can become fatigued in a fashion similar to that of any skeletal muscle when overloaded. The development of such fatigue can be detected by analysis of the EMG. The EMG signal is acquired by using intramuscular[392] or esophageal[393] electrodes and the frequency spectrum of the signal is analyzed. The median (centroid) frequency is determined; as fatigue develops, it is seen to shift to lower values.[394] Alternatively, the EMG signal is filtered into high- and low-frequency bands; the ratio of high over low frequency decreases as fatigue develops, predating the actual failure of force generation by the muscle.[316] Fatigue can be diagnosed noninvasively by measuring a decrease in the relaxation rate of the respiratory muscles; practically, this can be accomplished by measuring the rate of decline in esophageal pressure after a maximal sniff.[395, 396] Similarly, expiratory muscle fatigue can be detected by measuring the rate of decline of gastric pressure.[397]

The development of diaphragmatic fatigue can be predicted by measuring the tension-time index of the diaphragm during tidal breathing and relating this index to maximal transdiaphragmatic pressure. The tension-time index is calculated by multiplying the average transdiaphragmatic pressure per breath as a percentage of Pdi max by the inspiratory time; when the index approaches 15%, fatigue is likely to ensue.[317, 318] Obviously, the tension-time index can approach the critical value of 15% as a result of a decrease in maximal transdiaphragmatic pressure secondary to respiratory muscle weakness or an increase in tidal Pdi swings related to increased impedance of the respiratory system. The tension time index for all the respiratory muscles can be estimated by measuring mouth occlusion pressure as a percentage of maximal inspiratory mouth pressure multiplied by the inspiratory time as a percentage of total respiratory cycle time.[318a]

INHALATION CHALLENGE TESTS

Inhalation challenge tests can be broadly categorized into nonspecific and specific types. Nonspecific tests include aerosol challenge with nebulized agonists such as methacholine, histamine, prostaglandin F_2, leukotrienes, and aerosols of hypertonic saline, as well as protocols designed to produce cooling and drying of the airway mucosa by procedures such as exercise and isocapnic hyperventilation. Specific challenge refers to the inhalation of allergens to which the subject is known or suspected to be sensitive or exposure to dust or environmental agents that provoke idiosyncratic lung responses in some individuals.

Nonspecific Bronchial Reactivity

Although airway responsiveness to pharmacologic agonists was measured in the early[319, 320] and mid century,[321–323] it was not until the late 1970s that a number of investigators first described standardized methods to assess bronchial responsiveness;[324–326] since that time, systematic study of the phenomenon of nonspecific airway hyper-reactivity has progressed dramatically.

All the techniques used to measure nonspecific bronchial reactivity (NSBR) pharmacologically involve the inhalation of an aerosol containing a known bronchoconstrictive agent. Inhalation begins with a low concentration or dose of agonist, and the "dose" is progressively increased; an index of airway narrowing is measured at each step so that a "dose-response" relationship can be constructed. A variety of techniques of delivering agonists, measuring the response, and expressing the results have been developed[327] (Table 17–2). The most widely used technique involves the delivery of nebulized histamine or methacholine using a face mask during tidal breathing;[325, 328] two minute inhalations of increasing concentrations of histamine or methacholine are followed by measurements of FEV_1. Doubling concentrations of agonist are administered, beginning with 0.013 mg/ml and increasing to 16 mg/ml; the test is stopped when there is either a 20% or greater fall in FEV_1 or when the highest concentration of agonist is reached. The level of nonspecific reactivity is defined as the provocative concentration of inhaled agonist that results in a 20% fall in FEV_1 (PC_{20}). Minor modifications of the technique include the use of methacholine and a Bennett twin nebulizer with a higher output.[329]

In another technique that has been standardized and widely used, the nebulizer is coupled to a dosimeter that

Table 17–2. METHODS OF ASSESSING NONSPECIFIC BRONCHIAL REACTIVITY

AUTHOR	AGONIST	METHOD OF ADMINISTRATION	MEASURED VARIABLE	EXPRESSION OF RESULTS
Cockcroft et al.[325]	Histamine or methacholine	Face mask with nose clip, 2-min inhalations, tidal breathing, Wright nebulizer. Output, 0.13–0.16 ml/min; concentrations, 0.03, 16 mg/ml in doubling steps. AMMD = 0.87 ± 1.9 μm	FEV_1 before and after diluent and after each concentration until FEV_1 has decreased 20% or greater from postdiluent value	Provocative concentration producing a 20% fall in FEV_1 (PC_{20}) calculated by interpolation. Also slope = % change FEV_1 ÷ cumulative concentration
Chai et al.[324]	Histamine or methacholine	Devilbiss 646 neubulizer and Rosenthal French dosimeter model B-2A AMMD = 1.32 ± 2.5 μm, five vital capacity breaths per dose	FEV_1 after each dose until decreased 20% or greater *or* specific airway conductance after each dose until 35% or greater decrease occurs	Provocative dose producing a 20% fall in FEV_1 (PD_{20}) is calculated; or the dose resulting in a 35% decrease in specific airway conductance (PD_{35}-SGaw) is calculated. Also slope = % decrease ÷ cumulative dose
Lam et al.[329]	Methacholine	As for Cockcroft, except Bennett twin nebulizer with output of 0.25 ml/min AMMD = 3.1 μm	As for Cockcroft	As for Cockcroft, PC_{20}
Yan et al.[336]	Histamine	Handheld Devilbiss No. 40 glass nebulizer, bulb squeezed by technician to deliver 0.03 up to 0.6 mol in doubling steps at 1-min intervals, vital capacity breaths	FEV_1 60 sec after each dose until 20% fall in FEV_1 recorded	PD_{20} (cumulative dose calculation)
Smith and Anderson[349]	Hypertonic saline	Mistogen ultrasonic nebulizer. 4.5% saline aerosol. ~5 up to ~300 liters in doubling "doses" of tidal breathing with nose clip	FEV_1 60 sec after each inhalation until 20% fall in FEV_1	PD_{20} FEV_1: expressed as decrease in FEV_1 ÷ cumulative liters of hypertonic aerosol inhaled
Orehek et al.[331]	Carbachol	Different concentrations of carbachol solution nebulized into spirometer. Varying breath number. Breath volume, V_T: particle size, 0.1–5 μm	Specific airway resistance and specific airway conductance after each dose	Sensitivity = D_{25} dose causing a 25% rise (cumulative). Reactivity = arithmetic relationship of dose vs. specific airway conductance (%)

AMMD, aerodynamic mass median diameter of aerosol particles; FEV_1, forced expiratory volume in 1 second; V_T, tidal volume

delivers a known quantity of aerosol with each breath;[324] five VC breaths containing increasing concentrations of agonist are inhaled and the FEV_1 or specific airway conductance is measured after each dose. The dose that results in a 20% decrease in FEV_1 (PD_{20}) or a 35% decrease in specific airway conductance (PD_{35} SGaw) is calculated. Refinements of the dosimetric method that are faster and more accurate have been suggested.[330] For example, some investigators use carbachol, a longer-acting parasympathomimetic agent, to construct inhalation dose-response curves;[331] they measure specific airway conductance and calculate a threshold for response ("sensitivity") as the dose producing a 25% decrease in SGaw. Additional modifications of challenge tests include the use of respiratory system resistance—measured by forced oscillation or airway resistance by using the flow interruption technique—as the index of airway narrowing.[332–334] Abbreviated protocols in which fewer concentrations of agonist and a shorter time between inhalations are used have been reported to yield comparable results.[335] A rapid method for measuring bronchial responsiveness that uses a hand-held, bulb-operated glass nebulizer that delivers a known volume of aerosol with each squeeze of the bulb has also been described.[336]

The dose- or concentration-response curves generated by these techniques can be analyzed in a variety of ways to yield indices of airway responsiveness. "Sensitivity" is calculated as the dose or concentration that gives some predetermined magnitude of airway narrowing (e.g., PC_{20} and PD_{35} SGaw). Alternatively, sensitivity can be calculated as a threshold dose that causes a change in FEV_1 or resistance that is greater than 2 SD beyond the variability of baseline measurements. "Reactivity" is calculated as the slope of the dose-response curve obtained by plotting the cumulative dose of inhaled agonist against the per cent change in FEV_1 or specific conductance. It can be calculated over the steepest portion of the dose-response curve, as in classic pharmacology, or over the entire range of inhaled concentrations using only the first and last doses or using all the data and a least-squares curve-fitting method.[337, 338] The dose-response slope provides additional information since it allows an estimation of airway responsiveness in subjects who do not show a 20% decrease in FEV_1; it is especially useful in describing the distribution of airway responsiveness in population studies.[339] Many normal subjects and some patients who have airway disease display a plateau on the dose-response curve.[340–342] (A plateau is considered to be present when there is nonsignificant incremental airway narrowing despite increasing concentrations of agonist.[340, 343, 344]) The dose at which a plateau develops and the per cent change in the index of airway narrowing at the plateau can be calculated. Some evidence suggests that different factors contribute to the sensitivity and the maximal response; an increase in the maximal response may be a more important indicator of the severity of the airway disease.[341] The term *hyper-responsiveness* is used as a general description of exaggerated airway narrowing, *hypersensitivity* as an indication of a leftward shift in the dose-response curve, and *hyper-reactivity* as a measure of slope.[327]

For the most part, refinements in the challenge technique or the method of analysis have not proved more specific or sensitive in separating normal subjects from patients who have asthma than has measurement of changes in FEV_1.[328, 345, 346]

Another method that has been proposed as a measure of nonspecific airway responsiveness is the inhalation of aerosols of hypotonic or hypertonic solutions (water, hypertonic sodium or potassium chloride, and hypertonic dextrose).[347, 348] Although it is unclear exactly how hypotonic and hypertonic solutions induce bronchoconstriction, it is not by a direct action on smooth muscle; the altered tonicity probably releases inflammatory mediators from cells within the airway, which then act on the muscle to cause airway narrowing. The response to hypertonic saline aerosols is related to the responses to methacholine, exercise, and dry air hyperpnea.[349] A similar mechanism may explain the exaggerated airway narrowing that occurs in asthmatic subjects in response to aerosols of adenosine-5'-monophosphate (AMP). AMP is rapidly metabolized to adenosine and can act on purinergic receptors on mast cells and other inflammatory cells to release mediators that secondarily cause bronchoconstriction. Therefore, aerosols of altered tonicity and adenosine not only test the capacity of the airways to narrow but, in theory, may also reflect the number of inflammatory cells in the airways.[350] Bradykinin and sodium metabisulfite also cause exaggerated airway narrowing in asthmatic subjects, but their action is thought to be by stimulation of afferent nerves in the airway mucosa with subsequent reflex bronchoconstriction via efferent cholinergic and noncholinergic nerves.[351, 352]

The main variables determining PC_{20} are the output of the nebulizer, the inspiratory pattern during aerosol administration, and to a lesser extent, particle size.[353–356] To achieve reproducible and dependable results, patients must refrain from the use of inhaled β-adrenergic agonists for 8 hours prior to the study and from short- and long-acting theophylline preparations for 24 and 48 hours, respectively. Inhaled

or systemic steroids have no influence on the measurement of NSBR.[357] In stable patients, measurements of PC_{20} with histamine or methacholine show remarkable reproducibility over periods of weeks to months,[326, 358, 359] but they can change substantially over longer periods of follow-up.[360] Responses to the bronchoconstricting mast cell mediators leukotriene D_4 and prostaglandin D_2 are somewhat less reproducible.[361] A close correlation exists in airway responsiveness measured with histamine, methacholine, and prostaglandin F_2.[362–365] However, since histamine in high concentration tends to cause cough and flushing, prostaglandin F_2 causes cough and retrosternal irritation, and carbachol is a long-acting bronchoconstricting agent, methacholine is probably the agent of choice. Measurements of NSBR have been compared by using the tidal-breathing method and the more complex dose-metering device; the two have been found comparable and equally reproducible.[366] The more rapidly performed short test using a handheld nebulizer has also been shown to produce results comparable to the dosimeter method, and because of ease of performance, it may gain in popularity.[336]

A number of population studies have been carried out to assess the sensitivity of bronchial responsiveness in distinguishing asthmatic patients from normal subjects.[325, 367] PC_{20} is universally lower than 8 mg/ml in currently symptomatic asthmatic patients, whereas in subjects with normal pulmonary function and negative histories it is invariably greater than 16 mg/ml. This observation allows a clear separation of patients with reactive airway disease from normal subjects, although patients with chronic bronchitis, cystic fibrosis, or other chronic airway diseases may have intermediate values.

Although some agreement exists among investigators concerning methods of measuring NSBR and what represents normal and abnormal responsiveness, there is continued debate about the mechanisms that cause airway responsiveness. Dose-response curves to inhaled nonspecific agonists cannot be equated to the *in vitro* smooth muscle dose-response curve in which well-characterized parameters of receptor kinetics can be described. *In vivo*, the relationship between airway smooth muscle stimulation and airway narrowing is affected by smooth muscle shortening, mucosal edema, mucous plugs, and the starting airway caliber. These factors make it difficult or impossible to apply pharmacologic principles of dose-response relationships to *in vivo* dose-response curves. Nevertheless, there is an abundant literature in which the possible pathophysiologic significance of "sensitivity" and "reactivity" has been discussed.[331, 368–370] In fact, to date the distinction between sensitivity and reactivity has not been shown to be of any clinical significance.[371]

Methacholine and histamine inhalation challenges are useful in clinical practice. In doubtful cases, they can substantiate a diagnosis of asthma, especially when baseline spirometry is normal; in addition, patients whose primary complaint is cough frequently have underlying asthma that can be diagnosed by inhalation challenge testing. In patients with asthma, measurements of bronchial reactivity correlate well with the severity of symptoms and the need for medication (Fig. 17–9).[325] Bronchial responsiveness can change over time; for example, intensive therapy can result in a decrease in NSBR, whereas exposure to allergens or occupational sensitizers can increase it. Measures of NSBR are also

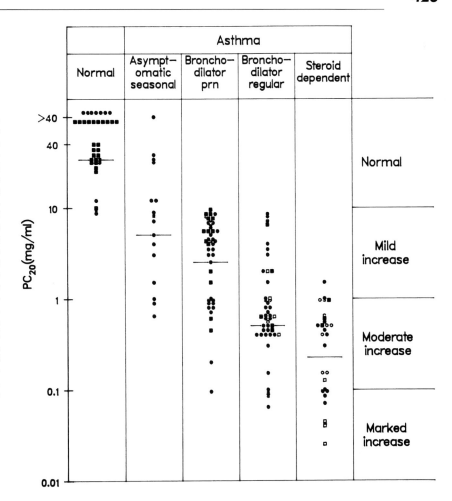

Figure 17–9. Bronchial Responsiveness in Relation to Symptoms and Medication Requirement in Asthmatics. The provocative concentration of inhaled histamine resulting in a 20% decrease in forced expiratory volume in 1 second (FEV$_1$) (PC$_{20}$) is plotted against clinical status. The data are from 35 normal subjects and 156 asthmatic patients of varying severity indicated by their medication usage. PC$_{20}$ is on a log scale. The *horizontal bars* are the geometric mean for each group; the *circles* indicate atopic subjects; the *squares* indicate nonatopic subjects. The *open symbols* represent those in whom baseline (prehistamine) FEV$_1$ was less than 70% predicted. There is some overlap in PC$_{20}$ values between normal and asymptomatic allergic asthmatic patients, but the PC$_{20}$ clearly separates normal patients from the more severely afflicted asthmatic patients. This nonspecific hyperresponsiveness is not related to atopic status, and although patients who have decreased starting FEV$_1$ tend to be more responsive (lower PC$_{20}$), marked airway hyper-responsiveness can occur despite normal starting expiratory flow rates. (Reprinted slightly modified from Cockcroft D, Killian D, Mellan J, et al: Clin Allergy 7:235, 1977.)

influenced by the pre-existing degree of airway narrowing; patients who have reduced air flow for whatever reason have increased airway responsiveness. However, airway responsiveness is more closely related to the starting FEV$_1$ in individual patients over time than between patients, which suggests that both measures reflect the severity of the underlying disease.[372] Serial measurements of PC$_{20}$ can be obtained to assess the efficacy of treatment or the detrimental effect of occupational exposure.

Specific Inhalation Challenge

Specific inhalation challenge tests are those performed on individuals who have or are suspected of having an allergy or sensitivity to specific allergens or chemical sensitizers. The techniques of inhalation challenge using antigen and occupational agents are less well standardized than are the nonspecific challenge tests using methacholine and histamine. In addition, allergy testing is time consuming and can induce severe and prolonged responses that are potentially hazardous. Before challenging any subject with an allergen or chemical sensitizer, it is important to know the level of nonspecific airway reactivity since the magnitude of response to the specific agent will be related to NSBR.[373] Inhalation of a specific antigen or chemical sensitizer can produce not only immediate bronchoconstriction but also a delayed response that can begin anywhere from 2 to 10 hours

after challenge. The delayed response may be prolonged and can result in altered NSBR in sensitized individuals. For these reasons allergen inhalation challenge is rarely indicated in clinical practice and should be reserved for special cases being investigated in larger centers where there is expertise in the methodology. However, inhalation challenge testing using agents suspected of causing allergic alveolitis or occupational asthma may be important in establishing proof of specific sensitivity to these agents and may be required for compensation purposes.

Exercise-Induced Bronchoconstriction and Isocapnic Hyperventilation

Exercise induces bronchoconstriction in subjects who have hyper-responsive airways and can be used as a clinical test of responsiveness. The pertinent stimulus is the volume of dry and/or cold air breathed per unit time rather than exercise *per se*. If the inspired air temperature and water content are constant, minute ventilation can be used as the "dose." Alternatively, total respiratory heat exchange (convective plus evaporative heat loss) can be used as a measure of the stimulus. Although there is a relationship between the airway response to exercise and histamine, some individuals respond to one and not the other, thus suggesting that the two challenges identify different abnormalities.[374–376]

Patients hyperventilate from a source of dry air, either

cold or at room temperature, and isocapnia is maintained by adding CO_2 to the inspired gas to maintain the end-tidal carbon dioxide content constant.[377, 378] Preserving eucapnia is important because hyperventilation in the absence of exercise would produce hypocapnia, which in itself produces bronchoconstriction. Expiratory flow is measured with progressively increasing levels of hyperventilation, and the level of ventilation or the calculated respiratory heat loss producing a given fall in FEV_1 can be calculated in a fashion similar to the PC_{20}. Although the mechanisms producing airway narrowing may differ, the sensitivity of isocapnic hyperventilation in detecting airway hyper-responsiveness is comparable to that of histamine and methacholine challenge.[379–381]

REFERENCES

1. Johns DP, Abramson M, Bowes G: Evaluation of a new ambulatory spirometer for measuring forced expiratory volume in one second and peak expiratory flow rate. Am Rev Respir Dis 147:1245, 1993.
2. Permutt S: Pulmonary function testing and the prevention of pulmonary disease (editorial). Chest 74:608, 1978.
3. Bunn AE, Vermaak JC, deKock MA: A comprehensive on-line computerised lung function screening test. Respiration 37:42, 1979.
4. Cary J, Huseby J, Culver B, et al: Variability in interpretation of pulmonary function tests. Chest 76:389, 1979.
5. Hubert H, Fabsitz R, Feinleib M, et al: Genetic and environmental influences on pulmonary function in adult twins. Am Rev Respir Dis 125:409, 1982.
6. Webster M, Lorimer G, Man S, et al: Pulmonary function in identical twins: Comparison of nonsmokers and smokers. Am Rev Respir Dis 119:223, 1979.
7. Sobol BJ, Sobol PG: Percent of predicted as the limit of normal in pulmonary function testing: A statistically valid approach. Thorax 34:1, 1979.
8. Becklake M, Crapo RO, Buist S, et al: Lung function testing: Selection of reference values and interpretative strategies. Am Rev Respir Dis 144:1202, 1991.
9. Crapo R, Morris A, Clayton P, et al: Lung volumes in healthy nonsmoking adults. Bull Eur Physiopathol Respir 18:419, 1982.
10. Statement on spirometry. Chest 83:547, 1983.
11. Hurwitz S, Allen J, Liben A: Lung function in young adults: Evidence for differences in the chronological age at which various functions start to decline. Thorax 35:615, 1980.
12. Schoenberg J, Beck G, Bouhuys A: Growth and decay of pulmonary function in healthy blacks and whites. Respir Physiol 33:367, 1978.
13. Bande J, Clement J, Van de Woestijne K: The influence of smoking habits and body weight on vital capacity and FEV_1 in male air force personnel: A longitudinal and cross-sectional analysis. Am Rev Respir Dis 122:781, 1980.
14. Woolcock AJ, Colman MH, Blackburn CRB: Factors affecting normal values for ventilatory lung function. Am Rev Respir Dis 106:692, 1972.
15. Dugdale AE, Bolton JM, Ganendran A: Respiratory function among Malaysian aboriginals. Thorax 26:740, 1971.
16. Yokoyama T, Mitsufuji M: Statistical representation of the ventilatory capacity of 2,247 healthy Japanese adults. Chest 61:655, 1972.
17. Wall M, Olson D, Bonn B, et al: Lung function in North American Indian children—reference standards for spirometry maximal expiratory flow volume curves, and peak expiratory flow. Am Rev Respir Dis 125:158, 1982.
18. Lam K, Pang S, Allan W, et al: Predictive nomograms for forced expiratory volume, forced vital capacity, and peak expiratory flow rate in Chinese adults and children. Br J Dis Chest 77:390, 1983.
19. Huang S, White D, Douglas N, et al: Respiratory function in normal Chinese: Comparison with Caucasians. Respiration 46:265, 1984.
20. Gonzalez-Camarena R, Carrasco-Sosa S, Gaitan MJ: Reliability of reference models for vital capacity in young Mexican males. Rev Invest Clin 45:29, 1993.
21. Pennock B, Rogers R, McCaffree DR: Changes in measured spirometric indices—what is significant? Chest 80:97, 1981.
22. Hutchison DCS, Revill S, Allen M, et al: Guidelines for the measurement of respiratory function. Respir Med 88:165, 1994.
23. Quanjer PH, Tammeling GJ, Cotes JE, et al: Lung volumes and forced ventilatory flows. Eur Respir J 16:5, 1993.
24. Pfaff J, Morgan W: Pulmonary function in infants and children. Respir Med 41:401, 1994.
25. Stocks J, Quanjer PH: Reference values for residual volume, functional residual capacity, and total lung capacity. Eur Respir J 8:492, 1995.
26. Crapo R, Hankinson J, Irvin C, et al: Standardization of Spirometry 1994 Update. Am J Respir Crit Care Med 152:1107, 1995.
27. Hutchison DCS, Barter CE, Martelli NA: Errors in the measurement of vital capacity: A comparison of three methods in normal subjects and in patients with pulmonary emphysema. Thorax 28:584, 1973.
28. Hughes J, Hutchinson D: Errors in the estimation of vital capacity from expiratory flow-volume curves in pulmonary emphysema. Br J Dis Chest 76:279, 1982.
29. Goldman HI, Becklake MR: Respiratory function tests: Normal values at median altitudes and the prediction of normal results. Am Rev Tuber 79:457, 1959.
30. Knudson R, Lebowitz M, Holberg C, et al: Changes in the normal maximal expiratory flow volume curve with growth and aging. Am Rev Respir Dis 127:725, 1983.
31. ACCP Scientific Section Recommendations: The determination of static lung volumes: Report of the Section on Respiratory Pathophysiology. Chest 86:471, 1984.
32. Heldt G, Peters M: A simplified method to determine functional residual capacity during mechanical ventilation. Chest 74:492, 1978.
33. Mashalla YJ, Quanjer PH: Validity of the forced rebreathing method in the measurement of residual volume in patients with airflow limitation. East Afr Med J 70:654, 1993.
34. Pino J, Teculescu D: Validity of total lung capacity determination by the single-breath nitrogen technique. Eur J Respir Dis 61:265, 1980.
35. Krumpe P, MacDannald J, Finley T, et al: Use of an acoustic helium analyzer for measuring lung volumes. J Appl Physiol 50:203, 1981.
36. Johansen B, Bjortuft O, Boe J: Static lung volumes in healthy subjects assessed by helium dilution during occlusion of one mainstem bronchus. Thorax 48:381, 1993.
37. Begin P, Peslin R: Plethysmographic measurements of thoracic gas volume: Back to the assumptions. Bull Eur Physiopathol Respir 19:247, 1983.
38. Paré PD: Breaking Boyle's law. Am Rev Respir Dis 119:684, 1979.
39. Habib M, Engel L: Influence of the panting technique on the plethysmographic measurement of the thoracic gas volume. Am Rev Respir Dis 117:265, 1978.
40. Brown R, Hoppin F Jr, Ingram R Jr, et al: Influence of abdominal gas on the Boyle's law determination of thoracic gas volume. J Appl Physiol 44:469, 1978.
41. Rodenstein D, Goncette L, Stanescu D: Extrathoracic airways changes during plethysmographic measurements of lung volume. Respir Physiol 52:217, 1983.
42. Rodenstein D, Stanescu D, Francis C: Demonstration of failure of body plethysmography in airway obstruction. J Appl Physiol 52:949, 1982.
43. Rodenstein D, Stanescu D: Reassessment of lung volume measurement by helium dilution and by body plethysmography in chronic airflow obstruction. Am Rev Respir Dis 126:1040, 1982.
44. Shore S, Milic-Emili J, Martin J: Reassessment of body plethysmographic technique for the measurement of thoracic gas volume in asthmatics. Am Rev Respir Dis 126:515, 1982.
45. Stanescu D, Rodenstein D, Cauberghs M, et al: Failure of body plethysmography in bronchial asthma. J Appl Physiol 52:939, 1982.
46. Knudson R, Knudson D: Frequency dependent phase and amplitude differences between simulated mouth and pleural pressures during panting: Demonstration with a mechanical model. Chest 86:589, 1984.
47. Paré PD, Coppin CA: Errors in the measurement of total lung capacity in patients with chronic obstructive pulmonary disease. Thorax 38:468, 1983.
48. Rodenstein D, Stanescu D: Frequency dependence of plethysmographic volume in healthy and asthmatic subjects. J Appl Physiol 54:159, 1983.
49. Bohadana A, Peslin R, Hannhart B, et al: Influence of panting frequency on plethysmographic measurements of thoracic gas volume. J Appl Physiol 52:739, 1982.
50. Shore S, Huk O, Mannix S, et al: Effect of panting frequency on the plethysmographic determination of thoracic gas volume in chronic obstructive pulmonary disease. Am Rev Respir Dis 128:54, 1983.
51. Begin P, Peslin R: Influence of panting frequency on thoracic gas volume measurements in chronic obstructive pulmonary disease. Am Rev Respir Dis 130:121, 1984.
52. Brown R, Ingram R Jr, McFadden E Jr: Problems in the plethysmographic assessment of changes in total lung capacity in asthma. Am Rev Respir Dis 118:685, 1978.
53. Garcia J, Hunninghake G, Nugent K: Thoracic gas volume measurement: Increased variability in patients with obstructive ventilatory defects. Chest 85:272, 1984.
54. Barnhard HJ, Pierce JA, Joyce JW, et al: Roentgenographic determination of total lung capacity: A new method evaluated in health, emphysema and congestive heart failure. Am J Med 28:51, 1960.
55. O'Brien R, Drizd T: Roentgenographic determination of total lung capacity: Normal values from a national population survey. Am Rev Respir Dis 128:949, 1983.
56. Stocks J, Quanjer PH: Reference values for residual volume, functional residual capacity, and total lung capacity. Eur Respir J 8:492, 1995.
57. Sackner J, Nixon A, Davis B, et al: Noninvasive measurement of ventilation during exercise using a respiratory inductive plethysmograph: I. Am Rev Respir Dis 122:867, 1980.
58. Cohen KP, Panescu D, Booske JH, et al: Design of an inductive plethysmograph for ventilation measurement. Physiol Meas 15:217, 1994.
59. Spier S, England S: The respiratory inductive plethysmograph—Bands versus Jerkins. Am Rev Respir Dis 127:784, 1983.
60. Cohn M, Rao A, Broudy M, et al: The respiratory inductive plethysmograph: A new non-invasive monitor of respiration. Bull Eur Physiopathol Respir 18:643, 1982.
61. Guyatt A, McBride M, Meanock C: Evaluation of the respiratory inductive plethysmograph in man. Eur J Respir Dis 64:81, 1983.
62. Tobin J, Jenouri G, Lind B, et al: Validation of respiratory inductive plethysmography in patients with pulmonary disease. Chest 83:615, 1983.
63. Chadha T, Watson H, Birch S, et al: Validation of respiratory inductive plethysmography using different calibration procedures. Am Rev Respir Dis 125:644, 1982.
64. Stromberg NO, Dahlback GO, Gustafsson PM: Evaluation of various models for respiratory inductance plethysmography calibration. J Appl Physiol 74:1206, 1993.
65. Sackner M, Rao A, Birch S, et al: Assessment of time-volume and flow-volume components of forced vital capacity. Chest 82:272, 1982.
66. Sackner M, Rao A, Birch S, et al: Assessment of density dependent flow-volume parameters in nonsmokers and smokers: Measurement with spirometry, body plethysmography, and respiratory inductive plethysmography. Chest 82:137, 1982.
67. Jackson E, Stocks J, Pilgrim L, et al: A critical assessment of uncalibrated respiratory inductance plethysmography (Respitrace) for the measurement of tidal breathing parameters in newborns and infants. Pediatr Pulmonol 20:119, 1995.
68. Valta P, Takala J, Foster R, et al: Evaluation of respiratory inductive plethysmography in the measurement of breathing pattern and PEEP-induced changes in lung volume. Chest 102:234, 1992.

69. Cantineau JP, Escourrou P, Sartene R, et al: Accuracy of respiratory inductive plethysmography during wakefulness and sleep in patients with obstructive sleep apnea. Chest 102:1145, 1992.

70. Becklake MR, White N: Sources of variation in spirometric measurements: Identifying the signal and dealing with noise. Occup Med 8:241, 1993.

71. Quanjer PH, Tammeling GJ, Cotes JE, et al: Lung volumes and forced ventilatory flows. Eur Respir J 16:5, 1993.

72. Peslin R, Bohadana A, Hannhart B, et al: Comparison of various methods for reading maximal expiratory flow-volume curves. Am Rev Respir Dis 119:271, 1979.

73. Medical Section, American Thoracic Society of the American Lung Association: ATS Statement, Snowbird Workshop on Standardization of Spirometry. Am Rev Respir Dis 119:831, 1979.

74. Ferris B Jr, Speizer F, Bishop G, et al: Spirometry for an epidemiologic study: Deriving optimum summary statistics for each subject. Bull Eur Physiopathol Respir 14:145, 1978.

75. Wise RA, Connett J, Kurnow K, et al: Selection of spirometric measurements in clinical trial: The Lung Health Study. Am J Respir Crit Care Med 151:675, 1995.

76. Suratt P, Hooe D, Owens D, et al: Effect of maximal versus submaximal expiratory effort on spirometric values. Respiration 42:233, 1981.

77. Stoller JK, Basheda S, Laskowski D, et al: Trial of standard versus modified expiration to achieve end-of-test spirometry criteria. Am Rev Respir Dis 148:275, 1993.

78. Enright PL, Connett JE, Kanner RE, et al: Spirometry in the Lung Health Study: II. Determinants of short-term intraindividual variability. Am J Respir Crit Care Med 151:406, 1995.

79. Shaw A, Fisher J: Reproducibility of the flow-volume loop (correspondence). Thorax 35:480, 1980.

80. Malmberg LP, Hedman J, Sovijarvi AR: Accuracy and repeatability of a pocket turbine spirometer: Comparison with a rolling seal flow-volume spirometer. Clin Physiol 13:89, 1993.

81. Rebuck DA, Hanania NA, D'Urzo AD, et al: The accuracy of a handheld portable spirometer. Chest 109:152, 1996.

82. Whitaker C, Chinn D, Lee W: Statistical reliability of indices derived from the closing volume and flow volume traces. Bull Eur Physiopathol Respir 14:237, 1978.

83. Ferris BG: Epidemiology standardization project. Am Rev Respir Dis 118(Part 2):1, 1978.

84. Lam S, Abboud R, Chan-Yeung M: Use of maximal expiratory flow-volume curve with air and helium-oxygen in the detection of ventilatory abnormalities in population surveys. Am Rev Respir Dis 123:234, 1981.

85. Rossoff L, Csima A, Zamel N: Reproducibility of maximum expiratory flow in severe chronic obstructive pulmonary disease. Bull Eur Physiopathol Respir 15:1129, 1979.

86. Knudson RJ, Lebowitz MD: Maximal mid-expiratory flow (FEF 25–75%): Normal limits and assessment of sensitivity. Am Rev Respir Dis 117:609, 1978.

87. Glindmeyer HW, Lefante JJ, McColloster C, et al: Blue-collar normative spirometric values for Caucasian and African-American men and women aged 18 to 65. Am J Respir Crit Care Med 151:412, 1995.

88. Sharp DS, Enright PL, Chiu D, et al: Reference values for pulmonary function tests of Japanese-American men aged 71 to 90 years. Am J Respir Crit Care Med 153:805, 1996.

89. Enright PL, Kronmal RA, Higgins M, et al: Spirometry reference values for women and men 65 to 85 years of age. Am Rev Respir Dis 147:125, 1993.

90. Boat RF, Tepper R, Stecenko A, et al: Assessment of lung function and dysfunction in studies of infants and children. Am Rev Respir Dis 148:1105, 1993.

91. Pfaff JK, Morgan WJ: Pulmonary function in infants and children. Pediatr Clin North Am 41:401, 1994.

92. American Thoracic Society/European Respiratory Society Statement: Respiratory mechanics in infants: Physiologic evaluation in health and disease. Am Rev Respir Dis 147:474, 1993

93. Hankinson JL, Das MK: Frequency response of portable PEF meters. Am J Respir Crit Care Med 152:702, 1995.

94. Hankinson JL, Crapo RO: Standard flow-time waveforms for testing of PEF meters. Am J Respir Crit Care Med 152:696, 1995.

95. Ewald FW Jr, Tenholder MF, Waller RF: Analysis of the inspiratory flow-volume curve: Should it always precede the forced expiratory maneuver? Chest 106:814, 1994.

96. Sourk R, Nugent K: Bronchodilator testing—confidence intervals derived from placebo inhalations. Am Rev Respir Dis 128:153, 1983.

97. Light RW, Conrad SA, George RB: Clinical significance of pulmonary function tests: The one best test for evaluating the effects of bronchodilator therapy. Chest 72:512, 1977.

98. Van Noord JA, Smeets J, Clement J, et al: Assessment of reversibility of airflow obstruction. Am J Respir Crit Care Med 150:551, 1994.

99. Gimeno F, Postma DS, van Altena R: Comparison of three normal breathing techniques to assess reversibility of airway obstruction. Ann Intern Med 69:513, 1992.

100. Brand PL, Quanjar PH, Postma DS, et al: Interpretation of bronchodilator response in patients with obstructive airways disease: The Dutch Chronic Non-Specific Lung Disease (CNSLD) Study Group. Thorax 47:429, 1992.

101. Paré PD, Lawson LM, Brooks LA: Patterns of response to inhaled bronchodilators in asthmatics. Am Rev Respir Dis 127:680, 1983.

102. Girard M, Light W: Should the FVC be considered in evaluating response to bronchodilator? Chest 84:87, 1983.

103. Ramsdell J, Tisi G: Determination of bronchodilation in the clinical pulmonary function laboratory—role in changes in static lung volumes. Chest 76:622, 1979.

104. Connolly MJ, Crowley JJ, Charan NB, et al: Impaired bronchodilator response to albuterol in healthy elderly men and women. Chest 108:401, 1995.

105. Chang JT, Moran MB, Cugell DW, et al: COPD in the elderly: A reversible cause of functional impairment. Chest 108:736, 1995.

106. Kradjan WA, Driesner NK, Abuan TH, et al: Effect of age on bronchodilator response. Chest 101:1545, 1992.

107. Despas PJ, Leroux M, Macklem PT: Site of airway obstruction in asthma as determined by measuring maximal expiratory flow breathing air and a helium-oxygen mixture. J Clin Invest 51:3235, 1972.

108. Hutcheon M, Griffin P, Levison H, et al: Volume of isoflow: A new test in detection of mild abnormalities of lung mechanics. Am Rev Respir Dis 110:458, 1974.

109. Teculescu D, Bohadana A, Peslin R, et al: One-second forced expiratory volume and density dependence in early airflow limitation. Respiration 44:433, 1983.

110. Knudson R, Bloom W, Lantenborn T, et al: Assessment of air versus helium-oxygen flow-volume curves as an epidemiologic screening test. Chest 86:419, 1984.

111. Teculescu D, Pino J, Sadoul P: Cigarette smoking and density dependence of maximal expiratory flow in asymptomatic men. Am Rev Respir Dis 122:651, 1980.

112. Spiro S, Bierman C, Petheram I: Reproducibility of flow rates measured with low-density gas mixtures in exercise-induced bronchospasm. Thorax 36:852, 1981.

113. Berend N, Nelson N, Rutland J, et al: The maximum expiratory flow-volume curve with air and a low-density gas mixture—an analysis of subject and observer variability. Chest 80:23, 1981.

114. Li K, Tan L, Chong P, et al: Between-technician variation in the measurement of spirometry with air and helium. Am Rev Respir Dis 124:196, 1981.

115. Dull W, Secker-Walker R: Helium-oxygen flow volume curves in young healthy adults. Respiration 38:18, 1979.

116. Loveland M, Corbin R, Ducic S, et al: Evaluation of the analysis and variability of the helium response. Bull Eur Physiopathol Respir 14:551, 1978.

117. Teculescu D, Pino J, Peslin R: Composite flow-volume curves matched at total lung capacity in the study of density dependence of maximal expiratory flows. Lung 159:127, 1981.

118. Zeck R, Solliday N, Celic L, et al: Variability of the volume of isoflow. Chest 79:269, 1981.

119. MacDonald J, Cole T: The flow-volume loop: Reproducibility of air- and helium-based tests in normal subjects. Thorax 35:64, 1980.

120. Mead J: Analysis of the configuration of maximum expiratory flow-volume curves. J Appl Physiol 44:156, 1978.

121. Castile R, Mead J, Jackson A, et al: Effects of posture on flow-volume curve configuration in normal humans. J Appl Physiol 53:1175, 1982.

122. Jansen M, Peslin R, Bohadana A, et al: Usefulness of forced expiration slope ratios for detecting mild airway abnormalities. Am Rev Respir Dis 122:221, 1980.

123. Jordanoglou J, Hadjistavrou C, Tatsis G, et al: Total effective time of the forced expirogram in disease: Sources of error and a correction factor. Thorax 37:304, 1982.

124. Vermaak J, Bunn A, de Kock M: A new lung function index. The area under the maximum expiratory flow-volume curve. Respiration 37:61, 1979.

125. Wall M, Misley M, Dickerson D: Partial expiratory flow-volume curves in young children. Am Rev Respir Dis 129:557, 1984.

126. Koulouris NG, Valta P, Lavoie A, et al: A simple method to detect expiratory flow limitation during spontaneous breathing. Eur Respir J 8:306, 1995.

127. Mahajan RP, Singh P, Murty GE, et al: Relationship between expired lung volume, peak flow rate and peak velocity time during a voluntary cough manoeuvre. Br J Anaesth 72:298, 1994.

128. Yernault J-C, De Troyer A, Rodenstein D: Sex and age differences in intrathoracic airways mechanics in normal man. J Appl Physiol 46:556, 1979.

129. Aldrich T, Arora N, Rochester D: The influence of airway obstruction and respiratory muscle strength on maximal voluntary ventilation in lung disease. Am Rev Respir Dis 126:195, 1982.

130. Lavietese M, Clifford E, Silverstein D, et al: Relationship of static respiratory muscle pressure and maximum voluntary ventilation in normal subjects. Respiration 38:121, 1979.

131. Martin B, Thomas C: Variation among normal persons in short-term ventilatory capacity. Respiration 43:23, 1982.

132. Kraemer R, Wiese G, Albertini M, et al: Elastic behaviour of the lungs in healthy children determined by means of an exponential function. Respir Physiol 52:229, 1983.

133. Colebatch H, Ng C, Nikov N: Use of an exponential function for elastic recoil. J Appl Physiol 46:387, 1979.

134. Gibson G, Pride N, Davis J, et al: Exponential description of the static pressure-volume curve of normal and diseased lungs. Am Rev Respir Dis 120:799, 1979.

135. Knudson R, Kaltenborn W: Evaluation of lung elastic recoil by exponential curve analysis. Respir Physiol 46:29, 1981.

136. Colebatch H, Greaves I, Ng C: Exponential analysis of elastic recoil and aging in healthy males and females. J Appl Physiol 47:683, 1979.

137. Yernault J, Noseda A, Van Muylem A, et al: Variability in lung elasticity measurements in normal humans. Rev Respir Dis 128:816, 1983.

138. McCuaig C, Vessal S, Coppin C, et al: Variability in measurements of pressure volume curves in normal subjects. Am Rev Respir Dis 131:656, 1985.

139. Paré PD, Brooks LA, Bates J, et al: Exponential analysis of the lung pressure-volume curve as a predictor of pulmonary emphysema. Am Rev Respir Dis 126:54, 1982.

140. Berend N, Skoog C, Thurlbeck W: Exponential analysis of lobar pressure-volume characteristics. Thorax 36:452, 1981.

141. Haber P, Colebatch H, Ng C, et al: Alveolar size as a determinant of pulmonary distensibility in mammalian lungs. J Appl Physiol 54:837, 1983.

142. Colebatch HJ, Ng CK: Estimating alveolar surface area during life. Respir Physiol 88:163, 1992.

143. McFadden ER Jr, Lyons HA: Airway resistance and uneven ventilation in bronchial asthma. J Appl Physiol 25:365, 1968.

144. Ingram RH Jr, Schilder DP: Association of a decrease in dynamic compliance with a change in gas distribution. J Appl Physiol 23:911, 1967.

145. Woolcock AJ, Vincent NJ, Macklem PT: Frequency dependence of compliance as a test for obstruction in the small airways. J Clin Invest 48:1097, 1969.

146. Cutillo A, Renzetti A Jr: Mechanical behaviour of the respiratory system as a function of frequency in health and disease. Bull Eur Physiopathol Respir 19:293, 1983.

147. Frey U, Schibler A, Kraemer R: The interrupter technique: A renaissance of noninvasive approach for lung function testing in infants and children. Agents Actions Suppl 40:64, 1993.

148. Chowiencyk PJ, Lawson CP, Lane S, et al: A flow interruption device for measurement of airway resistance. Eur Respir J 4:623, 1991.

149. Bates DV, Macklem PT, Christie RV: Respiratory Function in Disease: An Introduction to the Integrated Study of the Lung. 2nd ed. Philadelphia, WB Saunders, 1971.

150. Mead J, Whittenberger JL: Physical properties of human lungs measured during spontaneous respiration. J Appl Physiol 5:779, 1953.

151. Von Neergaard, Wirz K: Die Messung der Stromunswiederstande in den alem-vegen des Menschen, Insbesondere bei Asthma und Emphysem. Z Klin Med 51-82, 1927.

152. Lisboa C, Ross W, Jardim J, et al: Pulmonary pressure-flow curves measured by a data-averaging circuit. J Appl Physiol 47:621, 1979.

153. Clement J, Landser P, Van de Woestijne K: Total resistance and reactance in patients with respiratory complaints with and without airways obstruction. Chest 83:215, 1983.

154. Landser F, Clement J, Van de Woestijne K: Normal values of total respiratory resistance and reactance determined by forced oscillations—influence of smoking. Chest 81:586, 1982.

155. Bhansali P, Irvin C, Dempsey J, et al: Human pulmonary resistance: Effect of frequency and gas physical properties. J Appl Physiol 47:161, 1979.

156. Wouters EF: Total respiratory impedance measurement by forced oscillations: A noninvasive method to assess bronchial response in occupational medicine. Exp Lung Res 16:25, 1990.

157. Petro W, Nieding G, Boll W, et al: Determination of respiratory resistance by an oscillation method: Studies of long-term and short-term variability and dependence upon lung volume and compliance. Respiration 42:243, 1981.

158. Phagoo SB, Watson RA, Silverman M, et al: Comparison of four methods of assessing airflow resistance before and after induced airway narrowing in normal subjects. J Appl Physiol 79:518, 1995.

159. Ohrui T, Sekizawa K, Yanai M, et al: Partitioning of pulmonary responses to inhaled methacholine subjects with asymptomatic asthma. Am Rev Respir Dis 146:1501, 1992.

160. Fowler W: Lung function studies: II. The respiratory dead space. Am J Physiol 154:405, 1948.

161. Engel L: Intraregional ventilation distribution. Bull Eur Physiopathol Respir 18:181, 1982.

162. Comroe J, Fowler W: Lung function studies: VI. Detection of uneven alveolar ventilation during a single-breath of oxygen: A new test of pulmonary disease. Am J Med 10:408, 1951.

163. Cormier Y, Belanger J: The role of gas exchange in phase IV of the single-breath nitrogen test. Am Rev Respir Dis 125:396, 1982.

163a. Flores XF, Cruz JC: Single-breath, room-air method for measuring closing volume (phase 4) in the normal human lung. Chest 102:438, 1992.

164. Nichol G, Michels D, Guy H: Phase V of the single-breath washout test. J Appl Physiol 52:34, 1982.

165. Dollfuss RE, Milic-Emili J, Bates D: Regional ventilation of the lung, studied with boluses of 133 xenon. Respir Physiol 2:234, 1967.

166. Leblanc P, Ruff F, Milic-Emili J: Effects of age and body position on "airway closure" in man. J Appl Physiol 28:448, 1970.

167. McCarthy DS, Spencer R, Greene R, et al: Measurement of "closing volume" as a simple and sensitive test for early detection of small airway disease. Am J Med 52:747, 1972.

168. Green M, Travis DM, Mead J: A simple measurement of phase IV ("closing volume") using a critical orifice helium analyzer. J Appl Physiol 33:827, 1972.

169. Anthonisen NR, Danson J, Robertson PC, et al: Airway closure as a function of age. Respir Physiol 8:58, 1969.

170. Berend N, Skoog C, Thurlbeck W: Single-breath nitrogen test in excised human lungs. J Appl Physiol 51:1568, 1981.

171. Buist A, Ross B: Predicted values for closing volumes using a modified single-breath nitrogen test. Am Rev Respir Dis 107:744, 1973.

172. Buist A, Ross B: Quantitative analysis of the alveolar plateau in the diagnosis of early airway obstruction. Am Rev Respir Dis 108:1078, 1973.

173. Teculescu DB, Rebstock E, Caillier I, et al: Variability of the computerized single-breath nitrogen washout test in healthy adults: Results from a field survey in a French rural area. Clin Physiol 13:35, 1993.

174. Darling RC, Cournand A, Mansfield JS, et al: Studies on the intrapulmonary mixture of gases: I. Nitrogen elimination from blood and body tissues during high oxygen breathing. J Clin Invest 19:591, 1940.

175. Meneely GR, Kaltreider NL: The volume of the lung determined by helium dilution: Description of the method and comparison with other procedures. J Clin Invest 28:129, 1949.

176. Bates DV, Christie RV: Intrapulmonary mixing of helium in health and in emphysema. Clin Sci 9:17, 1950.

177. Hogg JC, Macklem PT, Thurlbeck WM: Site and nature of airway obstruction in chronic obstructive lung disease. N Engl J Med 278:1355, 1968.

178. Macklem PT, Mead J: Resistance of central and peripheral airways measured by a retrograde catheter. J Appl Physiol 22:395, 1967.

179. Becklake MR, Permutt S: Evaluation of tests of lung function for "screening" for early detection of chronic obstructive lung disease. In Macklem PT, Permutt S (eds): The Lung in Transition Between Health and Disease. Lung Biology in Health and Disease. New York, Marcel Dekker, 1979.

180. Buist AS, Ghezzo NR, Anthonisen RM, et al: Relationship between the single-breath N_2 test and age, sex, and smoking habit in three North American cities. Am Rev Respir Dis 120:305, 1979.

181. Hudgel D, Petty T, Baidwan B, et al: A community pulmonary disease screening effort—"Denver Lung Days." Chest 74:619, 1978.

182. Dosman JA, Cotton DJ: Interpretation of tests of early lung dysfunction. Chest 79:261, 1981.

183. Permutt S: Pulmonary function testing and the prevention of pulmonary disease (editorial). Chest 74:608, 1978.

184. Macklem P, Becklake M: Is screening for chronic limitation of airflow desirable? Chest 74:607, 1978.

185. Solomon D: Clinical significance of pulmonary function tests: Are small airway tests helpful in the detection of early airflow obstruction? Chest 74:567, 1978.

186. Van de Woestijne KP: Are the small airways really quiet? Eur J Respir Dis 63:19, 1982.

187. Gelb F, Williams J, Zamel N: Spirometry: FEV_1 versus FEF 25–75%. Chest 84:473, 1983.

188. Racineux J, Peslin R, Hannhart B: Sensitivity of forced expiration indices to induced changes in peripheral airway resistance. J Appl Physiol 50:15, 1981.

189. Lam S, Abboud R, Chan-Yeung M: Use of maximal expiratory flow-volume curves with air and helium-oxygen in the detection of ventilatory abnormalities in population surveys. Am Rev Respir Dis 123:234, 1981.

190. Krogh A, Krogh M: On the rate of diffusion of carbonic oxide into the lungs of man. Scand Arch Physiol 23:236, 1910.

191. Krogh M: The diffusion of gases through the lungs of man. J Physiol (Lond) 49:271, 1914.

192. Forster RE, Fowler WS, Bates DV, et al: The absorption of carbon monoxide by the lungs during breathholding. J Clin Invest 33:1135, 1954.

193. Ogilvie CM, Forster RE, Blakemore WS, et al: A standardized breath holding technique for the clinical measurement of the diffusing capacity of the lung for carbon monoxide. J Clin Invest 36:1, 1957.

194. Russell N, Bagg L, Dobrzynski J: Clinical assessment of a rebreathing method for measuring pulmonary gas transfer. Thorax 38:212, 1983.

195. Graham B, Mink J, Cotton D: Improved accuracy and precision of single-breath CO diffusing capacity measurements. J Appl Physiol 55:1306, 1981.

196. Cotton D, Newth C, Portner P, et al: Measurement of single-breath CO diffusing capacity by continuous rapid CO analysis in man. J Appl Physiol 46:1149, 1979.

197. Jones RS, Meade F: Pulmonary diffusing capacity: An improved single-breath method. Lancet 1:94, 1960.

198. Gaensler EA, Smith AA: Attachment for automated single breath diffusing capacity. Chest 63:136, 1973.

199. Make B, Miller A, Epler G, et al: Single-breath diffusing capacity in the industrial setting. Chest 82:351, 1982.

200. Crapo R, Hankinson J, Irvin C, et al: Single-breath carbon monoxide diffusing capacity (transfer factor). Am J Respir Crit Care Med 152:2185, 1995.

201. Cotes JE, Chinn DJ, Quanjer PH, et al: Standardization of the measurement of transfer factor (diffusing capacity). Eur Respir J 16:41, 1993.

202. Beck KC, Offord KP, Scanlon PD: Comparison of four methods for calculating diffusing capacity by the single breath method. Chest 105:594, 1994.

203. Turcotte RA, Perrault H, Marcotte JE, et al: A test for the measurement of pulmonary diffusion capacity during high-intensity exercise. J Sports Sci 10:229, 1992.

204. Graham B, Mink J, Cotton D: Improved accuracy and precision of single-breath CO diffusing capacity measurements. J Appl Physiol 55:1306, 1981.

205. Graham B, Mink J, Cotton D: Overestimation of the single-breath carbon monoxide diffusing capacity in patients with air-flow obstruction. Rev Respir Dis 129:403, 1984.

206. Cotton DJ, Taher F, Mink JT, et al: Effect of volume history on changes in DLcoSB-3EQ with lung volume in normal subjects. J Appl Physiol 73:434, 1992.

207. Newth C, Cotton D, Nadel J: Pulmonary diffusing capacity measured at multiple intervals during a single exhalation in man. J Appl Physiol 43:617, 1977.

208. Huang YC, Macintyre NR: Real-time gas analysis improves the measurement of single-breath diffusing capacity. Am Rev Respir Dis 146:946, 1992.

209. Huang YC, Helms MJ, MacIntyre NR: Normal values for single exhalation diffusing capacity and pulmonary capillary blood flow in sitting, supine positions, and during mild exercise. Chest 105:501, 1994.

210. Cotton DJ, Prabhu MB, Mink JT, et al: Effect of ventilation inhomogeneity on "intrabreath" measurements of diffusing capacity in normal subjects. J Appl Physiol 75:927, 1993.

211. Wilson AF, Hearne J, Matthew B, et al: Measurement of transfer factor during constant exhalation. Thorax 49:1121, 1994.

212. Siegler D, Zorab P: The influence of lung volume on gas transfer in scoliosis. Br J Dis Chest 76:44, 1982.

213. Ayers L, Ginsberg M, Fein J, et al: Diffusing capacity, specific diffusing capacity, and interpretation of diffusion defects. West J Med 123:255, 1975.

214. Crapo R, Morris A: Standardized single-breath normal values for carbon monoxide diffusing capacity. Rev Respir Dis 123:185, 1981.

215. Ogilvie CM, Forster RE: Single-breath transfer factor 25 years on: A reappraisal. Thorax 38:1, 1983.

216. Stam H, Hrachovina V, Stijnen T, et al: Diffusing capacity dependent on lung volume and age in normal subjects. J Appl Physiol 76:2356, 1994.

217. Finley T, Engelman E, Packer B, et al: Use of the R.C. time constant for CO in the measurement of diffusing capacity. Am Rev Respir Dis 109:682, 1974.

218. Macnaughton PD, Evans TW: Measurement of lung volume and DLCO in acute respiratory failure. Am J Respir Crit Care Med 150:770, 1994.

219. Hsia CC, McBrayer DG, Ramanathan M: Reference values of pulmonary diffusing capacity during exercise by a rebreathing technique. Am J Respir Crit Care Med 152:658, 1995.

220. Takahashi H, Iwabuchi K, Kudo Y, et al: Simultaneous measurement of pulmonary diffusing capacity for CO and cardiac output by a rebreathing method in patients with pulmonary diseases. Intern Med 34:330, 1995.

221. Macnaughton PD, Morgan CJ, Denison DM, et al: Measurement of carbon monoxide transfer and lung volume in ventilated subjects. Eur Respir J 6:231, 1993.

222. Bates DV, Woolf CR, Paul GI: Chronic bronchitis: A report on the first two stages of the coordinated study of chronic bronchitis in the Department of Veterans Affairs, Canada. Med Ser J Can 18:211, 1962.

223. Weinberger SE, Johnson TS, Weiss ST: Clinical significance of pulmonary function tests—use and interpretation of the single-breath diffusing capacity. Chest 78:483, 1980.

224. Crapo J, Crapo R: Comparison of total lung diffusion capacity and the membrane component of diffusion capacity as determined by physiologic and morphometric techniques. Respir Physiol 51:183, 1983.

225. Weibel ER, Federspiel WJ, Fryder-Doffey F, et al: Morphometric model for pulmonary diffusing capacity: I. Membrane diffusing capacity. Respir Physiol 93:125, 1993.

226. Harris E, Whitlock R: Fractional carbon monoxide uptake and "diffusing capacity" in models of pulmonary maldistribution. Bull Eur Physiopathol Respir 19:427, 1983.

227. Harris E, Whitlock R: Prediction equations for fractional CO uptake derived from 50 healthy subjects. Bull Eur Physiopathol Respir 19:433, 1983.

228. Mohsenifar Z, Tashkin D: Effect of carboxyhemoglobin on the single breath diffusing capacity: Derivation of an empirical correction factor. Respiration 37:185, 1979.

229. Sansores RH, Paré PD, Abboud RT: Acute effect of cigarette smoking on the carbon monoxide diffusing capacity of the lung. Am Rev Respir Dis 146:951, 1992.

230. Sansores RH, Paré PD, Abboud RT: Effect of smoking cessation on pulmonary carbon monoxide diffusing capacity and capillary blood volume. Am Rev Respir Dis 146:959, 1992.

231. Cotes J, Dabbs J, Elwood P, et al: Iron-deficiency anemia: Its effect on transfer factor for the lung (diffusing capacity) and ventilation and cardiac frequency during sub-maximal exercise. Clin Sci 42:325, 1972.

232. Mohsenifar Z, Brown H, Schnitzer B, et al: The effect of abnormal levels of hematocrit on the single breath diffusing capacity. Lung 160:325, 1982.

233. Greening A, Patel K, Goolden A: Carbon monoxide diffusing capacity in polycythaemia rubra vera. Thorax 37:528, 1982.

234. Riepl G: Effects of abnormal hemoglobin concentration in human blood on membrane diffusing capacity of the lung and on pulmonary capillary blood volume. Respiration 36:10, 1978.

235. Dinakara P, Blumenthal WS, Johnston RF, et al: The effect of anemia on pulmonary diffusing capacity with derivation of a correction equation. Am Rev Respir Dis 102:965, 1970.

236. Fisher J, Cerny F: Characteristics of adjustment of lung diffusing capacity to work. J Appl Physiol 52:1124, 1982.

237. Viegi G, Paoletti P, Carrozzi L, et al: CO diffusing capacity in a general population sample: Relationships with cigarette smoking and airflow obstruction. Respiration 60:155, 1993.

238. Cotton D, Mink K, Graham B: Effect of high-negative inspiratory pressure on single-breath CO diffusing capacity. Respir Physiol 54:19, 1983.

239. Nemery B, Piret L, Brasseur L, et al: Effect of nitroglycerin on D_L of normal subjects at rest and during exercise. J Appl Physiol 52:851, 1982.

240. Chang SC, Chang HI, Liu SY, et al: Effects of body position and age on membrane diffusing capacity and pulmonary capillary blood volume. Chest 102:139, 1992.

241. Prisk GK, Guy HJ, Elliott AR, et al: Pulmonary diffusing capacity, capillary blood volume, and cardiac output during sustained microgravity. J Appl Physiol 75:15, 1993.

242. Sansores RH, Abboud RT, Kennell C, et al: The effect of menstruation on the pulmonary carbon monoxide diffusing capacity. Am J Respir Crit Care Med 152:381, 1995.

243. Frans A, Lampert E, Kallay O, et al: Effect of cold pressor test on single-breath DLCO in normal subjects. J Appl Physiol 76:750, 1994.

244. Puri S, Baker BL, Dutka DP, et al: Reduced alveolar-capillary membrane diffus-

ing capacity in chronic heart failure: Its pathophysiological relevance and relationship to exercise performance. Circulation 91:2769, 1995.

245. Rasmussen J, Hanel B, Saunamaki K, et al: Recovery of pulmonary diffusing capacity after maximal exercise. J Sports Sci 10:525, 1992.

246. Manier G, Moinard J, Stoicheff H: Pulmonary diffusing capacity after maximal exercise. J Appl Physiol 75:2580, 1993.

247. Caillaud C, Serre-Cousine O, Anselme F, et al: Computerized tomography and pulmonary diffusing capacity in highly trained athletes after performing a triathlon. J Appl Physiol 79:1226, 1995.

248. Miller A, Thornton JC, Warshaw R, et al: Single-breath diffusing capacity in a representative sample of the population of Michigan, a large industrial state: Predicted values, lower limits of normal, and frequencies of abnormality by smoking history. Am Rev Respir Dis 127:270, 1983.

249. Hallenberg C, Holden W, Menzel T, et al: The clinical usefulness of a screening test to detect static pulmonary blood using a multiple-breath analysis of diffusing capacity. Am Rev Respir Dis 119:349, 1979.

250. Mohsenifar Z, Collier J, Belman MJ, et al: Isolated reduction in single-breath diffusing capacity in the evaluation of exertional dyspnea. Chest 101:965, 1992.

251. Steen VD, Graham G, Conte C, et al: Isolated diffusing capacity reduction in systemic sclerosis. Arthritis Rheum 35:765, 1992.

252. Yang SC, Yang SP, Lin PJ: Prediction equations for single-breath carbon monoxide diffusing capacity from a Chinese population. Am Rev Respir Dis 147:599, 1993.

253. Neas LM, Schwartz J: The determinants of pulmonary diffusing capacity in a national sample of U.S. adults. Am J Respir Crit Care Med 153:656, 1996.

254. Nasr SZ, Amato P, Wilmott RW: Predicted values for lung diffusing capacity in healthy children. Pediatr Pulmonol 10:267, 1991.

255. Rhodes CG, Hughes JM: Pulmonary studies using positron emission tomography. Eur Respir J 8:1001, 1995.

256. Brudin LH, Rhodes CG, Valind SO, et al: Interrelationships between regional blood flow, blood volume, and ventilation in supine humans. J Appl Physiol 76:1205, 1994.

257. Schuster DP, Kaplan JD, Gauvain K, et al: Measurement of regional pulmonary blood flow with PET. J Nucl Med 36:371, 1995.

258. Lopata M, Lourenco R: Evaluation of respiratory control. Clin Chest Med 1:33, 1980.

259. Cherniack N: Applied cardiopulmonary physiology: The clinical assessment of the chemical regulation of ventilation. Chest 70:274, 1976.

260. Derenne J, Macklem P, Roussos C: State of the art: The respiratory muscles—mechanics, control and pathophysiology: II. Am Rev Respir Dis 118:373, 1978.

261. Cherniack N, Dempsey J, Fencl V, et al: Workshop on assessment of respiratory control in humans: I. Methods of measurement of ventilatory responses to hypoxia and hypercapnia. Am Rev Respir Dis 115:177, 1977.

262. Rebuck A, Slutsky A: Measurement of ventilatory responses to hypercapnia and hypoxia. *In* Hornbein TF, Lenfant C (eds): Regulation of Breathing. Part II: Lung Biology in Health and Disease. New York, Marcel Dekker, 1981, p 745.

263. Read D: A clinical method for assessing the ventilatory response to carbon dioxide. Aust Ann Med 16:20, 1967.

264. Milic-Emili J: Clinical methods for assessing the ventilatory response to carbon dioxide and hypoxia. *In* Macklem PT (ed): Medical intelligence—current concepts—new tests to assess lung function. N Engl J Med 293:865, 1975.

265. Sullivan T, Yu P: Reproducibility of CO_2 response curves with 10 minutes separating each rebreathing test. Am Rev Respir Dis 129:23, 1984.

266. Rebuck AS, Read J: Patterns of ventilatory response to carbon dioxide during recovery from severe asthma. Clin Sci 41:13, 1971.

267. Arkinstall WW, Nirmel K, Klissouras V, et al: Genetic differences in the ventilatory response to inhaled CO_2. J Appl Physiol 36:6, 1974.

268. Douglas N, White D, Weil J, et al: Effect of breathing route on ventilation and ventilatory drive. Respir Physiol 51:209, 1983.

269. McBride BJ, Whitelaw WA: A physiological stimulus to upper airway receptors in humans. J Appl Physiol 51:1189, 1981.

270. Kochi T: Breathing route and ventilatory responses to inspiratory resistive loading in humans. Am J Respir Crit Care Med 150:742, 1994.

271. Hirshman C, McCullough R, Weil J: Normal values for hypoxic and hypercapnic ventilatory drives in man. J Appl Physiol 38:1095, 1975.

272. Khoo MC, Yang F, Shin JJ, et al: Estimation of dynamic chemoresponsiveness in wakefulness and non–rapid-eye-movement sleep. J Appl Physiol 78:1052, 1995.

273. Rebuck AS, Campbell EJM: A clinical method for assessing the ventilatory response to hypoxia. Am Rev Respir Dis 109:345, 1974.

274. Easton PA, Slykerman LJ, Anthonisen NR: Ventilatory response to sustained hypoxia in normal adults. J Appl Physiol 61:906, 1986.

274a. Easton PA, Slykerman LJ, Anthonisen NR: Recovery of the ventilatory response to hypoxia in normal adults. J Appl Physiol 64:521, 1988.

274b. Georgopoulos D, Bshouty Z, Younes M, et al: Hypoxic exposure and activation of the after-discharge mechanism in conscious humans. J Appl Physiol 69:1159, 1990.

275. Shaw R, Schonfeld S, Whitcomb M: Progressive and transient hypoxic ventilatory drive tests in healthy subjects. Am Rev Respir Dis 126:37, 1982.

276. Patakas D, Kakavelas H, Louridas G: Respiratory chemosensitivity evaluated by respiratory drive and breath holding. Respiration 40:256, 1980.

277. Whitelaw W, Derenne JP, Milic-Emili J: Occlusion pressure as a measure of respiratory centre output in conscious man. Respir Physiol 23:181, 1975.

278. Pourriat JL, Baud M, Lamberto C, et al: Measurement of CO_2 response with the breath-by-breath automatic acquisition of the breathing pattern and occlusion pressure. J Clin Monit 10:26, 1994.

279. Ward S, Agleh K, Poon C-S: Breath-to-breath monitoring of inspiratory occlusion pressures in humans. J Appl Physiol 51:520, 1981.

280. Scott GC, Piquette CA: Use of a face mask in the measurement of resting ventilatory parameters and mouth occlusion pressures. Sleep 16:668, 1993.

281. Grassino A, Derenne J, Almirall J, et al: Configuration of the chest wall and occlusion pressures in awake humans. J Appl Physiol 50:134, 1981.

282. Marazzini L, Cavestri R, Gori D, et al: Difference between mouth and esophageal occlusion pressure during CO_2 rebreathing in chronic obstructive pulmonary disease. Am Rev Respir Dis 118:1027, 1978.

283. Milic-Emili J, Whitelaw W, Grassino A: Measurement and testing of respiratory drive. *In* Hornbein TF, Lenfant C (eds): Regulation of Breathing. Part II: Lung Biology in Health and Disease. New York, Marcel Dekker, 1981, p 675.

284. Zackon H, Despas P, Anthonisen N: Occlusion pressure responses in asthma and chronic obstructive pulmonary disease. Am Rev Respir Dis 114:917, 1976.

285. Sassoon CS, Mahutte CK. Airway occlusion pressure and breathing pattern as predictors of weaning outcome. Am Rev Respir Dis 148:860, 1993.

286. Milic-Emili J: Recent advances in clinical assessment of control of breathing. Lung 160:1, 1982.

287. McKenzie DK, Gandevia SC: Electrical assessment of respiratory muscles. *In* Roussos C (ed): The Thorax. *In* Lenfant C (ed): Lung Biology in Health and Disease. New York, Marcel Dekker, 1995, pp 1029–1048.

288. Polkey MI, Green M, Moxham J: Measurement of respiratory muscle strength. Thorax 50:1131, 1995.

289. Gibson GJ: Measurement of respiratory muscle strength. Respir Med 89:529, 1995.

290. Black LF, Hyatt RE: Maximal respiratory pressures: Normal values and relationship to age and sex. Am Rev Respir Dis 99:696, 1969.

291. Hamnegard CH, Wragg S, Kyroussis D, et al: Portable measurement of maximum mouth pressures. Eur Respir J 7:398, 1994.

292. McKenzie DK, Gandevia SC, Gorman RB, et al: Software compensation for lung volume in assessment of inspiratory muscle strength and endurance. Thorax 50:230, 1995.

293. Ringqvist T: The ventilatory capacity in healthy subjects: An analysis of causal factors with special reference to the respiratory forces. Scand J Clin Lab Invest Suppl 18:5, 1966.

294. Aldrich TK, Spiro P: Maximal inspiratory pressure: Does reproducibility indicate full effort? Thorax 50:40, 1995.

294a. Fuso L, Di Cosmo V, Nardecchia B, Sammarro S, et al: Maximal inspiratory pressure in elite soccer players. J Sports Med Physical Fitness 36:67, 1996.

294b. Fiz JA, Aguilar J, Carreras A, et al: Maximum respiratory pressures in trumpet players. Chest 104:1203, 1993.

295. Enright PL, Kronmal RA, Manolio TA, et al: Respiratory muscle strength in the elderly: Correlates and reference values. Cardiovascular Health Study Research Group. Am J Respir Crit Care Med 149:430, 1994.

296. Tolep K, Kelsen SG: Effect of aging on respiratory skeletal muscles. Clin Chest Med 14:363, 1993.

297. Karvonen J, Saarelainen S, Nieminen MM: Measurement of respiratory muscle forces based on maximal inspiratory and expiratory pressures. Respiration 61:28, 1994.

298. Smyth R, Chapman K, Rebuck A: Maximal inspiratory and expiratory pressures in adolescents: Normal values. Chest 86:568, 1984.

299. Leech J, Ghezzo H, Stevens D, et al: Respiratory pressure and function in young adults. Am Rev Respir Dis 128:17, 1983.

300. Wilson S, Cooke N, Edwards R, et al: Predicted normal values for maximal respiratory pressure in Caucasian adults and children. Thorax 39:535, 1984.

301. Guleria R, Jindal SK: Normal maximal expiratory and inspiratory pressures in healthy teenagers. J Assoc Physicians India 40:108, 1992.

301a. Tolep K, Higgins N, Muza S, et al: Comparison of diaphragm strength between healthy adult elderly and young men. Am J Respir Crit Care Med 152:677, 1995.

302. Uldry C, Fitting JW: Maximal values of sniff nasal inspiratory pressure in healthy subjects. Thorax 50:371, 1995.

303. Heritier F, Rahm F, Pasche P, et al: Sniff nasal inspiratory pressure: A noninvasive assessment of inspiratory strength. Am J Respir Crit Care Med 150:1678, 1994.

303a. Heijdra YF, Dekhuijzen PN, van Herwaarden CL, Folgering HT: Differences between sniff mouth pressures and static maximal inspiratory pressure. Eur Resp J 6:541, 1993.

303b. Yan S, Gauthier AP, Similowski T, et al: Evaluation of human contractility using mouth pressure twitches. Am Rev Respir Dis 145:1064, 1992.

303c. Hamnegaard CH, Wragg S, Kyroussis D, et al: Mouth pressure in response to magnetic stimulation of the phrenic nerves. Thorax 50:620, 1995.

304. Loh L, Goldman M, Newsom D: The assessment of diaphragm function. Medicine (Baltimore) 56:165, 1977.

305. Gibson G, Clark E, Pride N: Static transdiaphragmatic pressures in normal subjects and in patients with chronic hyperinflation. Am Rev Respir Dis 124:685, 1981.

306. Vanmeenen M, Demedts M, Vaerenbergh H, et al: Transdiaphragmatic, esophageal, and gastric pressures during maximal static inspiratory and expiratory efforts in young subjects: Effects of maneuver and sex. Eur J Respir Dis 65:216, 1984.

307. Miller JM, Moxham J, Green M: The maximal sniff in the assessment of diaphragm function in man. Clin Sci 69:91, 1985.

308. Lisboa C, Paré PD, Pertuze J, et al: Inspiratory muscle function in unilateral diaphragmatic paralysis. Am Rev Respir Dis 134:488, 1986.

309. Laroche CM, Mier AK, Moxham J, et al: The value of sniff esophageal pressures

310. Newsom-Davis J: Phrenic nerve conduction in man. J Neurol Neurosurg Psychiatry 30:420, 1967.

310a. Mador MJ, Magalang UJ, Kufel TJ: Twitch potentiation following voluntary diaphragmatic contraction. Am J Respir Crit Care Med 149:739, 1994.

311. Machetanz J, Bischoff C, Pilchlmeier R, et al: Magnetically induced muscle contraction caused by motor nerve stimulation and not by direct muscle activation. Muscle Nerve 17:1170, 1994.

312. Nickerson B, Keens T: Measuring ventilatory muscle endurance in humans as sustainable inspiratory pressure. J Appl Physiol 52:768, 1982.

313. Martyn JB, Moreno RH, Paré PD, et al: Measurement of inspiratory muscle performance with incremental threshold loading. Am Rev Respir Dis 135:919, 1987.

314. Bardsley PA, Bentley S, Hall HS, et al: Measurement of inspiratory muscle performance with incremental threshold loading: A comparison of two techniques. Thorax 48:354, 1993.

315. Eastwood PR, Hillman DR: A threshold loading device for testing of inspiratory muscle performance. Eur Respir J 8:463, 1995.

316. Gross D, Grassino A, Ross W, et al: Electromyogram pattern of diaphragmatic fatigue. J Appl Physiol 46:1, 1979.

317. Bellemare F, Grassino A: Effect of pressure and timing of contraction on human diaphragm fatigue. J Appl Physiol 53:1190, 1982.

318. Ramonatxo M, Boulard P, Prefaut C: Validation of a noninvasive tension-time index of inspiratory muscles. J Appl Physiol 78:646, 1995.

318a. Ramonatxo M, Boulard P, Prefaut C: Validation of a noninvasive tension-time index of inspiratory muscles. J Appl Physiol 78:646, 1995.

319. Weiss S, Robb G, Blumgart H: The velocity of blood flow in health and disease as measured by the effect of histamine on the minute vessels. Am Heart J 4:664, 1929.

320. Weiss S, Robb G, Ellis L: The systemic effects of histamine in man with special reference to the responses of the cardiovascular system. Arch Intern Med 49:360, 1932.

321. Curry J: Comparative action of acetyl-beta-methylcholine and histamine on the respiratory tract in normals, patients with hay fever, and subjects with bronchial asthma. J Clin Invest 26:430, 1947.

322. Tiffeneau R: L'hyperexcitabilite acetylcholinique du poumon: Critere physiopharmacodynamique de la maladie asthmatique. Presse Med 63:227, 1955.

323. Van der Straeten M: Introduction, to Symposium on Bronchial Hyperreactivity, Ghent, 1980. Eur J Respir Dis 63:(Suppl 117):1, 1982.

324. Chai H, Farr RS, Froehlich LA, et al: Standardization of bronchial inhalation challenge procedures. J Allergy Clin Immunol 56:323, 1975.

325. Cockcroft D, Killian D, Mellon J, et al: Bronchial reactivity to inhaled histamine: A method and clinical survey. Clin Allergy 7:235, 1977.

326. Juniper EF, Frith PA, Dunnett C, et al: Reproducibility and comparison of response to inhaled histamine and methacholine. Thorax 33:705, 1978.

327. Sterk PJ, Fabbri LM, Quanjer PH, et al: Airway responsiveness: Standardized challenge testing with pharmacological, physical, and sensitizing stimuli in adults. Eur Respir J 16(Suppl):53, 1993.

328. Cockcroft D, Berscheid B, Murdock K: Measurement of responsiveness to inhaled histamine using FEV_1: Comparison of PC_{20} and threshold. Thorax 38:523, 1983.

329. Lam S, Wong R, Yeung M: Nonspecific bronchial reactivity in occupational asthma. J Allergy Clin Immunol 63:28, 1979.

330. Wouters EF: Total respiratory impedance measurement by forced oscillations: A noninvasive method to assess bronchial response in occupational medicine. Exp Lung Res 16:25, 1990.

331. Orehek J, Gayrard P, Smith A, et al: Airway response to carbachol in normal and asthmatic subjects: Distinction between bronchial sensitivity and reactivity. Am Rev Respir Dis 115:937, 1977.

332. Pairon JC, Iwatsubo Y, Hubert C, et al: Measurement of bronchial responsiveness by forced oscillation technique in occupational epidemiology. Eur Respir J 7:484, 1994.

333. Phagoo SB, Watson RA, Pride NB, et al: Accuracy and sensitivity of the interrupter technique for measuring airway calibre. Eur Respir J 6:996, 1993.

334. Sommer CW, Frey U, Schonli MH, et al: Specific approach on dose-response curves to inhaled carbachol assessed by the interruption technique in children. Pediatr Res 34:478, 1993.

335. Schmidt LE, Thorne PS, Watt JL, et al: Is an abbreviated bronchial challenge with histamine valid? Chest 101:141, 1992.

336. Yan K, Salome C, Woodcock A: Rapid method for measurement of bronchial responsiveness. Thorax 38:760, 1983.

337. O'Connor G, Sparrow D, Taylor D, et al: Analysis of dose-response curves to methacholine. Am Rev Respir Dis 136:1412, 1987.

338. Chinn S, Burney PG, Britton JR, et al: Comparison of $PD20$ with two alternative measures of response to histamine challenge in epidemiological studies. Eur Respir J 6:670, 1993.

339. Peat JK, Salome CM, Berry G, et al: Relation of dose-response slope to respiratory symptoms and lung function in a population study of adults living in Busselton, Western Australia. Am Rev Respir Dis 146:860, 1992.

340. Moore BJ. Hilliam CC, Verburgt LM, et al: Shape and position of the complete dose-response curve for inhaled methacholine in normal subjects. Am J Respir Crit Care Med 154:642, 1996.

341. Sterk PJ, Bel EH: Bronchial hyperresponsiveness: The need for a distinction between hypersensitivity and excessive airway narrowing. Eur Respir J 2:267, 1989.

342. Sterk PJ, Bel EH: The shape of the dose-response curve to inhaled bronchoconstrictor agents in asthma and in chronic obstructive pulmonary disease. Am Rev Respir Dis 143:1433, 1991.

343. Aerts JG, Bogaard JM, Overbeek SE, et al: Extrapolation of methacholine log-dose response curves with a cumulative Gaussian distribution function. Eur Respir J 7:895, 1994.

344. Sterk PJ, Daniel EE, Zamel N, et al: Limited bronchoconstriction to methacholine using partial flow-volume curves in nonasthmatic subjects. Am Rev Respir Dis 132:272, 1985.

345. Michoud M-C, Ghezzo H, Amyot R: A comparison of pulmonary function tests used for bronchial challenges. Bull Eur Physiopathol Respir 18:609, 1982.

346. Dehaut P, Rachiele A, Martin R, et al: Histamine dose-response curves in asthma: Reproducibility and sensitivity of different indices to assess response. Thorax 38:516, 1983.

347. Anderson S, Schoeffel R, Finney M: Evaluation of ultrasonically nebulized solutions for provocation testing in patients with asthma. Thorax 38:284, 1983.

348. Anderson SD, Smith CM: Osmotic challenges in the assessment of bronchial hyperresponsiveness. Am Rev Respir Dis 143(Suppl):43, 1991.

349. Smith CM, Anderson SD: Inhalational challenge using hypertonic saline in asthmatic subjects: A comparison with responses to hyperpnoea, methacholine, and water. Eur Respir J 3:144, 1990.

350. Daxun Z, Rafferty P, Richards R, et al: Airway refractoriness to adenosine 5'-monophosphate after repeated inhalation. J Allergy Clin Immunol 83:152, 1989.

351. Polosa R, Rajakulasingam K, Church MK, et al: Repeated inhalation of bradykinin attenuates adenosine 5'-monophosphate (AMP) induced bronchoconstriction in asthmatic airways. Eur Respir J 5:700, 1992.

352. Nichol GM, Nix A, Chung KF, et al: Characterisation of bronchoconstrictor response to sodium metabisulphite aerosol in atopic subjects with and without asthma. Thorax 44:1009, 1989.

353. Ryan G, Bolovitch M, Obminski G, et al: Standardization of inhalation provocation tests: Influence of nebulizer output, particle size, and the method of inhalation. J Allergy Clin Immunol 67:156, 1931.

354. Juniper E, Syty-Golda M, Hargreave F: Histamine inhalation tests: Inhalation of aerosol via a facemask versus a valve box with mouthpiece. Thorax 39:556, 1984.

355. Cockcroft DW, Berscheid BA: Effect of pH on bronchial response to inhaled histamine. Thorax 37:133, 1982.

356. Cockcroft D, Berscheid B: Standardization of inhalation provocation tests. Chest 82:572, 1982.

357. Hargreave F, Ryan G, Thomson N, et al: Bronchial responsiveness to histamine or methacholine in asthma measurement and clinical significance. J Allergy Clin Immunol 68:347, 1981.

358. Lowhagen O, Lindholm N: Short-term and long-term variation in bronchial response to histamine in asthmatic patients. Eur J Respir Dis 64:466, 1983.

359. Juniper E, Frith P, Hargreave F: Long-term stability of bronchial responsiveness to histamine. Thorax 37:288, 1982.

360. Rijcken B, Schouten JP, Weiss ST, et al: Long-term variability of bronchial responsiveness to histamine in a random population sample of adults. Am Rev Respir Dis 148:944, 1993.

361. Wood-Baker R, Town GI, Benning B, et al: The reproducibility and effect on non-specific airway responsiveness of inhaled prostaglandin D_2 and leukotriene D_4 in asthmatic subjects. Br J Clin Pharmacol 39:119, 1995.

362. Thomson N, Roberts R, Bandouvakis J, et al: Comparison of bronchial responses to prostaglandin F2-alpha and methacholine. J Allergy Clin Immunol 68:392, 1981.

363. Salome C, Schoeffel R, Woolcock A: Comparison of bronchial reactivity to histamine and methacholine in asthmatics. Clin Allergy 10:541, 1980.

364. Stick SM, Turner DJ, LeSouef PN: Lung function and bronchial challenges in infants: Repeatability of histamine and comparison with methacholine challenges. 16:177, 1993.

365. Weersink EJ, Elshout FJ, van Herwaarden CV, et al: Bronchial responsiveness to histamine and methacholine measured with forced expirations and with the forced oscillation technique. Respir Med 89:351, 1995.

366. Ryan G, Dolovich MB, Roberts RS, et al: Standardization of inhalation provocation tests: Two techniques of aerosol generation and inhalation compared. Am Rev Respir Dis 123:195, 1981.

367. Malo JL, Pineau L, Cartier A, et al: Reference values of the provocative concentrations of methacholine that cause 6% and 20% changes in forced expiratory volume in one second in a normal population. Am Rev Respir Dis 128:8, 1983.

368. Orehek J: The concept of airway "sensitivity" and "reactivity." Eur J Respir Dis 64(Suppl 131):27, 1983.

369. Eiser N: Calculation of data. Eur J Respir Dis 64(Suppl 131):241, 1983.

370. Walters E, Davies P, Smith A: Measurement of bronchial reactivity: A question of interpretation. Thorax 36:960, 1981.

371. Beaupre A, Malo J: Histamine dose-response curves in asthma: Relevance of the distinction between PC_{20} and reactivity in characterizing clinical state. Thorax 36:731, 1981.

372. Josephs LK, Gregg I, Mullee MA, et al: A longitudinal study of baseline FEV_1 and bronchial responsiveness in patients with asthma. Eur Respir J 5:32, 1992.

373. Cockcroft D, Ruffin R, Frith P, et al: Determinants of allergen-induced asthma: Dose of allergen, circulating IGE antibody concentration, and bronchial responsiveness to inhaled histamine. Am Rev Respir Dis 120:1053, 1979.

374. Haby MM, Anderson SD, Peat JK, et al: An exercise challenge protocol for epidemiological studies of asthma in children: Comparison with histamine challenge. Eur Respir J 7:43, 1994.

375. Steinbrugger B, Eber E, Modl M, et al: A comparison of a single-step cold-dry air challenge and a routine histamine provocation for the assessment of bronchial responsiveness in children and adolescents. Chest 108:741, 1995.

376. Backer V, Ulrik CS: Bronchial responsiveness to exercise in a random sample of 494 children and adolescents from Copenhagen. Clin Exp Allergy 22:741, 1992.

377. Deal E, McFadden E, Ingram R, et al: Hyperpnea and heat flux: Initial reaction sequence in exercise-induced asthma. J Appl Physiol 46:476, 1979.

378. O'Byrne P, Ryan G, Morris M, et al: Asthma induced by cold air and its relation to nonspecific bronchial responsiveness to methacholine. Am Rev Respir Dis 125:281, 1982.

379. Roach JM, Hurwitz KM, Argyros GJ, et al: Eucapnic voluntary hyperventilation as a bronchoprovocation technique: Comparison with methacholine inhalation in asthmatics. Chest 105:667, 1994.

380. de Benedictis FM, Canny GJ, MacLusky IB, et al: Comparison of airway reactivity induced by cold air and methacholine challenges in asthmatic children. Pediatr Pulmonol 19:326, 1995.

381. Modl M, Eber E, Steinbrugger B, et al: Comparing methods for assessing bronchial responsiveness in children: Single-step cold air challenge, multiple-step cold air challenge, and histamine provocation. Eur Respir J 8:1742, 1995.

382. Mills GH, Kyroussis D, Hamnegard CH, et al: Unilateral magnetic stimulation of the phrenic nerve. Thorax 50:1162, 1995.

383. Mador MJ, Rodis A, Magalang UJ, Ameen K: Comparison of cervical magnetic and transcutaneous phrenic nerve stimulation before and after threshold loading. Am J Respir Crit Care Med 154:448, 1996.

384. Silverman JL, Rodriquez AA: Needle electromyographic evaluation of the diaphragm. Electromyogr Clin Neurophysiol 34:509, 1994.

385. Saadeh PB, Crisafulli CF, Sosner J, Wolf E: Needle electromyography of the diaphragm: A new technique. Muscle Nerve 16:15, 1993.

385a. Gea J, Espadaler JM, Guiu R, et al: Diaphragmatic activity induced by cortical stimulation: Surface versus esophageal electrodes. J Appl Physiol 74:655, 1993.

386. Gandevia SC, Plassman BL: Responses in human intercostal and truncal muscles to motor cortical and spinal stimulation. Respir Physiol 73:325, 1988.

387. Gandevia SC, Rothwell JC: Activation of the human diaphragm from the motor cortex. J Physiol 384:109, 1987.

388. Zifko U, Remtulla H, Power K, et al: Transcortical and cervical magnetic stimulation with recording of the diaphragm. Muscle Nerve. 19:614, 1996.

389. Petitjean M, Bellemare F: Phonomyogram of the diaphragm during unilateral and bilateral phrenic nerve stimulation and changes with fatigue. Muscle Nerve 17:1201, 1994.

390. Muller-Felber W, Riepl R, Reimers CD, et al: Combined ultrasonographic and neurographic examination: A new technique to evaluate phrenic nerve function. Electromyogr Clin Neurophysiol 33:335, 1993.

391. Ueki J, De Bruin PF, Pride NB: *In vivo* assessment of diaphragm contraction by ultrasound in normal subjects. Thorax 50:1157, 1995.

392. Chen R, Collins SJ, Remtulla H, et al: Needle EMG of the human diaphragm: Power spectral analysis in normal subjects. Muscle Nerve 19:324, 1996.

393. Beck J, Sinderby C, Weinberg J, Grassino A: Effects of muscle-to-electrode distance on the human diaphragm electromyogram. J Appl Physiol 79:975, 1995.

394. Badier M, Guillot C, Lagier-Tessonnier F, et al: EMG power spectrum of respiratory muscles during static contraction in healthy man. Muscle Nerve 16:601, 1993.

395. Mador MJ, Kufel TJ: Effect of inspiratory muscle fatigue on inspiratory muscle relaxation rates in healthy subjects. Chest 102:1767, 1992.

396. Kyroussis D, Mills G, Hamnegard CH, et al: Inspiratory muscle relaxation rate assessed from sniff nasal pressure. Thorax 49:1127, 1994.

397. Kyroussis D, Mills GH, Polkey MI, et al: Effect of maximum ventilation on abdominal muscle relaxation rate. Thorax 51:510, 1996.

PART **III**

RADIOLOGIC SIGNS OF CHEST DISEASE

CHAPTER 18

Increased Lung Density

PREDOMINANTLY AIR-SPACE DISEASE, 434
  Radiologic Features of Air-Space Disease, 435
    Distribution Characteristics, 435
    Margination, 437
    The Air Bronchogram, 437
    The Air Bronchiologram and Air Alveologram, 438
    The Air-Space Nodule, 438
    The Time Factor, 438
    Absence of Atelectasis, 439
PREDOMINANTLY INTERSTITIAL DISEASE, 439
  Concepts of Radiologic Anatomy, 439
  Radiologic Patterns of Diffuse Interstitial Disease, 441
    Septal Pattern, 441
    Reticular Pattern, 444
    Nodular Pattern, 447
    Reticulonodular Pattern, 453
    Ground-Glass Pattern, 453
COMBINED AIR-SPACE AND INTERSTITIAL DISEASE, 454
LIMITATIONS OF THE PATTERN APPROACH, 455
  Modifying Factors, 455
  Nonspecific Radiologic Findings, 456
  Comparison of Chest Radiography and High-Resolution Computed Tomography, 456
GENERAL SIGNS IN DISEASES THAT INCREASE LUNG DENSITY, 457
  Characteristics of the Border of a Pulmonary Lesion, 457
  Change in Position of Interlobar Fissures, 459
  Cavitation, 461
  Calcification and Ossification, 463
    Local Parenchymal Calcification, 463
    Diffuse Parenchymal Calcification, 467
    Lymph Node Calcification, 474
    Calcification in Other Intrathoracic Sites, 474
  Distribution of Disease Within the Lungs, 474
  Radiologic Localization of Pulmonary Disease—The Silhouette Sign, 478
  The Time Factor in Radiologic Diagnosis, 479
LINE SHADOWS, 479
  Septal Lines, 480
  Tubular Shadows (Bronchial Wall Shadows), 483
  Linear Opacities Extending from Peripheral Parenchymal Lesions to the Hila or Visceral Pleura, 483
  Parenchymal Scarring, 483
  Linear Atelectasis, 483

The integration of information obtained from systematic interpretation of the chest radiograph and careful analysis of the clinical status of the patient yields a high degree of diagnostic accuracy in most chest diseases. As a rule, the radiologist should glean as much information as possible from an objective assessment of the radiograph *before* attempting clinical correlation; the radiographic pattern of disease may be sufficiently distinctive that an etiologic diagnosis can be made with reasonable certainty on that evidence alone. This diagnostic impression can then be confirmed by correlation with the information acquired from the clinical history and physical examination and, in selected cases, the results of laboratory tests and pulmonary function studies.

This chapter describes the basic radiologic signs associated with parenchymal opacification and includes a consideration of such features as the size, number, and density of pulmonary lesions; their homogeneity, sharpness of definition, and anatomic location and distribution; and the presence or absence of cavitation or calcification. Since knowledge of the pathogenesis and pathology of a disease process is necessary for an understanding of the radiologic images it creates, wherever possible we relate the signs to their gross and microscopic characteristics and to the mechanisms by which they occur (Fig. 18–1).

The various anatomic structures of the lung can be considered to consist of two functional units: that concerned with *conduction* (bronchi, blood vessels other than capillaries, and lymphatics) and that concerned with *gas exchange* (lung parenchyma, made up of peripheral air spaces, accompanying vessels, and extravascular interstitial tissue). Excluding the vascular system, it is obvious that all pulmonary disease that increases lung density involves change in one or both of two components, the air spaces and extravascular interstitial tissue. Although most diseases that increase lung density involve both the air spaces and interstitial tissue to a variable extent, it is helpful to divide these diseases into three general groups, depending on which component is predominantly involved: (1) *air spaces*, the air being replaced by liquid, cells, or a combination of the two (consolidation) or absorbed and not replaced (atelectasis, discussed separately on page 513); (2) *interstitial tissues*; and (3) *combined air spaces and interstitial tissues*.

The concept that pulmonary parenchymal opacities can be divided into those in which the involvement is predominantly interstitial or predominantly air space has been criticized on two grounds:[1–3] the majority of diseases affect both anatomic compartments to some degree, and the radiologic appearance may occasionally be misleading. Although these criticisms have some validity, we believe that the division is nevertheless useful if one accepts the proviso that the term *air-space pattern* indicates *predominant* involvement of the parenchymal air spaces and that a linear, reticular, or nodular pattern indicates *predominant* involvement of the intersti-

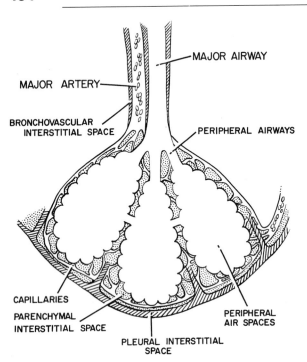

Figure 18–1. Diagrammatic Representation of the Lung. The diagram depicts the components of the lung that are involved in the majority of pulmonary diseases—the large and small airways; the peripheral air spaces (including communicating channels); the arteries, veins, and capillaries; and the bronchovascular, pleural, and parenchymal interstitial space. Throughout this and the following two chapters, this diagram of the normal lung is reproduced alongside diagrams depicting disturbances in morphology.

tium. Bearing this in mind, pattern recognition becomes a logical and useful technique in radiologic interpretation.

PREDOMINANTLY AIR-SPACE DISEASE

Parenchymal consolidation can be defined as the replacement of gas within the air spaces by liquid, cells, or a combination of the two (Fig. 18–2). Such air-space disease is characterized on radiographs and CT scans by the presence of one or more fairly homogeneous opacities associated with

obscuration of the pulmonary vessels and little or no volume loss (Fig. 18–3).[4, 5] The margins of the opacities are poorly defined except where the consolidation abuts the pleura. Air-containing bronchi (air bronchograms) are frequently visualized; localized small lucencies caused by nonopacified bronchioles (air bronchiolograms) or multiple nonopacified alveoli (air alveolograms) and localized round areas of consolidation measuring 10 mm in diameter or less (air-space nodules) may also be identified.

A number of terms have been used to describe the pattern of air-space disease, including consolidation, air-

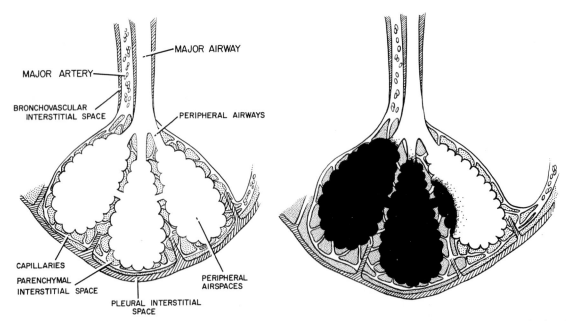

Figure 18–2. The Lung Diagram: Peripheral Air-Space Consolidation. Exudate has filled two of the air spaces and is flowing into the third via interacinar channels. Volume is unaffected, and the airways are patent. The parenchymal interstitial tissue is increased in amount around the consolidated air spaces.

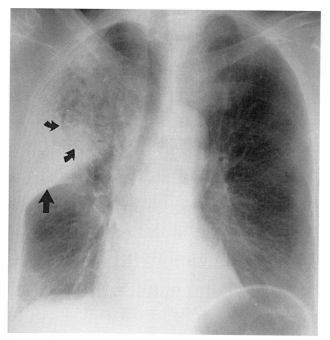

Figure 18–3. Air-Space Consolidation. A posteroanterior chest radiograph in a 64-year-old woman demonstrates extensive air-space consolidation in the right upper lobe. The findings consist of confluent fluffy opacities with poorly defined margins except where the consolidation abuts the horizontal fissure *(straight arrow)*. Note the presence of air bronchograms *(curved arrows)*. A small right pleural effusion is also evident. The patient had acute air-space pneumonia caused by *Streptococcus pneumoniae*.

space consolidation, parenchymal consolidation, air-space shadows, and air-space disease.[4] These terms represent inferred conclusions applicable when the visualized opacity can be attributed with reasonable certainty to air-space filling. Although the air space is usually filled with fluid or cells, occasionally extracellular material such as lipoprotein (as in alveolar proteinosis) fills the air spaces.

Radiologic Features of Air-Space Disease

The radiologic signs of air-space disease may result from filling of the air spaces or encroachment on them by an expanding interstitial process. Both these mechanisms can appear in an almost pure form, exemplified respectively by idiopathic pulmonary hemorrhage and lymphoma. On the other hand, in many situations both the interstitium and air spaces are involved simultaneously, in which case either an air-space or an interstitial pattern can predominate.

Distribution Characteristics

Air-space consolidation may be segmental or nonsegmental in distribution. In widely disseminated disease such as may be seen in acute pulmonary edema, adult respiratory distress syndrome, or diffuse pulmonary hemorrhage, such lack of segmental distribution is not unexpected (Fig. 18–4). However, intersegmental spread commonly occurs even in

Figure 18–4. "Bat's wing" Pattern of Pulmonary Edema. A posteroanterior radiograph demonstrates consolidation of the parahilar and "medullary" portions of both lungs, which creates a "bat's wing" or "butterfly" appearance; the "cortex" of both lungs is relatively unaffected. The consolidation is fairly homogeneous and is associated with a well-defined air bronchogram on both sides. This 59-year-old man had suffered a massive myocardial infarct 48 hours previously.

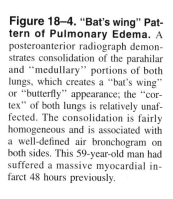

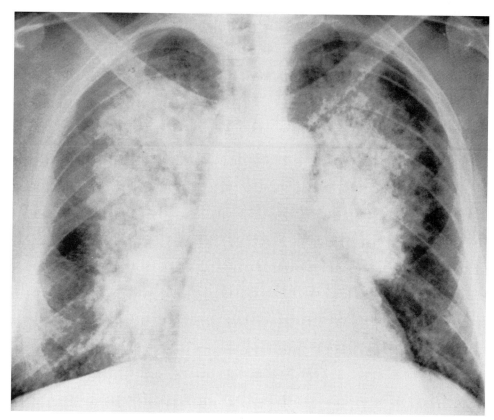

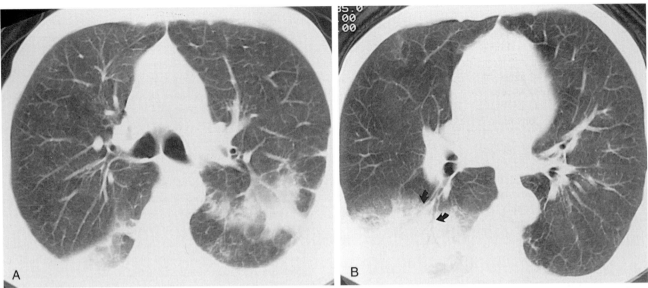

Figure 18–5. Aspiration Pneumonia. CT scans at the level of the right upper lobe bronchus *(A)* and the middle lobe bronchus *(B)* demonstrate foci of consolidation involving the apicoposterior segment of the left upper lobe and the superior segment of the right lower lobe. Note the presence of air bronchograms *(arrows)*. The patient was a 70-year-old man.

localized air-space disease; for example, in acute pneumococcal pneumonia, exudate typically spreads throughout the lung periphery via channels of collateral ventilation. Consequently, predominantly air-space diseases are characteristically *nonsegmental* in distribution, an observation of importance in establishing the pathogenesis of the disease process and in suggesting an etiologic diagnosis: nonsegmental or lobar pneumonia is most commonly caused by *Streptococcus pneumoniae* and less often by *Klebsiella pneumoniae, Legionella* species, or *Mycobacterium tuberculosis* (*see* Fig. 18–3).

By contrast with these conditions, processes that are intimately associated with the vascular or tracheobronchial tree usually display a striking *segmental* or peribronchial distribution. For example, large pleural-based pulmonary infarcts and foci of aspiration pneumonia typically have a segmental distribution; the latter usually affects multiple segments, the particular areas of lung involved being largely dependent on the patient's position at the time of aspiration (Fig. 18–5). Infection by *Staphylococcus aureus, Streptococcus pyogenes,* and various gram negative-organisms (bronchopneumonia) also characteristically has a patchy, predomi-

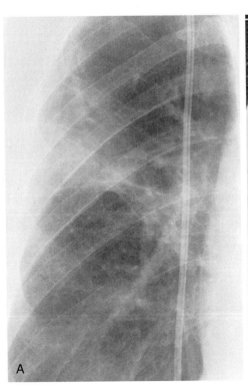

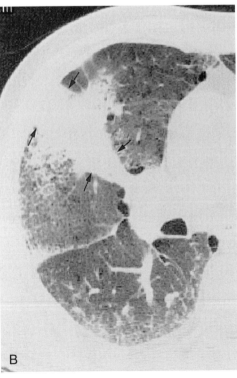

Figure 18–6. Subsegmental Consolidation. A view of the right lung from a posteroanterior chest radiograph *(A)* shows a wedge-shaped pleural-based area of consolidation in the right upper lobe. An HRCT scan *(B)* also demonstrates a subsegmental area of dense consolidation *(arrows)* that extends into the adjacent parenchyma. The appearance is consistent with a hemorrhagic infarct. The patient was an immunocompromised 54-year-old woman with angioinvasive aspergillosis.

nantly peribronchial distribution. It should be noted, however, that a particular organism may produce different patterns of consolidation. For example, although *S. pneumoniae* is characteristically associated with acute air-space pneumonia, it may also cause bronchopneumonia; similarly, infection by *Aspergillus* species may result in subsegmental or segmental hemorrhagic infarcts (Fig. 18–6) or predominantly peribronchial consolidation as a result of bronchopneumonia (Fig. 18–7).

On HRCT, areas of air-space consolidation can often be seen to be marginated by interlobular septa (Fig. 18–8).[6] Single or multiple spared lobules may be present within areas of massive consolidation.[6] Involvement of a secondary lobule or a cluster of lobules with normal adjacent parenchyma is particularly common in bronchopneumonia,[7] which is thus also known as lobular pneumonia.

Margination

The edge characteristics of air-space–filling processes often show poor margination on the chest radiograph.[8] This feature is a consequence of the spreading and coalescing wave of consolidation with partial filling of the air spaces so that the x-ray beam fails to detect a sharp border between involved and uninvolved parenchyma. The clearest example of this phenomenon is the "butterfly" or "bat's wing" appearance of acute air-space edema or hemorrhage.

The Air Bronchogram

In acute air-space pneumonia, consolidation usually begins in the subpleural parenchyma, the exudate rapidly spreading to surround bronchi as it advances towards the hilum. Since the consolidation is entirely parenchymal, air in the bronchi is not displaced. This situation results in contrast between the air within the bronchial tree and the surrounding airless parenchyma, so the normally invisible bronchial air column becomes visible on the radiograph (*see* Fig. 18–3, page 435). This important sign was described originally by Fleischner[9, 10] in 1927 and was aptly named the *air bronchogram* sign by Felson.[11]

Two situations must exist for an air bronchogram to be identified: the airways must contain air and the surrounding lung parenchyma must have a markedly reduced air content or be airless. The latter can occur as a result of either replacement of parenchymal air by liquid or tissue (consolidation) or its absorption (atelectasis); an air bronchogram

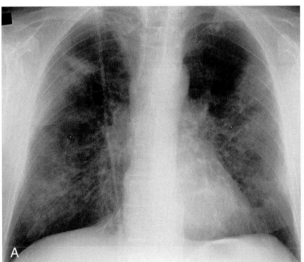

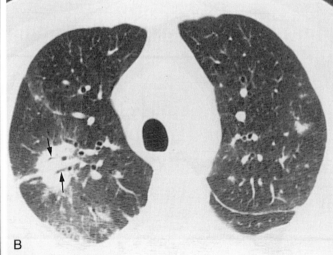

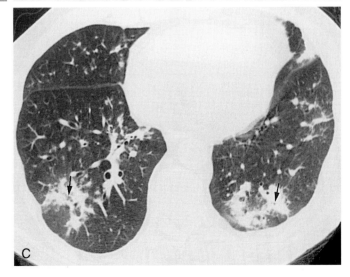

Figure 18–7. Bronchopneumonia. A posteroanterior chest radiograph *(A)* demonstrates patchy bilateral areas of consolidation. HRCT scans (*B* and *C*) demonstrate the predominant peribronchial distribution of the areas of consolidation. Air bronchograms are clearly identified within the areas of consolidation *(arrows)*. The patient was a 55-year-old man with acute myelogenous leukemia and pathologically proven bronchopneumonia caused by *Aspergillus*.

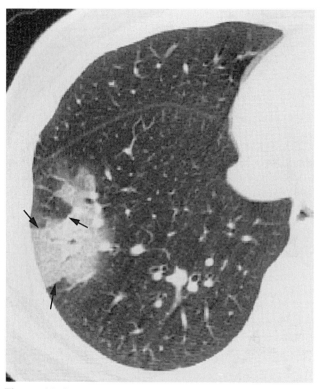

Figure 18–8. Pulmonary Hemorrhage. An HRCT scan in a 29-year-old woman demonstrates a focal area of consolidation in the right lower lobe caused by pulmonary hemorrhage. Several of the margins are clearly outlined by interlobular septa *(arrows)*, a feature leading to sharp demarcation between involved and uninvolved secondary pulmonary lobules.

may be seen in either circumstance, *but only when the supplying bronchus is not occluded.* Most diseases associated with air-space consolidation show this sign, although in some—for example, pulmonary infarction—it may be only temporary because of early filling of airways by blood or exudate.

It is important to recognize that although an air bronchogram is an almost invariable finding in air-space consolidation from whatever cause, it is not restricted to this state. As discussed in Chapter 20 (*see* page 513), four mechanisms can result in atelectasis, the most common being bronchial obstruction; in this situation, an air bronchogram cannot exist since the distal airways no longer communicate with the mouth. In the other three types of atelectasis—relaxation, cicatrization, and adhesive—bronchi are not obstructed; since the parenchyma surrounding air-containing bronchi is of reduced air content or airless, an air bronchogram is anticipated. For example, the collapsed lung associated with a large pneumothorax (relaxation atelectasis) invariably shows an air bronchogram; in fact, its absence indicates central bronchial obstruction associated with the pneumothorax. Similarly, both bronchiectasis and radiation fibrosis—varieties of cicatrization atelectasis—are often associated with air bronchograms. "Pure" interstitial lung disease of sufficient severity, such as talc granulomatosis accompanying long-standing intravenous drug abuse and the fibrotic stage of sarcoidosis, can also have prominent air bronchograms.[12]

The Air Bronchiologram and Air Alveologram

The identification of minute radiolucencies within an area of air-space consolidation relates histopathologically to incompletely filled bronchioles (air bronchiologram) and alveoli ("air alveologram") (Fig. 18–9). Although neither of these structures is normally visible on the chest radiograph or CT, when the air spaces become partly consolidated, some are rendered visible. Thus, the demonstration of such radiolucencies is analogous to an air bronchogram sign and carries the same pathogenetic implications. Despite what the term *air alveologram* might suggest—the depiction of air within an alveolus—this is clearly impossible: since there are at least 300 million of these structures in the human lung, their visibility must result from the air content of a multitude of adjacent alveoli.

The Air-Space Nodule

The presence of nodular lesions in air-space disease has been recognized since 1924 (Fig. 18–9).[13] Traditionally, such nodules have been classified into three types: acinar, subacinar, and spokewheel.[8, 14] An *acinar nodule* has been defined as a focal area of consolidation that shows the following three features: (1) a nodular shape measuring 4 to 10 mm in diameter; (2) poor margination (the lesion remaining discrete enough to permit individual identification); and (3) the presence of small radiolucencies caused by air within air spaces in the nodule.[14] A *subacinar nodule* has the same general characteristics as an acinar opacity except that many more radiolucencies are visible within it; thus, the two are distinguished by quantitative features.[14] The *spokewheel nodule*, the third and least frequent variety, measures 4 to 10 mm in diameter and shows a central, relatively large lucency from which smaller, linear radiolucencies radiate peripherally.[14]

Although small nodular opacities undoubtedly occur in air-space disease,[8, 14, 15] in practice it is not possible to determine on the radiograph whether they represent true acinar shadows or shadows that merely resemble acini. In fact, radiologic-pathologic correlation studies of bronchopneumonia have demonstrated that the "acinar nodules" seen on chest radiographs before death and on radiographs of postmortem lung slices represent consolidation of respiratory bronchioles and surrounding alveoli, the distal air spaces being spared.[15, 16] Similarly, air-space nodules related to endobronchial spread of tuberculosis have been shown to be characteristically centrilobular in distribution and affect the terminal and respiratory bronchioles and adjacent alveoli.[6, 15] Thus, so-called acinar nodules do not in fact represent true acinar consolidation, and we consider the more generic "air-space nodule" preferable to the terms acinar, subacinar, and spokewheel nodules. (It should also be noted that poorly defined 4- to 10-mm-diameter nodular opacities seen on the radiograph or CT are occasionally the result of interstitial rather than air-space disease [Fig. 18–10].[17])

The Time Factor

The rapidity with which consolidation resolves can be of great help in suggesting its etiology. For example, an air-space pattern that clears over a period of hours or several days is certain evidence of pulmonary edema or hemorrhage.

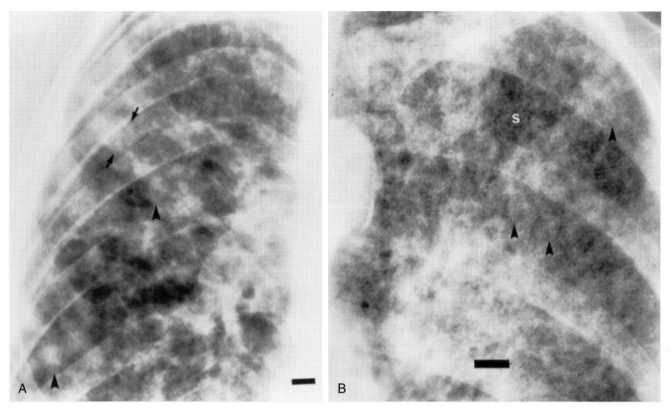

Figure 18–9. Air-Space Nodules. A detail view of the right lung from a posteroanterior (PA) chest radiograph of a patient with bronchioloalveolar carcinoma *(A)* shows several air-space nodules. An air-space nodule *(arrowheads)* is characterized by poor margination, nodular shape, 4- to 10-mm size, and intranodular radiolucencies caused by air within bronchioles and alveoli. Confluence of nodules creates a larger air-space opacity (between *arrows*). The *bar* represents 1 cm. A detail view of the left lung from a PA chest radiograph of a patient with acute air-space edema *(B)* demonstrates air-space nodules *(arrowheads)* containing radiolucencies (air alveolograms). Concomitant background stippling (S) is a prominent feature. The *bar* represents 1 cm.

By contrast, air-space disease that persists over time, sometimes for weeks or months, is usually caused by infection, aspiration, bronchioloalveolar carcinoma, or lymphoma.

Absence of Atelectasis

In distal air-space consolidation, lung volume is usually normal since air is replaced by an equal or almost equal quantity of liquid or tissue. Furthermore, since the pathogenetic process occurs predominantly within the parenchyma, airways leading to affected portions of lung remain patent; thus, there is no reason for collapse to occur before the air spaces are filled. Again, there are occasional exceptions to this rule; for example, in pulmonary infarction, volume is often lost despite patent airways, presumably because of regional surfactant deficit.

PREDOMINANTLY INTERSTITIAL DISEASE

A large number of pulmonary diseases are characterized by predominant involvement of the interstitium. In some, the associated radiographic pattern is so distinctive that a specific diagnosis can be strongly suggested on the basis of the appearance alone; however, in the majority, diagnosis by radiographic appearance alone is not possible.[2, 3] HRCT allows much better assessment of the pattern, distribution, and severity of interstitial abnormalities than is possible on the chest radiograph[18, 19] and often allows a specific diagnosis

even when the radiograph is normal or shows only nonspecific findings.[20–22] Nevertheless, it cannot be overemphasized that the findings on HRCT, similar to those of the chest radiograph, must always be interpreted in the context of the clinical history, laboratory findings, and pulmonary function tests. Moreover, although the procedure is superior to the chest radiograph in the differential diagnosis of interstitial lung diseases, lung biopsy may be required to establish a definitive diagnosis.

Concepts of Radiologic Anatomy

The interstitium consists of a continuum of connective tissue that provides support to the lungs. Anatomically and radiologically, it can be divided into three compartments: bronchoarterial (axial), parenchymal, and peripheral.[23, 24] The bronchoarterial (axial) interstitium surrounds the bronchoarterial bundles from the hila to the point at which bronchiolar walls become intimately related to lung parenchyma (i.e., alveolated). Pulmonary arteries and bronchi with their accompanying bronchial vessels, nerves, and lymphatics lie in this loose connective tissue. A similar sheath exists around the veins within the lung; this interstitial space is continuous with the interlobular septa and the pleural interstitial space. Together, these structures constitute the peripheral interstitium. Finally, there is a small interstitial space in the walls of the alveoli themselves that is referred to as the parenchymal

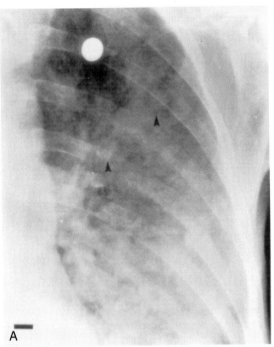

Figure 18–10. Interstitial Lung Disease Simulating Air-Space Disease. A close-up of the left upper lobe from a posteroanterior chest radiograph of a patient with metastatic calcification associated with chronic renal insufficiency *(A)* shows multiple air-space nodules *(arrowheads)*, some coalescent, and a faint air bronchogram against a background of fine reticulation or stippling. The features are those of a primary air-space process. However, low-power *(B)* and high-power *(C)* histologic sections obtained at autopsy reveal a normal complement of alveolar septa that are diffusely, although minimally thickened by interstitial calcification (dark linear staining material, *arrowheads*). The air spaces are normal. (From Genereux GP: Med Radiogr Photogr 61:2, 1985.)

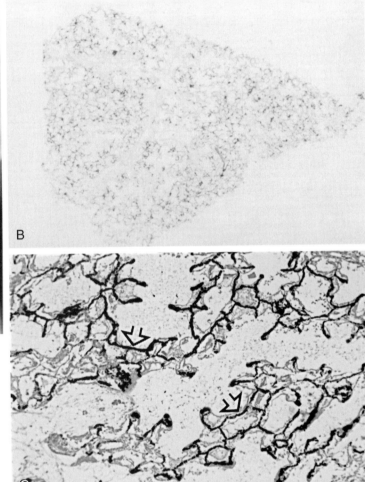

interstitial space, in keeping with our use of the term *parenchyma* to denote the gas-exchanging part of the lung.

Since interstitial diseases of the lung may affect all "compartments" to some degree, it might be argued that their subdivision is arbitrary and of little practical importance. From a diagnostic point of view, however, we have found their distinction to be of value, chiefly because their individual involvement usually produces distinguishable radiographic and HRCT patterns and therefore different diagnostic considerations. For example, one of the common abnormalities affecting the interstitial tissues of the lung is pulmonary edema. Studies of rapidly frozen dog lungs in which pulmonary venous pressures were raised by graded levels have shown a definite sequence of fluid accumulation in various pulmonary "compartments" (Fig. 18–11):[25] fluid appears first in the interstitial connective tissue compartment around the large blood vessels and airways and is followed

by thickening of the alveolar wall; it is not until the interstitial compartment is well filled that alveolar edema appears. This anatomic localization in the perivascular and interlobular septal interstitium produces the typical radiographic pattern of loss of the normal sharp definition of the pulmonary vascular markings and thickening of the interlobular septa (B lines of Kerley) (Fig. 18–12). Edema fluid that accumulates in the parenchymal interstitial tissues in these circumstances usually produces little or no discernible radiographic change. A similar distribution of disease occurs in lymphangitic spread of carcinoma,[26] some pneumoconioses,[27] and lymphoma (Fig. 18–13).[28]

Radiologic Patterns of Diffuse Interstitial Disease

Interstitial lung disease causes five radiologic patterns: septal, reticular, nodular, reticulonodular, and ground glass. Although these patterns can be clearly visualized on HRCT and correlate with specific histopathologic findings,[18, 19, 29] superimposition of structures makes interpretation considerably more difficult on the chest radiograph. For example, it might be logical to assume that a network of opacities forming a reticular pattern should be produced by linear accumulations of tissue within the lung or that a nodular pattern should be produced by multiple nodular lesions. However, such an assumption is only partly valid: the effect of *superimposition* of many abnormalities means that a reticular or nodular pattern on the radiograph can represent either a true or a summated image. For example, superimposition of small nodules can result in the formation of curvilinear and nodular opacities (i.e., false reticulonodularity).[30] Similarly, summation of linear opacities seen *en face* will appear radiographically as a reticular pattern but may simulate nodules when seen end-on. Thus, a reticulonodular pattern on the radiograph may result from a combination of a reticular pattern and nodules or be caused by linear opacities seen *en face* and end-on.[30]

A semiquantitative scheme that uses the terminology of the International Labor Office (ILO) for describing the pneumoconioses has been proposed for the assessment of diffuse interstitial lung disease.[2] Similar to that of the ILO, this scheme uses the designations p, q, and r to describe the various sizes of rounded opacities (corresponding to our nodular pattern) and s, t, and u to categorize irregular opacities (corresponding to our reticular pattern). It also includes a third group of opacities called *x, y,* and *z* that correspond to the reticulonodular pattern. Although this classification provides an understandable and quantifiable system of communication and a tool for teaching, clinical research, and epidemiologic studies, we believe that the more traditional nomenclature is preferable in daily clinical practice.

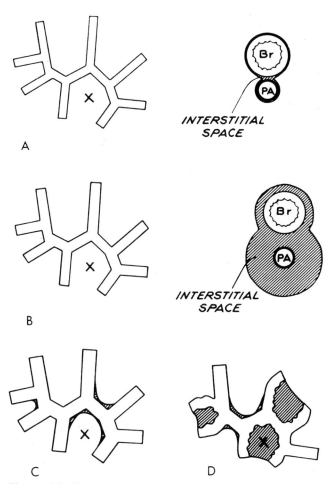

Figure 18–11. Schematic Representation of the Sequence of Fluid Accumulation in Acute Pulmonary Edema. *A,* Normal lung (alveolar wall and alveoli on the *left,* bronchovascular bundle on the *right*); *B,* interstitial edema in which fluid accumulates preferentially in the interstitial space around the conducting blood vessels and airways without affecting the alveolar walls; *C,* early alveolar edema showing the interstitial spaces filled and fluid overflowing into alveoli, preferentially at the corners at which the curvature is greatest; *D,* alveolar flooding in which individual alveoli have reached the critical configuration at which existing inflation pressure can no longer maintain stability and the alveolar gas volume rapidly passes to a new configuration with much reduced curvature. (Slightly modified from Staub NE, Nagano H, Pearce ML: J Appl Physiol 22:227, 1967, with permission.)

Septal Pattern

A septal pattern results from thickening of the interlobular septa, that is, the tissue that separates the secondary pulmonary lobules. Normally, no septal lines can be identified on the radiograph and only a few can be seen on HRCT, mostly in the anterior and lower aspects of the lower lobes.[31] When thickened, interlobular septa (septal lines) are visualized on the radiograph as short (1 to 2 cm) lines perpendicu-

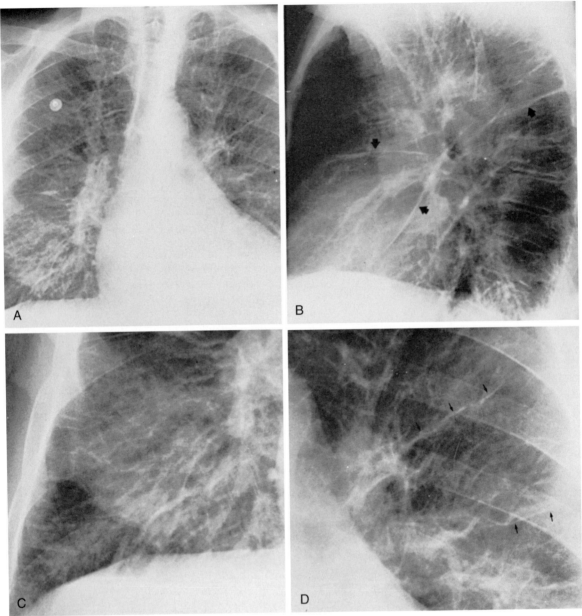

Figure 18–12. Interstitial Pulmonary Edema. Posteroanterior *(A)* and lateral *(B)* radiographs reveal multiple linear opacities throughout both lungs that are seen to better advantage in magnified views of the right lower *(C)* and left upper *(D)* lungs. These lines consist of a combination of long septal lines (Kerley A), predominantly in the midlung zones *(arrows in D),* and shorter peripheral septal lines (Kerley B). In lateral projection *(B),* the interlobar fissures are very prominent *(arrows)* and represent pleural edema. Twenty-four hours later, the edema had cleared completely.

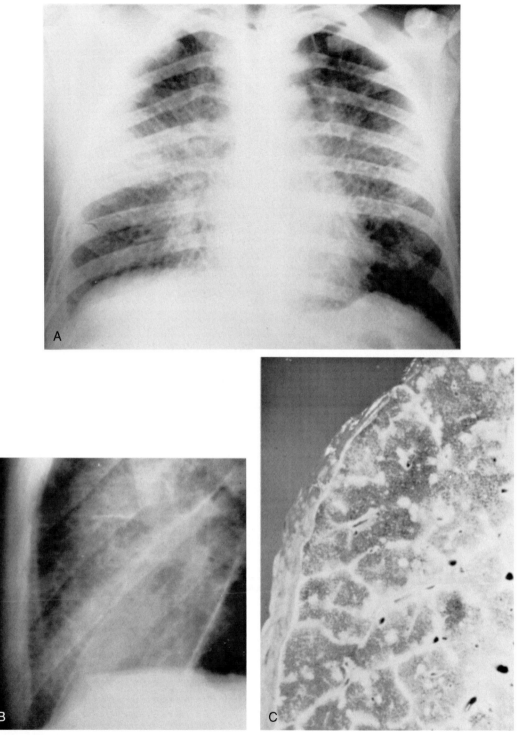

Figure 18–13. Interstitial Non-Hodgkin's Lymphoma. A posteroanterior radiograph *(A)* demonstrates extensive involvement of both lungs by a rather coarse reticular pattern. The severity of interstitial abnormality is reflected in a loss of definition of vascular markings throughout both lungs reminiscent of severe interstitial edema. A magnified view of the retrosternal area from a lateral radiograph *(B)* reveals a coarse network of linear opacities, many of which are oriented perpendicular to the plane of the sternum in the form of septal lines. A photograph of the anterior portion of the lung *(C)* removed at autopsy reveals extensive thickening of the interlobular septa and perivascular interstitial tissue. The patient was an 18-year-old man with non-Hodgkin's lymphoma.

lar to the pleura and continuous with it (Kerley B lines) or as longer (2 to 6 cm) lines oriented toward the hila (Kerley A lines) (Fig. 18–14). On HRCT they can be seen as short lines that extend to the pleura in the lung periphery and as polygonal arcades outlining one or more pulmonary lobules in more central lung regions (Fig. 18–15).[31, 32]

The presence of septal lines as the predominant radiologic abnormality effectively restricts the diagnostic considerations to hydrostatic pulmonary edema or malignancy (either lymphangitic spread of carcinoma or lymphoma), usually with simultaneous involvement of the bronchoarterial interstitium. The distinction between edema and cancer can often be determined on the basis of clinical findings; however, in cases in which there is doubt, the HRCT appearance may be helpful in differentiation—interlobular septal thickening as a result of pulmonary edema is usually smooth, whereas malignancy is frequently associated with a nodular component (Fig. 18–16).[18, 33, 34] Although septal thickening may also be seen in idiopathic pulmonary fibrosis, sarcoidosis, and alveolar proteinosis, it is usually not the main abnormality.[35–37] It should be noted that apparent thickening of interlobular septa on HRCT occasionally results from disease affecting the perilobular alveoli on both sides of a normal septum, particularly in idiopathic pulmonary fibrosis[6, 29] and less commonly in alveolar microlithiasis.[38]

Reticular Pattern

A reticular pattern consists of innumerable interlacing line shadows that suggest a mesh (Fig. 18–17).[5] The precise pattern depends on several variables, the two most important being the degree of interstitial thickening and its effect on the adjacent parenchymal air spaces. It is useful to subdivide the reticular pattern into three categories according to the size of the "mesh":[2, 5] (1) *fine reticulation*, which simulates a very fine mesh (e.g., as in a nylon stocking); (2) *coarse reticulation*, which is characterized by large cystic spaces 1 cm or more in diameter that are ringed by soft tissue; and (3) *medium reticulation*, which is characterized by 3- to 10-mm spaces between the reticular mesh.

A reticular pattern on the chest radiograph may be the result of summation of smooth or irregular linear opacities, cystic spaces, or both. Although distinction between these abnormalities is often difficult on the radiograph, it can be

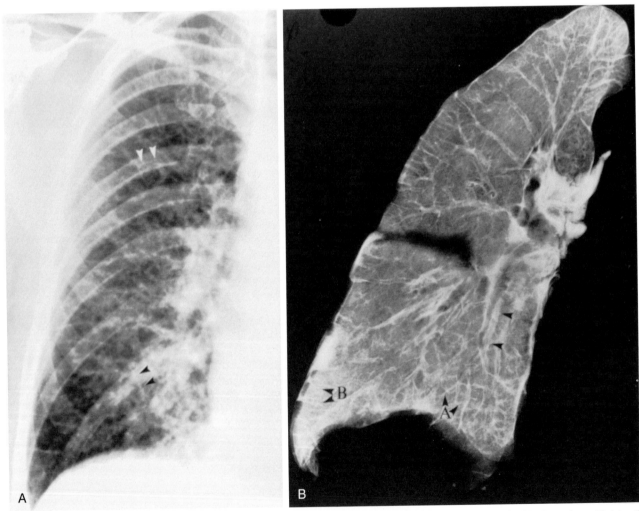

Figure 18–14. Septal Interstitial Pattern. A detail view of the right lung from a posteroanterior chest radiograph *(A)* of a patient with interstitial edema shows thickening and loss of definition of the bronchovascular bundles; Kerley A and B lines are visible *(arrowheads)*. A sliced, inflated postmortem specimen *(B)* from another patient with interstitial edema reveals enlargement of the bronchovascular bundles *(arrowheads)* and both A lines (A) and B lines (B).

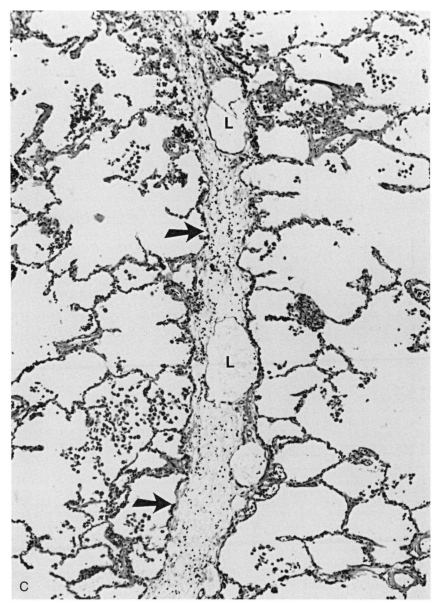

Figure 18–14 *Continued.* *C,* A histologic section shows thickening *(arrow)* of an interlobular septum. The radiologic demonstration of Kerley lines is related to a combination of widening of the septa as a result of accumulation of interstitial fluid and lymphatic (L) distention and maintenance of surrounding aerated lung (note the absence of edema within the alveoli). (*A* and *B* from Genereux GP: Med Radiogr Photogr 61:2, 1985. Reprinted courtesy Eastman Kodak Company.)

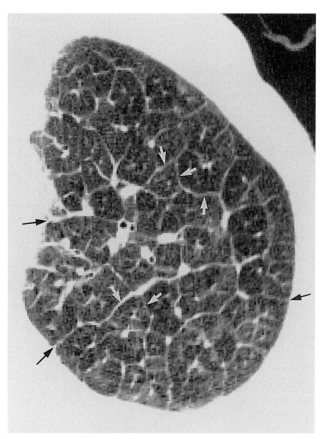

Figure 18–15. Interlobular Septal Thickening. An HRCT scan targeted to the left upper lobe demonstrates extensive interlobular septal thickening. The thickened septa can be identified as lines *(black arrows)* perpendicular to the pleura and extending to it and, more centrally, as polygonal arcades *(white arrows)* outlining the secondary pulmonary lobules. The patient was a 77-year-old woman with interstitial pulmonary edema as a result of congestive heart failure.

readily made on HRCT. A reticular pattern caused by smooth linear opacities is most commonly seen in interstitial pulmonary edema. Pulmonary fibrosis is most frequently associated with irregular thickening of interlobular septa and the presence of intralobular linear opacities (Fig. 18–18).[35, 39, 40] (The latter reflect thickening of the interstitium within the secondary pulmonary lobule and, when numerous, result in a fine reticular pattern.[41]) Cystic air spaces can be defined as enlarged foci of peripheral air-containing lung surrounded by a wall of variable thickness and composition.[5] They may be present without associated fibrosis, as in lymphangioleiomyomatosis (Fig. 18–19),[42] or may represent end-stage fibrosis (honeycombing), as in idiopathic pulmonary fibrosis, Langerhans' cell histiocytosis, asbestosis, and sarcoidosis.[5, 43]

Although pulmonary edema often leads to a predominant linear pattern characterized by the presence of septal (Kerley B) lines, a fine reticular pattern is also frequently seen. HRCT in patients with interstitial edema demonstrates thickening of the interlobular septal and bronchoarterial interstitium and intralobular linear opacities, changes that are usually most marked in the central and dependent lung regions.[44, 45] Summation of these abnormalities results in the fine reticular pattern seen on the chest radiograph. Other causes of a fine reticular pattern that develops acutely are viral and *Mycoplasma* pneumonia.

Chronic processes associated with a fine reticular pattern include chronic interstitial pulmonary edema (as may be seen in mitral stenosis), asbestosis, idiopathic pulmonary fibrosis, and interstitial pneumonitis associated with connective tissue diseases. The last two of these processes are characterized initially on the chest radiograph by a fine reticular pattern involving mainly the lower lung zones. As disease progresses, the reticular pattern becomes coarser and the process more diffuse. HRCT scans demonstrate intralobular linear opacities, irregular thickening of the interlobular septa, and honeycombing predominantly in the subpleural lung regions and the lung bases.[18, 39] Other findings associated with fibrosis include distortion of the underlying lung architecture and dilatation of the bronchi and bronchioles within the areas of fibrosis (traction bronchiectasis and bronchiolectasis).[39, 46]

A medium or coarse reticular pattern is seen most commonly in severe interstitial pulmonary fibrosis and often reflects the presence of honeycombing. The latter term was first used in 1949;[47] pathologically, it refers to an advanced stage of fibrosis in which normal lung is replaced by cystic spaces whose walls consist of a variable amount of fibrous tissue (Fig. 18–20). The spaces are usually 0.3 to 1 cm in diameter and represent mainly dilated respiratory bronchioles and alveolar ducts.[6, 48, 49] Honeycombing may be seen in the advanced stage of pulmonary fibrosis of any cause.[43, 50] The presence, distribution, and extent of honeycombing are much more readily assessed on HRCT than on the chest radiograph. For example, in a review of the radiographic and CT findings of 23 patients who had usual interstitial pneumonia,[51] honeycombing was identified on the radiograph in 7 (30%) and on CT in 21 (91%). The most common diseases that result in honeycombing are idiopathic pulmonary fibrosis, connective tissue disease, and sarcoidosis.[43]

The presence and severity of honeycombing vary considerably in different regions of the lung in different diseases, an observation of great importance in the differential diagnosis. Langerhans' cell histiocytosis and sarcoidosis usu-

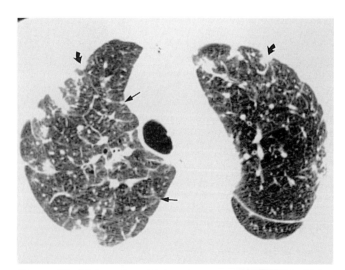

Figure 18–16. Lymphangitic Carcinomatosis. An HRCT scan demonstrates thickening of the interlobular septa *(straight arrows)* and several nodules *(curved arrows)* with irregular margins, predominantly in the subpleural lung regions. Lymphangitic carcinomatosis secondary to adenocarcinoma was proved at transbronchial biopsy.

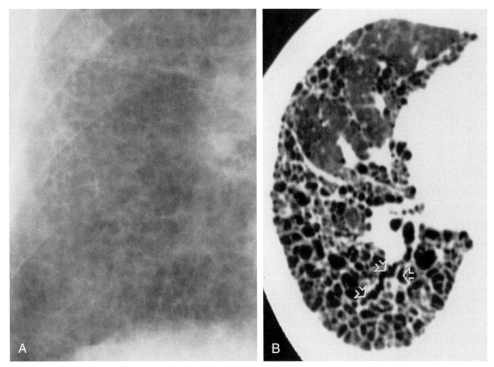

Figure 18–17. Reticular Pattern. A close-up of the right lower lung zone from a posteroanterior chest radiograph *(A)* demonstrates a reticular pattern. An HRCT scan *(B)* demonstrates honeycombing throughout the right lower lobe. Note the associated dilatation and distortion of the bronchi (traction bronchiectasis) *(arrows)*. Although the honeycombing is diffuse in the right lower lobe, it demonstrates a subpleural predominance in the right middle lobe. This pattern and distribution are consistent with an advanced stage of idiopathic pulmonary fibrosis.

ally show a predilection for the middle and upper lung zones, whereas idiopathic pulmonary fibrosis and interstitial pneumonitis associated with connective tissue diseases usually involve mainly the lower lung zones. On HRCT, the cystic spaces in Langerhans' cell histiocytosis have a random or diffuse distribution in the middle and upper lung zones with relative sparing of the lung bases, whereas the cystic spaces in sarcoidosis have a predominantly peribronchovascular and perihilar distribution.[43] The spaces in idiopathic pulmonary fibrosis and connective tissue diseases involve mainly the subpleural lung regions and the lower lung zones.[43]

Medium reticulation with cystic spaces ranging from approximately 3 to 10 mm in diameter is also seen in lymphangioleiomyomatosis.[42, 52, 53] The cystic spaces in this condition can be readily differentiated from honeycombing on HRCT because they are thin-walled and surrounded by normal lung parenchyma.[42, 52] They are usually distributed diffusely throughout the lungs, a feature allowing ready distinction from Langerhans' cell histiocytosis (which shows relative sparing of the lung bases) and from idiopathic pulmonary fibrosis (which characteristically involves mainly the subpleural lung regions and the lower lung zones).[43]

Nodular Pattern

A nodular pattern is produced when spherical lesions accumulate within the interstitium. The interstitial nodule differs from its air-space counterpart in that it is homogeneous and well circumscribed. In the setting of interstitial lung disease, nodules are defined as round opacities less than 1 cm in diameter.[2, 41] Some authors have used the term

micronodules to refer to nodules less than 7 mm,[54] 5 mm,[55] or 3 mm in diameter;[56, 57] although a consideration of the size of nodules is helpful in the differential diagnosis, because of this lack of standardization we believe that use of the term should be abandoned.

A purely nodular pattern in a febrile patient with acute disease is most suggestive of hematogenous infection, particularly miliary tuberculosis (Fig. 18–21). The nodules generally measure less than 3 mm in diameter and are usually diffusely distributed throughout the lungs (although they may have a lower lung zone predominance[58] (Fig. 18–22). A similar pattern may be seen in miliary fungal disease, silicosis, coal worker's pneumoconiosis, intravenous talcosis, pulmonary metastases (particularly from carcinoma of the thyroid),[59] and bronchioloalveolar carcinoma (Fig. 18–23).

In hematogenous infection such as miliary tuberculosis, the infecting organism reaches the lung via the circulation, from which it exits at the level of the capillary or venule; thus, at least initially, disease must be located within the parenchymal interstitium. Since the tubercles grow more or less uniformly in all directions, a small nodular pattern is eventually seen on the radiograph. Disseminated hematogenous metastases and the foci of inflammation related to intravenously injected talc particles *(see* Fig. 18–21) may have an identical pattern of growth and thus a virtually identical radiographic appearance. Some other diseases such as silicosis[60] and sarcoidosis[61] may also be manifested radiographically by discrete nodular lesions. However, the nodules in silicosis and coal worker's pneumoconiosis tend to involve mainly the middle and upper lung zones (Fig. 18–24),[2] whereas those resulting from hematogenous processes such as miliary tuberculosis and miliary metastases are dif-

Text continued on page 453

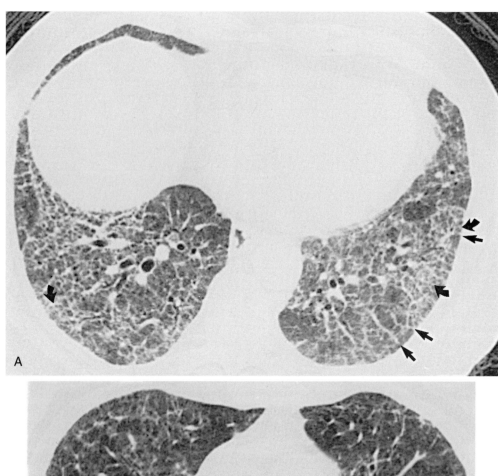

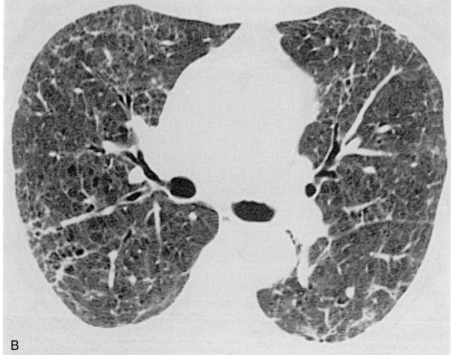

Figure 18–18. Fine Reticular Pattern on HRCT. An HRCT scan through the lower lung zone *(A)* demonstrates a diffuse fine reticular pattern resulting from a combination of irregular thickening of interlobular septa and intralobular lines. The interlobular septa are 1 to 2 cm in length and separated by 1 to 2 cm *(straight arrows)*, which corresponds to the diameter of the secondary lobule, whereas the intralobular linear opacities are smaller and only separated by a few millimeters *(curved arrows)*. An HRCT scan at the level of the right upper lobe bronchus demonstrates much less extensive fibrosis, *(B)* limited almost exclusively to the subpleural lung regions. This pattern and distribution are characteristic of idiopathic pulmonary fibrosis. Mild emphysema is also evident. The patient was a 58-year-old woman with idiopathic pulmonary fibrosis.

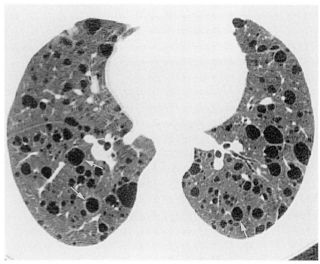

Figure 18–19. Cystic Spaces in Lymphangioleiomyomatosis. An HRCT scan through the lung bases demonstrates numerous cystic spaces with thin walls *(arrows)*. The lung parenchyma between the cysts is normal, and there is no evidence of fibrosis. The patient was a 50-year-old woman with lymphangioleiomyomatosis.

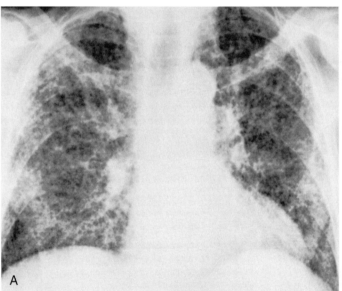

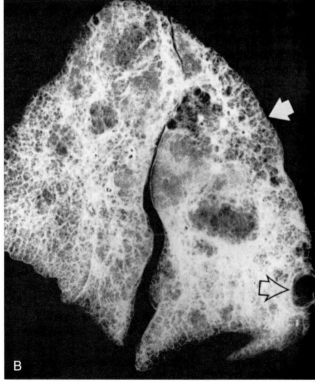

Figure 18–20. Advanced Idiopathic Pulmonary Fibrosis with Honeycombing. A posteroanterior radiograph *(A)* reveals a coarse reticular pattern without anatomic predominance. Honeycomb changes are present in several areas. A radiograph of a 1-cm-thick slice of left lung removed at autopsy *(B)* shows the honeycombing well *(solid arrows)* and also reveals a large subpleural bulla in the lower lobe *(open arrow)*.

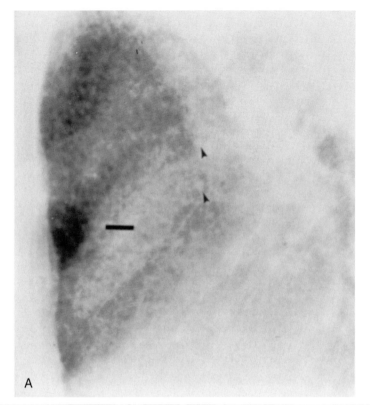

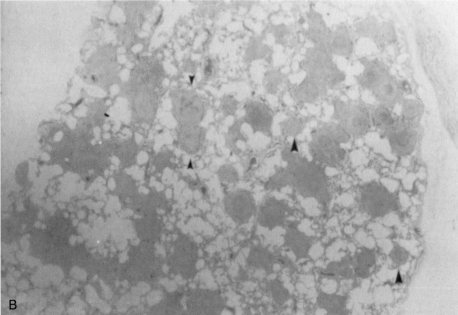

Figure 18–21. Nodular Interstitial Patterns. A detail view of the retrosternal lung from a lateral chest radiograph *(A)* shows isolated and confluent small nodular opacities; some of the nodules are denser (whiter) *(arrowheads)* than others, presumably as a result of summation. The *bar* denotes 1 cm. A section of a biopsy specimen *(B)* discloses isolated *(single arrowheads)* and confluent (between *arrowheads*) necrotizing granulomas consistent with miliary tuberculosis.

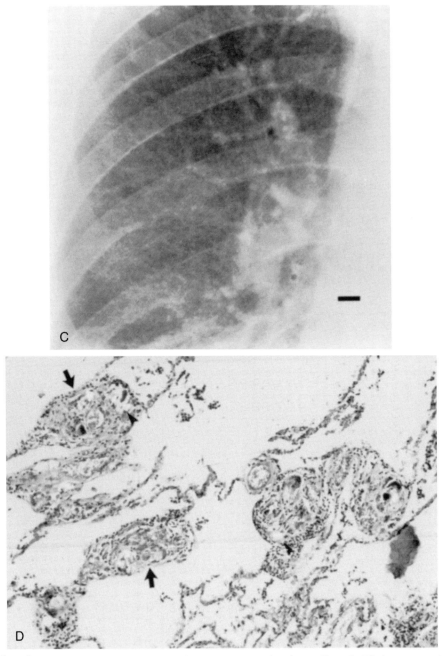

Figure 18–21 *Continued.* A detail view of the right lung from a posteroanterior chest radiograph *(C)* demonstrates innumerable micronodules measuring less than 1 mm in diameter. The *bar* denotes 1 cm. A section from a biopsy specimen *(D)* reveals isolated and coalescent nonnecrotizing interstitial granulomas *(arrows)*; polarized light examination revealed talc particles *(arrowheads)*. The appearance is that of intravenous talcosis. (From Genereux GP: Med Radiogr Photogr 61:2, 1985. Reprinted courtesy Eastman Kodak Company.)

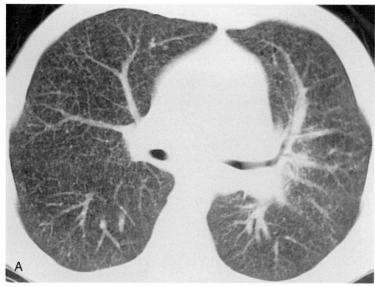

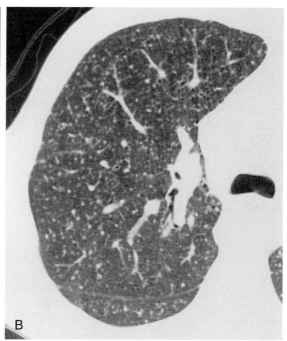

Figure 18–22. Miliary Nodules on CT. A conventional 10-mm-collimation CT scan *(A)* in a patient with miliary tuberculosis demonstrates numerous 1- to 2-mm-diameter nodules throughout both lungs. An HRCT scan targeted to the right lung in the same patient *(B)* better demonstrates the sharp margins of the nodules.

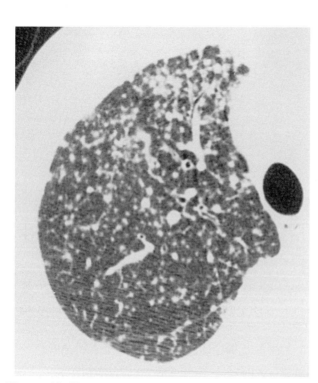

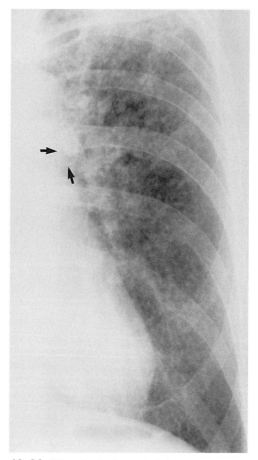

Figure 18–23. Bronchioloalveolar Carcinoma. An HRCT scan targeted to the right upper lobe demonstrates numerous sharply defined 1- to 3-mm-diameter nodules. Confluence of nodules is present anteriorly. Additional nodules were present throughout both lungs. The patient was a 38-year-old smoker with progressive shortness of breath.

Figure 18–24. Silicosis. A view of the left lung from a posteroanterior chest radiograph in a patient with silicosis demonstrates well-defined nodules, most numerous in the upper lobes. Also note the eggshell calcification of hilar and mediastinal nodes *(arrows)*, a finding virtually diagnostic of silicosis.

fuse or involve mainly the lower lung zones (where blood flow is greater).[62, 63] On HRCT, nodules resulting from hematogenous processes tend to have a random distribution in relation to lobular structures.[63, 64] By contrast, the nodules in silicosis and coal worker's pneumoconiosis frequently show a predominantly centrilobular distribution, a localization that corresponds to the accumulation of dust and fibrous tissue adjacent to respiratory bronchioles (Fig. 18–25).[65, 66] The nodules in sarcoidosis are characteristically distributed predominantly in the central peribronchovascular interstitium and lead to nodular thickening of bronchi and vessels.[19, 36]

Reticulonodular Pattern

Interlacing linear opacities result in a reticular pattern.[5] Orientation of some linear opacities parallel to the x-ray beam causes an additional nodular component and therefore results in a reticulonodular pattern.[67] Although in any given situation a reticulonodular pattern can be produced by this mechanism, it can also result from the presence of nodules superimposed on a reticular pattern as may be seen in sar-

coidosis, Langerhans' cell histiocytosis, and lymphangitic carcinomatosis (Fig. 18–26).

Ground-Glass Pattern

Ground-glass opacity is defined as the presence of hazy increased opacity without obscuration of underlying vascular markings.[5] (If vessels are obscured, the term *consolidation* should be used.) The abnormality is a frequent and important finding on HRCT, but is often difficult to recognize on the chest radiograph. With the former technique, ground-glass attenuation reflects the presence of abnormalities below the resolution limit. It may be seen in a number of situations, including interstitial disease, air-space disease, and increased capillary blood volume resulting from congestive heart failure or blood flow redistribution.[68–70] In one investigation of patients with chronic infiltrative lung disease in whom lung biopsy was performed in areas of ground-glass attenuation, the pattern was shown to be due to predominantly interstitial disease in 54% of cases, equal involvement of the interstitium and air spaces in 32%, and predominantly air-space disease in 14%.[69]

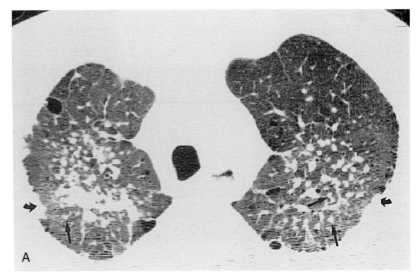

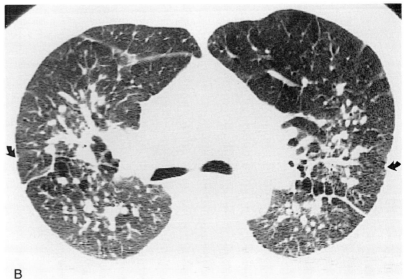

Figure 18–25. Silicosis. HRCT scans at the level of the upper *(A)* and middle *(B)* lung zones demonstrate numerous sharply defined nodules. Many have a centrilobular distribution *(straight arrows)*. Subpleural nodules *(curved arrows)* and evidence of emphysema are also evident. The patient was a 58-year-old male with long-standing silicosis.

A

B

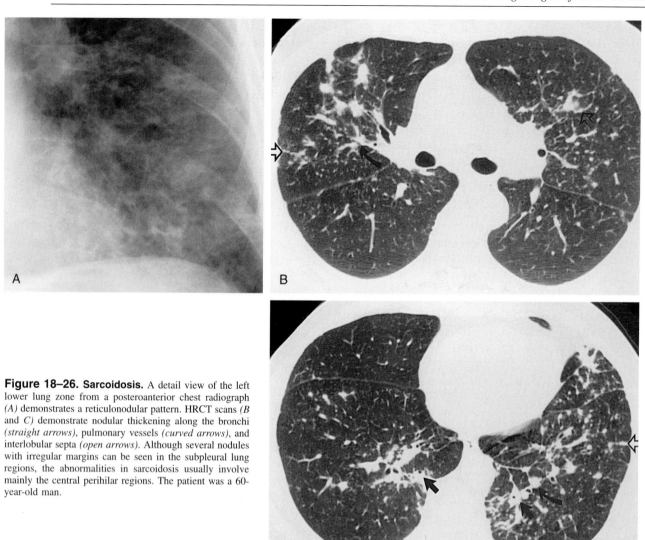

Figure 18–26. Sarcoidosis. A detail view of the left lower lung zone from a posteroanterior chest radiograph *(A)* demonstrates a reticulonodular pattern. HRCT scans *(B and C)* demonstrate nodular thickening along the bronchi *(straight arrows)*, pulmonary vessels *(curved arrows)*, and interlobular septa *(open arrows)*. Although several nodules with irregular margins can be seen in the subpleural lung regions, the abnormalities in sarcoidosis usually involve mainly the central perihilar regions. The patient was a 60-year-old man.

Acute lung diseases characteristically associated with a ground-glass pattern include *Pneumocystis carinii* pneumonia (Fig. 18–27),[70, 71] pulmonary hemorrhage,[72] and (occasionally) pulmonary edema.[33, 44] The first of these is particularly associated with ground-glass attenuation; in fact, in an individual infected with human immunodeficiency virus, the abnormality is highly suggestive of this diagnosis.[73]

Ground-glass opacification is frequently the main abnormality seen in the subacute phase of extrinsic allergic alveolitis (Fig. 18–28).[74, 75] It is also the predominant finding in patients who have desquamative interstitial pneumonia, in which it reflects the presence of mild interstitial thickening and filling of the air spaces with macrophages.[76, 78] The areas of ground-glass attenuation in pulmonary alveolar proteinosis usually have a patchy or geographic distribution.[37, 77] Although the abnormality consists mainly of filling of air spaces with proteinaceous material, on HRCT interlobular septal thickening is frequently identified in the areas of ground-glass attenuation.[37, 78]

COMBINED AIR-SPACE AND INTERSTITIAL DISEASE

In many pulmonary diseases, the radiologic and pathologic changes include a *combination* of the three basic abnormalities: air-space consolidation, atelectasis, and interstitial thickening. The combination may be the result of an acute process, such as bacterial bronchopneumonia (Fig. 18–29), or a more chronic process, such as endobronchial carcinoma with obstructive pneumonitis. These patterns are discussed in Chapter 20 *(see page 513)*.

The pattern created by combined air-space consolidation and interstitial thickening is best exemplified by pulmonary edema secondary to pulmonary venous hypertension. The radiographic manifestations of interstitial involvement are largely related to the presence of edema fluid within the perivascular connective tissue, with the edema resulting in increased size of the tissue and reduced definition of lung markings. Interstitial edema also leads to thickening of the

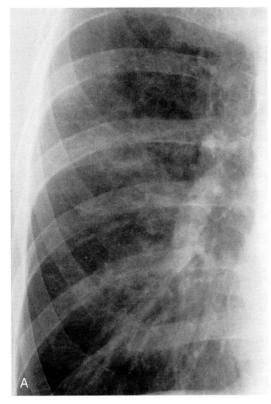

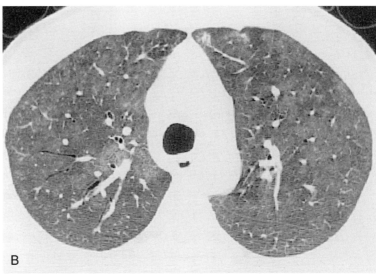

Figure 18–27. *Pneumocystis carinii* **Pneumonia.** A view of the right lung from a posteroanterior chest radiograph in a 28-year-old patient with acquired immunodeficiency syndrome *(A)* demonstrates a mild hazy increase in opacity (ground-glass opacity). An HRCT scan *(B)* reveals extensive bilateral areas of ground-glass attenuation. The latter can be readily recognized by comparing the attenuation of the involved lung with the attenuation within the bronchi ("black bronchus" sign).

interlobular septa (Fig. 18–30). The radiographic manifestations of edema fluid within the air spaces consist of confluent "fluffy" opacities characteristic of an air-space–filling process. Another example of combined involvement is acute pneumonitis of *Mycoplasma* or viral etiology. Either infection tends to be local rather than general in distribution and characteristically causes parenchymal interstitial inflammation and a pattern of fine to medium reticulation early in its course. This "pure" interstitial involvement is often of short duration, the inflammatory reaction soon extending into parenchymal air spaces and resulting in consolidation. Since involvement of the conducting airways is relatively insignificant, loss of volume is negligible in the acute stage of the disease.

LIMITATIONS OF THE PATTERN APPROACH

Modifying Factors

The pattern of parenchymal abnormality seen on the chest radiograph and HRCT may be modified by underlying parenchymal lung disease, particularly emphysema, and by secondary effects sometimes produced by diffuse interstitial disease. For example, on the radiograph, lobar pneumonia superimposed on emphysema may simulate interstitial lung disease, and conglomerate interstitial fibrosis may simulate air-space disease. Nevertheless, these modifications of the classic patterns may be fairly characteristic of specific diseases.

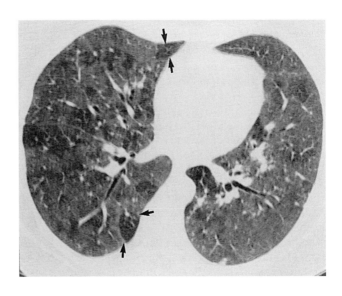

Figure 18–28. Extrinsic Allergic Alveolitis. An HRCT scan in a 59-year-old woman demonstrates extensive bilateral areas of ground-glass attenuation. Focal areas of lung parenchyma without ground-glass attenuation have the size and configuration of secondary pulmonary lobules *(arrows)*. This pattern of ground-glass attenuation with sparing of individual secondary pulmonary lobules is characteristic of the subacute stage of extrinsic allergic alveolitis.

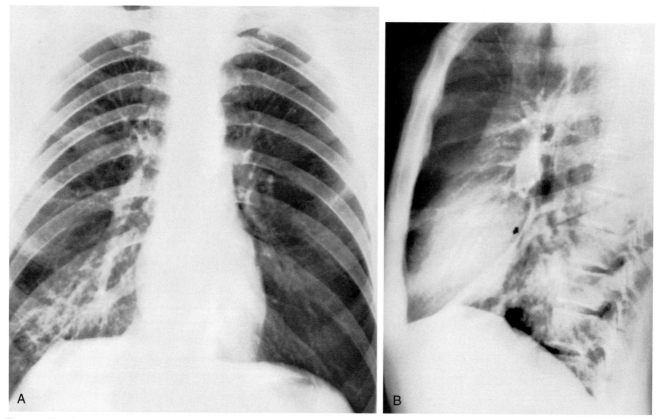

Figure 18–29. Bronchopneumonia, Right Lower Lobe. Posteroanterior *(A)* and lateral *(B)* radiographs demonstrate patchy consolidation of the anterior and lateral basal segments of the right lower lobe. The inhomogeneous nature of the disease suggests associated interstitial disease. Posterior bowing of the **major** fissure *(arrow)* indicates some degree of loss of volume.

Although a radiologic pattern of air-space consolidation occasionally is produced by confluent interstitial lung disease, in the vast majority of cases it represents either predominantly air-space disease or a combination of air-space and interstitial lung disease. Similarly, the presence of a predominant septal, reticular, small nodular, or reticulonodular pattern represents purely interstitial lung disease in the vast majority of cases. The pattern approach therefore usually allows correct classification of diseases into predominantly air-space or interstitial disease. As discussed previously, when more than one pattern of abnormality is present, the differential diagnosis should be based on the predominant pattern.

Nonspecific Radiologic Findings

The usefulness of recognizing patterns of parenchymal abnormality on the chest radiograph cannot be overemphasized: identification of the correct pattern, whether air-space, linear, reticular, nodular, or reticulonodular, in the appropriate clinical context often allows one to narrow the differential diagnosis to a relatively small number of entities and, occasionally, to make a specific diagnosis with a high degree of confidence. Nonetheless, in some cases it is impossible to determine the main pattern of abnormality on the chest radiograph, an observation that has led to recognition of the "I don't know pattern";[79] it is preferable to recognize the nonspecificity of the radiologic findings in some patients

rather than choose the wrong pattern for the differential diagnosis. It should also be noted that even experienced readers may disagree in interpretation of the radiographic pattern: for example, in one review of 360 chest radiographs in patients with biopsy-proven diffuse "infiltrative" disease,[2] two expert readers agreed that the predominant pattern was either nodular or linear in only 70% of cases. Furthermore, the presence of hazy increased opacity without obscuration of vascular markings (ground-glass opacity) may be readily missed on the chest radiograph.[14, 22] Ground-glass opacification is frequently seen on HRCT. This pattern, however, is nonspecific; it may indicate the presence of interstitial lung disease, air-space disease, or a combination of the two on both the radiograph and HRCT.

Comparison of Chest Radiography and High-Resolution Computed Tomography

Several groups have compared the diagnostic accuracy of HRCT with that of chest radiography in the differential diagnosis of chronic diffuse interstitial and air-space lung disease.[3, 20, 21, 80] In one investigation of 118 patients, radiographs and CT scans were assessed independently by three observers without knowledge of the clinical or pathologic data.[3] The observers made a confident diagnosis in 23% of radiographic and 49% of CT interpretations, the diagnosis being correct in 77% and 93% of the readings, respectively. Thus, a confident diagnosis was made more than twice as

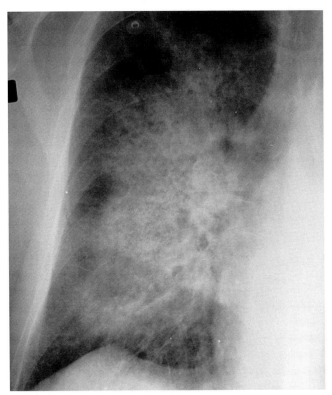

Figure 18–30. Interstitial and Air-Space Pulmonary Edema. A view of the right lung from an anteroposterior chest radiograph demonstrates extensive perihilar consolidation as well as thickening of the interlobular septa. The patient was a 49-year-old man with acute interstitial and air-space pulmonary edema secondary to mitral regurgitation.

often on the basis of CT scans than on the basis of chest radiographs, and the CT-based diagnosis was more often correct. In a second study of 140 patients, three independent observers listed the three most likely diagnoses and recorded the degree of confidence they had in their choice.[21] The percentages of high-confidence diagnoses by each of the three observers that were correct with chest radiography were 29%, 34%, and 19%, respectively, as compared with 57%, 55%, and 47% with HRCT. Interobserver agreement for the proposed diagnosis was also significantly better with HRCT than with conventional radiography.[21]

As might be expected, the diagnostic accuracy of both radiography and CT improves considerably when the findings are analyzed in the context of the clinical findings, pulmonary function tests, and laboratory data. The value of such combined information in classifying chronic diffuse lung disease was assessed in one investigation of 208 patients.[80] When clinical, chest radiographic, and CT findings were evaluated independently, a correct diagnosis with a high degree of confidence was made in 29% of the cases on the basis of clinical data, 9% on the basis of radiographic images, and 36% on the basis of the HRCT findings. Combining the clinical and radiographic data allowed a correct diagnosis with a high degree of confidence in 54% of cases. Combining the information provided by the clinical, radiographic, and CT findings allowed diagnosis with a high confidence level in 174 of the 208 patients (84%). This diagnosis was correct in 166 cases (95%). Therefore, in the appropriate clinical context, a specific diagnosis can often

be made with confidence, thus precluding the need for lung biopsy.

GENERAL SIGNS IN DISEASES THAT INCREASE LUNG DENSITY

In addition to the basic patterns and signs already described, several additional radiologic features may aid in determining the nature of a pathologic process within the lungs. The signs are described in general terms only, the intention being to indicate the mechanisms by which they are produced and the significance of each in radiologic interpretation.

Characteristics of the Border of a Pulmonary Lesion

The sharpness of definition of a consolidated area within the lungs gives some indication of the nature of the disease process causing the opacification. Acute air-space pneumonia (e.g., from *S. pneumoniae*) that has extended to an interlobar pleural surface has a sharply defined contour along that border; where it does not abut against a fissure, its margin is less distinct (*see* Fig. 18–3, page 435) since it is formed by a spreading zone of consolidation. Regardless of the etiology and extent of air-space consolidation, the margin between consolidated lung and contiguous air-containing parenchyma has the same definitive character whether the lesion is a small focus of exudative tuberculosis or massive consolidation produced by *Klebsiella pneumoniae*. The consolidation or ground-glass pattern in alveolar proteinosis, on the other hand, may be sharply demarcated from adjacent normal lung parenchyma without any apparent anatomic boundary to account for the sharp edge.[77]

The margin of a pulmonary nodule may be smooth, lobulated, or spiculated (Fig. 18–31). These margin characteristics are of some help in predicting whether the nodule is more likely to be benign or malignant. In general, smooth margins suggest benignity and spiculation suggests malignancy; lobulation is seen with approximately equal frequency in benign and malignant nodules.[81–83] In a review of the CT findings of 634 solitary nodules, 52 of 66 (79%) that had sharply defined, smooth nonlobulated margins were benign and 14 (21%) were malignant.[84] Of 218 nodules that had spiculated margins, 184 (84%) represented primary pulmonary carcinoma and 9 metastases; only 25 (11%) were benign. Of 359 nodules with smooth but lobulated margins, 202 (56%) were benign whereas 148 were malignant (either primary pulmonary carcinoma or metastasis). In another multicenter study of patients with lung nodules not considered to be calcified on chest radiography, 130 nodules were classified as having smooth margins, 48 as having lobulated margins, and 91 as having spiculated margins;[85] 80 (62%) of the nodules with smooth margins were benign, 28 (22%) represented metastases, 9 were carcinoid tumors, and only 13 (10%) were primary pulmonary carcinomas. Twenty (42%) of the 48 nodules with lobulated margins were benign and 28 were malignant. On the other hand, only 11 of the 91 nodules (12%) with spiculated margins were benign. Correlation of HRCT with pathologic findings has shown

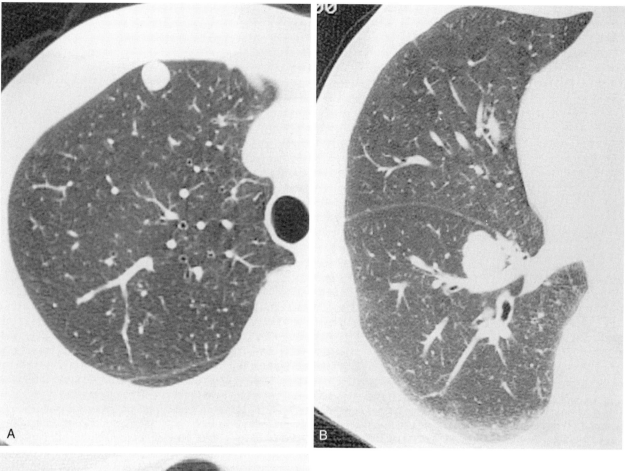

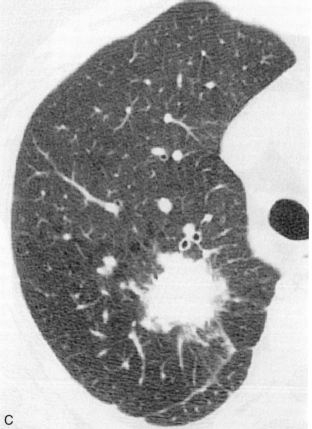

Figure 18–31. Characteristics of the Border of Three Pulmonary Nodules on HRCT. A smooth, nonlobulated border of a solitary nodule *(A)* is most suggestive of a benign lesion (proven hamartoma). A smooth, lobulated contour of a solitary nodule *(B)* is seen with approximately equal frequency in benign and malignant lesions (proven adenocarcinoma). A spiculated border of a nodule *(C)* is most suggestive of a malignant lesion (proven adenocarcinoma).

that spiculation may result from irregular fibrosis, localized lymphatic spread of tumor, or infiltrative tumor growth.[82]

A discussion of "satellite lesions" is conveniently included here since they are closely related to the margins of a pulmonary lesion. These abnormalities can be defined as small nodular opacities in close proximity to a larger lesion, usually a solitary peripheral nodule. They usually indicate an infectious, particularly tuberculous, etiology; in two studies they were observed in 5 of 52 patients[86] and 10 of 122 patients[87] with tuberculoma. However, in the latter series, satellite lesions were also found in 3 of 280 cases of primary carcinoma—an admittedly very low incidence but one that belies the validity of assuming an infectious origin for a peripheral lesion on the strength of satellite lesions alone.

The contour of an opacity that relates to the pleura, either over the convexity of the thorax or contiguous to the mediastinum or diaphragm, can provide a useful clue about whether the process is intrapulmonary or extrapulmonary in origin. A mass that originates within the pleural space or extrapleurally displaces the pleura and underlying lung inward such that the angle formed by the margins of the mass and the chest wall is obtuse; by contrast, an intrapulmonary mass tends to relate to contiguous pleura in an acute angle (Fig. 18–32). It should be obvious that these general rules apply when such lesions are viewed tangentially; when viewed *en face*, the extrapulmonary mass will be indistinctly defined because of the obtuse angle of its margins, whereas an intrapulmonary mass will tend to be more sharply defined. As with all other radiologic signs, this sign is fallible: occasionally an extrapulmonary mass relates to the lung in an acute angle, particularly when it is 4 cm or more in diameter, and an intrapulmonary mass in an obtuse angle.

Change in Position of Interlobar Fissures

Displacement of fissures toward a zone of increased opacity constitutes a reliable sign of atelectasis. An equally valuable but less frequent sign is displacement of interlobar fissures in the *opposite* direction from the involved lobe—in other words, bulging of a fissure. Clearly, this displacement is evidence of expansion of the involved lobe; since diseases of increased density that are capable of increasing the volume of a lobe are relatively few, recognition of such displacement frequently permits a specific etiologic diagnosis.

Bulging of a fissure occurs most often in infections caused by organisms that produce an abundant exudate, the most common of which are *K. pneumoniae* and *S. pneumoniae*;[88] the abnormality has been reported in 30% to 60% of infections caused by the former organism and in 10% to 15% with the latter.[88, 89] Because *S. pneumoniae* pneumonia is much more common than *Klebsiella* pneumonia, it accounts for approximately 80% of cases overall.[88] Less common organisms associated with the abnormality are *M. tuberculosis*, *Acinetobacter*, and *Haemophilus influenzae*.[88, 90, 91] Although rapid and massive air-space filling by inflammatory exudate is probably the most common cause of a bulging fissure in pulmonary infection, the appearance can also be seen with an acute lung abscess in which air trapping by a check-valve mechanism in the communicating airway distends the abscess cavity (Fig. 18–33).

In addition to acute pneumonia, any space-occupying mass within a lobe may displace a fissure if the lesion occupies significant volume and if it is contiguous to the fissure; peripheral pulmonary carcinoma is the most common of these masses (Fig. 18–34). A central tumor that causes

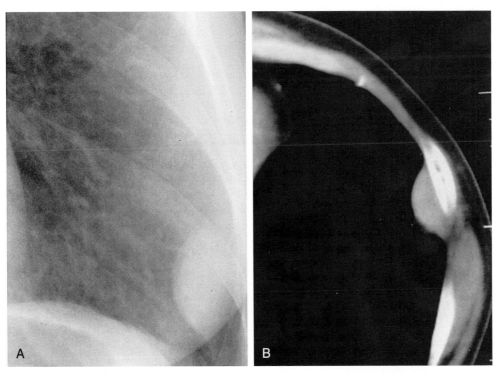

Figure 18–32. Extrapulmonary Sign. A view of the left lower hemithorax from a posteroanterior chest radiograph *(A)* shows the characteristic features of an extrapulmonary mass: a smooth convex border where it abuts the lung and tapering superiorly and inferiorly; the lateral margin, where it abuts the soft tissues of the chest wall, is obscured. A CT scan *(B)* demonstrates tapering anterior and posterior margins. The patient was a 46-year-old woman with a fibrous tumor of the pleura.

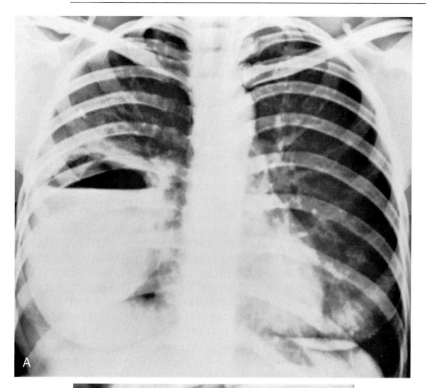

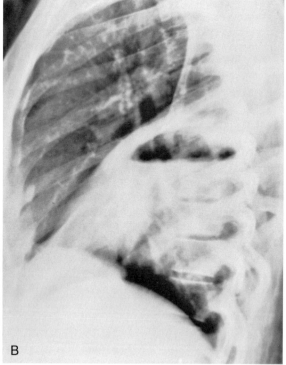

Figure 18–33. Bulging of Interlobar Fissures: Acute Staphylococcal Lung Abscess. Radiographs in posteroanterior *(A)* and lateral *(B)* projection reveal a large abscess in the right lower lobe producing anterior and upward bulging of the major fissure.

bronchial obstruction may be associated with focal convexity of the interlobar fissure because of the mass itself and concavity of the fissure distally as a result of atelectasis, the shape of the fissure thus resembling the letter S.[92] This finding—known eponymously as the S sign of Golden—is most suggestive of obstructive pneumonitis and lobar atelectasis secondary to bronchogenic carcinoma.

Fissures are ordinarily an efficient barrier to the interlobar spread of parenchymal disease. However, a few condi-

tions have a propensity for crossing pleural boundaries, thus creating a helpful sign in differential diagnosis. Such pleural transgression is particularly common in actinomycotic infection, in which organisms can cross both interlobar fissures and the visceral and parietal pleura over the convexity of the lung, and they may incite abscesses and osteomyelitis in the chest wall. Pulmonary tuberculosis, particularly in children, may also transgress pleural boundaries; pulmonary carcinoma seldom does. One caveat to the unwary: these

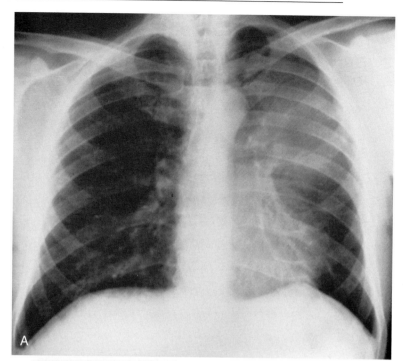

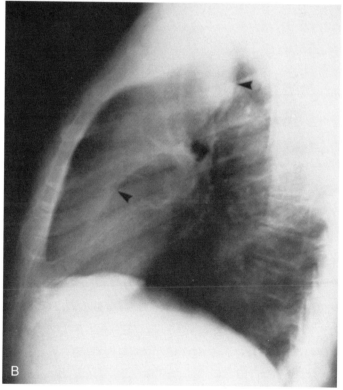

Figure 18–34. Bulging of Interlobar Fissures: Pulmonary Carcinoma. Radiographs in posteroanterior *(A)* and lateral *(B)* projection reveal obliteration of much of the left border of the heart; the opacity is homogeneous and does not contain an air bronchogram. Anterior displacement of the major fissure *(arrowheads)* and elevation of the left hemidiaphragm indicate considerable loss of volume. The lower half of the major fissure is concave posteriorly, the upper half convex posteriorly. This bulging of the upper portion of the fissure is caused by a large peripheral carcinoma. Lymph node metastases produced upper lobe bronchial obstruction and atelectasis.

statements apply to complete interlobar fissures; the frequency with which fissures are incomplete introduces a situation that may cause confusion—the extension of a pathologic process from one lobe to a contiguous lobe through a parenchymal bridge (Fig. 18–35).

Cavitation

A cavity is defined radiologically as a gas-containing space within the lung surrounded by a wall whose thickness is greater than 1 mm.[93] The term generally implies that the central portion of the lesion has undergone necrosis and been expelled via the bronchi, with a gas-containing space remaining.[93] A bulla is defined as a gas-containing space with a wall 1 mm or less in diameter;[93, 94] the term is usually reserved for a space that occurs in a background of emphysema.[94] A gas-containing space with a well-defined wall not related to emphysema is commonly referred to as a cyst (whether or not it has an epithelial lining, as would be implied pathologically).[94] Neither the presence of a fluid

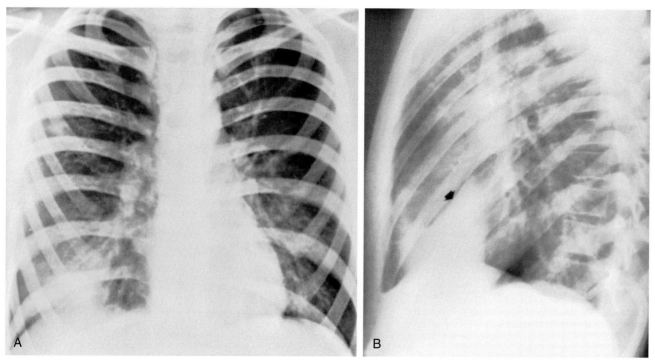

Figure 18–35. Acute Air-Space Pneumonia. Posteroanterior _(A)_ and lateral _(B)_ radiographs reveal consolidation of the anterior basal zone of the right lower lobe; the shadow is homogeneous except for an air bronchogram (visualized in _A_). Where the consolidation abuts against the major fissure _(arrow)_, it is sharply defined, but its definition posteriorly, medially, and laterally is less sharp because of the spreading nature of the inflammatory reaction. A small area of parenchymal consolidation is also visible in the medial segment of the middle lobe in _B_, possibly representing spread across an incomplete fissure.

level nor the size of the cavity is necessary for the definition of cavity. The terms _cavity_ and _abscess_ are not synonymous: an intrapulmonary abscess without communication with the bronchial tree is radiographically opaque; only when the abscess cavity communicates with the bronchial tree and allows air to replace necrotic material should "cavity" be applied.

The mechanism by which necrosis occurs varies according to the underlying disease. In infectious processes such as acute staphylococcal pneumonia, bacterial toxins and enzymes released by dead or dying leukocytes may lead directly to tissue death; the necrosis of neoplasms is probably related at least partly to deficient blood supply. In septic emboli, it is likely that both vascular deficiency and bacterial toxins are operative.

The radiographic demonstration of pulmonary cavitation may be simple or exceedingly difficult. If the cavity contains fluid, as is frequently the case, the identification of a fluid level is clearly pathognomonic. However, diagnostic difficulty may be present when cavities have no fluid level, particularly when they are small or are situated either among an inhomogeneous group of opacities or in anatomic regions ordinarily difficult to see, such as the paramediastinal zones. In these circumstances, CT is essential to confirm the diagnosis. (Perhaps more commonly, CT results in the identification of cavitary disease that was not even remotely suspected on plain radiography.)

Although the nature of cavity formation within specific disease groups varies considerably, in most cases the general appearance gives some indication of the underlying etiology, particularly whether the lesion is benign or malignant (Fig.

18–36). The specific radiologic features that should be noted with respect to this distinction include the thickness of the cavity wall, the smoothness or irregularity of its inner lining, the presence and character of its contents, whether lesions are solitary or multiple, and when multiple, the number that have cavitated. The following discussion indicates the findings that are suggestive of a specific etiology for each of these features; it should be remembered that there are occasional exceptions to the general rule in each category.

Cavity Wall. The cavity wall is usually thick in acute lung abscess (Fig. 18–37), primary (Fig. 18–38) and metastatic carcinoma, and Wegener's granulomatosis (Fig. 18–39) and often thin in chronic infection such as coccidioidomycosis and paragonimiasis. Assessment of cavity wall thickness is perhaps most useful in distinguishing between a benign and a malignant lesion: in one study of 65 solitary cavities in the lung, all lesions in which the thickest part of the cavity wall was 1 mm or less were benign;[95] of the lesions whose thickest measurement was 4 mm or less, 92% were benign; of cavities that were 5 to 15 mm in their thickest part, benign and malignant lesions were equally divided; and when the cavity wall was over 15 mm in thickness, 92% of the lesions were malignant.

Character of the Inner Lining. The inner lining is usually nodular in carcinoma (_see_ Fig. 18–38), shaggy in acute lung abscess (_see_ Fig. 18–33), and smooth in most other cavitary lesions.

Nature of the Cavitary Contents. In the majority of cases, the contents are liquid and have no distinctive characteristics. Fluid levels that are visible on conventional chest radiographs obtained in the erect position on fixed equipment

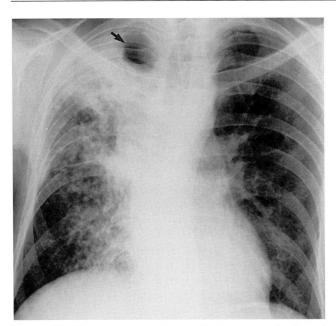

Figure 18–36. Tuberculous Cavity with Bronchogenic Spread. A posteroanterior chest radiograph demonstrates a 3-cm cavity in the apical segment of the right upper lobe *(arrow)*, extensive consolidation in the right upper lobe, and 3- to 7-mm-diameter nodules throughout the right lung. The findings are characteristic of tuberculosis with associated endobronchial spread. The patient had a positive smear and culture for *Mycobacterium tuberculosis.*

should be perfectly horizontal and parallel to the upper or lower borders of the film; however, this rule clearly does not apply to radiographs exposed with mobile apparatus at a patient's bedside. In addition, very occasionally a fluid level is tilted slightly from the horizontal even with fixed equipment, a peculiar finding that may be caused by displacement of the fluid by cardiac pulsation; in one fluoroscopic study of three patients with hydropneumothorax in whom the fluid interface was tilted, the interface was found to "seesaw" synchronously with the heartbeat.[96]

In contrast to the nonspecific character of a flat, smooth fluid level, the presence of intracavitary material in the fluid is so typical in some diseases as to be virtually diagnostic. Examples include the intracavitary fungus ball, which may form a freely mobile intracavitary mass (Fig. 18–40), and the collapsed membranes of a ruptured *Echinococcus* cyst, which float on top of the fluid within the cyst and create the characteristic "water-lily" sign[97] or the "sign of the camalote"[98] (a water plant found in South American rivers) (Fig. 18–41). The latter sign is seen on the radiograph or CT in approximately 75% of patients with ruptured pulmonary echinococcal cysts.[97] Another rare but characteristic intracavitary mass is that associated with pulmonary gangrene, in which irregular pieces of sloughed necrotic lung parenchyma float like icebergs in the cavity fluid (Fig. 18–42); although this complication can be seen with virtually any organism, it is most common with *Klebsiella pneumoniae.*[99, 100]

Multiplicity of Lesions. Some cavitary disease is characteristically solitary—for example, primary pulmonary carcinoma, acute lung abscess, and post-traumatic lung cyst; other diseases are characteristically multiple—for example, metastatic neoplasm, Wegener's granulomatosis,[101] and septic emboli.[101a, b]

Bubble Lucencies (Pseudocavitation). On CT, particularly HRCT, round or oval areas of low attenuation usually measuring 5 mm or less in diameter (Fig. 18–43) may be visible within lung nodules.[82, 102] Such "bubble" lucencies (pseudocavitation) can be identified on HRCT in approximately 60% of bronchioloalveolar carcinomas, in 30% of acinar adenocarcinomas, and less commonly in other malignant lung tumors.[82, 102] They can also be identified in benign lesions (albeit uncommonly, as shown in one study in which they were found in only 1 of 11 [9%] such nodules).[82] Correlation with pathologic findings has shown that the lucencies usually represent patent bronchi or small air-containing cystic spaces associated with papillary tumor growth.[82] Rarely, "cystic spaces" resembling cavities and measuring more than 5 mm in diameter are visible on conventional radiographs and on CT in bronchioloalveolar carcinoma (Fig. 18–44).[103] These larger spaces have been shown to represent paracicatricial emphysema, localized bronchiectasis, or tumor developing in an area of fibrosis and honeycombing.[103] These cystic spaces cannot be differentiated radiologically from true cavitation, which has been reported in as many as 7% of 136 bronchioloalveolar carcinomas in some studies.[104]

Calcification and Ossification

The presence, absence, and site of calcification of pulmonary lesions as detected by chest radiographs or CT are important diagnostic signs. In the majority of cases, the calcification is dystrophic (calcium deposition in damaged or dead cells or tissue); less commonly, it is metastatic (calcification of vital tissues). Although the latter is frequent in cases of severe hypercalcemia, presumably because of the relatively alkaline pH of lung tissue, it is seldom visible on the chest radiograph. (In addition to the simple tissue deposition of calcium, lamellar bone can also be identified radiologically or pathologically in some patients, in which case the term *ossification* is more appropriate; however, since distinction between the two is not usually possible radiologically, we use "calcification" to refer to both processes.)

Both the distribution and character of calcification should be noted since each has diagnostic significance. It is convenient to consider intrathoracic calcification under five headings, depending on its anatomic location and distribution: local parenchymal, diffuse parenchymal, lymph node, pleural, and other.

Local Parenchymal Calcification

The most common form of pulmonary calcification is a single, often densely calcified nodule situated anywhere in the lungs and representing a healed focus of granulomatous inflammation (Fig. 18–45). It is most frequently caused by tuberculosis, except in areas endemic for histoplasmosis, where this organism accounts for the majority of cases; it is seen only occasionally in coccidioidomycosis and rarely in blastomycosis.[105] Such foci of calcification are believed to occur in approximately one third of patients who react to the histoplasmin test, but in only one tenth of those who are PPD positive.[105] The focus of parenchymal calcification (Ghon focus) is usually part of a duo (the Ranke complex),

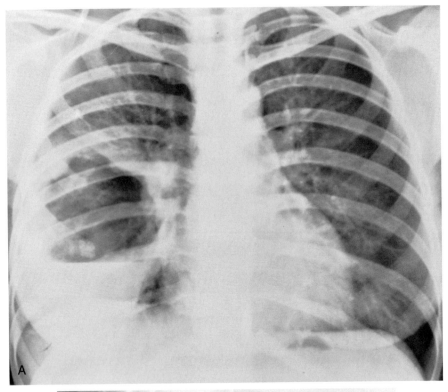

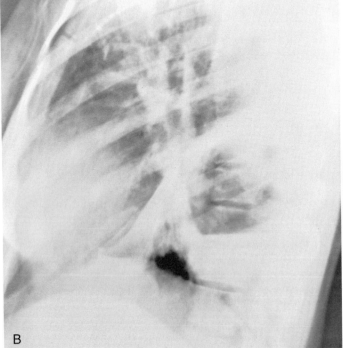

Figure 18–37. Acute Staphylococcal Lung Abscess. Radiographs in posteroanterior *(A)* and lateral *(B)* projection reveal a large cavity in the right lower lobe. The thickness of its wall and the shaggy irregular nature of its inner lining suggest an acute lung abscess.

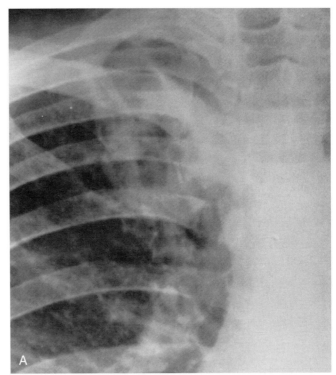

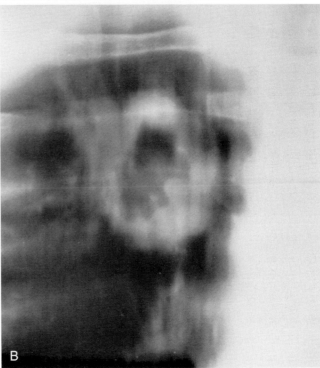

Figure 13–38. Cavitated Pulmonary Carcinoma. Views of the upper half of the right lung from a posteroanterior radiograph *(A)* and an anteroposterior tomogram *(B)* reveal a rather poorly defined cavitated mass. The thickness of the wall and irregular nodular character of the inner lining are highly suggestive of carcinoma. Squamous cell carcinoma was identified on biopsy.

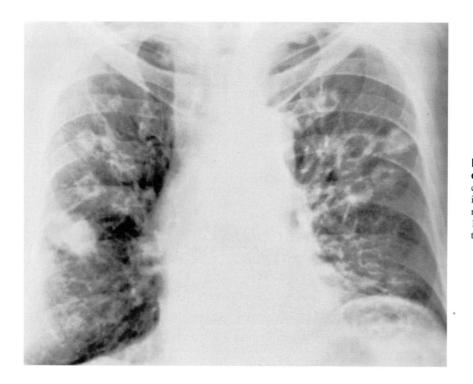

Figure 18–39. Multiple Cavities in Wegener's Granulomatosis. A posteroanterior chest radiograph shows multiple thick-walled cavities scattered throughout both lungs but predominantly in the upper zones. The lesions range from 1.5 to 3 cm and are rather thick walled. At least three lesions show no evidence of cavitation.

Figure 18–40. Intracavitary Fungus Ball. Views of the upper half of the right lung from a posteroanterior radiograph *(A)* and an anteroposterior tomogram *(B)* reveal a rather thin-walled but irregular cavity in the paramediastinal zone. Situated within it is a smooth oblong shadow of homogeneous density whose relationship to the wall of the cavity changes from the erect *(A)* to the supine *(B)* position. The cavity was of tuberculous etiology and the loose body was composed of *Aspergillus* hyphae.

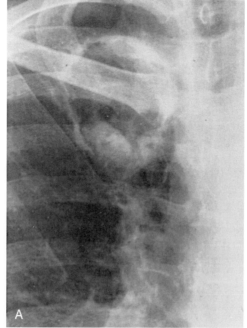

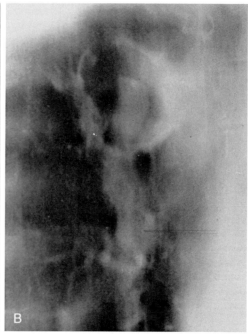

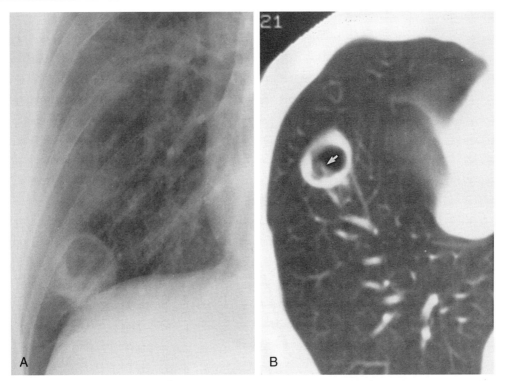

Figure 18–41. Hydatid Cyst with "Water-Lily" Sign. A view of the right lower lung from a posteroanterior radiograph *(A)* shows a smoothly marginated cavity in the right lower lobe containing an air-fluid level. A CT scan *(B)* demonstrates the presence of a floating membrane *(arrow)*. Visualization of the membrane (the "water-lily" sign) is a characteristic finding of a ruptured hydatid cyst with bronchial communication. (From Müller NL: J Respir Dis 11:933, 1990, with permission.)

the other component being a calcified hilar or mediastinal lymph node. Calcification in the pulmonary lesion is usually homogeneous, whereas that in the lymph node generally consists of scattered punctate deposits. Identification of the Ranke complex fairly conclusively establishes previous infection by either *Histoplasma capsulatum* or *M. tuberculosis*. A decision regarding which is the more likely may be aided by the radiographic demonstration of multiple punctate calcifications within the spleen, which are almost always due to histoplasmosis.[105] The presence of calcification is much more readily detected on CT[84, 85, 106] and on dual-energy computed radiography[107] than on conventional radiography.

Calcification within a solitary pulmonary nodule is the most reliable single piece of evidence that a lesion is benign;[108, 109] although it is also seen in malignant tumors in 10% to 15% of cases,[110, 85] the pattern of calcification allows distinction of benign from malignant nodules in the vast majority of cases.[110, 109] Four patterns of calcification are characteristically associated with benign lesions: diffuse, central nidal, laminated, and popcorn (Fig. 18–46).[110] The diffuse or laminated forms are virtually diagnostic of a granuloma. A small central nidus of calcification is most commonly seen with granulomatous lesions, although it also occurs in some hamartomas. Popcorn calcification is characteristic of hamartoma. Such benign patterns of calcification are rarely seen in malignant tumors. In one study of 634 nodules assessed with CT, 153 were correctly diagnosed as benign based on the presence of central or diffuse calcification;[84] although focal areas of calcification were identified in 13% of the primary lung tumors, only 1 carcinoid tumor had a benign pattern of calcification, the other malignant tumors having neither central nor diffuse calcification.

Calcification in malignant tumors may be seen in several circumstances: (1) most important from a differential diagnostic point of view is the isolated instance of a peripheral primary carcinoma engulfing an existing calcified granuloma, in which case the calcification is usually eccentric; (2) a solitary metastasis of osteogenic sarcoma or chondrosarcoma (Fig. 18–47), in which there is bone formation in the osteoid or calcification of the malignant cartilage;[111] (3) other metastatic malignancies such as medullary carcinoma of the thyroid,[111] in which there is stromal calcification; (4) the rare instance of a primary squamous cell carcinoma or primary or metastatic mucin-secreting adenocarcinoma, in which there is dystrophic calcification of necrotic tumor or mucus;[112] (5) rare cases of primary or metastatic papillary adenocarcinoma, which appear calcified as a result of the presence of psammoma bodies;[113] and (6) occasional pulmonary carcinoid tumors, in which there is ossification of the stroma.[84, 114]

Diffuse Parenchymal Calcification

Four types of diffuse parenchymal calcification are recognized—punctate, nodular, dendriform, and interstitial—each of which is usually fairly distinctive. Tiny punctate calcifications are characteristic of alveolar microlithiasis. Multiple nodular foci of calcification are seen frequently on the radiograph or CT in silicosis,[115] talcosis,[116] and certain healed disseminated infectious diseases such as tuberculosis,[105] histoplasmosis, and varicella pneumonitis (Fig. 18–48);[117, 118] they are identified less commonly in sarcoidosis[54] and amyloidosis[119, 120] and rarely in adult respiratory distress syndrome.[121] Nodular foci of true ossification may occur in

Text continued on page 474

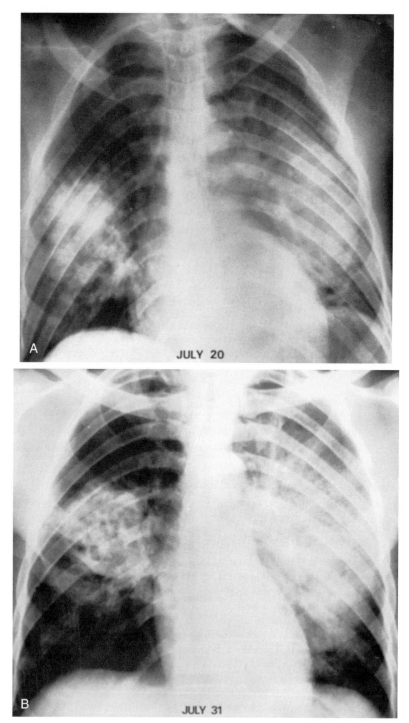

Figure 18–42. Acute Lung Gangrene in *Klebsiella* Pneumonia. On admission to the hospital, an anteroposterior radiograph in the supine position *(A)* revealed massive air-space consolidation throughout much of the left lung and the midportion of the right lung. *Klebsiella pneumoniae* was grown from the sputum; blood cultures were negative. Although 11 days later his clinical condition had improved somewhat, a radiograph *(B)* revealed a change in the texture of the consolidation in that its homogeneity was disturbed by a multitude of poorly defined air-containing spaces, better visualized in the right than the left lung.

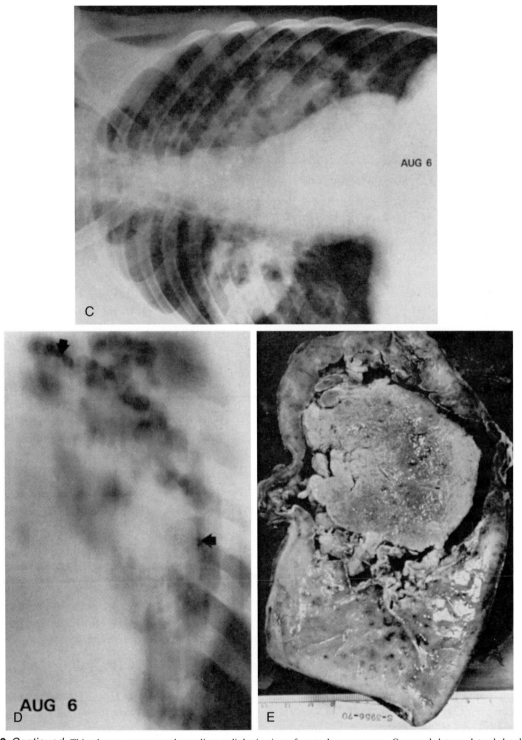

Figure 18–42 *Continued.* This change represents the earliest radiologic sign of acute lung gangrene. One week later, a lateral decubitus radiograph *(C)* revealed a large, irregular shaggy mass within a huge cavity in the left lung, indicated to better advantage in an anteroposterior tomogram *(arrows in D)*. The left lower lobe was resected and the specimen *(E)* showed a large necrotic mass lying within a huge cavity and completely separated from the cavity walls. (From Knight L, Fraser RG, Robson HG: Can Med Assoc J 112:196, 1975.)

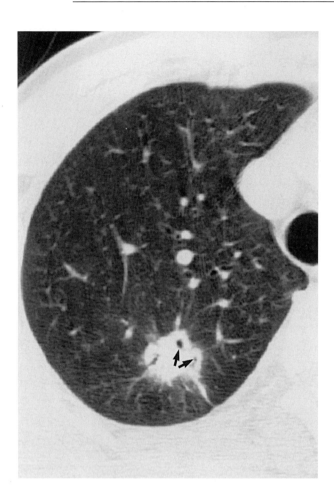

Figure 18–43. Bubble Lucencies. An HRCT scan through a 2-cm-diameter nodule in the right upper lobe demonstrates focal lucencies measuring less than 5 mm in diameter *(arrows)*. The patient underwent right upper lobectomy. Pathologic assessment demonstrated bronchioloalveolar carcinoma. The bubble lucencies were shown to represent patent bronchi within the tumor.

Figure 18–44. Pseudocavitation. An HRCT scan through a 3.5-cm-diameter nodule in the left lower lobe demonstrates several lucencies, the largest measuring 1 cm in diameter. The patient underwent left lower lobectomy. Pathologic assessment showed that the lucencies were the result of bronchiectasis within a bronchioloalveolar carcinoma. There was no evidence of cavitation.

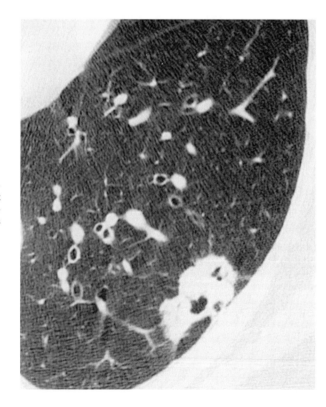

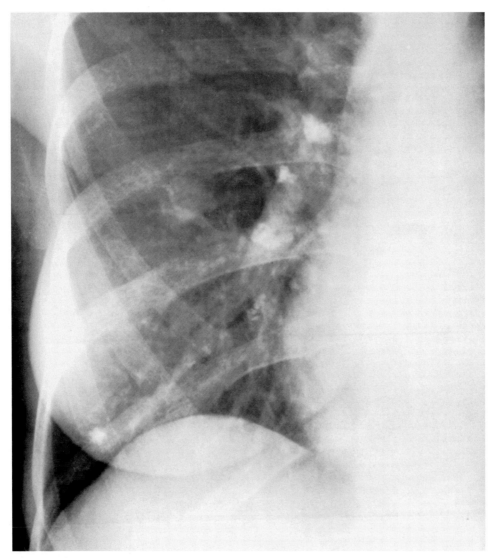

Figure 18–45. The Ranke Complex. A view of the lower half of the right lung from a posteroanterior chest radiograph demonstrates a solitary, densely calcified nodule just above the right costophrenic sulcus (the Ghon lesion); the calcification is homogeneous, although irregular. Situated in the right hilum are three or four lymph nodes containing scattered punctate calcium deposits. (The solitary nodule in the right midlung proved to be metastatic adenocarcinoma of the uterus.)

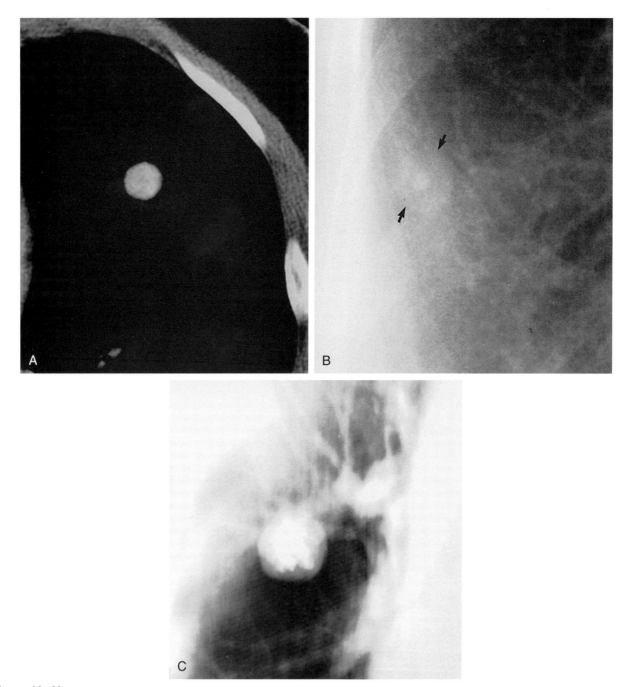

Figure 18–46. Benign Patterns of Calcification. A CT scan *(A)* demonstrates diffuse calcification in a tuberculoma. A view of the right lung from a posteroanterior chest radiograph *(B)* demonstrates a tuberculoma *(arrows)* with a central nidus of calcification. A view from the right upper lobe *(C)* demonstrates a large central area of so-called popcorn ball calcification characteristic of hamartoma.

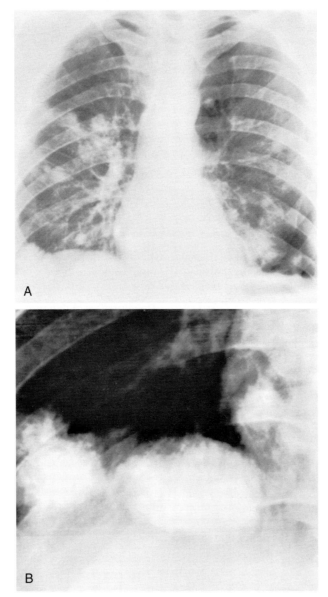

Figure 18–47. Calcified Metastases from Osteogenic Sarcoma. A posteroanterior *(A)* radiograph reveals multiple nodular shadows throughout both lungs varying considerably in size. A pneumothorax is present on the left, a remarkably frequent complication of metastatic osteogenic sarcoma. A detail view of the lower right lung from an overexposed radiograph *(B)* reveals extensive calcification (ossification?) of the two largest metastatic lesions.

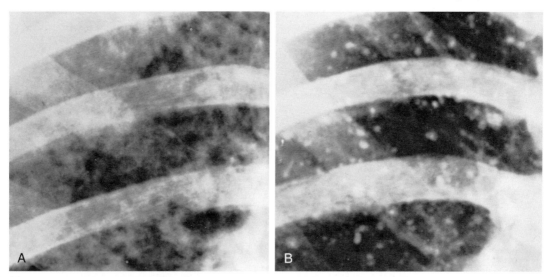

Figure 18–48. Multiple Punctate Calcifications Following Acute Varicella-Zoster Pneumonia. Widespread air-space pneumonia in association with classic cutaneous chickenpox developed in this 28-year-old woman. A chest radiograph revealed multiple air-space nodules, seen to advantage in a magnified view of the right midlung zone *(A)*. Eight years later, a posteroanterior radiograph *(B)* revealed multiple tiny punctate calcifications throughout both lungs. (Courtesy of Dr. Max Palayew, Jewish General Hospital, Montreal.)

mitral stenosis[122, 123] (Fig. 18–49) and other diseases associated with increased left atrial pressure such as hypertrophic cardiomyopathy.[124] Dendriform pulmonary ossification is a rare disorder characterized by branching and sometimes tubular foci of bone most often in the lower lobes. Interstitial (metastatic) calcification is a complication of hypercalcemia, usually secondary to chronic renal failure. It is not often detected radiographically despite its demonstration at autopsy. The last two forms of calcification are discussed more fully in Chapter 68 (*see* page 2699).

Lymph Node Calcification

Lymph node calcification is usually amorphous and irregular in distribution (*see* Fig. 18–45). It results most commonly from healed granulomatous infection, usually tuberculosis or histoplasmosis, in which case it constitutes part of the Ranke complex. Such calcified lymph nodes are usually an incidental finding of little or no clinical significance; however, they may serve as foci for reactivation of infection and occasionally erode a contiguous airway and lead to broncholithiasis (*see* page 2287).

A ring of calcification around the periphery of a lymph node ("eggshell" calcification) is uncommon. Several criteria have been proposed for diagnosis:[125] (1) a shell-like zone of calcification up to 2 mm thick must be present in the peripheral zone of at least two lymph nodes; (2) although the ringlike shadow may be solid or broken, it must be complete in at least one of the lymph nodes; (3) the central part of the lymph node may or may not show additional calcification; and (4) one of the affected lymph nodes must be at least 1 cm in greatest diameter.

The bronchopulmonary nodes are affected most frequently, but involvement of mediastinal and even retroperitoneal nodes has been described.[126] The abnormality is most often seen in silicosis (*see* Fig. 18–24) or coal worker's pneumoconiosis; other rare causes include sarcoidosis, Hodgkin's disease (following mediastinal irradiation), blasto-

mycosis, histoplasmosis, amyloidosis,[125] and tuberculosis (Fig. 18–50).

Calcification in Other Intrathoracic Sites

Calcification or ossification of the cartilage plates of the trachea and major bronchi appears to be a physiologic concomitant of aging (Fig. 18–51); curiously, it is far more common in elderly women than in men.[105] Rarely, the abnormality occurs in younger patients with hypercalcemia. In contrast to these relatively innocuous forms of degenerative or metastatic calcification is tracheobronchopathia osteochondroplastica, a rare condition characterized by nodules or spicules of cartilage and bone that develop in the submucosa of the trachea and bronchi and may result in symptoms of chronic obstructive pulmonary disease (*see* page 2042). Occasionally, the complication occurs in tracheobronchial amyloidosis.

Calcification of the walls of the central pulmonary arteries occurs in a high percentage of patients with severe long-standing pulmonary arterial hypertension, particularly those with a left-to-right shunt. The calcification may be localized to the main pulmonary artery or may extend into the major hilar and even lobar branches;[127] the arteries are invariably severely dilated. Somewhat similar calcification occurs in the walls of aneurysms involving the main pulmonary artery or its hilar branches. Rarely, calcification affects the pulmonary arteries in association with an organized thrombus, as in one case in which a cylindrical, branching, V-shaped calcification was detected in a hilar pulmonary artery approximately 30 years after pulmonary embolization.[128]

Distribution of Disease Within the Lungs

For several reasons, some known and others obscure, many lung diseases tend to develop in certain anatomic locations. Knowledge of such anatomic bias is of obvious

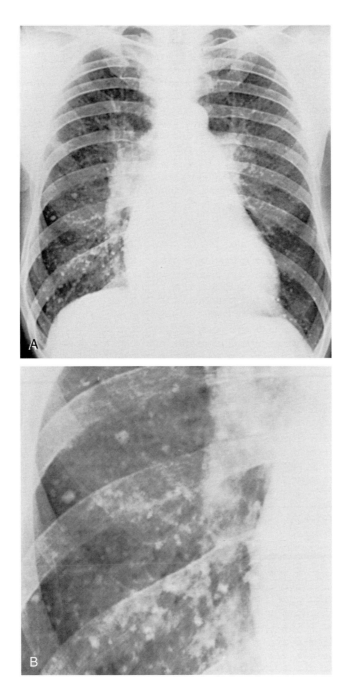

Figure 18–49. Pulmonary Ossification in Mitral Stenosis. A posteroanterior radiograph *(A)* of a 46-year-old man with long-standing mitral stenosis and severe pulmonary arterial hypertension reveals multiple densely calcified nodular shadows ranging in diameter from 1 to 5 mm and situated predominantly in the lower half of the right lung *(B)*. Lesions of this type and localization are highly suggestive of long-standing mitral stenosis. They should not be confused with hemosiderosis.

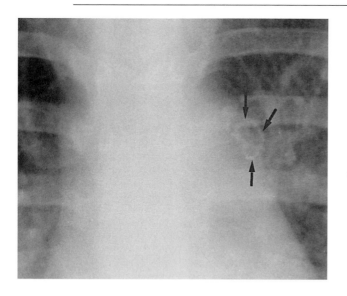

Figure 18–50. "Eggshell" Calcification in Tuberculosis. A view from an anteroposterior chest radiograph in a 4-year-old girl demonstrates eggshell calcification in an aortopulmonary window node *(arrows)*. Smaller calcified nodes can be seen lateral to the aortic arch and in the left hilum. The patient had been treated for primary tuberculosis 2 years previously.

diagnostic importance; the following selected examples indicate how such knowledge can be used in the differential diagnosis.

Aspiration pneumonia is a typical example in which the influence of gravity largely establishes the anatomic distribution of disease *(see* Fig. 18–5). If aspiration occurs when the patient is supine (during the postoperative period, for instance), the upper lobes are involved more often than the lower and their posterior portions more frequently than their anterior;[129] conversely, if aspiration occurs when the patient is erect, involvement of the lower lobes predominates.[130] Whether the patient is recumbent or erect, aspiration

occurs more readily into the right than the left lung because of the more direct origin of the right main bronchus from the trachea.

Gravity also may play a significant role in the localization of pneumonia: the results of an experimental study in dogs showed that the anatomic site in which pneumonia developed could be controlled by altering the position of a dog's thorax so that bacteria-laden exudate flowed into specific segments under the influence of gravity.[131] That this effect is operative in humans is lent support by the tendency of acute air-space pneumonia to occur predominantly in the posterior portions of lobes.[132]

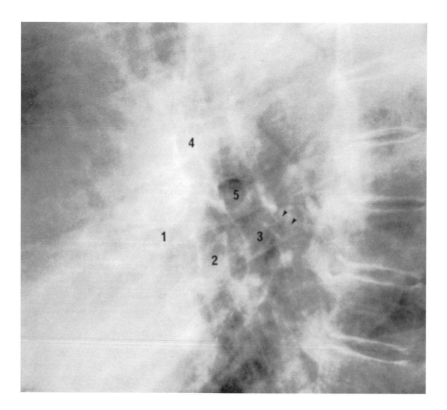

Figure 18–51. Calcification of the Cartilage of the Trachea and Major Bronchi. A detail view from a lateral chest radiograph reveals calcification within the cartilage of the trachea and major bronchi that permitted enhanced perception of the middle lobe bronchus (1), the anterior and posterior walls of the right (2) and left (3) lower lobe bronchi, and the orifices of the right (4) and left (5) upper lobe bronchi. Note the clarity with which the superior segmental bronchus of the left lower lobe is seen *(arrowheads)*. The patient was an elderly woman.

Gravity also explains the observation that pulmonary infarction occurs much more frequently in lower than in upper lobes.[133] This anatomic bias undoubtedly reflects the disparity in blood flow to the base and apex of the lung in erect humans, a disparity amounting to approximately 5 to 1. For the same reason, metastatic tumors occur more frequently in lower lobes; in fact, a solitary mass in an upper lobe is unlikely to be metastatic. This preponderance of metastatic neoplastic involvement of the lower lobes reflects the longer duration in the erect posture (the average adult spends only one third of the time recumbent in bed); in bedridden patients, metastatic deposits do not show the usual anatomic bias and may in fact predominate in the upper zones (Fig. 18–52).

In contrast to the bias for lower lung zones displayed by metastatic neoplasms, primary pulmonary carcinoma has a clear predilection for the upper lung zones.[134] Cavitary carcinoma particularly shows a strong anatomic bias for the upper lobes; for example, of 8 cases of radiographically apparent cavitation among 80 cases of pulmonary carcinoma, 7 were in the upper lobes and 1 in the apex of a lower lobe.[135] It has been postulated that the greater tendency for such upper zone lesions to undergo cavitation is attributable to the relatively greater stress to which the lungs are subject at this site.[136]

Pulmonary tuberculosis provides a singular opportunity to apply anatomic bias to the differential diagnosis. In postprimary tuberculosis in adults, susceptibility of the apical and posterior bronchopulmonary segments of the upper lobes and the superior segment of the lower lobes is well recognized; these three segments were involved in *all* 100 cases in one series[137] and in most (93%) or in part (3.4%) of 500 cases in another.[138] These segments are characterized by a high $\dot{V}/\dot{Q}$ ratio and relatively high Po_2 levels, which favors growth of mycobacteria. The rarity with which the anterior bronchopulmonary segment of an upper lobe is affected *to the exclusion* of other segments is sufficient to make the diagnosis of postprimary tuberculosis in this area extremely unlikely (only 1 case was reported in the series of 100).[137] Predominant involvement of the lower lung zones occurs in only 0.5% to 4% of patients with postprimary tuberculosis.[139] (In contrast to the situation in postprimary disease, primary tuberculosis shows no significant difference in the frequency of involvement of the upper and lower lung zones in either children[140, 141] or adults.[142])

Pulmonary sequestration occurs almost exclusively in

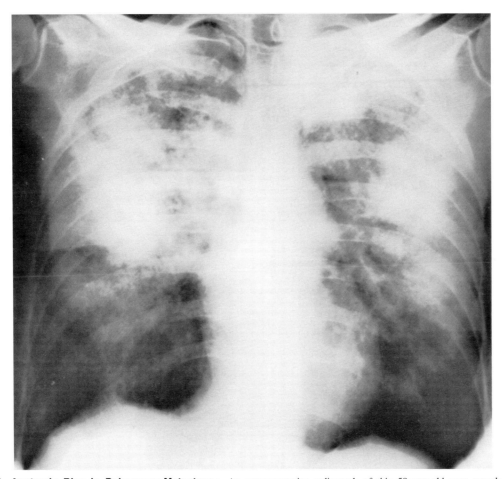

Figure 18–52. Anatomic Bias in Pulmonary Metastases. An anteroposterior radiograph of this 59-year-old man reveals extensive disease predominantly affecting the upper two thirds of both lungs. Although there is some superimposed pneumonia, most of the opacities are due to metastases from carcinoma of the colon. The unusual anatomic distribution of metastases in the patient was related to two factors: (1) emphysema predominantly affecting both lower lung zones and (2) a recumbent position necessitated by long-standing quadriplegia.

the lower lobes, most commonly in the posterior basilar bronchopulmonary segment and more commonly on the left side than the right.[143, 144] Intrapulmonary bronchogenic cysts have a similar but lesser predilection for the lower lobes; two thirds of 32 cases in one study were so located.[145]

Radiologic Localization of Pulmonary Disease— The Silhouette Sign

The anatomic location of the great majority of pulmonary diseases associated with increased density can be established precisely from posteroanterior and lateral radiographs. In two situations, however, localization may be difficult: (1) when multiple segments of both lungs are involved, with resultant confusion of superimposed shadows in the lateral projection; and (2) when only an anteroposterior projection is available for evaluation (for example, in the immediate postoperative period or when the patient is too ill for standard radiography). In these circumstances, the "silhouette sign" may be useful in disease localization. Felson and Felson,[146] who popularized the term, credited Dunham with first reference to this invaluable sign in the mid 1930s.

The silhouette sign is an extremely valuable radiologic sign in both localizing and identifying local pulmonary disease. It can best be defined in the words of Felson:[11] "an intrathoracic lesion touching a border of the heart or aorta will obliterate that border on the roentgenogram; an intrathoracic lesion not anatomically contiguous with a border of the heart or aorta will not obliterate the border."

The mediastinal and diaphragmatic contours are rendered radiographically visible by their contrast with contiguous air-containing lung. Thus, when an opacity is situated in any portion of lung adjacent to a mediastinal or diaphragmatic border, that border can no longer be seen radiographically (Fig. 18–53). The corollary is that an opacity within the lungs that does *not* obliterate the mediastinal or diaphragmatic contour cannot be situated within lung contiguous to these structures (Fig. 18–54). Clearly, this sign is apparent only when structures have been adequately exposed; for example, in an underexposed radiograph, massive consolidation of the right lower lobe may prevent identification of the right border of the heart merely because the x-ray photons have attained insufficient penetration to reproduce the heart shadow through the massive lower lobe density—despite the presence of air-containing lung contiguous to the heart.

Although the silhouette sign is most useful in the differentiation of middle lobe and lingular disease from lower lobe disease, it may also provide precise anatomic information in many other sites—for example, obliteration of the aortic arch on the left side by airlessness of the apical-posterior segment of the left upper lobe, obliteration of the ascending arch of the aorta and the superior vena cava by consolidation of the anterior pulmonary segment of the right upper lobe, and obliteration of the posterior paraspinal line by contiguous airless lung in the left posterior gutter.

Although this sign is used chiefly to localize pulmonary disease, we have found it almost as useful for identifying disease processes. For example, the increased opacity produced by total collapse of the right middle lobe may be impossible to appreciate on a posteroanterior radiograph; however, the silhouette sign invariably accompanies such

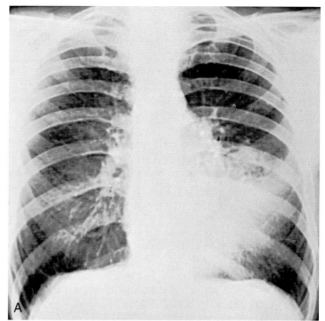

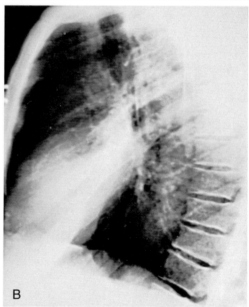

Figure 18–53. The Silhouette Sign. Posteroanterior *(A)* and lateral *(B)* radiographs reveal obliteration of the left heart border by a shadow of homogeneous density situated within the lingula; such obliteration inevitably indicates lingular disease (provided that there is adequate radiographic exposure). Squamous cell carcinoma of the lingular bronchus with distal obstructive pneumonitis was diagnosed.

collapse (apparent as loss of sharp definition of the right heart border) and should permit a categorical statement that disease is present in the right middle lobe (a lateral or lordotic projection will be confirmatory). (An uncommon exception to this rule is severe pectus excavatum, which is occasionally associated with loss of definition of the right heart border.) It may also be very difficult to identify the shadow of minor consolidation or atelectasis in a posterior basal segment of a lower lobe as an area of increased density; however, invisibility of the posterior portion of the hemidiaphragm in lateral projection often permits identification of disease in that segment.

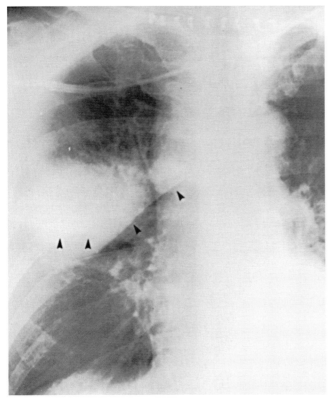

Figure 18–54. Application of the Silhouette Sign for Disease Localization. A detail view of the right hemithorax from an anteroposterior chest radiograph demonstrates an area of air-space consolidation in the right lung caused by acute bacterial pneumonia. The process does not obliterate any portion of the right mediastinal contour and is sharply delineated by the superomedial portion of the right major fissure *(oblique arrowheads)* and the lateral aspect of the minor fissure *(vertical arrowheads)*. These three features thus localize the pneumonia to the posterior and lateral portions of the right upper lobe.

The Time Factor in Radiologic Diagnosis

In clinical practice, radiographic signs may be such that only differential diagnostic possibilities can be suggested at the first examination; if the diagnosis cannot be established by the integrated clinical evidence and results of laboratory and pulmonary function tests, serial films showing changes over the subsequent days, weeks, or months often provide valuable clues to the diagnosis. For example, the progression of changes after pulmonary thromboembolism allows significant deductions concerning the underlying pathologic process: consolidation that clears fairly rapidly within 4 to 7 days indicates pulmonary hemorrhage without tissue necrosis; persistence of the opacity with progressive retraction and loss of volume supports a diagnosis of infarction. The rapidity with which diffuse interstitial pulmonary edema may appear and disappear (often within hours) allows immediate differentiation from pneumonia or irreversible interstitial disease, which it may otherwise closely mimic. Moreover, it is surprising how frequently a small area of parenchymal consolidation in an upper lobe radiographically typical of tuberculosis or a nodule mimicking carcinoma disappears in a few days (indicating a less significant etiology).

In all these examples it is clearly preferable to suggest the correct diagnosis at the time of the first radiograph so that appropriate treatment can be instituted immediately. When initial radiographic diagnosis is impossible, however, and clinical and laboratory evidence is inconclusive, the observation of progression or regression of radiographic abnormalities draws attention not only to the need for discontinuation of useless therapy in the face of an erroneous diagnosis but also to the necessity of instituting suitable treatment when the true nature of the process becomes known.

The time over which a peripheral pulmonary nodule is seen to grow ("doubling time"*) may also be useful information in the differential diagnosis of benignity and malignancy.[147] For example, in one study of 218 pulmonary nodules, 177 of which were malignant and 41 were benign, almost all nodules with a doubling time of 7 days or less or more than 465 days (Fig. 18–55) were benign.[148] The growth rate principle is perhaps most useful in assessing solitary nodules in patients over 40 years of age, a group in which the incidence of malignancy increases significantly. In this group, nearly all solitary nodules that doubled in less than 37 days were benign; the longest doubling time of 72 malignant nodules was 200 days.[149] It therefore seems that pulmonary nodules whose rate of growth falls outside these "benign" limits should be considered malignant.

Whatever practical use is made of doubling time, it is clear that information derived from it enables one to give a more accurate assessment of the underlying nature of the disease than does a simple increase in the size of a nodule. It has also been shown that pulmonary carcinomas with long doubling times tend to have a better prognosis than do carcinomas with a short doubling time.[149, 150] However, since benign lesions such as hamartoma and histoplasmoma may grow slowly, an increase in size *per se* should not be the sole consideration in determining therapy for a pulmonary nodule. Furthermore, lack of growth, even over a 2-year period, does not guarantee that a nodule is benign.[151] Although widely accepted as a criterion of benignity, the concept of 2-year stability as a reliable criterion for benignity is based on a single report published in 1958.[152] Careful review of the data revealed that 2-year stability had only a 65% predictive value for the diagnosis of benign nodules.[151] Therefore, close follow-up is recommended for noncalcified lung nodules, even if they have been stable for 2 years.[151, 153]

LINE SHADOWS

A linear opacity (line shadow, linear shadow, band shadow) can be defined most simply as a shadow resembling a line, i.e., any elongated opacity of approximately uniform width. The normal substratum of all chest radiographs—the vascular markings and interlobar fissures—is formed by such shadows; the radiologic appearance of these structures is described in Chapters 2 and 6 (*see* pages 77 and 154). Other linear opacities can be considered in five categories: septal lines, tubular shadows (bronchial wall shadows), linear opacities extending from peripheral parenchymal lesions

---

*Doubling in this context refers to volume, not diameter. Assuming a nodule to be spherical, multiplication of its diameter by 1.25 yields the diameter of a sphere whose volume is double; e.g., the volume of a nodule 2 cm in diameter is doubled by the time its diameter reaches 2.5 cm.

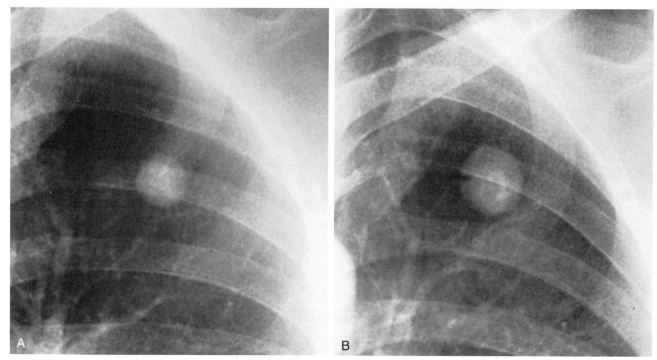

Figure 18–55. Solitary Nodule: Enlarging Histoplasmoma. When initially examined *(A)* a solitary nodule in the left upper lobe of this 61-year-old asymptomatic man measured 17 mm in diameter; it was sharply circumscribed and showed questionable central calcification. Two years later *(B)*, the diameter of the lesion had reached 21 mm, almost a doubling of the volume. Faint central calcification is present. Despite the appearance of calcification, the lesion was resected; organisms consistent with *Histoplasma capsulatum* were identified histologically.

to the hila or visceral pleura, parenchymal scars, and linear atelectasis.

Septal Lines

Septal lines are caused by thickening of the interstitial tissue and, to a lesser extent, by lymphatic dilatation in the interlobular septa and around deep parenchymal veins and anastomotic lymphatic channels.[4, 154, 155] They were first described in 1933 by Kerley,[156] who subsequently categorized them into three types: "A" lines, "B" lines, and "C" lines.[157–159]

Kerley A lines are straight or almost straight linear opacities within the lung substance, seldom more than 1 mm thick and 2 to 6 cm long; their course bears no definite relationship to the anatomic distribution of bronchoarterial bundles (Fig. 18–56). They never extend to the visceral pleura, although their medial extension is usually to a hilum. In one radiologic-pathologic correlation study, they were shown to correspond to the connective tissue within the lung that contains veins and anastomotic lymphatics crossing from perivenous to peribronchial locations.[154] Depending on the disease process that causes them, Kerley A lines may be reversible (as in pulmonary edema) or irreversible (as in pneumoconiosis or lymphangitic carcinomatosis).

Kerley B lines are less than 2 cm long and, in contrast to A lines, are located in the lung periphery; they are short and straight, seldom more than 1 mm thick, and lie roughly perpendicular to the pleural surface (Fig. 18–57). Their outer ends invariably abut the visceral pleura, although this relationship may not be apparent on a posteroanterior radio-

graph. Kerley B lines are caused by thickening of the interlobular septa that abut the visceral pleura; because of this anatomic location, they are often referred to as "septal lines." Care is needed to avoid mistaking them for small vascular shadows in the lung periphery; the latter branch, a characteristic never seen with the former. The most common cause of Kerley B lines is interstitial pulmonary edema secondary to pulmonary venous hypertension (as in mitral stenosis or left ventricular failure). In such circumstances, the influence of gravity on pulmonary hemodynamics gives rise to interlobular septal edema in the lower portions of the lungs and not in the upper; thus, these shadows are seen to best advantage just above the costophrenic angles on posteroanterior and lateral radiographs. When the edema is transient, septal lines appear and disappear sporadically with each episode of decompensation; with repeated insults of this character or in the presence of chronic and severe pulmonary venous hypertension, fibrosis within the interlobular septa may result in irreversible B lines. In diseases other than edema, the anatomic distribution of B lines may be entirely different. For example, in pneumoconiosis,[160] sarcoidosis,[161] lymphangitic carcinomatosis,[162] lipid pneumonia,[163] and lymphoma,[164] the lines may be visible anywhere in the lung periphery where septa normally occur.

Kerley C lines consist of a fine network of interlacing linear shadows projected on the anterior portion of both lungs, their size and configuration corresponding to those of the secondary lobules. They are sometimes seen in cases of interstitial pulmonary edema (Fig. 18–58) and, like B lines, have been shown to be caused by thickening of the interlobular septa.[155] Thickening of septa in adjacent secondary lobules results in a pattern of polygonal arcades on HRCT[34, 56] and corresponds to the presence of C lines on the radiograph.

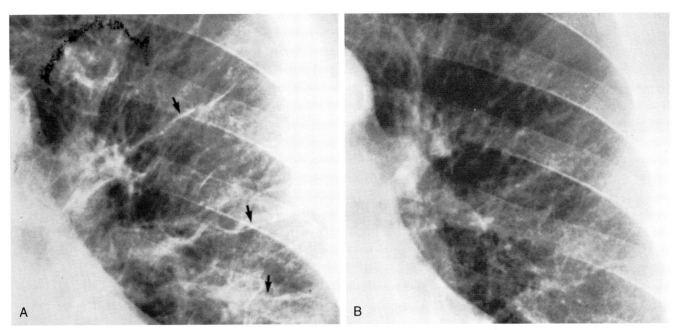

Figure 18–56. Line Shadows: Kerley A Lines. A view of the left lung from a posteroanterior radiograph *(A)* reveals a coarse network of linear strands widely distributed throughout the lung. Several long line shadows measuring up to 4 cm in length can be identified in the central zone approximately midway between the axillary lung margin and the heart *(arrows)*; the orientation of these lines does not conform to the distribution of bronchovascular bundles. These are Kerley A lines and represent edema of central pulmonary septa. A radiograph several days later *(B)* shows complete clearing. Cardiac decompensation was diagnosed.

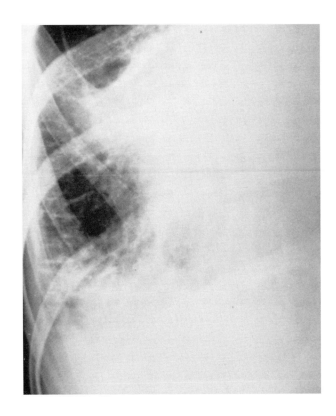

Figure 18–57. Line Shadows: Septal (Kerley B) Lines. A magnified view of the lower portion of the right lung from a posteroanterior chest radiograph reveals several line shadows approximately 1 cm in length oriented in a horizontal plane perpendicular to the axillary pleura (there is a small pleural effusion as well). These are Kerley B lines caused by edema of the interlobular septa.

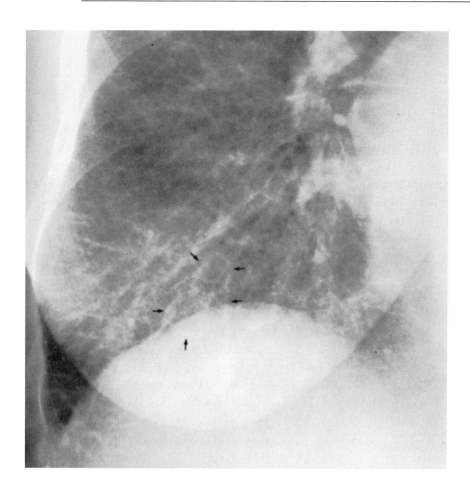

Figure 18–58. The Nature of Kerley C Lines. A view of the lower half of the right lung from a posteroanterior radiograph reveals numerous septal (Kerley B) lines in the axillary lung zone. In addition, at least three or four roughly circular ring shadows *(arrows)* can be seen in the midlung zone and represent the boundaries of secondary lobules thickened by edema fluid. These Kerley C lines are thus another manifestation of septal edema and are no more than Kerley B lines perceived *en face*.

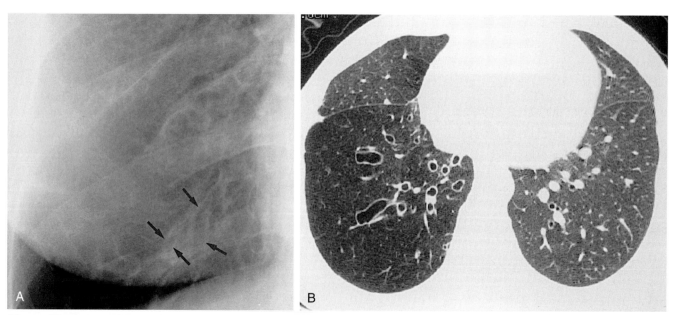

Figure 18–59. Line Shadows: Tubular. A view of the lower half of the right lung from a posteroanterior chest radiograph *(A)* reveals several tubular shadows *(arrows)*, some of whose walls are parallel and others divergent. An HRCT scan *(B)* demonstrates extensive bronchiectasis in the right lower lobe. Also note the decreased vascularity in comparison to the normal left lower lobe. The patient was a 43-year-old woman with bronchiectasis presumed to be related to childhood viral infection.

Tubular Shadows (Bronchial Wall Shadows)

Tubular shadows are double-line shadows that may be parallel or slightly tapered as they proceed distally and always have a bronchovascular distribution (Fig. 18–59); they may branch in a manner typical of the bronchial tree. When one of the paired lines is contiguous to a vessel, it casts no radiographic shadow; however, identification of a single line paralleling a vessel has the same significance as a tubular shadow.

The air columns of the trachea, main bronchi, right intermediate bronchus, and left lower lobe bronchus are normally visible on a well-exposed radiograph. These structures are in contact with air-containing parenchyma, and their walls are also visible, their thickness being sufficient to cast a radiographic shadow. Beyond the immediate confines of the hilar shadows, however, neither the bronchial walls nor their air columns should be visible normally (except when viewed end-on [*see* further on]); thus, when tubular shadows are identified outside the hilar limits, they constitute a definite sign of disease.

The most common cause of tubular shadows is bronchiectasis (*see* Fig. 18–59), in which case the line shadows are roughly parallel and measure 1 mm or slightly more in width. The width of the air column separating them depends on the severity of the bronchial dilatation. Since chronic bronchiectasis is often associated with atelectasis, multiple tubular shadows may be crowded together with little air-containing parenchyma separating them. Pathologically, these line shadows are caused by thickened bronchial walls as a result of fibrosis and chronic inflammation. When bronchiectatic segments become filled with mucus or pus, their tubular appearance is transformed into homogeneous, band-like opacities known as the "gloved-finger" shadow (Fig. 18–60).[165] Of a similar nature but more proximal in the bronchial tree are the mucous plugs of mucoid impaction or allergic bronchopulmonary aspergillosis; these plugs vary from a broad linear shadow to a Y or V configuration depending on the length of airway involved and whether a bronchial bifurcation is affected.

Tubular shadows ("tram lines") can occasionally be identified as an isolated abnormality, usually in the right lower lobe, in persons without bronchiectasis. They may occur in patients with chronic bronchitis[166] and asthma[167] (Fig. 18–61). Bronchial walls can also be identified in the parahilar zones in a large number of healthy individuals and patients with bronchial wall thickening when they are viewed end-on (Fig. 18–62).[168] The resulting shadows range in diameter from 3 to 7 mm and usually represent segmental or subsegmental bronchi in the anterior segment of an upper lobe or the superior segment of a lower lobe, where they are seen end-on. The reason for the visibility of a bronchial wall when viewed *en face* as opposed to end-on is related to the different absorptive power of its tissue "in tangent." Since the image of the tangential wall thickness fades off at the margins, loss of definition precludes accurate appreciation of total wall thickness; by contrast, when the same tube is viewed end-on, a substantially greater amount of tissue is traversed by the x-ray beam, particularly at its periphery, thus reducing the effect of subliminal absorption (Fig. 18–63). Normal bronchial wall thickness ranges from approximately 10% to 15% of the diameter of the bronchus.[169, 170]

Linear Opacities Extending from Peripheral Parenchymal Lesions to the Hila or Visceral Pleura

Line shadows of varying width can often be seen extending from a peripheral parenchymal opacity to the hilum. They are usually uneven in width and their course may be interrupted for varying distances. Their conformity to the pattern of vascular distribution establishes their anatomic location within bronchovascular bundles. Such communicating strands have been described in both infectious and neoplastic processes and are thus of no value in the differential diagnosis. In active tuberculosis, the shadows are produced by an admixture of granulomatous inflammatory tissue, fibrous tissue, thickened lymphatics, and thickened bronchial walls; in neoplasms, they may be related to the presence of carcinoma in lymphatic and perilymphatic interstitial tissue (lymphangitic carcinomatosis).

When a parenchymal mass of almost any etiology is situated near the periphery of the lung, a line shadow extending from the mass to the visceral pleura is sometimes visible and commonly associated with local indrawing of the pleura ("tail sign" or "pleural tag") (Fig. 18–64). This sign was initially observed in bronchioloalveolar carcinoma and was considered to be highly suggestive of that diagnosis.[171] However, in one study of 18 patients with the "tail sign," 9 had benign disease (granulomas of varying etiology);[172] moreover, of the 9 cancers, 5 were bronchioloalveolar carcinoma, 2 were adenocarcinoma, 1 was squamous cell carcinoma, and 1 was metastatic carcinoma of the colon. In a more extensive study, the tail sign was found to be an entirely nonspecific feature of peripherally located pulmonary lesions, whether benign or malignant.[173]

Parenchymal Scarring

A segment of lung that was the site of infectious disease and has undergone healing through fibrosis may be manifested as a linear shadow. The width of the shadow largely depends on the amount of lung originally involved. Healed upper lobe postprimary tuberculosis is a common example of this type of linear shadow. In some cases the shadow is related to the presence of fibrous tissue in the peribronchovascular interstitium or lung adjacent to the initial focus of granulomatous inflammation; occasionally, the latter itself has a linear rather than a round appearance. Several shadows may be fairly closely grouped, commonly extending from the hilum to the visceral pleural surface and diverging slightly toward the periphery. In many cases, there is compensatory overinflation of adjacent lung parenchyma.

The line shadow created by healed pulmonary infarction represents fibrous scarring secondary to lung necrosis. These linear shadows always extend to a pleural surface, and it has been suggested that this relationship is caused, at least in part, by indrawing of the pleura by the scar (Figs. 18–65 and 18–66).[174]

Linear Atelectasis

Atelectasis frequently results in linear opacities measuring 1 to 3 mm in thickness and 4 to 10 cm in length that are visible on both the chest radiograph and CT. Such linear atelectasis, also known as platelike or discoid atelectasis, is discussed in Chapter 20 (*see* page 554).

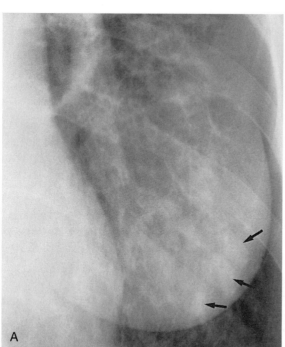

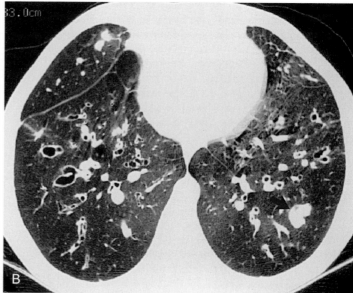

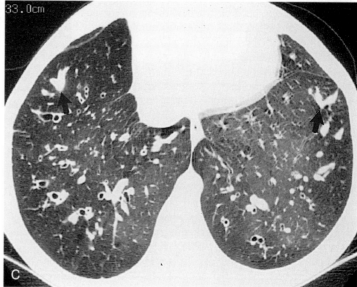

Figure 18–60. Cystic Fibrosis with Bronchiectasis and Mucoid Impaction. *(A)* A view of the lower half of the left lung from a posteroanterior chest radiograph demonstrates several tubular, branching opacities *(arrows)*. HRCT scans *(B and C)* demonstrate extensive bilateral bronchiectasis as well as several branching opacities *(arrows)* typical of mucoid impaction. The patient was a 39-year-old woman.

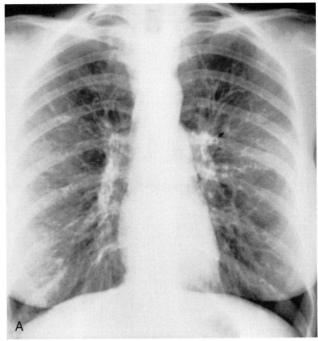

Figure 18–61. Line Shadows Caused by Thickened Bronchial Walls: Tram Lines. A posteroanterior radiograph *(A)* reveals prominent markings throughout both lungs. In the left upper zone, parallel or slightly tapering line shadows can be identified in the bronchial distribution of the left upper lobe, seen to better advantage on the anteroposterior tomogram in *B (arrows)*. These "tram lines" represent thickened bronchial walls, an abnormality more easily appreciated by viewing a bronchus end-on *(arrow in A)*. The patient is a 17-year-old girl with chronic asthma.

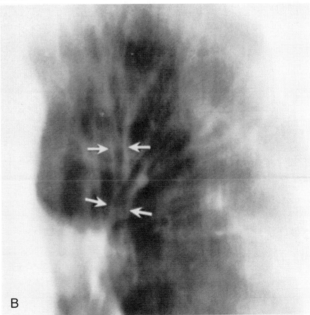

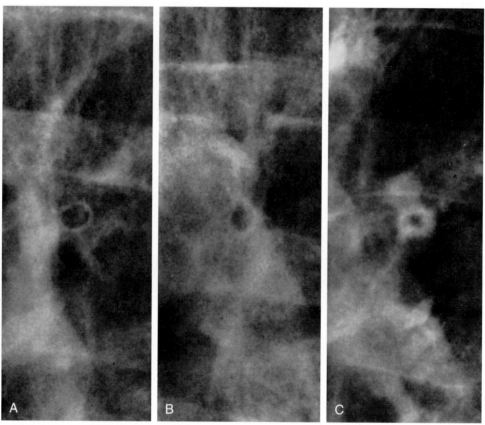

Figure 18–62. Bronchial Wall Thickening as Assessed from Parahilar Bronchi Viewed End-on. Views of the left parahilar zone from posteroanterior chest radiographs of three different patients show a normal bronchus *(A)*, a bronchus with moderate wall thickening *(B)*, and a bronchus with marked wall thickening *(C)*. (From Fraser RG, Fraser RS, Renner JW, et al: Radiology 120:1, 1976.)

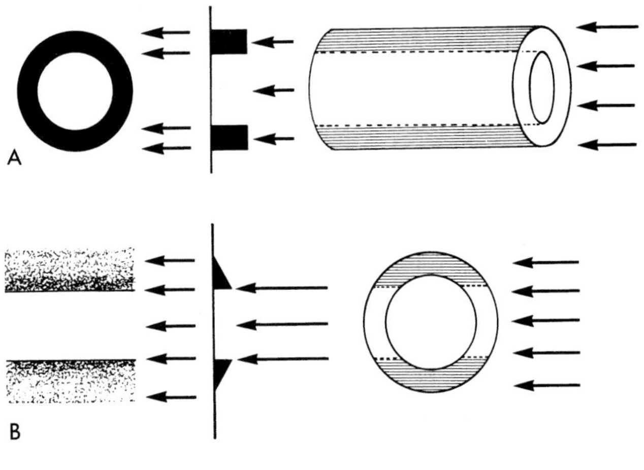

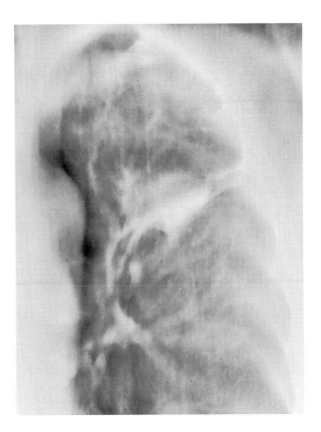

Figure 18–63. Diagram of a Hollow Tube. A hollow tube is in cross section (end-on) *(A)* and in tangent (longitudinally) *(B).* See the text. (From Fraser RG, Fraser RS, Renner JW, et al: Radiology 120:1, 1976.)

Figure 18–64. Line Shadows: Communication Between a Peripheral Mass and the Visceral Pleura. A view of the upper half of the left lung reveals a rather indistinctly defined homogeneous mass lying in the midlung zone. A prominent line shadow extending from the lateral margin of the mass to the pleura resulted in a V-shaped deformity of the pleura caused by indrawing. Histoplasmosis was diagnosed.

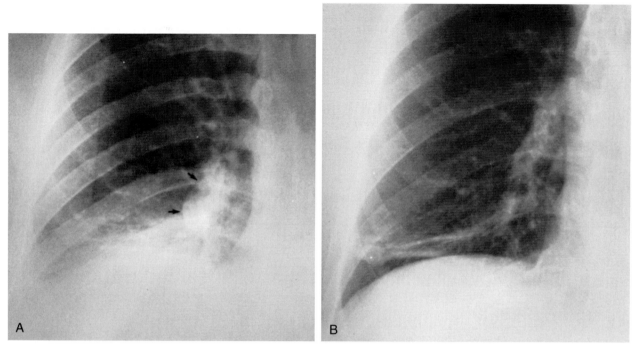

Figure 18–65. Linear Scarring Secondary to Pulmonary Thromboembolism. Two days before the radiograph illustrated in *A*, this 33-year-old man had experienced a sudden onset of right chest pain and hemoptysis. This view of the right lung in anteroposterior projection reveals bulging of the right interlobar artery *(arrows)*, "knuckling" of this vessel, a poorly defined opacity in the right lower lobe, and elevation of the right hemidiaphragm. This combination of changes is highly suggestive of pulmonary thromboembolism and infarction. Ten days later, a detail view of the right lower zone *(B)* demonstrates a horizontally oriented linear opacity at the right base that subsequently underwent little change in appearance over the next several months. The scar was presumed to be secondary to infarction.

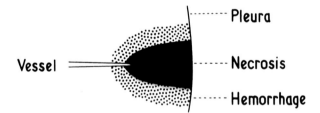

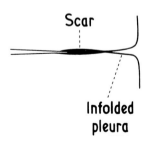

Figure 18–66. Diagrammatic Representation of Indrawn Pleura. Possible mechanism of the production of a line shadow with a pleural component, specifically following an infarct. (Reprinted from Br J Radiol, 43:327, 1970, with permission of Dr. Lynne Reid and the editor.)

REFERENCES

1. Felson B: A new look at pattern recognition of diffuse pulmonary disease. Am J Roentgenol 133:183, 1979.
2. McLoud TC, Carrington CB, Gaensler EA: Diffuse infiltrative lung disease: A new scheme for description. Radiology 149:353, 1983.
3. Mathieson JR, Mayo JR, Staples CA, Müller NL: Chronic diffuse infiltrative lung disease: Comparison of diagnostic accuracy of CT and chest radiography. Radiology 171:111, 1989.
4. Glossary of terms for thoracic radiology: Recommendations of the nomenclature committee of the Fleischner Society. Am J Roentgenol 143:509, 1984.
5. Austin JHM, Müller NL, Friedman PJ, et al: Glossary of terms for CT of the lungs: Recommendations of the nomenclature committee of the Fleischer Society. Radiology 200:327, 1996.
6. Itoh H, Murata K, Konishi J, et al: Diffuse lung disease: Pathologic basis for the high-resolution computed tomography findings. J Thorac Imaging 8:176, 1993.
7. Heitzman ER, Markarian B, Berger I, et al: The secondary pulmonary lobule: A practical concept for interpretation of chest radiographs. Radiology 93:513, 1969.
8. Genereux GP: Pattern recognition in diffuse pulmonary disease: A review of theory and practice. Med Radiogr Photogr 61:2, 1985.
9. Reed JC, Madewell JE: The air bronchogram in interstitial disease of the lungs: A radiological-pathological correlation. Radiology 116:1, 1975.
10. Fleischner FG: Der sichtbare Bronchialbaum, ein differentialdiagnostisches Symptom im Röntgenbild der Pneumonie. Fortschr Roentgenstr 36:319, 1927.
11. Felson B: Chest Roentgenology. Philadelphia, WB Saunders, 1973.
12. Reed JC, Madewell JE: The air bronchogram in interstitial disease of the lungs: A radiological-pathological correlation. Radiology 116:1, 1975.
13. Aschoff L: In Lectures on Pathology. New York, Hoeber, 1924, pp 42–43, 53–57.
14. Genereux GP: The Fleischner lecture: Computed tomography of diffuse pulmonary disease. J Thorac Imaging 4:50, 1989.
15. Itoh H, Tokunaga S, Asamoto H, et al: Radiologic-pathologic correlations of small lung nodules with special reference to peribronchiolar nodules. Am J Roentgenol 130:223, 1978.
16. Murata K, Itoh H, Todo G, et al: Centrilobular lesions of the lung: Demonstration by high-resolution CT and pathologic correlation. Radiology 161:641, 1986.
17. Naidich DP, Zerhouni EA, Hutchins GM, et al: Computed tomography of the pulmonary parenchyma. Part 1: Distal air-space disease. J Thorac Imaging 1:39, 1985.
18. Müller NL, Miller RR: State of the art: Computed tomography of chronic diffuse infiltrative lung disease. I. Am Rev Respir Dis 142:1206, 1990.
19. Müller NL, Miller RR: State of the art: Computed tomography of chronic diffuse infiltrative lung disease. II. Am Rev Respir Dis 142:1440, 1990.
20. Padley SPG, Hansell DM, Flower CDR, et al: Comparative accuracy of high-resolution computed tomography and chest radiography in the diagnosis of chronic diffuse infiltrative lung disease. Clin Radiol 44:222, 1991.
21. Grenier P, Valeyre D, Cluzel P, et al: Chronic diffuse interstitial lung disease: Diagnostic value of chest radiography and high-resolution CT. Radiology 179:123, 1991.
22. Müller NL: Clinical value of high-resolution CT in chronic diffuse lung disease. Am J Roentgenol 157:1163, 1991.
23. Weibel ER: Looking into the lung: What can it tell us? Am J Roentgenol 133:1021, 1979.
24. Bergin CJ, Müller NL: CT of interstitial lung disease: A diagnostic approach. Am J Roentgenol 148:9, 1987.
25. Staub NC, Nagano H, Pearce ML: Pulmonary edema in dogs, especially the sequence of fluid accumulation in lungs. J Appl Physiol 22:227, 1967.
26. Levin B: Subpleural interlobular lymphectasis reflecting metastatic carcinoma. Radiology 72:682, 1959.
27. Trapnell DH: Septal lines in pneumoconiosis. Br J Radiol 37:805, 1964.
28. Stolberg HO, Patt NL, MacEwen KF, et al: Hodgkin's disease of the lung: Roentgenologic-pathologic correlation. Am J Roentgenol 92:96, 1964.
29. Colby TV, Swensen SJ: Anatomic distribution and histopathologic patterns in diffuse lung disease: Correlation with HRCT. J Thorac Imaging 11:1, 1996.
30. Genereux GP: Pattern recognition in diffuse lung disease: A review of theory and practice. Med Radiogr Photogr 61:2, 1985.
31. Stein MG, Mayo J, Müller N, et al: Pulmonary lymphangitic spread of carcinoma: Appearance on CT scans. Radiology 162:371, 1987.
32. Hirakata K, Nakata H, Nakagawa T: CT of pulmonary metastases with pathological correlation. Semin Ultrasound CT MR 16:379, 1995.
33. Bessis L, Callard P, Gotheil C, et al: High-resolution CT of parenchymal lung disease: Precise correlation with histologic findings. Radiographics 12:45, 1992.
34. Munk PL, Müller NL, Miller RR, et al: Pulmonary lymphangitic carcinomatosis: CT and pathologic findings. Radiology 166:705, 1988.
35. Webb WR, Stein MG, Finkbeiner WE, et al: Normal and diseased isolated lungs: High-resolution CT. Radiology 166:81, 1988.
36. Müller NL, Kullnig P, Miller RR: The CT findings of pulmonary sarcoidosis: Analysis of 25 patients. Am J Roentgenol 152:1179, 1989.
37. Murch CR, Carr DH: Computed tomography appearances of pulmonary alveolar proteinosis. Clin Radiol 40:240, 1989.
38. Kang EY, Grenier P, Laurent F, et al: Interlobular septal thickening: Patterns at high-resolution CT. J Thorac Imaging 11:260, 1996.
39. Nishimura K, Kitaichi M, Izumi T, et al: Usual interstitial pneumonia: Histologic correlation with high-resolution CT. Radiology 182:337, 1992.
40. Meziane MA: High-resolution computed tomography scanning in the assessment of interstitial lung diseases. J Thorac Imaging 7:13, 1992.
41. Webb WR, Müller NL, Naidich DP: High-Resolution CT of the Lung. 2nd ed. Philadelphia, Lippincott-Raven, 1996, pp 41–108.
42. Müller NL, Chiles C, Kullnig P: Pulmonary lymphangiomyomatosis: Correlation of CT with radiographic and functional findings. Radiology 175:335, 1990.
43. Primack SL, Hartman TE, Hansell DM, et al: End-stage lung disease: CT findings in 61 patients. Radiology 189:681, 1993.
44. Primack SL, Müller NL, Mayo JR, et al: Pulmonary parenchymal abnormalities of vascular origin: High-resolution CT findings. Radiographics 14:739, 1994.
45. Storto ML, Kee ST, Golden JA, et al: Hydrostatic pulmonary edema: High-resolution CT findings. Am J Roentgenol 165:817, 1995.
46. Remy-Jardin M, Giraud F, Remy J, et al: Importance of ground-glass attenuation in chronic diffuse infiltrative lung disease: Pathologic-CT correlation. Radiology 189:693, 1993.
47. Oswald N, Parkinson T: Honeycomb lungs. Q J Med 18:1, 1949.
48. Pimentel JC: Three-dimensional photographic reconstruction in a study of the pathogenesis of honeycomb lung. Thorax 22:444, 1967.
49. Hogg JC: Chronic interstitial lung disease of unknown cause: A new classification based on pathogenesis. Am J Roentgenol 156:225, 1991.
50. Genereux GP: The end-stage lung: Pathogenesis, pathology, and radiology. Radiology 116:279, 1975.
51. Staples CA, Müller NL, Vedal S, et al: Usual interstitial pneumonia: Correlation of CT with clinical, functional, and radiologic findings. Radiology 162:377, 1987.
52. Templeton PA, McLoud TC, Müller NL, et al: Pulmonary lymphangioleiomyomatosis: CT and pathologic findings. J Comput Assist Tomogr 13:54, 1989.
53. Heppleston AG: The pathology of honeycomb lung. Thorax 11:77, 1956.
54. Remy-Jardin M, Beuscart R, Sault MC, et al: Subpleural micronodules in diffuse infiltrative lung diseases: Evaluation with thin-section CT scans. Radiology 177:133, 1990.
55. Remy-Jardin M, Remy J, Wallaert B, et al: Subacute and chronic bird breeder hypersensitivity pneumonitis: Sequential evaluation with CT and correlation with lung function tests and bronchoalveolar lavage. Radiology 189:111, 1993.
56. Zerhouni EA, Naidich DP, Stitik FP, et al: Computed tomography of the pulmonary parenchyma: II. Interstitial disease. J Thorac Imaging 1:54, 1985.
57. Brauner MW, Lenoir S, Grenier P, et al: Pulmonary sarcoidosis: CT assessment of lesion reversibility. Radiology 182:349, 1992.
58. Kwong JS, Carignan S, Kang EY, et al: Miliary tuberculosis: Diagnostic accuracy of chest radiography. Chest 110:339, 1996.
59. Coppage L, Shaw C, Curtis AM: Metastatic disease to the chest in patients with extrathoracic malignancy. J Thorac Imaging 2:24, 1987.
60. Gough J, Wentworth JE: The use of thin sections of entire organs in morbid anatomical studies. J R Microbiol Soc 69:231, 1949.
61. Ellis K, Renthal G: Pulmonary sarcoidosis: Roentgenographic observations on course of disease. Am J Roentgenol 88:1070, 1962.
62. Kwong JS, Carignan S, Kang EY, et al: Miliary tuberculosis: Diagnostic accuracy of chest radiography. Chest 110:339, 1996.
63. Hirakata K, Nakata H, Nakagawa T: CT of pulmonary metastases with pathological correlation. Semin Ultrasound CT MR 16:379, 1995.
64. Murata K, Takahashi M, Mori M, et al: Pulmonary metastatic nodules: CT-pathologic correlation. Radiology 182:331, 1992.
65. Remy-Jardin M, Degreef JM, Beuscart R, et al: Coal worker's pneumoconiosis: CT assessment in exposed workers and correlation with radiographic findings. Radiology 177:363, 1990.
66. Bégin R, Bergeron D, Samson L, et al: CT assessment of silicosis in exposed workers. Am J Roentgenol 148:509, 1987.
67. Kattan KR, Eyler WR, Felson B: The juxtaphrenic peak in upper lobe collapse. Semin Roentgenol 15:187, 1980.
68. Remy-Jardin M, Remy J, Giraud F, et al: Computed tomography assessment of ground-glass opacity: Semiology and significance. J Thorac Imaging 8:249, 1993.
69. Leung AN, Miller RR, Müller NL: Parenchymal opacification in chronic infiltrative lung diseases: CT-pathologic correlation. Radiology 188:209, 1993.
70. Bergin CJ, Wirth RL, Berry GJ, et al: Pneumocystis carinii pneumonia: CT and HRCT observations. J Comput Assist Tomogr 14:756, 1990.
71. Moskovic E, Miller R, Pearson M: High-resolution computed tomography of Pneumocystis carinii pneumonia in AIDS. Clin Radiol 42:239, 1990.
72. Primack SL, Miller RR, Müller NL: Diffuse pulmonary hemorrhage: Clinical, pathologic, and imaging features. Am J Roentgenol 164:295, 1995.
73. Hartman TE, Primack SL, Müller NL, et al: Diagnosis of thoracic complications in AIDS: Accuracy of CT. Am J Roentgenol 162:547, 1994.
74. Silver SF, Müller NL, Miller RR, et al: Hypersensitivity pneumonitis: Evaluation with CT. Radiology 173:441, 1989.
75. Hansell DM, Moskovic E: High-resolution computed tomography in extrinsic allergic alveolitis. Clin Radiol 43:8, 1991.
76. Hartman TE, Primack SL, Swensen SJ, et al: Desquamative interstitial pneumonia: Thin-section CT findings in 22 patients. Radiology 187:787, 1993.
77. Godwin JD, Müller NL, Takasugi JE: Pulmonary alveolar proteinosis: CT findings. Radiology 169:609, 1988.
78. Müller NL, Colby TV: Idiopathic interstitial pneumonias: High-resolution CT and histologic findings. RadioGraphics 17:1016, 1997.
79. Felson B: A new look at pattern recognition of diffuse pulmonary disease. Am J Roentgenol 133:183, 1979.

80. Grenier P, Chevret S, Beigelman C, et al: Chronic diffuse infiltrative lung disease: Determination of the diagnostic value of clinical data, chest radiography, and CT with Bayesian analysis. Radiology 191:383, 1994.

81. Bateson EM: An analysis of 155 solitary lung lesions illustrating the differential diagnosis of mixed tumours of the lung. Clin Radiol 16:51, 1965.

82. Zwirewich CV, Vedal S, Miller RR, Müller NL: Solitary pulmonary nodule: High-resolution CT and radiologic-pathologic correlation. Radiology 179:469, 1991.

83. Theros EG: Varying manifestations of peripheral pulmonary neoplasms: A radiologic-pathologic correlative study. Am J Roentgenol 128:893, 1977.

84. Siegelman SS, Khouri NF, Leo FP, et al: Solitary pulmonary nodules: CT assessment. Radiology 160:307, 1986.

85. Zerhouni EA, Stitik FP, Siegelman SS, et al: CT of the pulmonary nodule: A cooperative study. Radiology 160:319, 1986.

86. Bleyer JM, Marks JH: Tuberculomas and hamartomas of the lung: Comparative study of 66 proved cases. Am J Roentgenol 77:1013, 1957.

87. Steele JD: The Solitary Pulmonary Nodule. Springfield, IL, Charles C Thomas, 1964.

88. Barnes DJ, Naraqi S, Igo JD: The diagnostic and prognostic significance of bulging fissures in acute lobar pneumonia. Aust N Z J Med 18:130, 1988.

89. Felson B, Rosenberg LS, Hamburger M: Roentgen findings in acute Friedlander's pneumonia. Radiology 53:559, 1949.

90. Moon WK, Im JG, Yeon KM, et al: Complications of *Klebsiella* pneumonia: CT evaluation. J Comput Assist Tomogr 19:176, 1995.

91. Francis JB, Francis PB: Bulging (sagging) fissure sign in *Hemophilus influenzae* lobar pneumonia. South Med J 71:1452, 1978.

92. Golden R: The effect of bronchostenosis upon the roentgen-ray shadows in carcinoma of the bronchus. Am J Roentgenol 13:21, 1925.

93. Glossary of terms for thoracic radiology: Recommendations of the Nomenclature Committee of the Fleischner Society. Am J Roentgenol 143:519, 1984.

94. Austin JHM, Müller NL, Friedman PJ, et al: Glossary of terms for CT of the lungs: Recommendations of the Nomenclature Committee of the Fleischner Society. Radiology 200:327, 1996.

95. Woodring JH, Fried M, Chuang VP: Solitary cavities of the lung: Diagnostic implications of cavity wall thickness. Am J Roentgenol 135:1269, 1980.

96. Jackson H, Stark P: Tilted air-fluid interfaces on chest radiographs. Am J Roentgenol 144:37, 1985.

97. Lewall DB, McCorkell SJ: Rupture of echinococcal cysts: Diagnosis, classification, and clinical implications. Am J Roentgenol 146:391, 1986.

98. Fainsinger MH: Pulmonary hydatid disease: The sign of the camalote. S Afr Med J 23:723, 1949.

99. Danner PK, McFarland DR, Felson B: Massive pulmonary gangrene. Am J Roentgenol 103:548, 1968.

100. Penner C, Maycher B, Long R: Pulmonary gangrene: A complication of bacterial pneumonia. Chest 105:567, 1994.

101. Cordier JF, Valeyre D, Guillevin L, et al: Pulmonary Wegener's granulomatosis: A clinical and imaging study of 77 cases. Chest 97:906, 1990.

101a. Huang RM, Naidich DP, Lubat E, et al: Septic pulmonary emboli: CT-radiographic correlation. Am J Roentgenol 153:41, 1989.

101b. Kuhlman JE, Fishman EK, Tiegen C: Pulmonary septic emboli: Diagnosis with CT. Radiology 174:211, 1990.

102. Kuhlman JE, Fishman EK, Kuhajda FP, et al: Solitary bronchioloalveolar carcinoma: CT criteria. Radiology 167:379, 1988.

103. Weisbrod GL, Chamberlain D, Herman SJ: Cystic change (pseudocavitation) associated with bronchioloalveolar carcinoma: A report of four patients. J Thorac Imaging 10:106, 1995.

104. Hill CA: Bronchioloalveolar carcinoma: A review. Radiology 150:15, 1984.

105. Salzman E: Lung Calcifications in X-ray Diagnosis. Springfield, IL, Charles C Thomas, 1968.

106. Bhalla M, Shepard JAO, Nakamura K, Kazerooni EA: Dual kV CT to detect calcification in solitary pulmonary nodule. J Comput Assist Tomogr 19:44, 1995.

107. Kelcz F, Zing FE, Peppler WW, et al: Conventional chest radiography versus dual-energy computed radiography in the detection and characterization of pulmonary nodules. Am J Roentgenol 162:271, 1994.

108. Good CA: The solitary pulmonary nodule: A problem of management. Radiol Clin North Am 1:429, 1963.

109. Gurney JW: Determining the likelihood of malignancy in solitary pulmonary nodules with Bayesian analysis: I. Theory. Radiology 186:405, 1993.

110. O'Keefe ME Jr, Good CA, McDonald JR: Calcification in solitary nodules of the lung. Am J Roentgenol 77:1023, 1957.

111. Maile CW, Rodan BA, Godwin JD, et al: Calcification in pulmonary metastases. Br J Radiol 55:108, 1982.

112. Stewart JG, MacMahon H, Vyborny CJ, et al: Dystrophic calcification in carcinoma of the lung: Demonstration by CT (case report). Am J Roentgenol 148:29, 1987.

113. London SB, Winter WJ: Calcification within carcinoma of the lung: Report of a case with isolated pulmonary nodule. Arch Intern Med 94:161, 1954.

114. Zwiebel BR, Austin JHM, Grimes MM: Bronchial carcinoid tumors: Assessment with CT of location and intratumoral calcification in 31 patients. Radiology 179:483, 1991.

115. Felson B: Thoracic calcifications. Dis Chest 56:330, 1969.

116. Padley SPG, Adler BD, Staples CA, et al: Pulmonary talcosis: CT findings in three cases. Radiology 186:125, 1993.

117. Abrahams EW, Evans C, Knyvett AF, et al: Varicella pneumonia: A possible cause of subsequent pulmonary calcification. Med J Aust 2:781, 1964.

118. Knyvett AF: Pulmonary calcifications following varicella. Am Rev Respir Dis 92:210, 1965.

119. Graham CM, Stern EJ, Finkbeiner WE, et al: High-resolution CT appearance of diffuse alveolar septal amyloidosis. Am J Roentgenol 158:265, 1992.

120. Utz JP, Swensen SJ, Gertz MA: Pulmonary amyloidosis: The Mayo Clinic experience from 1980 to 1993. Ann Intern Med 124:407, 1996.

121. Hamrick-Turner J, Abbitt PL, Harrison RB, et al: Diffuse lung calcifications following fat emboli and adult respiratory distress syndromes: CT findings. J Thorac Imaging 9:47, 1994.

122. Whitaker W, Black A, Warrack AJN: Pulmonary ossification in patients with mitral stenosis. J Fac Radiol 7:29, 1955.

123. Galloway RW, Epstein EJ, Coulshed N: Pulmonary ossific nodules in mitral valve disease. Br Heart J 23:297, 1961.

124. Buja LM, Roberts WC: Pulmonary parenchymal ossific nodules in idiopathic hypertrophic subaortic stenosis. Am J Cardiol 25:710, 1970.

125. Gross BH, Schneider HJ, Proto AV: Eggshell calcification of lymph nodes: An update. Am J Roentgenol 135:1265, 1980.

126. Bellini F, Ghislandi E: "Egg-shell" calcifications at extrahilar sites in a silicotuberculotic patient. Med Lav 51:600, 1960.

127. Mallamo JT, Baum RS, Simon AL: Diffuse pulmonary artery calcifications in a case of Eisenmenger's syndrome. Radiology 99:549, 1971.

128. McAlister WH, Blatt E: Calcified pulmonary artery thrombus. Am J Roentgenol 87:908, 1962.

129. Baker GL, Heublein GW: Postoperative aspiration pneumonitis. Am J Roentgenol 80:42, 1958.

130. Brown BJ, Ma H, Dunbar JS, et al: Foreign bodies in the tracheobronchial tree in childhood. J Can Assoc Radiol 14:158, 1963.

131. Robertson OH, Hamburger M: Studies on the pathogenesis of experimental pneumococcus pneumonia in dogs: II. Secondary pulmonary lesions. Their production by intratracheal and intrabronchial injection of fluid pneumonic exudate. J Exp Med 72:275, 1940.

132. Fraser RG, Wortzman G: Acute pneumococcal lobar pneumonia: The significance of non-segmental distribution. J Can Assoc Radiol 10:37, 1959.

133. Fleischner FG: Roentgenology of the pulmonary infarct. Semin Roentgenol 2:61, 1967.

134. Garland LH: Bronchial carcinoma: Lobar distribution of lesions in 250 cases. Calif Med 94:7, 1961.

135. Rutishauser M: Die maligne Lungencaverne. [The malignant pulmonary cavity.] Schweiz Med Wochenschr 95:349, 1965.

136. West JB: Regional Differences in the Lung. New York, Academic Press, 1977, pp 313–319.

137. Lentino W, Jacobson HG, Poppel MH: Segmental localization of upper lobe tuberculosis: The rarity of anterior involvement. Am J Roentgenol 77:1042, 1957.

138. Poppius H, Thomander K: Segmentary distribution of cavities: A radiologic study of 500 consecutive cases of cavernous pulmonary tuberculosis. Ann Med Int Fenn 46:113, 1957.

139. Segarra F, Sherman DS, Rodriguez-Aguero J: Lower lung field tuberculosis. Am Rev Respir Dis 87:37, 1963.

140. Starke JR, Taylor-Watts KT: Tuberculosis in the pediatric population of Houston, Texas. Pediatrics 84:28, 1989.

141. Leung AN, Müller NL, Pineda PR, et al: Primary tuberculosis in childhood: Radiographic manifestations. Radiology 182:87, 1992.

142. Choyke PL, Sostman HD, Curtis AM, et al: Adult onset pulmonary tuberculosis. Radiology 148:357, 1983.

143. Ranniger K, Valvasorri GE: Angiographic diagnosis of intralobar pulmonary sequestration. Am J Roentgenol 92:540, 1964.

144. Witten DM, Clagett OT, Woolner LB: Intralobar bronchopulmonary sequestration involving the upper lobes. J Thorac Cardiovasc Surg 43:523, 1962.

145. Rogers LF, Osmer JC: Bronchogenic cyst: A review of 46 cases. Am J Roentgenol 91:273, 1964.

146. Felson B, Felson H: Localization of intrathoracic lesions by means of the postero-anterior roentgenogram: The silhouette sign. Radiology 55:363, 1950.

147. Collins VP, Loeffler RK, Tivey H: Observations on growth rates of human tumors. Am J Roentgenol 76:988, 1956.

148. Nathan MH, Collins VP, Adams RA: Differentiation of benign and malignant pulmonary nodules by growth rate. Radiology 79:221, 1962.

149. Weiss W: Tumor doubling time and survival of men with bronchogenic carcinoma. Chest 65:3, 1974.

150. Mizuno T, Masaoka A, Ichimura H, et al: Comparison of actual survivorship after treatment with survivorship predicted by actual tumor-volume doubling time from tumor diameter at first observation. Cancer 53:2716, 1984.

151. Yankelevitz DF, Henschke CI: Does 2-year stability imply that pulmonary nodules are benign? Am J Roentgenol 168:325, 1997.

152. Good CA, Wilson TW: The solitary circumscribed pulmonary nodule: Study of seven hundred five cases encountered roentgenologically in a period of three and one-half years. JAMA 166:210, 1958.

153. Viggian RW, Swensen SJ, Rosenow EC: Evaluation and management of solitary and multiple pulmonary nodules. Clin Chest Med 13:83, 1992.

154. Trapnell DH: The differential diagnosis of linear shadows in chest radiographs. Radiol Clin North Am 11:77, 1973.

155. Heitzman ER, Ziter FM Jr, Makarian B, et al: Kerley's interlobular septal lines: Roentgen pathologic correlation. Am J Roentgenol 100:578, 1967.

156. Kerley P: Radiology in heart disease. BMJ 2:594, 1933.

157. Twining EW (revised by Kerley P): Respiratory system. *In* Shanks SC, Kerley P (eds): A Textbook of X-Ray Diagnosis. Vol 2. 2nd ed. Philadelphia, WB Saunders, 1951, p 414.

158. Kerley P: *In* Shanks SC, Kerley P (eds): A Textbook of X-Ray Diagnosis. Vol 2. 2nd ed. Philadelphia, WB Saunders, 1951, p 241.

159. Kerley P: *In* Shanks SC, Kerley P (eds): A Textbook of X-Ray Diagnosis. Vol 2. 2nd ed. Philadelphia, WB Saunders, 1951, p 404.
160. Trapnell DH: Septal lines in pneumoconiosis. Br J Radiol 37:805, 1964.
161. Trapnell DH: Septal lines in sarcoidosis. Br J Radiol 37:811, 1964.
162. Levin B: Subpleural interlobular lymphectasia reflecting metastatic carcinoma. Radiology 72:682, 1959.
163. Brody JS, Levin B: Interlobular septal thickening in lipid pneumonia. Am J Roentgenol 88:1061, 1962.
164. Stolberg HO, Patt N, MacEwen KF, et al: Hodgkin's disease of the lung: Roentgenologic/pathologic correlation. Am J Roentgenol 92:96, 1964.
165. Simon G: Principles of Chest X-ray Diagnosis. 3rd ed. London, Butterworth, 1971.
166. Bates DV, Gordon CA, Paul GI, et al: Chronic bronchitis: Report on the third and fourth stages of the coordinated study of chronic bronchitis in the Department of Veterans Affairs, Canada. Med Serv J Can 22:5, 1966.
167. Hodson CJ, Trickey SE: Bronchial wall thickening in asthma. Clin Radiol 11:183, 1960.
168. Fraser RG, Fraser RS, Renner JW, et al: The roentgenographic diagnosis of chronic bronchitis: A reassessment with emphasis on parahilar bronchi seen end-on. Radiology 120:1, 1976.
169. Weibel ER, Taylor CR: Design and structure of the human lung. *In* Fishman AP (ed): Pulmonary Diseases and Disorders. New York, McGraw-Hill, 1988, p 11.
170. Webb WR, Müller NL, Naidich D: High-Resolution CT of the Lung. 2nd ed. New York, Lippincott-Raven, 1996, p 1.
171. Rigler LG: Personal communication, 1965.
172. Webb WR: The pleural tail sign. Radiology 127:309, 1978.
173. Hill CA: "Tail" signs associated with pulmonary lesions: Critical reappraisal. Am J Roentgenol 139:311, 1982.
174. Reid L: [Quoted by Simon G as a personal communication.] Br J Radiol 43:327, 1970.

CHAPTER *19*

Decreased Lung Density

ALTERATION IN PULMONARY VOLUME, 494
General Excess of Air, 495
Local Excess of Air, 497
Static Signs, 498
Dynamic Signs, 499
ALTERATION IN PULMONARY VASCULATURE, 499
General Reduction in Vasculature, 500
Local Reduction in Vasculature, 503
BULLAE, BLEBS, PNEUMATOCELES, AND CYSTS, 504

The diseases that cause a decrease in lung density result in increased radiolucency (hyperlucency) on the chest radiograph and decreased attenuation on computed tomography (CT). Just as lung density may be increased by a change in the relative amounts of air, blood, and interstitial tissue, so may decreased density result from alteration of these three elements in the opposite direction. As with diseases of increased density, it is useful to subdivide those of decreased density on the basis of the *predominant* component that is modified.

It is emphasized that here we are dealing only with the diseases of the lung that cause increased radiolucency. However, any assessment of chest radiographs must take into consideration the contribution that abnormalities of extrapulmonary tissue might make to reduced density. Thus, certain pleural diseases (e.g., pneumothorax) and some congenital and acquired abnormalities of the chest wall (e.g., congenital absence of the pectoral muscles, mastectomy, and poliomyelitis) produce unilateral radiolucency that might easily be mistaken for pulmonary disease unless this possibility is borne in mind (Fig. 19–1). Because it eliminates the influence of superimposition of density from the chest wall, CT is superior to the chest radiograph in demonstrating both focal and diffuse decreases in lung density.

In clinical practice, assessment of a change in lung density on the chest radiograph is purely subjective. In diseases of increased density, such assessment may be relatively simple since the variation in density from normal lung to consolidated lung is approximately 10-fold—from the average density of lung parenchyma (0.12 gm/ml) to that of consolidated lung (1.1 gm/ml). By contrast, the reduction in lung density in diseases that increase radiolucency may be very slight, probably amounting to no more with 0.01 or 0.02 gm/ml. Thus, the physician is faced with the difficulty of trying to classify a group of diseases on the basis of a radiologic sign that may be very subtle. The reasons by which this approach can be justified are twofold.

Subjective assessment of a general reduction in lung density is often unreliable because of the wide variation in exposure factors that characterizes much of chest radiography. However, recognition of diseases that cause reduced density is often possible by identification of secondary signs such as overinflation (flattening of the diaphragm and increased retrosternal air space), increased sharpness and branching angles of pulmonary vessels, loss of their normal sinuosity, and paucity of peripheral vascular markings.

In localized diseases that reduce lung density (e.g., lobar emphysema or a large bulla), a region of lung is present in which the density can be compared with that of normal tissue in the same or opposite lung. Thus, this form of disease can be classified according to relative change in density, an advantage lacking in generalized disease. This is not to imply that secondary signs are not as valuable in local as in general disease; as will be discussed, signs of overinflation and alteration in vasculature play an integral

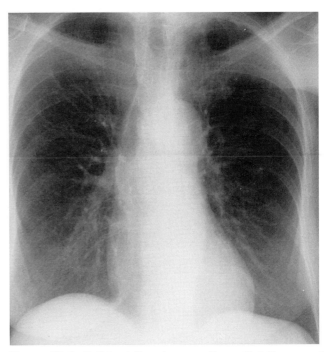

Figure 19–1. Unilateral Hyperlucency: Congenital Absence of the Pectoralis Muscle. A posteroanterior chest radiograph demonstrates marked asymmetry of radiolucency of the hemithoraces. The pulmonary vascular markings in the right and left lungs are similar. The patient was a 67-year-old woman with congenital absence of the left pectoralis; she had not undergone any previous surgery. Note that the breast shadows are symmetric.

role in the diagnosis and differential diagnosis of all diseases characterized by reduced density.

If it is accepted that diseases that reduce density are characterized by an altered ratio of the three components of air, blood, and interstitial tissue, four combinations of change can reduce lung density.

Increased Air with Unchanged Blood and Tissue. This group of disorders (Fig. 19–2) is exemplified by obstructive overinflation without lung destruction. The overinflation may be either local (e.g., compensatory overinflation secondary to pulmonary resection or atelectasis) or general (e.g., asthma).

Increased Air with Decreased Blood and Tissue. Localized abnormalities include bullae and pneumatoceles. Generalized abnormalities are epitomized by diffuse emphysema, in which the lungs are overdistended and have a decreased amount of alveolar wall tissue and capillary blood (Fig. 19–3).

Normal Amount of Air with Decreased Blood and Tissue. This group is characterized by a reduction in the quantity of blood and tissue in the absence of pulmonary overinflation (Fig. 19–4). Local diseases include lobar or unilateral emphysema and pulmonary embolism without infarction. (However, in both these conditions the volume of air may also be reduced, in the former because of incomplete maturation of lung parenchyma and in the latter because of surfactant deficit.) Examples of generalized abnormalities include diseases characterized by diminished pulmonary artery flow (e.g., tetralogy of Fallot) and diseases affecting the peripheral vascular system (e.g., primary pulmonary hypertension).

Reduction in All Three Components. This situation is rare and probably occurs in only one abnormality or variants thereof—proximal interruption (absence) of the right or left pulmonary artery (Fig. 19–5). In this abnormality, the lung is reduced in volume and derives its vascular supply solely from the systemic circulation; the resultant density is usually (albeit not always) reduced.[1]

On the basis of these concepts and using the radiologic signs to be described, one can fairly confidently diagnose most cases of pulmonary disease that decrease lung density. In the following section, no attempt is made to describe the radiologic characteristics of individual disease entities, specific affections being cited only to illustrate points under discussion.

ALTERATION IN PULMONARY VOLUME

Lung diseases that cause decreased density are characterized by overinflation, with the exception of unilateral pulmonary artery interruption (absence), unilateral or lobar emphysema (Swyer-James syndrome), partly obstructing endobronchial lesions, and pulmonary embolism without infarction. Before considering the radiologic signs of overinflation, it is well to briefly review the mechanisms that keep the lung expanded and the alterations in these mechanisms that increase lung volume.

The lung has a natural tendency to collapse and normally does so when removed from the thoracic cavity. This tendency stems from its inherent elastic recoil properties, which are partly related to the presence of collagen and elastic tissue and partly to alveolar surface tension. When the lung's elastic properties are decreased, as in emphysema, the organ can be inflated beyond its normal maximal volume (hyperinflation).

Similarly, the lung's compliance—the change in volume per unit change in pressure—is increased; in other words, a given pressure will produce a greater volume change than in normal lung. Although loss of lung elastic recoil is the major cause of hyperinflation, there is evidence that dynamic hyperinflation is an additional mechanism in some patients with asthma or chronic obstructive pulmonary disease. Dynamic hyperinflation occurs during tidal breathing when a patient breaths in before the lungs have emptied to their static equilibrium volume (i.e., the volume at which the

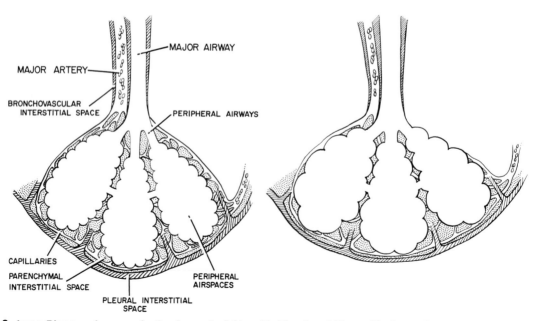

Figure 19–2. Lung Diagram: Increase in the Amount of Air, with Blood and Tissue Unchanged. The only abnormality depicted is an increase in size of the peripheral air spaces.

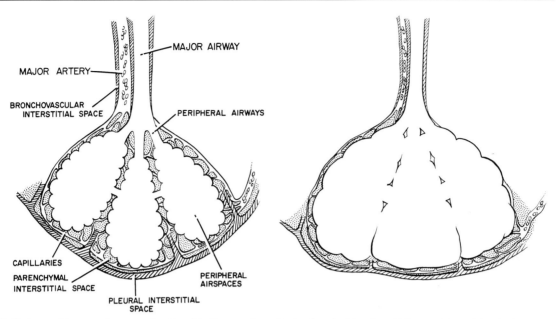

Figure 19–3. Lung Diagram: Increase in Air with Concomitant Reduction in Blood and Tissue. The peripheral air spaces are markedly dilated, with dissolution of their walls. The major artery and vein are reduced in caliber and the capillaries greatly diminished.

balance of the lung and chest wall recoil normally set functional residual capacity). This situation happens when maximal expiratory flow from the lung is markedly decreased to the extent that the patient is exhaling with maximal flow during normal tidal breathing. The presence of dynamic hyperinflation implies that alveolar pressure remains positive throughout expiration. At the end of the expiration, this positive pressure is termed "intrinsic positive end-expiratory pressure" (PEEPi or "auto-PEEP").

General Excess of Air

Radiologic signs that can be observed in association with a general increase in intrapulmonary air relate to the

diaphragm, the retrosternal space, and the cardiovascular silhouette (Fig. 19–6); by far the most important is the diaphragm. In patients with severe emphysema, the diaphragm is depressed at total lung capacity (TLC), often to the level of the 7th rib anteriorly and the 11th interspace or the 12th rib posteriorly; the normal "dome" configuration is concomitantly flattened. The low position of the diaphragm increases the angle of the costophrenic sinuses, sometimes almost to a right angle. In this situation, costophrenic muscle slips extending from the diaphragm to the posterior and posterolateral aspect of the ribs may be prominent; however, these slips are occasionally seen in healthy adults who have taken an exceptionally deep breath and should therefore not be regarded as diagnostic of hyperinflation.

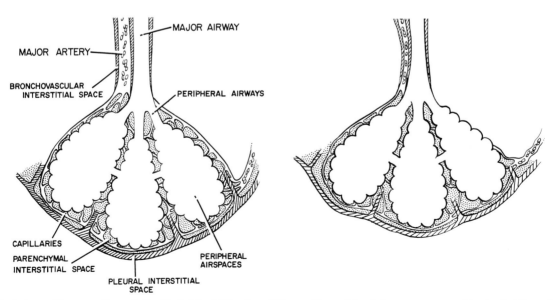

Figure 19–4. Lung Diagram: Normal Air, Diminished Blood and Tissue. The peripheral air spaces are normal in size, but the major artery and vein are reduced in caliber and the capillaries diminished in number.

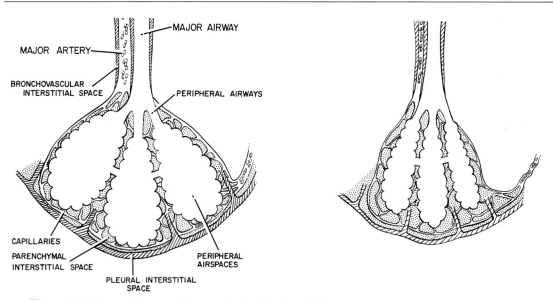

Figure 19–5. Lung Diagram: Decrease in Air, Blood, and Tissue. All elements of the lung are diminished.

Although diaphragmatic flattening is often assessed subjectively, direct measurement is clearly more accurate. This is best performed on the lateral chest radiograph by drawing a straight line from the sternophrenic junction to the posterior costophrenic junction. The dome of the hemidiaphragm should be 2.6 cm or more above this line; measurements less than 2.6 cm indicate overinflation.[2] A height less than 2.6 cm correlates with functional measurements of airway obstruction and air trapping; in one study, it identified 68% of patients with airway obstruction.[2] Flattening of the diaphragm can also be assessed on the posteroanterior (PA) radiograph by drawing a line from the costophrenic to the costovertebral angle and measuring the height of the dome of each hemidiaphragm;[2] however, this measurement is less sensitive than that from a lateral radiograph.[2, 3] In one study designed to test the accuracy of a variety of measurements from PA and lateral radiographs in discriminating normal and overinflated lungs, the best criterion was found to be the sum of the height of each diaphragmatic dome measured in PA and lateral projections.[4]

The severity of diaphragmatic flattening is of some value in the differential diagnosis, invariably being most marked in emphysema; in fact, the overinflation in this disease may render the diaphragmatic contour actually concave rather than convex upward (Fig. 19–6). In asthma, the upper surface is nearly always convex (this observation applies to adults only—severe air trapping in infants and children may be associated with remarkable depression and flattening of the diaphragmatic domes).

Another helpful sign in the detection of overinflation is an increase in the retrosternal air space on the lateral chest radiograph.[5, 3] Again, direct measurement is preferred to subjective assessment; a distance greater than 2.5 cm between the posterior of the sternum and the most anterior margin of the ascending aorta is indicative of overinflation.[5, 6]

Alteration in the size and contour of the thoracic cage is a variable and usually undependable sign of excess air in the lungs. Although a barrel-shaped chest is commonly regarded as indicative of emphysema, often its radiologic expression as an increase in the anteroposterior diameter of

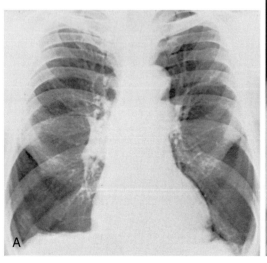

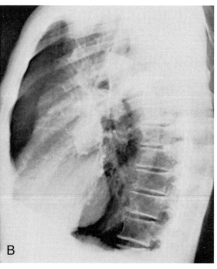

A   B

Figure 19–6. Diffuse Emphysema. A posteroanterior chest radiograph *(A)* reveals a low position and somewhat flattened contour of both hemidiaphragms. The lungs are oligemic. In lateral projection *(B)*, the superior aspect of the diaphragm is concave rather than convex and the retrosternal air space deepened.

the chest is inconspicuous. The anteroposterior chest diameter measured as the horizontal distance at the level of the top of the right hemidiaphragm from the sternum to the posterior of the ribs correlates poorly with lung volume.[2]

When the diaphragm is depressed, the heart tends to be elongated, narrow, and central in position. However, this configuration is of little value as a radiologic sign; in fact, it creates difficulty in the assessment of cardiac enlargement when pulmonary hypertension has given rise to right ventricular hypertrophy.

Local Excess of Air

Overinflation of a segment of a lobe or one or more lobes, the remainder of the lungs being normal, may occur with or without air trapping; distinction between the two circumstances is of major diagnostic importance.

Overinflation *with air trapping* results from obstruction of the egress of air from affected lung parenchyma. It may be seen in neonatal lobar hyperinflation (congenital lobar emphysema),[7, 8] in congenital bronchial atresia (Fig. 19–7),[9, 10] or distal to an endobronchial lesion as a result of check-valve obstruction. Such obstructive hyperinflation may develop distal to obstructing tumors of the main, lobar, or segmental bronchi and may be useful in diagnosis;[11] however, in our experience and that of others, it is a rare manifestation. For example, in a study of the radiographic patterns of 600 cases of bronchogenic carcinoma, overinflation distal to a partly obstructing endobronchial lesion was not seen in any case.[12–14] By contrast, in our experience, the volume of lung behind a partly obstructing endobronchial lesion is almost invariably reduced at TLC. Overinflation of

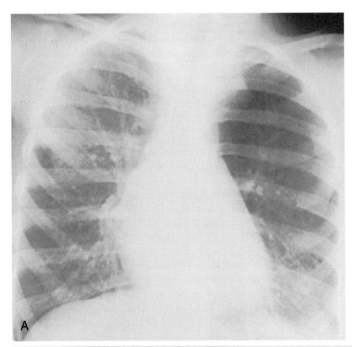

Figure 19–7. Congenital Bronchial Atresia of the Left Upper Lobe. A posteroanterior chest radiograph *(A)* demonstrates decreased vascularity and hyperlucency of the upper two thirds of the left lung; the mediastinum is displaced slightly to the right. The resected left upper lobe viewed from the lateral aspect *(B)* shows the apical (AP) and anterior (A) segments to remain hyperinflated whereas the posterior (P) segment has collapsed normally. The specimen was inflated and barium injected into the only patent bronchus (the posterior segmental bronchus); the lung was sectioned in the sagittal plane and radiographed *(C)*. Marked overinflation is seen in the apical and anterior segments (more severe in the latter). The atretic bronchi *(arrowheads)* are filled with mucus. (From Genereux GP: J Can Assoc Radiol 22:71, 1971.)

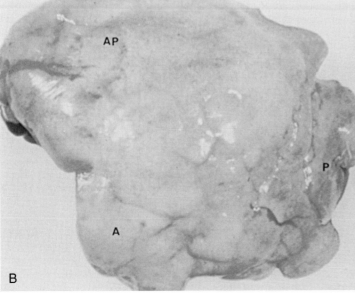

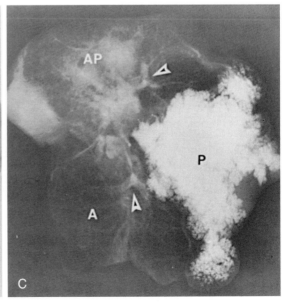

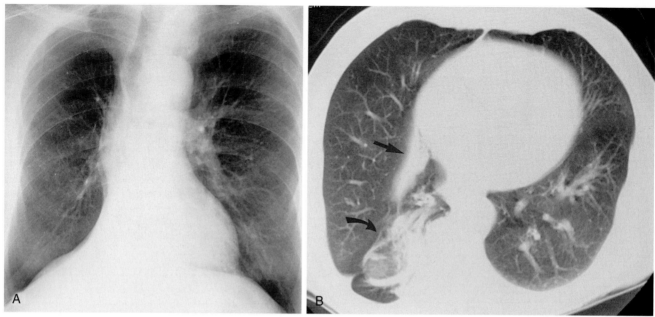

Figure 19–8. Hyperinflation Without Air Trapping Secondary to Combined Atelectasis of the Right Middle and Lower Lobes. A posteroanterior chest radiograph *(A)* demonstrates increased radiolucency of the right hemithorax as a result of compensatory hyperinflation of the right upper lobe secondary to combined atelectasis of the right middle and lower lobes. A CT scan *(B)* shows right middle *(straight arrow)* and lower lobe *(curved arrow)* atelectasis and hyperinflation of the right upper lobe. Note the decreased vascularity and attenuation of the right lung when compared with the left. The patient was a 69-year-old man with long-standing right middle and lower lobe atelectasis of unknown etiology.

the lung at TLC must be distinguished from air trapping on expiration, a vital distinction considered in greater detail farther on.

Hyperinflation *without air trapping* is a compensatory process: parts of the lung assume a larger volume than normal in response to loss of volume elsewhere in the thorax. Such hyperinflation may occur after surgical removal of lung tissue or as a result of atelectasis (Fig. 19–8) or parenchymal scarring; in any event, the remaining lung contains more than its normal complement of air. Since there is no airway obstruction, the radiologic signs are different from those of conditions in which air trapping plays a significant role. Thus, it is important to consider the radiologic signs of local excess of air under two headings, static and dynamic,* according to the presence or absence of airway obstruction.

Static Signs

Alteration in Lung Density. The fact that the excess of air is local permits comparison with normal density in the remainder of the same lung or in the contralateral lung; thus, in contrast to diseases in which there is a generalized excess of air, altered density is a significant and reliable sign. The increased radiolucency is caused mainly by an increase in air in relation to blood *content*. In the case of a partly obstructing endobronchial lesion, the situation is somewhat different: as discussed earlier, our experience is that the

volume of lung behind a partly obstructing endobronchial lesion is almost invariably reduced, not increased, at TLC. Despite this smaller volume, the density of affected parenchyma is typically *less* than that of the opposite lung rather than greater as might be anticipated. This decreased density is caused by a reduction in perfusion (oligemia) resulting from hypoxic vasoconstriction in response to alveolar hypoventilation. The overall effect is an increase in radiolucency despite the reduction in volume (Fig. 19–9).

Alteration in Volume. The volume of the affected lung depends entirely on whether the excess of air is compensatory (i.e., secondary to resection or atelectasis) or caused by airway obstruction. Since compensatory overinflation is the expansion of lung tissue beyond its normal volume to fill a limited space, the volume that the expanded lung tissue occupies cannot exceed the volume for which it compensates. However, when the alteration in lung volume results from bronchial obstruction, the volume of affected lung may be normal, less than normal, or greater than normal. Conditions in which the volume is greater than normal include congenital bronchial atresia and neonatal lobar hyperinflation; as already stated, a partly obstructing endobronchial lesion is usually associated with a lung volume that is less than normal (Fig. 19–10).

The main radiologic sign of increased volume is displacement of structures contiguous to overinflated lung, the degree varying with the amount and location of affected lung tissue: if in a lower lobe, the hemidiaphragm may be depressed and the mediastinum shifted to the contralateral side; if in an upper lobe, the mediastinum may be displaced and the thoracic cage expanded. If a whole lung is involved, the hemithorax in general is enlarged, the diaphragm depressed, the mediastinum shifted, and the thoracic cage enlarged. One of the more reliable signs of *lobar* overinflation is bulging of the interlobar fissure.

*For our purposes, the term *static* implies the changes apparent on standard radiographs or CT scans performed at TLC; *dynamic* implies changes that occur during respiration. Although the latter are most readily apparent on fluoroscopy or dynamic expiratory CT, these are seldom performed in this situation. Dynamic hyperinflation can also be inferred by comparing radiographs or CT scans performed at full inspiration and maximal expiration.

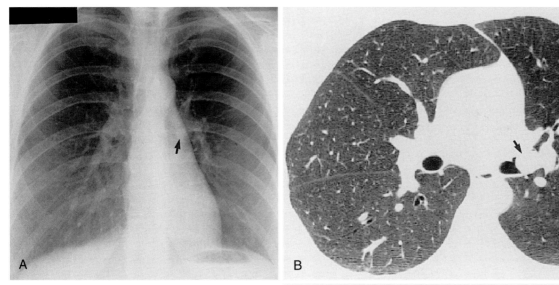

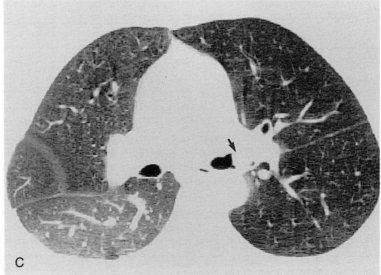

Figure 19–9. Decreased Vascularity and Lung Volume Caused by Endobronchial Tumor. A posteroanterior chest radiograph *(A)* in a 35-year-old woman reveals increased radiolucency of the left hemithorax and decreased vascularity. An endobronchial tumor *(arrow)* is present in the distal left main bronchus. Also note the decrease in size of the left lung. An HRCT scan *(B)* shows the endobronchial tumor *(arrow)*, decreased vascularity of the left lung, and a slight decrease in attenuation. Note the decrease in size of the left lung with shift of the mediastinum and anterior junction line to the left. An HRCT scan at end-expiration *(C)* demonstrates air trapping in the left lung with shift of the mediastinum and anterior junction line to the right.

Alteration in Vascular Pattern. The linear markings throughout the affected lung are splayed out in a distribution consistent with the extent of overinflation, and their angles of bifurcation are increased. Provided that blood flow is maintained at normal or almost normal levels, vessel caliber is little altered.

Dynamic Signs

When local hyperlucency is caused by compensatory overinflation, the volume of the overinflated lobe decreases proportionately with normal lung tissue during expiration: airway obstruction being absent, the affected lung parenchyma deflates normally. Since the overinflated lung tissue contains more air than normal at TLC, it still contains a greater than normal complement of air at residual volume and is therefore still relatively more radiolucent.

In the presence of partial airway obstruction, regardless of whether distal lung parenchyma is overinflated or underinflated, radiologic signs are vastly different from those seen in compensatory overinflation. During expiration, air is trapped within the affected lung parenchyma and volume changes

little, whereas the remainder of the lung deflates normally. The radiologic signs depend on both the volume and the anatomic location of affected lung. Since there is less change in the amount of air within the obstructed lung parenchyma during expiration, density is little altered and the contrast between affected areas and normally deflated lung is maximally accentuated at residual volume (Fig. 19–11). Because the hyperinflated parenchyma occupies space within the hemithorax, contiguous structures are displaced away from the affected lobe during expiration: the mediastinum shifts toward the contralateral side and elevation of the hemidiaphragm is restricted. The distribution of the vascular pattern throughout the hyperinflated lobe changes little.

It cannot be overemphasized that evidence of a local excess of air may be extremely subtle on radiographs exposed at full inspiration (Fig. 19–11); when such changes are suspected, expiratory radiographs should be obtained.

ALTERATION IN PULMONARY VASCULATURE

Just as overinflation may reflect an abnormality of the conducting airways of the lung, so may alteration in the

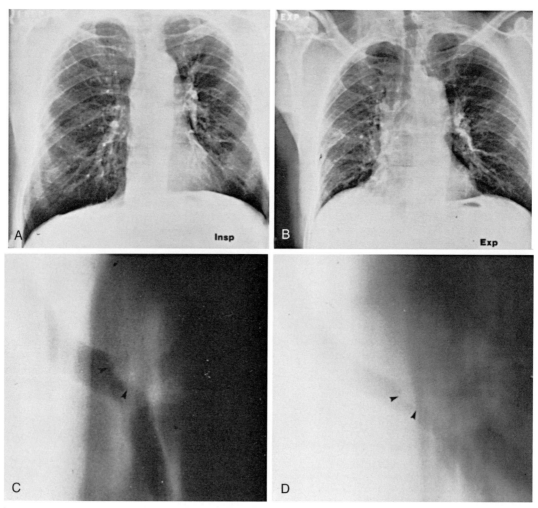

Figure 19–10. Small Cell Carcinoma with Expiratory Air Trapping. A posteroanterior radiograph exposed at full inspiration *(A)* reveals decreased size of the left lung in comparison to the right; the left hemidiaphragm is moderately elevated and the mediastinum is shifted to the left. Despite this loss of volume, no opacities can be identified in the left lung to suggest a cause of the collapse. The left lower lobe vessels are obviously smaller than the corresponding vessels on the right, indicative of reduced perfusion. A radiograph exposed at maximal expiration *(B)* reveals little change in volume of the left lung from inspiration, indicative of air trapping; by contrast, the right hemidiaphragm has elevated considerably and the mediastinum has swung to the right, indicative of good air flow from the right lung. Tomograms of the left main bronchus in inspiration *(C)* and expiration *(D)* reveal a smooth, well-defined soft tissue mass protruding into the air column of the bronchus near its bifurcation *(arrowheads)*; the caliber of the bronchial air column is markedly reduced on expiration.

vascular pattern indicate abnormality of perfusion. Vascular loss may be central or peripheral, in the former instance produced by vascular obstruction (for example, pulmonary artery thrombosis) and in the latter by peripheral vascular obliteration (for example, emphysema). Like overinflation, the alteration in lung vasculature may be either general or local; since the radiologic signs differ somewhat, it is desirable to describe them separately.

General Reduction In Vasculature

Diffuse pulmonary oligemia is characterized by a reduction in caliber of the arteries throughout the lungs. Appreciation of such vascular change is a subjective process based on thorough familiarity with the normal lung and is clearly subject to observer error. Since reduction in the size of peripheral vessels constitutes the main criterion of diagnosis of all diseases in this category, reliance must be placed on

secondary signs for their differentiation. Two ancillary signs are of major importance: the size and configuration of the central hilar vessels and the presence or absence of general pulmonary overinflation. Three combinations of changes are possible.

Small Peripheral Vessels, No Overinflation, and Normal or Small Hila. This combination indicates reduced pulmonary blood flow from central causes and is almost always the result of congenital heart disease. A reduction in pulmonary blood flow in congenital heart disease usually results from a combination of a right-to-left cardiac shunt and obstruction of blood flow at the level of the tricuspid valve, right ventricle, or pulmonary valve; in both adults and children, the most common cause is the tetralogy of Fallot.[15, 16] Another congenital heart disease associated with decreased pulmonary blood flow that may be seen in adults is Ebstein's anomaly (Fig. 19–12).[15, 17] This anomaly is characterized by malformation of the tricuspid valve, with downward displacement of the posterior and septal leaflets into the right

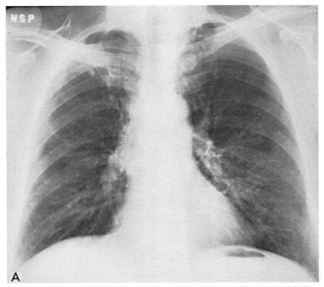

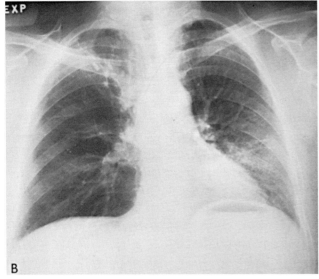

Figure 19–11. Expiratory Air Trapping Caused by Endobronchial Obstruction. A posteroanterior chest radiograph exposed at full inspiration *(A)* shows a slight decrease in volume and vascularity of the right lung. On expiration *(B)*, the left hemidiaphragm has elevated normally whereas the right has maintained its inspiratory position; the mediastinum has shifted to the left. Bronchoscopy revealed granulation tissue causing partial obstruction of the right main bronchus. *Mycobacterium tuberculosis* was identified on smear and culture.

ventricle resulting in a functionally small right ventricle, tricuspid regurgitation, and right atrial enlargement. Decreased pulmonary blood flow is frequently related to the presence of a right-to-left shunt through an atrial septal defect.

The combination of small peripheral vessels, no overinflation, and normal or small hila may also occasionally be seen in acquired conditions such as cardiac tamponade and inferior vena cava obstruction.[18]

Small Peripheral Vessels, No Overinflation, and Enlarged Hilar Pulmonary Arteries. This combination may result from peripheral or central causes. The former include primary pulmonary hypertension,[19, 20] chronic thromboembolic pulmonary hypertension,[20] and pulmonary hypertension secondary to chronic schistosomiasis.[21] In each of these conditions,

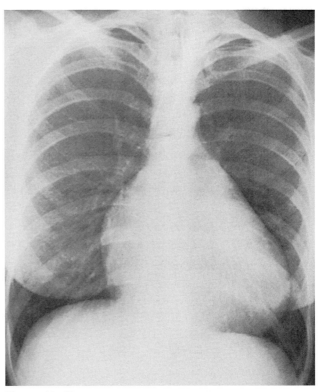

Figure 19–12. Diffuse Oligemia Without Overinflation: Ebstein's Anomaly. The peripheral pulmonary markings are diminished in caliber and the hila are diminutive; the lungs are not overinflated. The contour of the enlarged heart is consistent with Ebstein's anomaly.

the major changes apparent radiographically are the consequence of pulmonary arterial hypertension and consist of enlargement of the hilar pulmonary arteries and diminution of the peripheral vessels (Fig. 19–13). Pulmonary hypertension resulting from chronic thromboembolic disease is often

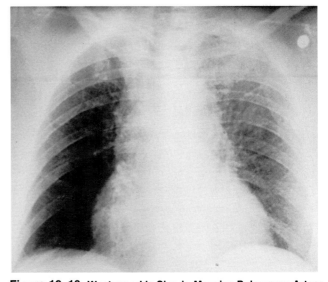

Figure 19–13. Westermark's Sign in Massive Pulmonary Artery Thromboembolism. An anteroposterior chest radiograph obtained at the patient's bedside discloses hyperlucency and oligemia of the right lung. The heart is moderately enlarged. The patient was a 69-year-old woman with acute dyspnea and circulatory collapse. At autopsy, a massive saddle embolus obstructed the right pulmonary artery and its two major branches.

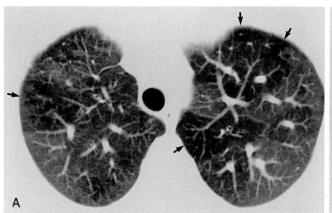
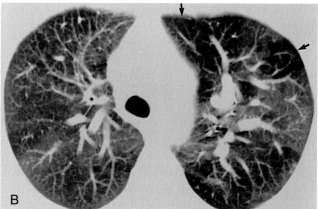

Figure 19–14. Mosaic Attenuation Caused by Recurrent Pulmonary Thromboembolism. CT scans (*A* and *B*) demonstrate a pattern of mosaic perfusion and attenuation. Focal areas of decreased perfusion and attenuation *(arrows)* are present in both lungs, whereas the vessels in the remainder of the lungs are increased in size. The patient was a 38-year-old woman with progressive shortness of breath and pulmonary arterial hypertension. The diagnosis of chronic pulmonary thromboembolism was proved by selective pulmonary angiography.

associated with disparity in the size of segmental vessels and a mosaic pattern of perfusion that can be readily identified on CT (Fig. 19–14).[22, 23] This pattern results from decreased vascularity and attenuation in the areas of lung supplied by vessels containing thrombus and increased vascularity and attenuation in other regions (as a result of blood flow redistribution).[23, 24]

The most common central cause of the combination of small peripheral vessels, no overinflation, and enlarged hilar pulmonary arteries is massive thromboembolism without infarction.[25, 26] In this situation, the reduction in peripheral

pulmonary artery flow results from mechanical obstruction in the large hilar vessels, the latter being ballooned out by thrombus within them; severe cardiac enlargement caused by acute cor pulmonale is usually present (Fig. 19–15).

Small Peripheral Vessels, General Pulmonary Overinflation, and Normal or Enlarged Hilar Pulmonary Arteries. This combination is characteristic of diffuse emphysema (Fig. 19–16).[27–29] Since diffuse hyperinflation may also occur in asthma, recognition of peripheral vascular deficiency is important in the differentiation of these two conditions. Enlargement of the hilar pulmonary arteries may be present; it indicates pulmonary arterial hypertension resulting from chronically increased vascular resistance and is usually seen

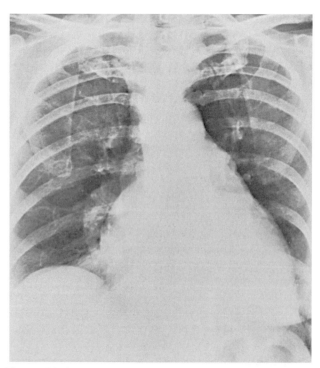

Figure 19–15. Diffuse Oligemia Without Overinflation: Massive Pulmonary Artery Thromboembolism Without Infarction. Marked oligemia of both lungs is associated with moderate enlargement of both hila and rapid tapering of the pulmonary arteries as they proceed distally. The cardiac contour is typical of cor pulmonale. There is no overinflation.

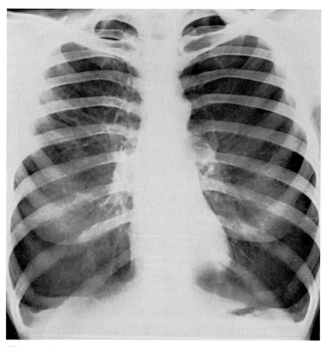

Figure 19–16. Diffuse Oligemia with Generalized Overinflation: Emphysema. A posteroanterior chest radiograph demonstrates decreased vascularity of both lungs and hyperinflation. Despite the severe oligemia, the hilar pulmonary arteries are not enlarged.

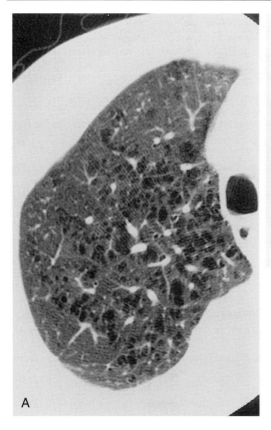

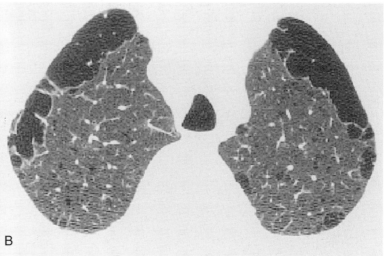

Figure 19–17. Emphysema. An HRCT scan *(A)* in a 73-year-old patient demonstrates characteristic features of centrilobular emphysema with sharply defined focal areas of low attenuation within the lung parenchyma. An HRCT scan *(B)* in a 71-year-old patient demonstrates characteristic features of paraseptal emphysema with bullae involving mainly the subpleural lung regions. Also noted is mild centrilobular emphysema.

only in advanced emphysema. In such circumstance, the rapid tapering of pulmonary vessels distally is accentuated by the hilar enlargement.

In addition to a decrease in the size of peripheral vessels, emphysema is associated with a variety of other vascular changes, including curvilinear displacement, increased branching angles, loss of normal sinuosity and side branches, and increased sharpness with a reduction in caliber.[30] Even when severe, emphysema is seldom uniform in distribution. It should be suspected in the presence of focal areas of increased radiolucency[31] and uneven distribution of vascular markings.[32] Decreased vascularity predominantly involving the upper lobes suggests centrilobular emphysema; decreased vascularity in the lower lung zone suggests panacinar emphysema.[29, 33] On CT, emphysema is characterized by the presence of areas of abnormally low attenuation; the procedure has been shown to provide images that closely reflect the macroscopic pathologic findings (Fig. 19–17).[34, 35]

Local Reduction in Vasculature

The same three combinations of changes apply as in a general reduction in vasculature; the major difference lies in their effects on pulmonary hemodynamics. In the following examples the affected portion of lung may be segmental, lobar, or multilobar.

Small Peripheral Vessels, Normal or Subnormal Inflation, and Normal or Small Hilum. This combination is epitomized by lobar or unilateral hyperlucent lung, variously known by the eponyms Swyer-James syndrome[36] and Macleod's syndrome (Fig. 19–18).[37] This uncommon abnormality is characterized by normal or slightly reduced lung volume at TLC, severe airway obstruction during expiration, oligemia, and a diminutive hilum.[38, 39] The increased vascular resistance in affected areas results in a redistribution of blood flow to the contralateral lung or unaffected lobes. The condition is believed to be related to acute bronchiolitis during infancy since the volume of the lung in adulthood is associated with the age at which the bronchiolar damage occurred.[37, 39] Although the hyperlucency is usually confined to one lobe or lung on the radiograph, on CT and on radionuclide scans the abnormality is often patchy in distribution:[40, 41] the hyperlucent lung may show foci of normal attenuation on CT (Fig. 19–19), and the normal lung may show foci of decreased attenuation.

Radiographic changes identical to those of Swyer-James syndrome may result from a clinically more important situation. Consider an endobronchial lesion incompletely obstructing the lumen of a main bronchus (*see* Fig. 19–10): the reduced ventilation of distal parenchyma results in local hypoxia, which leads to reflex vasoconstriction and consequently a reduced caliber of vessels in affected bronchopulmonary segments. The volume of affected lung is generally *reduced* rather than *increased* (*see* Fig. 19–9). Since the endobronchial lesion invariably causes expiratory air trapping, it may be extremely difficult to radiologically differentiate this combination of changes from Swyer-James syndrome. Therefore, whenever such changes are present, it is imperative to exclude an endobronchial lesion.

The site of hypoxic vasoconstriction was assessed in an investigation on greyhound dogs in which the pulmonary lobes were exteriorized.[42] In response to hypoxia, arteriography revealed vasoconstriction that was maximal (approxi-

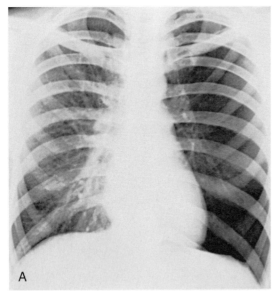

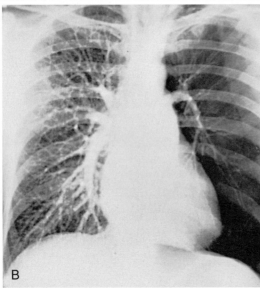

Figure 19–18. Unilateral Hyperlucent Lung: Swyer-James Syndrome. A posteroanterior chest radiograph exposed at total lung capacity *(A)* reveals a marked discrepancy in radiolucency of the two lungs, the left showing severe oligemia. The left hilar shadow is diminutive. In the pulmonary angiogram *(B)*, the discrepancy in blood flow to the two lungs is readily apparent; note that the left pulmonary artery is present, although diminutive.

mately 20% reduction) in vessels 0.3 mm in diameter; no significant change in caliber occurred in vessels exceeding 2 mm in diameter. Reversal of the vascular response occurred promptly after withdrawal of the hypoxic stimulus.

A picture somewhat similar to that produced by Swyer-James syndrome may be seen in patients with proximal interruption (absence) of the right or left pulmonary artery, a condition in which the pulmonary artery is interrupted in the region of the hilum so that the lung is devoid of pulmonary artery perfusion.[43] On plain radiographs, the two can be distinguished by the virtual absence of a hilar shadow in the proximal interruption of the pulmonary artery and a diminutive hilar shadow in Swyer-James syndrome; in the former, there is also no expiratory airway obstruction. In

pulmonary artery interruption, linear markings throughout the affected lung are caused by a greatly increased bronchial arterial circulation. The pulmonary vessels in the contralateral lung are often enlarged as a result of associated intracardiac left-to-right shunt. Contrast-enhanced CT or magnetic resonance imaging can accurately differentiate the two if standard radiography leaves the diagnosis in doubt.[44–46]

A combination of radiographic changes similar to that of proximal interruption of the pulmonary artery sometimes occurs when pulmonary arterial flow has been reduced by compression or obstruction of a pulmonary artery by a contiguous (usually neoplastic) abnormality (Fig. 19–20). Generally speaking, however, such a process results in enlargement or increased radiopacity of the involved hilum.

Small Peripheral Vessels, Normal or Subnormal Lung Volume, and Enlarged Hilar Pulmonary Arteries (or an Enlarged Hilum). This combination is nearly always caused by unilateral pulmonary artery thromboembolism without infarction (Fig. 19–21). The occluding embolus may lead to enlargement of the involved artery (Fleischner's sign).[47] However, the vascular dilatation at the site of the embolus is usually small and difficult to detect on the radiograph: in one study of the chest radiographs of 1,063 patients with suspected pulmonary thromboembolism (embolism subsequently being confirmed angiographically in 383 and excluded in 680), an enlarged hilum was interpreted as being present in 26 patients (7%) with embolism and in 42 (6%) without.[48] Oligemia distal to the obstructing embolus—Westermark's sign[49]—is also a relatively uncommon finding.[48] Since bronchial obstruction is not a feature, there is no overinflation—on the contrary, lung volume may be reduced. A similar radiographic picture may be produced by neoplastic obstruction of a pulmonary artery secondary to either invasion by a contiguous carcinoma or intravascular growth of a primary sarcoma; in each case, the hilar enlargement is caused by the neoplasm itself.

Small Peripheral Vessels, Overinflation, and Normal Hilar Pulmonary Arteries. This combination is characteristic of emphysema. The radiographic appearance of the vascular deficiency of emphysema is often local rather than general; for example, 13 of 26 patients with established emphysema in one study had predominantly local involvement.[32] The lower or upper lobes or almost any combination of individual lobes may be predominantly affected (Fig. 19–22). The involved portions of lung show a combination of overinflation and severely diminished peripheral vasculature; less involved areas tend to be pleonemic as a result of the redistribution of blood to them caused by the increased resistance to pulmonary blood flow in emphysematous areas. Since the lack of increase in vascular resistance in uninvolved lung prevents the development of pulmonary artery hypertension, the hilar pulmonary arteries do not enlarge.

BULLAE, BLEBS, PNEUMATOCELES, AND CYSTS

Bullae. A bulla is a sharply demarcated, air-containing space 1 cm or more in diameter that possesses a smooth wall 1 mm or less in thickness. The space may be unilocular or separated into several compartments by thin septa (Fig. 19–23). Bullae may arise *de novo*, in which case the sur-

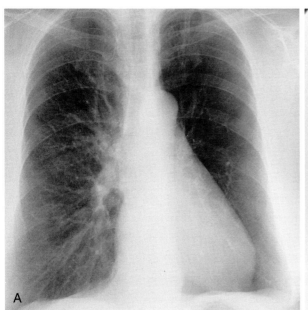

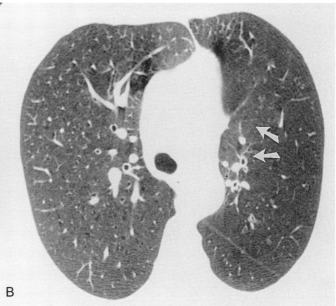

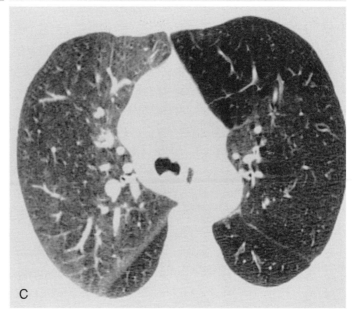

Figure 19–19. Unilateral Hyperlucent Lung: Swyer-James Syndrome. A posteroanterior chest radiograph *(A)* demonstrates increased radiolucency, decreased vascularity, and a slight decrease in size of the left lung. An HRCT scan *(B)* at end-inspiration also shows decreased vascularity of the left lung and an associated decrease in attenuation. A focal area with normal lung attenuation is present in the otherwise hyperlucent lung *(arrows)*. Also note the decrease in volume of the left lung with associated shift of the mediastinum and the anterior junction line to the left. An HRCT scan *(C)* performed at end-expiration reveals air trapping in the left lung. The mediastinum and junction line have shifted to the midline. The patient was a 61-year-old woman.

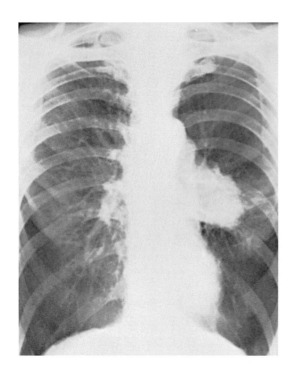

Figure 19–20. Unilateral Pulmonary Oligemia: Compression of Hilar Pulmonary Arteries by Bronchogenic Carcinoma. A posteroanterior chest radiograph reveals a discrepancy in radiolucency of the two lungs, the left being oligemic and comparatively more radiolucent. The large hilar mass proved to be primary squamous cell carcinoma encasing the left pulmonary artery.

Figure 19–21. Lobar Oligemia Without Hyperinflation: Thromboembolism Without Infarction. An anteroposterior radiograph exposed in the supine position demonstrates a marked increase in radiolucency of the lower half of the right lung. The vascular markings are diminished in caliber, and the descending branch of the right pulmonary artery is dilated and sharply defined; the vessel tapers rapidly as it proceeds distally. Lobar oligemia as a result of thromboembolism without infarction constitutes Westermark's sign.

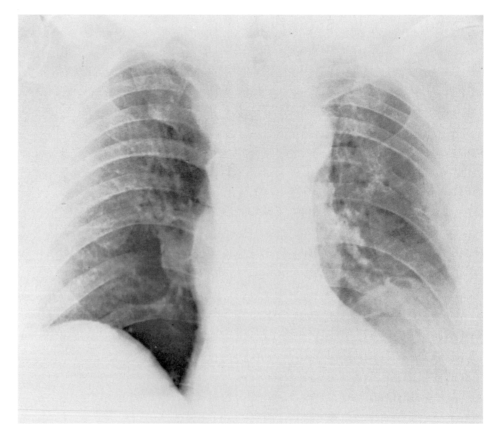

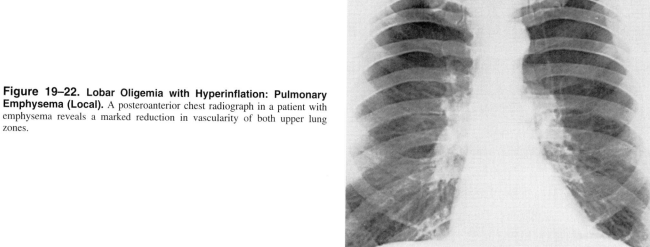

Figure 19–22. Lobar Oligemia with Hyperinflation: Pulmonary Emphysema (Local). A posteroanterior chest radiograph in a patient with emphysema reveals a marked reduction in vascularity of both upper lung zones.

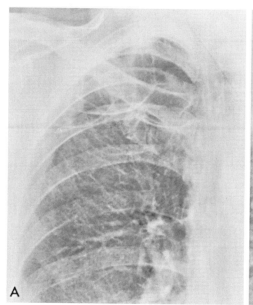
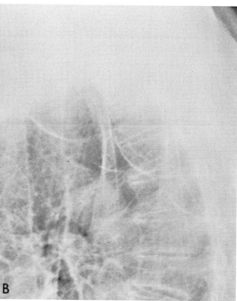

Figure 19–23. Bullae. Views of the upper half of the right lung in posteroanterior *(A)* and lateral *(B)* projections reveal several spaces in the lung apex sharply separated from contiguous lung by curvilinear, hairline shadows. The appearance suggests multiple bullae rather than a single space separated into compartments by thin septa.

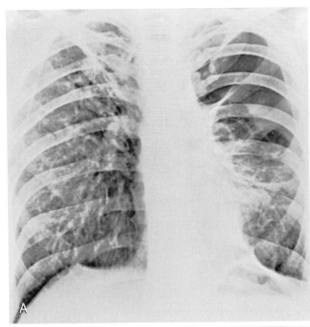

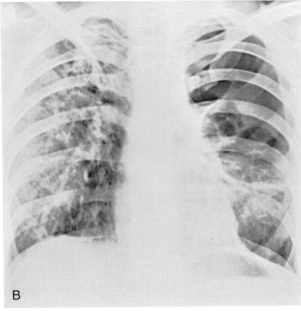

Figure 19–24. Bulla Associated with Pulmonary Scarring. A poster-oanterior chest radiograph exposed at total lung capacity (TLC) *(A)* demonstrates a large, well-defined space occupying the upper half of the left hemithorax and sharply demarcated from contiguous lung. Extensive bilateral parenchymal disease is present as a result of tuberculosis. A radiograph exposed at residual volume (RV) *(B)* reveals marked air trapping within the bulla; in fact, by actual measurement the space is larger at RV than at TLC. *See* the text.

rounding lung tissue is normal. However, they occur more commonly in association with other disease, usually emphysema or infection; in the latter situation, adjacent parenchymal scarring is frequent (Fig. 19–24). Secondary signs may be present, depending on the size of the bulla; for example, when a large bulla occupies most of the volume of one hemithorax (Fig. 19–25), signs of air trapping are apparent on radiographs taken following maximal expiration—the mediastinum is displaced to the side of the normal lung during expiration, and ipsilateral hemidiaphragmatic excursion and movements of the thoracic wall are restricted. When a bulla occupies most of one lobe, lobar expansion may be apparent by outward bulging of the interlobar fissure. Bullae are characteristically poorly ventilated and unperfused.[50] They usually decrease in size or (less commonly) remain unchanged in size during expiration.[50a] However, studies of

their mechanical properties have shown that they sometimes inflate during expiration (pendelluft) (Fig. 19–24);[51] the mechanism of this phenomenon is uncertain.

Bleb. A bleb is a localized collection of air located within the pleura. It develops most frequently over the lung apices and seldom exceeds 1 cm in diameter. The mechanism of bleb development has been attributed to the dissection of air from a ruptured alveolus through interstitial tissue into the thin fibrous layer of visceral pleura, where it accumulates in the form of a "cyst."[52, 53]

Pneumatocele. A pneumatocele is a thin-walled gas-filled space within the lung that usually occurs in association with infection; it characteristically increases in size over a period of days to weeks and almost invariably resolves. The pathogenesis is believed to relate either to check-valve obstruction of a small bronchus or bronchiole with distention

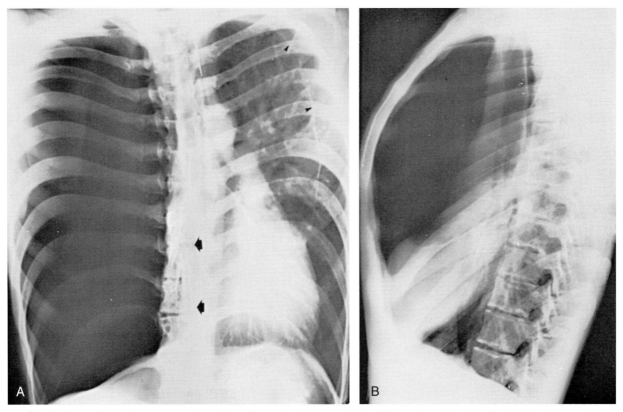

Figure 19–25. Huge Bulla. An anteroposterior radiograph reveals a bulla completely filling and overdistending the right hemithorax and extending across the anterior mediastinal septum almost as far as the left axillary pleura (the line shadow indicated by *arrowheads* is formed by four layers of pleura). The right lung is compressed into a small nubbin of tissue situated in the midline; note the markedly crowded right bronchial tree *(thick arrows)*. In lateral projection *(B)*, herniation of the bulla across the anterior mediastinal septum has resulted in a marked increase in depth of the retrosternal air space and posterior displacement of the heart and major vessels.

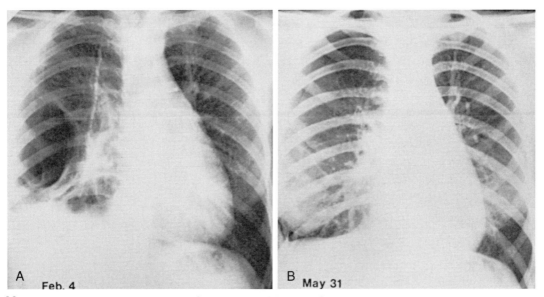

Figure 19–26. Pneumatocele Formation in Acute Staphylococcal Pneumonia. This 16-year-old girl was admitted to the hospital with an acute respiratory illness. Her original radiograph *(A)* reveals an inhomogeneous opacity in the lower portion of the right lung associated with a large cystic space (pneumatocele) laterally and several smaller air-containing spaces inferiorly. The mediastinum is shifted to the left. Several weeks later *(B)*, much of the parenchymal reaction in the right lung had resolved, and the large pneumatocele originally identified had almost completely disappeared.

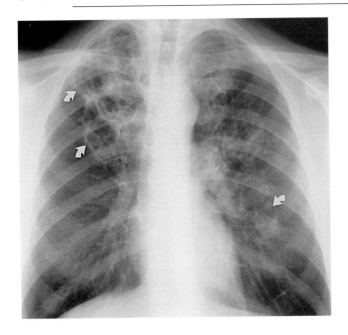

Figure 19–27. Pneumatoceles in *Pneumocystis carinii* Pneumonia. A posteroanterior chest radiograph in a 53-year-old man with AIDS demonstrates numerous cystic lesions *(arrows)* involving mainly the right upper lobe. The pneumatoceles had not been present on a chest radiograph performed 3 months previously when *P. carinii* was identified in BAL fluid.

of the lung distal to the obstruction or to local necrosis of a bronchial wall with dissection of air into the bronchovascular interstitial space.[54] It is usually caused by *Staphylococcus aureus* in infants and children or *Pneumocystis carinii* in patients with acquired immunodeficiency syndrome (Figs. 19–26 and 19–27). The abnormality can also occur following trauma (Fig. 19–28).

Cysts. Cysts can be defined as gas-containing spaces within the lung whose walls are greater than 1 mm in thickness. By pathologic criteria, a cyst has an epithelial lining; however, when used to refer to a radiologic abnormality, an epithelial lining is not necessarily implied. Numerous disease processes can be manifested in whole or in part by cyst formation, including developmental abnormalities and infections. Although rare, primary pulmonary or metastatic carcinoma can be manifested as a thin-walled cyst (Fig. 19–29),[55] which points out the hazard of dismissing every cystic pulmonary lesion as benign.

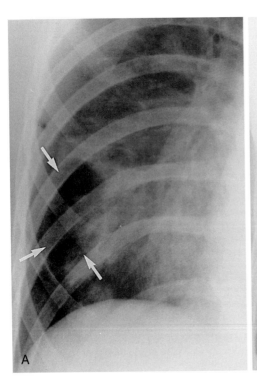
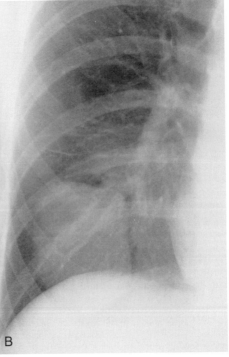

Figure 19–28. Traumatic Pneumatocele. A view of the right lower lung from an anteroposterior chest radiograph *(A)* in a 25-year-old patient following a motor vehicle accident demonstrates a focal radiolucent area *(arrows)* caused by pulmonary laceration (traumatic pneumatocele) and consolidation secondary to contusion. A view from a chest radiograph obtained 11 days later *(B)* demonstrates a post-traumatic hematoma, the radiolucent area seen on the admission chest radiograph having been filled with blood.

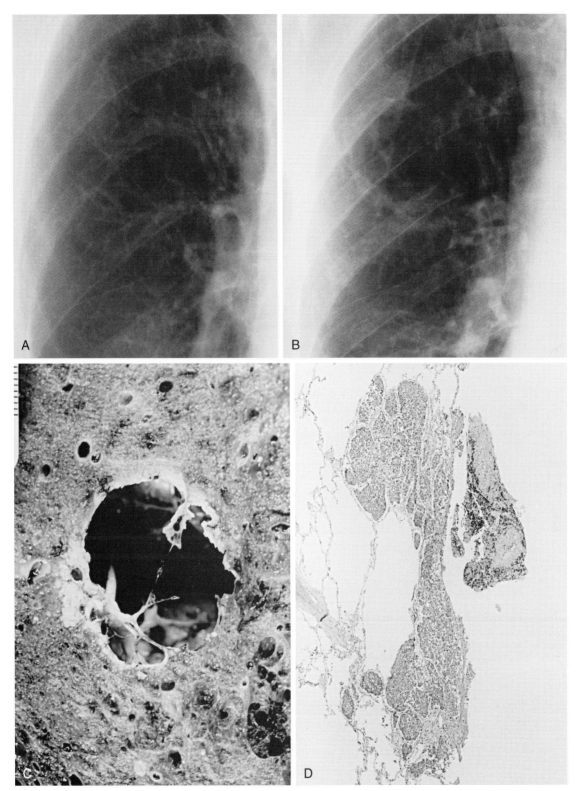

Figure 19–29. Metastatic Carcinoma to a Bulla. A view of the right lung on a posteroanterior radiograph *(A)* shows evidence of emphysema. A view of the same region several years later *(B)* shows a thin-walled bulla with local areas of nodular thickening. A magnified view of a slice of the upper lobe *(C)* shows the lesion to be approximately 2.5 cm in diameter. Mild emphysema present in the adjacent lung and thin fibrovascular strands extending into and across the bulla indicate its emphysematous nature. The wall is thickened by a tumor that extends 0.5 to 5 mm into the adjacent lung; tumor can also be seen on the surface of the fibrovascular strands. A section through the bulla "wall" *(D)* shows the presence of carcinoma irregularly infiltrating parenchymal air spaces. The patient had a high-grade transitional cell carcinoma of the urinary bladder, histologically identical to the tumor surrounding the bulla. Focal intravascular metastases were evident elsewhere in the lungs.

REFERENCES

1. Sherrick DW, Kincaid OW, DuShane JW: Agenesis of a mainbranch of the pulmonary artery. Am J Roentgenol 87:917, 1962.
2. Reich SB, Weinshelbaum A, Yee J: Correlation of radiographic measurements and pulmonary function tests in chronic obstructive pulmonary disease. Am J Roentgenol 144:695, 1985.
3. Kilburn KH, Warshaw RH, Thornton JC: Do radiographic criteria for emphysema predict physiologic impairment? Chest 197:1225, 1995.
4. Thomson KR, Eyssen GE, Fraser RG: Discrimination of normal and overinflated lungs and prediction of total lung capacity based on chest film measurements. Radiology 119:721, 1976.
5. Sutinen S, Christoforidis AJ, Klugh GA, et al: Roentgenologic criteria for the recognition of nonsymptomatic pulmonary emphysema: Correlation between roentgenologic findings and pulmonary pathology. Am Rev Respir Dis 91:69, 1965.
6. Pratt PC: Role of conventional chest radiography in diagnosis and exclusion of emphysema. Am J Med 82:998, 1987.
7. Franken EA, Buehl I: Infantile lobar emphysema: Report of two cases with the usual roentgenographic manifestation. Am J Roentgenol 98:354, 1966.
8. Kennedy CD, Habibi P, Matthew DJ, et al: Lobar emphysema: Long-term imaging follow-up. Radiology 180:189, 1991.
9. Simon G, Reid L: Atresia of an apical bronchus of the left upper lobe: Report of three cases. Br J Dis Chest 57:126, 1963.
10. Jederlinic PJ, Sicilian LS, Baigelman W, et al: Congenital bronchial atresia: A report of four cases and a review of the literature. Medicine (Baltimore) 65:73, 1986.
11. Woodring JH: Pitfalls in the radiologic diagnosis of lung cancer. Am J Roentgenol 154:1165, 1990.
12. Byrd RB, Miller WE, Carr DT, et al: The roentgenographic appearance of squamous cell carcinoma of the bronchus. Mayo Clin Proc 43:327, 1968.
13. Byrd RB, Miller WE, Carr DT, et al: The roentgenographic appearance of large cell carcinoma of the bronchus. Mayo Clin Proc 43:333, 1968.
14. Byrd RB, Miller WE, Carr DT, et al: The roentgenographic appearance of small cell carcinoma of the bronchus. Mayo Clin Proc 43:337, 1968.
15. Steiner RM, Gross GW, Flicker S, et al: Congenital heart disease in the adult patient: The value of plain film chest radiology. J Thorac Imaging 10:1, 1995.
16. Abraham KA, Cherian G, Rao VD, et al: Tetralogy of Fallot in adults: A report on 147 patients. Am J Med 66:811, 1979.
17. Giuliani ER, Fuster V, Brandenburg RO, et al: Ebstein's anomaly: The clinical features and natural history of Ebstein's anomaly of the tricuspid valve. Mayo Clin Proc 54:163, 1979.
18. Templeton AW, Garotto LJ: Acquired extracardiac causes of pulmonary ischemia. Dis Chest 51:166, 1967.
19. Rich S, Pietra GG, Kieras K, et al: Primary pulmonary hypertension: Radiographic and scintigraphic patterns of histologic subtypes. Ann Intern Med 105:499, 1986.
20. Randall PA, Heitzman ER, Bull MJ, et al: Pulmonary arterial hypertension: A contemporary review. Radiographics 9:905, 1989.
21. Farid Z, Greer JW, Ishak KG, et al: Chronic pulmonary schistosomiasis. Am Rev Respir Dis 79:119, 1959.
22. Bergin CJ, Rios G, King MA, et al: Accuracy of high-resolution CT in identifying chronic pulmonary thromboembolic disease. Am J Roentgenol 166:1371, 1996.
23. Remy-Jardin M, Remy J, Giraud F, et al: Computed tomography assessment of ground glass opacity: Semiology and significance. J Thorac Imaging 8:249, 1993.
24. Primack SL, Müller NL, Mayo JR, et al: Pulmonary parenchymal abnormalities of vascular origin: High-resolution CT findings. Radiographics 14:739, 1994.
25. Keating DR: Thrombosis of pulmonary arteries. Am J Surg 90:447, 1955.
26. Ball KP, Goodwin JF, Harrison CV: Massive thrombotic occlusion of the large pulmonary arteries. Circulation 14:766, 1956.
27. Simon G: Radiology and emphysema. Clin Radiol 15:293, 1964.
28. Pratt PC: Radiographic appearance of the chest in emphysema. Invest Radiol 22:927, 1987.
29. Thurlbeck WM, Müller NL: Emphysema: Definition, imaging, and quantification. Am J Roentgenol 163:1017, 1994.
30. Miniati M, Filippi E, Falaschi F, et al: Radiologic evaluation of emphysema in patients with chronic obstructive pulmonary disease. Am J Respir Crit Care Med 151:1359, 1995.
31. Foster WL, Gimenez EI, Roubidoux MA, et al: The emphysemas: Radiologic-pathologic correlations. Radiographics 13:311, 1993.
32. Fraser RG, Bates DV: Body section roentgenography in the evaluation and differentiation of chronic hypertrophic emphysema and asthma. Am J Roentgenol 82:39, 1959.
33. Thurlbeck WM, Simon G: Radiographic appearance of the chest in emphysema. Am J Roentgenol 130:429, 1978.
34. Miller RR, Müller N, Vedal S, et al: Limitations of computed tomography in the assessment of emphysema. Am Rev Respir Dis 139:980, 1989.
35. Gevenois PA, De Vuyst P, Sy M, et al: Pulmonary emphysema: Quantitative CT during expiration. Radiology 199:825, 1996.
36. Swyer PR, James GCW: A case of unilateral pulmonary emphysema. Thorax 8:133, 1953.
37. MacLeod WM: Abnormal transradiancy of one lung. Thorax 9:147, 1954.
38. Margolin HN, Rosenberg LS, Felson B, et al: Idiopathic unilateral hyperlucent lung: A roentgenologic syndrome. Am J Roentgenol 82:63, 1959.
39. Reid L, Simon G: Unilateral lung transradiancy. Thorax 17:230, 1962.
40. Moore ADA, Godwin JD, Dietrich PA, et al: Swyer-James syndrome: CT findings in eight patients. Am J Roentgenol 158:1211, 1992.
41. Reid L, Simon G, Zorab PA, et al: The development of unilateral hypertransradiancy of the lung. Respir Med 61:190, 1967.
42. Allison DJ, Stanbrook HS: A Radiologic and Physiologic Investigation into Hypoxic Pulmonary Vasoconstriction in the Dog. George Simon Memorial Fellowship Award, No 3, 1979, p 178.
43. Kieffer SA, Amplatz K, Anderson RC, et al: Proximal interruption of a pulmonary artery: Roentgen features and surgical correction. Am J Roentgenol 95:592, 1965.
44. Harris KM, Lloyd DCF, Morrissey B, et al: The computed tomographic appearances in pulmonary artery atresia. Clin Radiol 45:382, 1992.
45. Debatin JF, Moon RE, Spritzer CE, et al: MRI of absent left pulmonary artery. J Comput Assist Tomogr 16:641, 1992.
46. Morgan PW, Foley DW, Erickson SJ: Proximal interruption of a main pulmonary artery with transpleural collateral vessels: CT and MR appearances. J Comput Assist Tomogr 15:311, 1991.
47. Fleischner FG: Unilateral pulmonary embolism with increased compensatory circulation through the unoccluded lung: Roentgen observations. Radiology 73:591, 1959.
48. Worsley DF, Alavi A, Aronchick JM, et al: Chest radiographic findings in patients with acute pulmonary embolism: Observations from the PIOPED study. Radiology 189:133, 1993.
49. Westermark N: On the roentgen diagnosis of lung embolism. Acta Radiol 19:357, 1938.
50. Laurenzi GA, Turino GM, Fishman AP: Bullous disease of the lung. Am J Med 32:361, 1962.
50a. Worthy SA, Brown MJ, Müller NL: Technical Note: Cystic air spaces in the lung: Change in size on expiratory high-resolution CT in 23 patents. Clin Radiol 53:515, 1998.
51. Ting EY, Klopstock R, Lyons HA: Mechanical properties of pulmonary cysts and bullae. Am Rev Respir Dis 87:538, 1963.
52. Grimes OF, Farber SM: Air cysts of the lung. Surg Gynecol Obstet 113:720, 1961.
53. Feraru F, Morrow CS: Surgery of subpleural blebs: Indications and contraindications. Am Rev Respir Dis 79:577, 1959.
54. Quigley MJ, Fraser RS: Pulmonary pneumatocele: Pathology and pathogenesis. Am J Roentgenol 150:1275, 1988.
55. Peabody JW Jr, Rupnick EJ, Hanner JM: Bronchial carcinoma masquerading as a thin-walled cyst. Am J Roentgenol 77:1051, 1957.

CHAPTER *20*

Atelectasis

MECHANISMS OF ATELECTASIS, 513
   Resorption Atelectasis, 513
   Relaxation Atelectasis, 517
     Round Atelectasis, 521
   Adhesive Atelectasis, 522
   Cicatrization Atelectasis, 522
RADIOLOGIC SIGNS OF ATELECTASIS, 525
   Direct Signs, 525
   Indirect Signs, 526
PATTERNS OF ATELECTASIS, 534
   Total Pulmonary Atelectasis, 539
   Lobar Atelectasis, 539
     Right Upper Lobe, 539
     Left Upper Lobe, 543
     Right Middle Lobe, 549
     Lower Lobes, 552
   Combined Lobar Atelectasis, 552
     Combined Right Middle and Lower Lobe Atelectasis, 554
     Combined Right Upper and Middle Lobe Atelectasis, 554
     Combined Right Upper and Lower Lobe Atelectasis, 554
   Segmental Atelectasis, 554
   Linear (Platelike) Atelectasis, 554

The term *atelectasis* is derived from the Greek words *ateles* (incomplete) and *ektasis* (stretching). In this text we use it specifically to denote diminished gas within the lung associated with reduced lung volume. (Although the term *collapse* is often used synonymously with atelectasis, it should be reserved for complete atelectasis.[1]) It is important to note that the definition just given implies simply loss of volume, not necessarily an increase in radiopacity; significant atelectasis can occur without change in radiographic density. For example, pulmonary thromboembolism may be accompanied by considerable volume loss of the affected lobe or segment manifested only by diaphragmatic elevation and displacement of the interlobar fissure without an increase in radiopacity; in fact, the lung may be *radiolucent* because of the oligemia resulting from arterial obstruction. Thus, it is important to regard atelectasis as a process in which the only direct radiologic sign is loss of lung volume, and it is in this context that the term is used throughout this book.

MECHANISMS OF ATELECTASIS

Since we have described atelectasis essentially in terms of lung volume, it is important to consider the mechanisms that keep the lung expanded. Alterations in these mechanisms provide a basis for classifying atelectasis into four types: resorption, relaxation, adhesive, and cicatrization.

The lung has a natural tendency to collapse and does so when removed from the chest. While the lungs are in the thoracic cavity, this tendency is opposed by the chest wall; at the resting respiratory position (functional residual capacity), the tendency for the lung to collapse and the chest wall to expand is equal and opposite. When the thorax contains a space-occupying process (e.g., pneumothorax), the lung retracts and its volume decreases; this condition is *relaxation (passive) atelectasis*. A similar mechanism exists at the edge of a local space-occupying lesion; because of its inherent elastic recoil properties, the parenchyma for some distance contiguous to the mass or cyst is reduced in volume. Although this mechanism of volume loss has been termed *compression atelectasis*, from a conceptual point of view we consider it preferable to regard it as a variant of relaxation atelectasis. We also consider gravity-dependent atelectasis—characteristically seen on computed tomography (CT) as an area of increased attenuation in the dependent lung regions (dependent opacity)—a form of relaxation atelectasis.

In a static system, the volume attained by the lung depends on the balance between the applied force and the opposing elastic forces. It follows that when the lung is stiffer than normal—i.e., when compliance is decreased—lung volume is decreased. This condition classically occurs with pulmonary fibrosis and can be termed *cicatrization atelectasis*. The pressure-volume behavior of the lung also depends on the forces acting at the air-tissue interface of the alveolar wall. As alveoli diminish in volume, the surface tension of the interface is diminished by the surfactant. When the action of surfactant is interfered with, as may occur in respiratory distress syndrome (RDS), there may be widespread collapse of alveoli. This type of atelectasis has been referred to as "microatelectasis" or "nonobstructive" atelectasis, but we prefer to refer to it as *adhesive atelectasis*.

The most common form of atelectasis—and the most complex—is caused by the resorption of gas from the alveoli, as commonly occurs in bronchial obstruction. Since we have classified other forms of atelectasis on the basis of mechanism rather than etiology, this type of atelectasis is best termed *resorption atelectasis*.

Resorption Atelectasis

Resorption atelectasis occurs when communication between alveoli and the trachea is obstructed (Fig. 20–1). The

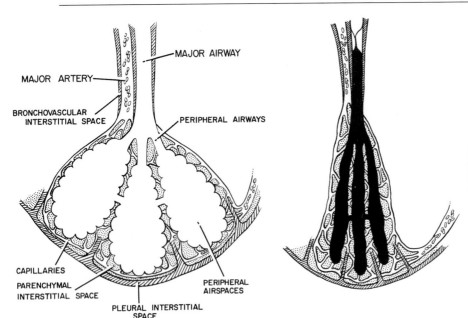

Figure 20–1. Lung Diagram: Resorption Atelectasis. The major airway is obstructed, and the peripheral airways and air spaces are airless and collapsed.

mechanism of resorption is straightforward. The total partial pressure of gases is lower in mixed venous blood than in alveolar air; as blood passes through the alveolar capillaries, the partial pressures of its gases equilibrate with alveolar pressure. The alveoli diminish in volume corresponding to the quantity of oxygen absorbed, their pressure remaining atmospheric; consequently, the partial pressures of carbon dioxide and nitrogen in the alveoli rise relative to capillary blood, and both gases diffuse into blood to maintain equilibrium. Thus, alveolar volume is further reduced, with a consequent rise in the alveolar-capillary blood P_{O_2} gradient; oxygen diffuses into capillary blood, and the cycle is repeated until all alveolar gas is absorbed.

In a previously healthy lobe, all gas disappears after 18 to 24 hours of airway obstruction.[2] Since oxygen is absorbed much more rapidly than nitrogen, when a lobe is filled with oxygen at the moment of occlusion (a situation that might pertain during anesthesia), collapse occurs much more rapidly and may be radiologically apparent within an hour (Fig. 20–2).[3, 4] In one study, the lobar bronchi of dogs were obstructed with a balloon catheter following 100% oxygen breathing for 5 minutes.[5] The affected lobe became airless in 5 minutes or less; in fact, continuous cinefluorography of the events in one dog showed unequivocally that opacity in the obstructed lobe was increased after three respiratory cycles! The same effect may be observed in a patient in whom malposition of an endotracheal tube has caused bronchial occlusion; it is important that the physician be aware of the exceptional rapidity with which an obstructed lung or lobe can collapse in such circumstances. Resorption atelectasis can also occur very rapidly when a one-way valve allows air to escape from a lobe but prevents its entrance: in one study, lobar collapse was produced approximately 50 minutes after inserting such a valve in a dog's bronchus.[2] Lobar collapse has also been reported in a human patient within a few minutes of assuming the supine position because a mobile bronchial tumor impacted at the orifice of a bronchus and acted as a one-way valve.[6]

It is important to realize that resorption atelectasis is not the inevitable or only accompaniment of bronchial obstruction, nor is obstruction of a major bronchus the only cause of resorption atelectasis. The effect of obstruction of the airways depends on the site and extent of bronchial or bronchiolar obstruction, the pre-existing condition of the lung tissue, the rapidity of the obstruction, and collateral ventilation.

It is clear that considerable collateral ventilation can occur in the normal lung, predominantly between segments but sometimes even between upper and lower lobes when fissures are incomplete (*see* page 59). Such collateral ventilation may result in air trapping (Fig. 20–3). In one study of 160 children who had foreign bodies in the tracheobronchial tree, air trapping was by far the most common radiographic finding, being present in 109 patients (68%);[7] atelectasis was the initial radiographic finding in only 22 (14%). This large discrepancy between the number of cases of air trapping and atelectasis could be attributable to collateral ventilation. The observation that overinflation occurs distal to bronchial atresia also illustrates the remarkable ability of collateral ventilation to maintain lung inflation.[8] Despite these findings, we suspect that partial obstruction is a more important cause of air trapping in these patients.

If collateral ventilation is such a potent force in preventing parenchymal collapse, under what circumstances does collapse occur? The conditions leading to collapse depend chiefly on the site of obstruction: if at the level of a lobar bronchus, the development of atelectasis is readily explained by the absence of a parenchymal bridge from the involved lobe to a contiguous lobe; if the obstruction is in a segmental or subsegmental bronchus, collapse must be caused by some influence *preventing* collateral ventilation,[8] probably inflammatory exudate.

Even excluding the effect of collateral ventilation, the end result of bronchial obstruction is not necessarily a collapsed lobe, particularly if the obstructing process is prolonged (as, for example, with bronchogenic carcinoma); in this situation, "obstructive pneumonitis" frequently leads to consolidation severe enough to limit loss of volume (Fig.

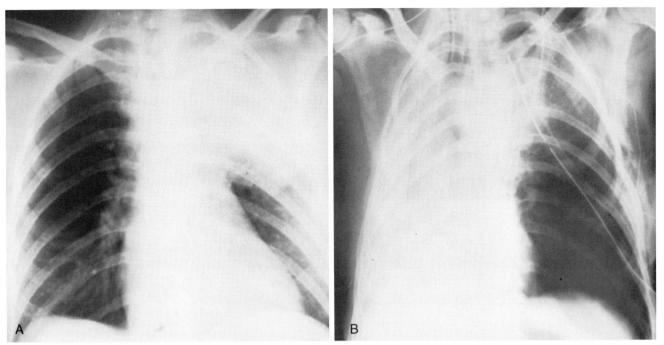

Figure 20–2. Acute Atelectasis of the Right Lung: Influence of Contained Gas on Rapidity of Atelectasis. The initial radiograph *(A)* of this 44-year-old man reveals a large mass in the left upper lobe that proved on biopsy to be adenocarcinoma; at thoracotomy, the lesion was unresectable. Shortly after his return to the recovery room, the patient became short of breath; a radiograph *(B)* showed complete collapse of the right lung associated with marked shift of the mediastinum into the right hemithorax. Bronchoscopy revealed a large mucous plug in the right main bronchus, and this was removed; 3 hours later the right lung had completely re-expanded. The rapidity with which the right lung underwent complete atelectasis resulted from the presence within it of 100% oxygen or other readily soluble anesthetic gas at the time the bronchial occlusion occurred.

20–4). It is important to realize that the pathologic counterpart of such radiologically evident obstructive pneumonitis is actually a combination of atelectasis, bronchiectasis with mucous plugging, and parenchymal inflammation and fibrosis.[9] In the vast majority of cases, the inflammation is not caused by bacterial infection: in parenchyma that has recently been obstructed, the principal histologic finding is filling of alveolar air spaces by proteinaceous fluid con-

taining scattered macrophages (Fig. 20–5); the polymorphonuclear leukocytes and necrosis that would be expected in infection are not evident and cultures are usually sterile.[9] In later stages, fluid is typically replaced by foamy macrophages (Fig. 20–5); although there is still no evidence of an acute inflammatory cellular response, the alveolar interstitium is frequently thickened by a combination of fibrous tissue and a lymphocytic infiltrate. When infection does

Figure 20–3. Lung Diagram: Collateral Ventilation Associated with Air Trapping. The airway on the *left* is obstructed, that on the *right*, patent; the parenchyma distal to the obstructed airway is being ventilated by collateral ventilation. The diagram depicts a situation in which air enters the obstructed segment more easily than it leaves, thus resulting in air trapping.

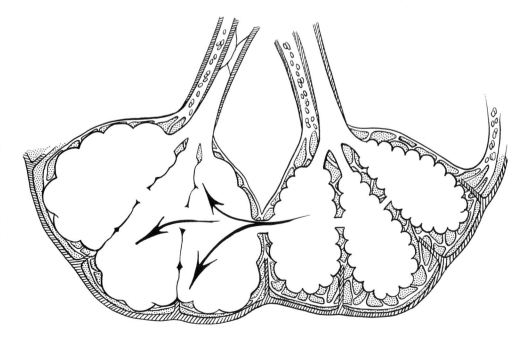

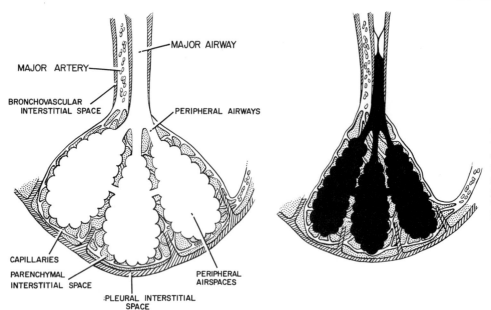

Figure 20–4. Lung Diagram: Obstructive Pneumonitis. Although the major airway is completely obstructed, loss of volume of the peripheral air spaces is only moderate; accumulated fluid and alveolar macrophages within the air spaces have prevented complete atelectasis, depicted in Figure 20–1.

occur distal to bronchial obstruction, it is almost always superimposed on these underlying noninfectious parenchymal changes. In most cases it is not possible to determine whether infection is present from the radiologic findings alone. Nevertheless, the characteristic radiographic picture of obstructive pneumonitis—homogeneous opacification without air bronchograms—should immediately alert the physician to the presence of an obstructing endobronchial lesion (Fig. 20–6).

The pathogenesis of these postobstructive pathologic changes is not clear. It is possible, however, that the early findings are related to the development of intra-alveolar edema. Since intrapleural pressure represents the balance of forces between inward recoil of the lung and outward recoil

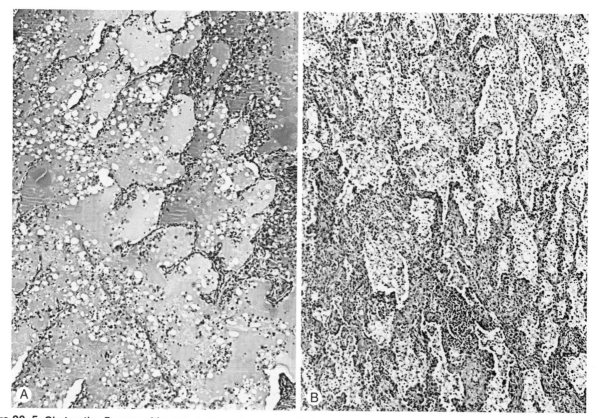

Figure 20–5. Obstructive Pneumonitis. *A,* Early obstructive pneumonitis showing alveoli filled with proteinaceous fluid and occasional macrophages. *B,* Later stage, with absence of fluid and numerous intra-alveolar foamy macrophages. Moderate interstitial fibrosis and chronic inflammation are also present.

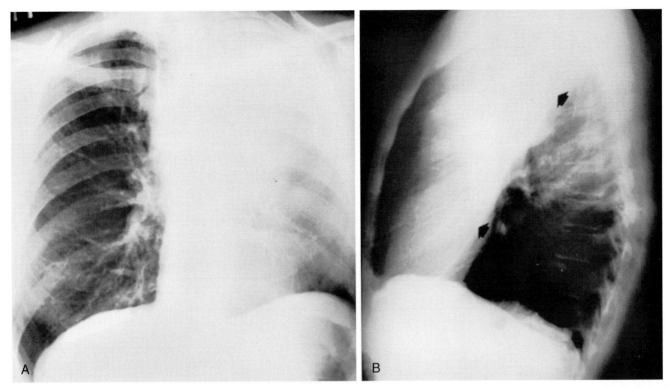

Figure 20–6. Obstructive Pneumonitis—Left Upper Lobe. Posteroanterior *(A)* and lateral *(B)* radiographs reveal homogeneous opacification of the left upper lobe; there is no air bronchogram. The major fissure *(arrows)* is not displaced forward, and the only signs indicating loss of volume are slight mediastinal shift and hemidiaphragmatic elevation. Collapse was prevented by the accumulation of fluid and alveolar macrophages within distal air spaces and chronic inflammatory cells and fibrous tissue within the interstitium—obstructive pneumonitis. The patient had squamous cell carcinoma originating in the left upper lobe bronchus.

of the chest wall, intrapleural pressure becomes more negative when air is resorbed and collapse results. This negative pressure is transmitted to the interstitial space of the lungs; when the negative pressure is of sufficient magnitude, hydrostatic pressure is increased and transudation of fluid from the alveolar capillaries takes place. In an experimental investigation on dogs, atelectasis of each pulmonary lobe was selectively produced following a period of 100% oxygen breathing; when the lobe was completely airless, the animal was sacrificed, frozen, and sectioned in a transverse axial or coronal plane.[5] Planimetric volume determinations of the collapsed and contralateral lobes showed an approximately 50% reduction in the former; in three animals, the wet weight–dry weight ratio was approximately 7 in the collapsed lobes and 5 in the normal lobes. This study thus showed that acute bronchial obstruction rapidly renders an oxygen-filled lobe airless, not only from gas absorption but also from air replacement by edema fluid.

Such fluid exudation occurs to some extent in all cases of acute obstructive atelectasis and is euphemistically termed *drowned lung* (*see* Fig. 20–6). If the obstruction persists and the obstructed lobe remains sterile, excess edema fluid and blood within the "drowned lobe" are gradually reabsorbed. Eventually, the collapsed lobe may be so small that it is almost invisible on the chest radiograph, in which case the radiologist must rely heavily on evidence of compensatory phenomena to appreciate the underlying atelectasis.

Resorption atelectasis caused by peripheral airway obstruction generally results in an opacity that is less uniform than the opacity seen when a major airway is obstructed.

Another difference between resorption atelectasis produced by central obstruction and that produced by peripheral obstruction is the presence of an air bronchogram in the latter if there is sufficient parenchymal collapse since the obstruction is peripheral to the major bronchial tree (Fig. 20–7).

Relaxation Atelectasis

Relaxation (passive) atelectasis denotes loss of lung volume in the presence of pneumothorax or hydrothorax or adjacent to a space-occupying lesion (Fig. 20–8). Provided that the pleural space is free (i.e., without adhesions), atelectasis of any portion of lung is proportional to the amount of air or fluid in the adjacent pleural space. In upright human beings, the tendency for air to pass to the upper portion of the pleural space results in a relatively greater degree of atelectasis of the upper lobe than the lower.

It might be thought that shrinkage of a lung to half its normal area on the radiograph would double its density. That this is not so is illustrated by the difficulty commonly experienced in identifying the lung edge in cases of spontaneous pneumothorax, even of moderate degree (*see* Fig. 20–8). In fact, as a lung shrinks adjacent to a pneumothorax, its density does not increase notably until its projected area is reduced to about one tenth its normal area at total lung capacity.[10] The probable explanation for this apparently anomalous situation is twofold: first, the reduction in lung volume is approximately balanced by a reduction in blood content, net lung density being altered only slightly; and

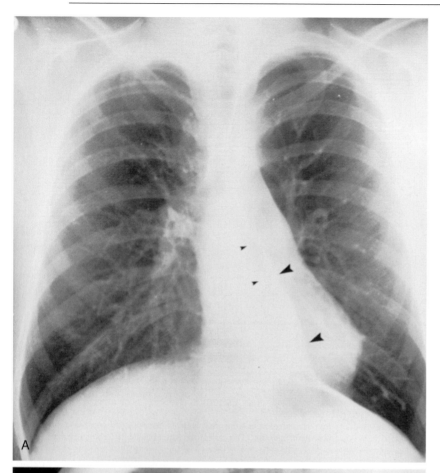

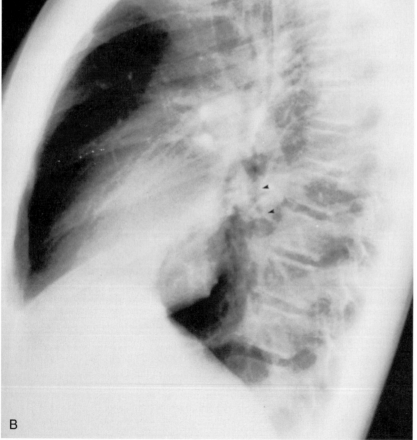

Figure 20–7. Effects of Peripheral Obstruction. Conventional posteroanterior *(A)* and lateral *(B)* radiographs disclose a triangular homogeneous opacity *(large arrowheads)* behind the heart. A faint central air bronchogram *(small arrowheads)* is present. The patient was a young woman with bronchiectasis. Although the large central airways were patent, atelectasis occurred because of obstruction of small peripheral airways and destruction of lung parenchyma.

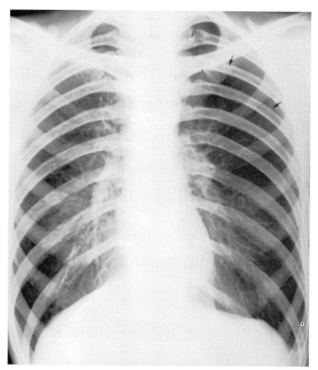

Figure 20–8. Spontaneous Pneumothorax. A posteroanterior radiograph reveals a small left pneumothorax (*arrows* point to the visceral pleural line). Although the left lung is partly atelectatic, the left hemithorax is more radiolucent than the right. Note the increased size of the left hemithorax as a result of removal of the influence of the lung's elastic recoil on the chest wall.

second, air in the pleural space, both anteriorly and posteriorly, serves as a nonabsorbing medium that contributes to the overall radiolucency of the radiographic image.

The pulmonary collapse that occurs in association with total pneumothorax presents an opportunity for appreciating how small a volume the lung may occupy when its parenchyma is completely airless: a lung whose volume at total lung capacity approximates 3.5 liters may shrink to a size no larger than a tennis ball (Fig. 20–9). Even when pneumothorax-induced collapse is total, the lung mass is not completely airless, the lobar and larger segmental bronchi being sufficiently stable structurally to resist collapse and remain filled with air; although reduced in caliber, these structures should therefore be apparent as an air bronchogram (Fig. 20–9). It is essential that this sign be sought carefully in any case of total or almost total pneumothorax; absence of an air bronchogram should immediately arouse suspicion of endobronchial obstruction.[11]

Although pleural effusion has been cited as a cause of compression atelectasis,[12, 13] the response of the lung to a large pleural effusion is similar to that of a pneumothorax of the same volume: the lung undergoes relaxation atelectasis, which if complete should be associated with an identifiable air bronchogram (Fig. 20–10). The term *compression atelectasis* has also been used to designate parenchymal atelectasis contiguous to a space-occupying mass within the thorax (Fig. 20–11) and therefore local rather than general atelectasis as in pneumothorax. Any intrathoracic space-occupying process, such as a bronchogenic cyst, an emphysematous bulla, or a peripheral neoplasm, induces airlessness

of a thin layer of contiguous lung parenchyma; although this situation could reasonably be regarded as "compression," the lung's elastic recoil properties render a concept of "relaxation" more logical. Thus we prefer to regard this process as a form of passive atelectasis.

The pathologist is accustomed to seeing a thin zone of collapsed lung adjacent to a pulmonary mass; in most cases, however, the airless lung is contiguous to tissue of identical density, and radiographic differentiation of the basic lesion from adjacent collapsed tissue is often impossible. Only when the loss of volume occurs contiguous to a zone of relative radiolucency, such as a bulla or bleb, is the atelectatic lung recognizable as a distinct shadow of increased density. Even then, the wall of a bulla, however large, may be no more than a hairline shadow, thus indicating the extremely small volume of completely collapsed lung parenchyma.

On CT, atelectasis is commonly seen in the dependent lung regions as an ill-defined area of increased attenuation or subpleural curvilinear opacities (Fig. 20–12).[14–16] The former measures from a few millimeters to 1 cm or more in thickness and has been called *dependent opacity* or *dependent density*.[14, 15] Subpleural curvilinear opacities, also known as subpleural lines, are linear areas of increased attenuation measuring several centimeters in length and located within 1 cm of the pleura and parallel to it.[17] Both manifestations of dependent atelectasis characteristically disappear when the patient changes position (Fig. 20–12); differentiation of dependent atelectasis from true interstitial or air-space disease can therefore be easily established by scanning the patient in both the supine and prone positions.[14, 18] Dependent atelectasis results in radiologic changes that are distinct from the normal gradient in attenuation seen between dependent and nondependent portions of lungs.[19]

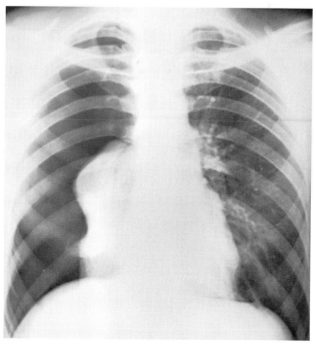

Figure 20–9. Pneumothorax with Pulmonary Collapse. A posteroanterior radiograph following spontaneous pneumothorax reveals the small volume occupied by a whole lung when totally collapsed. The well-defined air bronchogram indicates airway patency.

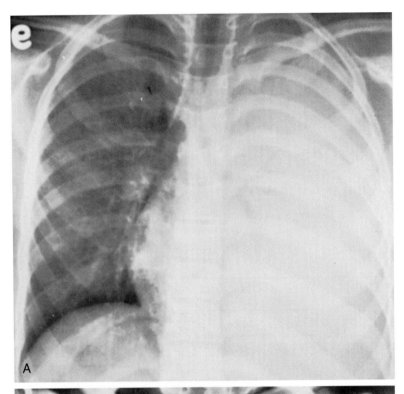

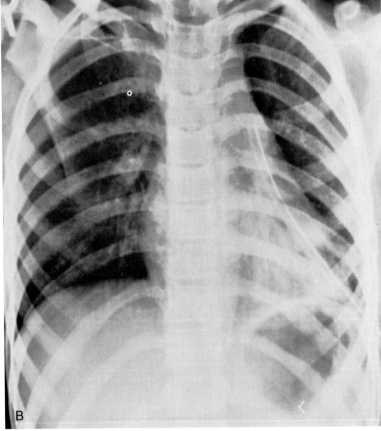

Figure 20–10. Atelectasis in the Presence of Massive Pleural Effusion. *A*, An air bronchogram is clearly visible within the opacity caused by a massive left pleural effusion, analogous to the atelectasis that accompanies a large pneumothorax. *B*, Shortly following insertion of a chest tube and removal of the fluid, the lung had almost completely reinflated.

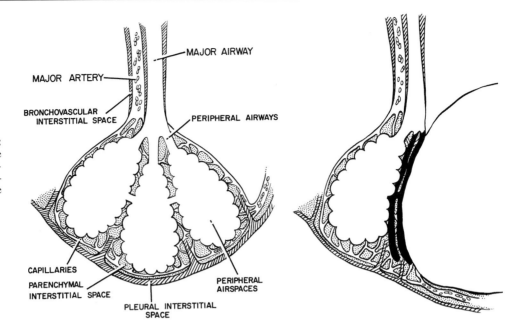

Figure 20–11. Lung Diagram: Relaxation Atelectasis. A large "bulla" situated on the right has permitted relaxation of contiguous parenchyma and subsequent complete atelectasis.

Alveoli and small airways in the dependent lung regions are smaller than in nondependent regions because of a gravity-dependent decrease in transpulmonary pressure.[20, 21] A reduction in lung volumes—such as may be seen during anesthesia or in bedridden patients with prolonged shallow breathing—therefore predisposes to *dependent* atelectasis.[22–24] In one study, the CT findings in anesthetized rabbits were assessed under conditions of reduced lung volume caused by pneumoperitoneum.[22] Homogeneous increased attenuation shown pathologically to be the result of atelectasis developed in the dependent lung regions. In another investigation involving the same experimental model, small airways in the areas of dependent atelectasis were shown histologically to remain patent;[23] the authors concluded that the dependent atelectasis was due to a reduction in alveolar volume rather than small airway collapse.

Such gravity-dependent atelectasis is commonly seen during anesthesia and in the early postoperative period[25, 26] and may be associated with considerable venous/arterial shunting and hypoxemia.[27, 28] The complication is more common in patients with increased blood volume, pulmonary edema, impaired mucociliary transport, and intrinsic airway abnormalities such as seen in smokers.[24, 29, 30] In one study, dependent atelectasis was seen on HRCT in 6 of 51 (12%) nonsmokers, 11 of 26 (42%) ex-smokers, and 33 of 98 (34%) of smokers.[30]

Round Atelectasis

Round atelectasis (rounded atelectasis, folded lung) is a distinct form of atelectasis characteristically associated with focal pleural thickening.[31, 32] On conventional radiographs, the lesion is seen as a fairly homogeneous, round, oval, wedge-shaped, or irregularly shaped subpleural mass.[31, 32] It usually measures 2.5 to 5 cm in greatest diameter, althoughit may reach up to 10 cm[33, 34] and involve an entire lobe.[35] The bronchovascular bundles in the vicinity of the mass are gathered together in a curvilinear fashion as they pass toward the mass, similar to the tail of a comet, a feature best appreciated on CT. The abnormality occurs most

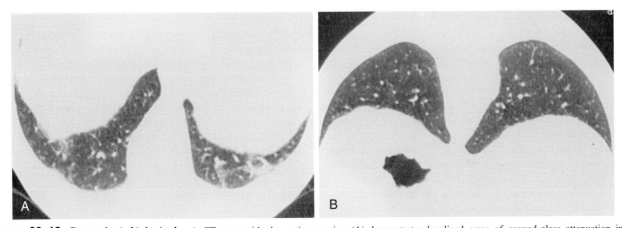

Figure 20–12. Dependent Atelectasis. A CT scan with the patient supine *(A)* demonstrates localized areas of ground-glass attenuation in the dependent portions of both lower lobes. A repeat scan with the patient prone *(B)* is normal. Reversibility from supine to prone positions allows distinction of passive dependent atelectasis from air-space or interstitial disease.

commonly in the lower lobes: in a literature review of 100 cases, 74 occurred in this location, 21 in the middle lobe or lingula, and only 5 in the upper lobes.[36]

The pathogenesis of round atelectasis has been debated. According to one theory, the abnormality begins when a pleural effusion "floats" the lower lobe upward and compresses it into a finger-like projection.[37] The atelectatic portion of lung then becomes adherent to the parietal pleura through fibrin deposition; as the pleural fluid is resorbed, the central part of the collapsed lung reinflates while the peripheral part remains atelectatic and tends to roll into a ball, thus resulting in the round appearance characteristic of the abnormality. We consider it more likely that the majority of cases are related to a focus of pleural fibrosis that contracts as it develops, causing invaginations of pleura into contiguous lung and compression of its parenchyma.[38] In a number of patients on whom thoracotomy has been performed for a mistaken diagnosis of cancer, the collapsed pulmonary parenchyma has re-expanded following decortication of the region of pleural fibrosis; as a consequence, it is reasonable to regard this form of atelectasis as relaxation in type.

The characteristic CT features consist of bronchi and vessels curving and converging towards a round or oval mass that abuts an area of pleural thickening and is associated with evidence of volume loss in the affected lobe (Fig. 20–13).[39–41] The hilar (central) aspect of the mass usually has indistinct margins as a result of blurring by the entering vessels.[40, 41] Air bronchograms are identified within the mass in approximately 60% of cases.[40, 41] Subpleural fat may be identified within the mass,[42] a feature that undoubtedly reflects chronicity and is therefore not be seen in all cases; however, it is our opinion that this finding is highly suggestive of the diagnosis and that its presence argues strongly against other more serious processes such as infection or neoplasia. Vessels and bronchi curve into the periphery of the mass, which forms the basis for the "comet tail" sign. Although this sign is commonly seen, bronchi and blood vessels are sometimes oriented obliquely or in the cephalocaudal plane and are thus not readily apparent on conventional cross-sectional CT images; multiplanar reconstructions using spiral CT or multiplanar imaging using magnetic resonance imaging may be helpful in better determining the course of the blood vessels and bronchi in these cases.[34, 43] Lung parenchyma adjacent to the mass is hyperinflated and oligemic. The lung adjacent to pleural invaginations can occasionally be visible as radiolucent areas within the atelectatic lung.

In most patients, the CT findings are sufficiently characteristic that neither biopsy nor further investigative procedures are necessary to exclude more ominous disease.[15, 40, 41] However, one case has been described of a patient with the typical radiologic features of round atelectasis, which on subsequent biopsy proved to be an infiltrating, poorly differentiated carcinoma;[44] it was concluded that the carcinoma probably abutted a zone of round atelectasis and that the benign nature of such lesions cannot always be guaranteed from their radiologic appearance. From a practical point of view, however, such an event must be exceptional, and careful radiographic follow-up rather than transthoracic needle aspiration or thoracotomy is probably the best course of action in these patients.

The majority of cases of round atelectasis are seen in patients exposed to asbestos.[36] Other causes include pleural effusion from tuberculosis, therapeutic pneumothorax, congestive heart failure, infections other than tuberculosis,[45] pulmonary infarction, and malignant tumor.[36] We have also seen a case developing after cardiac surgery (Fig. 20–14).

Follow-up of patients who have round atelectasis has shown that the majority of lesions are stable for many years.[34, 36] Occasionally, a lesion decreases in size or resolves within a few weeks to several years[36, 46] or enlarges.[47, 48] Regression occurs mainly in patients who do not have a history of asbestos exposure,[36, 49] although it has been reported in those who have after benign asbestos-related pleural effusion.[50]

Adhesive Atelectasis

The term *adhesive atelectasis* is used to described atelectasis caused, at least in part, by surfactant deficiency.[24, 51] As discussed previously (*see* page 54), surfactant reduces the surface tension of an alveolus as its surface area or volume decreases; thus the critical closing pressure of an alveolus occurs at a lower volume and distending pressure, effectively protecting against collapse. Absence of surfactant has been reported in studies of atelectatic lungs, both with[52] and without[53] associated pneumonia.

The best examples of adhesive atelectasis are RDS of newborn infants and acute radiation pneumonitis (Fig. 20–15); other causes include adult respiratory distress syndrome, smoke inhalation, pneumonia, prolonged shallow breathing, and pulmonary thromboembolism.[24, 54, 55] In newborn and adult forms of RDS, smoke inhalation, and prolonged shallow breathing, the atelectasis is frequently diffuse throughout both lungs.[24, 54] By contrast, atelectasis in acute radiation pneumonitis is usually limited to the irradiated portions of the lungs (Fig. 20–16);[56, 57] occasionally, it is seen outside the regions of the radiation ports, particularly on CT.[56] The radiographic and CT findings consist of areas of ground-glass opacification or consolidation with associated loss of volume.[56–58] Adult respiratory distress syndrome with diffuse bilateral consolidation has been described in some patients who have undergone treatment for lung cancer;[59] at autopsy, hyaline membranes were found within irradiated and nonirradiated lung. The radiologic manifestations of radiation pneumonitis usually occur approximately 1 to 6 months following the completion of radiation therapy.[56–58] Focal ischemia distal to pulmonary thromboembolism may lead to a local reduction in surfactant that results in subsegmental, segmental, or less commonly, lobar atelectasis.[24, 60]

It is likely that adhesive atelectasis also plays a part in loss of volume postoperatively and accounts for the marked arteriovenous shunting that may occur even when chest radiographs are relatively normal.[61–63] Atelectasis is seen in the majority of patients following coronary artery bypass surgery.

Cicatrization Atelectasis

Although for the sake of completeness we have included loss of volume associated with pulmonary fibrosis in the section on atelectasis, the term *atelectasis* is seldom used

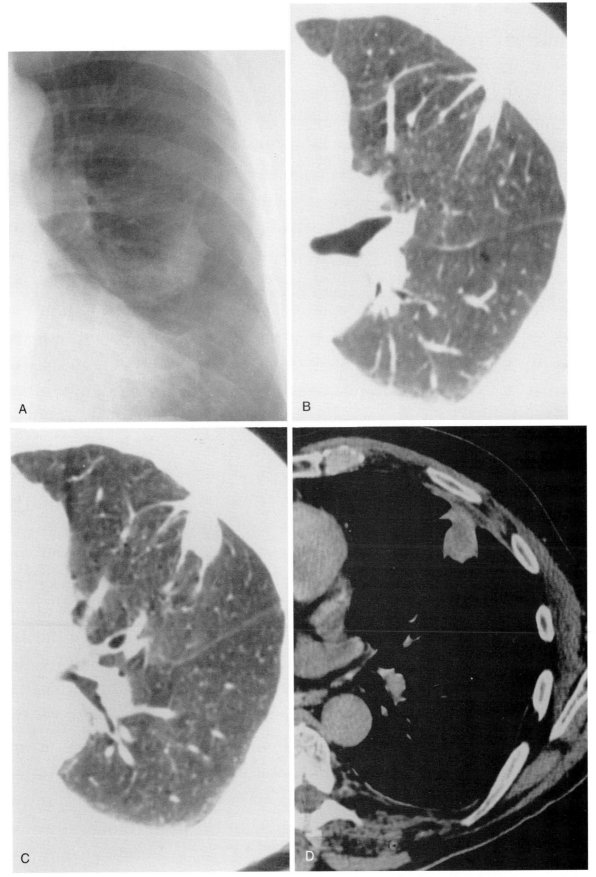

Figure 20–13. Round Atelectasis. A view of the left lung from a posteroanterior chest radiograph *(A)* demonstrates an oval soft tissue nodule measuring 3 cm in maximal diameter. CT scans *(B* and *C)* show vessels converging toward the nodule. Note the evidence of volume loss, with the vessels and the left major fissure curving toward the area of atelectasis. CT photographed at soft tissue windows *(D)* demonstrates that the nodule abuts a focal area of pleural thickening. The patient was a 70-year-old man who had a history of asbestos exposure.

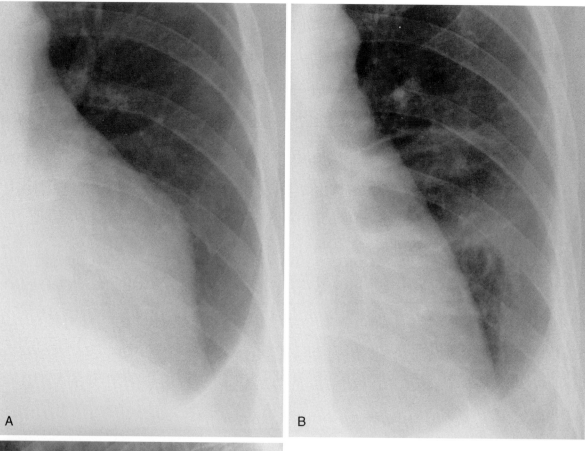

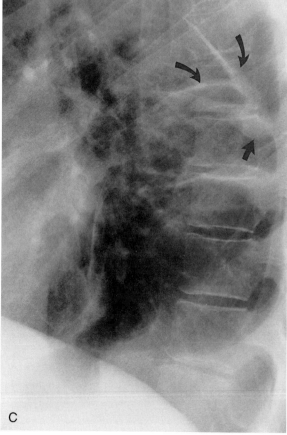

Figure 20–14. Round Atelectasis Following Surgery. A view of the left lung from a posteroanterior chest radiograph *(A)* performed 1 week after open-heart surgery demonstrates a small left pleural effusion. The lung is normal. A follow-up radiograph *(B)* performed 15 months later demonstrates poorly defined linear opacities associated with mild loss of volume as well as a small pleural effusion. A view of the posterior aspect of the chest from a lateral radiograph *(C)* shows characteristic features of round atelectasis: a focal round opacity *(straight arrow)* abutting an area of pleural thickening associated with broad curvilinear opacities *(curved arrows)* that extend toward the area of atelectasis.

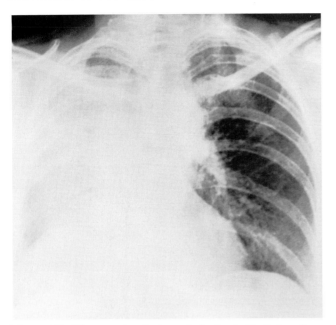

Figure 20–15. Adhesive Atelectasis in Acute Radiation Pneumonitis. A posteroanterior radiograph reveals opacification and loss of volume of the right lung associated with mediastinal shift and hemidiaphragmatic elevation (the oblique shadow across the left upper lung is an artefact). A faint air bronchogram can be seen in the right lower lung zone.

in this context. The fundamental pathologic process is one of fibrosis, the fibrous tissue undergoing retraction as it matures and resulting in loss of volume of the affected portion of lung. The radiologic signs depend on whether the process is local or generalized.

Localized cicatrization atelectasis is best exemplified by chronic infection, often granulomatous in nature, and epitomized by long-standing tuberculosis (Fig. 20–17). The bronchi and bronchioles within the affected lung are dilated because of the increased elastic recoil from the surrounding pulmonary fibrosis, a phenomenon known as *traction bronchiectasis and bronchiolectasis*.[64] The radiologic signs are as might be expected (Fig. 20–18): a segment or lobe occupying a volume smaller than normal, with a density rendered inhomogeneous by dilated, air-containing bronchi and with irregular thickened strands extending from the atelectatic segment to the hilum. Compensatory signs of chronic loss of volume are usually evident, including local mediastinal shift (frequently manifested by a sharp deviation of the trachea when segments of the upper lobe are involved), displacement of the hilum (which may be severe in upper lobe disease), and compensatory overinflation of the remainder of the affected lung. The loss of volume may be so severe as to render the atelectatic lung almost invisible on a standard posteroanterior (PA) radiograph, particularly if involvement of apical or apical-posterior segments of an upper lobe results in incorporation of the shadow of the atelectatic lung into that of the mediastinum; in this circumstance, correct diagnosis depends on identification of the compensatory signs of atelectasis (Fig. 20–19).

Generalized fibrotic disease of the lungs may also be associated with loss of volume (Fig. 20–20). For example, patients who have idiopathic pulmonary fibrosis commonly show elevation of the diaphragm and an overall reduction in

lung size. In fact, a gradual reduction in thoracic volume in cases of diffuse interstitial disease is a useful indicator of the fibrotic nature of the underlying pathologic process (Fig. 20–21). Other diseases associated with pulmonary fibrosis may produce entirely different radiologic patterns.

In summary, atelectasis may occur by four mechanisms acting independently or in combination.

1. *Resorption atelectasis* occurs when communication between the trachea and alveoli is obstructed; the obstruction may be in a major bronchus or in multiple small bronchi or bronchioles.

2. *Relaxation atelectasis* denotes loss of volume accompanying an intrathoracic space-occupying process, particularly pneumothorax or hydrothorax. Atelectasis contiguous to a local space-occupying process such as a pulmonary mass or bulla is of the same nature and does not warrant the separate designation of compression atelectasis. Round atelectasis is a variant of relaxation atelectasis that is characteristically associated with an area of pleural thickening.

3. *Adhesive atelectasis* is related to a deficiency of surfactant. As with relaxation and cicatrization atelectasis, it is associated with patent large airway communications.

4. *Cicatrization atelectasis* results from contraction of interstitial fibrous tissue as it matures.

RADIOLOGIC SIGNS OF ATELECTASIS

The radiologic signs of atelectasis may be classified into direct and indirect signs (Table 20–1). The former include displacement of the interlobar fissures and crowding of bronchi and vessels within the area of atelectasis; the latter include pulmonary opacification and signs related to shift of other structures to compensate for the loss of volume.

Direct Signs

Displacement of Interlobar Fissures. Displacement of the fissures that form the boundary of an atelectatic lobe is one of the most dependable and easily recognized signs of

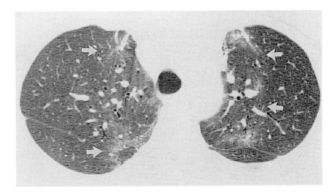

Figure 20–16. Adhesive Atelectasis in Radiation Pneumonitis. An HRCT scan demonstrates areas of ground-glass attenuation in a distribution conforming to the radiation portals for treatment of Hodgkin's disease *(arrows)*. Evidence of loss of volume is present, with bronchi and vessels being closer to the mediastinum than normal, particularly on the left side. The patient was a 28-year-old woman who had undergone radiation therapy 5 months previously.

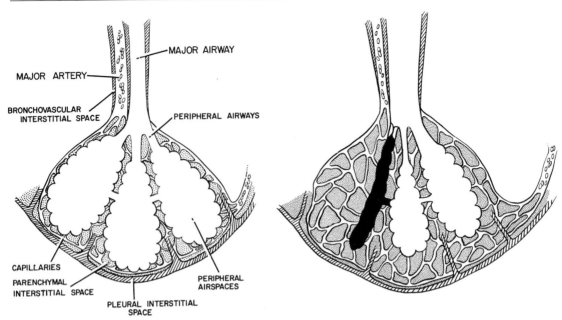

Figure 20–17. Lung Diagram: Local Cicatrization Atelectasis. The interstitial space is increased in amount and density as a result of fibrosis. The left air space is totally obliterated, and those to the right show different degrees of loss of volume. The major airway is dilated (bronchiectasis), as is the peripheral airway on the right (bronchiolectasis).

atelectasis (Fig. 20–22). For each lobe, the position and configuration of the displaced fissures are predictable for a given loss of volume; these factors are considered later in relation to patterns of specific lobar and segmental atelectasis.

Crowding of Vessels and Bronchi. As the lung loses volume, the vessels and bronchi in the atelectatic area become crowded together. Such crowding is one of the earliest signs of atelectasis and can be most readily recognized when comparison is made with previous radiographs.[24] Increased opacification of the atelectatic lobe may result in obscuration

of the vessels; however, except in patients with resorptive atelectasis, crowded air bronchograms will be visible within the area of atelectasis on the radiograph or CT (*see* Fig. 20–22).

Indirect Signs

Apart from the presence of a local opacity, the main indirect radiologic signs of atelectasis are those that are related to mechanisms that compensate for the reduction in

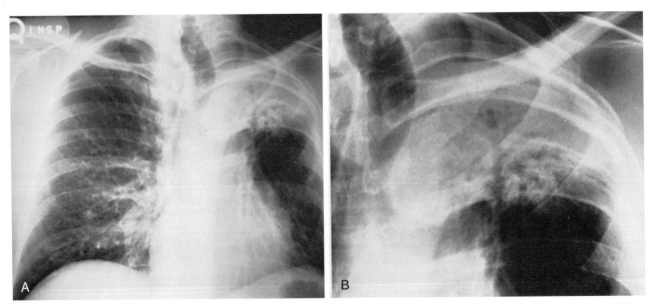

Figure 20–18. Local Cicatrization Atelectasis: Postirradiation Fibrosis. One and one-half years previously, this 48-year-old man was found to have inoperable squamous cell carcinoma of the left upper lobe, for which he had received an intensive course of radiotherapy. A posteroanterior radiograph *(A)* reveals considerable loss of volume of the left upper lung, with displacement of the trachea to the left, approximation of the left upper ribs, and elevation of the left hilum. A magnified view *(B)* shows a prominent air bronchogram in an otherwise homogeneous opacity.

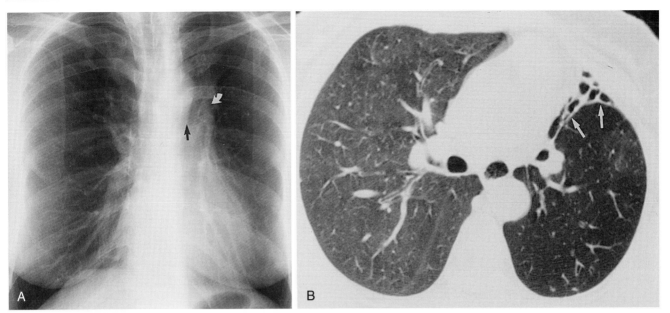

Figure 20–19. Severe Cicatrization Atelectasis. A posteroanterior chest radiograph *(A)* in a 41-year-old woman demonstrates volume loss of the left upper lobe with elevation of the left main bronchus *(straight black arrow)* and left hilum *(curved white arrow)* and shift of the mediastinum. Note the decreased vascularity of the left lung in comparison to the right. Although the left upper lobe is collapsed, it has not resulted in any increase in opacity. An HRCT scan *(B)* confirms the presence of complete atelectasis of the left upper lobe. All that remains are markedly ectatic bronchi outlined by the major fissure *(arrows)*, which is displaced cephalad, anteriorly and medially. Note the marked hyperinflation of the left lower lobe and decreased size of the left hemithorax. The findings are the result of previous tuberculosis.

intrapleural pressure—diaphragmatic elevation, mediastinal shift, approximation of ribs, and overinflation of the remainder of the lung *(see* Fig. 20–22). The part played by each compensatory mechanism in any given situation is somewhat unpredictable, although predominance is dictated largely by the anatomic position of the collapsed lobe; all four mechanisms may operate fairly equally, or one or two may predominate to the exclusion of others. Two general rules deserve emphasis. (1) Displacement of the diaphragm and mediasti-

num is maximal contiguous to the area of atelectasis; for example, lower lobe atelectasis tends to elevate the posterior more than the anterior portion of the hemidiaphragm and displace the inferior more than the superior mediastinum. Conversely, upper lobe atelectasis is associated with upper mediastinal displacement, often with little hemidiaphragmatic elevation. (2) The more acute the atelectasis, the greater the predominance of diaphragmatic and mediastinal displacement (Fig. 20–23); the more chronic the atelectasis,

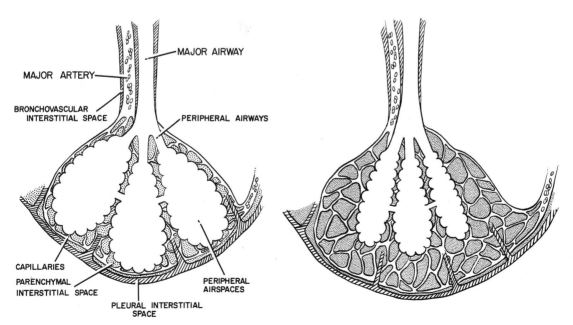

Figure 20–20. Lung Diagram: General Cicatrization Atelectasis. There is a marked increase in interstitial tissue with a uniform reduction in the volume of all air spaces as a result of fibrosis. The dilatation of the major airway seen in local cicatrization atelectasis is not a prominent part of the picture, although peripheral airway dilatation may occur.

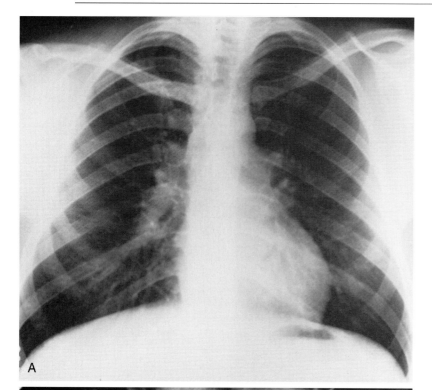

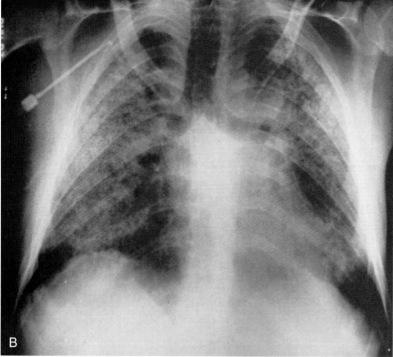

Figure 20–21. General Cicatrization Atelectasis Secondary to Intravenous Talcosis. At the time of a normal chest radiograph *(A)*, this 19-year-old man had been taking drugs (both heroin and methadone) intravenously for over 2 years. Six years later, a radiograph *(B)* reveals diffuse interstitial disease throughout both lungs associated with loss of lung volume (as evidenced by elevation of the diaphragm and smallness of the thoracic cage). This loss of volume is the result of diffuse interstitial fibrosis caused by intravenously injected talc.

the more that compensatory overinflation of nonatelectatic lung predominates (*see* Fig. 20–22).

Local Increase in Opacity. Undoubtedly the most important indirect sign of atelectasis, a local increase in opacity is caused by a combination of resorption of air and accumulation of fluid.[5] The volume of an airless lobe or segment depends not only on which order of bronchus is obstructed but also on the amount of sequestered fluid within the obstructed parenchyma. Because the lung contains a large

amount of air and normal lung density is only 0.12 gm/ml, the lung must become almost completely collapsed before increased opacification from loss of volume is apparent on the chest radiograph.

Elevation of the Hemidiaphragm. As already stated, hemidiaphragmatic elevation is always a more prominent feature of lower than upper lobe atelectasis (compare Figures 20–23*A* and *B*). In the lower lung zones, elevation tends to occur in the area contiguous to the lobe involved—posterior

Table 20–1. RADIOLOGIC SIGNS OF ATELECTASIS

Direct
1. Displacement of the interlobar fissures
2. Crowding of vessels and bronchi

Indirect
1. Local increase in opacity
2. Elevation of the hemidiaphragm
3. Displacement of the mediastinum
4. Compensatory overinflation
5. Displacement of the hila
6. Approximation of the ribs
7. Absence of an air bronchogram (in cases of resorption atelectasis only)
8. Absence of visibility of the interlobar artery (in cases of lower lobe atelectasis only)

elevation in lower lobe atelectasis and anterior elevation in middle lobe or lingular atelectasis (although in the latter two situations, the diaphragmatic displacement is seldom severe).

When assessing diaphragmatic elevation, one should take into consideration possible variations in the relationship of the two hemidiaphragms. Although the right dome is normally 1 to 2 cm higher than the left, deviation from normal was observed in 11% of 500 normal subjects in one study;[65] in 9%, the two hemidiaphragms were level or the left was slightly higher than the right, and in 2% the right hemidiaphragm was more than 3 cm higher than the left.

Mediastinal Displacement. The normal mediastinum is a surprisingly mobile structure and reacts promptly to differences in pressure between the two halves of the thorax (*see* Fig. 20–23). The anterior and middle compartments are less stable than the posterior and therefore shift to a greater extent.

As with the diaphragm, normal variations in configura-tion of the mediastinum should be recognized; this variation is less of a problem with the trachea and upper mediastinum than with the heart, since the trachea is consistently a midline structure. The amount of cardiac silhouette that projects to the right of the spine varies in normal subjects, however, and a central position of the heart does not necessarily indicate displacement.

Compensatory Overinflation. Overinflation of the remainder of the ipsilateral lung is one of the most important and reliable indirect signs of atelectasis. It seldom occurs rapidly and, in the early stages of lobar atelectasis, is usually of less diagnostic help than the other compensatory phenomena such as diaphragmatic elevation and mediastinal displacement. As the period of atelectasis lengthens, however, overinflation becomes more prominent and the diaphragmatic and mediastinal changes regress. The degree to which the lung can be overinflated without its functional capabilities being significantly affected is truly remarkable. In one of our patients, a young woman whose entire left lung and right lower and middle lobes were removed because of severe bronchiectasis, the remaining right upper lobe overinflated and filled the whole thorax (Fig. 20–24); her pulmonary function, although obviously impaired, was approximately what might be predicted for one fifth the normal complement of pulmonary tissue.

Radiologic evidence of compensatory overinflation may be extremely subtle. In particular, it may be difficult to estimate the increase in radiolucency resulting from the greater air-blood ratio on the radiograph. More reliable evidence for overinflation on the radiograph is supplied by the alteration in vascular markings (*see* Fig. 20–22),[66] the vessels typically being more widely spaced and sparser than in the normal contralateral lung. The densitometric capabilities and the ability for transverse display of the pulmonary vessels

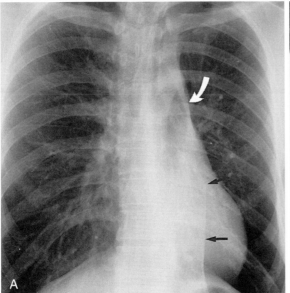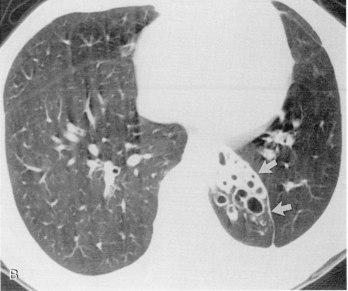

Figure 20–22. Left Lower Lobe Atelectasis. A posteroanterior chest radiograph *(A)* demonstrates caudad and medial displacement of the left major fissure *(black arrows)* characteristic of left lower lobe atelectasis. Crowding of ectatic bronchi within the atelectatic lobe can also be seen. Indirect signs of left lower lobe atelectasis include overinflation of the left upper lobe, overinflation of the right lung with displacement of the anterior junction line *(curved white arrow)* to the left, and shift of the mediastinum. An HRCT scan *(B)* demonstrates caudad and medial displacement of the major fissure *(straight white arrows)* and left lower lobe bronchiectasis. Note that even though the lobe is markedly atelectatic, there is little opacification of the lung parenchyma, presumably because of reflex vasoconstriction. The patient was a 23-year-old man who had a history of childhood viral pneumonia.

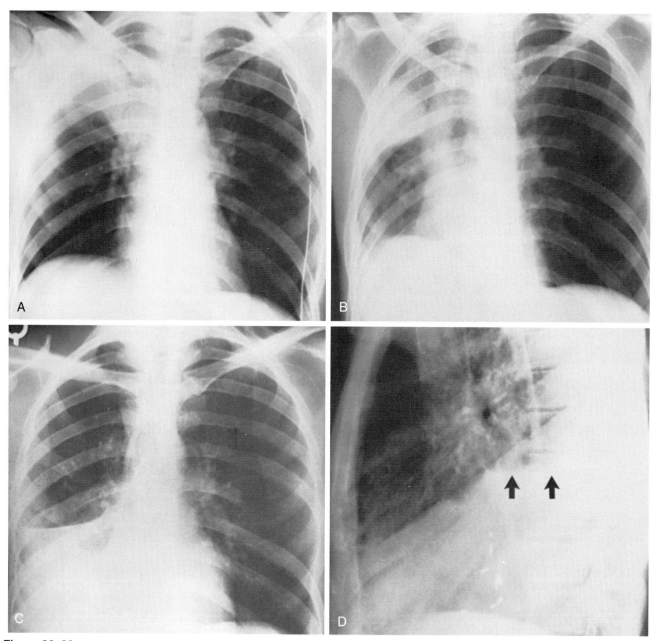

Figure 20–23. Radiologic Signs of Atelectasis. A radiograph of the chest in anteroposterior projection, supine position *(A)*, reveals a homogeneous shadow in the upper portion of the right hemithorax whose concave lower margin is formed by the upwardly displaced horizontal fissure; the right hemidiaphragm is slightly elevated. The features are indicative of right upper lobe atelectasis; the patient had undergone surgical repair of a hiatus hernia via a thoracoabdominal approach 24 hours earlier. Twenty-four hours later *(B)*, the right upper lobe atelectasis is clearing, but the diaphragmatic elevation has increased and the mediastinum has shifted markedly to the right; note the approximation of ribs. These signs indicate acute obstruction of the right intermediate bronchus with progressing atelectasis of the middle and lower lobes. Twenty-four hours later, posteroanterior (PA) *(C)* and lateral *(D)* views reveal the right middle and lower lobes to be virtually airless; the right upper lobe has completely re-expanded. The roughly horizontal interface in *C* is the major fissure, not the minor as might be thought; in the lateral projection, note that the upper portion of the major fissure has swung caudally to a roughly horizontal position *(arrows)*, thus making it tangential to the x-ray beam and creating the sharp interface in PA projection. Following this examination, a mucous plug was removed from the intermediate bronchus.

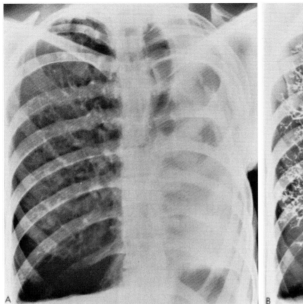

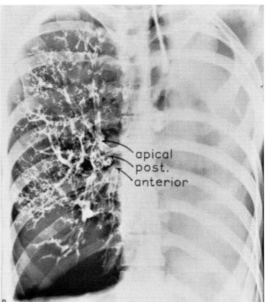

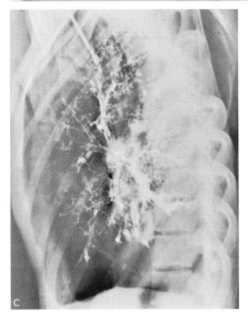

Figure 20–24. Compensatory Overinflation: The One-Lobe Thorax. Over a span of several years, thoracotomy was performed on this 28-year-old woman on three different occasions for advanced incapacitating bronchiectasis: on the first, the left lower lobe and lingula were removed; on the second, the left upper lobe; and on the third, the right middle and lower lobes. At the time of each thoracotomy, the bronchial tree was found to be normal bronchographically in those areas subsequently affected. A right bronchogram (*B* and *C*) reveals only three segmental bronchi of the right upper lobe, at least one of which shows moderately advanced bronchiectasis. *See* the text.

make CT an ideal technique for the combined detection of increased lung radiolucency and spatial redistribution of the pulmonary vessels.

When only a relatively small volume of one lung is atelectatic, compensatory overinflation is usually restricted to the remainder of that lung. However, when the atelectasis is more extensive, there is a greater tendency for overinflation to involve the contralateral lung; such involvement may progress to the point at which the opposite lung displaces the mediastinum either generally or locally. These local displacements occur in the three "weakest" areas of the mediastinum, where the two lungs are separated only by loose connective tissue:[67] (1) the anterior mediastinum at the level of the first three or four costal cartilage, limited anteriorly by the sternum and posteriorly by the great vessels; (2) the posterosuperior mediastinum at the level of the third to fifth thoracic vertebrae, limited anteriorly by the esophagus and trachea and posteriorly by the vertebral column (the

supra-aortic triangle); and (3) the posteroinferior mediastinum, limited anteriorly by the heart and posteriorly by the vertebral column and aorta (the retrocardiac space). Anterior mediastinal displacement is usually easy to appreciate radiologically through identification of the displaced anterior junction line; the curvilinear opacity of the apposed pleural surfaces is usually seen on a PA radiograph to protrude into the involved hemithorax; in lateral projection the anterior mediastinum appears exceptionally radiolucent and increased in depth. Appreciation of displacement of the posterior mediastinal weak areas is more difficult and relies on detection of displacement of the posterior junction line and azygoesophageal recess interface.

The term *mediastinal herniation* is commonly used to refer to mediastinal displacement by overinflated lung compensating for atelectasis of all or part of the contralateral lung. We dislike the word "herniation" in this context, since it is defined as displacement of a viscus from one chamber into another through a defect or hiatus in the intervening septum. In fact, the mediastinum is intact; the effect of atelectasis and compensatory overinflation is that of displacement, either local or general, and not herniation.[67]

When an entire lung becomes atelectatic following obstruction of a main bronchus, the resultant loss of volume of the hemithorax must be compensated for largely by overinflation of the contralateral lung (similar to the situation after pneumonectomy) (*see* Fig. 20–24). In this situation, the mediastinal shift may be large; since the mediastinum is less stable anteriorly than elsewhere, the anterior septum is rotated laterally and posteriorly, the normal lung overinflating to such an extent that it occupies the whole anterior portion

of the thorax. Thus the heart and the collapsed lung are displaced into the posterior portion of the ipsilateral hemithorax. The radiologic appearance in lateral projection is distinctive:[68] both the depth and radiolucency of the retrosternal air space are increased, the heart and great vessels are displaced posteriorly, and there is a general increase in density posteroinferiorly (Fig. 20–25); the margin of the collapsed lung may be sharply delineated where it comes in contact with the opposite overinflated lung. Such an appearance enhances differentiation of massive collapse from massive unilateral pneumonic consolidation or pleural effusion (Fig. 20–25).[68]

Displacement of the Hila. The hila are often displaced in

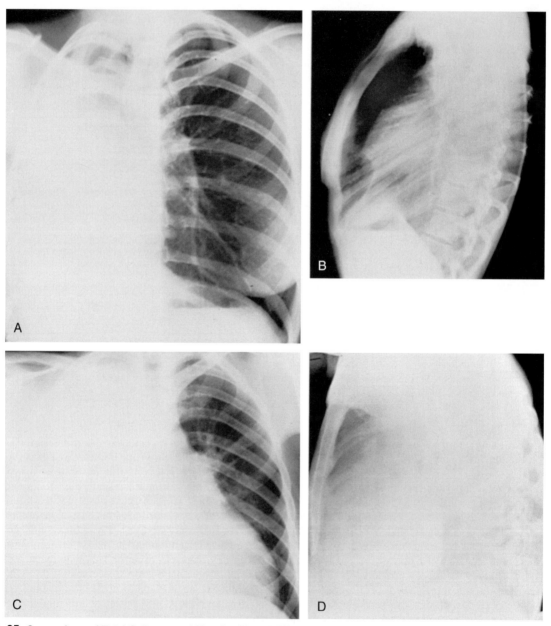

Figure 20–25. Comparison of Total Collapse and Massive Pleural Effusion. Radiographs of the chest in posteroanterior and lateral projections (*A* and *B*) of a patient whose right lung has been removed (analogous to total right pulmonary collapse) reveal a marked shift of the mediastinum into the posterior portion of the right hemithorax, with herniation of the overinflated left lung across the midline into the anterior portion of the right side of the chest (note the clear retrosternal space). In *C* and *D* (radiographs of another patient), a massive right pleural effusion has resulted in a shift of the mediastinum to the left; in lateral projection, the opacity of the thorax is more or less homogeneous (the uniform filter effect). Compare the appearance of the retrosternal space in the two patients.

the presence of atelectasis. Such displacement occurs more commonly in atelectasis of the upper than the lower lobes and is usually more marked the more chronic the atelectasis; for example, scarring of the upper lobes as a result of tuberculosis commonly causes severe upward displacement of the ipsilateral hilum (Fig. 20–26). Downward displacement of the right hilum in cases of lower lobe atelectasis is seldom as clearly appreciated. Downward displacement of only the left hilum, however, is more readily apparent, particularly if it brings the left hilum level with the right—an appearance seen in only 3% of normal individuals.[65]

Assessment of the position of the air columns of the trachea and major bronchi in lateral projection can also be helpful in detecting the presence of atelectasis.[69] On a well-aligned lateral radiograph of the chest, the trachea, both main bronchi, and both upper lobe bronchi are normally in vertical alignment; any alteration in this relationship should be considered abnormal. Since the upper lobes are situated mainly anteriorly, atelectasis of these lobes will displace their respective main bronchi forward; similarly, with atelectasis of the lower lobes, the posterior position of these lobes will displace their major bronchi backward (Fig. 20–27). Although we have seen this sign repeatedly in cases of lower lobe atelectasis, we have found it seldom to be very clear when the upper lobes are affected. Posterior displacement of the left upper lobe bronchus may also result from distention of the left superior pulmonary vein (Fig. 20–28) in cases of left atrial and pulmonary venous hypertension[70] and (occasionally) from a prominent but normal common left pulmonary venous confluence; it is of obvious importance to distinguish such displacement from that caused by lower lobe atelectasis.

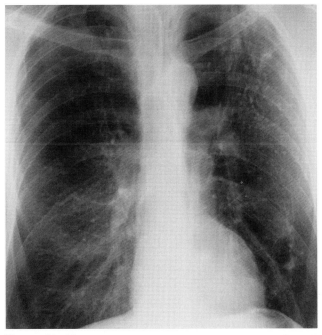

Figure 20–26. Unilateral Hilar Elevation Secondary to Chronic Left Upper Lobe Fibrosis. A posteroanterior chest radiograph in a 47-year-old man demonstrates elevation of the left hilum and left main bronchus. Extensive fibrocalcific changes are present in the left upper lobe and lingula, consistent with previous tuberculosis. Other secondary signs of volume loss include shift of the mediastinum and mild elevation of the left hemidiaphragm.

Of equal importance to displacement of the hila as a sign of atelectasis is redistribution of the vascular shadows that form these structures. The right hilum normally possesses a concave lateral aspect formed by the superior pulmonary vein above and the descending pulmonary artery below. Atelectasis of the right upper lobe is associated with rotation of the superior pulmonary vein medially and flattening of the right hilar concavity.[71] However, the concavity can also be flattened by distention of the superior pulmonary vein in cases of severe pulmonary venous hypertension.

A cardinal sign of lower lobe atelectasis is loss of visibility of the interlobar artery; since the lung parenchyma adjacent to the artery is airless, the air-tissue interface is lost and the vessel becomes invisible. A helpful sign in detecting lower lobe atelectasis is medial displacement of the interlobar and lower lobe pulmonary arteries (Fig. 20–29). This sign is particularly valuable on the left side, where pleural effusion sometimes creates a triangular shadow in the posterior paravertebral zone that simulates total left lower lobe atelectasis. Preservation of the shadow of the interlobar artery establishes the pleural origin of the opacity, whereas its obliteration indicates lobar atelectasis.

Changes in the Chest Wall. In our experience, approximation of the ribs is the least dependable of all compensatory radiographic signs of atelectasis. Even a slight degree of rotation of the patient may produce an asymmetry of the two sides of the rib cage that renders assessment of abnormal approximation difficult. The difficulty may be further compounded by alterations in rib angulation produced by even minor degrees of scoliosis. Thus, although approximation of ribs as a sign of smallness of a hemithorax may be of some value in cases of chronic loss of volume, we believe that it should not be relied on as an accurate indicator of reduction in hemithoracic volume in cases of acute disease.

Absence of an Air Bronchogram. For the most part, resorption atelectasis cannot be present if air is visible in the bronchial tree; if the bronchial obstruction is severe enough to cause absorption of air from the parenchyma of the affected lobe, it must also cause absorption of gas from the airways themselves. Thus, particularly when pneumonitis behind the obstruction is so severe that consolidation exceeds atelectasis, absence of an air bronchogram is a radiologic sign of vital importance since it may be the only clue in differentiating between an obstructing bronchogenic carcinoma and a consolidative process such as bacterial pneumonia. Although there are rare exceptions to this rule—e.g., an endobronchial lesion that causes peripheral pneumonitis but incomplete obstruction of the bronchial lumen—the true nature of the underlying pathologic process should become evident either when the lesion completely obstructs the bronchus or when serial radiographs reveal nonresolution of the pneumonia despite appropriate therapy. Another exception to the general rule is acute confluent bronchopneumonia, such as from *Staphylococcus aureus*, in which a lobe or segment becomes homogeneously opaque and the bronchi are filled with inflammatory exudate; obviously, an air bronchogram would not be anticipated.

The preceding statements apply only to resorption atelectasis; in the relaxation and adhesive forms particularly, an air bronchogram is virtually always present. In fact, as discussed previously, absence of an air bronchogram—for example, in a lung collapsed behind a pneumothorax—indi-

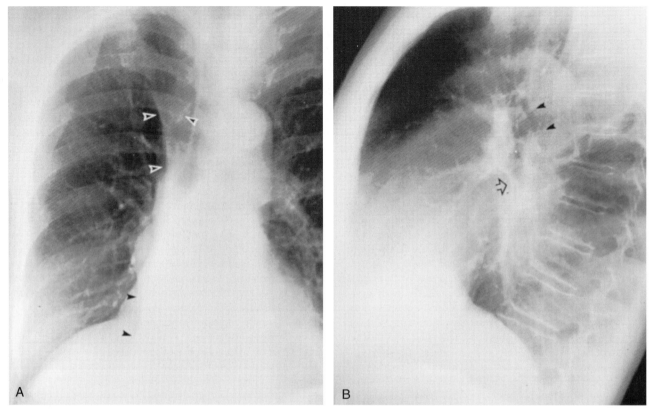

Figure 20–27. Posterior Displacement of the Intermediate and Lower Lobe Bronchi Associated with Atelectasis of the Right Lower Lobe. In posteroanterior projection *(A)*, the right lower lobe is collapsed and airless *(small arrowheads* point to the interface between the downward-displaced major fissure and the overinflated right upper lobe). The anterior junction line and mediastinal triangle *(arrowheads)* are displaced to the right *(upper triangle sign)*. Note that the right interlobar artery is no longer visible because of obscuration by the airless lower lobe. In lateral projection *(B)*, collapse of the lower lobe is manifested by a vague triangular opacity overlying the lower thoracic vertebrae and by posterior displacement of the air column of the intermediate and right lower lobe bronchi *(arrowheads)*. Normally, the lower lobe bronchus is aligned with the tracheal air column, slightly in front of the anterior wall of the left lower lobe bronchus *(open arrow)*. The patient was a 55-year-old man with a centrally obstructing carcinoma.

cates endobronchial obstruction in addition to the passive atelectasis.

Miscellaneous Signs. An interesting although very uncommon indirect sign of atelectasis is the "shifting granuloma."[72] A pulmonary nodule whose position shifts from one examination to another is almost certainly related to loss of volume of either the lobe in which the nodule is situated or a contiguous lobe; it thus represents an internal marker of atelectasis. Of a similar nature is a nodule or mass that disappears from one examination to another as a result of being surrounded by airless lung in an atelectatic lobe (Fig. 20–30).

PATTERNS OF ATELECTASIS

The radiographic manifestations of lobar and segmental atelectasis were first described in 1945.[73–79] Since then, several authors have further clarified the findings and made additional observations.[80–83] The CT characteristics of lobar atelectasis have also been documented by several groups.[35, 51, 84, 85] The typical radiologic patterns of atelectasis may be influenced by several variables, including pre-existing disease within the involved lobe or elsewhere in the lungs, a relatively fixed thoracic cage or mediastinum, pleural adhesions, pleural fluid, or pneumothorax. The effects of these

variables are not discussed here, the patterns described being those that typically occur in atelectasis of previously normal pleuropulmonary tissue.

Since the degree of atelectasis of a lobe is governed to a large extent by the amount of fluid and cells it contains, the radiographic image varies from a consolidated lobe with only minimal loss of volume to a state of total collapse; therefore the anatomic-spatial relationships in each lobe are described from a state of normal volume through all stages to total atelectasis.

Provided that there is no pneumothorax or hydrothorax, it is a general rule that the visceral pleura covering an atelectatic lobe continues to relate intimately to the parietal pleura, regardless of the severity of atelectasis; in other words, the visceral pleural surface usually maintains contact with the parietal pleura over either the convex or mediastinal surface of the hemithorax (Fig. 20–31). Two exceptions to this rule are noteworthy: occasionally in lower lobe atelectasis (Fig. 20–31*C*) and frequently in severe middle lobe atelectasis (Fig. 20–31*D*), the convex pleural contact may be lost as the lobe foreshortens in a triangular fashion toward the hilum. Maintenance of visceral and parietal pleural contiguity with the mediastinum is also generally maintained, although in severe middle lobe atelectasis this contact may be lost.

In the majority of cases, therefore, maintenance of con-

Text continued on page 539

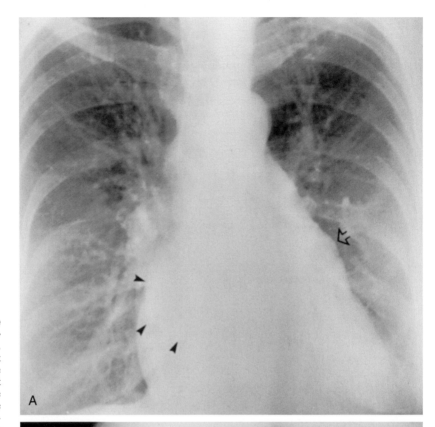

Figure 20–28. Posterior Displacement of the Left Main and Lower Lobe Bronchi in Postcapillary Pulmonary Venous Hypertension. Conventional posteroanterior *(A)* and lateral *(B)* chest radiographs disclose an abnormal cardiac silhouette consistent with right ventricular enlargement; the left atrium (three *arrowheads*) and left atrial appendage *(open arrow)* are also enlarged. The left upper lobe (LU) and lower lobe (LL) bronchi are displaced posteriorly; this feature is usually caused by enlargement of the left superior pulmonary vein or confluence rather than by the left atrium *per se*. Note the flow redistribution into the arteries and veins of the upper lobes, loss of the normal right hilar concavity, and lack of definition of the lower zone vasculature, features indicative of postcapillary (venous) hypertension. The patient was a 47-year-old women with mitral stenosis.

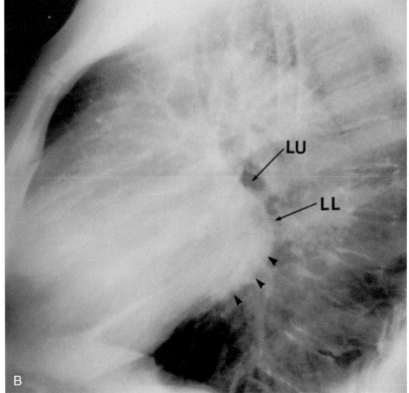

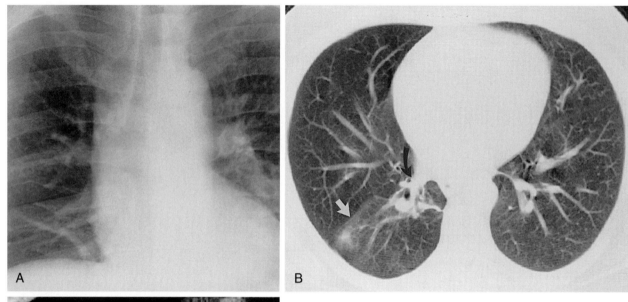

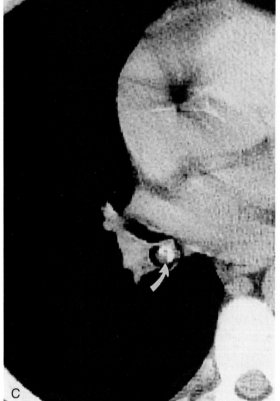

Figure 20–29. Right Lower Lobe Atelectasis Caused by Endobronchial Hamartoma. A view from a posteroanterior chest radiograph *(A)* in a 44-year-old man demonstrates poor visualization of the right hilum. The right interlobar and lower lobe arteries are displaced medially and thus obscured by the heart border. The combination of poor visualization of the right hilum, relatively vertical course of the right main bronchus, and medial displacement of the right interlobar and lower lobe pulmonary arteries is characteristic of right lower lobe atelectasis. A CT scan *(B)* demonstrates posterior displacement of the right major fissure *(straight white arrow)* and posterior orientation of the right inferior pulmonary vein *(curved black arrow)*, signs also indicative of right lower lobe atelectasis. Soft tissue windows *(C)* demonstrate a partly calcified nodule *(curved white arrow)* in the right lower lobe bronchus. This nodule was removed bronchoscopically and shown to be an endobronchial hamartoma.

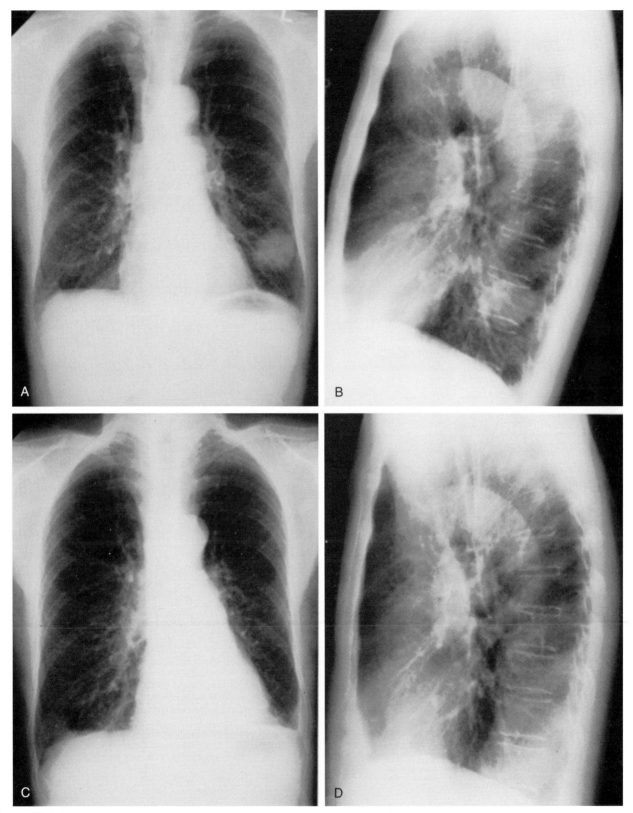

Figure 20–30. "Disappearance" of a Lung Mass as a Result of Lobar Atelectasis. Posteroanterior *(A)* and lateral *(B)* radiographs reveal a 5-cm mass in the posterior portion of the left lower lobe. Several days later, similar projections *(C* and *D)* show the mass to have disappeared. In the interval, the left lower lobe has undergone total atelectasis as a result of bronchial compression by lymph nodes containing metastatic carcinoma; the mass has become invisible because the surrounding parenchyma has become airless.

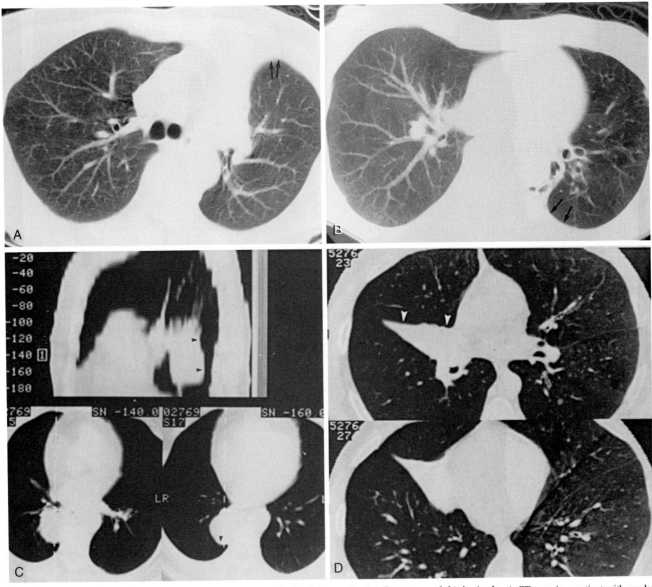

Figure 20–31. Relationship Between the Visceral and Parietal Pleura in the Presence of Atelectasis. A CT scan in a patient with marked left upper lobe atelectasis *(A)* demonstrates that the contiguity between visceral and parietal pleura is maintained anteriorly *(arrows)*. Another scan in a patient with complete left lower lobe atelectasis *(B)* shows that contiguity of the two pleurae is also maintained over the lobe's convex (posterior) surface *(arrows)*. *C,* In contrast to these two cases, a sagittal CT reformation *(top)* and representative transverse images *(bottom)* in a patient with right lower lobe atelectasis reveal the visceral pleura *(arrowheads)* to have lost all contact with the parietal pleura of the posterior chest wall but not the mediastinum. Similarly, transverse CT scans *(D)* of a patient with right middle lobe atelectasis *(arrowheads)* show the visceral pleura over the convex (anterior) surface of the lobe to have lost contact with the parietal pleura; however, a thin linear opacity is still visible between the lateral point of the collapsed lobe and the chest wall, which conceivably could be caused by either contact between the upper and lower lobes or airless lung at the extreme periphery of the middle lobe. Loss of contiguity between the visceral and parietal pleura over the convex surface of a lobe is most apt to occur with atelectasis of the middle lobe, occasionally in a lower lobe, and rarely if ever in an upper lobe.

tiguity of the pleural surfaces restricts movement toward the hilum; since the medial aspect of the lobe is relatively fixed at the hilum, the forms that the atelectatic lobe must adopt are limited. The resultant shape is partly affected by the relatively rigid components of the lung (bronchi, arteries, and veins), which can be crowded together in very close apposition in one plane but have a limited capacity to foreshorten. Thus, any pulmonary lobe in its fully inflated state may be likened to a pyramid with its apex at the hilum and its base contiguous to the parietal pleura; as the lobe loses volume, two surfaces of the pyramid approximate, the end result of total atelectasis being a flattened triangle or triangular "pancake" whose apex and base tend to maintain contiguity with the hilum and parietal pleura, respectively.[86]

On CT, atelectatic lobes become wedge shaped rather than hemispheric in cross section, with the apex situated at the origin of the affected bronchus (*see* Fig. 20–31).[35, 51] The atelectatic lobe tapers smoothly towards the hilum except when the atelectasis is due to a large central tumor, in which case there is a focal lateral convexity (S sign of Golden) (*see* farther on).[51, 87] Other signs suggestive of an obstructive tumor on CT include the presence of an endobronchial or peribronchial soft tissue mass and absence of air bronchograms within the atelectatic lobe.[51, 85] Delineation of the extent of a central obstructing tumor on CT requires administration of intravenous contrast, preferably by power injector.[88]

Total Pulmonary Atelectasis

When an entire lung becomes atelectatic because of obstruction of a main bronchus, the compensatory phenomena are identical in character to those that develop with less severe pulmonary atelectasis, but are obviously greater in degree and, in some respects paradoxically, less readily apparent (Fig. 20–32). Elevation of the ipsilateral hemidiaphragm is recognizable only on the left side, the stomach bubble indicating its position. The hemithorax usually shows evidence of retraction. As the normal contralateral lung overinflates, the whole mediastinum moves to the affected side, the greatest shift occurring anteriorly, where the mediastinum is most mobile. In PA projection, the uniform opacity caused by the superimposed cardiovascular structures and atelectatic lung is interrupted by the radiolucency of overinflated contralateral lung that has passed across the midline of the thorax. The margin of the overinflated lung is usually seen to extend into the involved hemithorax.

Atelectasis of an entire lung is usually secondary to complete obstruction of a main bronchus and is associated with increased opacity of the atelectatic lung (Fig. 20–32). However, in patients with partial obstruction, previous tuberculosis, or pneumothorax, loss of volume may occur with normal or even increased radiolucency of the atelectatic lung (Fig. 20–33; *see* also Fig. 20–8, page 519).

Lobar Atelectasis

The patterns created by atelectasis of the right and left upper lobes differ and are therefore described separately; the lower lobes have almost identical patterns and are considered together.

Right Upper Lobe

The minor fissure and the upper half of the major fissure approximate by shifting upward and forward, respectively (Fig. 20–34). On lateral projection, both fissures appear gently curved, the minor fissure assuming a concave configuration inferiorly whereas the major fissure may be convex, concave, or flat;[89] the minor fissure shows roughly the same curvature in PA projection. As volume diminishes further, the visceral pleural surface sweeps upward over the apex of the hemithorax so that the lobe comes to occupy a flattened position contiguous to the superior mediastinum. When completely atelectatic, its volume is so small that in PA projection its shadow creates no more than a slight widening of the superior mediastinum (Fig. 20–35). In lateral projection, the collapsed lobe may appear as an indistinctly defined triangular shadow with its apex at the hilum and its base contiguous to the parietal pleura just posterior to the extreme apex of the hemithorax ("the mediastinal wedge"). The atelectatic lobe is usually contiguous to the mediastinum, so no air shadow separates them; occasionally, however, a part of the overinflated lower lobe is interposed between the mediastinum and the medial edge of the atelectatic upper lobe, a feature seen much more often with left upper lobe atelectasis (*see* farther on). In approximately 50% of patients with atelectasis of the right upper lobe and 80% of those with atelectasis of the left, an array of parallel or divergent tubular or linear opacities can be seen in the perihilar region.[90] This finding is the result of reorientation of vessels within the overinflated lower lobe.[90, 91]

Another sign commonly associated with right or left upper lobe atelectasis (less commonly with middle lobe atelectasis) is the *juxtaphrenic peak*.[92] This consists of a small, sharply defined triangular opacity that projects upward from the medial half of the hemidiaphragm at or near the highest point of the dome (Fig. 20–36). It was initially believed that the peak was related to upward displacement of the diaphragmatic component of the pulmonary ligament.[92] However, studies correlating radiographic with CT findings have demonstrated that it is related to an inferior accessory fissure in the vast majority of cases.[93, 94] For example, in one investigation of 12 patients, surgical clips were placed along the inferior pulmonary ligament at the time of upper lobectomy;[93] juxtaphrenic peaks developed in 4 patients and were shown to be associated with inferior accessory fissures remote from the clips.[93] Less common causes of a juxtaphrenic peak include accessory fissures other than the inferior accessory fissure, a parenchymal scar, and extrapleural fat drawn into a reoriented major fissure.[85, 94]

The mechanism behind the development of a juxtaphrenic peak is not clear. It has been suggested that the negative pressure caused by upper lobe atelectasis may lead to upward retraction of the portion of the visceral pleura (and associated extrapleural fat) that protrudes into a recess on the basal surface of the lung.[92] The tethering effect is presumably greater at this pleural extension into the inferior accessory fissure because the pleural extension is less distensible than the adjacent lung parenchyma.[94]

Right upper lobe atelectasis caused by large hilar tu-

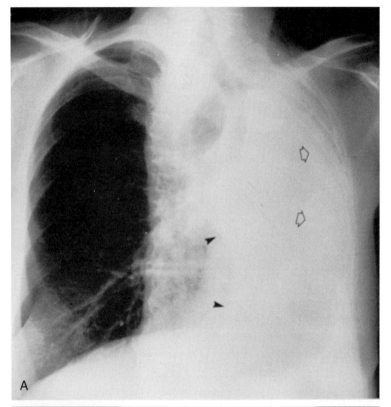

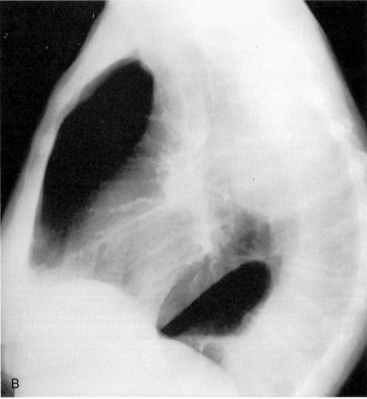

Figure 20–32. Total Atelectasis of the Left Lung. Posteroanterior *(A)* and lateral *(B)* chest radiographs disclose an opaque and shrunken left hemithorax. The right lung is markedly overinflated and has displaced the mediastinum to the left both posteriorly *(arrowheads)* and anteriorly *(open arrows)*. The cardiac silhouette is obscured except for its anterior surface, which is clearly visible in the lateral projection; curvilinear calcification in the upper left hemithorax identifies the aortic arch. The patient was a 73-year-old woman with total atelectasis of the left lung caused by a centrally obstructing carcinoma.

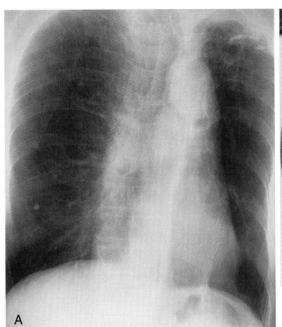

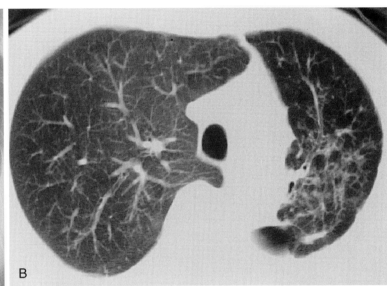

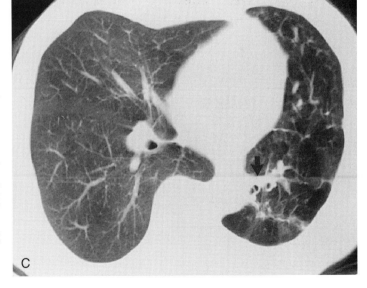

Figure 20–33. Loss of Volume of the Left Lung as a Result of Previous Tuberculosis. A posteroanterior chest radiograph *(A)* in an 80-year-old man demonstrates marked loss of volume of the left lung with shift of the mediastinum and compensatory overinflation of the right lung. Areas of scarring are present in the left upper and left lower lobes. Also noted are elevation of the left hilum, left apical pleural thickening, and a calcified granuloma in the right lung. Although reduced in volume, the left lung is more radiolucent than the right. An HRCT scan at the level of the aortic arch *(B)* reveals a marked decrease in vascularity and an associated decrease in attenuation of the left lung. Note the hyperinflation of the right upper lobe with a shift of the anterior junction line to the left. Areas of scarring and mild bronchiectasis are evident in the left upper lobe. An HRCT scan through the lower lung zones *(C)* demonstrates decreased vascularity and attenuation in the lingula and left lower lobe. Scarring is present in the left lower lobe with associated posterior displacement of the left inferior pulmonary vein *(arrow)* and basal segmental bronchi.

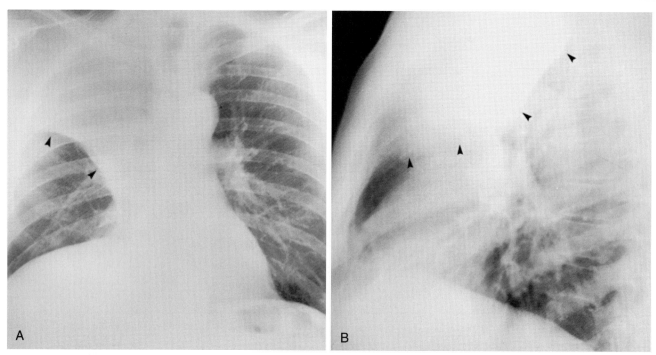

Figure 20–34. Right Upper Lobe Atelectasis (Moderate). Posteroanterior *(A)* and lateral *(B)* radiographs reveal a homogeneous opacity *(arrowheads)* occupying the anterosuperior portion of the right hemithorax. In lateral projection, the opacity is sharply defined on its posterior and anteroinferior margins. The right hemidiaphragm is elevated and there is slight displacement of the trachea to the right. The patient was a 51-year-old man with a large squamous cell carcinoma in the right upper lobe. The atelectasis was caused by bronchial compression from involved lymph nodes.

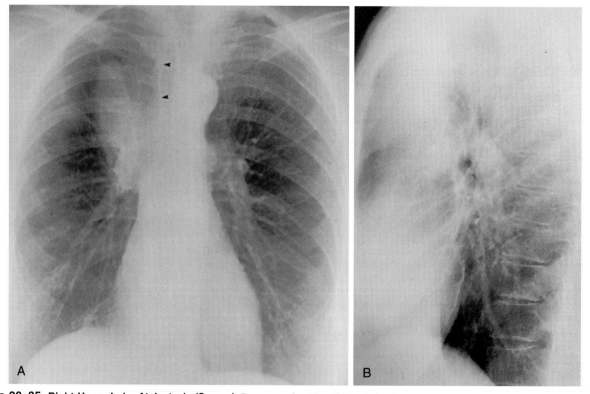

Figure 20–35. Right Upper Lobe Atelectasis (Severe). Posteroanterior *(A)* and lateral *(B)* chest radiographs disclose a reduction in volume of the right hemithorax, elevation of the right hemidiaphragm, and a peaked appearance to the superomedial contour of the right hemidiaphragm. The trachea is displaced minimally to the right, but the tracheal stripe is maintained *(arrowheads)*. Note the slight lucency immediately lateral to the trachea. This lucency is the result of an overinflated superior segment of the right lower lobe and represents a right-sided Luftsichel sign. An opacity extends from an elevated right hilum superiorly toward the apex of the right lung. The patient was a 68-year-old woman with a central squamous carcinoma.

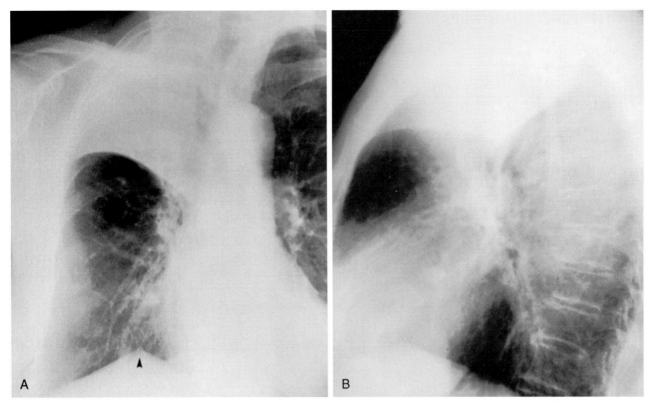

Figure 20–36. The Juxtaphrenic Peak in Upper Lobe Atelectasis. Posteroanterior *(A)* and lateral *(B)* chest radiographs in a patient with right upper lobe atelectasis show the normally smooth contour of the right hemidiaphragm to be interrupted by a triangular opacity *(arrowhead)*, with its apex pointing cephalad. This juxtaphrenic peak is the result of an inferior accessory fissure that can be seen extending obliquely cephalad and medial from the juxtaphrenic peak.

mors may be associated with a characteristic downward bulge in the medial portion of the minor fissure. This feature, combined with the concave appearance of the lateral aspect of the minor fissure, results in a reverse S configuration of the minor fissure and is known as the *S sign of Golden* (Fig. 20–37).[82, 95] The sign is highly suggestive of bronchogenic carcinoma as the cause of atelectasis on both radiographs[24, 82] and CT.[87] Although initially described for right upper lobe atelectasis, Golden's S sign is in fact applicable to atelectasis of any lobe.[24, 82]

On CT, the medial margin of the atelectatic right upper lobe abuts the mediastinum and is associated with superior and medial displacement of the minor fissure *(see Fig. 20–37)*. With elevation of the minor fissure, the overinflated middle lobe shifts upward laterally alongside the atelectatic upper lobe. Compensatory overinflation of the right lower lobe results in superior, anterior, and medial displacement of the major fissure.[35, 51]

Left Upper Lobe

The major difference between atelectasis of the left and right upper lobes is related to the absence of a minor fissure on the left; all lung tissue anterior to the major fissure is involved (Fig. 20–38). This fissure—which is slightly more vertical than the major fissure on the right—is displaced forward in a plane roughly parallel to the anterior chest wall, a relationship depicted particularly well on a lateral radiograph (Fig. 20–38). As volume loss increases, the fissure moves further anteriorly and medially, until on lateral

projection the shadow of the lobe is no more than a broad linear opacity contiguous and parallel to the anterior chest wall (Fig. 20–39). The contiguity of the atelectatic lobe to the anterior mediastinum obliterates the left cardiac border in frontal projection (the "silhouette sign").

As the apical segment moves downward and forward, the space it vacates is occupied by the overinflated superior segment of the lower lobe; the apex of the hemithorax thus contains aerated lung (Fig. 20–39).[96] Sometimes, this lower lobe segment inserts itself medially between the apex of the atelectatic upper lobe and the mediastinum, thereby creating a sharp interface with the medial edge of the atelectatic lobe and allowing visualization of the aortic arch. The overinflated superior segment is seen as a crescent of hyperlucency, hence the term *Luftsichel* ("air crescent") in the German literature.[97] This feature is more often seen on the left *(see Fig. 20–38)* than on the right *(see Fig. 20–35)*.[89] CT assessment in such circumstances almost invariably shows a V-shaped or peaked appearance of the posteromedial fissural surface between the atelectatic upper lobe and the overinflated lower lobe segment (Fig. 20–40).[89] The superior segment of the lower lobe is pulled forward along both the medial and lateral limbs of the V, the medial limb forming a tongue of aerated lung between the mediastinum and the atelectatic left upper lobe and accounting for the periaortic lucency.

On CT, the atelectatic left upper lobe can be seen to abut the anterior chest wall and mediastinum (Fig. 20–41). The major fissure is shifted cephalad and anteriorly. The posterior margin of the atelectatic left upper lobe has a V-

Text continued on page 549

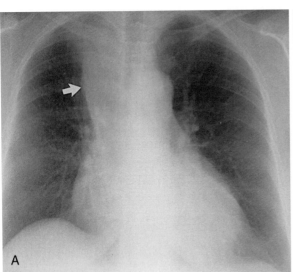

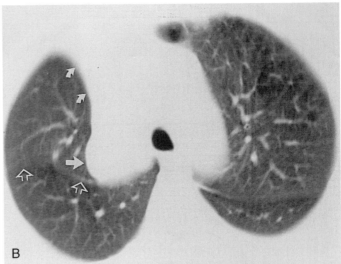

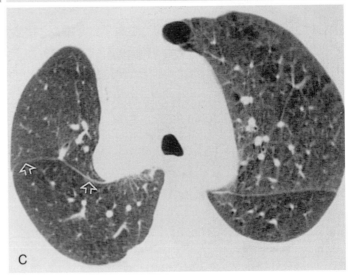

Figure 20–37. Right Upper Lobe Atelectasis with Golden's S Sign. A posteroanterior chest radiograph *(A)* reveals right upper lobe atelectasis with elevation and medial displacement of the minor fissure. Note the focal convexity caused by a central tumor (Golden's S sign) *(arrow)*. A CT scan at the level of the tracheal carina *(B)* demonstrates upward and medial displacement of the minor fissure *(curved arrows)* with a localized convexity (Golden's S sign) *(straight arrow)* and upward and forward displacement of the right major fissure *(open arrows)*. The reorientation of the major fissure is easier to appreciate on the HRCT image *(C)* *(open arrows)*. The patient was a 55-year-old woman with right upper lobe obstruction by squamous cell carcinoma.

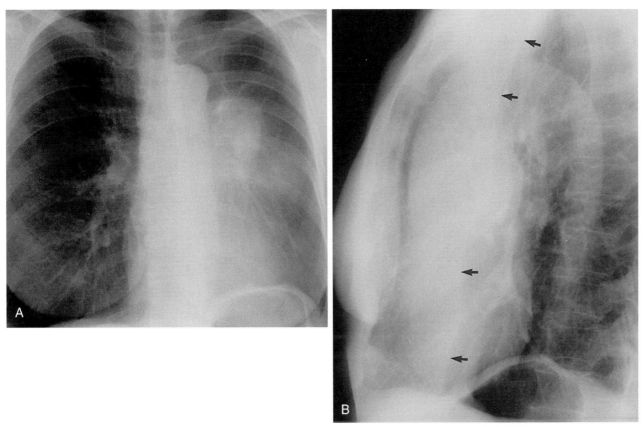

Figure 20–38. Left Upper Lobe Atelectasis with the Luftsichel Sign. A posteroanterior (PA) chest radiograph *(A)* demonstrates elevation of the left hilum and left main bronchus and a poorly defined increased opacity in the left perihilar region. A crescent of aerated lung outlines the aortic arch ("Luftsichel" sign). The lateral radiograph *(B)* reveals anterior displacement of the major fissure *(arrows)*. Note that the overinflated superior segment of the left lower lobe outlines the aortic arch and accounts for the area of increased lucency lateral to the aortic arch on the PA radiograph.

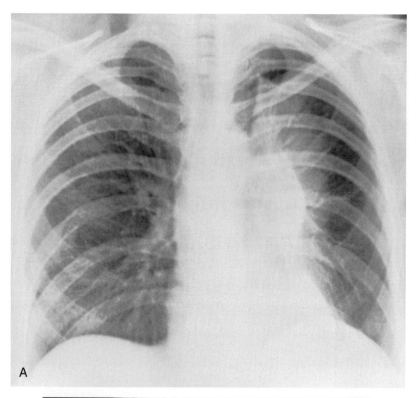

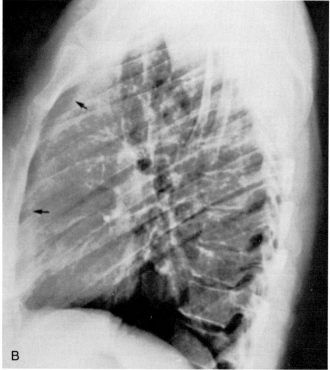

Figure 20–39. Atelectasis of the Left Upper Lobe (Severe). The homogeneous shadow created by the almost complete collapse of the left upper lobe occupies the anteromedial portion of the left hemithorax contiguous to the mediastinum. In posteroanterior projection *(A)*, the apex of the hemithorax is occupied by the overinflated lower lobe. In lateral projection *(B)*, the major fissure has swept far anteriorly and can be identified as a rather indistinctly defined shadow of increased opacity paralleling the anterior chest wall *(arrows)*. The "mediastinal wedge" can be only vaguely distinguished.

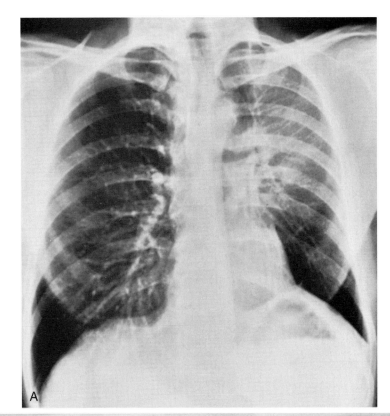

Figure 20–40. Left Upper Lobe Atelectasis with the Luftsichel Sign. A posteroanterior chest radiograph *(A)* reveals elevation of the left hilum and a crescent of radiolucency (Luftsichel sign) between the aortic arch and the atelectatic left upper lobe. A CT scan *(B)* shows a V-shaped contour of the left upper lobe fissure. The peak *(curved arrow)* is caused by tethering of the major fissure by the hilar structures. The portion of the superior segment medial to the pleural reflection accounts for the Luftsichel sign.

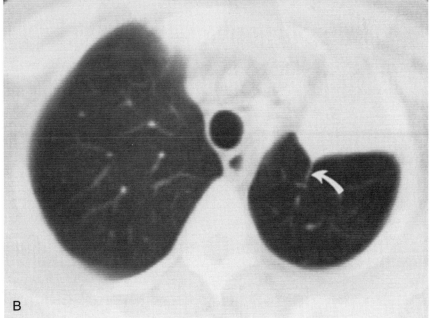

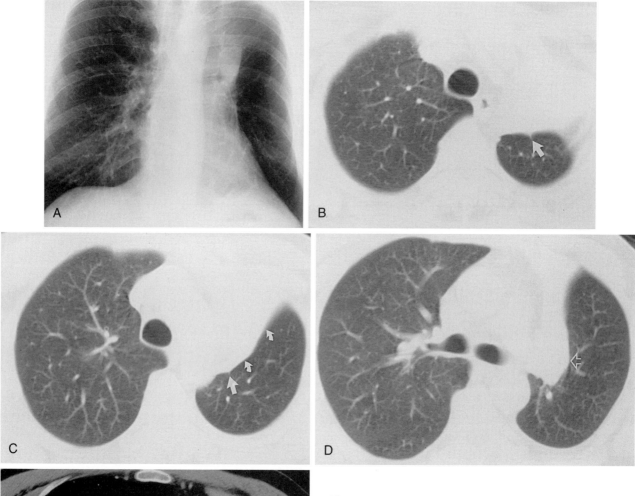

Figure 20–41. Left Upper Lobe Atelectasis. A posteroanterior chest radiograph *(A)* demonstrates elevation of the left hilum and opacification of the left upper lobe. A CT scan near the lung apex *(B)* reveals anterior and cephalad displacement of the major fissure. Note the slightly peaked appearance of the posterior surface of the major fissure *(straight arrow)* caused by tethering from the hilar structures. A CT scan at the level of the aortic arch *(C)* shows anterior and medial displacement of the interlobar fissure *(curved arrows)* with a focal peak *(straight arrow).* Also note the peaked appearance of the posterior fissural surface *(arrow)* and lack of air bronchograms indicative of resorptive atelectasis. A CT scan at the level of the left main bronchus *(D)* reveals a focal convexity *(open arrow)* characteristic of a central obstructive tumor (S sign of Golden). A CT scan photographed at soft tissue windows *(E)* demonstrates central tumor *(arrows)* associated with complete obstruction of the left upper lobe bronchus. The patient was a 58-year-old man with squamous cell carcinoma.

shaped contour or a small peak from the lung apex to the hilum as a result of tethering of the major fissure by the hilum (Fig. 20–41). A focal convexity in the hilar region indicates the presence of a central obstructing tumor (S sign of Golden) (Fig. 20–41).

Atelectasis of the upper division of the left upper lobe with sparing of the lingula results in findings similar to those of right upper lobe atelectasis.[82] The interface between the atelectatic upper division and the overinflated lingula is usually arcuate and bowed in an upward direction, even in the absence of a left minor fissure.[24, 82] Lingular atelectasis resembles right middle lobe atelectasis and is associated with obscuration of the left heart border on the PA radiograph and a triangular opacity with the apex at the hilum on the lateral view.[82] The inferior margin of the atelectatic segment is well defined, being bordered by the major fissure; however, because a left minor fissure is uncommon, the superior margin is usually irregular or poorly defined.[24, 82]

Right Middle Lobe

The diagnosis of right middle lobe atelectasis is one of the easiest to make on a lateral radiograph and one of the

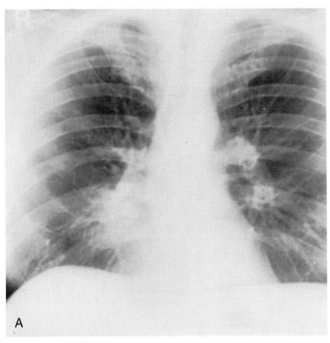

A

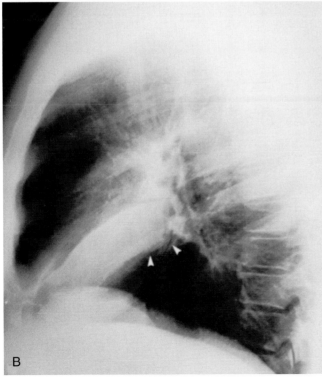

B

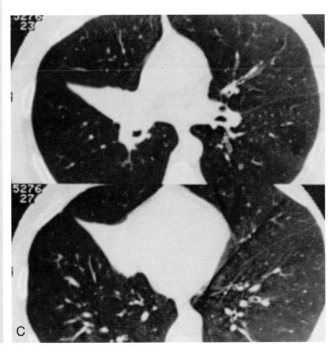

C

Figure 20–42. Right Middle Lobe Atelectasis. A posteroanterior radiograph *(A)* reveals a vague opacity in the right lower hemithorax obliterating the right cardiac border, whereas a lateral projection of the same patient *(B)* shows the characteristic triangular opacity of middle lobe atelectasis. Note the convex inferior configuration of the major fissure at the hilum *(arrowheads)*, indicative of an underlying mass. The opacity of the middle lobe has a sharp oblique orientation downward, which constitutes the "tipped-down" pattern of middle lobe atelectasis. CT scans *(C)* show the typical triangular opacity with its apex pointing peripherally. Contiguity between the visceral and parietal pleura over the anterolateral aspect of the lobe has been lost. The right middle lobe bronchus was obstructed by carcinoma.

Illustration continued on following page

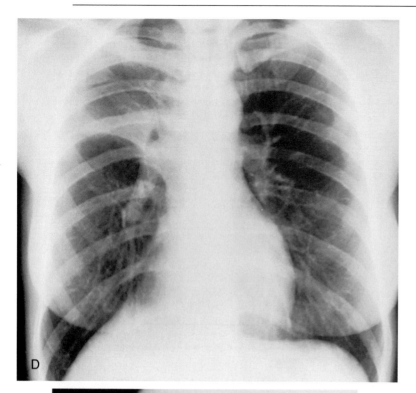

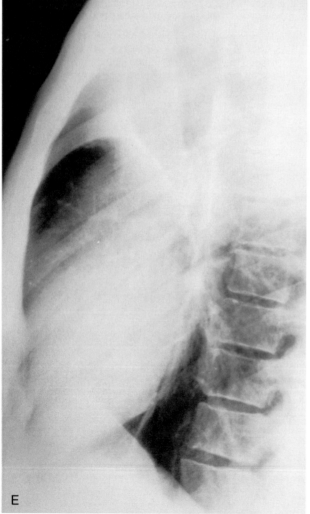

Figure 20–42 *Continued.* Conventional posteroant-erior *(D)* and lateral *(E)* radiographs of another patient with an obstructing middle lobe carcinoid tumor show that the atelectatic middle lobe is in a "tipped-up" con-figuration, a pattern that closely simulates anterior seg-mental disease of the right upper lobe.

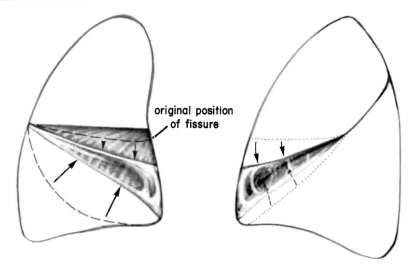

Figure 20–43. Patterns of Lobar Atelectasis: Right Middle Lobe. *See* the text for a description.

original position of fissure

most difficult on PA projection (Fig. 20–42). With progressive loss of volume, the minor fissure and the lower half of the major fissure approximate and are almost in contact when collapse is complete (Fig. 20–43). The resultant triangular "pancake" of tissue has its apex at the hilum and its base apparently contiguous to the parietal pleura over the anterolateral convexity of the thorax. As indicated previously, CT may demonstrate that this apparent contiguity with the parietal pleura is deceptive, since the visceral pleura can be retracted almost completely from the anterior chest wall (Fig. 20–42).

In PA projection there may be no discernible increase in opacity, the only evidence of disease being obliteration of part of the right cardiac border as a result of contiguity of the right atrium with the medial segment of the atelectatic lobe (the silhouette sign). The difficulty in detecting atelectasis in this projection is related to the obliquity of the atelectatic lobe in a superoinferior plane and the thickness of the collapsed lobe itself. The obliquity is variable and undoubtedly relates in large measure to fixation of the lobe at the hilum: in lateral projection, it may be almost horizontal in orientation and/or oblique, at times paralleling the plane of the major fissure. The horizontal and sharp oblique patterns of middle lobe atelectasis have been described as "tipped up" and "tipped down," respectively (*see* Fig. 20–42).[98] Severe atelectasis of the right middle lobe in the tipped-down position may result in an opacity that is insufficiently thick to cause a discernible radiographic shadow in PA projection. However, when the patient assumes a lordotic position or the middle lobe collapses in a tipped-up direction, the downwardly displaced minor fissure becomes oriented in a plane parallel to the x-ray beam on PA projection so that the atelectatic lobe appears as a thin, triangular ("sail-like") opacity; the apex of this opacity is directed away from the hilum, whereas the base abuts the right cardiac border.

The CT appearance of right middle lobe atelectasis is characteristic and consists of a broad triangular or trapezoidal opacity with the apex directed toward the hilum (Fig. 20–44). The anterior margin of the atelectatic lobe tends to retract towards the hilum, whereas the overinflated right upper lobe parenchyma intrudes anteromedially. As the lobe loses volume, the minor and major fissures move toward each other, the former downward and the latter upward and forward. The posterior border of the atelectatic middle lobe is usually defined because the major fissure is almost perpendicular to the plane of section. The interface between the right middle and upper lobes is often indistinct because of the dome-shaped contour of the minor fissure. In the tipped-up pattern, the atelectatic lobe tends to parallel the plane of the x-ray beam; consequently, the atelectasis is usually identified as a broad opacity on only one or two of the scans. By contrast, in the tipped-down position the triangular configuration is much smaller, but is identified over a span of 3 or 4 cm. In both patterns of atelectasis, contiguity with a portion or all of the cardiac silhouette is usually maintained (although unusual configurations of these more typical patterns may result from pleural adhesions).[99]

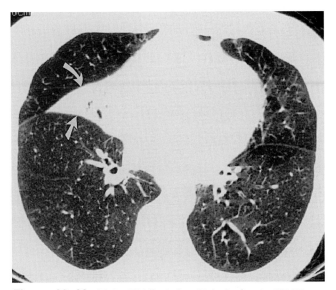

Figure 20–44. Right Middle Lobe Atelectasis. An HRCT scan demonstrates anterior displacement of the right major fissure *(straight arrow)* and posterior displacement of the minor fissure *(curved arrow).* Patent bronchi can be seen within the atelectatic lobe. The patient was a 72-year-old woman with recurrent right middle lobe atelectasis secondary to bronchiectasis.

Lower Lobes

The configuration adopted by the lower lobes in the presence of atelectasis is modified by the fulcrum-like effect exerted on the lung by the hilum and pulmonary ligament,[100] the fissures approximating in such a manner that the upper half of the major fissure swings downward and the lower half backward (Fig. 20–45; *see* also Fig. 20–29, page 536). This displacement is best appreciated in lateral projection when the lobe is only partly atelectatic and the major fissure is tangential to the x-ray beam and thus visible as a well-defined interface. During its downward displacement, the upper half of the fissure usually becomes clearly evident in PA projection as a well-defined interface extending obliquely downward and laterally from the region of the hilum (Fig. 20–45).[101, 102]

As atelectasis progresses, the lobe moves posteromedially to occupy a position in the posterior costophrenic gutter and medial costovertebral angle. Since the flat surface of the triangular "pancake" lies against the mediastinum, the thickness of tissue traversed by the x-ray beam in lateral projection may be insufficient to cast a shadow; indeed, when atelectasis is severe, the only abnormal feature may be a subtle increase in opacity of the lower thoracic vertebrae (Fig. 20–46) (normally, the vertebrae become relatively more radiolucent from above downward). The "mediastinal wedge" (consisting of the bronchoarterial bundle and adjacent parenchyma) may be apparent as a narrow triangular band of increased opacity extending downward and posteriorly from the hilum. Provided that exposure factors ensure

adequate penetration of the heart, the atelectatic lobe should be plainly visible in frontal projection as a diminutive triangular or round opacity in the costovertebral angle.[100] As noted previously, the interlobar artery is not identifiable because of obscuration by surrounding airless lung; therefore, a localized convex bulge in the expected location of the interlobar artery should suggest an underlying mass.

The variable appearance of lower lobe atelectasis is thought to be the result of the different forms that the pulmonary ligament may assume. When the ligament is complete, the lung is tethered to the mediastinum and hemidiaphragm so that the atelectatic lobe maintains a close relationship to both, which accounts for the triangular configuration. On the other hand, when the ligament is incomplete, the base of the lobe is not adherent to the hemidiaphragm and consequently the shape that the atelectatic lobe assumes depends primarily on the mediastinal attachment; as a result, the lobe assumes a more rounded configuration.[100]

On CT, atelectatic lower lobes can be seen to lose volume in a posteromedial direction and to subsequently pull the major fissure down (*see* Figs. 20–22 and 20–29). The lateral portion of the major fissure demonstrates a greater degree of mobility because the medial aspect is fixed to the mediastinum by the hilar structures and the pulmonary ligament (Fig. 20–46).

Combined Lobar Atelectasis

Since involvement of the two lobes of the left lung results in total pulmonary collapse, atelectasis of two lobes

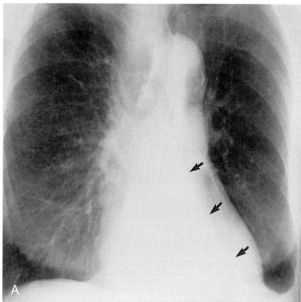

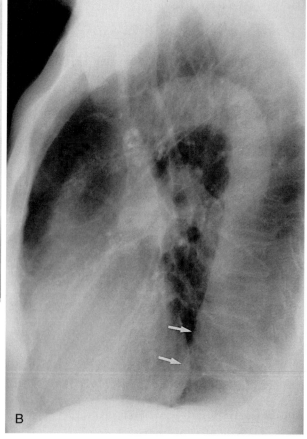

Figure 20–45. Left Lower Lobe Atelectasis. A posteroanterior chest radiograph *(A)* demonstrates caudad and medial shift of the left major interlobar fissure *(arrow)*. Also note the caudad displacement of the left hilum, compensatory overinflation of the left upper lobe and right lung, and shift of the mediastinum. A lateral radiograph *(B)* reveals posterior displacement of the interlobar fissure. The atelectatic left lower lobe is associated with increased opacity in the paravertebral region. A small left pleural effusion is also evident. The patient was a 74-year-old man with left lower lobe atelectasis as a result of a mucous plug.

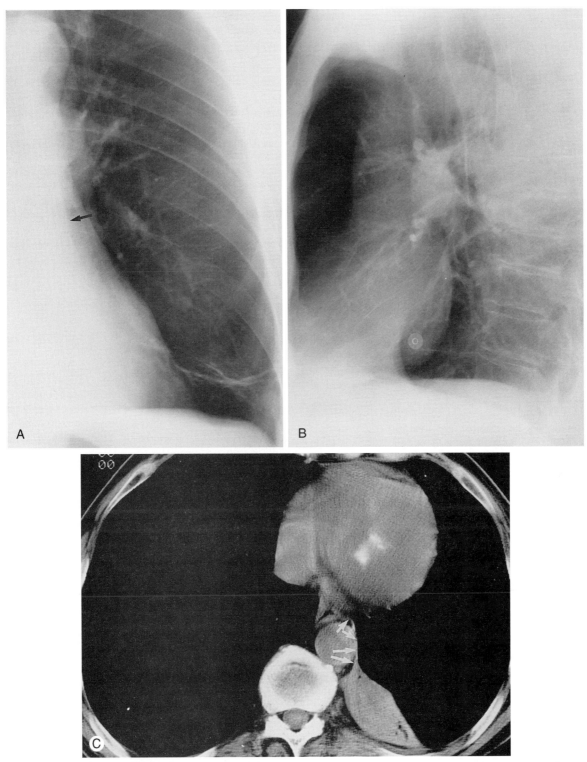

Figure 20–46. Left Lower Lobe Atelectasis. A view of the left side of the chest from a posteroanterior (PA) radiograph *(A)* reveals a caudad shift of the left interlobar fissure *(arrow)*. The inferior portion of the interlobar fissure is not visualized. On the lateral radiograph *(B)*, the atelectatic left lower lobe results in a subtle increase in opacity in the paravertebral region. A CT scan *(C)* demonstrates the atelectatic lobe to be displaced medially and tethered *(arrows)* by the inferior pulmonary ligament. The oblique orientation of the major fissure accounts for the lack of a clearly defined interface on the PA and lateral radiographs.

simultaneously produces a distinctive radiologic pattern only in the right lung.

Combined Right Middle and Lower Lobe Atelectasis

Combined atelectasis of the right middle and lower lobes results from obstruction of the bronchus intermedius.[103] On a PA radiograph, an atelectatic right lower lobe obscures the right hemidiaphragm whereas an atelectatic right middle lobe obscures the right heart border (Fig. 20–47). The major and minor fissures are displaced downward and backward so that the opacity occupies the posteroinferior portion of the hemithorax. The opacity may possess an upper surface that is concave or convex upward.[81]

Combined atelectasis of the right middle and lower lobes may be confused with isolated atelectasis of the right lower lobe on the PA radiograph and with right subpulmonic effusion on the lateral radiograph.[81, 82] The presence of increased opacity extending to the right costophrenic angle favors the diagnosis of combined atelectasis rather than atelectasis limited to the right lower lobe.[81] Visualization of the right minor fissure should suggest a diagnosis of isolated atelectasis of the right lower lobe. On the lateral view, the upper border of a subpulmonic effusion usually has a flat surface and appears to terminate at the major fissure anteriorly, whereas the upper border of combined atelectasis extends from front to back.[103] The most useful sign in differentiating subpulmonic effusion from atelectasis, however, is identification of the major and minor fissures in their normal locations.

On CT, the atelectatic right middle and lower lobes occupy the lower hemithorax and abut the right cardiac border medially and the right hemidiaphragm inferiorly (Fig. 20–47). The right major fissure borders the lateral margin of the atelectatic lobes, and the minor fissure borders the anteromedial margin.[89, 103]

Combined Right Upper and Middle Lobe Atelectasis

Because of the independent and sometimes remote origin of the lobar bronchi of these lobes, such an occurrence is uncommon. Separate etiologies or a single etiology operating at two anatomic locations must be invoked to explain coincidental involvement; it has been described most commonly with mucous plugs and primary bronchogenic carcinoma and, less commonly, with carcinoid tumors, metastatic tumors, and inflammatory processes.[89, 95, 103, 104]

The radiographic findings of combined atelectasis of the right upper and middle lobes are similar to those of left upper lobe atelectasis (Fig. 20–48). On the PA radiograph, it appears as an opacity that obscures the outline of the mediastinum and fades laterally.[103] Cephalad and lateral displacement as well as rotation of the hilar vessels may be apparent and is usually associated with obscuration of the silhouettes of the ascending aorta and right atrium. On the lateral radiograph, the major fissure can be seen to be displaced anteriorly (Fig. 20–48). The major fissure may be straight, convex anteriorly, or convex posteriorly.[103]

On CT, there is anterior displacement of the major fissure, with the hyperinflated lower lobe filling most of the right hemithorax.[103] The atelectatic lobes cause a wedge-shaped area of soft tissue attenuation that abuts the chest wall anteriorly and the ascending aorta and right heart border medially.[103]

Combined Right Upper and Lower Lobe Atelectasis

Combined atelectasis of the right upper and lower lobes is rare. It may result from mucous plugs occurring simultaneously in the bronchi of the right upper and lower lobes. We have also seen an example in a patient with bronchioloalveolar carcinoma without any CT or bronchoscopic evidence of bronchial obstruction (Fig. 20–49).[103]

The radiologic and CT findings of combined atelectasis of the right upper and lower lobes are similar to those of isolated atelectasis of either lobe. Upper lobe atelectasis is associated with elevation of the minor fissure, whereas lower lobe atelectasis leads to downward and medial deviation of the major fissure. On CT, the minor fissure is higher than normal because of the right upper lobe atelectasis and more posterior than normal because of the right lower lobe atelectasis.[103] The middle lobe is overinflated.

Segmental Atelectasis

Segmental atelectasis usually results from bronchial obstruction and is associated with obstructive pneumonitis. Thus, a homogeneous opacity that conforms to the anatomic distribution of a bronchopulmonary segment and in which no air bronchogram is identifiable should immediately alert the physician to the presence of an obstructing endobronchial lesion associated with obstructive pneumonitis and atelectasis (Fig. 20–50). As might be anticipated, the opacity resulting from segmental obstructive pneumonitis depends not only on the original volume of lung parenchyma affected but also on the volume of inflammatory tissue that has replaced it. Thus, the shadow can vary from a large conical opacity in which there is very little loss of volume to little more than a broad linear opacity in which atelectasis has predominated.

Linear (Platelike) Atelectasis

Few would dispute the statement that of all pathologic linear opacities observed on chest radiographs, the most common are those that tend to occur in the lung bases and that for many years have been called *platelike atelectasis* (discoid atelectasis, plate atelectasis, Fleischner lines). Because they are visualized as linear opacities, we believe that the term *linear atelectasis* is the most appropriate. First described in 1936,[105] these opacities are of unit density and range from 1 to 3 mm in thickness and 4 to 10 cm in length; they are situated in the mid and lower lung zones, most commonly the latter (Fig. 20–51). Although usually oriented in a roughly horizontal plane, they may be obliquely oriented depending on the zone of lung affected; in the midlung zones particularly, they may be angled more than 45 degrees to the horizontal. They may be single or multiple, unilateral or bilateral (Fig. 20–52).

The anatomic basis of linear atelectasis was elucidated in a detailed radiologic/pathologic correlative study of 10

Text continued on page 559

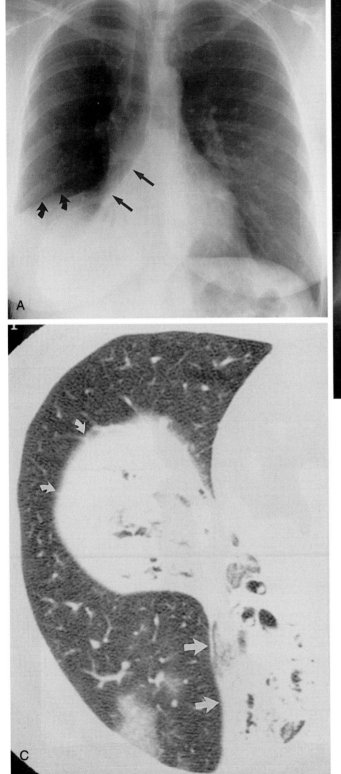

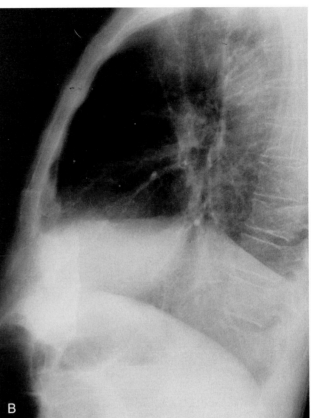

Figure 20–47. Combined Atelectasis of the Middle and Lower Lobes. A posteroanterior chest radiograph *(A)* reveals caudad displacement of the right major *(straight arrows)* and minor *(curved arrows)* fissures. Caudad displacement of the right hilum and overinflation of the right upper lobe are also evident. The silhouette of the right atrium is obscured by the atelectatic middle lobe. A lateral view *(B)* reveals increased opacity throughout the right lower lung zone with obscuration of the right hemidiaphragm. The upper border of the opacity is outlined anteriorly by the minor fissure and posteriorly by the major fissure. An HRCT scan *(C)* demonstrates major *(straight arrows)* and minor *(curved arrows)* interlobar fissures bordering the posterior and anterior margins, respectively, of the atelectatic lobes. A focal area of consolidation is present in the overinflated right upper lobe. The patient was a 29-year-old woman with a carcinoid tumor obstructing the bronchus intermedius. (From Lee KS, et al: Am J Roentgenol 163:43, 1994, with permission.)

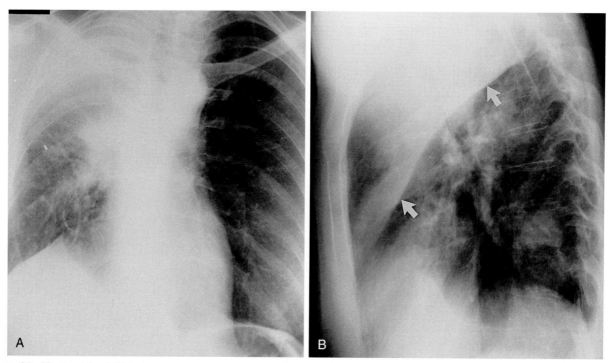

Figure 20–48. Combined Right Upper and Middle Lobe Atelectasis. A posteroanterior chest radiograph *(A)* reveals opacification of the right upper half of the chest with cephalad displacement of the right hilum and obscuration of the right heart border. Also note the right juxtaphrenic peak caused by tethering of the inferior accessory fissure. A lateral view *(B)* shows marked anterior and cephalad displacement of the major fissure *(arrows)*. Elevation of the right hemidiaphragm and a small right pleural effusion are also evident. The patient was a 51-year-old woman with obstruction of the right middle and upper lobe bronchi by small cell carcinoma.

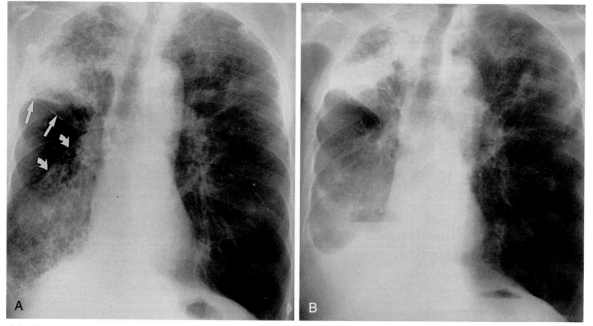

Figure 20–49. Combined Right Upper Lobe and Right Lower Lobe Atelectasis. A posteroanterior chest radiograph *(A)* reveals opacification of the right upper and lower lobes with mild elevation of the right minor fissure *(straight arrows)* and caudad and medial displacement of the major fissure *(curved arrows)*. There is compensatory overinflation of the right middle lobe. A posteroanterior chest radiograph obtained 2 weeks later *(B)* reveals further volume loss of the upper lobe. A right pleural effusion and a loculated hydropneumothorax related to recent open-lung biopsy are also evident. The patient had no evidence of bronchial obstruction at CT or bronchoscopy. A diagnosis of bronchioloalveolar carcinoma was made at open-lung biopsy.

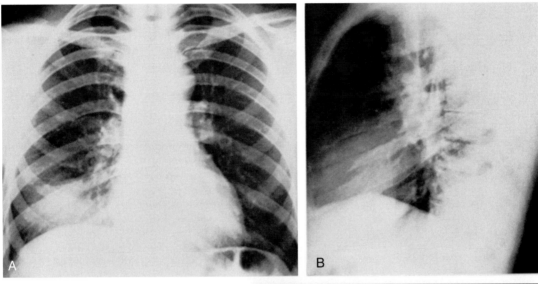

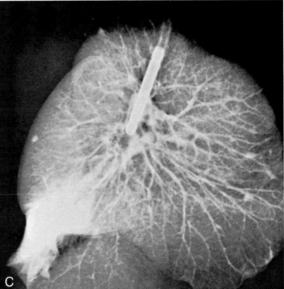

Figure 20–50. Segmental Atelectasis and Consolidation, Posterior Basal Segment, Right Lower Lobe. Posteroanterior *(A)* and lateral *(B)* radiographs reveal a homogeneous opacity localized to the posterior bronchopulmonary segment of the right lower lobe; no air bronchogram is present. The process is both consolidative and atelectatic, the latter evidenced by posterior displacement of the major fissure. A lateral radiograph of the resected lung *(C)* shows the precise segmental nature of the disease; as a result of preoperative chemotherapy, the bronchial obstruction had been partly relieved, so the operative specimen shows a well-defined air bronchogram. Squamous cell carcinoma of the posterior basal bronchus was diagnosed.

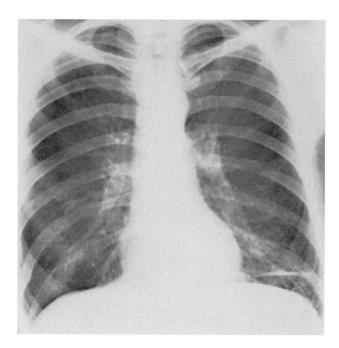

Figure 20–51. Linear Atelectasis. A posteroanterior radiograph reveals a line shadow measuring 3 mm in width and 9 cm in length situated in a plane just above the left hemidiaphragm and roughly horizontal in position; the left hemidiaphragm is slightly elevated. The shadow was present 2 days after laparotomy; it had disappeared 4 days later.

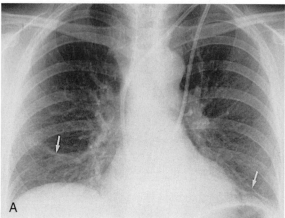

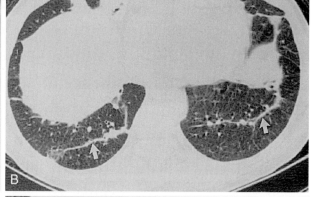

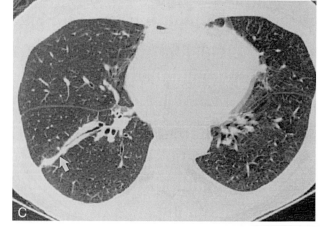

Figure 20–52. Linear Atelectasis. An anteroposterior chest radiograph *(A)* reveals linear opacities *(arrows)* in both lower lobes. HRCT scans *(B* and *C)* demonstrate several linear opacities in the lower lobes *(arrows)*. These opacities extend to the pleura, are associated with patent bronchi, and do not respect segmental boundaries. The patient was a 51-year-old woman undergoing chemotherapy for acute leukemia. The abnormalities resolved spontaneously and are consistent with linear (platelike) atelectasis.

patients in whom a linear opacity was present on their last antemortem radiograph and who subsequently underwent autopsy.[106] In all 10 patients, the linear areas of atelectasis extended to the pleural surface and were associated with invagination of the overlying pleura. All 10 revealed pathologic foci of subpleural parenchymal collapse associated with invagination of the adjacent pleura. The atelectasis was either deep to an incomplete fissure or extended to pre-existing pleural clefts; in either case, the surface of the lung

appeared folded in at the site of atelectasis. This frequent association with congenital pleural clefts, indentations, scars, and incomplete fissures suggested to the investigators that linear atelectasis develops preferentially at sites of pre-existing pleural invagination. The bronchi supplying the areas of atelectasis were not obstructed. Of considerable interest was the observation that in 9 of the 10 patients, prominent interlobular septa were observed either within or bordering the linear atelectasis, a finding that may in part explain the

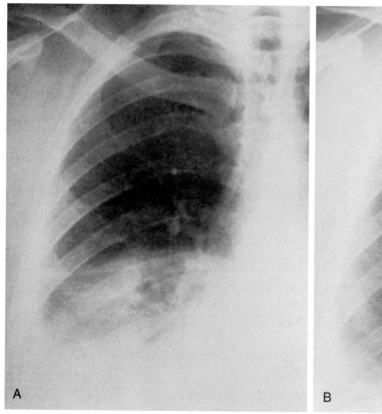

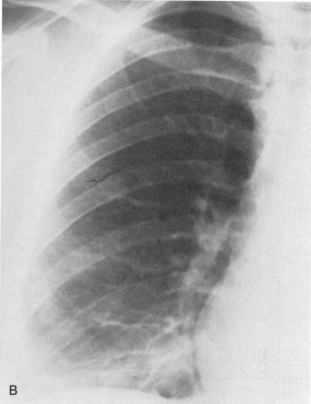

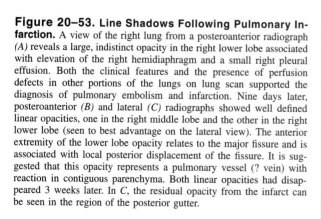

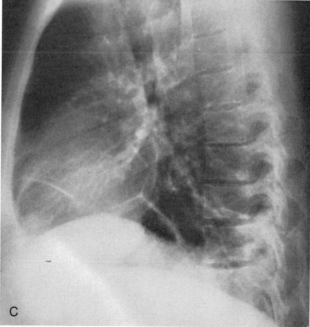

Figure 20–53. Line Shadows Following Pulmonary Infarction. A view of the right lung from a posteroanterior radiograph *(A)* reveals a large, indistinct opacity in the right lower lobe associated with elevation of the right hemidiaphragm and a small right pleural effusion. Both the clinical features and the presence of perfusion defects in other portions of the lungs on lung scan supported the diagnosis of pulmonary embolism and infarction. Nine days later, posteroanterior *(B)* and lateral *(C)* radiographs showed well defined linear opacities, one in the right middle lobe and the other in the right lower lobe (seen to best advantage on the lateral view). The anterior extremity of the lower lobe opacity relates to the major fissure and is associated with local posterior displacement of the fissure. It is suggested that this opacity represents a pulmonary vessel (? vein) with reaction in contiguous parenchyma. Both linear opacities had disappeared 3 weeks later. In *C*, the residual opacity from the infarct can be seen in the region of the posterior gutter.

absence of collateral ventilation in preventing the atelectasis. The linear opacities were caused by atelectasis alone in 6 patients, atelectasis associated with edema in 3, and atelectasis combined with "alveolitis" in 1.[106]

The pathogenesis of linear atelectasis is probably related to several mechanisms. The opacities are almost invariably associated with conditions that diminish diaphragmatic excursion, such as intra-abdominal surgery or inflammatory disease. Such conditions may promote atelectasis by several means, including: (1) restriction of diaphragmatic excursion leading to decreased ventilation of the lungs, especially in the bases; (2) inhibition of coughing by the pain and the discomfort that it engenders, which results in the accumulation of bronchial secretions in the dependent portions of the lungs and obstruction of small airways; (3) stagnation of secretions and the development of pneumonia, which leads to obstruction of channels of collateral ventilation by inflammatory exudate; and (4) reduction in surfactant production resulting from diminished perfusion secondary to decreased ventilation.

The postoperative clinical setting just described is also commonly complicated by pulmonary thromboembolism (Fig. 20–53). We therefore believe that the presence of linear opacities on a chest radiographs should alert the referring physician or surgeon to the possibility of thromboembolic disease despite the fact that in many of these cases the radiographic opacity represents atelectasis unassociated with vascular abnormality.

REFERENCES

1. Glossary of terms for thoracic radiology: Recommendations of the Nomenclature Committee of the Fleischner Society. Am J Roentgenol 143:509, 1984.
2. Coulter WW Jr: Experimental massive pulmonary collapse. Dis Chest 18:146, 1950.
3. Lansing AM: Radiological changes in pulmonary atelectasis. Arch Surg 90:52, 1965.
4. Rahn H: The role of N_2 gas in various biological processes, with particular reference to the lung. Harvey Lect 55:173, 1960.
5. Stein LA, McLoud TC, Vidal JJ, et al: Acute lobar collapse in canine lungs. Invest Radiol 11:518, 1976.
6. Henry WJ, Miscall L: Rapidly reversible atelectasis due to change in position. J Thorac Cardiovasc Surg 41:686, 1961.
7. Brown BStJ, Ma H, Dunbar JS, et al: Foreign bodies in the tracheobronchial tree in childhood. J Can Assoc Radiol 14:158, 1963.
8. Culiner MM, Reich SB: Collateral ventilation and localized emphysema. Am J Roentgenol 85:246, 1961.
9. Burke M, Fraser R: Obstructive pneumonitis: A pathologic and pathogenetic reappraisal. Radiology 166:699, 1988.
10. Dornhorst AC, Pierce JW: Pulmonary collapse and consolidation: The role of collapse in the production of lung field shadows and the significance of segments in inflammatory lung disease. J Fac Radiol 5:276, 1954.
11. Nelson SW: Large pneumothorax and associated massive collapse of the homolateral lung due to intrabronchial obstruction: A case report. Radiology 68:411, 1957.
12. Reed JC: Chest Radiology: Plain Film Patterns and Differential Diagnoses. 3rd ed. St. Louis, Mosby–Year Book, 1991, pp 167–193.
13. Freundlich IM: Atelectasis. In Freundlich IM, Bragg DG, (eds): A Radiologic Approach to Diseases of the Chest. Baltimore, Williams & Wilkins, 1992, pp 60–71.
14. Aberle DR, Gamsu G, Ray CS, et al: Asbestos-related pleural and parenchymal fibrosis: Detection with high-resolution CT. Radiology 166:729, 1988.
15. Gamsu G, Aberle DR, Lynch D: Computed tomography in the diagnosis of asbestos-related thoracic disease. J Thorac Imaging 4:61, 1989.
16. Bergin CJ, Castellino RA, Blank N, et al: Specificity of high-resolution CT findings in pulmonary asbestosis: Do patients scanned for other indications have similar findings? Am J Roentgenol 163:551, 1994.
17. Yoshimura H, Hatakeyama M, Otsuji H, et al: Pulmonary asbestosis: CT study of curvilinear shadow. Radiology 158:653, 1986.
18. Primack SL, Remy-Jardin M, Remy J, et al: High-resolution CT of the lung: Pitfalls in the diagnosis of infiltrative lung disease. Am J Roentgenol 167:413, 1996.
19. Verschakelen JA, Van Fraeyenhoven L, Laureys G, et al: Differences in CT density between dependent and nondependent portions of the lung: Influence of lung volume. Am J Roentgenol 161:713, 1993.
20. West JB: Regional differences in the lung. Chest 74:426, 1978.
21. Forgacs P: Gravitation stress in lung disease. Br J Dis Chest 68:1, 1974.
22. Morimoto S, Takeuchi N, Imanaka H, et al: Gravity-dependent atelectasis: Radiologic, physiologic, and pathologic correlation in rabbits on high-frequency oscillation ventilation. Invest Radiol 24:522, 1989.
23. Tomiyama N, Takeuchi N, Imanaka H, et al: Mechanism of gravity-dependent atelectasis: Analysis by nonradioactive xenon-enhanced dynamic computed tomography. Invest Radiol 28:633, 1993.
24. Woodring JH, Reed JC: Types and mechanisms of pulmonary atelectasis. J Thorac Imaging 11:92, 1996.
25. Strandberg A, Tokics L, Brismar B, et al: Atelectasis during anaesthesia and in the postoperative period. Acta Anaesthesiol Scand 30:154, 1986.
26. Klingstedt C, Hedenstierna G, Lundquist H, et al: The influence of body position and differential ventilation on lung dimensions and atelectasis formation in anaesthetized man. Acta Anaesthesiol Scand 34:315, 1990.
27. Bendixen HH, Hedley-Whyte J, Chir B, et al: Impaired oxygenation in surgical patients during general anesthesia with controlled ventilation: A concept of atelectasis. N Engl J Med 269:991, 1963.
28. Diament ML, Palmer KNV: Venous/arterial pulmonary shunting as the principal cause of postoperative hypoxaemia. Lancet 1:15, 1967.
29. Gamsu G, Singer MM, Vincent HH, et al: Postoperative impairment of mucous transport in the lung. Am Rev Respir Dis 114:673, 1976.
30. Remy-Jardin M, Remy J, Boulenguez C, et al: Morphologic effects of cigarette smoking on airways and pulmonary parenchyma in healthy adult volunteers: CT evaluation and correlation with pulmonary function tests. Radiology 186:107, 1993.
31. Schneider HJ, Felson B, Gonzalez LL: Rounded atelectasis. Am J Roentgenol 134:225, 1980.
32. Cho S-R, Henry DA, Beachley MC, et al: Round (helical) atelectasis. Br J Radiol 54:643, 1981.
33. Hayashi K, Kohzaki S, Uetani M, et al: Rounded atelectasis with emphasis on its wide spectrum. Nippon Acta Radiol 53:1020, 1993.
34. Batra P, Brown K, Hayashi K, et al: Rounded atelectasis. J Thorac Imaging 11:187, 1996.
35. Lee KS, Ahn JM, Im JG, Müller NL: Lobar atelectasis: Typical and atypical radiographic and CT findings. Postgrad Radiol 15:203, 1995.
36. Hillerdal G: Rounded atelectasis: Clinical experience with 74 patients. Chest 95:836, 1989.
37. Hanke R, Kretzschmar R: Round atelectasis. Semin Roentgenol 15:174, 1980.
38. Menzies R, Fraser R: Round atelectasis. Pathologic and pathogenetic features. Am J Surg Pathol 11:674, 1987.
39. Doyle TC, Lawler GA: CT features of rounded atelectasis of the lung. Am J Roentgenol 143:225, 1984.
40. McHugh K, Blaquiere RM: CT features of rounded atelectasis. Am J Roentgenol 153:257, 1989.
41. Carvalho PM, Carr DH: Computed tomography of folded lung. Clin Radiol 41:86, 1990.
42. Hilgenberg AD, Mark EJ: Case records of the Massachusetts General Hospital. N Engl J Med 308:1466, 1983.
43. Verschakelen JA, Demaerel P, Coolen J, et al: Rounded atelectasis of the lung: MR appearance. Am J Roentgenol 152:965, 1989.
44. Greyson-Fleg RT: Lung biopsy in rounded atelectasis (letter). Am J Roentgenol 144:1316, 1985.
45. Stancato-Pasik A, Mendelson DS, Marom Z: Rounded atelectasis caused by histoplasmosis. Am J Roentgenol 155:275, 1990.
46. Hanke R, Kretzschmar R: Round atelectasis. Semin Roentgenol 15:174, 1980.
47. Menzies R, Fraser R: Round atelectasis: Pathologic and pathogenetic features. Am J Surg Pathol 11:674, 1987.
48. Silverman SP, Marino PL: Unusual case of enlarging pulmonary mass. Chest 91:457, 1987.
49. Smith LS, Schillaci RF: Rounded atelectasis due to acute effusion: Spontaneous resolution. Chest 85:830, 1984.
50. Geremia G, Mintzer RA: An unusual case of rounded atelectasis. Chest 86:485, 1984.
51. Naidich DP, McCauley DI, Khouri NF, et al: Computed tomography of lobar collapse: I. Endobronchial obstruction. J Comput Assist Tomogr 7:745, 1983.
52. Sutnick AI, Soloff LA: Atelectasis with pneumonia: A pathophysiologic study. Ann Intern Med 60:39, 1964.
53. Sutnick AI, Soloff LA: Surface tension reducing activity in the normal and atelectatic human lung. Am J Med 35:31, 1963.
54. Putman CE, Loke J, Matthay RA, et al: Radiographic manifestations of smoke inhalation. Am J Roentgenol 129:865, 1977.
55. Iannuzzi M, Petty TL: The diagnosis, pathogenesis, and treatment of adult respiratory distress syndrome. J Thorac Imaging 1:1, 1986.
56. Ikezoe J, Takashima S, Morimoto S, et al: CT appearance of acute radiation-induced injury in the lung. Am J Roentgenol 150:765, 1988.
57. Davis SD, Yankelevitz DF, Henschke CI: Radiation effects on the lung: Clinical features, pathology, and imaging findings. Am J Roentgenol 159:1157, 1992.
58. Ikezoe J, Morimoto S, Takashima S, et al: Acute radiation-induced pulmonary injury: Computed tomography evaluation. Semin Ultrasound CT MR 11:409, 1990.
59. Byhardt RW, Abrams R, Almagro U: The association of adult respiratory distress syndrome (ARDS) with thoracic irradiation (RT). Int J Radiat Oncol Biol Phys 15:1441, 1988.
60. Kerr IH, Simon G, Sutton GC: The value of the plain radiograph in acute massive pulmonary embolism. Br J Radiol 44:751, 1971.
61. Benjamin JJ, Cascade PN, Rubenfire M, et al: Left lower lobe atelectasis and consolidation following cardiac surgery: The effect of topical cooling on the phrenic nerve. Radiology 142:11, 1982.
62. Wilcox P, Baile EM, Hards J, et al: Phrenic nerve function and its relationship to atelectasis after coronary artery bypass surgery. Chest 93:693, 1988.
63. Wheeler WE, Rubis LJ, Jones CW, et al: Etiology and prevention of topical cardiac hypothermia-induced phrenic nerve injury and left lower lobe atelectasis during cardiac surgery. Chest 88:680, 1985.
64. Westcott JL, Cole SR: Traction bronchiectasis in end-stage pulmonary fibrosis. Radiology 161:665, 1986.
65. Felson B: Chest Roentgenology. Philadelphia, WB Saunders, 1973.
66. Cranz HJ, Pribam HFW: The pulmonary vessels in the diagnosis of lobar collapse. Am J Roentgenol 94:665, 1965.
67. Lodin H: Mediastinal herniation and displacement studied by transversal tomography. Acta Radiol 48:337, 1957.
68. Lubert M, Krause GR: Total unilateral pulmonary collapse: A study of the roentgen appearance in the lateral view. Radiology 67:175, 1956.
69. Whalen JP, Lane EJ Jr: Bronchial rearrangements in pulmonary collapse as seen on the lateral radiograph. Radiology 93:285, 1969.
70. Lane EJ Jr, Whalen JP: A new sign of left atrial enlargement: Posterior displacement of the left bronchial tree. Radiology 93:279, 1969.
71. Simon G: Principles of Chest X-ray Diagnosis. 3rd ed. London, Butterworth, 1971.
72. Rohlfing BM: The shifting granuloma: An internal marker of atelectasis. Radiology 123:283, 1977.
73. Robbins LL, Hale CH: Roentgen appearance of lobar and segmental collapse of the lung: Preliminary report. Radiology 44:107, 1945.
74. Robbins LL, Hale CH, Merrill OE: Roentgen appearance of lobar and segmental collapse of the lung: Technic of examination. Radiology 44:471, 1945.
75. Robbins LL, Hale CH: The roentgen appearance of lobar and segmental collapse of the lung: II. The normal chest as it pertains to collapse. Radiology 44:543, 1945.
76. Robbins LL, Hale CH: The roentgen appearance of lobar and segmental collapse

of the lung: III. Collapse of an entire lung or the major part thereof. Radiology 45:23, 1945.

77. Robbins LL, Hale CH: The roentgen appearance of lobar and segmental collapse of the lung: IV. Collapse of the lower lobes. Radiology 45:120, 1945.

78. Robbins LL, Hale CH: The roentgen appearance of lobar and segmental collapse of the lung: V. Collapse of the right middle lobe. Radiology 45:260, 1945.

79. Robbins LL, Hale CH: The roentgen appearance of lobar and segmental collapse of the lung: VI. Collapse of the upper lobes. Radiology 45:347, 1945.

80. Krause GR, Lubert M: Cross anatomico-spatial changes occurring in lobar collapse: A demonstration by means of three-dimensional plastic models. Am J Roentgenol 79:258, 1958.

81. Lubert M, Krause GR: Further observations on lobar collapse. Radiol Clin North Am 1:331, 1963.

82. Proto AV, Tocino I: Radiographic manifestations of lobar collapse. Semin Roentgenol 15:117, 1980.

83. Woodring JH, Reed JC: Radiographic manifestations of lobar atelectasis. J Thorac Imaging 11:109, 1996.

84. Naidich DP, McCauley DI, Khouri NF: Computed tomography of lobar collapse: II. Collapse in the absence of endobronchial obstruction. J Comput Assist Tomogr 7:758, 1983.

85. Raasch BN, Heitzman ER, Carsty EW, et al: A computed tomographic study of bronchopulmonary collapse. Radiographics 4:195, 1985.

86. Lubert M, Krause GR: Patterns of lobar collapse as observed radiographically. Radiology 56:165, 1951.

87. Reinig JW, Ross P: Computed tomography appearance of Golden's "S" sign. J Computed Tomogr 8:219, 1984.

88. Shepard JO, Dedrick CG, Spizarni DL, et al: Technical note: Dynamic incremental computed tomography of the pulmonary hila using a flow-rate injector. J Comput Assist Tomogr 10:369, 1986.

89. Khoury MB, Godwin JD, Halvorsen RA Jr, et al: CT of obstructive lobar collapse. Invest Radiol 20:708, 1985.

90. Proto AV: Conventional chest radiographs: Anatomic understanding of newer observations. Radiology 183:593, 1992.

91. Proto AV, Moser ES: Upper lobe volume loss: Divergent and parallel patterns of vascular reorientation. Radiographics 7:875, 1987.

92. Kattan KR, Eyler WR, Felson B: The juxtaphrenic peak in upper lobe collapse. Semin Roentgenol 15:187, 1980.

93. Cameron DC: The juxtaphrenic peak (Katten's [sic] sign) is produced by rotation of an inferior accessory fissure. Australas Radiol 37:332, 1993.

94. Davis SD, Yankelevitz DF, Wand A, et al: Juxtaphrenic peak in upper and middle lobe volume loss: Assessment with CT. Radiology 198:143, 1996.

95. Golden R: The effect of bronchostenosis upon the roentgen-ray shadows in carcinoma of the bronchus. Am J Roentgenol Radiat Ther 13:21, 1925.

96. Zdansky E: Bemerkung zur atelektatischen Retraktion des linken Oberlappens. [Atelectatic retraction of the left upper lobe.] Fortschr Roentgenstr 100:725, 1964.

97. Webber M, Davies P: The Luftsichel: An old sign in upper lobe collapse. Clin Radiol 32:271, 1981.

98. Raasch BN, Heitzman ER, Carsky EW, et al: A computed tomographic study of bronchopulmonary collapse. Radiographics 4:195, 1984.

99. Naidich DP, McCauley DI, Khouri NF, et al: Computed tomography of lobar collapse: I. Endobronchial obstruction. J Comput Assist Tomogr 7:745, 1983.

100. Cohen BA, Rabinowitz JG, Mendleson DS: The pulmonary ligament. Radiol Clin North Am 22:659, 1984.

101. Fisher MS: Significance of a visible major fissure on the frontal chest radiograph. Am J Roentgenol 137:577, 1981.

102. Friedman PJ: Radiology of the superior segment of the lower lobe: A regional perspective, introducing the B⁶ bronchus sign. Radiology 144:15, 1982.

103. Lee KS, Logan PM, Primack SL, Müller NL: Combined lobar atelectasis of the right lung: Imaging findings. Am J Roentgenol 163:43, 1994.

104. LeRoux BT: Opacities of the middle and upper lobes in combination. Thorax 26:55, 1971.

105. Fleischner F: Uber das Wesen der basalan horizontalen Schattenstreifen im Lungenfeld. Wien Arch Inn Med 28:461, 1936.

106. Westcott JL, Cole S: Plate atelectasis. Radiology 155:1, 1985.

CHAPTER 21

Pleural Abnormalities

RADIOLOGIC SIGNS OF PLEURAL EFFUSION, 563
   General Considerations, 563
   Typical Configuration of Free Pleural Fluid, 564
   Subpulmonary Effusion, 566
   Distribution of Pleural Effusion in the Supine
     Patient, 572
   Computed Tomographic Manifestations of Pleural
     Effusion, 572
   Atypical Distribution of Free Pleural Fluid, 577
   Loculation of Pleural Fluid, 579
RADIOLOGIC SIGNS OF PLEURAL THICKENING, 582
   Pleural Fibrosis, 582
   Pleural Calcification or Ossification, 583
   Pleural Neoplasms, 584
RADIOLOGIC SIGNS OF PNEUMOTHORAX, 587
   Pneumothorax in the Upright Patient, 587
   Pneumothorax in the Supine Patient, 587
   Hydropneumothorax, 589
   Tension Pneumothorax and Hydrothorax, 589

RADIOLOGIC SIGNS OF PLEURAL EFFUSION

General Considerations

Despite the usually effective action of oncotic and hydrostatic forces and lymphatic drainage, small amounts of pleural fluid can accumulate and be identified radiographically in a significant percentage of healthy individuals. For example, in one study in which a modification of the lateral decubitus projection was used with a horizontal x-ray beam, pleural fluid was identified in 15 (12%) of 120 healthy adults.[1] The authors performed thoracentesis on some of these subjects and concluded that the smallest amount of fluid identifiable by their technique was 3 to 5 ml; the largest amount found was 15 ml. In another investigation of 300 healthy adults using a similar technique, conclusive radiographic evidence of fluid was found in 12 individuals (4%) and suggestive evidence in an additional 19 (6%).[2] The thickness of the fluid layer ranged from 1 to 10 mm and averaged 5 mm. Fluid was identified unilaterally in some subjects and bilaterally in others; in some, the amount varied from one examination to another. It was often observed during repeated examinations of the same subjects, suggesting that a fluid accumulation was an inherent feature of the individual's physiologic status.[2] It is of interest that in 92 women studied a few days postpartum, convincing evidence of pleural fluid was found in 21 (23%) and the possibility of fluid in another 14 (15%).[2] A study based on the injection of 5-ml increments of saline or plasma into the pleural space in cadavers showed that even 5 ml of fluid was clearly visible on radiographs exposed in the unmodified lateral decubitus position.[3] These studies are of obvious practical importance insofar as they indicate that small amounts of pleural fluid may be demonstrated radiologically in the absence of disease; thus, they point out a potential source of error in the diagnosis of clinically significant pleural effusion.

Conventional posteroanterior (PA) and lateral chest radiographs are considerably less sensitive than the lateral decubitus view in the detection of pleural effusions: Accumulation of at least 175 ml of fluid is necessary to cause detectable blunting of the lateral costophrenic sulcus on the PA radiograph.[4] Moreover, although the majority of effusions greater than 200 ml are evident on the PA radiograph, up to 500 ml of fluid may be present without any blunting of the costophrenic sulcus on this view (Fig. 21–1).[4] In the supine patient, pleural fluid layers posteriorly making it difficult to detect even moderately large effusions, particularly if they are bilateral;[5] for example, in one prospective study, anteroposterior supine chest radiographs had a sensitivity of only 67% and a specificity of 70% in the detection of pleural effusions, compared with lateral decubitus radiographs.[6] Because the posterior costophrenic sulcus is deeper than the lateral sulcus, small effusions are more readily detected on a lateral radiograph than on the frontal view.[7, 8]

Ultrasonography, computed tomography (CT), and magnetic resonance (MR) imaging allow more effective detection of small or loculated effusions and distinction of effusions from pleural thickening.[5] Because of its ready availability and ability for bedside imaging, ultrasonography has become a particularly important imaging modality, not only in determining the presence of pleural fluid but also as a guide to therapeutic and diagnostic aspiration (*see* Fig. 21–1).[9, 10] The technique also has been shown to be superior to lateral decubitus radiography in the quantification of pleural fluid.[11] In one study of 51 patients who underwent complete aspiration of the pleural fluid in the sitting position, effusion was quantified on ultrasonography by measuring the maximal perpendicular distance between the posterior surface of the lung and the posterior chest wall during maximal inspiration with the patient supine;[11] an effusion with a maximal width of 20 mm had a mean volume of 380 $\pm$ 130 ml, whereas that with 40 mm had a mean volume of 1,000 $\pm$ 330 ml. Patients with no evidence of fluid on ultrasound had a mean of 5 $\pm$ 15 ml (range, 0 to 90 ml) of fluid.

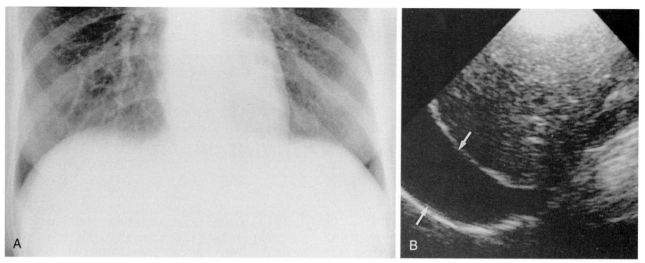

Figure 21–1. Right Pleural Effusion. A view of the lower thorax from an anteroposterior chest radiograph *(A)* is essentially normal except for questionable minimal blunting of the right costophrenic sulcus. Ultrasound *(B)* reveals right pleural effusion *(arrows).*

Typical Configuration of Free Pleural Fluid

As discussed previously, the negative pressure normally present within the pleural cavity is the result of the difference between the elastic forces of the chest wall and the lungs: Lung tissue has a natural tendency to recoil but is prevented from doing so beyond a certain point by the tendency of the chest wall to expand outward with an equal and opposite force. Thus, in the normal state, intimate contact between the visceral and parietal pleural surfaces is maintained. When liquid or gas is introduced into the pleural space, the lung can recoil inward toward its fixed moorings at the hilum. the amount of retraction depending on the quantity of liquid or gas introduced. The site of retraction depends on the nature of the material introduced into the pleural space, as illustrated by the different effects of hydrothorax and pneumothorax. In the upright subject, the effect of gravity causes gas to rise and liquid to fall in the pleural space; therefore with pneumothorax, the upper portions of the lung retract, and with hydrothorax, the lower portions retract.

As it loses volume, the lung tends to maintain its original shape, a characteristic known as *form elasticity*:[12] When a complete pneumothorax is present or the thoracic cage is opened at thoracotomy or autopsy, the shape of the lung in its completely collapsed state is a miniature replica of its shape in the fully distended form. The same feature is seen with pleural effusion, except that the collapse may be local rather than general.

These two influences—gravity and elastic recoil—are the major forces that control the configuration of free fluid in the pleural space.[7, 12] Fluid gravitates first to the base of the hemithorax, where it comes to lie between the inferior surface of the lung and the hemidiaphragm.[7, 13] When the amount of fluid in the subpulmonary pleural space reaches a certain level, it spills over into the posterior costophrenic sulcus, which is thus obliterated in lateral radiographic projection. The normally sharp costophrenic angle is replaced by a shallow, homogeneous shadow whose upper surface is meniscus shaped. This radiographic appearance—pseudo-diaphragmatic elevation as a result of subpulmonic localization, with or without obliteration of the posterior costo-

phrenic sulcus—may be unaccompanied by other discernible evidence of pleural effusion; because the evidence supplied by blunting of the posterior costophrenic sinus sulcus may be subtle, lateral radiographs of excellent technical quality are necessary.

As a result of pleural capillarity, fluid in the posterior costophrenic sulcus extends up the adjacent pleural space, resulting in increased width of the pleural line along the posterior thoracic wall. With increasing amounts of fluid, the radiologic signs develop in predictable fashion: obliteration of the lateral and eventually anterior costophrenic sulci and greater extension of fluid up the chest wall in a mantle distribution.

On the basis of this description, it is easy to picture the typical radiographic appearance of pleural effusion. Consider the hypothetical situation of a large pleural effusion (Fig. 21–2): Such an amount of fluid completely obscures the hemidiaphragm and the costophrenic sulci and extends upward around the anterior, lateral, and posterior thoracic wall. Because the mediastinal surface of the lung is not free to move owing to its fixation at the hilum and pulmonary ligament, less fluid accumulates along this surface than around the convexity. Thus, in PA projection, the radiopacity of the effusion is high laterally and curves gently downward and medially with a smooth meniscus-shaped upper border, terminating along the midcardiac border. In lateral projection, because the fluid has ascended along the anterior and posterior thoracic wall to roughly an equal extent, the upper surface of the fluid density is semicircular, being high anteriorly and posteriorly and curving smoothly downward to its lowest point in the midaxillary line. Comparison of the maximal height of the fluid density in the PA and lateral projections shows that this height is identical posteriorly, laterally, and anteriorly (*see* Fig. 21–2)—that is, the top of the fluid accumulation is *horizontal*; the meniscus shape is caused by the fact that the layer of fluid is of insufficient depth to cast a discernible shadow when viewed *en face*.[12, 14]

A distinctive radiologic manifestation of pleural effusion develops when the major interlobar fissures are incomplete medially.[15] In this circumstance, fluid that extends into the major fissures creates a sharp concave line, medial to

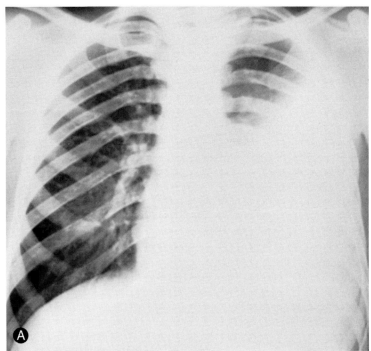

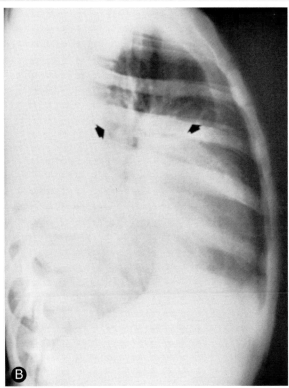

Figure 21–2. Large Pleural Effusion: Typical Arrangement. Posteroanterior *(A)* and lateral *(B)* radiographs exposed in the upright position demonstrate uniform opacification of the lower two thirds of the left hemithorax. The upper level of the fluid is meniscus shaped in both posteroanterior and lateral projections *(arrows on B)*. Note that only the right hemidiaphragm is visualized in the lateral projection, the left being obscured by fluid (the silhouette sign).

which the lung is of normal or almost normal lucency and peripheral to which the presence of fluid results in a uniform opacity (Fig. 21–3).

The effects on the thorax as a whole of the accumulation of large amounts of fluid in the pleural space depend largely on the condition of the ipsilateral lung. Even small amounts of fluid produce compression atelectasis of contiguous lung, in much the same manner as when air is present in pneumothorax. When the effusion is massive, collapse of the ipsilateral lung may be almost complete. Despite severe

atelectasis, however, the overall effect of a massive effusion almost invariably is that of a space-occupying process, with enlargement of the ipsilateral hemithorax, displacement of the mediastinum to the contralateral side, and depression and flattening of the ipsilateral hemidiaphragm; in fact, the hemidiaphragm may be depressed so severely as to be concave superiorly (Fig. 21–4).[16]

When one hemithorax is totally opacified, appreciation of the balance of forces between the two sides of the thorax is of obvious importance. If the mediastinum shows no

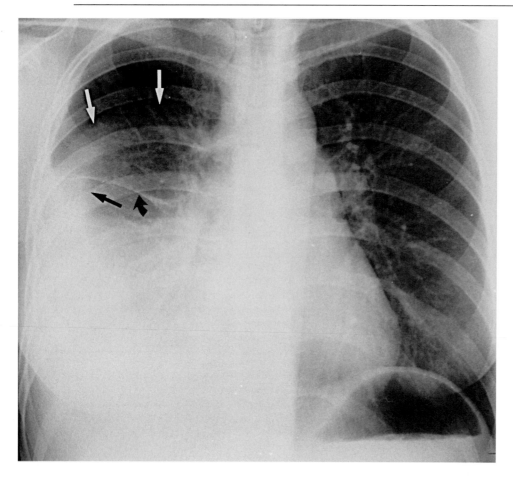

Figure 21–3. Pleural Effusion Extending into the Major Fissure. A posteroanterior chest radiograph in a 25-year-old woman demonstrates a moderate-sized right pleural effusion. Note the characteristic curvilinear opacity *(straight arrows)* due to fluid extension into the major fissure. Fluid has also extended into the minor fissure *(curved arrow).* The effusion was caused by primary tuberculosis.

shift and the hemidiaphragm is only slightly depressed, the presence of disease within the ipsilateral lung can be inferred with reasonable confidence (Fig. 21–5). The possibility of an obstructing endobronchial lesion (e.g., pulmonary carcinoma with pleural metastases) is obvious; in fact, total opacification of one hemithorax without mediastinal or diaphragmatic displacement is highly suggestive of this diagnosis or extensive mesothelioma.

Subpulmonary Effusion

As indicated previously, the first place fluid accumulates in the erect patient is between the inferior surface of the lower lobe and the diaphragm; in effect, the lung "floats" on a layer of fluid (Fig. 21–6). If the amount of fluid is small, it may occupy only this position without spilling over into the dependent costophrenic sulci (Fig. 21–7). In this circumstance, the configuration of the hemidiaphragm is maintained, and the appearance on PA and lateral radiographs suggests no more than slight elevation of that hemidiaphragm.[17] Bearing in mind the variation in the height of the diaphragm in normal subjects, it is readily apparent that such small accumulations of fluid in the pleural space can be easily missed on the PA and lateral radiographs. Only if the observer is alert to the possibility of a small pleural effusion can the diagnosis be confirmed by radiography in the lateral decubitus position with a horizontal x-ray beam. A subpulmonary location of fluid is *usual* in the normal pleural space[2, 7] (although it would be reasonable to consider subpulmonary accumulation of a large amount of fluid as atypical).

Subpulmonary effusion causes a configuration in the erect subject that closely simulates diaphragmatic elevation (thus the designation *pseudodiaphragmatic contour*) *(see* Fig. 21–6). It may be unilateral or bilateral, the former more commonly on the right.[18] Several signs are helpful in the detection of subpulmonic effusions on PA and lateral radiographs of the erect patient.

1. In PA projection (Fig. 21–8), the peak of the pseudodiaphragmatic configuration is lateral to that of the normal hemidiaphragm, being situated near the junction of the middle and lateral thirds rather than near the center, and slopes down sharply toward the lateral costophrenic sulcus.[7, 12, 19]

2. On the left side, the pseudodiaphragmatic contour is separated farther than normal from the gastric air bubble (Fig. 21–9), and effusion should be suspected when there is a greater than 2-cm distance between the two.[2] Care is needed to detect interposition of the spleen or the left lobe of the liver and to exclude the presence of gross ascites, which can occasionally simulate subpulmonic effusion.[20]

3. On lateral projection (Fig. 21–10), a characteristic configuration is frequently seen anteriorly where the convex upper margin of the fluid meets the major fissure. In these cases, the contour anterior to the fissure is flattened, this portion of the pseudodiaphragmatic contour descending abruptly to the anterior costophrenic sulcus.[7, 12]

4. On lateral projection, a small amount of fluid is

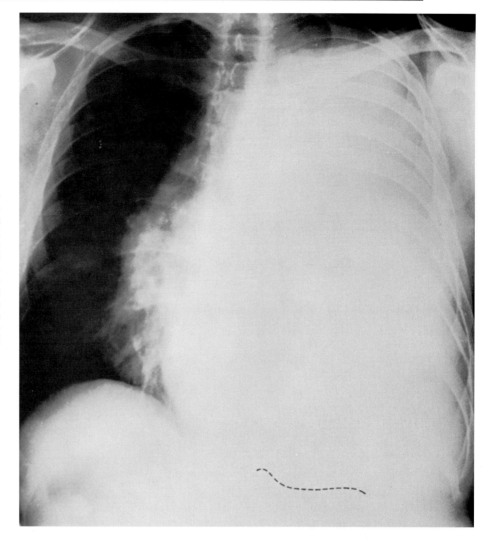

Figure 21–4. Massive Effusion, Underlying Lung Normal. A posteroanterior radiograph reveals total opacification of the left hemithorax by a massive pleural effusion. The mediastinum is displaced to the right. The stomach bubble *(dotted line)* is displaced inferiorly, and its upper surface is concave rather than convex, suggesting that the hemidiaphragm possesses the same contour. A faint air bronchogram can be visualized through the fluid in the medial portion of the left lung; the underlying lung was normal. Metastatic pleural carcinoma from the maxillary antrum.

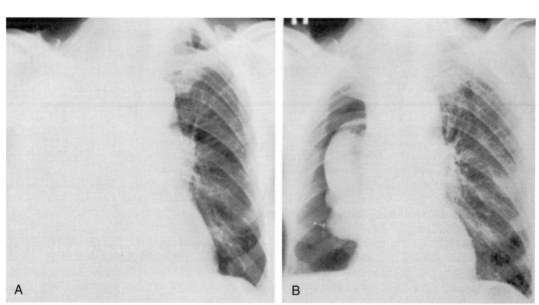

Figure 21–5. Massive Pleural Effusion Associated with Obstructive Atelectasis of the Underlying Lung. A posteroanterior radiograph *(A)* shows total opacification of the right hemithorax; in contrast with the situation in Figure 21–4, the mediastinum is central in position. After removal of almost all the fluid and replacement with an equal quantity of air (without air replacement, the patient became severely dyspneic), the right lung *(B)* can be seen to be totally collapsed and airless (with the exception of small quantities of air in the upper lobe). In such a situation, the absence of an air bronchogram constitutes absolute evidence of endobronchial obstruction. At thoracotomy, the intermediate bronchus was found to be compressed by enlarged lymph nodes replaced by adenocarcinoma.

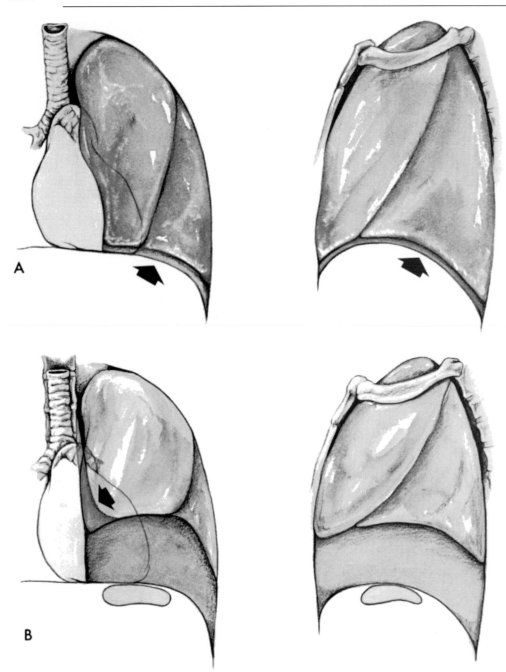

Figure 21–6. Subpulmonary Accumulation of Pleural Fluid. These drawings depict two degrees of subpulmonary effusion: (1) the situation in *A* is typical, in that it represents the *usual* anatomic location of small amounts of fluid (up to 500 ml); and (2) the amount of fluid is large in *B* (e.g., 1,500 ml), and the local subpulmonary accumulation is thus atypical. *See* text.

usually apparent in the lower end of the major fissure where it joins the infrapulmonary collection.

5. In PA projection, a thin, triangular opacity may be observed in the left paramediastinal zone, with its apex approximately halfway up the mediastinum and its base contiguous to the pseudodiaphragmatic contour inferiorly. This shadow—which represents mediastinal extension of the infrapulmonary fluid collection—was observed in 8 of 39 patients in one study;[18] because it is situated posteriorly, it obliterates or causes an apparent widening of the left paraspinal line.[18] It must not be mistaken for left lower lobe atelectasis, which it closely resembles. The ability to identify clearly the left interlobar artery permits ready distinction.

6. Pulmonary vessels, which are normally visible below the diaphragmatic contour, cannot be seen through the

pseudodiaphragmatic contour of a subpulmonic effusion.[21] Care should be taken to exclude underexposed radiographs, lower lobe consolidation, and ascites, which may cause similar findings.[7]

When a subpulmonic effusion is suspected, lateral decubitus radiography should be performed, both to confirm the diagnosis and to permit assessment of the quantity of fluid more accurately than is possible with the patient erect. Sonography can also be useful in identifying subpulmonic collections of fluid; if at all possible, the examination should be carried out in the erect rather than in the supine position because effusions clearly identifiable in the erect position may be missed on ultrasound performed with the patient supine.[22]

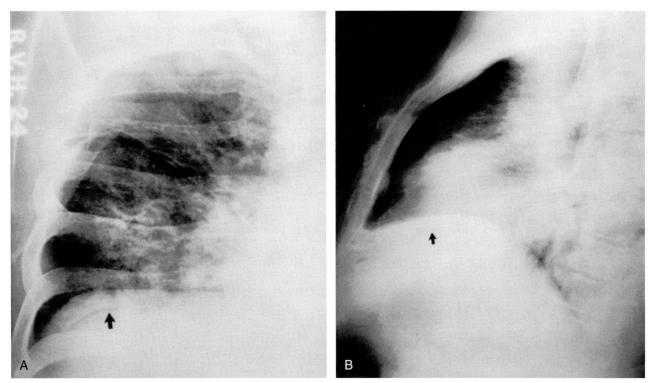

Figure 21–7. Subpulmonary Pleural Effusion Associated with Pneumoperitoneum. Views of the right hemithorax from posteroanterior *(A)* and lateral *(B)* radiographs (exposed in the erect position post mortem) demonstrate a thin line of air density *(arrow)* situated approximately 1 cm below the base of the right lung, roughly parallel to the right hemidiaphragm. Since this gas is situated within the peritoneal space, it outlines the undersurface of the right hemidiaphragm, indicating the presence of a layer of fluid approximately 1 cm in thickness between the diaphragm and the undersurface of the right lung. By multiplying the anteroposterior and lateral dimensions of the right hemidiaphragm by the thickness of fluid (1 cm), it was estimated that the amount of fluid in the pleural space was approximately 400 ml. At autopsy, the right pleural space was found to contain 450 ml. This study demonstrates the large quantity of fluid that may accumulate in an infrapulmonary location without producing convincing radiologic evidence of its presence.

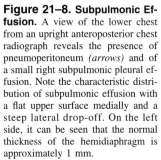

Figure 21–8. Subpulmonic Effusion. A view of the lower chest from an upright anteroposterior chest radiograph reveals the presence of pneumoperitoneum *(arrows)* and of a small right subpulmonic pleural effusion. Note the characteristic distribution of subpulmonic effusion with a flat upper surface medially and a steep lateral drop-off. On the left side, it can be seen that the normal thickness of the hemidiaphragm is approximately 1 mm.

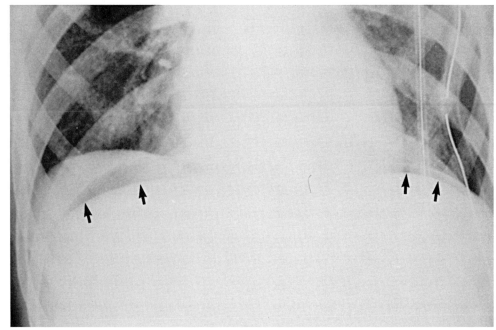

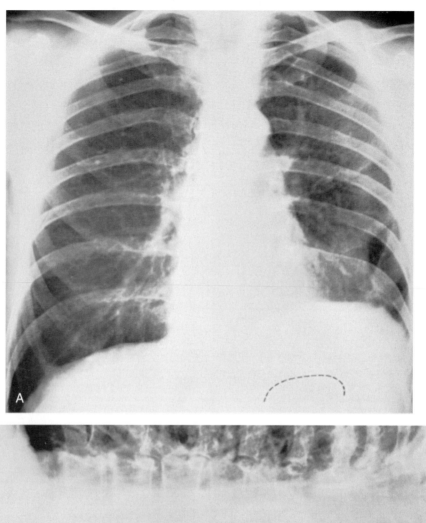

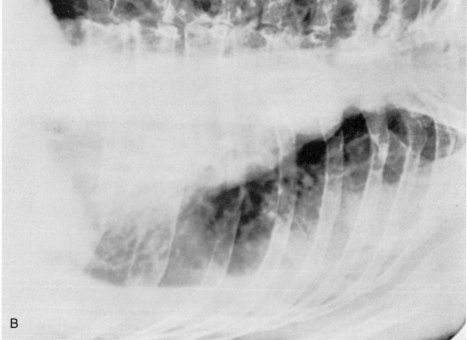

Figure 21–9. Subpulmonary Pleural Effusion. A posteroanterior radiograph exposed in the upright position *(A)* shows a high left pseudodiaphragm whose peak is more laterally situated than that of a normal hemidiaphragm. It is situated several centimeters from the stomach bubble *(dotted line).* The costophrenic sulcus is sharp. A radiograph exposed in the left lateral decubitus position with a horizontal x-ray beam *(B)* shows the fluid to have extended along the axillary lung zone. Following removal of approximately 1,000 ml of fluid, a posteroanterior radiograph in the erect position *(C)* shows normal apposition of the gastric air bubble to the left hemidiaphragm.

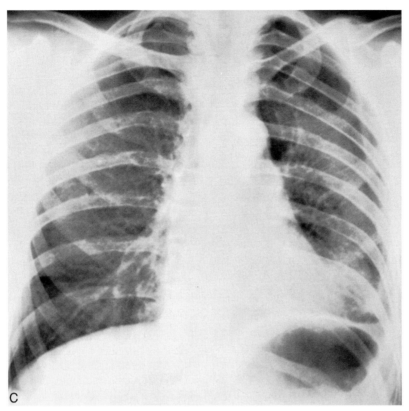

Figure 21–9 *Continued.*

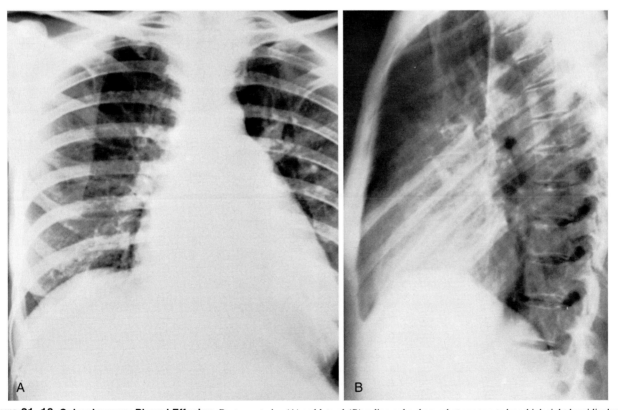

Figure 21–10. Subpulmonary Pleural Effusion. Posteroanterior *(A)* and lateral *(B)* radiographs show what appears to be a high right hemidiaphragm; both the lateral and the posterior costophrenic sulci are sharp, although minimal thickening of the pleural line immediately above the lateral sulcus suggests that the shadow may be caused by a subpulmonary effusion. This suspicion is heightened by the characteristic configuration of the shadow in lateral projection: Its anterior portion ascends abruptly and in almost a straight line to the region of the *major* fissure; a "dome" configuration is present posterior to this point. The major fissure is slightly thickened by fluid.

Distribution of Pleural Effusion in the Supine Patient

In the supine patient, free pleural fluid layers posteriorly and produces a hazy increase in opacity without obscuration of the bronchovascular markings.[2, 12] With small pleural effusions, the increase in opacity is limited to the lower lung zones; as the amount of fluid increases, there is progressive cephalad extension of the increased opacity until the entire hemithorax is involved (Fig. 21–11).[23] An apical fluid cap is seen on supine radiographs in approximately 50% of patients who have large effusions.[23] Occasionally, relatively small effusions also form apical caps,[7] presumably because the superior and lateral aspects of the apex can be the most dependent portion of the thorax tangential to the x-ray beam. Blunting of the lateral costophrenic sulcus (meniscus sign) in the supine position occurs when the amount of fluid is sufficient to fill the posterior hemithorax up to the level of the sulcus.[23] Other helpful signs in the diagnosis of pleural effusion on the supine radiograph include obscuration of the hemidiaphragm, apparent elevation of the hemidiaphragm, decreased visibility of the lower lobe vessels below the level of the apparent dome of the diaphragm, and thickening of the right minor fissure.[6, 23]

Compared with lateral decubitus radiographs, supine radiographs have a relatively low sensitivity and specificity in the diagnosis of pleural effusions.[6] In a prospective analysis of anteroposterior supine radiographs, pleural effusions were correctly identified on supine radiographs in 24 of 36 cases (sensitivity 67%) and correctly excluded in 18 of 26 cases (specificity 70%). The most helpful diagnostic findings were increased opacity of the hemithorax, blunting of the costophrenic angle, and obscuration of the hemidiaphragm.[6]

Computed Tomographic Manifestations of Pleural Effusion

Pleural effusions are characterized on CT by attenuation values between those of water (0 HU) and soft tissue (approximately 100 HU); therefore except when small,[24] effusions can usually be readily distinguished from pleural thickening or pleural masses (Fig. 21–12).[25] On CT of a supine patient, free pleural fluid first accumulates in the posterior pleural sulci. Because the lung tends to maintain its shape as it loses volume, the fluid has a concave or meniscoid anterior margin. As the effusion increases in size, fluid extends cephalad and anteriorly and may track into the major and right minor fissures.

Because of the dome-shaped curvature of the diaphragm and the cross-sectional imaging of CT, fluid collections in the posterior pleural sulci may cause an appearance resembling that of intra-abdominal fluid. The two can usually be readily distinguished by means of careful analysis of four signs.[5, 26]

1. Because the diaphragm has soft tissue attenuation similar to that of liver and spleen, it cannot be identified on CT where it abuts these viscera; however, its position can be inferred because it is located immediately lateral and cephalad to these structures (Fig. 21–13). The *diaphragm sign* refers to the different distribution of pleural effusion compared with that of intra-abdominal fluid in relation to the diaphragmatic dome: the lungs and pleura lie adjacent and peripheral to the convexity of the hemidiaphragm, whereas the abdominal structures and fluid lie adjacent and central to it (Fig. 21–14).[26, 27]

2. The *interface sign* refers to the different appearance

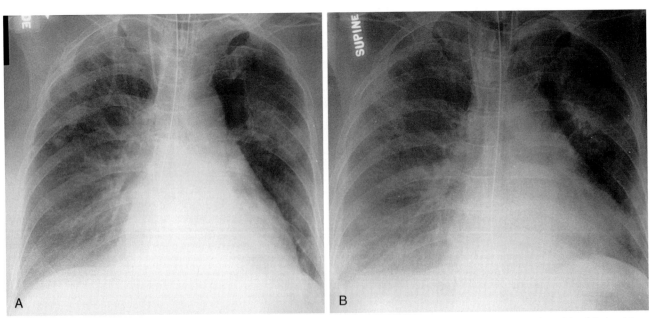

Figure 21–11. Pleural Effusion in the Supine Patient. An anteroposterior supine view *(A)* demonstrates hazy opacification of the right hemithorax. A supine view of the chest 24 hours later *(B)* demonstrates further increase in opacity of the right hemithorax, obscuration of the lateral border of the right hemidiaphragm, blunting of the right costophrenic sulcus, and fluid extending cephalad along the lateral chest wall. The patient was a 60-year-old woman who developed a large right pleural effusion following liver transplantation.

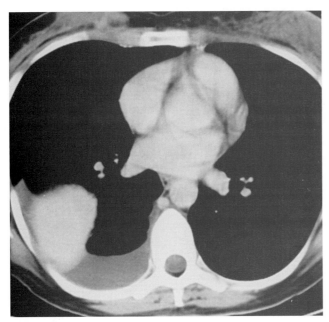

Figure 21–12. Pleural Effusion. Contrast-enhanced CT scan demonstrates a small right pleural effusion. The near water density of pleural fluid allows ready distinction from the pleural-based mass. The patient was a 35-year-old woman with right pleural effusion associated with a localized fibrous tumor of the pleura.

of the interface between fluid and the adjacent liver or spleen depending on whether the fluid is pleural or intra-abdominal in location. In the former situation, the interface between the fluid and the liver or spleen is ill-defined, presumably because the diaphragm is interposed between the fluid and these structures; by contrast, in ascites, it is sharply defined (Fig. 21–15).[26, 28]

3. The fluid in pleural effusion is interposed between the crus and the vertebral column and therefore tends to displace the diaphragmatic crus anteriorly (*displaced crus sign*) (Fig. 21–16).[26, 29] By contrast, intra-abdominal collections are situated anterior to the crus and therefore displace this structure posteriorly.

4. The bare area of the liver is that region of the right lobe that lacks peritoneal covering and is directly apposed to the posterior abdominal wall. As a consequence of this anatomic feature, ascites is prevented from extending behind the posteromedial surface of the right lobe of the liver; however, effusion in the posterior pleural sulcus frequently extends behind the liver at this level (the *bare area sign*) (Fig. 21–17).[27, 30]

Distinction of pleural effusions from intra-abdominal fluid collections requires careful assessment of all four signs. Used individually, any sign may be indeterminate or misleading;[26] however, in combination, the signs have a high degree of accuracy. In one review of 52 patients with pleural effusion, ascites, or both, four independent radiologists correctly identified the presence and location of all fluid collections when using all four signs.[26]

Occasionally, pleural effusion associated with left lower lobe atelectasis or inversion of the hemidiaphragm mimics intra-abdominal fluid.[5] Compressive atelectasis of the lower lobe associated with pleural effusion may result in a curvilinear band at the lung base, which may be confused with the hemidiaphragm (Fig. 21–18).[31] In patients with subsegmental basilar areas of atelectasis and subpulmonic effusion, the pleural fluid anterior to the atelectasis may cause a false impression of peritoneal fluid.[31] Correct diagnosis can usually be readily made by careful analysis of contiguous CT sections and by noting continuity of the areas of subsegmental atelectasis with the adjacent lung and the presence of gas within the atelectatic lung.[26, 31] Although pleural effusion is normally adjacent and peripheral to the hemidiaphragm, with inversion of this structure it is central and may thus mimic intraperitoneal fluid.[5, 27] Such diaphragmatic inversion is usu-

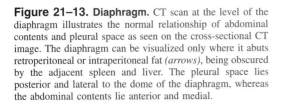

Figure 21–13. Diaphragm. CT scan at the level of the diaphragm illustrates the normal relationship of abdominal contents and pleural space as seen on the cross-sectional CT image. The diaphragm can be visualized only where it abuts retroperitoneal or intraperitoneal fat *(arrows)*, being obscured by the adjacent spleen and liver. The pleural space lies posterior and lateral to the dome of the diaphragm, whereas the abdominal contents lie anterior and medial.

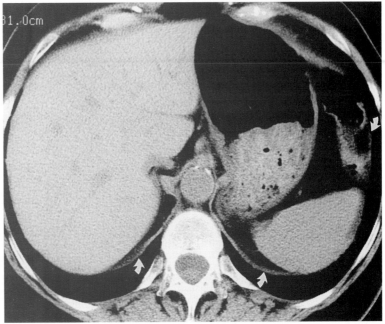

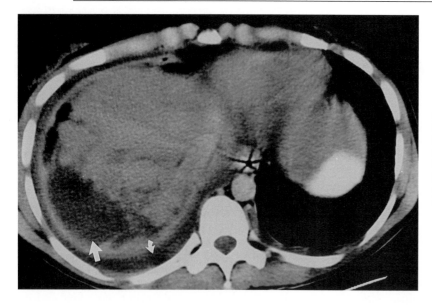

Figure 21–14. Diaphragm Sign. Contrast-enhanced CT scan in a 25-year-old woman with extensive liver injury due to a motor vehicle accident. Fluid outlines the right hemidiaphragm. Intra-abdominal fluid lies central to the right hemidiaphragm *(straight arrow)*, whereas pleural fluid lies posterior and peripheral *(curved arrow)*. Also noted is a small left pleural effusion. (From Müller NL: Imaging of the pleura. Radiology 186:297, 1993.)

ally the result of a large pleural effusion (Fig. 21–19); correct diagnosis can therefore be readily made by evaluation of contiguous CT sections.

Assessment of the attenuation of pleural fluid is of limited value in differentiating transudates, exudates, and chylous effusions.[5, 32] Although the presence of fat in chylothorax might be expected to produce attenuation values lower than those of water, the high-protein content usually causes attenuation values slightly greater; however, attenuation values as low as −17 HU are occasionally seen with chylous effusions.[33] Acute hemorrhage into the pleural space may be identified on CT as a result of increased attenuation of the pleural fluid (Fig. 21–20) or by layering of fluids with different CT attenuation, giving a fluid-fluid level.[34, 35] The

former manifestation is related to the high hemoglobin content of retracted clot or sedimented blood.[34]

Although the attenuation of pleural fluid is of limited value in distinguishing an exudate from a transudate, this distinction can often be suggested by measurement of pleural thickness or assessment of enhancement of the pleura after intravenous administration of contrast material:[36, 37] exudates are frequently associated with pleural thickening and enhancement, findings that are seldom identified in patients with transudates (Fig. 21–21).[36, 37] The enhancement is presumably related to the increased vascular supply of the inflamed pleura.[36, 38] In one study of 80 patients with 86 pleural effusions, 59 of the effusions were exudates, and 27 were transudates.[37] Thirty-six (61%) of the 59 exudates were associated with parietal pleural thickening (usually 2 to 4 mm); of these, 12 showed diffuse, smooth, parietal pleural

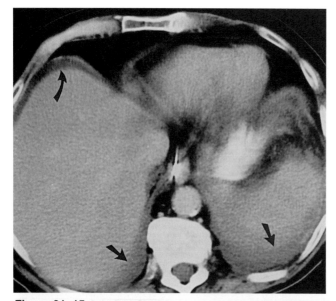

Figure 21–15. Interface Sign. Intravenous contrast–enhanced CT scan in a 64-year-old man reveals bilateral effusions and ascites due to pancreatitis. Note that the interface between the pleural effusion, liver, and spleen is ill-defined *(straight arrows)*, whereas the interface between ascites and liver *(curved arrow)* is well-defined. (From Müller NL: Imaging of the pleura. Radiology 186:297, 1993.)

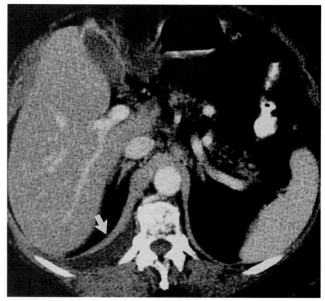

Figure 21–16. Displaced Crus Sign. CT scan in a 76-year-old woman demonstrates anterior and lateral displacement of the right crus *(arrow)* due to a small right pleural effusion.

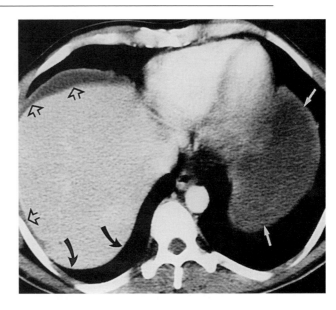

Figure 21–17. Bare Area Sign. CT scan in a 36-year-old man with ascites demonstrates sharp interface between the fluid and the liver (interface sign) *(open arrows)*. Also noted is ascites central to the left hemidiaphragm *(straight arrows)*. Ascites, however, is prevented from extending behind the posteromedial aspect of the right lobe of the liver (bare area) *(curved arrows)*.

thickening, 2 had diffuse, irregular thickening, and 22 had irregular or smooth focal thickening. Parietal pleural thickening was visible in all 10 empyemas but in only 10 (56%) of 18 parapneumonic exudates and in 11 (48%) of 23 malignant exudates. Only 1 of the 27 transudates showed parietal pleural thickening (specificity 96%).

In a second study, the parietal pleura was analyzed on CT in 35 patients with empyema, 30 patients with malignant effusion, and 20 patients with pleural transudates.[36] Of the patients with empyema, 86% had pleural thickening, 60% had thickening of the extrapleural subcostal tissues, and 35% had increased attenuation of the extrapleural fat. Enhancement of the parietal pleura was present in 96% of the 25 patients with empyema who underwent contrast-enhanced CT. These findings were not seen in any of the 20 patients

with transudates. Only 10% of patients with malignant pleural effusions who had not undergone sclerotherapy and who had no associated findings such as empyema showed evidence of pleural enhancement.[36] On the basis of the results of these two investigations, it seems reasonable to conclude that the presence of parietal pleural thickening at contrast-enhanced CT almost always indicates the presence of an exudate; the finding is particularly suggestive of empyema and is seen less commonly in exudates associated with malignancy.[37]

Increased attenuation and thickness of the extrapleural tissues on the undersurface of the ribs are also seen relatively commonly in patients with empyema and seldom in patients with malignant effusions or transudates (Fig. 21–22).[36, 37] In one investigation of 35 patients with empyema, 11 (31%)

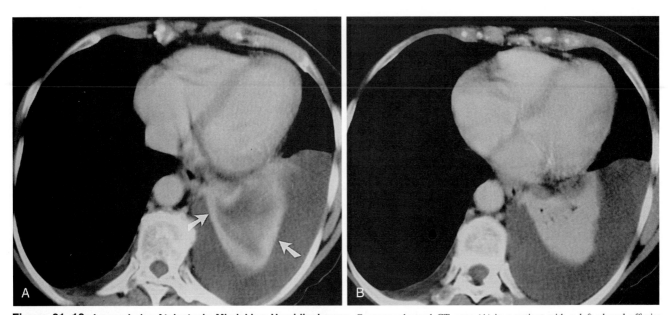

Figure 21–18. Lower Lobe Atelectasis Mimicking Hemidiaphragm. Contrast-enhanced CT scan *(A)* in a patient with a left pleural effusion demonstrates compressive atelectasis of the left lower lobe *(arrows)*. The configuration of the atelectatic lobe mimics the configuration of the dome of the left hemidiaphragm. The low attenuation centrally may therefore be confused with ascites. The correct diagnosis of pleural fluid anterior and posterior to the atelectatic lobe, however, can be easily made by identification of air within the atelectatic lobe on the contiguous cephalad image *(B)*.

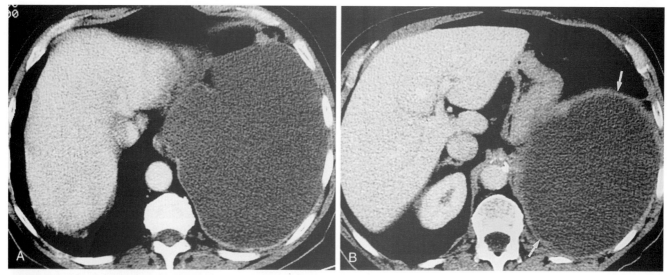

Figure 21–19. Large Pleural Effusion with Inversion of the Hemidiaphragm. Contrast-enhanced CT scan *(A)* demonstrates a large left pleural effusion. CT scan through the upper abdomen *(B)* reveals fluid central to the left hemidiaphragm *(straight arrows)* indicating the presence of inversion. Although at this single level the finding may be confused with intraperitoneal fluid, the correct diagnosis of a large pleural effusion with inversion of the diaphragm is readily made by assessment of contiguous cephalad sections. The patient was a 69-year-old man with a large malignant pleural effusion due to pulmonary carcinoma.

showed increased attenuation of the extrapleural tissues intermediate between that of fat and that of soft tissue.[36] With the exception of one patient who had a history of malignant effusion complicated by empyema, none of the patients with malignant exudates or with transudates showed increased thickness or attenuation of extrapleural subcostal tissues.[36] In this investigation, the thickness of the extrapleural subcostal tissues was also measured in the posterior subcostal area at least 5 cm lateral to the midline to avoid the variability of the paraspinal tissues. (The normal thickness of extrapleural tissues in this area is ≤ 2 mm.[39]) Sixty per cent of the patients with empyema showed extrapleural tissues 3 mm

thick or thicker in this area, compared to only 10% of patients with malignant effusion and 5% of patients with transudates.[36] In another study of 36 patients who had exudative effusions associated with parietal pleural thickening, 20 also showed thickening of the extrapleural soft tissues;[37] 8 were empyemas and 8 parapneumonic effusions. Only 1 of the 23 patients who had exudative effusions without parietal pleural thickening had thickening of the extrapleural fat or soft tissue.

Thickening of the visceral pleura is seen less commonly in association with effusion than thickening of the parietal pleura. In one study, it was seen in 13 (22%) of 59 patients

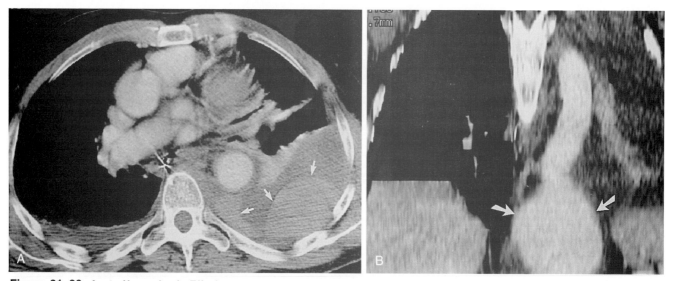

Figure 21–20. Acute Hemorrhagic Effusion. Contrast-enhanced CT scan *(A)* demonstrates a moderate-sized left pleural effusion with localized areas of increased attenuation *(arrows)* characteristic of acute hemorrhage into the pleural space. Note near water density of the right pleural effusion. Coronal reconstruction from spiral CT *(B)* reveals large focal aneurysm of the aorta *(arrows)*. The patient was a 77-year-old man with surgically proven acute hemorrhage into the pleural space from rupture of the low thoracic portion of the thoracoabdominal aneurysm.

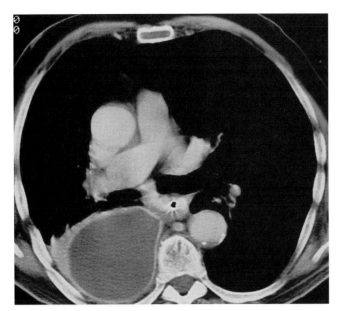

Figure 21–21. Empyema. Contrast-enhanced CT scan demonstrates right pleural fluid collection associated with enhancement and thickening of the parietal and visceral pleura and compressive atelectasis of the adjacent right lower lobe. The patient was an 82-year-old man with empyema following rupture of the esophagus.

with exudates resulting from parapneumonic effusion, empyema, or malignancy and in 1 (4%) of 27 patients with transudates.[37]

Administration of an intravenous bolus of contrast material is useful not only in helping to distinguish pleural exudates from transudates but also to distinguish pleural from parenchymal lung disease.[38, 40] The procedure allows direct demonstration of the blood vessels within the lung parenchyma, the most reliable finding in distinguishing pulmonary from pleural disease (Fig. 21–23).[40] This is particularly important in the presence of pulmonary parenchymal abnormalities, such as resorptive atelectasis or extensive consolidation.

Atypical Distribution of Free Pleural Fluid

The typical arrangement of fluid in the free pleural space (i.e., a pleural space without adhesions) requires that the underlying lung be free of disease and thus capable of preserving its shape even while recoiling from the chest wall—that is, able to maintain its *form elasticity.* An alteration in this recoiling tendency is the primary explanation for atypical configuration or distribution of pleural fluid (excluding the restriction of free movement occasioned by pleural adhesions and fibrosis). It has been suggested that pulmonary parenchymal disease, particularly atelectasis, modifies the retractility of the affected portion of the lung so that pleural fluid is attracted to it.[12, 41, 42] Support for this hypothesis is provided by a study in dogs in which lobar collapse was shown to be associated with a more negative pleural pressure around the collapsed lobe than around uncollapsed lobes.[43] Moreover, a radiographic investigation in dogs in which atelectasis of selected lobes was produced and fluid injected into the pleural space showed that when

lower lobes were collapsed, fluid tended to move to the area of maximal parenchymal distortion, where negative pleural pressure was greatest.[42] In the presence of upper lobe collapse, free pleural fluid tended to remain in its typical location in an infrapulmonary position.

Regardless of the mechanism by which fluid accumulates in atypical locations within the pleural space, there is little doubt that in the majority of cases it relates to underlying pulmonary disease. Thus, the major radiologic significance of an atypical location of pleural effusion is that it alerts the physician to the presence of both parenchymal and pleural disease. The radiographic appearance of atypical pleural fluid accumulation in disease affecting individual lobes has been described in detail.[2, 12]

Because radiography in other than the erect position can detect any change in distribution of *free* pleural fluid, examination in the supine or, preferably, lateral decubitus position can show displacement of the fluid over the posterior or lateral pleural space. Use of these procedures enables clarification of the nature of unusual patterns of effusion, such as an effusion simulating lower lobe consolidation. In addition, these procedures permit clearer identification and

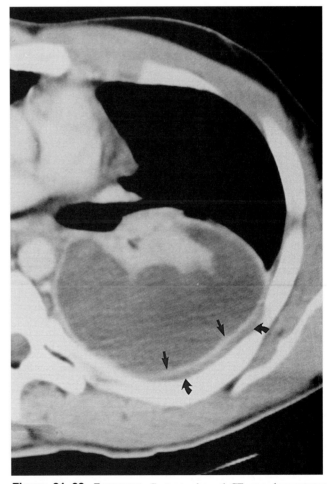

Figure 21–22. Empyema. Contrast-enhanced CT scan demonstrates left pleural effusion with associated enhancement and smooth thickening of the parietal pleura *(straight arrows)* and compressive atelectasis of the left lower lobe. Also note increased thickness and attenuation of the extrapleural tissues *(curved arrows)*, a finding highly suggestive of empyema. The patient was a 23-year-old man. Cultures from the left pleural fluid at needle aspiration and at surgical decortication grew *Streptococcus viridans.*

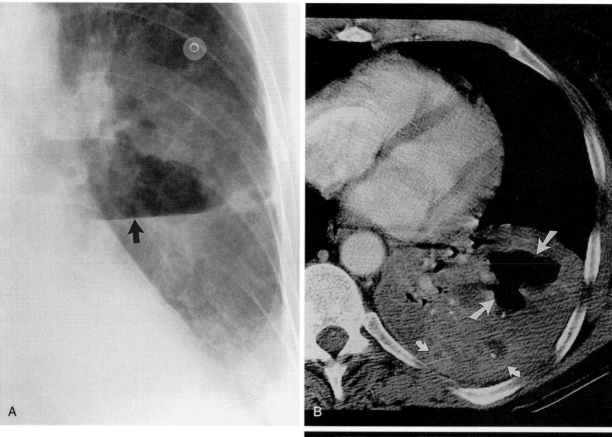

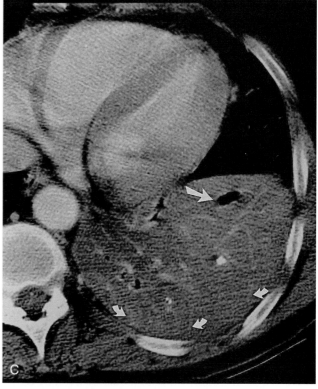

Figure 21–23. Distinction of Parenchymal from Pleural Disease. A view of the left chest from a posteroanterior radiograph *(A)* in a 59-year-old man demonstrates a large cavity with an air-fluid level *(black arrow)* in the left lower lobe. Increased opacity in the costophrenic sulcus is suggestive of a pleural effusion. Contrast-enhanced CT scans *(B and C)* demonstrate a large cavity *(straight arrows)* and dense consolidation. Contrast enhancement of the vessels *(curved arrows)* and pulmonary parenchyma allows confident diagnosis of consolidation and exclusion of pleural effusion. The patient was shown to have left lower lobe pneumonia and abscess formation due to gram-negative and anaerobic organisms.

more accurate assessment of the underlying parenchymal disease.

Loculation of Pleural Fluid

A loculated effusion may occur anywhere in the pleural space, either between the parietal and visceral pleura over the periphery of the lung or between visceral layers in the interlobar fissures. Loculation is caused by adhesions between contiguous pleural surfaces and therefore tends to occur during or after episodes of pleuritis, often associated with pyothorax or hemothorax. Over the convexity of the thorax, the loculated effusion appears as a smooth, sharply demarcated, homogeneous opacity protruding into the hemithorax and compressing contiguous lung (Fig. 21–24).

The precise location and nature of loculated collections of pleural fluid can be readily assessed using ultrasonography or CT. Ultrasonography not only allows assessment of the amount of fluid within a pleural pocket but also can be used as a guide to identify the optimal anatomic site to perform thoracentesis. CT scanning is particularly useful in differentiating pleural from pulmonary lesions;[44] when combined with intravenous injection of contrast medium, it allows accurate assessment of complex combined pulmonary and pleural disease[40] and distinction of empyema from a peripheral pulmonary abscess.[38, 45]

Empyemas usually have sharply defined margins delineated by the visceral and parietal pleura and are associated with displacement of vessels and bronchi.[38] Visualization of intravenous contrast-enhancing thickened visceral and parietal pleura surrounding the fluid (the *split-pleura sign*) allows confident distinction of loculated empyema from a peripheral lung abscess (*see* Fig. 21–24); for example, in one study, the sign was seen in 39 (68%) of 57 patients with empyema and in 0 of 10 patients with lung abscess.[38] In the same investigation, lung compression with displacement of bronchi and vessels was also seen on CT in 47% of empyemas and in none of the lung abscesses (Fig. 21–25).[38] Another helpful feature in distinguishing loculated empyema from a peripheral lung abscess is the shape of the fluid collection: in one study, 63% of empyemas and none of the lung abscesses were lenticular in shape.[38] However, a round collection may be seen in empyemas and lung abscesses. Findings that are not helpful in distinguishing empyema from lung abscesses include the angle of the collection with the chest wall, the presence or absence of air within the lesion, septation, multiple lesions, or free pleural fluid. Although CT allows confident distinction in the majority of cases, it is occasionally impossible to differentiate parenchymal from pleural fluid collections.[46, 47]

Interlobar loculated effusions are typically elliptical when viewed tangentially on the chest radiograph, and their extremities blend imperceptibly with the interlobar fissure (Fig. 21–26). In some conditions, particularly cardiac decompensation, the effusion may simulate a mass radiographically

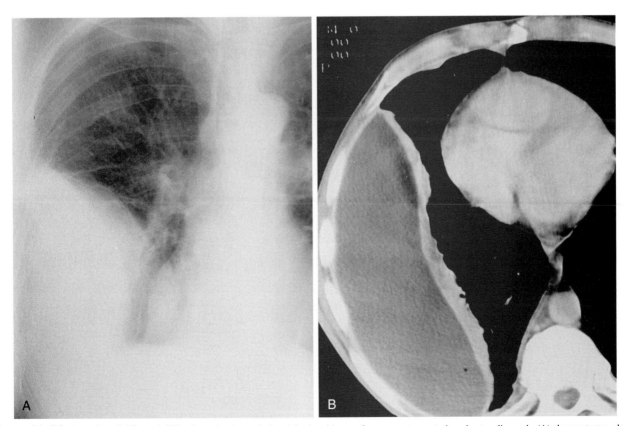

Figure 21–24. Loculated Pleural Effusion. A view of the right hemithorax from a posteroanterior chest radiograph *(A)* demonstrates sharply demarcated, homogeneous opacity having convex borders with the lung and displacing the adjacent parenchyma. Contrast-enhanced CT scan *(B)* reveals right pleural effusion associated with enhancement and thickening of the visceral and parietal pleura and compressive atelectasis of the adjacent lung. The findings are characteristic of a loculated empyema. Visualization of enhancing thickened visceral and parietal pleura surrounding pleural fluid is known as the *split-pleura* sign.

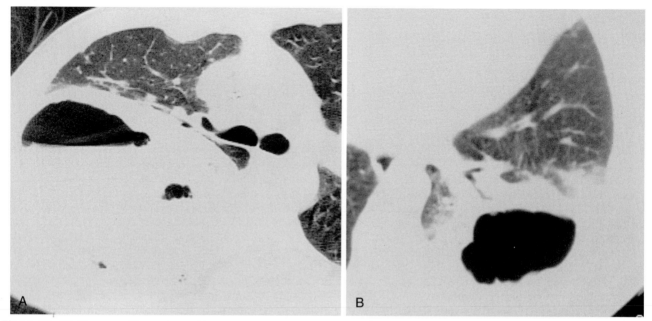

Figure 21–25. Empyema Versus Lung Abscess. CT scan in a 39-year-old man with empyema *(A)* reveals a fluid collection in the right hemithorax with associated air-fluid level. Note anterior displacement of the right main and upper lobe bronchi. Displacement of the parenchyma and bronchi is characteristic of pleural fluid collections. CT scan of a 53-year-old man with a lung abscess *(B)* demonstrates no displacement of the adjacent lung parenchyma, bronchi, or vessels. Focal areas of consolidation are present surrounding the left lower lobe abscess. (From Müller NL: Imaging of the pleura. Radiology 186:297, 1993.)

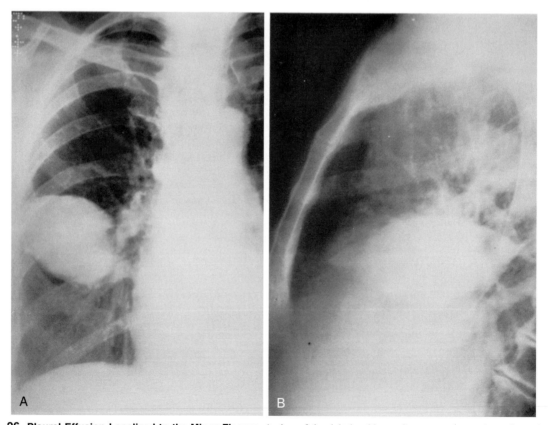

Figure 21–26. Pleural Effusion Localized to the Minor Fissure. A view of the right hemithorax from a posteroanterior radiograph *(A)* reveals a sharply circumscribed, homogeneous opacity in the right midlung zone. In lateral projection *(B)*, the true nature of the opacity can be appreciated: the mass is elliptical in shape, its pointed extremities being situated anteriorly and posteriorly in keeping with the position of the minor fissure. This unusual collection of pleural fluid developed during a recent episode of cardiac decompensation. With appropriate therapy, it disappeared completely in 3 weeks ("vanishing tumor").

and be misdiagnosed as a pulmonary neoplasm;[48, 49] however, its distinctive configuration in either PA or lateral projection should establish the diagnosis in the majority of cases. Occasionally, CT or sonography is required for definitive diagnosis (Fig. 21–27). These fluid accumulations tend to be absorbed spontaneously when the heart failure is relieved and therefore have been called *vanishing tumor* (*phantom tumor*, *pseudotumor*). In one series of 41 patients, the effusion was localized to the minor fissure in 32 (78%).[50]

It is sometimes difficult to differentiate loculated fluid in the lower half of the major fissure from atelectasis or combined atelectasis and consolidation of the right middle lobe on the chest radiograph. Three points should be borne in mind in this differentiation: (1) if the minor fissure is visible as a separate shadow, the diagnosis of loculated fluid is certain; (2) loculated fluid tends not to obscure the right heart border, whereas middle lobe atelectasis almost invariably does (silhouette sign); and (3) in lateral projection, a loculated effusion usually has a bulging surface on one or both sides, whereas the borders of the shadow tend to be straight or slightly concave in disease of the right middle lobe.

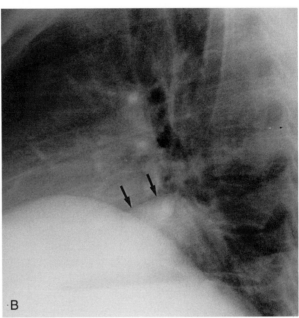

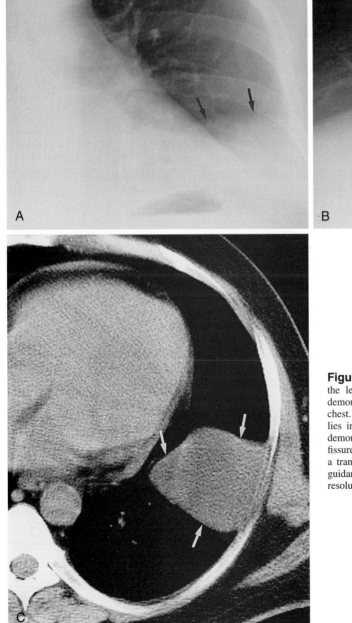

Figure 21–27. Loculated Interlobar Effusion. A view of the left hemithorax from a posteroanterior *(A)* chest radiograph demonstrates a poorly defined opacity *(arrows)* in the left lower chest. View from the lateral radiograph *(B)* reveals that the opacity lies in the region of the interlobar fissure *(arrows)*. CT scan *(C)* demonstrates characteristic appearance of fluid within the left major fissure *(arrows)*. The fluid collection tapers medially. Diagnosis of a transudate was made by fine needle aspiration under ultrasound guidance. Follow-up chest radiographs 6 months later demonstrated resolution of the fluid collection.

RADIOLOGIC SIGNS OF PLEURAL THICKENING

Pleural Fibrosis

Thickening of the pleural line over the convexity of the thorax and occasionally in the interlobar fissures is fairly common. The thickness may increase from 1 to 10 mm, usually after an episode of pleuritis and almost exclusively as a result of fibrosis of the visceral pleural surface. The major exception is the pleural plaque formation characteristic of asbestos-related disease, which occurs almost exclusively on the parietal pleura; the latter condition is considered in detail elsewhere (*see* pages 2433 and 2796). Severe thickening may markedly restrict pulmonary expansion, in which case surgical removal of the "peel" may be curative. Although sometimes local, pleural fibrosis is more often diffuse over the costal lung surface, presenting as a thin line of soft tissue opacity separating air-containing lung from contiguous ribs. The costophrenic sulci often are partly or completely obliterated, particularly laterally, and radiography in the lateral decubitus position may be necessary to differentiate such fibrosis from a small pleural effusion; in cases of pleural thickening, however, the obliterated costophrenic sulcus usually is sharply angulated rather than meniscus shaped, and the two can often be distinguished on this evidence alone (Fig. 21–28).

Several radiologic features are helpful in differentiating the various causes of fibrothorax on radiographs and on CT scans.[5] Evidence of underlying parenchymal disease is usually seen in patients with previous tuberculosis or empyema. Extensive calcification of the fibrothorax also favors these conditions and is seldom seen with asbestos-related diffuse pleural thickening.[51] Pleural plaques are identified radiologically as circumscribed areas of pleural thickening, whereas diffuse asbestos-related pleural thickening is considered present when there is a smooth uninterrupted pleural opacity extending over at least one fourth of the chest wall with or without associated obliteration of the costophrenic sulci.[5, 52] Hemorrhagic effusion, tuberculosis, and empyema usually lead to unilateral pleural abnormalities, whereas asbestos-related pleurisy is usually associated with bilateral disease, whether as diffuse thickening or plaques.[53, 54] Even when extensive pleural fibrosis is present, it seldom involves the mediastinal pleura (*see* Fig. 21–28).[53] This feature is helpful in the differential diagnosis of benign from malignant causes of pleural thickening. For example, in one study, only 1 (12%) of 8 patients with fibrothorax had mediastinal pleural thickening compared to 8 (72%) of 11 with mesothelioma.[53]

A curved shadow of soft tissue opacity frequently is identified in the apex of one or both lungs, in the concavity formed by the first and second ribs (Fig. 21–29). Sometimes called the *apical cap*, this abnormality has been erroneously ascribed to tuberculosis.[55] In one study of 113 left lungs obtained at autopsy, the commonest pathologic finding (in 20% of cases) was nonspecific fibrosis of apical lung parenchyma, which merged with the visceral pleura;[56] in no case was there histologic evidence of tuberculosis. Calcification (and occasionally ossification) was present in some cases. Radiologic-pathologic correlation showed a surprising incidence of false-negative and false-positive radiologic interpretations, which were considerably more frequent with minor degrees of subpleural scarring. The frequency of pathologically observed scarring increased significantly with age.

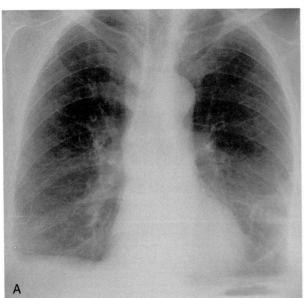
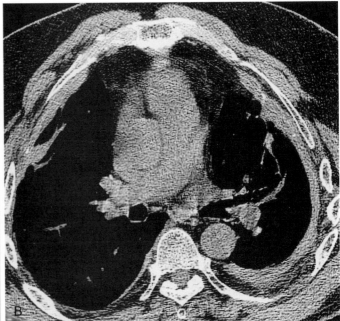

Figure 21–28. Pleural Fibrosis. A posteroanterior chest radiograph *(A)* demonstrates extensive bilateral pleural thickening. The blunted costophrenic angles are sharply angulated rather than meniscus shaped, a finding helpful in distinguishing pleural thickening from effusion. Also note the curved bands of increased opacity extending from the left lung to the pleural thickening, a feature most commonly related to asbestos. A CT scan *(B)* reveals marked bilateral pleural thickening with small areas of calcification. Although there is marked thickening of the costal and paravertebral pleura, the mediastinal pleura is free. The patient was a 53-year-old man with a history of exposure to asbestos.

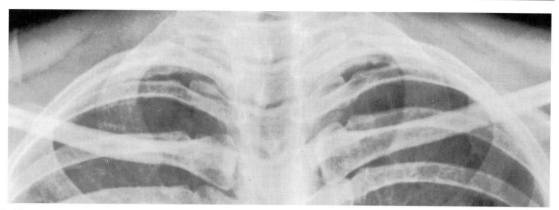

Figure 21–29. Apical Pleural Thickening. A view of the apical zones from a posteroanterior radiograph reveals irregular, symmetric thickening of the apical pleura. The irregularity serves to differentiate this thickening from companion shadows of the ribs.

Pleural Calcification or Ossification

Pleural calcification is most often the result of a remote hemothorax, pyothorax, or tuberculous effusion and commonly is associated with extensive thickening of the pleura. The calcification may be in the form of a broad continuous sheet or of multiple discrete plaques. It usually extends from about the level of the midthorax posteriorly, around the lateral lung margin in a generally inferior direction, roughly paralleling the major fissure (Fig. 21–30). The calcium may be deposited on the inner surface of the thickened pleura, either visceral or parietal; if only the former is calcified, a thick soft tissue opacity exists between the calcium and the thoracic wall. CT studies have shown that extrapleural fat may be deposited adjacent to the thickened parietal pleura, so the assumption that the pleura is markedly thickened because of fibrosis or calcification is not always valid (Fig. 21–31). Enlargement of the ribs adjacent to a focus of thickened and calcified pleura is common (Fig. 21–31).[57]

Pleural calcification of an entirely different form is seen following exposure to asbestos and talc.[58–60] Although the latency period between exposure and development of plaques is approximately 15 years, that for radiologically visible calcified pleural plaques is usually 20 years or more.[59, 61] The prevalence of plaques correlates with the intensity of asbestos exposure and the time interval from initial exposure.[62, 63] Some patients develop calcified plaques after a short exposure to asbestos; for example, they were reported in two patients approximately 20 years after 8 and 11 months of exposure.[64]

The radiologic characteristics of calcified asbestos-related pleural plaques are sufficiently different from calcification secondary to empyema or hemothorax that there should be no difficulty in differentiating the two (Fig. 21–32). The former are typically seen as circumscribed small areas of calcification, whereas the latter is continuous and usually extensive. In addition, the calcification in plaques usually forms along the diaphragmatic and costal pleura and almost invariably occurs in the parietal pleura, whereas that secondary to pyothorax or hemothorax may be confined to the visceral pleura. Differentiation of parietal from visceral pleural calcification can be reliably made radiologically only in the presence of pneumothorax or pleural effusion, unless the thickening involves the interlobar fissures. Pleural calcifica-

tion related to asbestos exposure is most often bilateral, although it may be asymmetric or unilateral.[65]

Pleural Neoplasms

The most common local pleural tumors are lipoma, fibrous tumor, and pulmonary carcinoma.[5] Although mesothelioma, pleural metastases, and lymphoma may also cause a focal abnormality, they are usually associated with diffuse involvement.[5, 53]

Localized pleural tumors present radiographically as smoothly marginated, homogeneous opacities, which, when viewed en face, characteristically have a sharply defined medial edge and an ill-defined lateral margin (Fig. 21–33).[5] Similar to chest wall lesions, they are convex with respect to the lung and displace adjacent lung parenchyma.[5] Particularly if small, these tumors frequently form obtuse angles with the chest wall; those that are large or pedunculated often form acute angles.[35, 66] Although the majority of pleural tumors have relatively nonspecific soft tissue attenuation on CT, the diagnosis of lipoma can be readily made by the presence of homogeneous fat attenuation (*see* Fig. 21–33).[67, 68]

Localized fibrous tumors of the pleura may originate in either the parietal or the visceral pleural surface. They usually arise over the convexity of the lung. When associated with a fissure, they may simulate an intrapulmonary nodule or an encapsulated interlobar effusion; in either case, CT should help establish the true nature of the lesion. Tumors may be sessile or pedunculated[69] and almost invariably have smoothly tapering margins.[35, 70] If small, they may form obtuse angles with the chest wall; however, large or pedunculated lesions frequently form acute angles.[66] Pedunculated tumors may be mobile, changing in position with respiration, posture, or on serial radiographs (Fig. 21–34).[71, 72]

Mesotheliomas are typically diffuse and accompanied by pleural effusion (Fig. 21–35). Even when the effusion is massive, however, there tends to be little displacement of the mediastinum away from the affected hemithorax. The reasons for this are twofold: In some cases, it results from *compression* of lung by extensive neoplastic involvement of the pleural surface; in others, it occurs as a result of fixation of the mediastinum by tumor. Regardless of the mechanism,

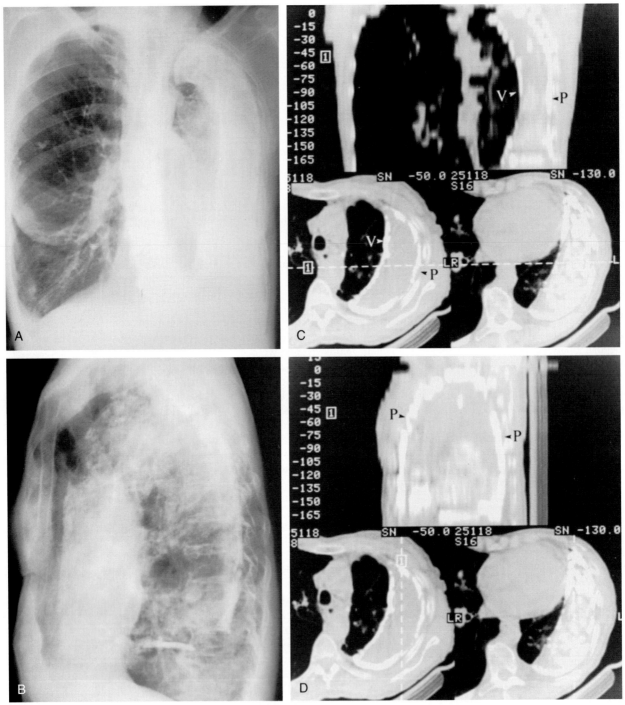

Figure 21–30. Pleural Fibrosis and Calcification (Calcific Fibrothorax). Posteroanterior *(A)* and lateral *(B)* chest radiographs reveal a thick calcific rind separated by a broad band of intervening soft tissue. The most lateral portion of the calcification relates closely to hypertrophied ribs. Coronal *(C)* and sagittal *(D)* CT reformations *(top)* with appropriate cross-sectional CT scans *(bottom)* illustrate a thick mantle of calcification delineating the visceral (V) and parietal (P) pleura; the tissue between the pleural layers is both fibrous and calcific in nature. The patient was a middle-aged woman with a history of previous tuberculous empyema.

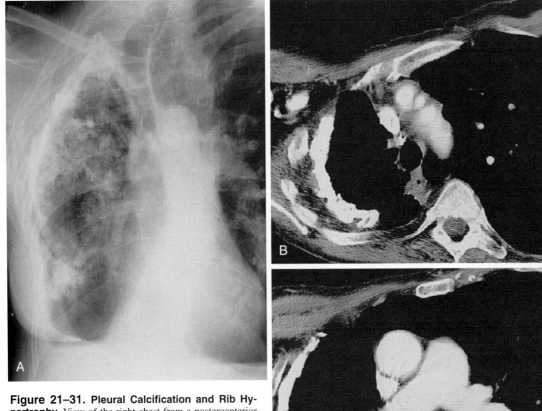

Figure 21–31. Pleural Calcification and Rib Hypertrophy. View of the right chest from a posteroanterior chest radiograph *(A)* demonstrates extensive right pleural calcification with associated loss of volume. Note increased thickness of the extrapleural soft tissues. Contrast-enhanced CT scans *(B and C)* reveal marked calcification of the right costal pleura. On CT, it can be seen that the increased thickness of the extrapleural tissues is mainly the result of accumulation of extrapleural fat *(arrows)*. Although there is marked loss of volume of the right hemithorax, the right ribs are considerably thicker than the ones on the left. The patient was a 71-year-old woman with long-standing right pleural calcification due to previous tuberculosis.

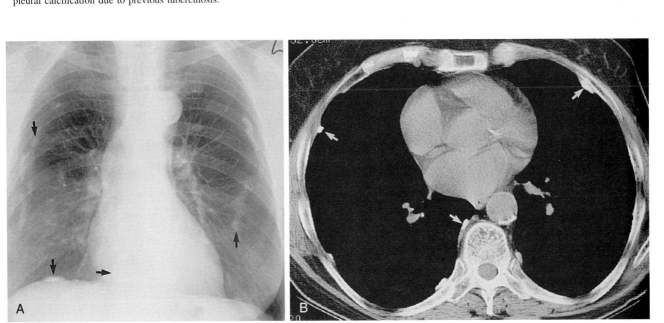

Figure 21–32. Calcified Asbestos-Related Pleural Plaques. Posteroanterior chest radiograph *(A)* and CT scan *(B)* reveal multiple bilateral, discrete, calcified pleural plaques *(arrows)* involving the costal, diaphragmatic, and paravertebral pleura. The patient was a 79-year-old man with previous occupational asbestos exposure.

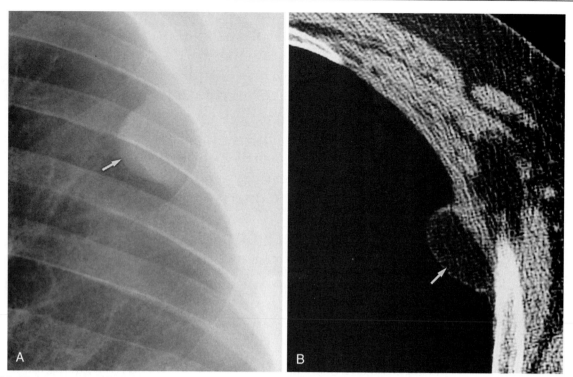

Figure 21–33. Pleural Lipoma. A view of the left upper chest from a posteroanterior radiograph *(A)* demonstrates homogeneous opacity *(arrow)* with smooth margins, sharply defined medial edge, and ill-defined lateral border characteristic of a pleural-based lesion. A view from the HRCT scan *(B)* demonstrates characteristic homogeneous fat attenuation of a pleural lipoma *(arrow)*. The patient was a 55-year-old man.

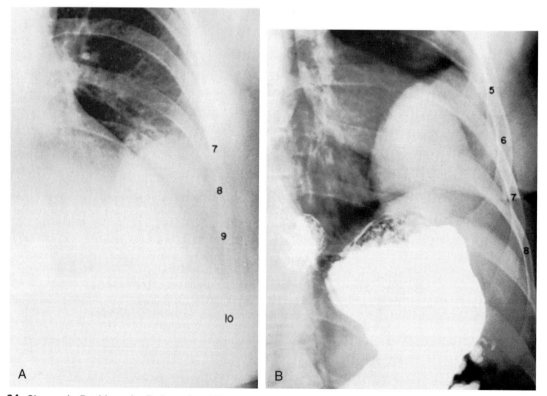

Figure 21–34. Change in Position of a Pedunculated Tumor. A view of the lower half of the left hemithorax from a posteroanterior radiograph exposed in the erect position *(A)* reveals a rather poorly defined homogeneous mass lying in the posterior portion of the thorax contiguous to the diaphragm and lateral chest wall; in this body position, it relates to the axillary portion of ribs 7 to 10. A view of the same area with the patient in the prone position *(B)* shows the mass to relate to the axillary portion of ribs 5 to 8. Such movement establishes the fact that the mass is not attached to the rib cage. At thoracotomy, the mass was found to arise from the costal surface of the visceral pleura to which it was attached by a long pedicle. Pathologic diagnosis was localized fibrous tumor of the pleura.

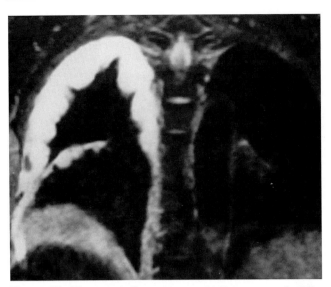

Figure 21–35. Mesothelioma. A coronal MR image reveals diffuse nodular thickening of the right pleura with involvement of the mediastinal pleura and interlobar fissure. The patient was a 37-year-old man with no occupational history of asbestos exposure. MR image was obtained using 1.5 T, spin-echo technique, TR 2118, TE 100.

the lack of displacement is important to the radiologic diagnosis, although it should be borne in mind that a similar radiographic picture may be produced by pulmonary carcinoma with obstructive atelectasis and effusion caused by pleural metastases.

Diffuse pleural abnormalities usually consist of various degrees of thickening, calcification, and effusion. Therefore there is an overlap of the radiologic manifestations of benign and malignant pleural thickening.[5] Findings on CT that are suggestive of malignancy include circumferential or nodular thickening, parietal pleural thickening greater than 1 cm, mediastinal pleural thickening,* and evidence of chest wall or mediastinal invasion (Fig. 21–36).[5] The value of various CT findings in the differential diagnosis was assessed in one study of 74 patients (including 39 who had a malignant process and 35 who had a benign abnormality).[53] The presence of circumferential pleural thickening (pleural rind) had 100% specificity in identifying malignancy; however, the sensitivity was only 41%. Nodular pleural thickening was present in 51% of malignant cases and 6% of benign ones. The most sensitive sign was thickening of the mediastinal pleura, which was seen in 56% of patients who had malignant pleural involvement; this finding was also present in 12% of patients who had diffuse benign pleural disease.

RADIOLOGIC SIGNS OF PNEUMOTHORAX

Pneumothorax in the Upright Patient

The previous discussion concerning the influence on underlying lung of material within the pleural space applies

---

*The *mediastinal pleura* is defined as the pleura that abuts the mediastinum, the posterior extent of which is demarcated by the anterior aspect of the vertebrae.[5, 73] The parietal pleura abutting the paravertebral sulci is not part of the anatomic mediastinal pleura and is most commonly referred to as the *paravertebral pleura*.[5, 39]

as well to air as to fluid. The only difference is the effect of gravity: in the erect individual, air rises to the apex of the hemithorax and causes relaxation atelectasis of the upper portion of the lung, whereas fluid falls to the bottom of the hemithorax and permits relaxation of the lower lobe. When pneumothorax is present, the weight of the lung in its gaseous surroundings causes it to drop to its most dependent position, slung by its fixed attachment at the pulmonary ligament. For this reason, a pneumothorax must be large to produce collapse of an entire lung. Although for most practical clinical purposes it usually suffices to designate the size of a pneumothorax as small, medium, or large, various methods have been described by which size can be more precisely quantified.[74, 75]

A radiologic diagnosis of pneumothorax can be made only by identifying the visceral pleural line. The latter is visualized as a sharply defined line of increased opacity that can be readily distinguished from the black line owing to Mach effect, which may be seen outlining a skin fold (Fig. 21–37). Because the lung is partly collapsed by the pneumothorax, it might be anticipated that its density would be increased and that this altered density, compared with that of the normal lung, should be sufficient to suggest the diagnosis; in fact, this is often not the case. As the lung progressively collapses with increasing size of the pneumothorax, blood flow through it diminishes; therefore the ratio of air to tissue and blood is not materially altered, and the overall density of the collapsing lung is not changed (Fig. 21–38).[76]

In the erect individual, pneumothorax is first evident near the apex of the chest (Fig. 21–39); a subpulmonic location has been reported occasionally in patients with chronic obstructive pulmonary disease[77] or penetrating injury to the thorax.[78] The visceral pleural line is usually readily identifiable, even on radiographs exposed at total lung capacity. In the vast majority of cases, the inspiratory chest radiograph is the only imaging modality required for diagnosis. When pneumothorax is strongly suspected clinically but a pleural line is not identified (possibly obscured by an overlying rib), gas in the pleural space can be detected by either of two procedures: (1) radiography in the erect position in full expiration (the rationale being that lung density is increased and volume of gas in the pleural space is constant, thus making it easier to detect the pneumothorax); and (2) radiography in the lateral decubitus position with a horizontal x-ray beam (the rationale here being obvious—air rises to the highest point in the hemithorax and is more clearly visible over the lateral chest wall than over the apex, where overlying bony shadows may obscure fine linear shadows). Although upright expiratory radiographs are obtained in most patients in whom pneumothorax is suspected clinically, the lateral decubitus view provides an excellent alternative when this cannot be obtained or when the upright view provides equivocal findings.[79–81]

Pneumothorax in the Supine Patient

When patients with suspected pneumothorax must be examined in the supine position, as is so often the case in the intensive care unit, gas within the pleural space rises to the vicinity of the diaphragm, the highest point in the hemi-

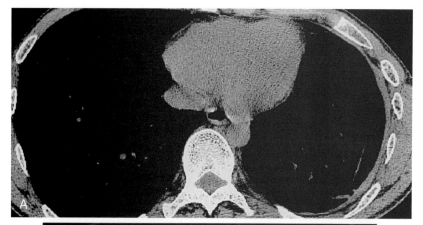

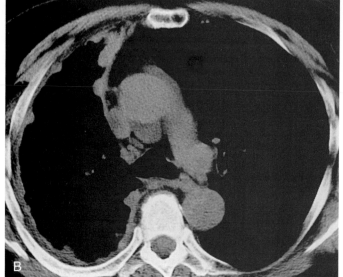

Figure 21–36. Benign Versus Malignant Pleural Thickening. Benign pleural thickening is shown in *A*. CT scan demonstrates smooth thickening of the left costal pleura with no associated pleural effusion or involvement of the mediastinal pleura. The patient was a 32-year-old man with surgically proven benign fibrothorax, presumably due to previous pleurisy. Malignant pleural thickening is shown in *B*. CT scan reveals pleural thickening that is diffuse and nodular in nature. At surgical biopsy, this was shown to represent a mesothelioma. Note that in both cases the size of the affected hemithorax is decreased, a finding that is not helpful in distinguishing benign from malignant pleural thickening.

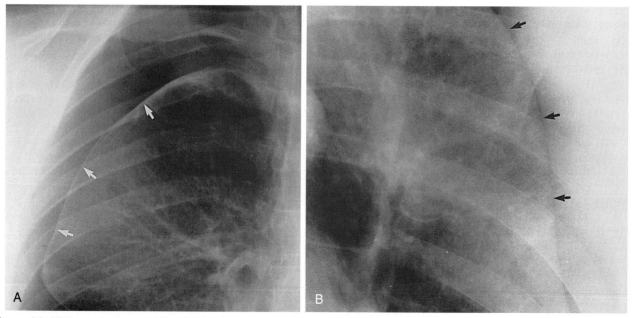

Figure 21–37. Pneumothorax Versus Skin Fold. A view of the right chest from a posteroanterior radiograph *(A)* demonstrates the sharply defined pleural line *(arrows)* characteristic of a pneumothorax. A view of the left chest from an anteroposterior radiograph *(B)* reveals a skin fold. The black line *(arrows)* seen at the edge of the skin fold is the result of the Mach effect.

thorax in this position. Depending on the size of the pneumothorax, the result can be an exceptionally deep radiolucent costophrenic sulcus *(deep sulcus sign)* (Fig. 21–40),[2] a lucency over the right or left upper quadrant,[83] or a much sharper than normal appearance of the hemidiaphragm with or without the presence of a visceral pleural line visible above it.[84] Other findings include visualization of the anterior costophrenic sulcus, increased sharpness of the cardiac border, collection of air within the minor fissure, and depression of the ipsilateral hemidiaphragm.[84, 85]

The distribution of pneumothorax in the supine and semirecumbent patient was reviewed in one study of 88 critically ill patients who had 112 pneumothoraces.[86] The pneumothorax most commonly involved the anteromedial (38% of cases), subpulmonic (26%), or apicolateral (22%) pleural sulci. Thirty-four (30%) of the 112 pneumothoraces were initially missed on the radiograph by clinicians, radiologists, or, most commonly, both.

When a pneumothorax is suspected in a supine patient, confirmation can be most readily obtained by performing a lateral decubitus view with the involved hemithorax uppermost.[79–81] CT has also been shown to be useful and is superior to frontal chest radiography.[86] To minimize the possibility of missing a pneumothorax, some investigators recommend CT in patients who have head trauma and require emergency surgery or mechanical ventilation.[86, 87]

Hydropneumothorax

Hydropneumothorax should be immediately apparent on radiographs exposed in the erect position because of the almost invariable air-fluid level. Loculated hydropneumothorax may occur as single or multiple collections, some of which may contain air-fluid levels. Radiography of a patient in various body positions sometimes shows the passage of fluid from one apparently loculated space into another, indicating their communication.

Hydropneumothorax in the supine patient can be diagnosed on radiographs by recognition of the pleural line—as a result of the pneumothorax—and an increased opacity lateral to it—caused by fluid in the pleural space (Fig. 21–41).[88] If there is more fluid than air in the pleural space, the lateral aspect of the visceral pleura tangent to the x-ray beam may be immersed in fluid and therefore obscured;[88] in this situation, pleural effusion is suspected, but the pneumothorax is missed. Confirmation of hydropneumothorax can be readily obtained by performing lateral decubitus or upright views of the chest or CT.[88]

Tension Pneumothorax and Hydrothorax

The detection of tension pneumothorax may be exceedingly difficult by chest radiography. Shift of the mediastinum

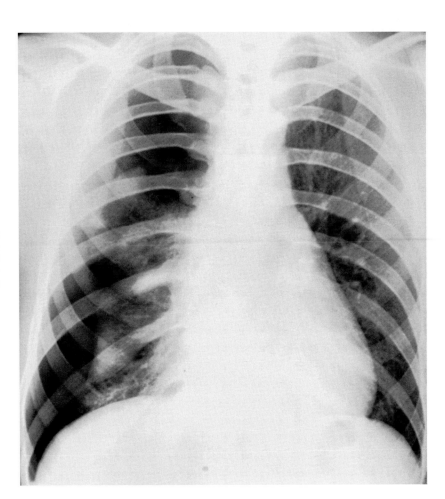

Figure 21–38. Effect of Pneumothorax on Lung Density. A posteroanterior radiograph reveals a moderate right pneumothorax; despite the fact that the right lung has been reduced in volume by approximately 50%, its density (except in local areas) differs little from that of the left lung. *See* text.

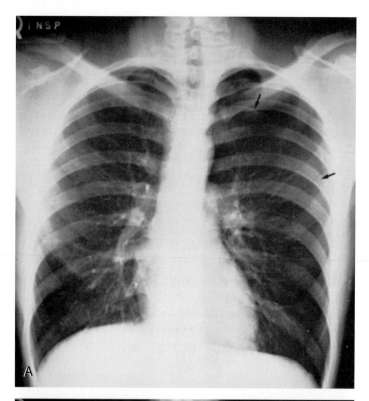

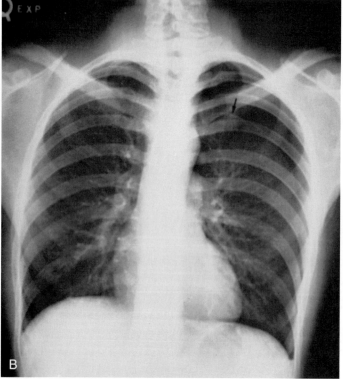

Figure 21–39. Inspiratory-Expiratory Radiographs in Spontaneous Pneumothorax Showing Little Change in Lung Volume on Expiration. A posteroanterior radiograph exposed at full inspiration *(A)* shows a 10% to 15% left pneumothorax (the visceral pleura is indicated by *arrows*). On expiration *(B)*, the volumes of the pneumothorax and of the left lung have reduced roughly proportionately, suggesting that equilibrium is present between the two compartments and that the pleural defect thus is open.

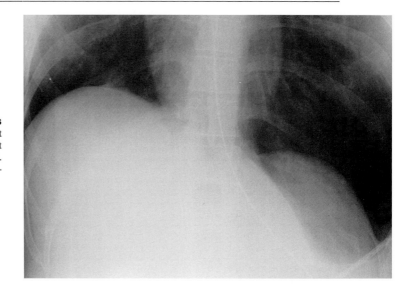

Figure 21–40. Pneumothorax with Deep Sulcus Sign. A view of the lower chest from an anteroposterior chest radiograph with the patient supine reveals a radiolucent left costophrenic sulcus and a sharply defined left hemidiaphragm. These findings are characteristic of a pneumothorax in a supine patient.

away from the side of a pneumothorax of any size is inevitable, pressure in the contralateral (normal) hemithorax being relatively more negative; such a shift must not be mistaken for evidence of tension pneumothorax. For the volume of a pneumothorax to increase, air must flow from the lung parenchyma or external environment (where pressure is atmospheric) through the pleural defect and into the pleural space; obviously, such flow cannot occur if pleural pressure is greater than atmospheric pressure throughout the respiratory cycle, unless the patient is on positive-pressure ventilation. Thus, for a pneumothorax to increase in volume, pressure within the pleural space must be relatively negative *during inspiration*; if a check-valve mechanism exists, allowing air to enter the pleural space during inspiration but preventing its egress during expiration, pressure within the pleural space is positive only during the latter phase of

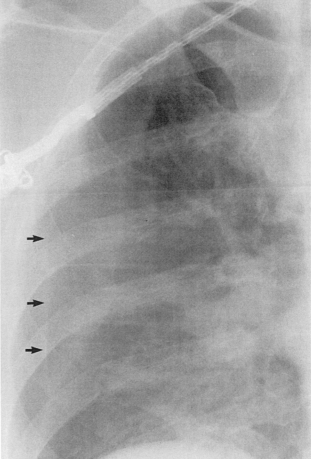

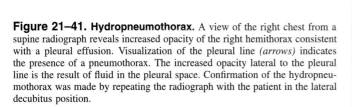

Figure 21–41. Hydropneumothorax. A view of the right chest from a supine radiograph reveals increased opacity of the right hemithorax consistent with a pleural effusion. Visualization of the pleural line *(arrows)* indicates the presence of a pneumothorax. The increased opacity lateral to the pleural line is the result of fluid in the pleural space. Confirmation of the hydropneumothorax was made by repeating the radiograph with the patient in the lateral decubitus position.

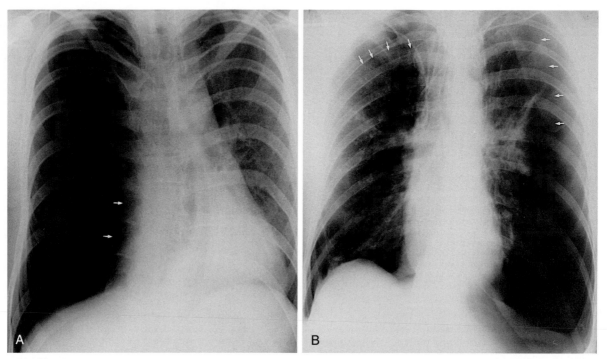

Figure 21–42. Tension Pneumothorax. An anteroposterior chest radiograph in a 26-year-old man *(A)* demonstrates a large right pneumothorax. The presence of complete collapse of the right lung, marked mediastinal shift to the left, and areas of atelectasis in the left lower lobe is consistent with tension pneumothorax. An anteroposterior chest radiograph in a 73-year-old woman with emphysema *(B)* demonstrates a large left pneumothorax *(arrows)*. Although the left lung is not completely collapsed, the presence of tension pneumothorax can be recognized by inversion of the left hemidiaphragm and contralateral shift of the mediastinum (even though there is also a small right pneumothorax *[arrows]*).

respiration. In clinical practice, a tension pneumothorax is considered present when there is excessive shift of the mediastinum accompanied by evidence of hemodynamic compromise (Fig. 21–42). A tension pneumothorax should not be diagnosed radiologically if the underlying lung remains partially expanded, unless the patient has adult respiratory distress syndrome[89] or airway obstruction, in which case the lung may not collapse even when the surrounding pressure is atmospheric or above. Tension pneumothorax is uncommon except in patients undergoing mechanical ventilation or after cardiopulmonary resuscitation.[90]

Tension hydrothorax, although rare, constitutes as much of a danger as tension pneumothorax—perhaps more so because the possibility of its occurrence is not generally recognized. In one case of a 23-year-old woman with meta-static carcinoma, pleural effusion increased greatly and rapidly and caused severe dyspnea and eventual circulatory collapse.[91] At thoracotomy, serosanguineous fluid spurted to a height of about 25 cm; several liters were removed. The explanation suggested by the investigators for this unusual circumstance seems reasonable: serum albumin was severely diminished, amounting to 1.4 gm/dl, and the protein content of the pleural fluid was 4.8 gm/dl. Thus, the colloid osmotic pressure difference between blood and pleural space was reversed, creating an alteration of pleural space dynamics that favored massive accumulation of fluid. Although such a set of circumstances must be rare, it is well to bear in mind the possibility in any patient with a massive pleural effusion, disproportionately increasing symptoms, and progressive deterioration in condition.

REFERENCES

1. Müller R, Löfstedt S: The reaction of the pleura in primary tuberculosis of the lungs. Acta Med Scand 122:105, 1945.
2. Hessén I: Roentgen examination of pleural fluid: A study of the localization of free effusion: The potentialities of diagnosing minimal quantities of fluid and its existence under physiological conditions. Acta Radiol 86(Suppl), 1951.
3. Moskowitz H, Platt RT, Schachar R, et al: Roentgen visualization of minute pleural effusion: An experimental study to determine the minimum amount of pleural fluid visible on a radiograph. Radiology 109:33, 1973.
4. Collins JD, Burwell D, Furmanski S, et al: Minimal detectable pleural effusions. Radiology 105:51, 1972.
5. Müller NL: Imaging of the pleura. Radiology 186:297, 1993.
6. Ruskin JA, Gurney JW, Thorsen MK, et al: Detection of pleural effusions on supine chest radiographs. Am J Roentgenol 148:681, 1987.
7. Raasch BN, Carsky EW, Lane EJ, et al: Pleural effusion: Explanation of some typical appearances. Am J Roentgenol 139:899, 1982.
8. Henschke CI, Davis SD, Romano PM, et al: The pathogenesis, radiologic evaluation, and therapy of pleural effusions. Radiol Clin North Am 27:1241, 1989.
9. Lipscomb DJ, Flower CDR, Hadfield JW: Ultrasound of the pleura: An assessment of its clinical value. Clin Radiol 32:289, 1981.
10. O'Moore PV, Mueller PR, Simeone JF, et al: Sonographic guidance in diagnostic and therapeutic interventions in the pleural space. Am J Roentgenol 149:1, 1987.
11. Eibenberger KL, Dock WI, Ammann ME, et al: Quantification of pleural effusions: Sonography versus radiography. Radiology 191:681, 1994.
12. Fleischner FG: Atypical arrangement of free pleural effusion. Radiol Clin North Am 1:347, 1963.
13. Petersen JA: Recognition of infrapulmonary pleural effusion. Radiology 74:34, 1960.
14. Davis S, Gardner F, Ovist G: The shape of a pleural effusion. BMJ 1:436, 1963.
15. Dandy WE Jr: Incomplete pulmonary interlobar fissure sign. Radiology 128:21, 1978.
16. Mulvey RB: The effect of pleural fluid on the diaphragm. Radiology 84:1080, 1965.
17. Collins JD, Burwell D, Furmanski S, et al: Minimal detectable pleural effusions: A roentgen pathology model. Radiology 105:51, 1972.
18. Dunbar JS, Favreau M: Infrapulmonary pleural effusion with particular reference to its occurrence in nephrosis. J Can Assoc Radiol 10:24, 1959.
19. Rigler LG: Roentgen diagnosis of small pleural effusion: A new roentgenographic position. JAMA 96:104, 1931.
20. Kafura PJ, Barnhard HJ: Ascites simulating subpulmonary pleural effusion. Radiology 101:525, 1971.
21. Schwartz MI, Marmorstein BL: A new radiologic sign of subpulmonic effusion. Chest 67:176, 1975.
22. Connell DG, Crothers G, Cooperberg PL: The subpulmonic pleural effusion: Sonographic aspects. J Can Assoc Radiol 33:101, 1982.
23. Woodring JH: Recognition of pleural effusion on supine radiographs: How much fluid is required? Am J Roentgenol 142:59, 1984.
24. Pugatch RD, Faling LJ, Robbins AH, et al: Differentiation of pleural and pulmonary lesions using computed tomography. J Comput Assist Tomogr 2:601, 1978.
25. Maffessanti M, Tommasi M, Pellegrini P: Computed tomography of free pleural effusions. Eur J Radiol 7:87, 1987.
26. Halvorsen RA, Fedyshin PJ, Korobkin M, et al: Ascites or pleural effusion? RadioGraphics 6:135, 1986.
27. Naidich DP, Megibow AJ, Hilton S, et al: Computed tomography of the diaphragm: Peridiaphragmatic fluid localization. J Comput Assist Tomogr 7:641, 1983.
28. Teplick JG, Teplick SK, Goodman L, et al: The interface sign: A computed tomographic sign for distinguishing pleural and intra-abdominal fluid. Radiology 144:359, 1982.
29. Dwyer A: The displaced crus: A sign for distinguishing between pleural fluid and ascites on computed tomography. J Comput Assist Tomogr 2:598, 1978.
30. Griffin DJ, Gross BH, McCracken S, et al: Observation on CT differentiation of pleural and peritoneal fluid. J Comput Assist Tomogr 8:24, 1984.
31. Silverman PM, Baker ME, Mahony BS: Atelectasis and subpulmonic fluid: A CT pitfall in distinguishing pleural from peritoneal fluid. J Comput Assist Tomogr 9:763, 1985.
32. Vock P, Effmann EL, Hedlung LW, et al: Analysis of the density of pleural fluid analogs by computed tomography. Invest Radiol 19:10, 1984.
33. Sullivan KL, Steiner RM, Wexler RJ: Lymphaticopleural fistula: Diagnosis by computed tomography. J Comput Assist Tomogr 8:1005, 1984.
34. Wolverson MK, Crepps LF, Sundaram M, et al: Hyperdensity of recent hemorrhage at body computed tomography: Incidence and morphologic variation. Radiology 148:779, 1983.
35. McLoud TC, Flower CDR: Imaging the pleura: Sonography, CT and MR imaging. Am J Roentgenol 156:1145, 1991.
36. Waite RJ, Carbonneau RJ, Balikian JP, et al: Parietal pleural changes in empyema: Appearances at CT. Radiology 175:145, 1990.
37. Aquino SL, Webb WR, Gushiken BJ: Pleural exudates and transudates: Diagnosis with contrast-enhanced CT. Radiology 192:803, 1994.
38. Stark DD, Federle MP, Goodman PC, et al: Differentiating lung abscess and empyema: Radiography and computed tomography. Am J Roentgenol 141:163, 1983.
39. Im JG, Webb WR, Rosen A, et al: Costal pleura: Appearance at high-resolution CT. Radiology 171:125, 1989.
40. Bressler EL, Francis IR, Glazer GM, et al: Bolus contrast medium enhancement for distinguishing pleural from parenchymal lung disease: CT features. J Comput Assist Tomogr 11:436, 1987.
41. Hinson KFW, Kuper SWA: The diagnosis of lung cancer by examination of sputum. Thorax 18:350, 1963.
42. Rigby M, Zylak CJ, Wood LDH: The effect of lobar atelectasis on pleural fluid distribution in dogs. Radiology 136:603, 1980.
43. Zidulka A, Nadler S, Antonisen NR: Pleural pressure with lobar obstruction in dogs. Respir Physiol 26:239, 1976.
44. Pugatch RD, Faling LJ, Robbins AH, et al: Differentiation of pleural and pulmonary lesions using computed tomography. J Comput Assist Tomogr 2:601, 1978.
45. Baber CE, Hedlund LW, Oddson TA, et al: Differentiating empyemas and peripheral pulmonary abscesses: The value of computed tomography. Radiology 135:755, 1980.
46. Zinn WL, Naidich DP, Whelan CA, et al: Fluid within preexisting air-spaces: A potential pitfall in the CT differentiation of pleural from parenchymal disease. J Comput Assist Tomogr 11:441, 1987.
47. Naidich DP, Zerhouni EA, Siegelman SS: Pleura and chest wall. In Naidich DP, Zerhouni EA, Siegelman SS (eds): Computed Tomography and Magnetic Resonance of the Thorax. 2nd ed. New York, Raven, 1991, pp 407–471.
48. Feldman DJ: Localized interlobar pleural effusion in heart failure. JAMA 146:1408, 1951.
49. Weiss W, Boucot KR, Gefter WI: Localized interlobular effusion in congestive heart failure. Ann Intern Med 38:1177, 1953.
50. Higgins JA, Juergens JL, Bruwer AJ, et al: Loculated interlobar pleural effusion due to congestive heart failure. Arch Intern Med 96:180, 1955.
51. Friedman AC, Fiel SB, Radecki PD, et al: Computed tomography of benign pleural and pulmonary parenchymal abnormalities related to asbestos exposure. Semin Ultrasound CT MR 11:393, 1990.
52. McLoud TC, Woods BO, Carrington CB, et al: Diffuse pleural thickening in an asbestos-exposed population: Prevalence and causes. Am J Roentgenol 144:9, 1985.
53. Leung AN, Müller NL, Miller RR: CT in differential diagnosis of diffuse pleural disease. Am J Roentgenol 154:487, 1990.
54. Aberle DR, Gamsu G, Ray CS, et al: Asbestos-related pleural and parenchymal fibrosis: Detection with high-resolution CT. Radiology 166:729, 1988.
55. Fraser RG, Paré JAPP: Diagnosis of Diseases of the Chest: An Integrated Study Based on the Abnormal Roentgenogram. Philadelphia, WB Saunders, 1970.
56. Renner RR, Markarian B, Pernice NJ, et al: The apical cap. Radiology 110:569, 1974.
57. Eyler WR, Monsein LH, Beute GH, et al: Rib enlargement in patients with chronic pleural disease. Am J Roentgenol 167:921, 1996.
58. Schneider L, Wimpfheimer F: Multiple progressive calcific pleural plaque formation: A sign of silicatosis. JAMA 189:328, 1964.
59. Schwartz DA: New developments in asbestos-related pleural disease. Chest 99:191, 1991.
60. Hillerdal G: Pleural plaques in a health survey material: Frequency, development and exposure to asbestos. Scand J Respir Dis 59:257, 1978.
61. Fletcher DE, Edge JR: The early radiological changes in pulmonary and pleural asbestosis. Clin Radiol 21:355, 1970.
62. Harries PG, Mackenzie FAF, Sheers G, et al: Radiological survey of men exposed to asbestos in naval dockyards. Br J Indust Med 29:274, 1972.
63. Greene R, Boggis C, Jantsch H: Asbestos-related pleural thickening: Effect of threshold criteria on interpretation. Radiology 152:569, 1984.
64. Sargent EN, Jacobson G, Wilkinson EE: Diaphragmatic pleural calcification following short occupational exposure to asbestos. Am J Roentgenol 115:473, 1972.
65. Hu H, Beckett L, Kelsey K, et al: The left-sided predominance of asbestos-related pleural disease. Am Rev Respir Dis 148:981, 1993.
66. Mendelson DS, Meary E, Buy JN, et al: Localized fibrous pleural mesothelioma: CT findings. Clin Imaging 15:105, 1991.
67. Epler GR, McLoud TC, Munn CS, et al: Pleural lipoma: Diagnosis by computed tomography. Chest 90:265, 1986.
68. Buxton RC, Tan CS, Khine NM, et al: Atypical transmural thoracic lipoma: CT diagnosis. J Comput Assist Tomogr 12:196, 1988.
69. Berne AS, Heitzman ER: The roentgenologic signs of pedunculated pleural tumors. Am J Roentgenol 87:892, 1962.
70. Dedrick CG, McLoud TC, Shepard JAO, et al: Computed tomography of localized pleural mesothelioma. Am J Roentgenol 144:275, 1985.
71. Weisbrod GL, Yee AC: Computed tomographic diagnosis of a pedunculated fibrous mesothelioma. J Can Assoc Radiol 34:147, 1983.
72. Soulen MC, Greco-Hunt VT, Templeton P: Cases from A³CR²: Migratory chest mass. Invest Radiol 25:209, 1990.
73. Platzer W: Pernkopf Anatomy: Atlas of Topographic and Applied Human Anatomy. Vol 2. Thorax, Abdomen, and Extremities. Baltimore, Urban & Schwarzenberg, 1989, p 63.
74. Axel L: A simple way to estimate the size of a pneumothorax. Invest Radiol 16:165, 1981.
75. Rhea JT, DeLuca SA, Greene RE: Determining the size of pneumothorax in the upright patient. Radiology 144:733, 1982.

76. Dornhorst AC, Pierce JW: Pulmonary collapse and consolidation: The role of collapse in the production of lung field shadows and the significance of segments in inflammatory lung disease. J Fac Radiol 5:276, 1954.

77. Christensen EE, Dietz GW: Subpulmonic pneumothorax in patients with chronic obstructive pulmonary disease. Radiology 121:33, 1976.

78. Schulman A, Dalrymple RB: Subpulmonary pneumothorax. Br J Radiol 51:494, 1978.

79. Carr JJ, Reed JC, Choplin RH, et al: Conventional film and computed radiography of experimentally induced pneumothoraces in cadavers: Implications for detection in patients. Radiology 183:193, 1992.

80. Beres RA, Goodman LR: Pneumothorax: Detection with upright versus decubitus radiography. Radiology 186:19, 1993.

81. Beres RA, Goodman LR: Pneumothorax detection: Clarifications and additional thoughts. Radiology 186:25, 1993.

82. Gordon R: The deep sulcus sign. Radiology 136:25, 1980.

83. Rhea JT, vanSonnenberg E, McLoud TC: Basilar pneumothorax in the supine adult. Radiology 133:595, 1979.

84. Ziter FMH, Westcott JL: Supine subpulmonary pneumothorax. Am J Roentgenol 137:699, 1981.

85. Spizarny DL, Goodman LR: Air in the minor fissure: A sign of right-sided pneumothorax. Radiology 160:329, 1986.

86. Tocino IM, Miller MH, Fairfax WR: Distribution of pneumothorax in the supine and semirecumbent critically ill adult. Am J Roentgenol 144:901, 1985.

87. Tocino IM, Miller MH, Frederick PR, et al: CT detection of occult pneumothorax in head trauma. Am J Roentgenol 143:987, 1984.

88. Onik G, Goodman PC, Webb WR, et al: Hydropneumothorax: Detection on supine radiographs. Radiology 152:31, 1984.

89. Gobien RP, Reines HD, Schabel SI: Localized tension pneumothorax: Unrecognized form of barotrauma in adult respiratory distress syndrome. Radiology 142:15, 1982.

90. Ludwig J, Kienzle GD: Pneumothorax in a large autopsy population. Am J Clin Pathol 70:24, 1978.

91. Rabinov K, Stein M, Frank H: Tension hydrothorax—an unrecognized danger. Thorax 21:465, 1966.

PART IV

DEVELOPMENTAL LUNG DISEASE

Developmental Anomalies Affecting the Airways and Lung Parenchyma

PULMONARY AGENESIS, APLASIA, AND
HYPOPLASIA, 598
    Etiology and Pathogenesis, 598
      Agenesis and Aplasia, 598
      Secondary Hypoplasia, 598
      Primary Hypoplasia, 599
    Pathologic Characteristics, 599
    Radiologic Manifestations, 599
    Clinical Manifestations and Prognosis, 601
BRONCHOPULMONARY SEQUESTRATION, 601
    Pathogenesis, 601
  Intralobar Sequestration, 602
    Pathologic Characteristics, 602
    Radiologic Manifestations, 604
    Clinical Manifestations, 609
  Extralobar Sequestration, 609
CONGENITAL BRONCHOGENIC CYSTS, 609
    Pathologic Characteristics, 610
  Pulmonary Bronchogenic Cysts, 611
    Radiologic Manifestations, 611
    Clinical Manifestations, 612
  Mediastinal Bronchogenic Cysts, 612
    Radiologic Manifestations, 614
    Clinical Manifestations, 614
CONGENITAL BRONCHIECTASIS, 615
CONGENITAL CYSTIC ADENOMATOID
MALFORMATION, 615
CONGENITAL TRACHEOBRONCHIAL STENOSIS, 618
CONGENITAL BRONCHIAL ATRESIA, 620
NEONATAL LOBAR HYPERINFLATION, 621
    Pathogenesis and Pathologic Characteristics, 623
    Radiologic Manifestations, 624
    Clinical Manifestations, 625
ANOMALOUS TRACHEOBRONCHIAL BRANCHING, 625
  Abnormal Bronchial Number, 626
  Abnormal Origin of Lobar or Segmental Bronchi, 626
  Bronchial Isomerism, 626
  Tracheobronchial Diverticula, 626
ANOMALOUS TRACHEOBRONCHIAL
COMMUNICATION, 627
  Tracheobronchial-Esophageal Fistula, 627
  Bronchobiliary Fistula, 628
MISCELLANEOUS BRONCHOPULMONARY
ANOMALIES, 628
  Accessory and Heterotopic Pulmonary Tissue, 628
  Heterotopic Tissue Within the Lung, 628
  Horseshoe Lung, 628

For purposes of discussion, developmental anomalies of the lungs can be divided into two major groups, depending on the *predominant* structure affected: (1) those originating in the primitive foregut or its lung bud (bronchopulmonary or foregut anomalies, discussed in this chapter) and (2) those arising from the sixth aortic arch or venous radicals and their derivatives (pulmonary vascular anomalies, discussed in Chapter 23). Despite the convenience of this division and the use of specific terms for various anatomic patterns of disease, it should be appreciated that considerable overlap exists between conditions in both groups[1–3] and that multiple lesions are occasionally identified in the same patient.[4–6] The presence of significant pathogenetic differences and the reliability of precise morphologic classification can thus be questioned.

For obvious reasons, the majority of developmental abnormalities that affect the lungs are manifested at or soon after birth.[7] Occasional examples of most anomalies have been reported in adolescents or adults, however, and it is important for the respiratory physician to be aware of them, even if his or her practice does not include children. It is also important to recognize that abnormalities of pulmonary development and growth during childhood may have significant effects on pulmonary function in adult life.[8, 9]

Although knowledge of the pathogenesis of bronchopulmonary anomalies is incomplete, embryologic evidence is consistent with the hypothesis that it is related to interference with normal development of the lungs between the 3rd and the 24th weeks of gestation—during the embryonic, pseudoglandular, and canalicular periods (although an insult between the 24th week and term could interfere with development during the terminal sac period and could affect postnatal development). A variety of abnormalities of growth factors, cell receptors, neuropeptides, extracellular matrix molecules, maternal or fetal hormones, and other substances presumably underlie this altered development.[10] Clinical, radiologic, and pathologic criteria permit designation of a specific disease process in most cases; in some, however, it is impossible to categorize an anomaly precisely. In addition, certainty that one is dealing with a developmental defect rather than an acquired lesion may be lacking at times.

Although strictly speaking not developmental in nature,

a variety of abnormalities of pulmonary mesenchymal tissue that affect its structure and function and that have a hereditary basis are also discussed in this section (*see* Chapter 24).

PULMONARY AGENESIS, APLASIA, AND HYPOPLASIA

Arrested development of the lung can be classified into three types:[11] (1) *agenesis*, in which there is complete absence of one or both lungs, with no trace of bronchial or vascular supply or of parenchymal tissue; (2) *aplasia*, in which there is suppression of all but a rudimentary bronchus that ends in a blind pouch, with no evidence of pulmonary vasculature or parenchyma; and (3) *hypoplasia*, in which the gross morphology of the lung is essentially unremarkable but in which there is a decrease in the number or size of airways, vessels, and alveoli.

In practice, an etiologic, pathogenetic, and clinical distinction between agenesis and aplasia is seldom apparent, and the two conditions are usually considered together.[12] By contrast, hypoplasia is often associated with other congenital anomalies, many of which are thought to be important in pathogenesis, and it is likely that most of these cases represent a disease state that is qualitatively different from either agenesis or aplasia. Hypoplasia usually involves the whole lung; when it affects only one lobe,[11] it is often accompanied by anomalies of the ipsilateral pulmonary artery and anomalous pulmonary venous drainage (hypogenetic lung syndrome; *see* page 653). Rare cases have been reported in which apparently isolated lobar hypoplasia has been identified in otherwise normal individuals.[13, 14]

The incidence of unilateral agenesis is low;[15] for example, chest radiography has been reported to show it in only 1 of 10,000 individuals.[16] There is no clear-cut predominance in either men or women, and neither the right nor the left lung is more commonly affected.[17] Hypoplasia of the lung may be regarded as primary (idiopathic) or secondary (when it occurs in association with environmental factors or other congenital anomalies that may be implicated in its pathogenesis).[18, 19] The incidence of the secondary form is difficult to determine; however, because of its association with a variety of other abnormalities and the difficulty of pathologic diagnosis in some cases, it is likely to be more common than generally recognized. The incidence of primary hypoplasia has been estimated to be 1 to 2 per 12,000 births.[20]

Etiology and Pathogenesis

Agenesis and Aplasia

Unilateral pulmonary agenesis (aplasia) has occasionally been described in twins and in infants with chromosomal abnormalities, suggesting a genetic basis for the anomaly.[21, 22] The abnormality has also been described in association with anomalies of the chest wall and skeleton[23] or the ipsilateral face,[24] leading some to hypothesize an underlying abnormality in development of the aortic arches.[24] Bilateral agenesis is sometimes associated with anomalies of the trachea and esophagus,[25] suggesting a defect in the formation of the primary lung bud.

Secondary Hypoplasia

Several mechanisms have been implicated in secondary pulmonary hypoplasia, including decreased hemithoracic volume, decreased pulmonary vascular perfusion, decreased fetal respiratory movement, and decreased lung fluid.[26]

Decreased Volume of the Ipsilateral Hemithorax. This is the most frequent abnormality associated with pulmonary hypoplasia. The most common cause is a space-occupying mass within the pleural cavity, usually abdominal contents that have been displaced through a congenital diaphragmatic hernia.[27, 28] Thoracic neuroblastoma, sequestered lung,[27] accessory diaphragm,[29] and pleural effusion[12, 30] have also been reported; occasionally, intra-abdominal tumors or fluid collections can be large enough to have the same effect. The importance of the space-occupying nature of the abnormal intrathoracic contents is shown by the development of pulmonary hypoplasia after the production of experimental diaphragmatic hernias in lambs.[31] A variety of musculoskeletal deformities of the thoracic cage,[27, 32–34] diaphragm,[35] and abdominal wall[36] have also been associated with pulmonary hypoplasia; although it is likely that these abnormalities also act by reducing the size of the thoracic cavity, it is possible that decreased intrauterine respiratory movements secondary to diminished chest wall compliance or decreased respiratory muscle mass may be of greater significance (*see* farther on).[37]

Another relatively common group of developmental anomalies associated with pulmonary hypoplasia involves the kidney and urinary tract. Of these, Potter's syndrome (renal agenesis, abnormal facies, limb abnormalities, and pulmonary hypoplasia) is the most frequent. It has been suggested that the presence of oligohydramnios in these conditions leads to hypoplasia as a result of thoracic compression by the closely applied uterine wall.[18, 27, 38] Although this is theoretically possible, the occasional cases in which both renal and pulmonary abnormalities are present and amniotic fluid is either normal or excessive in amount[27] suggest that other factors, such as the loss of the ability of the lungs to retain their normally produced fluid (*see* farther on), may be more important.[39, 40]

Decreased Pulmonary Vascular Perfusion. Although the effects on the developing lung of a decrease of pulmonary arterial flow are not known in detail, there is evidence that such a decrease may result in pulmonary hypoplasia; for example, in some patients with tetralogy of Fallot[41] and in pigs with experimental unilateral ligation of a pulmonary artery,[42] the number and size of alveoli have been shown to be decreased. It is possible, therefore, that some of the abnormal parenchymal development in the hypogenetic lung syndrome is the result of hypoplasia of the pulmonary artery.

Decreased Fetal Respiratory Movements. Lung hypoplasia has been shown to occur in rabbits[40, 43] and sheep[44] subjected to intrauterine cervical cord injury and in fetal lambs in which bilateral phrenic nerve section had been performed.[45] As a result, it has been speculated that the central nervous system may play an important role in lung development, possibly by maintaining normal fetal respiratory movements;[43, 44] it is conceivable, therefore, that some neurologic abnormality could result in human pulmonary hypoplasia. It is also possible that a decrease in respiratory muscle movement is important in the hypoplasia associated with a thoracic mass or deformed chest wall or with diaphragmatic muscle dysfunction.[37, 46]

Decreased Lung Fluid. There is compelling evidence that lung hypoplasia associated with oligohydramnios is related to a decrease in intrapulmonary fluid;[40, 47] because such fluid normally exerts positive pressure within the developing lung, its deficiency could theoretically result in the loss of an internal template about which the lung can form. In support of this hypothesis are observations in fetal animals that drainage of pulmonary fluid results in lung hypoplasia[48] and that tracheal ligation is followed by accelerated lung growth and maturation.[48a] Moreover, some (albeit not all[49]) human neonates with laryngeal atresia, in which there may be an increased amount of lung fluid, have been shown to have pulmonary *hyperplasia*.[50–52] Finally, a monoamniotic twin with normal kidney function appears to be able to produce sufficient amniotic fluid to prevent the development of pulmonary hypoplasia in the twin with renal abnormality.[53]

Miscellaneous Associations. In addition to these known or potential mechanisms for pulmonary hypoplasia, several authors have described fairly consistent associations between pulmonary hypoplasia and other abnormalities that do not clearly fit into the previously discussed pathogenetic mechanisms. These include rhesus isoimmunization,[54] anencephaly and hydranencephaly,[55] and a variety of congenital syndromes (e.g., Down's syndrome,[56] Klippel-Feil syndrome,[57] Wolcott-Rallison syndrome,[49] Matthew-Wood syndrome,[58] Fryns syndrome,[59] and an unnamed syndrome that includes ankylosis and multiple facial anomalies[60, 61]). Pulmonary hypoplasia has also been sporadically associated with a variety of other chromosomal and developmental anomalies[27, 49] and, rarely, has occurred in families.[62]

Primary Hypoplasia

The pathogenesis of primary hypoplasia is even less clear than the secondary form.[27, 63] By definition unassociated with other anomalies, it may represent an intrinsic defect in lung development. Conceivably, unrecognized abnormalities in central nervous system control of fetal respiratory movements might also be a causative factor.

Pathologic Characteristics

As noted earlier, the morphologic distinction between aplasia and agenesis is the presence in the former of a rudimentary bronchus of variable length unassociated with pulmonary vessels or parenchyma. It has been suggested that poor clearance of secretions from this pouch may be responsible, in part, for the increased risk of infection in the contralateral lung.[64] In one study of a 3-month-old infant with pulmonary aplasia, the single lung was found to be twice the normal volume and to have twice the number of alveoli expected for one lung;[65] its airways and blood vessels were hypoplastic, possibly from the same event that had severely inhibited development of the aplastic lung. These findings are similar to those that have been described if one lung is removed from a dog in the neonatal period; the remaining lung undergoes marked hyperplasia with an increase in the number of alveoli, but the size of the airways remains unchanged, rendering them relatively hypoplastic.[66]

Although the pathologic diagnosis of pulmonary hypoplasia can be made on formalin-inflated, routinely processed lungs on the basis of a combination of fresh lung weight, fixed lung volume, radial alveolar count, and estimates of tissue maturity,[67] precise characterization of the morphologic changes is best performed by morphometric measurement after inflation of the lungs to a known transpulmonary pressure. Hypoplastic lungs are typically smaller and weigh less than normally expected for their age. Detailed morphologic changes have been studied in association with thoracic dystrophy,[68, 69] diaphragmatic hernia,[39, 70–72] scoliosis,[73] bilateral renal agenesis and dysplasia,[39, 74, 75] rhesus isoimmunization,[54] Down's syndrome,[56, 76] and several vascular anomalies.[41, 77] Although there is variation in the severity and type of change between different cases, the most consistent finding is a decrease in the number of airway generations, ranging from about 50% to 75% of normal.[54, 74, 78] In addition, there is frequently a decrease in the number of alveoli,[56] estimated by one group of investigators to be about one third normal.[78] This is often associated with a decrease in alveolar size. Some investigators have shown normal airway and alveolar maturation for gestational age; others have found an immature appearance.[39, 54, 55, 72, 79] Abnormalities of the pulmonary arterial system have also been identified,[35, 54, 74, 78] consisting of decreased elastic tissue in the larger arteries, increased muscle in normally muscular arteries, and extension of muscle into normally nonmuscular arteries.

The basis for the variation in morphologic findings may be related to the severity and cause of the hypoplasia as well as to the timing of the etiologic events that led to the anomaly.[35, 79] For example, in one study of three patients with unilateral lung hypoplasia and vascular anomalies, quantification of the structural changes showed the pulmonary artery to be hypoplastic in one patient;[80] bronchial artery distribution was normal, but its volume was increased, and the number of airways was normal, a combination that suggested onset in late intrauterine life or early infancy. In the other two patients, the number of airways was subnormal, and the blood supply was from the systemic circulation only, suggesting onset in the early weeks of intrauterine development.

Morphologic changes in cases of primary hypoplasia have not been as thoroughly investigated. In one study of four neonates with unexplained respiratory distress, the lungs were found to be significantly decreased in weight-to-body weight and weight-to-gestational age ratios;[63] because no other anomalies were found, it was assumed that the lungs were examples of primary hypoplasia. Histologic examination showed no detectable architectural abnormalities; however, in a limited morphometric analysis, alveolar number was found to be considerably reduced. Histologic examination of an additional case of apparently primary hypoplasia showed severe deficiency of normal pulmonary structures distal to the bronchi; morphometric measurements were not obtained.[81]

Radiologic Manifestations

The radiographic findings in cases of agenesis, aplasia, or severe hypoplasia are similar and are characterized principally by total or almost total absence of aerated lung in one hemithorax. The markedly reduced volume is indicated by approximation of the ribs, elevation of the ipsilateral hemidiaphragm, and shift of the mediastinum (Fig. 22–1). In most cases, the contralateral lung is greatly overinflated and dis-

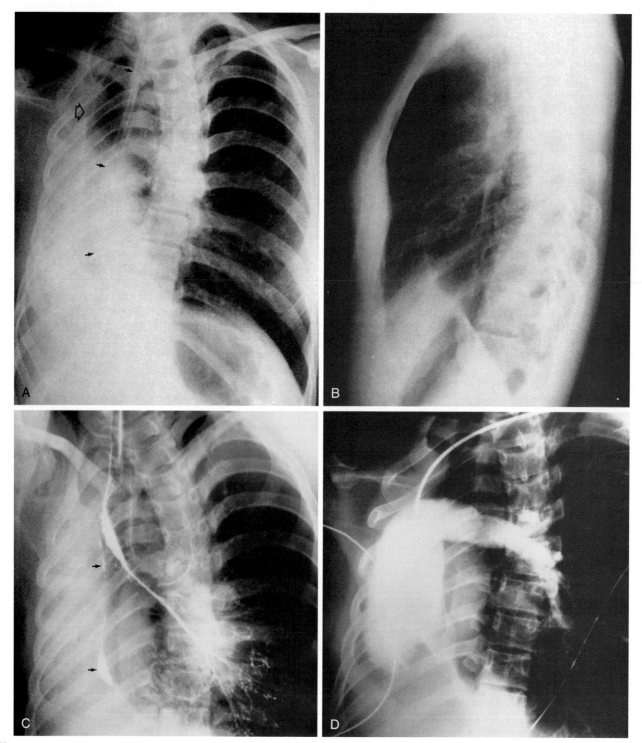

Figure 22–1. Agenesis of the Right Lung. A posteroanterior chest radiograph *(A)* shows marked displacement of the mediastinum to the right, both the heart and the esophagus being entirely within the right hemithorax (the latter indicated by the position of the nasogastric tube—*solid arrows*). The left lung is severely overinflated, as indicated by the displaced anterior mediastinal junction line in posteroanterior projection *(open arrow)* and by the large retrosternal air space in lateral projection *(B)*. A bronchogram *(C)* shows no vestige of a right main bronchus *(arrows* point to contrast medium in the displaced esophagus). A pulmonary angiogram *(D)* reveals total absence of a right pulmonary artery. (Courtesy of Dr. David Stephen, Royal Prince Albert Hospital, Sydney, Australia.)

placed, along with the anterior mediastinum, into the involved hemithorax;[82–85] this displacement of air-containing lung to the side of the agenesis may lead to some confusion in diagnosis. Computed tomography (CT) may be required to establish the degree of underdevelopment[85] or to differentiate agenesis from other conditions that may closely mimic it radiographically: total atelectasis from any cause, severe bronchiectasis with collapse, and advanced fibrothorax (Fig. 22–2). In patients with aplasia, CT can demonstrate the rudimentary bronchus as well as absence of the ipsilateral pulmonary artery;[85] in those with hypoplasia, it can demonstrate the patent bronchus, the pulmonary artery, and the hypoplastic lung.[85]

The main differential diagnosis of hypoplastic lung is Swyer-James syndrome (*see* page 2337). Although both conditions are associated with unilateral low lung volume, patients with Swyer-James syndrome demonstrate air trapping on radiographs or HRCT scans performed at the end of maximal expiration.[86, 87]

Clinical Manifestations and Prognosis

Clinical findings depend on the degree of pulmonary abnormality and the presence of congenital malformations elsewhere, particularly of the kidneys, diaphragm, and chest wall. In patients who are asymptomatic, physical examination characteristically reveals asymmetry of the two sides of the thorax, reduction in respiratory movement, and absence of air entry into the affected side. Infants who have primary pulmonary hypoplasia may present with respiratory distress and are prone to pneumothorax.[63] The condition has been recognized in occasional adults with chronic respiratory failure.[88]

Although most evidence suggests that patients with unilateral pulmonary agenesis usually die in the neonatal period, survival into adulthood, sometimes without symptoms, is clearly possible.[15, 89] The number of individuals who survive with hypoplasia, especially the less severe forms, is undoubtedly much greater. Despite this, the anomalies appear to predispose to respiratory infections,[12, 15, 27] and some patients die before they reach their teens. Among those who

survive, many have mild pulmonary function abnormalities, including increased residual volume and airway responsiveness to methacholine.[90]

BRONCHOPULMONARY SEQUESTRATION

Bronchopulmonary sequestration is a congenital malformation in which a portion of pulmonary tissue is detached from the remainder of the normal lung and receives its blood supply from a systemic artery. The anomaly may be intralobar or extralobar: the former lies contiguous with normal lung parenchyma and within the same visceral pleural envelope; the latter is enclosed within its own pleural membrane, usually in close proximity to the normal lung but sometimes within or below the diaphragm. (Although intralobar sequestration is sometimes referred to as an *accessory lung*, we prefer to restrict the use of this term to the rare cases of ectopic pulmonary tissue that maintains its connection to the tracheobronchial and pulmonary vascular tree [*see* page 628].)

Although discussed here as a specific entity, bronchopulmonary sequestration possesses anatomic features that overlap with a variety of other congenital anomalies, and the distinctiveness of the condition has been questioned.[1–3, 91] In fact, some investigators consider it to represent a spectrum of malformations characterized by abnormal connections of one or more pulmonary components (airways, arteries, or veins).[2, 92] Occasional cases have also been reported in which pulmonary abnormalities otherwise characteristic of intralobar sequestration have been unassociated with systemic arterial supply;[77, 93] whether these are part of the spectrum of sequestration or a different entity is not clear. Despite these observations, we believe that the majority of cases—particularly those seen in adults—can be readily classified into *intralobar* and *extralobar sequestration* and favor the continued use of these diagnostic terms.

Sequestration is one of the more common congenital pulmonary abnormalities; in a review of 70 patients with such malformations from the Children's National Medical Center in Washington, DC, it was identified in 20.[7]

Pathogenesis

Most authors believe that both extralobar and intralobar sequestration represent developmental anomalies, the pathogenesis of which has been related to a variety of potential mechanisms, including[94–99] (1) a primary abnormality of an anomalous systemic artery associated with traction and eventual displacement of a developing bronchial bud;[94] (2) failure of pulmonary arterial development with persistence of systemic arterial supply and secondary postnatal cystic changes in the involved parenchyma;[96] (3) coincidental abnormal development of lung cysts and a systemic arterial supply;[99] (4) interference with "embryonic organization" of various thoracic structures;[93] and (5) an anomaly of tracheobronchial branching with persistence and localized development of a separate branch fragment and retention of its embryonic systemic vascular supply.[95] The last is currently the most widely accepted theory.

As discussed previously (*see* page 136), the lung bud arises as an outpouching of the foregut in the 3-week-old

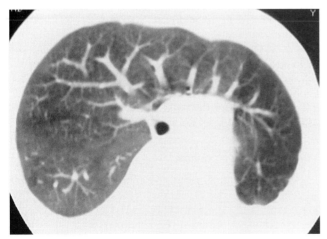

Figure 22–2. Pulmonary Agenesis. CT scan at the level of the bronchus intermedius in an 18-year-old male patient demonstrates absence of the left lung with compensatory overinflation of the right lung. No left bronchus or pulmonary artery was identified on CT.

embryo and subsequently undergoes repeated divisions to produce the primitive bronchial tree. Separation of a portion of the developing lung with continuing branching and parenchymal growth could thus result in a segment "sequestered" from the otherwise normal lung in its fully developed stage. When separation occurs in the earliest stage of foregut development, the sequestered tissue may communicate with the esophagus through a muscular, epithelium-lined tube; at a later stage, this connection may be no more than a thin, fibrous strand without a lumen. In the great majority of bronchopulmonary sequestrations, however, an esophagobronchial connection is not evident, the only evidence of foregut origin of the sequestration being the anomalous blood supply.

Normally, when the pulmonary artery develops from the sixth embryonic arch and invaginates its branches into the primitive pulmonary tissue, the branches of the splanchnic plexus that supply the lung bud remain as the bronchial arteries. According to the fifth theory enumerated earlier, additional branches persist, resulting in the anomalous systemic arterial supply to the sequestered lung. The reason for this hypothesized persistence is not clear but may be related to failure of normal pulmonary vascular ingrowth caused by the abnormal position of the sequestered fragment.

There has also been dispute concerning the differences between intralobar and extralobar sequestration, some authors[100] postulating a different embryogenesis of the two forms and others[77, 95] believing that the two are variations of the same pathogenetic process. According to the latter viewpoint, the location of the sequestered tissue may reflect the time at which the developmental insult occurred: fragments of the developing bronchial tree that separate at an early stage from the primitive outpouching itself or from a separate foregut diverticulum may acquire a separate pleural investment and develop within the mediastinum, thus forming an extralobar sequestration; by contrast, separated bronchial fragments of the partially developed lung might be expected to continue their development within the already developing lung tissue and thus be recognized as an intralobar form.

Although most investigators believe that the intralobar form of bronchopulmonary sequestration represents a developmental anomaly, some have proposed that it is an acquired lesion, pathogenetically different from the extralobar variety.[97, 98, 101] According to this view, the initial event in the formation of intralobar sequestration is focal bronchial obstruction, possibly as a result of bronchial infection or foreign body aspiration.[98] Persistence of the obstruction (or perhaps the effects of an associated pneumonitis) leads to the characteristic cystic and fibrotic changes in lung parenchyma. The initial inflammatory process also interrupts pulmonary blood flow into the affected lung segment; hypertrophy of systemic arteries then results in the "anomalous" vascular supply. The existence of this sequence of events is supported by the following observations: (1) the demonstration in some children of systemic arteries arising in the esophageal plexus, coursing through the pulmonary ligaments, and supplying a portion of the visceral pleura of the lower lobe;[98] (2) the observation that systemic vessels can undergo marked hypertrophy and supply portions of abnormal lung in clearly acquired conditions; (3) the rarity of intralobar sequestration in neonates; and (4) the occasional cases that resemble intralobar sequestration but in which there is a clearly defined acquired pathogenesis.[102–104] Despite

these observations, cases of intralobar sequestration have been identified at birth or in utero,[105–107] in families,[108] and in association with bronchogenic cysts[109, 110] or other bronchopulmonary malformations,[110, 111] suggesting that at least some are truly abnormalities of pulmonary development.

Intralobar Sequestration

Intralobar sequestration accounts for approximately 75% of bronchopulmonary sequestrations.[101, 112] Although most commonly diagnosed in children and young adults, it may be recognized at any age: in one review of 16 cases, the patients included 1 newborn, 5 children, and 10 adults ranging from 20 to 71 years of age.[113] The majority of patients present with a history of pneumonia.[92] A delay of 3 months to 7 years between the onset of symptoms and the diagnosis was found in one study.[114]

The abnormal tissue invariably derives its arterial supply from the aorta or one of its branches, most commonly the descending thoracic aorta and less often the abdominal aorta or one of its branches;[112] a coronary artery origin has been reported rarely.[115] The following origins were documented in one study of 105 cases:[116] descending thoracic aorta, 74; abdominal aorta, 25; intercostal artery, 5; and aortic arch, 1. Multiple tributary vessels, sometimes as many as six, were identified in some cases. Venous drainage is generally via the pulmonary venous system, producing a left-to-left shunt; occasionally, there is drainage into the inferior vena cava or azygos system.[116–118]

In approximately two thirds of cases, the sequestered portion of lung is situated in the paravertebral gutter within the posterior bronchopulmonary segment of the left lower lobe; in most others, it occupies the same anatomic region of the right lower lobe.[116, 119, 120] The upper lobes are uncommonly affected;[112, 116, 121] in these cases, the anomalous vessel commonly arises from the ascending thoracic aorta or one of its major branches, and associated cardiac malformations are common.[122] Except for these uncommon upper lobe lesions, intralobar sequestration is infrequently associated with other anomalies (in approximately 15% of cases in one review),[112] the most common being diaphragmatic hernia and a variety of skeletal and cardiac anomalies. Exceptionally, a lesion is located in the abdomen.[122a] Rarely, both intralobar and extralobar sequestration are identified in the same patient,[112] or separate sequestra are present in the right and left lungs.[123] As indicated previously, communication of the sequestered lung with the gastrointestinal tract (usually the esophagus) has been reported by several investigators.[95, 123–125] An association between intralobar sequestration and gastric duplication has also been documented in one case.[125]

Pathologic Characteristics

Morphologic findings in the affected lung are variable and depend on the degree of development of the sequestered lung tissue[77] and on the presence and severity of secondary infective changes. Grossly the abnormal tissue is usually well demarcated from surrounding lung parenchyma and consists of one or more cystic spaces with a variable amount of intervening more solid tissue (Fig. 22–3). It may have a pale or tan color in comparison with surrounding paren-

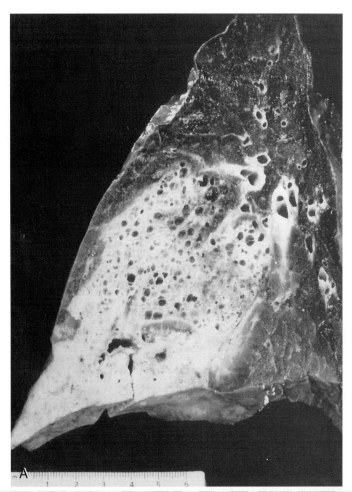

Figure 22–3. Intralobar Pulmonary Sequestration. The posterior basal region of this resected left lower lobe *(A)* shows a poorly defined area of consolidation containing numerous cystic spaces measuring 1 to 5 mm; its blood supply originated in the intra-abdominal aorta. Section through the affected lung *(B)* shows thick-walled intercommunicating cystic spaces containing numerous macrophages and cellular debris. Incidental finding in an asymptomatic 19-year-old woman. (×60.)

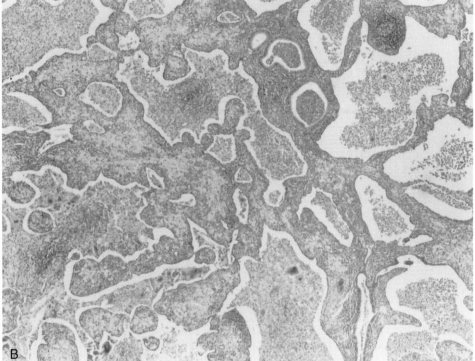

chyma owing to an absence of anthracotic pigment. The cysts are filled with mucus or, when infection is present, with pus.

Microscopically the cysts resemble dilated bronchi, with respiratory epithelium and occasional mural cartilage plates; the epithelium may be attenuated or focally absent, especially in the presence of infection. The amount of intervening parenchymal tissue varies from scanty to abundant and generally is composed of alveoli that contain intraluminal macrophages and show interstitial fibrosis and a mononuclear inflammatory infiltrate (obstructive pneumonitis). The sequestered tissue may be separated from normal lung by a well-developed fibrous capsule, or there may be an indistinct transition from one to the other, without a well-defined boundary.[122]

The sequestered segment may or may not be connected to the normal bronchial tree; in the former situation, there is usually infection in the sequestered and surrounding lung tissue. For example, in one study of 11 cases, communication between the cystic areas and branches of the bronchial tree was demonstrated in 7;[77] in all 7, the bronchial tree in the vicinity of the sequestration showed acute and chronic inflammation. Despite these observations, it appears that infection is not essential for the abnormal lung to become air containing. Of five surgical specimens studied morphologically in another investigation, three showed small communications between the cystic areas and the normal bronchial tree;[126] histologic study of the transition from the normal airways to the cysts revealed no evidence of inflammation to indicate an infectious cause of the fistulous communication, suggesting to the authors that congenital bronchocystic communications pre-existed within the pulmonary sequestration. In addition to providing a pathway for air flow, these communications may also be important in the pathogenesis of infection. In other reports in which resected specimens revealed total absence of inflammation, the authors showed that collateral ventilation had aerated the sequestered parenchyma.[127, 128]

The anomalous vessel often enters the lung by way of the lower part of the pulmonary ligament and is much larger than would be expected for the volume of tissue supplied; aneurysmal dilation has been seen in some cases.[129] It may supply only the sequestered tissue, or it may overlap with apparently normal parenchyma.[94, 122] Histologically the vessel is usually an elastic artery that shows intimal thickening and atherosclerotic changes; muscular arteries may also be seen.[112] Within the sequestration, the arteries frequently are tortuous and thick walled and usually possess distinct internal and incomplete or absent external elastic laminae. Sometimes, histologic determination of whether such vessels are systemic or pulmonary is difficult.[130] Plexogenic arteriopathy has been described in some cases.[131]

Radiologic Manifestations

The most common radiographic presentation of intralobar sequestration is as a homogeneous opacity in the posterior basal segment of a lower lobe (usually the left and almost invariably contiguous with the hemidiaphragm) (Fig. 22–4); less commonly, it presents as a cystic mass or prominent vessels (Fig. 22–5).[92, 101, 113, 132] Bilateral sequestration is exceptional.[112, 113, 124, 133, 134] In one case, the sequestration

involved an entire lung;[135] although the bronchial tree in this patient communicated with the lower end of the esophagus, the affected parenchyma was completely airless because collateral ventilation from contiguous lung was not possible.

The appearance varies somewhat depending on the volume of lung tissue sequestered, the presence or absence of infection, and the space-occupying nature of the process. The last-named feature often creates a characteristic radiographic sign that in many cases permits a presumptive diagnosis: the bronchoarterial and venous bundles of the normal lung are displaced away from or festooned around the periphery of the sequestered lobe. In instances in which no communication exists between the sequestration and the contiguous normal lung, the anomalous tissue appears as a homogeneous, sharply defined opacity. Calcification within the sequestered tissue is rare[136] but can be readily identified with CT.[113, 137, 138]

When infection has resulted in communication with the bronchial tree, the radiographic presentation consists of an air-containing cystic mass, with or without fluid levels (Fig. 22–6).[139–141] The cysts can be single or multiple and are of variable size.[122, 142] Cases have been reported in which serial radiographs have shown a transition from homogeneity to multiple cystic spaces, presumably as a result of infection (Fig. 22–7).[143] The pneumonia usually affects the surrounding parenchyma, thereby obscuring the underlying anomaly; in fact, the cystic nature of the mass may not become manifest until the pneumonia resolves. The size of the lesion can vary considerably with time, depending on the amount of gas and fluid within it; sometimes a rapidly changing radiologic pattern occurs over a short period of time.[144] Other findings that have been described in a small number of cases include decreased lung volume with mediastinal shift, prominence of the hilum, focal bronchiectasis, and cavitation.[92, 101, 109]

Definitive radiologic diagnosis is based on the demonstration of the anomalous systemic arterial supply to the sequestered lobe. This diagnosis has traditionally been made with aortography, a procedure that allows assessment of the origin of the arterial supply, the presence of one or more tributary vessels, and the assessment of the venous drainage.[116, 132] Identification of the systemic arterial supply can also be made in the majority of cases by CT (*see* Figs. 22–4 and 22–5).[101, 113, 145–147] In one review of the CT findings in 16 cases, the parenchymal abnormalities consisted of cysts with or without fluid in 7, areas of low attenuation surrounding cysts or nodules in 6, multiple dilated vessels in 2, and a soft tissue mass in 1.[113] The systemic arterial supply was identified in 13 cases (80%); however, in 2 patients in whom only one systemic artery was identified on CT, two or more anomalous systemic arteries were demonstrated at angiography or surgery. The anomalous vessel may be seen in cross-section or as an enhancing linear or tubular structure coursing from the lower thoracic or upper abdominal aorta through the inferior pulmonary ligament into the sequestered lung.[101, 113, 145, 148] The demonstration of the origin and course of the anomalous systemic vessel supplying the sequestered lung has been improved considerably with the advent of spiral CT, which allows overlapping slice reconstruction and multiplanar display.[101, 147]

The presence of areas of low attenuation in some cases (*see* Fig. 22–5) is presumably explained by collateral ventila-

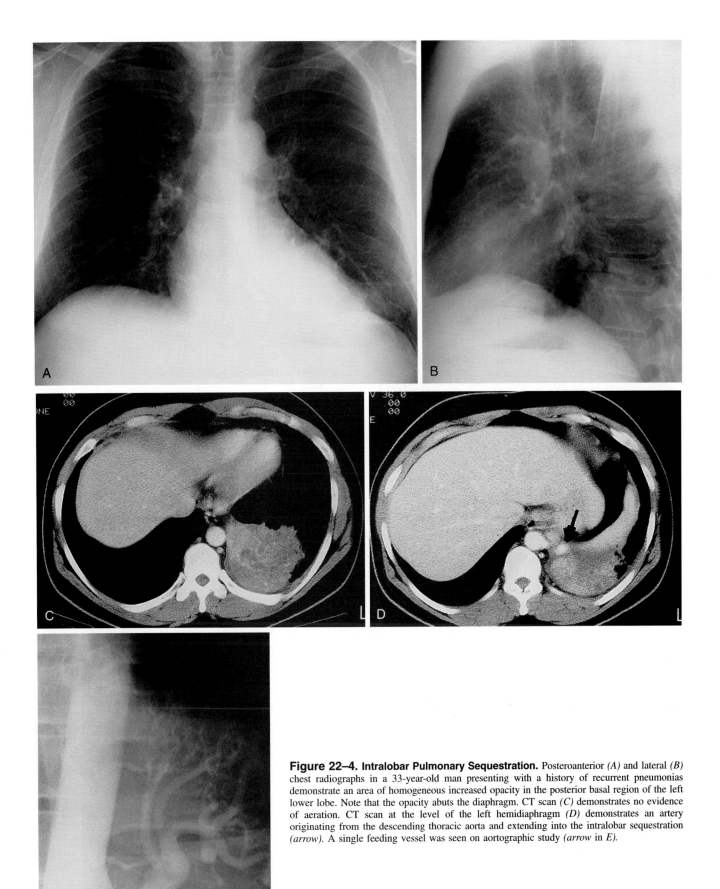

Figure 22–4. Intralobar Pulmonary Sequestration. Posteroanterior *(A)* and lateral *(B)* chest radiographs in a 33-year-old man presenting with a history of recurrent pneumonias demonstrate an area of homogeneous increased opacity in the posterior basal region of the left lower lobe. Note that the opacity abuts the diaphragm. CT scan *(C)* demonstrates no evidence of aeration. CT scan at the level of the left hemidiaphragm *(D)* demonstrates an artery originating from the descending thoracic aorta and extending into the intralobar sequestration *(arrow)*. A single feeding vessel was seen on aortographic study *(arrow in E)*.

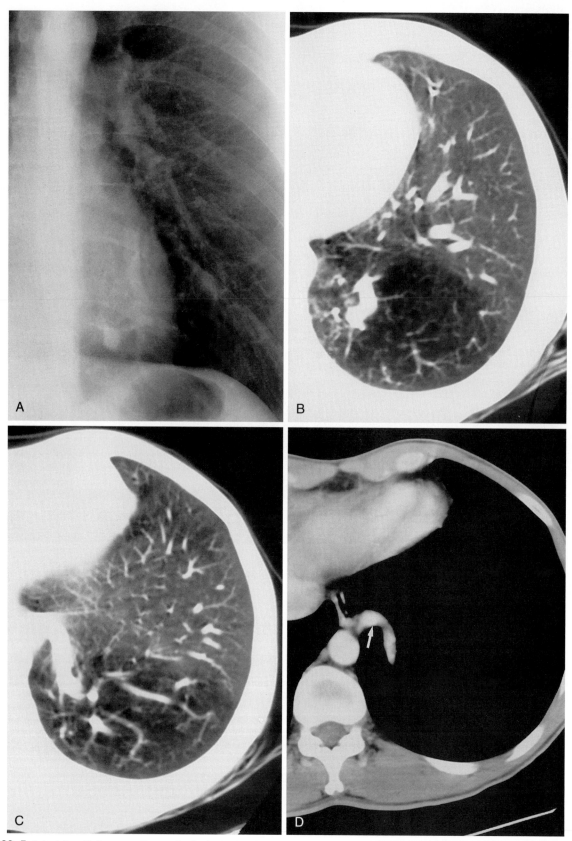

Figure 22–5. Intralobar Pulmonary Sequestration. A posteroanterior chest radiograph *(A)* in a 35-year-old man demonstrates enlarged vessels in the left lower lobe. CT scans *(B* and *C)* demonstrate an area of decreased attenuation in the posterior left lung with associated anterior displacement of the left lower lobe vessels. Contrast-enhanced CT *(D)* demonstrates that the feeding vessel *(arrow)* originates from the descending thoracic aorta.

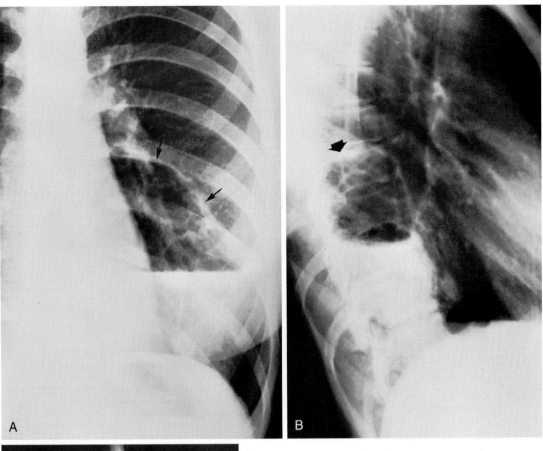

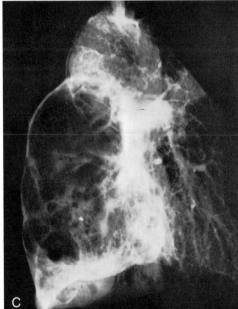

Figure 22–6. Intralobar Pulmonary Sequestration. Views of the left hemithorax in posteroanterior *(A)* and lateral *(B)* projections demonstrate a large, sharply circumscribed mass in the posteroinferior portion of the left hemithorax, containing a well-defined air-fluid level. The wall of the cavity is thin and sharply circumscribed *(arrows* in both projections). At thoracotomy, the anomalous systemic artery supplying the sequestered portion of lung was found to arise directly from the descending thoracic aorta. In a radiograph *(C)* in lateral projection of the resected left lower lobe, the cyst appears to be multiloculated.

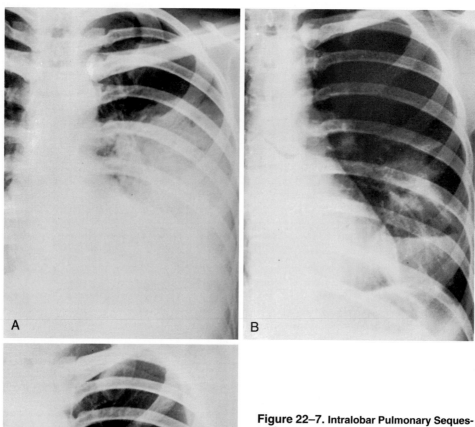

Figure 22–7. Intralobar Pulmonary Sequestration. A view of the left hemithorax from a posteroanterior radiograph *(A)* reveals massive airspace consolidation of the lower two thirds of the left lung; note the air bronchogram in the upper portion of the consolidation. Three weeks later *(B),* there is almost complete resolution of the pneumonia, but there remains a rather well-defined mass lying contiguous to the left hemidiaphragm and possessing a prominent air-fluid level. Two months later *(C),* the fluid has disappeared, leaving a thin-walled cyst measuring several centimeters in diameter and showing an irregular nubbin of tissue in its superior portion. At thoracotomy, an anomalous systemic vessel was seen to enter the sequestered mass from the diaphragm.

tion and air trapping[149] or fistulous bronchial communications after an episode of infection.[150] HRCT may demonstrate small air-containing cysts within the pulmonary sequestration.[150] Dynamic HRCT performed in one patient with multiple thin-walled cysts showed a delayed and diminished increase in lung attenuation during exhalation, indicating communication with air-containing lung and air trapping during rapid exhalation;[150] because no bronchial connection to the sequestration was demonstrated on pathologic examination, its aeration was presumably the result of collateral ventilation.

Although magnetic resonance (MR) imaging has been performed in a relatively small number of cases, it has been shown to allow excellent visualization of vessels in multiple imaging planes and therefore may obviate the need for angiography.[92, 101, 151–153] The procedure also may demonstrate vessels not visualized at arteriography.[154] Although the aberrant vessel can often be seen on conventional cardiac-gated spin-echo MR imaging, it is likely that the delineation of the feeding vessel can be improved with the use of newer gradient-echo techniques.[101, 155] Both CT and MR imaging may fail to demonstrate small aberrant vessels; thus, angiography may still be required to confirm the diagnosis and to demonstrate the course of the vessels that supply the sequestered tissue.[101]

The diagnosis should be considered in any child or young adult with persistent or recurrent lower lobe pneumonia.[92, 101] The radiologic differential diagnosis includes bronchiectasis, lung abscess, empyema, primary or metastatic neoplasm, hernia of Bochdalek, bronchogenic cyst, and congenital cystic adenomatoid malformation.[84, 141, 156]

Clinical Manifestations

Most patients are asymptomatic until an acute respiratory infection develops; in many cases, this does not happen until adulthood.[119, 156] Signs and symptoms are then usually those of acute lower lobe pneumonia, the basic defect becoming apparent only through radiologic observation of the sequence of changes during resolution of the infection. Infections are usually caused by nontuberculous bacteria; however, tuberculous,[100, 157, 158] nocardial,[159] and fungal[158, 160] causes have also been reported. A case of fungus ball formation has also been documented.[161]

Other clinical manifestations are seen occasionally. In one report of two infants, the clinical presentation was of breathlessness;[162] huge space-occupying cysts were found, apparently under tension. Similar symptoms may be caused by spontaneous pneumothorax resulting from rupture of a cyst.[163] An unusual complication, seen most commonly in children if not unique to this age group, is cardiac decompensation,[164, 165] presumably caused by a voluminous left-to-left shunt from systemic artery to pulmonary vein. A continuous murmur related to the anomalous vessel has occasionally been reported.[156] Hemorrhage (sometimes massive) can occur into the bronchi,[166] esophagus,[167] or pleural cavity.[168, 169] Rarely, neoplasms—including carcinoma,[170, 171] carcinoid tumor,[172] and solitary fibrous tumor[173]—have been found to arise within the sequestered tissue.

Extralobar Sequestration

Extralobar pulmonary sequestration is less common than intralobar sequestration, accounting for approximately 25% of cases.[101, 112] It is related to the left hemidiaphragm in 90% of cases[174] and may be situated between the inferior surface of the lower lobe and the diaphragm, immediately beneath or within the substance of the diaphragm,[175] or in the mediastinum or retroperitoneum.[176, 177] The systemic arterial supply is commonly from the abdominal aorta or one of its branches; the vessels may be multiple and small.[119] In contrast to intralobar sequestration, drainage is usually via the systemic venous system—the inferior vena cava, the azygos or hemiazygos veins, or the portal venous system[178, 179]—resulting in a left-to-right shunt.

The anomaly is most often seen in neonates, in many cases associated with other congenital anomalies.[119, 163, 174, 180–182] Eventration or paralysis of the ipsilateral hemidiaphragm is present in approximately 60% of cases and left-sided diaphragmatic hernias in approximately 30%;[57, 112, 183] this high incidence has been attributed to interference with normal closure of the pleuroperitoneal canal by the sequestered mass.[95] Depending on the volume of sequestered tissue and presence of associated diaphragmatic abnormalities, a variable degree of ipsilateral pulmonary hypoplasia is usually present.

Morphologically the sequestered tissue is completely enclosed in a pleural sac, which may have prominent lymphatic channels.[184] The cut surface has a spongy, tan-colored

appearance with two or more vessels often more prominent at one end of the specimen. Airways are usually few in number and show only sparse cartilage and seromucinous glands. Some lesions (particularly those situated in the abdomen) resemble congenital cystic adenomatoid malformation (type 2).[185] Parenchymal tissue is often immature but corresponds roughly to the expected architecture for age. Fibrosis and inflammation may be seen in older children and adults. Rarely, necrotizing vasculitis unassociated with similar changes in other systemic or pulmonary vessels has been demonstrated;[186, 187] although the pathogenesis of this is uncertain, it has been regarded as an effect of systemic pressure on vessels in the sequestered segment.

The radiographic findings typically consist of a sharply defined, triangular-shaped opacity in the posterior costophrenic angle, as indicated previously, usually adjacent to the left hemidiaphragm.[112, 174, 183] It may also appear as a small bump on the left hemidiaphragm.[183] Less commonly, the abnormality presents as a mass in the upper thorax, mediastinum, paravertebral region, or (rarely) subdiaphragmatic region.[176, 183, 188] Aortography usually demonstrates the anomalous systemic arterial supply;[112, 183] multiple feeding vessels can be demonstrated in about 20% of cases.[183] Identification of the venous drainage may necessitate selective catheterization of the feeding vessel(s).[183]

The CT findings consist most commonly of a homogeneous opacity or well-circumscribed mass.[113, 183] Cystic areas are occasionally seen within the sequestration.[113] In one study of eight patients, areas of low attenuation in the surrounding nonsequestered lung were described in seven.[113] CT is of limited value in demonstrating the vascular supply; in one review of 24 cases of sequestration, an anomalous systemic artery was identified on CT in 13 of 16 (81%) that were intralobar but only 3 of 8 (37%) that were extralobar.[113]

Because an extralobar sequestered segment is enveloped in its own pleural sac, the chances of its becoming infected are small unless there is communication with the gastrointestinal tract.[95] Consequently the chief mode of presentation is as an asymptomatic soft tissue mass discovered during investigation of an infant with other congenital anomalies. Rarely the chest radiograph is initially normal, sequestration subsequently becoming evident as a result of an acute episode, such as spontaneous hemorrhage.[188] Other complications include infarction,[189] arteriovenous shunt,[190] or respiratory distress secondary to the sequestered tissue itself[191] or to an associated pleural effusion or hemothorax.[192, 193] Because of symptoms related to associated congenital anomalies, most cases are discovered in early childhood (approximately 60% in the first 6 months of life).[183]

CONGENITAL BRONCHOGENIC CYSTS

Intrathoracic cysts derived from the foregut may be classified into three major categories depending on their presumed embryologic derivation:[194] (1) *paravertebral (enteric) cysts*, arising from a primordial foregut that has herniated through a split in the notochord and is often associated with spinal anomalies (split notochord syndrome) (*see* page 2979); (2) *esophageal cysts (esophageal duplication)*, resulting from failure of the originally solid esophagus to produce a hollow tube completely (*see* page 2943); and (3) *bronchogenic cysts*, resulting from abnormal budding of the developing tracheobronchial tree. Rare examples of intrapulmonary enteric cysts lined by gastric or duodenal epithelium and presumably derived from intrapulmonary foregut buds that retain the capacity for this form of differentiation have also been reported.[195, 196]

As indicated, bronchogenic cysts are believed to represent localized portions of the tracheobronchial tree that become separated from normal airways during the branching process and do not undergo further development. They are thought by some authors to represent one end of a spectrum of pathogenetically similar conditions, including extralobar and intralobar sequestration and (possibly) congenital cystic bronchiectasis.[125, 197, 198] The great majority probably develop between the 26th and the 40th day of intrauterine life, during the most active period of airway development. As in bronchopulmonary sequestration, the timing of the abnormal budding may determine the eventual location of the cyst: if it occurs at an early stage when there is little tissue surrounding the developing airways, the anomalous bud is likely to remain in the mediastinum; if later, the abnormal branch is more apt to be contained within lung tissue already present and thus have an intrapulmonary location.

Approximately 65% to 90% of bronchogenic cysts occur in the mediastinum; almost all the remainder are present in the lungs.[199–202] Rare examples are also found in the pericardium, thymus, diaphragm, retroperitoneum, or cervical region.[202–206] In one unusual case, a cyst arising in relation to the right hemidiaphragm had a dumbbell configuration, one part being within the thorax and readily visible radiographically and the other part being intra-abdominal and visible only by CT.[207]

Although they have been observed in fetuses and newborns,[99, 208] the majority of cysts come to attention in early adult life. In two reviews, the average age at thoracotomy was 24 and 35 years (range, 1 to 48 and 8 to 62 years).[197, 202] The anomaly appears to have a predilection for males[209, 210] and for Yemenite Jews.[211, 212]

Pathologic Characteristics

Bronchogenic cysts are usually solitary, thin-walled, unilocular, and roughly spherical in shape (Figs. 22–8 and 22–9). They are filled with either mucoid or serous fluid and do not communicate with the tracheobronchial tree unless they become infected, in which case the cyst fluid may be replaced by pus or by pus and air. Aspiration of the cyst may yield mucus and bronchial epithelial cells, confirming the diagnosis.[213] A case has also been reported in which both the serum and the cyst contents contained high levels of the tumor marker CA 19-9.[214]

Histologically the cyst wall is lined by a pseudostratified, ciliated epithelium, often with focal (occasionally ex-

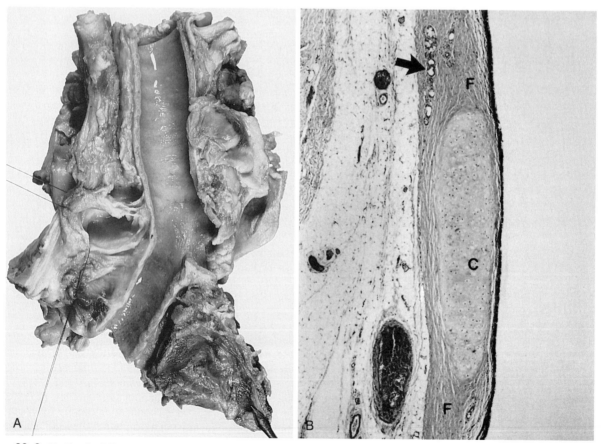

Figure 22–8. Mediastinal Bronchogenic Cyst. A unilocular cyst approximately 2 cm in greatest dimension is present in the connective tissue adjacent to the trachea just above the origin of the left main bronchus *(A)*. A histologic section of cyst wall *(B)* shows cartilage (C), seromucinous glands *(arrow)*, and fibrous tissue (F). At this magnification, the respiratory epithelial lining is evident only as a dark line to the right of the cartilage. Incidental finding in a 65-year-old woman.

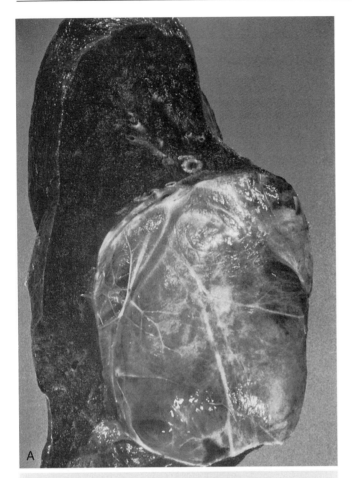

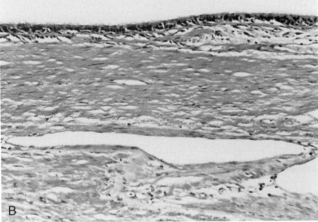

Figure 22–9. Pulmonary Bronchogenic Cyst. A slice of lower lobe of the patient whose radiograph is shown in Figure 22–10. A well-circumscribed cyst with a smooth inner surface is shown *(A)*. A histologic section *(B)* shows the cyst to be lined by respiratory epithelium overlying fibrous tissue; occasional foci of smooth muscle were identified elsewhere.

tensive) areas of metaplastic squamous or attenuated cuboidal epithelium.[215] The wall typically contains cartilage and strands of smooth muscle; sometimes, seromucinous bronchial-type glands are also evident (*see* Fig. 22–8). The presence of these structures, especially cartilage, is important for the diagnosis: although intrapulmonary cysts that do not contain cartilage and glands in their wall may represent bronchogenic cysts, the walls of healed abscess cavities may

have an epithelial lining, sometimes ciliated and pseudostratified, presumably as a result of ingrowth from communicating airway epithelium.[216] On the other hand, the epithelium and other cyst wall components of a bronchogenic cyst may be destroyed if it becomes secondarily infected, so that their absence does not exclude a congenital origin in the presence of inflammation. In practice, therefore, it may be impossible to differentiate an infected intrapulmonary bronchogenic cyst from an acquired infected bulla or abscess solely on morphologic criteria, and prior radiographic evidence may be necessary for precise classification.

Although the morphologic features of mediastinal bronchogenic cysts are much less likely to be altered by infection, difficulty in precise diagnosis of a "bronchial" origin may also occur. Because esophageal epithelium is ciliated and pseudostratified in early embryonic development and because seromucinous glands similar to bronchial glands may exist in the normal esophagus, it is possible that a mediastinal cyst that does not contain cartilage and that is situated posteriorly may be of esophageal derivation.[215] Because of these potential diagnostic difficulties, mediastinal cysts that contain only respiratory-type epithelium without additional structures that indicate a bronchial origin are probably best classified imprecisely as simple or nonspecific cysts.[199, 215]

Pulmonary Bronchogenic Cysts

Radiologic Manifestations

The typical appearance of an intrapulmonary bronchogenic cyst is a sharply circumscribed, round or oval nodule or mass, usually in the medial third of the lungs. There is a predilection for the lower lobes: in one report of 32 cases, almost two thirds were in this location with equal distribution in the two lungs.[217] Serial radiographs usually show little change in the size and shape of the mass with time, although previous radiographs show an abnormality in only about 50% of symptomatic patients.[218] In one exceptional case, multiple cysts were observed to develop over a 2-year period.[219]

Characteristically, the lesions do not communicate with the tracheobronchial tree until they become infected, a complication that occurs in about 75% of cases recognized clinically. When communication is established, the cyst contains air, with or without fluid (Fig. 22–10).[217] If the patient presents initially with an infected cyst, the usual sharp definition of the lesion may be obscured by consolidation of surrounding parenchyma, the true nature of the abnormality becoming apparent only when the pneumonitis has resolved. Air-containing cysts may increase in size as a result of a check-valve mechanism (Fig. 22–11).[220] Rarely, a cyst is large enough to compress an adjacent airway and cause atelectasis.[208] Calcification of the cyst wall can be seen in some cases (Fig. 22–12).[215, 221] Occasionally, the cyst fluid itself contains sufficient calcium to be seen radiographically;[222] in one case, this appeared as an opacity that changed position within the cyst when the patient changed position.[208]

As discussed previously, it may be difficult to differentiate bronchogenic from acquired cysts; because most of the latter are the residua of remote lung abscesses, a history of an acute respiratory episode may be helpful in suggesting

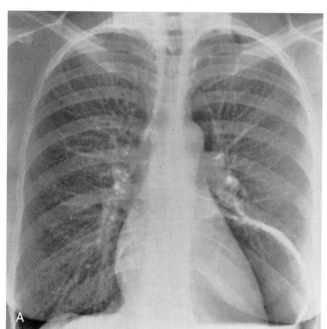
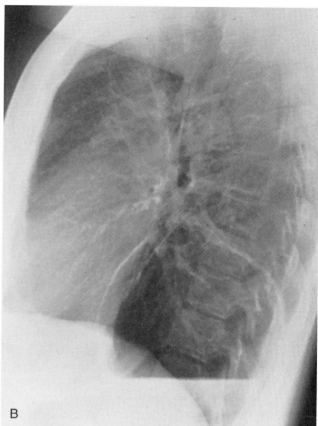

Figure 22–10. Congenital Bronchogenic Cyst. Posteroanterior *(A)* and lateral *(B)* radiographs reveal a large cystic space in the left lower lobe containing a prominent fluid level. The cyst wall measured a maximum of 3 mm in width. Same patient as Figure 22–9.

the latter diagnosis. A bulla may also have an identical appearance as that of a communicating bronchogenic cyst; unless pulmonary emphysema is present to suggest this, pathologic examination may be necessary to differentiate the two.

In some cases, a confident diagnosis can be made on CT based on the presence of nonenhancing homogeneous attenuation at or near water density (0 to 20 HU) and a smooth thin wall.[85, 148, 202] In approximately 50% of cases, the cysts have higher than water density as a result of the presence of proteinaceous material or calcium (Fig. 22–13).[223, 224] When infected, the cysts may have inhomogeneous enhancement and resemble an abscess.[225] The cysts may also be air filled and multilocular.[202] MR imaging is superior to CT in diagnosis.[225, 226] The characteristic appearance on T2-weighted spin-echo images consists of homogeneous high-signal intensity approximating that of cerebrospinal fluid. The signal intensity on T1-weighted images is intermediate between that of muscle and subcutaneous fat.[226] Infected cysts may have intermediate signal intensity on both T1-weighted and T2-weighted images and be indistinguishable from an abscess.[225]

Clinical Manifestations

In adults, the majority of uninfected bronchogenic cysts cause no symptoms and are discovered by accident on a screening chest radiograph.[227] Symptoms—of which hemoptysis is perhaps the most common—are almost always sec-

ondary to infection in and around the cyst.[210, 229, 230] Organisms cultured from such sites are usually bacteria (including rare examples of *Mycobacteria*).[218] Other, rare complications include pneumothorax, air embolism (in one case during decompression after construction work in a tunnel and in another during air travel[228, 231]), and adenocarcinoma.[232] As indicated previously, communication between a cyst and the tracheobronchial tree may incorporate a check-valve mechanism that results in rapid expansion of the cyst;[220] such an air space may become so large as to compress the mediastinum, causing cardiac embarrassment and even death.[233]

Mediastinal Bronchogenic Cysts

Mediastinal bronchogenic cysts may be classified into five types depending on their site of origin: paratracheal, carinal, hilar, paraesophageal, and miscellaneous;[234] the first two are the most common.[202, 217] Among the miscellaneous sites are the thymus, pericardium, and anterolateral surface of a thoracic vertebral body.[202] Cysts within the pericardium usually arise between the root of the aorta and the superior vena cava and thus may displace the mediastinal vessels and the heart.[221, 235] Coexistence of a bronchogenic cyst with a partial pericardial defect has been documented in some patients.[236] The vast majority of mediastinal bronchogenic cysts are solitary; in one patient, two cysts were identified, one in relation to the left hilum and the other in the posterior mediastinum caudally.[237]

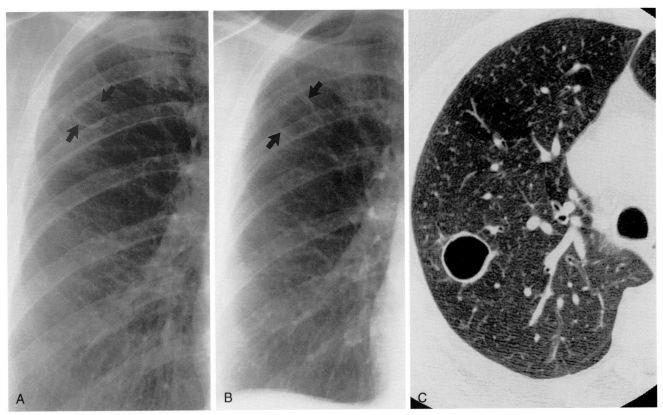

Figure 22–11. Pulmonary Bronchogenic Cyst. A view of right lung from a posteroanterior chest radiograph *(A)* in a 54-year-old woman who presented with a single episode of productive, foul-smelling sputum demonstrates a thin-walled 1.5-cm-diameter cyst *(arrows)* in the right upper lobe. A posteroanterior chest radiograph obtained 5 months later *(B)* demonstrates increase in size of the cyst *(arrows)*. HRCT *(C)* essentially confirms the radiographic findings.

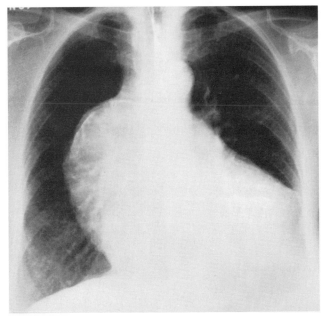

Figure 22–12. Mediastinal Bronchogenic Cyst with a Calcified Wall. A posteroanterior radiograph reveals a large anterior mediastinal mass projecting chiefly to the right of the midline and showing prominent calcification on its superior and lateral aspects. The resected specimen proved to be a huge bronchogenic cyst with a partially calcified wall.

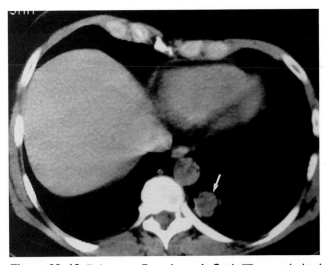

Figure 22–13. Pulmonary Bronchogenic Cyst. CT scan at the level of the diaphragm shows a 2.5-cm-diameter nodule with soft tissue attenuation *(arrow)* in the left lower lobe. The patient was a 48-year-old woman in whom the nodule was detected incidentally on the chest radiograph. At surgery, it was shown to be a bronchogenic cyst associated with hypoplasia of the posterior basal segmental bronchus.

Radiologic Manifestations

Mediastinal bronchogenic cysts usually present as clearly defined masses of homogeneous density in the right paratracheal region (Fig. 22–14) or just inferior to and slightly to the right of the carina, overlapping the right hilar shadow (Fig. 22–15). The majority are oval or round; the shape may vary with inspiration and expiration. In contrast to pulmonary bronchogenic cysts, the mediastinal variety rarely communicates with the tracheobronchial tree.[238] Thus, infection is less likely, and the cysts may grow to a large size before being recognized. In one report, a cyst measured 5 × 15 × 23 cm, almost completely filling the right thoracic cavity;[239] of some interest is the fact that 5 years earlier the cyst measured only 5 × 5 × 10 cm. Such cysts may compress adjacent structures (Fig. 22–16) and (rarely) rupture (Fig. 22–17);[240] the latter complication may result in pneumothorax.[241] Calcification of the cyst wall is uncommon[221] but can occasionally be seen radiographically (*see* Fig. 22–12).[215] Pleural effusion is rare.[242]

The cysts can be identified on the chest radiograph in about 90% to 95% of cases;[202, 243] those not visible are usually in the subcarinal region.[202] As might be expected, CT is even more sensitive; in two series of surgically treated cysts, it allowed visualization of all lesions.[223, 243] The procedure also confirms the cystic and benign nature of the lesion in 50% to 60% of cases. A diagnosis of a benign cyst can be confidently made on CT when it demonstrates a homogeneous attenuation at or near water density (0 to 20 HU) (*see* Fig. 22–14).[202, 223] In approximately 50% of patients, the cysts have higher attenuation (ranging up to 130 HU) and therefore are indistinguishable from soft tissue lesions (*see* Fig. 22–16). This increase in attenuation is the result of a high protein level or calcium oxalate in the mucoid cyst contents.[223, 244]

The difficulty in distinguishing a soft tissue lesion from a cystic one may be resolved by MR imaging. With this procedure, bronchogenic cysts demonstrate variable signal intensity on T1-weighted images but characteristically have high signal intensity on T2-weighted sequences (*see* Fig. 22–16).[225, 226] The signal intensity on T1-weighted images is influenced by the specific gravity of the fluid: if the fluid within a cyst is mainly serous and has a low specific gravity, it has a lower signal intensity on T1-weighted images; cysts with a large amount of proteinaceous material have high signal intensity on T1-weighted images.[202] Thus, bronchogenic cysts with soft tissue density on CT have high signal intensity on T1-weighted images. Regardless of the protein content, the fluid nature of the cyst results in high signal intensity on the T2-weighted images. When the cysts abut the chest wall or esophagus, the cystic nature of the lesion may also be determined using ultrasonography.[202, 244a]

Clinical Manifestations

Many patients with mediastinal bronchogenic cysts are asymptomatic;[227, 245] however, in one surgical review of 69 patients, almost two thirds complained of a symptom attributable to the cyst.[246] The location of the cyst appears to be more important than size in this respect;[246] those in the carinal area particularly may cause pressure symptoms even when quite small and radiographically invisible.[247] Signs and symptoms are more common in infants and children than adults and may simulate those related to a vascular ring (sling), tracheal or bronchial stenosis (sometimes resembling asthma), an aspirated foreign body, or bronchiolitis.[248]

Symptoms include dyspnea on effort, stridor, persistent cough, and chest pain.[214, 249] Symptomatic compression of the heart or great vessels can also occur, as exemplified by cysts that caused paroxysmal atrial fibrillation,[250] superior vena cava syndrome,[227] and pulmonary artery stenosis.[251, 252] Rarely, symptoms related to vascular or airway compression progress rapidly and seriously compromise the patient.[245, 246, 252] The cyst may recur after partial resection,[253, 254] sometimes after many years.[255] As with pulmonary bronchogenic cysts,

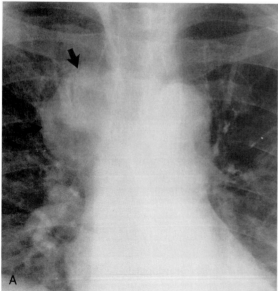
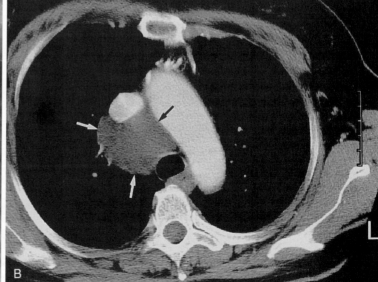

Figure 22–14. Mediastinal Bronchogenic Cyst. A view from a posteroanterior chest radiograph *(A)* in a 60-year-old woman demonstrates a right paratracheal mass *(arrow)*. Contrast-enhanced CT scan *(B)* demonstrates that the lesion *(arrows)* has homogeneous water density characteristic of a bronchogenic cyst. The attenuation value was 9 HU.

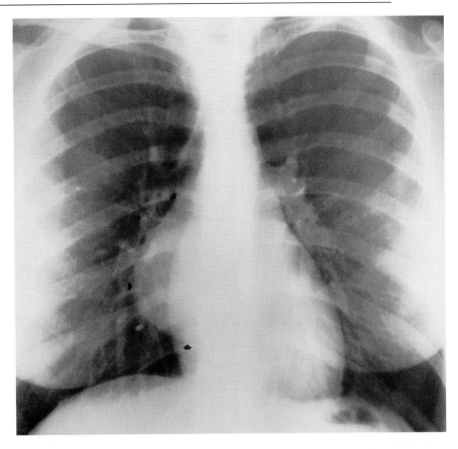

Figure 22–15. Mediastinal Bronchogenic Cyst. A conventional posteroanterior chest radiograph discloses a homogeneous soft tissue mass beneath the carina *(arrowheads)*. The anatomic location, shape, and radiographic features are highly suggestive of a mediastinal bronchogenic cyst.

the development of carcinoma is a rare complication in a mediastinal cyst.[255a]

CONGENITAL BRONCHIECTASIS

Congenital bronchiectasis is much rarer than the acquired disease and has been hypothesized to be secondary to incomplete branching of the developing bronchial tree.[256, 257] Morphologically, there is tubular dilation of almost all bronchi in a lobe or lung extending to a level just beneath the pleural surface.[257] Microscopically the bronchi end abruptly in a small amount of peripheral parenchymal tissue, which is itself abnormal, containing only scattered alveoli, abnormal bundles of smooth muscle, and small foci of lymphangiectasis; inflammation is typically mild.

Several patients have also been described with bronchiectasis that became manifest in infancy or early childhood and that was associated with otherwise normal lung.[258, 259] Some of these patients have a familial history of the abnormality, suggesting a genetic defect.[260, 261] Histologic analysis of some affected lungs has shown a marked deficiency of cartilage in segmental and subsegmental airways, considered to be the result of a developmental defect.[258, 259] Patients usually present in infancy with cough and recurrent respiratory tract infection.

CONGENITAL CYSTIC ADENOMATOID MALFORMATION

The term *congenital cystic adenomatoid malformation* refers to a group of several pathologically distinct abnormalities characterized by architecturally abnormal pulmonary tissue with or without gross cyst formation. When present, the cysts can usually be shown to communicate with normal airways. Most often, the vascular supply is via the pulmonary circulation; however, some cases have been shown to have a systemic blood supply.[262, 263] Although three major types of malformation have been described (*see* farther on), the pathologic and clinical differences between them and the lack of overlap forms suggest that their grouping together under a single term may not have an etiologic or pathogenetic basis.

As might be expected, the majority of cases are discovered in the very young. In one review of 142 cases from the literature and 17 new cases, 62% of patients presented between birth and 1 month of age;[264] an additional 24% of cases became manifest after 1 month, mostly in the first 5 years of life. Cases have also been discovered in adults up to about 60 years of age.[265, 265a, 265b]

The cause and pathogenesis are unknown. The anomaly has been considered by some authors to represent a hamartoma;[266] however, most believe that it results from localized arrested development of the fetal bronchial tree.[267, 268] Occasional cases are associated with bronchial atresia of the affected lobe,[269, 270] and it has also been suggested that the abnormality may be related to bronchial obstruction.[267]

The condition has been divided into three major morphologic subtypes.[264, 266, 271, 272] The *Type I* (cystic) form consists of a large, often multiloculated cyst sometimes associated with several smaller cysts in the adjacent parenchyma. This is the most common type, comprising 29 (53%) of the 55 cases in two series.[264, 271] The cyst wall contains smooth muscle but usually no cartilage and is lined mostly by

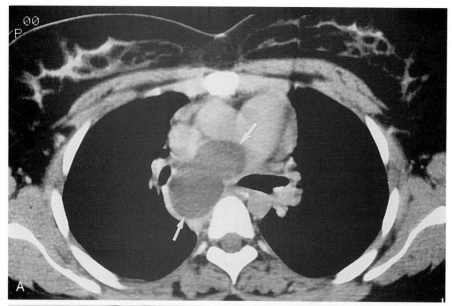

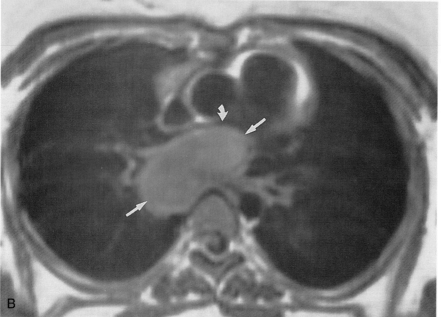

Figure 22–16. Mediastinal Broncho-genic Cyst. Contrast-enhanced CT scan *(A)* in a 26-year-old woman demonstrates a dumbbell-shaped mass *(arrows)* with inhomogeneous attenuation in the subcarinal region. The attenuation values within the mass were greater than 20 HU. Transverse T1-weighted (TR 645, TE 20) MR image *(B)* demonstrates a slightly inhomogeneous mass *(straight arrows)* with a signal similar to that of chest wall muscle. Note marked narrowing of the right pulmonary artery *(curved arrow)*. Transverse T2-weighted (TR 2581, TE 90) spin-echo MR image *(C)* demonstrates homogeneous high-signal intensity *(arrows)* characteristic of a fluid-filled cyst. At surgery, the lesion was shown to be a mediastinal bronchogenic cyst associated with a partial pericardial defect.

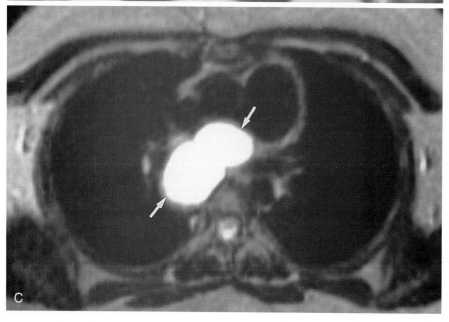

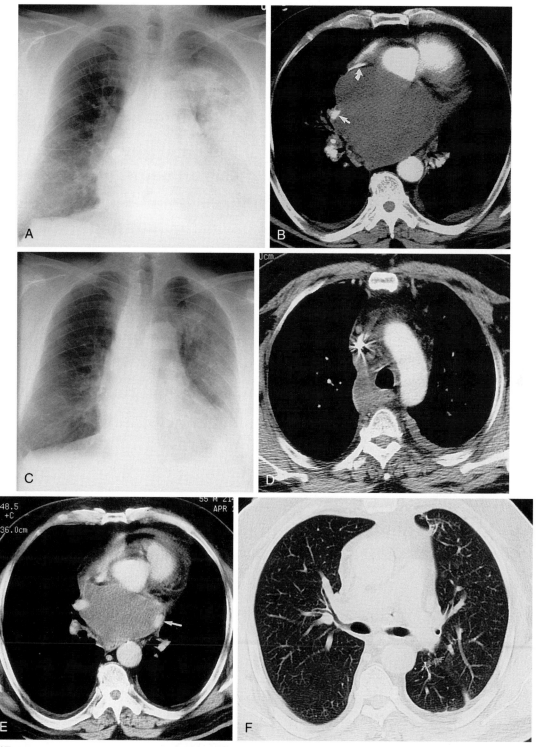

Figure 22–17. Mediastinal Bronchogenic Cyst with Spontaneous Rupture. Posteroanterior chest radiograph *(A)* in a 55-year-old man demonstrates extensive consolidation in the left upper lobe and small bilateral pleural effusions. CT scan *(B)* demonstrates a large cystic mass with homogeneous water density in the subcarinal region consistent with a mediastinal bronchogenic cyst. Note that the right superior pulmonary vein is seen *(straight arrow)* but that the left superior pulmonary vein is not being compressed by the mass. Note displacement of the superior vena cava *(curved arrow)*. Also noted are small bilateral pleural effusions. Chest radiograph performed 3 days later *(C)* shows marked improvement in the left upper lobe consolidation. In the interval, the patient has developed increased opacity in the right paratracheal region with associated displacement of the trachea. Contrast-enhanced CT scan *(D)* at the level of the aortic arch demonstrates fluid in the right paratracheal region. CT scan at a lower level *(E)* demonstrates marked decrease in size of the subcarinal cyst. Note that the left superior pulmonary vein is now seen *(arrow)*. CT scan 3 days later *(F)* shows resolution of the consolidation in the left upper lobe. At this time, the fluid in the paratracheal region had been almost completely resorbed, and the subcarinal cyst had shown further decrease in size. The consolidation in the left upper lobe presumably represented pulmonary edema due to compression of the left superior pulmonary vein. This edema resolved after spontaneous rupture of the cyst. (Case courtesy of Dr. Carole Dennie, Department of Radiological Sciences, Ottawa Civic Hospital, Ottawa, Canada.)

bronchiolar-type epithelium; foci of columnar mucus-secreting epithelium are also commonly present and may be seen in lung tissue adjacent to the cyst where they appear in a lepidic pattern identical to that of bronchioloalveolar carcinoma (Fig. 22–18).[273] The *Type II* (intermediate) form (21 [38%] of 55 cases) is composed of solid areas separated by numerous, fairly evenly spaced cysts measuring 1 to 10 mm and lined by ciliated columnar or cuboidal epithelium. In some[271] but not all[264] studies, a large proportion of patients with Type II lesions have had coexistent congenital anomalies that often masked pulmonary symptoms. The *Type III* (solid) form (5 [9%] of 55 cases) is manifested by a bulky, more-or-less solid mass of tissue without gross cyst formation. Microscopically the abnormal tissue is composed primarily of irregularly shaped bronchiolar and alveolar-like structures that resemble terminal air spaces of the pseudoglandular period of fetal development.

In the newborn, the radiographic findings consist of a homogeneous opacity, which, in the case of Type I and II lesions, usually becomes air filled over a few days to several weeks.[274] The abnormality has been reported to involve the upper lobes slightly more commonly than the lower lobes, multilobar involvement being present in approximately 15%

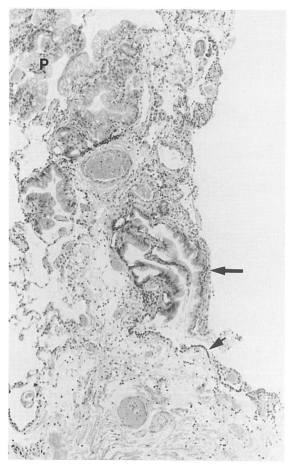

Figure 22–18. Congenital Cystic Adenomatoid Malformation. A section through the cyst wall illustrated in Figure 22–21 shows it to be lined by a low cuboidal *(short arrow)* or columnar, mucus-secreting *(long arrow)* epithelium. The latter epithelium is also present in the lung parenchyma adjacent to the cyst (P), where it lines alveolar septa and resembles bronchioloalveolar carcinoma. (Courtesy of Dr. L. Bouchard, Verdun General Hospital, Montreal, Canada.)

of cases;[264] rare cases involve an entire lung.[275] In older children and adults, the lesion presents most commonly as a lower lobe mass composed of numerous air-containing cysts scattered irregularly through tissue of unit density (Fig. 22–19). It is space occupying, expanding the ipsilateral hemithorax and shifting the mediastinum to the contralateral side. Occasionally, one cyst preferentially expands, creating a single lucent area (Fig. 22–20).[271] The cysts may contain fluid or air, or both, and occasionally fluid levels may be seen (Fig. 22–21); only rarely does fluid completely fill the cysts, resulting in complete radiographic opacification.[271] Owing to the absence of cystic spaces in the Type III lesion, radiographs reveal only a large homogeneous mass.[276]

CT is superior to chest radiography in demonstrating both the cystic and the solid components of the abnormality.[277–279] In one review of seven adult cases, the findings consisted of multiple thin-walled, complex cystic masses ranging from 4 to 12 cm in diameter.[278] Five of the patients had Type I lesions with at least one cyst greater than 2 cm in diameter. Two patients had Type II malformation with multiple thin-walled cysts ranging from 2 to 20 mm in diameter. In all seven cases, the abnormality involved the lower lobes and was associated with displacement and splaying of vessels in an area of adjacent hyperlucent lung. In another review of the CT findings in 21 children, the malformation involved a total of 26 lobes, including the lower lobes in 69% of cases, the upper lobes in 27%, and the right middle lobe in 4%.[279]

Clinically the majority of patients present with increasing respiratory distress in the neonatal period, the severity being related chiefly to the volume of lung involved. A minority of patients—approximately 15% in one study[264]—present with cough and fever, with or without recurrent respiratory infections;[278] most of these are older than 1 month of age. Spontaneous pneumothorax occurs occasionally.[57, 278] Lesions are sometimes discovered in asymptomatic patients by routine chest radiography. Some cases, particularly of the Type I form, are complicated by mucin-secreting bronchioloalveolar carcinoma.[280–282] The incidence of maternal hydramnios and neonatal anasarca is fairly high; the latter has been thought to result from obstruction of venous return by the expanding mass.[272]

CONGENITAL TRACHEOBRONCHIAL STENOSIS

Several intrinsic anomalies of the tracheobronchial tree can result in airway narrowing. Abnormalities of the cartilaginous skeleton can occur either alone or in association with a variety of systemic osteocartilaginous defects.[283] Localized absence of tracheal cartilage usually results in tracheomalacia, with resultant expiratory airway obstruction and repeated bouts of bronchopneumonia. Incomplete segmentation of the tracheal cartilage rings may be focal or diffuse and can result in defective formation of the posterior membranous sheath and transformation of the trachea into a cartilaginous tube. This can be either cylindrical or tapered caudally, forming the so-called funnel or carrot-shaped trachea. Rarely, these changes are of sufficient severity to result in clinically significant tracheal stenosis,[283] frequently associated with anomalous origin of the left pulmonary artery (*see* page 638).

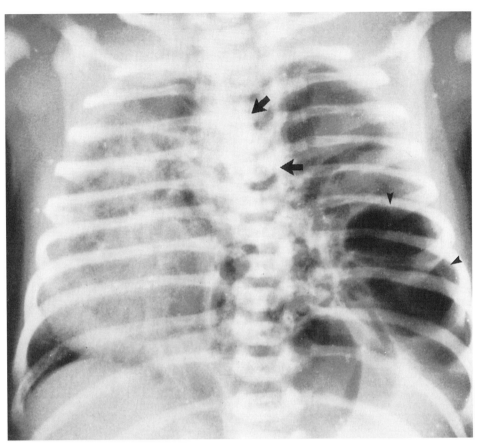

Figure 22–19. Congenital Cystic Adenomatoid Malformation of the Lung. An anteroposterior chest radiograph of a male infant reveals a gas-filled lucency in the left lower hemithorax caused by the gastric fundus *(arrowheads)* protruding through a congenital diaphragmatic hernia. Projected superiorly and medially is a vaguely defined cystic and solid lesion *(arrows)* overlying the thoracic spine that was ultimately shown at surgery to represent an adenomatoid malformation of the left lung. Note the extreme mediastinal displacement to the right occasioned by the combined diaphragmatic and pulmonary abnormalities.

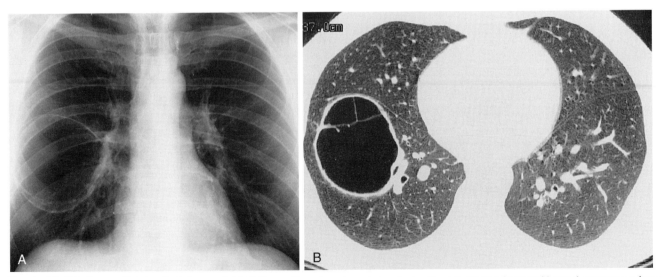

Figure 22–20. Congenital Cystic Adenomatoid Malformation. A posteroanterior chest radiograph *(A)* in a 31-year-old man demonstrates a large cystic lesion in the right lower lobe. HRCT scan *(B)* shows a few septations within the thin-walled cyst. At surgery, this was shown to be a Type I cystic adenomatoid malformation.

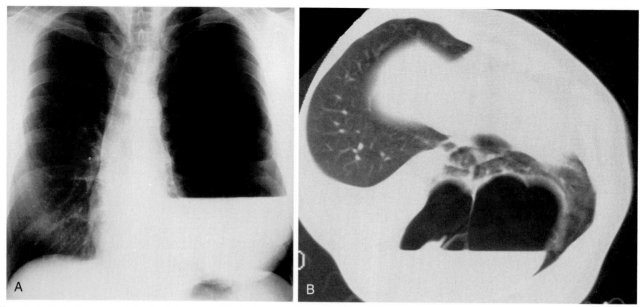

Figure 22–21. Congenital Cystic Adenomatoid Malformation. A posteroanterior chest radiograph *(A)* in a 34-year-old man demonstrates a large air-fluid level in the left lower lobe. The volume of the left lung is increased and associated with mild contralateral mediastinal shift. A CT scan *(B)* demonstrates thin-walled cystic lesions with air-fluid levels in the basal segments of the left lower lobe. The diagnosis of congenital cystic adenomatoid malformation was confirmed at surgery. (Courtesy of Dr. L. Bouchard, Verdun General Hospital, Montreal, Canada.)

Similar quantitative and qualitative cartilaginous abnormalities that result in localized airway narrowing can occasionally occur within main, lobar, or segmental bronchi.[283a–c] Other causes of localized bronchial stenosis include atresia (*see* farther on), apparent hypoplasia,[283c] and occlusive fibrous webs.[283c] All these anomalies usually manifest themselves early in the neonatal period by respiratory distress, stridor, or recurrent pneumonia. They are often associated with other congenital anomalies, the most common being the skeletal dysplasia syndromes.[57] They may also be associated with neonatal lobar hyperinflation (*see* farther on) and (possibly) with sudden death.[299]

CONGENITAL BRONCHIAL ATRESIA

Congenital bronchial atresia consists of atresia or stenosis of a lobar, segmental, or subsegmental bronchus at or near its origin; the apicoposterior segmental bronchus of the left upper lobe is most commonly affected, followed by segmental bronchi of the right upper lobe, middle lobe, and (rarely) lower lobe.[289] It is usually an isolated finding; occasionally, it is associated with other congenital bronchopulmonary,[290] skeletal,[291] or cardiovascular[292] anomalies. The condition is rare, only 86 cases having been reported by 1986.[291] Approximately 50% are discovered after the patient reaches 15 years of age;[293] occasionally, it is first noted at birth.[294]

Two pathogenetic theories have been proposed:[295] (1) an island of multiplying cells at the tip of a bronchial bud loses its connection with the bud itself but continues to branch independently, resulting in a normal distal bronchial branch pattern without a connection between distal and central airways; and (2) a localized intrauterine interruption of the bronchial artery blood supply results in bronchial wall ischemia and secondary luminal obliteration. Whatever the

mechanism of airway interruption, mucus secreted within the patent airways distal to the point of atresia cannot pass the stenosis and accumulates in the form of a plug or mucocele. Air can enter the affected bronchopulmonary segments only via collateral channels, resulting in overinflation and expiratory air trapping.[296, 297] This has been documented in one case, assessed both radiographically[294] and physiologically,[298] in which the lesion was discovered at birth and the involved parenchyma was observed to undergo progressive hyperinflation.

Pathologically the bronchial tree peripheral to the point of obliteration is patent, and the complement of bronchi and bronchioles is normal or near normal. Depending on the amount of inspissated mucus, the intrabronchial plug may be linear, branched, ovoid, or cystlike (Fig. 22–22). In two cases, histologic examination of the blind bronchus showed normal architecture except for thinning of the wall and abnormalities of cartilage staining as a result of decreased acid mucopolysaccharides;[295] no fibrosis was present between the blind bronchus and distal airways.

Chest radiographs reveal an area of pulmonary hyperlucency in 90% of cases, a hilar mass in 80%, and a combination of both findings in 70%.[300] The hyperlucency results from a combination of oligemia and an increase in the volume of air within the affected parenchyma (Fig. 22–23).[300] Adjacent normal lung is compressed and displaced; the mediastinum may or may not show displacement. Accumulation of secretions and mucoid impaction distal to the bronchial atresia result in ovoid, round, branching opacities near the hilum in most cases (Fig. 22–24).[289] Dynamic inspiratory and expiratory films reveal air trapping that is indistinguishable from that caused by a partly or completely obstructing endobronchial lesion; in the authors' experience, however, endobronchial lesions are rarely if ever associated with overinflation of affected bronchopulmonary segments at total lung capacity (TLC), an almost invariable finding in bronchial atresia.

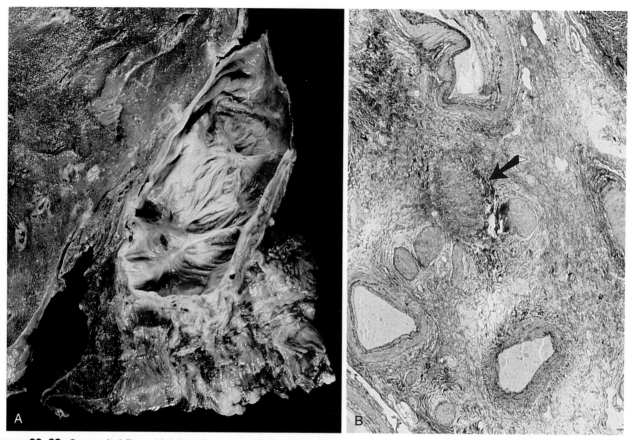

Figure 22–22. Congenital Bronchial Atresia. A midsagittal slice of right lower lobe *(A)* shows an oval cyst in the superior segment; the cyst was filled with thick mucus that was washed out to expose its wall. (The abnormal tissue below the cyst is fibrotic pleura; the basal lung parenchyma—a portion of which is seen at the left—was essentially normal.) Dissection of the lower lobe bronchi showed a normal complement of basal segmental branches; however, the superior segmental branch narrowed abruptly just after its origin. A section through this area *(B)* shows fibrous and elastic tissue surrounded by bronchial and pulmonary vessels and nerves without evidence of a residual bronchus *(arrow* indicates the approximate site at which it should have been located). The patient was a 25-year-old man without respiratory symptoms.

CT allows excellent visualization of the mucoid impaction and segmental overinflation and hypovascularity,[85, 301] a combination of findings that is generally considered diagnostic.[148] Mucoid impaction is readily recognized by the presence of branching soft tissue densities in a bronchial distribution, usually associated with bronchial dilation (Fig. 22–25).[301, 302] Although a similar appearance has been reported on MR,[303, 304] CT is the imaging modality of choice.

The majority of patients are asymptomatic. Some present with a history of recurrent pneumonia.[291, 300] Pectus excavatum has been noted in some individuals.[291]

NEONATAL LOBAR HYPERINFLATION

Neonatal lobar hyperinflation (congenital lobar emphysema) is characterized by variably severe overinflation of a pulmonary lobe, almost always presenting in infancy and causing marked respiratory distress. Although the condition possesses fairly characteristic radiologic and clinical manifestations, the cause and pathogenesis of the overinflation are varied, and the abnormality should be regarded as a clinicopathologic syndrome rather than as a specific disease entity. Although many cases undoubtedly are associated with developmental anomalies and therefore should be regarded

as truly congenital, others are related to acquired bronchial obstruction.[305, 306] For these reasons, it is probably preferable to employ the designation *neonatal* or *infantile* rather than congenital. In addition, although the use of the term *emphysema* is well established in the literature, not all cases represent true emphysema (air space enlargement accompanied by tissue destruction): histologic examination of lung sections has yielded conflicting results, some authors finding no structural evidence of alveolar wall damage and others describing significant alveolar fragmentation and coalescence.[306] Thus, the relative importance of emphysema versus hyperinflation is not well established, and the word "emphysema" should be used with this understanding; in fact, the authors believe that it should preferably be replaced with the more nonspecific descriptor, "overinflation."

In many instances, the abnormality is associated with congenital cardiac anomalies, estimated by some to occur in approximately 50% of cases[307, 308] but found in only 15% of the 106 cases reviewed in one series.[309] A male-to-female ratio of 3:1 was observed in the large review cited.[309] There is a distinct predilection for the left upper lobe and a slightly lesser one for the right middle lobe;[307, 310] the lower lobes are rarely affected.[309] The abnormality is almost always unilateral.[311, 312] Familial cases have been documented rarely.[313]

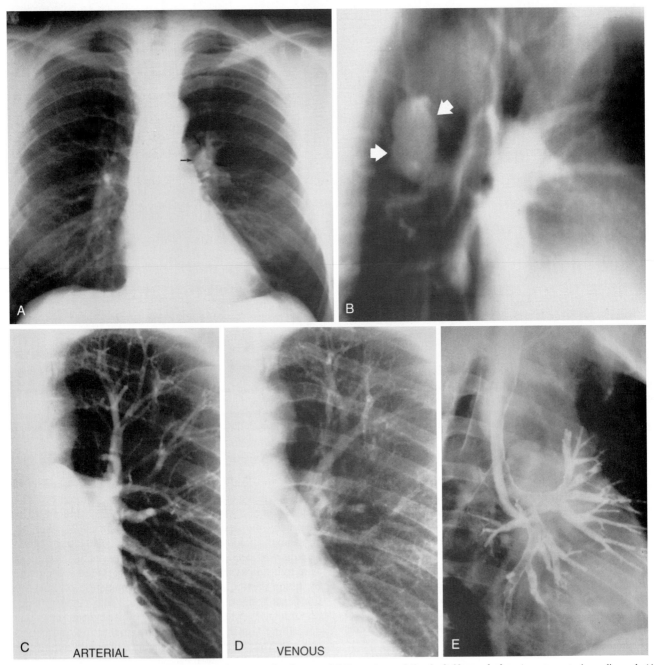

Figure 22–23. Congenital Atresia of the Apicoposterior Segmental Bronchus of the Left Upper Lobe. A posteroanterior radiograph *(A)* reveals increased radiolucency, overinflation, and sparse vasculature (oligemia) of the upper half of the left lung. An oval mass of homogeneous density is present just above and behind the left hilum, seen to better advantage on a lateral tomogram *(B) (arrows* in both *A* and *B)*. Because the differential diagnosis included a vascular malformation, a pulmonary arteriogram was obtained, but neither the arterial *(C)* nor venous *(D)* phase showed evidence of opacification of the mass. A left bronchogram *(E)* shows only the lingular and anterior segmental bronchi arising from the left upper lobe bronchus, there being no evidence of an apicoposterior bronchus. The elliptical mass relates to the expected position of origin of the apicoposterior bronchus and represents inspissated mucus within the lumen of the affected bronchus distal to atresia. The affected bronchopulmonary segment is air containing as a result of collateral air draft from contiguous, normally ventilated segments. Oligemia is the result of reflex vasoconstriction secondary to diminished ventilation.

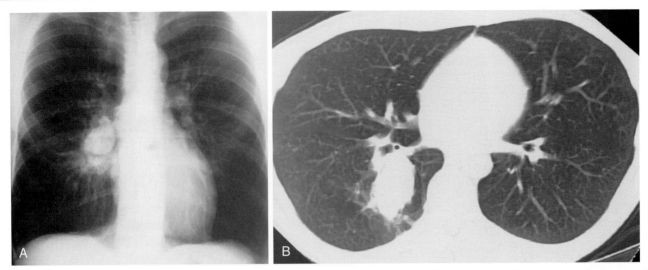

Figure 22–24. Bronchial Atresia. A posteroanterior chest radiograph *(A)* in a 25-year-old man demonstrates a soft tissue mass projecting over the right hilum. A CT scan *(B)* demonstrates a soft tissue mass in the region of the superior segment of the right lower lobe. The superior segmental bronchus could not be visualized separate from this lesion. At surgery, this was shown to represent mucoid impaction distal to bronchial atresia of the superior segmental bronchus of the right lower lobe. (Same patient as in Fig. 22–22.)

Pathogenesis and Pathologic Characteristics

An anatomic cause for neonatal lobar hyperinflation has been identified in about 50% of cases and may be the result of either airway or parenchymal abnormalities.[306] In the former situation, the pathogenesis is related to partial airway obstruction with secondary overinflation; it can be caused by extrinsic, intramural, or intraluminal disease.

Extrinsic (extramural) compression can result from a variety of abnormalities. Probably the most common is an anomalous vessel, such as a large patent ductus arteriosus, an anomalous pulmonary vein, or a left pulmonary artery that arises on the right. This mechanism has been estimated to account for about 5% of all cases of lobar hyperinflation.[314] Other, less common compressive abnormalities include intrathoracic neoplasms, extralobar sequestration,[306] and kinking of the bronchus secondary to lobar herniation through an anterior mediastinal defect.[315]

Intramural abnormalities are invariably characterized by a deficiency of the cartilaginous skeleton with resultant airway collapse and secondary parenchymal overinflation. Some form of cartilaginous defect has been documented in about two thirds of cases with a presumed obstructive pathogenesis;[306] these include a local absence of cartilage in the lobar bronchus,[316] a decrease in peripheral airway cartilage only,[317] or a generalized deficiency of cartilage throughout lobar airways.[318, 319] In cases in which the changes are localized, cartilage morphology can be quite variable. In one series of eight patients whose segmental and subsegmental airways were studied by a microdissection technique, patchy loss of cartilage was found in some cases, and a generalized reduction in plate number and size throughout all airways was found in others.[318] Other investigators have found irregularly shaped and unevenly distributed cartilaginous plates.[319]

Intraluminal obstruction may be either developmental or acquired, the former consisting of mucosal folds or localized bronchostenosis[306] and the latter of mucus plugs[306] or infectious bronchiolitis. Some cases have also been described after prolonged neonatal respiratory support, apparently as a result of masses of endobronchial granulation tissue formed in response to the repeated mechanical trauma of endotracheal tube suctioning.[305]

Although an intrinsic abnormality of the pulmonary parenchyma as a cause for the hyperinflation is theoretically possible, it has rarely been documented. In one detailed morphometric and pathologic study of single lobes resected from three infants who showed the classic radiologic and clinical features of neonatal lobar hyperinflation, the number of alveoli was found to be increased rather than reduced in each case.[320] In one, a 17-day-old infant, they were increased fivefold but of normal size; the number and structure of the airways and vessels were normal for the infant's age, suggesting that the condition represented "giantism" of the pulmonary acinus. In the other two patients, not only were the alveoli increased in number, but also in size. These two patients were older at the time of surgical resection, and the "emphysema" may have developed postnatally; in fact, it was suggested that the large air spaces may have been caused by interference with alveolar multiplication after birth.

Morphometric analysis of the resected lobe of another case of a 2-month-old infant showed normal alveolar, bronchial, and vascular parameters except for a four to five times increase in alveolar size.[321] At the time of surgery, the upper lobe appeared to have been rotated by 180 degrees within the thoracic cavity, suggesting that the hyperinflation may have been secondary to the lobar torsion with partial bronchial obstruction; the cause of the rotation was not apparent. Another variation was reported in a lobe in which alveolar size was markedly increased, but the absolute size of the lobe was smaller than normal (i.e., hypoplastic);[322] although this appearance is not likely to be confused with typical neonatal lobar hyperinflation, the authors of the study suggested that the case represented a variant of that condition.

Approximately 50% of reported cases of neonatal lobar hyperinflation have not been associated with any of the above-mentioned morphologic findings. It is possible that

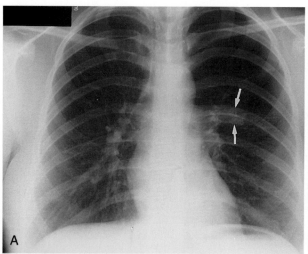

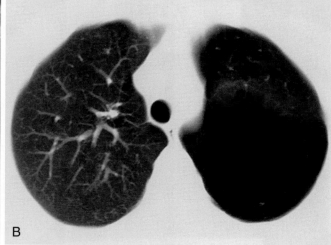

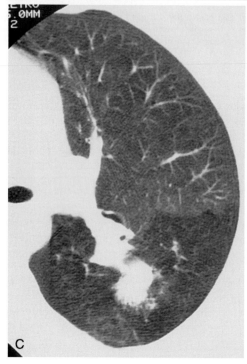

Figure 22–25. Bronchial Atresia. A posteroanterior chest radiograph *(A)* in a 14-year-old girl demonstrates marked lucency and decreased vascularity in the left upper lobe. An ill-defined opacity is evident near the left hilum *(arrows).* A conventional 10-mm collimation CT scan *(B)* shows marked decrease in attenuation and vascularity in the region of the apical posterior segment of the left upper lobe. HRCT scan *(C)* demonstrates focal opacity near the origin of the apicoposterior segmental bronchus and decreased attenuation of the adjacent lung.

this deficiency is simply a technical matter, as careful morphometric studies are necessary to show an abnormality in alveolar size and as airway microdissection techniques and special stains are usually necessary to identify intramural cartilaginous abnormalities. In many early case reports, neither of these procedures was carried out, and it is possible that the etiologic basis for the overinflation was not recognized. It is also possible that partial bronchial obstruction as the result of focal cartilaginous abnormality or a mucosal web may have been left behind in the bronchial stump at surgery, thus precluding morphologic examination.

Radiologic Manifestations

The radiologic manifestations of neonatal lobar hyperinflation are distinctive, and there is usually little difficulty in diagnosis. The cardinal features are overinflation and air trapping, the former manifested by markedly increased vol-

ume of the affected lobe, even at TLC, depressing the ipsilateral hemidiaphragm and displacing the mediastinum into the contralateral hemithorax (Fig. 22–26). The distended lobe may lead to compression (relaxation) atelectasis of the lung's other lobes.[323] Vascular markings in the affected lobe tend to be widely separated and attenuated, the lobe appearing more radiolucent than other lung tissue. Identification of vascular markings is important, permitting differentiation from congenital air cysts, postpneumonic pneumatocele, and loculated pneumothorax.[307, 311, 324] Air trapping is manifested by the usual radiographic signs: displacement of the heart and mediastinum toward the normal (contralateral) hemithorax during expiration and their partial return toward the midline during inspiration.

Infrequently, the overinflated lobe shows uniformly increased density rather than translucency, possibly the result of impaired fluid drainage secondary to bronchial obstruction.[325–327] The fetal lung normally is filled with fluid; some

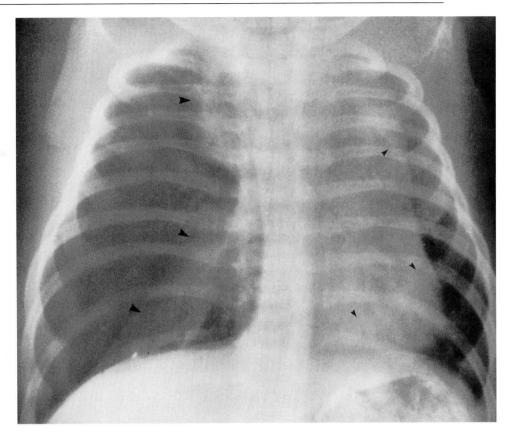

Figure 22–26. Neonatal Lobar Hyperinflation. An anteroposterior chest radiograph of a male infant demonstrates a grossly overinflated right lung that has displaced the mediastinum markedly to the left *(small arrowheads)*. The hyperexpanded right middle lobe is devoid of recognizable vascularity, and the right upper and lower lobes *(large arrowheads)* are compressed and displaced medially. After surgical resection, the middle lobe was found to possess a narrowed bronchus associated with malarranged and deficient cartilage plates.

is squeezed out as the infant passes through the birth canal, and the remainder is cleared by the pulmonary lymphatics and veins and perhaps by the airways themselves. Thus, an obstruction in a lobar bronchus might interfere with removal of fluid from that lobe. The radiographic manifestations resemble those of the usual form of lobar hyperinflation except that the affected lobe is opaque rather than radiolucent. The fluid may be cleared within 24 hours to 2 weeks;[327] the appearance of the thorax then is typical of the usual form of lobar hyperinflation.

The classic form of neonatal lobar hyperinflation can usually be diagnosed easily on the chest radiograph. CT may be helpful in confirming the diagnosis and in ruling out mediastinal and bronchial masses.[328] $\dot{V}/\dot{Q}$ scans demonstrate abnormalities in the affected lobe and are particularly helpful in assessing the function of the adjacent lung, which may appear to be atelectatic and nonfunctioning on the chest radiograph but well perfused and ventilated on scans.[328]

The majority of patients are diagnosed and treated surgically during infancy. Even in patients treated medically, the radiographs usually become essentially normal between 10 to 20 years of age.[314, 329]

Clinical Manifestations

Respiratory distress usually develops during the neonatal period;[307] in only 5% does it develop after 6 months of age.[330] Rarely, the condition is first recognized in an adult (Fig. 22–27). A small percentage of patients are asymptomatic.[331] Physical examination may reveal thoracic asymme-

try, an increased percussion note, reduced breath sounds, crackles, a local wheeze, and an increased respiratory rate.

In some cases, the course is rapid and progressive, ending fatally unless the lobe is resected;[324] in one series, all nine patients required emergency operation to relieve dyspnea and cyanosis.[310] The urgency of treatment depends on the severity of respiratory embarrassment, and, in many cases, the clinical and radiographic manifestations regress spontaneously without the need for thoracotomy and lobar resection.[332] For example, in one study of 12 patients followed for 6 months to 12 years (median, 3 years), investigators documented less hyperinflation of the affected lobe and (in 6 cases) improvements in $\dot{V}/\dot{Q}$ scans paralleling gradual improvement in clinical symptoms.[328]

ANOMALOUS TRACHEOBRONCHIAL BRANCHING

Many variations in the tracheobronchial branching pattern have been described.[330, 333–336] Some represent an isolated alteration of normal bronchial development, whereas others are associated with anomalies in other organs or tissues and are discovered in early neonatal life or in stillbirths or abortions as part of a spectrum of abnormalities. Although most of these abnormal branches are of no radiologic, functional, or clinical consequence, pathologic effects are occasionally produced, usually related to recurrent infection. One group of investigators found a high incidence of bronchial anomalies (including accessory and absent bronchi) in patients who had a history of spontaneous pneumothorax compared with subjects in a control group.[337]

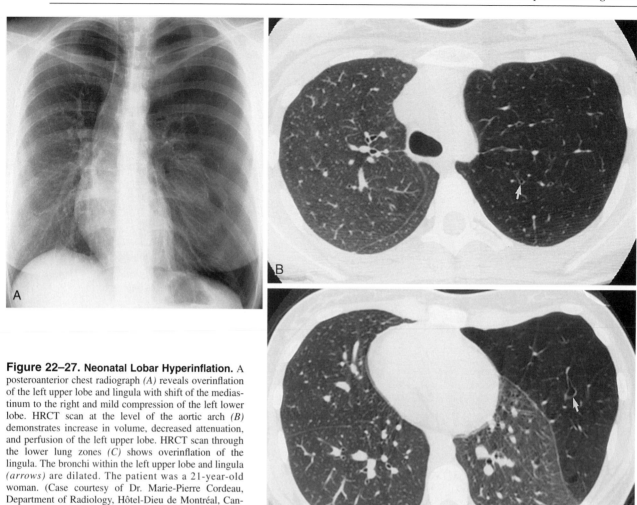

Figure 22–27. Neonatal Lobar Hyperinflation. A posteroanterior chest radiograph *(A)* reveals overinflation of the left upper lobe and lingula with shift of the mediastinum to the right and mild compression of the left lower lobe. HRCT scan at the level of the aortic arch *(B)* demonstrates increase in volume, decreased attenuation, and perfusion of the left upper lobe. HRCT scan through the lower lung zones *(C)* shows overinflation of the lingula. The bronchi within the left upper lobe and lingula *(arrows)* are dilated. The patient was a 21-year-old woman. (Case courtesy of Dr. Marie-Pierre Cordeau, Department of Radiology, Hôtel-Dieu de Montréal, Canada.)

Abnormal Bronchial Number

Abnormal bronchial number is usually characterized by more than one lobar or segmental bronchi;[335, 338] occasionally, an airway branch is absent.

Abnormal Origin of Lobar or Segmental Bronchi

The most common of abnormal origins is tracheal origin of the right upper lobe bronchus, sometimes known as *tracheal* or *pig bronchus (bronchus suis).* The reported prevalence ranges from 0.1% in studies of adults to 2% in children.[339, 340] The bronchus usually arises from the right lateral wall of the trachea less than 2 cm above the carina.[341] It usually is seen as an incidental finding at bronchoscopy, chest radiography, or CT (Fig. 22–28);[342] occasionally, it has been associated with recurrent infection[343, 344] or dyspnea.[345]

In one study of 1,500 bronchograms, 7 cases were identified in which the left apicoposterior bronchus had its origin from the left main bronchus;[346] 4 of the 7 patients showed radiographic and pathologic evidence of airway obstruction isolated to the bronchopulmonary territory of this bronchus (including emphysema, bronchiectasis, and chronic

pneumonia). Pathologic examination showed no structural abnormality of the segmental bronchus that would explain the obstruction, and the authors of the study postulated that the effects may have been caused by pressure on the anomalous bronchus by the left pulmonary artery.

A *bridging bronchus* is a rare anomaly in which air flow to and from the right middle or right lower lobe passes via an airway that crosses the mediastinum and joins the left main bronchus.[347, 348]

Bronchial Isomerism

Bronchial isomerism is characterized by a pattern of bronchial branching and pulmonary lobe formation that is identical in the two lungs. Although it may be an isolated finding, it is frequently associated with a variety of cardiac, splenic, and other anomalies.[349–351]

Tracheobronchial Diverticula

The most common location of an airway diverticulum is probably the inferior medial wall of the right main or intermediate bronchi. The abnormality (sometimes termed the *accessory cardiac bronchus*) may end blindly or be associated with

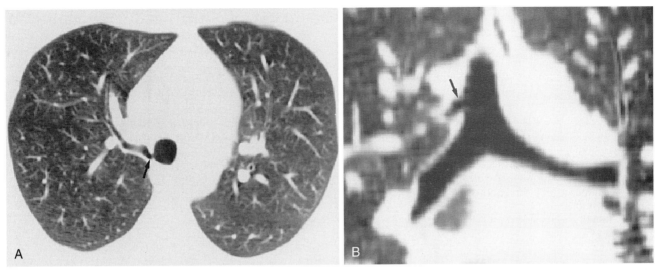

Figure 22–28. Tracheal Bronchus. A 3-mm collimation spiral CT scan at the level of the aortic arch *(A)* demonstrates the right upper lobe bronchus *(arrow)* originating directly from the trachea. Coronal reconstruction *(B)* demonstrates the lower trachea and right upper lobe bronchus *(arrow)* originating from the trachea rather than from the right main bronchus. The patient was a 42-year-old man with no symptoms related to the airways or lung parenchyma.

small amounts of abnormal pulmonary parenchyma.[54] The frequency of the anomaly ranges from 0.09% to 0.5% in the general population.[352, 353] The diagnosis can be readily made with CT, which demonstrates a distinct airway originating in the medial wall of the main bronchus or bronchus intermedius cephalad to the origin of the middle lobe bronchus (Fig. 22–29).[354, 355] In one CT study of six cases, associated pulmonary parenchymal tissue was identified in four.[354]

Although usually an incidental finding in an asymptomatic patient, an accessory cardiac bronchus may serve as a potential reservoir of infectious organisms; inflammation in the bronchial pouch or spillage of infectious material may result in hemorrhage, productive cough, or recurrent pneumonia.[353, 354] Purulent material can sometimes be identified bronchoscopically within the bronchial pouch.[355] In one ex-

ceptional case, a squamous cell carcinoma was found to arise from the bronchus.[356] Airway diverticula have also been identified in the trachea[357–359] and main bronchi. They have been associated with recurrent pneumonia and, in one case, perforation during endotracheal intubation with subsequent pneumomediastinum.[360]

ANOMALOUS TRACHEOBRONCHIAL COMMUNICATION

Tracheobronchial-Esophageal Fistula

Extralaryngeal communication of the normal tracheobronchial tree is most often seen as a tracheoesophageal

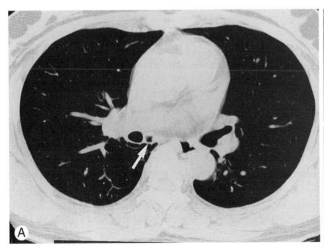
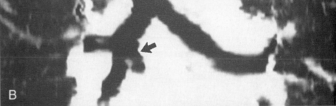
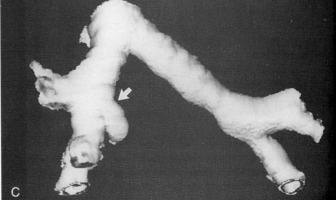

Figure 22–29. Spiral CT with Coronal and Three-Dimensional Reconstruction of an Accessory Cardiac Bronchus. A cross-sectional spiral CT image *(A)* demonstrates a localized area of air density *(arrow)* medial to the bronchus intermedius. A coronal reconstruction *(B)* demonstrates that this localized abnormality communicates with the distal right main bronchus *(arrow)*. The diagnosis of an accessory cardiac bronchus can be readily made on the coronal reconstruction. Three-dimensional reconstruction *(C)* more clearly defines the bronchial anatomy and the cardiac bronchus. The patient was a 39-year-old woman with recurrent respiratory infections. (Case courtesy of Dr. Kyung Soo Lee, Department of Radiology, Samsung Medical Center, Seoul, Korea.)

fistula.[361, 362] Two clinicopathologic subtypes have been described.[362] In the first, constituting approximately 85% of cases, the esophagus ends blindly in a dilated pouch (esophageal atresia).[363] The trachea can communicate with the proximal or distal esophageal segments (or both); numerous minor anatomic variations have been described.[364] Other congenital anomalies, particularly of the gastrointestinal and cardiovascular systems, are present in approximately 50% of patients.[362] The presence of a blind (proximal) esophageal ending leads to regurgitation and aspiration of oropharyngeal secretions and milk, resulting in cough and pneumonia. The condition is thus invariably detected in the neonatal period.

Congenital tracheoesophageal and bronchoesophageal communications can also occur in association with an otherwise normal esophagus.[365] In this situation, survival into adult life is possible because of the lack of early signs and symptoms related to regurgitation and aspiration.[363, 366, 367] In one review of 260 cases of tracheoesophageal fistula without esophageal atresia (66 of which were in adults), 189 (72%) showed communication with the trachea and the remainder with the bronchi.[368] Of the bronchi, the right main is most commonly affected; however, the left main[369] and even segmental airways[368] are sometimes involved. Although some of these cases may represent inflammatory fistulas secondary to congenital or acquired esophageal diverticula, in most the absence of inflammation and the presence of intramural muscle in the communication implies a true developmental anomaly.

Anatomically the fistulas are usually obliquely oriented, the esophageal end being distal to the upper airway communication. It has been proposed that this arrangement—possibly aided by contraction of mural smooth muscle during swallowing—explains the frequent mildness of respiratory symptoms and the delay in diagnosis until adulthood.[370] Occlusive membranes and mucosal folds at the esophageal origin of the fistulas may act as check-valves, providing further protection against aspiration.[372]

Chest radiographs of neonates with tracheoesophageal fistula and esophageal atresia frequently show acute airspace pneumonia consistent with aspiration. Total opacification of the right lung associated with deviation of the esophagus to the right and a normal position of the trachea should lead to the suspicion of "esophageal lung," in which the right main bronchus originates from the esophagus.[373, 374] In older patients without esophageal atresia, evidence of bronchiectasis may be present. The diagnosis of fistula is best confirmed by identification of contrast medium within the tracheobronchial tree after its ingestion.

Symptoms in neonatal tracheoesophageal fistula are usually prominent and consist of "excessive salivation" (representing drooling of normal oropharyngeal secretions) and choking on feeding. As indicated, when a fistula is unassociated with esophageal atresia, the diagnosis often is not made until adulthood; however, careful questioning often reveals a history of coughing when eating or drinking or of recurrent pneumonia, sometimes for many years.[370, 375] Hemoptysis occurs in some patients. Young adults may be suspected of having cystic fibrosis or asthma[376] and older ones chronic obstructive pulmonary disease.[377] Neither bronchography nor esophagoscopy is of much value in diagnosis, although bronchoscopy may reveal the orifice of the communication.

In adults, the prognosis is good after reparative surgery.[367] Similarly, in otherwise healthy term infants in whom a blind proximal esophageal pouch is present, the survival rate after surgery is greater than 90%; however, this rate drops to 55% in premature infants and in neonates with major medical problems.[378] Some infants who have undergone successful surgery are still prone to acute and chronic respiratory complications, presumably as a result of gastroesophageal reflux secondary to an incompetent lower esophageal sphincter;[379] the latter, in turn, may be caused by a congenital defect of tracheal and esophageal innervation.[380, 381]

Bronchobiliary Fistula

Congenital communication between the biliary tree and the carina or main bronchi (bronchobiliary fistula) is rare; only 12 cases had been reported by 1987.[382] Characteristically, the anomaly results in neonatal pneumonia and the production of greenish, bile-containing sputum;[57, 383] in one report, the lesion was recognized in an adult with chronic cough.[382] In such patients, an acquired communication secondary to biliary tract disease must be excluded.[384]

MISCELLANEOUS BRONCHOPULMONARY ANOMALIES

Accessory and Heterotopic Pulmonary Tissue

Accessory pulmonary tissue may be defined as the presence of lung parenchyma over and above the normal complement of left and right lungs, supplied by branches of the pulmonary arterial and venous systems and connected by an airway to some portion of the tracheobronchial tree. Compared with extralobar sequestration (in which the pulmonary parenchyma is supplied by a systemic artery), the condition is quite rare. Individual lobes and occasionally a reduplicated whole lung can be completely enclosed in their own pleural cavity.[385, 386]

Heterotopic pulmonary tissue outside the thorax is extremely rare. Most cases represent extralobar sequestration; however, in one instance a small focus of pulmonary tissue was located in the skin and had no pleural envelope or obvious large systemic artery supply.[386a]

Heterotopic Tissue Within the Lung

Heterotopic skeletal muscle,[387] adrenal tissue (occasionally with cytomegalic change),[388] hepatic tissue,[389] thyroid tissue, and glial tissue[390] can be found occasionally within lung parenchyma.[391] Most cases are of no consequence; rarely, they serve as the source for the development of a pulmonary neoplasm or choristoma.[391] An unusual case of neonatal respiratory distress related to glial heterotopia has also been reported.[392]

Horseshoe Lung

Horseshoe lung is a rare congenital malformation in which an isthmus of pulmonary parenchyma extends from the right lung base across the midline behind the pericardium and joins the posterobasal segments of the right and left lungs. Thirty-six cases had been reported by 1997.[393–395] The majority (30 of the 36)[395] have been associated with the hypogenetic lung (scimitar) syndrome (*see* page 653); in one review, the abnormality was identified in 6 of 147 (4%) cases of this anomaly.[393] Associated findings include hypoplastic right pulmonary artery, anomalous connections of some or all of the right pulmonary veins to the inferior vena cava–right atrial junction, abnormal systemic arterial supply from the descending thoracic or abdominal aorta to the right lung, and a variable degree of bronchial sequestration.[396] Rarely, left-sided pulmonary hypoplasia[394] or pulmonary sequestration[393] has been described.

The radiographic findings typically consist of a variable degree of right hemithorax hypoplasia, dextrocardia, and a large left lung.[396] The diagnosis can be made by pulmonary angiography, which reveals a branch of the right pulmonary artery originating from its proximal but inferior aspect and coursing into the left hemithorax, or by CT.[393, 397]

REFERENCES

1. Clements BS, Warner JO, Shinebourne EA: Congenital bronchopulmonary vascular malformations: Clinical application of a simple anatomical approach in 25 cases. Thorax 42:409, 1987.
2. Clements BS, Warner JO: Pulmonary sequestration and related congenital bronchopulmonary-vascular malformations: Nomenclature and classification based on anatomical and embryological considerations. Thorax 42:401, 1987.
3. Panicek DM, Heitzman ER, Randall PA, et al: The continuum of pulmonary developmental anomalies. RadioGraphics 7:747, 1987.
4. Williams S, Burton EM, Day S, et al: Combined sequestration, bronchogenic cyst, and dysgenetic lung simulating congenital lobar emphysema. South Med J 89:1220, 1996.
5. Grewal RG, Yip CK: Intralobar pulmonary sequestration and mediastinal bronchogenic cyst. Thorax 49:615, 1994.
6. Vevecka E, De Boeck K, Moerman P, et al: Tracheal bronchus associated with congenital cystic adenomatoid malformation. Pediatr Pulmonol 20:413, 1995.
7. Schwartz MZ, Ramachandran P: Congenital malformations of the lung and mediastinum—a quarter century of experience from a single institution. J Pediatr Surg 32:44, 1997.
8. Shaheen S, Barker DJ: Early lung growth and chronic airflow obstruction. Thorax 49:533, 1994.
9. Helms PJ: Lung growth: Implications for the development of disease. Thorax 49:440, 1994.
10. Warburton D, Lee M, Berberich MA, et al: Molecular embryology and the study of lung development. Am J Respir Cell Mol Biol 9:5, 1993.
11. Boyden EA: Developmental anomalies of the lungs. Am J Surg 89:79, 1955.
12. Landing BH: Congenital malformations and genetic disorders of the respiratory tract (larynx, trachea, bronchi, and lungs): State of the art. Am Rev Respir Dis 120:151, 1979.
13. Hepburn D: Note on a right lung which resembled a left lung in presenting only apical and basal lobes. J Anat 59:326, 1924–25.
14. Della Pona C, Rocco G, Rizzi A, et al: Lobar hypoplasia. Eur Respir J 4:1140, 1991.
15. Maltz DL, Nadas AS: Agenesis of the lung: Presentation of eight new cases and review of the literature. Pediatrics 42:175, 1968.
16. Hülsoff TH, Kalvelage H: Ein Beitrag zur Diagnose und zur Frage der Häufigkeit des angeborenen Lungenmangels. [Contribution to the diagnosis and frequency of congenital lung aplasia.] Fortschr Rontgenstr 91:725, 1959.
17. Valle AR: Agenesis of the lung. Am J Surg 89:90, 1955.
18. Swischuk LE, Richardson CJ, Nichols MM, et al: Bilateral pulmonary hypoplasia in the neonate. Am J Roentgenol 133:1057, 1979.
19. Hussain AN, Heggler RG: Neonatal pulmonary hypoplasia: An autopsy study of 25 cases. Pediatr Pathol 13:475, 1993.
20. Fagan DG, Emery JL: A review and restatement of some problems in histological interpretation of the infant lung. Semin Diagn Pathol 9:13, 1992.
21. Warkany J: The lung. In Warkany M (ed): Congenital Malformations. Chicago, Year Book Medical Publishers, 1971, p 604.
22. Lurie IW, Ilyina HG, Gurevich DB, et al: Trisomy 2p: Analysis of unusual phenotypic findings. Am J Med Genet 55:229, 1995.
23. Mardini MK, Nyhan WL: Agenesis of the lung: Report of four patients with unusual anomalies. Chest 87:522, 1985.
24. Cunningham ML, Mann N: Pulmonary agenesis: A predictor of ipsilateral malformations. Am J Med Genet 70:391, 1997.
25. Oster AG, Stillwell R, Fortune DW: Bilateral pulmonary agenesis. Pathology 10:243, 1978.
26. Lauria MR, Gonik B, Romero R: Pulmonary hypoplasia: Pathogenesis, diagnosis, and antenatal prediction. Obstet Gynecol 86:466, 1995.
27. Page DV, Stocker JT: Anomalies associated with pulmonary hypoplasia. Am Rev Respir Dis 125:216, 1982.
28. Vanamo K: A 45-year perspective of congenital diaphragmatic hernia. Br J Surg 83:1758, 1996.
29. Becmeur F, Horta P, Donato L, et al: Accessory diaphragm—review of 31 cases in the literature. Eur J Pediatr Surg 5:43, 1995.
30. Dresler S: Massive pleural effusion and hypoplasia of the lung accompanying extralobar pulmonary sequestration. Hum Pathol 12:862, 1981.
31. deLorimier AA, Tierney DF, Parker HR: Hypoplastic lungs in fetal lambs with surgically produced congenital diaphragmatic hernia. Surgery 62:12, 1967.
32. Finegold MJ, Katzew H, Genieser NB, et al: Lung structure in thoracic dystrophy. Am J Dis Child 122:153, 1971.
33. Johnson VP, Keppen LD, Carpenter MS: New syndrome of spondylospinal thoracic dysostosis with multiple pterygia and arthrogryposis. Am J Med Genet 69:73, 1997.
34. Thibeault DW, Pettett G, Mabry SM, et al: Osteogenesis imperfecta Type IIA and pulmonary hypoplasia with normal alveolar development. Pediatr Pulmonol 20:301, 1995.
35. Goldstein JD, Reid LM: Pulmonary hypoplasia resulting from phrenic nerve agenesis and diaphragmatic amyoplasia. J Pediatr 97:282, 1980.
36. Argyle JC: Pulmonary hypoplasia in infants in giant abdominal wall defects. Pediatr Pathol 9:43, 1987.
37. Liggins GC, Vilos GA, Campos GA, et al: The effect of bilateral thoracoplasty on lung development in fetal sheep. J Dev Physiol 3:275, 1981.
38. Thomas IT, Smith DW: Oligohydramnios, cause of the nonrenal features of Potter's syndrome, including pulmonary hypoplasia. Pediatrics 84:811, 1974.
39. Wigglesworth JS, Desai R, Guerrini P: Fetal lung hypoplasia: Biochemical and structural variations and their possible significance. Arch Dis Child 56:606, 1981.
40. Adzick NS, Harrison MR, Glick PL, et al: Experimental pulmonary hypoplasia and oligohydramnios: Relative contributions of lung fluid and fetal breathing movements. J Pediatr Surg 19:658, 1984.
41. Johnson RJ, Haworth SG: Pulmonary vascular and alveolar development in tetralogy of Fallot: A recommendation for early correction. Thorax 37:893, 1982.
42. Haworth SG, McKenzie SA, Fitzpatrick ML: Alveolar development after ligation of left pulmonary artery in newborn pig: Clinical relevance to unilateral pulmonary artery. Thorax 36:938, 1981.
43. Wigglesworth JS, Winston RML, Bartlett K: Influence of the central nervous system on fetal lung development. Arch Dis Child 52:965, 1977.
44. Liggins GC, Vilos GA, Campos GA, et al: The effect of spinal cord transection on lung development in fetal sheep. J Dev Physiol 3:267, 1981.
45. Fewell JE, Lee CC, Kitterman JA: Effects of phrenic nerve section on the respiratory system of fetal lambs. J Appl Physiol 51:293, 1981.
46. van Noort G, Straks W, Van Diggelen OP, et al: A congenital variant of glycogenosis type IV. Pediatr Pathol 13:685, 1993.
47. Harding R, Hooper SB: Regulation of lung expansion and lung growth before birth. J Appl Physiol 81:209, 1996.
48. Alcorn D, Adamson TM, Lambert TE, et al: Morphological effects of chronic tracheal ligation and drainage in the fetal lamb lung. J Anat 123:649, 1977.
48a. de Paepe ME, Johnson BD, Papadakis K, et al: Temporal pattern of accelerated lung growth after tracheal occlusion in the fetal rabbit. Am J Pathol 152:179, 1998.
49. Thornton CM, Carson DJ, Stewart FJ: Autopsy findings in the Wolcott-Rallison syndrome. Pediatr Pathol Lab Med 17:487, 1997.
50. Wigglesworth JS, Desai R, Hislop AA: Fetal lung growth in congenital laryngeal atresia. Pediatr Pathol 7:515, 1987.
51. Silver MM, Thurston WA, Patrick JE: Perinatal pulmonary hyperplasia due to laryngeal atresia. Hum Pathol 19:110, 1988.
52. Stevens CA, McClanahan C, Steck A, et al: Pulmonary hyperplasia in the Fraser cryptophthalmos syndrome. Am J Med Genet 52:427, 1994.
53. McNamara MF, McCurdy CM, Reed KL, et al: The relation between pulmonary hypoplasia and amniotic fluid volume: Lessons learned from discordant urinary tract anomalies in monoamniotic twins. Obstet Gynecol 85:867, 1995.
54. Chamberlain D, Hislop A, Hey E, et al: Pulmonary hypoplasia in babies with severe rhesus isoimmunisation: A quantitative study. J Pathol 122:43, 1977.
55. Cooney TP, Thurlbeck WM: Lung growth and development in anencephaly and hydranencephaly. Am Rev Respir Dis 132:596, 1985.
56. Cooney TP, Thurlbeck WM: Pulmonary hypoplasia in Down's syndrome. N Engl J Med 307:1170, 1982.
57. Landing BH, Dixon LG: Congenital malformations and genetic disorders of the respiratory tract (larynx, trachea, bronchi, and lungs). Am Rev Respir Dis 120:151, 1979.
58. Seller MJ, Davis TB, Fear CN, et al: Two sibs with anophthalmia and pulmonary hypoplasia (the Matthew-Wood syndrome). Am J Med Genet 62:227, 1996.
59. Van Hove JL, Spiridigliozzi GA, Heinz R, et al: Fryns syndrome survivors and neurologic outcome. Am J Med Genet 59:334, 1995.
60. Punnett HH, Kistenmacher ML, Valdes-Dapena M, et al: Syndrome of ankylosis, facial anomalies, and pulmonary hypoplasia. J Pediatr 85:375, 1974.
61. Pena SDJ, Shokeir MHK: Syndrome of camptodactyly, multiple ankyloses, facial anomalies, and pulmonary hypoplasia: A lethal condition. J Pediatr 85:373, 1974.
62. Frey B, Fleischhauer A, Gersbach M: Familial isolated pulmonary hypoplasia: A case report, suggesting autosomal recessive inheritance Eur J Pediatr 153:460, 1994.
63. Swischuk LE, Richardson CJ, Nichols MM, et al: Primary pulmonary hypoplasia in the neonate. Pediatrics 95:573, 1979.
64. Borja AR, Ransdell HT Jr, Villa S: Congenital developmental arrest of the lung. Ann Thorac Surg 10:317, 1970.
65. Ryland D, Reid L: Pulmonary aplasia—a quantitative analysis of the development of the single lung. Thorax 26:602, 1971.
66. Georgopoulos D, Mink SN, Oppenheimer L, et al: How is maximal expiratory flow reduced in canine postpneumonectomy lung growth? J Appl Physiol 71:834, 1991.
67. Husain AN, Hessel RG: Neonatal pulmonary hypoplasia: An autopsy study of 25 cases. Pediatr Pathol 13:475, 1993.
68. Finegold MJ, Katzew H, Genieser NB, et al: Lung structure in thoracic dystrophy. Am J Dis Child 122:153, 1971.
69. Williams AJ, Vawter G, Reid LM: Lung structure in asphyxiating thoracic dystrophy. Arch Pathol Lab Med 108:658, 1984.
70. Areechon W, Reid L: Hypoplasia of lung with congenital diaphragmatic hernia. BMJ 1:230, 1963.
71. Boyden EA: The structure of compressed lungs in congenital diaphragmatic hernia. Am J Anat 134:497, 1972.
72. George DK, Cooney TP, Chiu BK, et al: Hypoplasia and immaturity of the terminal lung unit (Acinus) in congenital diaphragmatic hernia. Am Rev Respir Dis 136:947, 1987.
73. Boffa P, Stovin P, Shneerson J: Short reports: Lung developmental abnormalities in severe scoliosis. Thorax 39:681, 1984.
74. Hislop A, Hey E, Reid L: The lungs in congenital bilateral renal agenesis and dysplasia. Arch Dis Child 54:32, 1979.

75. Reale FR, Esterly JR: Pulmonary hypoplasia: A morphometric study of the lungs of infants with diaphragmatic hernia, anencephaly, and renal malformations. Pediatrics 51:91, 1973.

76. Schloo BL, Vawter GF, Reid LM: Down syndrome: Patterns of disturbed lung growth. Hum Pathol 22:919, 1991.

77. Iwai K, Shindo G, Hajikano H, et al: Intralobar pulmonary sequestration, with special reference to developmental pathology. Am Rev Respir Dis 107:911, 1973.

78. Kitagawa M, Hislop A, Boyden EA, et al: Lung hypoplasia in congenital diaphragmatic hernia: A quantitative study of airway, artery, and alveolar development. Br J Surg 58:342, 1971.

79. Rutledge JC, Jensen P: Acinar dysplasia: A new form of pulmonary maldevelopment. Hum Pathol 17:1290, 1986.

80. Hislop A, Sanderson M, Reid L: Unilateral congenital dysplasia of lung associated with vascular anomalies. Thorax 28:435, 1973.

81. Mendelsohn G, Hutchins G: Primary pulmonary hypoplasia: Report of a case with polyhydramnios. Am J Dis Child 131:1220, 1977.

82. Steiner HA: Aplasia of the lung: A case report. Radiology 67:751, 1956.

83. Brünner S, Nissen E: Agenesis of the lung. Am Rev Respir Dis 87:103, 1963.

84. Soulen RL, Cohen RV: Plain film recognition of pulmonary agenesis in the adult. Chest 60:185, 1971.

85. Mata JM, Cáceres J, Lucaya J, et al: CT of congenital malformations of the lung. RadioGraphics 10:651, 1990.

86. Greenspan RH, Sagel S, McMahon J, et al: Timed expiratory chest films in detection of air-trapping. Invest Radiol 8:264, 1973.

87. Moore ADA, Godwin JD, Dietrich PA, et al: Swyer-James syndrome: CT findings in eight patients. Am J Roentgenol 158:1211, 1992.

88. Mas A, Mirapeix RM, Domingo C: Pulmonary hypoplasia presenting in adulthood as a chronic respiratory failure: Report of two cases: Embryology, clinical symptoms and diagnostic procedures. Respiration 64:240, 1997.

89. Mardini MK, Nyhan WL: Agenesis of the lung: Report of four patients with unusual anomalies. Chest 87:522, 1985.

90. Ijsselstijn H, Tibboel D, Hop WJ, et al: Long-term pulmonary sequelae in children with congenital diaphragmatic hernia. Am J Respir Crit Care Med 155:174, 1997.

91. Sade RM, Clouse M, Ellis FH: The spectrum of pulmonary sequestration. Ann Thorac Surg 18:644, 1974.

92. Felker RE, Tonkin ILD: Imaging of pulmonary sequestration. Am J Roentgenol 154:241, 1990.

93. Blesovsky A: Pulmonary sequestration: A report of an unusual case and a review of the literature. Thorax 22:351, 1967.

94. Pryce DM: Lower accessory pulmonary artery with intralobar sequestration of lung: A report of seven cases. J Pathol Bacteriol 58:457, 1946.

95. Gerle RD, Jaretzi A III, Ashley CA, et al: Congenital bronchopulmonary-foregut malformation: Pulmonary sequestration communicating with the gastrointestinal tract. N Engl J Med 278:1413, 1968.

96. Smith RA: A theory of the origin of intralobar sequestration of the lung. Thorax 11:10, 1956.

97. Gebauer PW, Mason CB: Intralobar pulmonary sequestration associated with anomalous pulmonary vessels: A nonentity. Dis Chest 35:282, 1959.

98. Stocker JT, Malczak HT: A study of pulmonary ligament arteries: Relationship to intralobar pulmonary sequestration. Chest 86:611, 1984.

99. Boyden EA: Bronchogenic cysts and the theory of intralobar sequestration: New embryologic data. J Thorac Surg 35:604, 1958.

100. Smith R: Intralobar sequestration of the lung. Thorax 10:142, 1955.

101. Frazier AA, Rosado de Christenson ML, Stocker JT, et al: Intralobar sequestration: Radiologic-pathologic correlation. RadioGraphics 17:725, 1997.

102. Scully RE, Mark EJ, McNeely BU: Case 48-1983. Case Records of the Massachusetts General Hospital. N Engl J Med 309:1374, 1983.

103. Schlesinger AE, Lee VW, Chapiro JH: Scintiangiographic demonstration of parasitization of systemic blood supply by inflammatory lung disease. Clin Nucl Med 10:204, 1985.

104. Sheffield EA, Addis BJ, Corrin B, et al: Epithelial hyperplasia and malignant change in congenital lung cysts. J Clin Pathol 40:612, 1987.

105. Ng KJ, Hasan N, Gray ES, et al: Intralobar bronchopulmonary sequestration: Antenatal diagnosis. Thorax 49:379, 1994.

106. Kolls JK, Kiernen MP, Ascuitto RJ, et al: Intralobar pulmonary sequestration presenting as congestive heart failure in a neonate. Chest 102:974, 1992.

107. Nicolette LA, Kosloske AM, Bartow SA, et al: Intralobar pulmonary sequestration: A clinical and pathological spectrum. J Pediatr Surg 28:802, 1993.

108. Abuhamad AZ, Bass T, Katz ME, et al: Familial recurrence of pulmonary sequestration. Obstet Gynecol 87:843, 1996.

109. Croyle P, Estrera AS: Bronchogenic cyst and intralobar sequestration mimicking thoracic aortic aneurysm. South Med J 75:1267, 1982.

110. Hruban RH, Shumway SJ, Orel SB, et al: Congenital bronchopulmonary foregut malformations: Intralobar and extralobar pulmonary sequestrations communicating with the foregut. Am J Clin Pathol 91:403, 1989.

111. Trigaux JP, Jamart J, Van Beers B, et al: Pulmonary sequestration: Visualization of an enlarged azygos system by CT. Acta Radiol 36:265, 1995.

112. Savic B, Birtel FJ, Tholen W, et al: Lung sequestration: Report of seven cases and review of 540 published cases. Thorax 34:96, 1979.

113. Ikezoe J, Murayama S, Godwin JD, et al: Bronchopulmonary sequestration: CT assessment. Radiology 176:375, 1990.

114. Gustafson RA, Murray GF, Warden HE, et al: Intralobar sequestration: A missed diagnosis. Ann Thorac Surg 47:841, 1989.

115. Silverman ME, White CS, Ziskind AA: Pulmonary sequestration receiving arterial supply from the left circumflex coronary artery. Chest 106:948, 1994.

116. Turk LN, Lindskog GE: The importance of angiographic diagnosis in intralobar pulmonary sequestration. J Thorac Cardiovasc Surg 41:299, 1961.

117. Köhler R: Pulmonary sequestration. Acta Radiol [Diagn] (Stockholm) 8:337, 1969.

118. Krishnan M, Snelling MRJ: Lobar pulmonary sequestration. Aust N Z J Surg 39:362, 1970.

119. Ranniger K, Valvassori GE: Angiographic diagnosis of intralobar pulmonary sequestration. Am J Roentgenol 92:540, 1964.

120. Allison RS, Chirnside AM: Pulmonary sequestration: A review of 12 cases. N Z Med J 96:381, 1983.

121. Hoeffel J-C, Bernard C: Pulmonary sequestration of the upper lobe in children. Radiology 160:513, 1986.

122. Jensen V, Wolff A: Congenital intralobar pulmonary sequestration with anomalous artery from the aorta. Acta Radiol 45:357, 1956.

122a. Fraggetta F, Cacciaguerra S, Nash R, et al: Intra-abdominal pulmonary sequestration associated with congenital cystic adenomatoid malformation of the lung. Pathol Res Prac 194:209, 1998.

123. Halasz NA, Lindskog GE, Liebow AA: Esophago-bronchial fistula and bronchopulmonary sequestration: Report of a case and review of the literature. Ann Surg 155:215, 1962.

124. Felson B: The many faces of pulmonary sequestration. Semin Roentgenol 7:3, 1972.

125. Heithoff KB, Sane SM, Williams HJ, et al: Bronchopulmonary foregut malformations: A unifying etiological concept. Am J Roentgenol 126:46, 1976.

126. Takahashi M, Ohno M, Mihara K, et al: Intralobar pulmonary sequestration: With special emphasis on bronchial communication. Radiology 114:543, 1975.

127. Culiner MM, Wall CA: Collateral ventilation in "intralobar pulmonary sequestration": Report of a case. Dis Chest 47:118, 1965.

128. Hopkins RL, Levine SD, Waring WW: Intralobar sequestration: Demonstration of collateral ventilation by nuclear lung scan. Chest 82:192, 1982.

129. Janssen DP, Schilte PP, De Graaff CS, et al: Bronchopulmonary sequestration associated with an aneurysm of the aberrant artery. Ann Thorac Surg 60:193, 1995.

130. Wagenvoort CA, Heath D, Edwards JE: The Pathology of the Pulmonary Vasculature. Springfield, IL, Charles C Thomas, 1964.

131. Tandon M, Warnock ML: Plexogenic angiopathy in pulmonary intralobar sequestrations: Pathogenetic mechanisms. Hum Pathol 24:263, 1993.

132. Felson B: Pulmonary sequestration revisited. Med Radiogr Photogr 64:1, 1988.

133. Karp W: Bilateral sequestration of the lung. Am J Roentgenol 128:513, 1977.

134. Roe JP, Mack JW, Shirley JH: Bilateral pulmonary sequestrations. J Thorac Cardiovasc Surg 80:8, 1980.

135. Bates M: Total unilateral pulmonary sequestration. Thorax 23:311, 1968.

136. Turner RJ, Hayward RW: Calcification in pulmonary sequestration. Radiology 124:15, 1977.

137. Wojtowycz M, Gould HR, Atwell DT, et al: Calcified bronchopulmonary sequestration in a 76-year-old female. J Comput Tomogr 8:171, 1984.

138. Dyke JA, Sagel SS: Calcified pulmonary sequestration: CT demonstration. J Comput Assist Tomogr 9:372, 1985.

139. Kilman JW, Battersby JS, Taybi H, et al: Pulmonary sequestration. Arch Surg 90:648, 1965.

140. Gerard FP, Lyons HA: Anomalous artery in intralobar bronchopulmonary sequestration: Report of two cases demonstrated by angiography. N Engl J Med 259:662, 1958.

141. Symbas PN, Hatcher CR Jr, Abbott OA, et al: An appraisal of pulmonary sequestration: Special emphasis on unusual manifestations. Am Rev Respir Dis 406:99, 1969.

142. Fuller DN: Congenital intra-lobar sequestration of the lung: Report on four cases. S Afr Med J 29:987, 1955.

143. Simopoulos AP, Rosenblum DJ, Mazumdar H, et al: Intralobar bronchopulmonary sequestration in children: Diagnosis by intrathoracic aortography. Am J Dis Child 97:796, 1959.

144. O'Connell DJ, Kelleher J: Congenital intrathoracic bronchopulmonary foregut malformations in childhood. J Can Assoc Radiol 30:1979, 1979.

145. Miller PA, Williamson BRJ, Minor GR, et al: Pulmonary sequestration: Visualization of the feeding artery by CT. J Comput Assist Tomogr 6:828, 1982.

146. Paul DJ, Mueller CF: Pulmonary sequestration. J Comput Assist Tomogr 6:163, 1982.

147. Frush DP, Donnelly LF: Pulmonary sequestration spectrum: A new spin with helical CT. Am J Roentgenol 169:679, 1997.

148. Rappaport DC, Herman SJ, Weisbrod GL: Congenital bronchopulmonary diseases in adults: CT findings. Am J Roentgenol 162:1295, 1994.

149. Culiner M, Wall C: Collateral ventilation in intralobar pulmonary sequestration. Dis Chest 47:118, 1965.

150. Stern EJ, Webb WR, Warnock ML, et al: Bronchopulmonary sequestration: Dynamic, ultrafast, high-resolution CT evidence of air trapping. Am J Roentgenol 157:947, 1991.

151. Oliphant L, McFadden RG, Carr TJ, et al: Magnetic resonance imaging to diagnose intralobar pulmonary sequestration. Chest 91:500, 1987.

152. Naidich DP, Rumancik WM, Lefleur RS, et al: Intralobar pulmonary sequestration: MR evaluation. J Comput Assist Tomogr 11:531, 1987.

153. Pessar ML, Soulen RL, Kan JS, et al: MR imaging demonstration of pulmonary sequestration. Pediatr Radiol 18:229, 1988.

154. Doyle AJ: Demonstration of blood supply to pulmonary sequestration by MR angiography. Am J Roentgenol 258:989, 1992.

155. Stannard PA, Sivananthan MU, Robertson RJH: Case report: The use of turbo-

FLASH MR imaging for delineating vascular anatomy in bronchopulmonary sequestration. Clin Radiol 49:286, 1994.

156. Durnin RE, Lababidi Z, Butler C, et al: Bronchopulmonary sequestration. Chest 57:454, 1970.

157. Schachter EN, Karpick RJ: Bronchopulmonary sequestration and pulmonary tuberculosis. Chest 62:331, 1972.

158. Mattila SP, Ketonen PES, Kyllönen KEJ, et al: Pulmonary sequestration associated with tuberculosis, aspergillosis and pseudomycosis. Ann Chir Gynaecol Fenn 64:30, 1975.

159. Charbonneau R, Jodoin G, Bernier J: Une lesion congenitale vasculaire pulmonaire: la sequestration. Observation d'un cas typique. Union Med Can 96:158, 1967.

160. Samuels T, Morava-Protzner I, Youngson B, et al: Calcification in bronchopulmonary sequestration. Can Assoc Radiol J 40:106, 1989.

161. Uppal MS, Kohman LJ, Katzenstein AL: Mycetoma within an intralobar sequestration: Evidence supporting acquired origin for this pulmonary anomaly. Chest 103:1627, 1993.

162. Jensen FO, Maclean AD: Intralobar sequestration of the lung with tension cysts: An unusual presentation of two cases with clinical and radiological evidence of tension phenomena. Australas Radiol 14:269, 1970.

163. Kilman JW, Battersby JS, Taybi H, et al: Pulmonary sequestration. Arch Surg 90:648, 1965.

164. O'Connell DJ, Kelleher J: Congenital intrathoracic bronchopulmonary foregut malformations in childhood. J Can Assoc Radiol 30:103, 1979.

165. Choplin RH, Siegel MJ: Pulmonary sequestration: Six unusual presentations. Am J Radiol 134:695, 1980.

166. Rubin EM, Garcia H, Horowitz MD, et al: Fatal massive hemoptysis secondary to intralobar sequestration. Chest 106:954, 1994.

167. Arroyo JG, James G: Bronchopulmonary sequestration as a rare cause of acute, massive intraesophageal bleeding. South Med J 76:241, 1983.

168. Zapatero J, Baamonde C, Bellan JM, et al: Hemothorax as rare presentation of intralobar pulmonary sequestration. Scand J Thorac Cardiovasc Surg 17:177, 1983.

169. Pratter MR, Kaemmerlen JT, Erickson AD: Bloody pleural effusion associated with an intralobar pulmonary sequestration. Chest 75:394, 1979.

170. Bell-Thomson J, Missier P, Sommers SC: Lung carcinoma arising in bronchopulmonary sequestration. Cancer 44:334, 1979.

171. Gatzinsky P, Olling S: A case of carcinoma in intralobar pulmonary sequestration. Thorac Cardiovasc Surg 36:290, 1988.

172. Juettner FM, Pinter HH, Friehs GB, et al: Bronchial carcinoid arising in intralobar bronchopulmonary sequestration with vascular supply from the left gastric artery. J Thorac Cardiovasc Surg 90:25, 1985.

173. Paksoy N, Demircan A, Altiner M, et al: Localised fibrous mesothelioma arising in an intralobar pulmonary sequestration. Thorax 47:837, 1992.

174. Wier JA: Congenital anomalies of the lung. Ann Intern Med 52:330, 1960.

175. Williams AO, Enumah FI: Extralobar pulmonary sequestration. Thorax 23:200, 1968.

176. Sippel JM, Ravichandran PS, Antonovic R, et al: Extralobar pulmonary sequestration presenting as a mediastinal malignancy. Ann Thorac Surg 63:1169, 1997.

177. Nelson JB, Blum MD, Cook WA: Retroperitoneal pulmonary sequestration: A rare congenital anomaly in a 71-year-old man. J Urol 152:2341, 1994.

178. Bliek AJ, Mulholland DJ: Extralobar lung sequestration associated with fatal neonatal respiratory distress. Thorax 26:125, 1971.

179. Shuford WH, Sybers RG: Bronchopulmonary sequestration with venous drainage to the portal vein. Am J Roentgenol 106:118, 1969.

180. Sutton D, Samuel RH: Thoracic aortography in intralobar lung sequestration. Clin Radiol 14:317, 1963.

181. Campbell JA: The diaphragm in roentgenology of the chest. Radiol Clin North Am 1:395, 1963.

182. Tharion J, Das PB, Gupta RP, et al: Sequestration of lung associated with achalasia cardia. Chest 65:222, 1974.

183. Rosado de Christenson ML, Frazier AA, Stocker JT, et al: Extralobar sequestrations: Radiologic-pathologic correlation. RadioGraphics 13:425, 1993.

184. Stocker JT, Kagan-Halett K: Extralobar pulmonary sequestration. Am J Clin Pathol 72:917, 1978.

185. Aulicino MR, Reis ED, Dolgin SE, et al: Intra-abdominal pulmonary sequestration exhibiting congenital cystic adenomatoid malformation: Report of a case and review of the literature. Arch Pathol Lab Med 118:1034, 1994.

186. Heath D, Watts GT: The significance of vascular changes in an accessory lung presenting as a diaphragmatic cyst. Thorax 12:142, 1957.

187. Mahadevia PS: Necrotizing vasculitis in an extralobar sequestrated lung. Arch Pathol Lab Med 104:114, 1980.

188. Reichert JR, Winkler SS: Spontaneous hemorrhage into an extralobar bronchopulmonary sequestration. Radiology 110:359, 1974.

189. Maull KI, McElvein RB: Infarcted extralobar pulmonary sequestration. Chest 68:98, 1975.

190. Goldblatt E, Vimpani G, Brown JH: Extralobar pulmonary sequestration: Presentation as an arteriovenous aneurysm with cardiac failure in infancy. Am J Cardiol 29:100, 1972.

191. Werthammer JW, Hatten HP Jr, Blake WB Jr: Upper thoracic extralobar pulmonary sequestration presenting with respiratory distress in a newborn. Pediatr Radiol 9:116, 1980.

192. Lucaya J, Carcia-Conesa JA, Bernado L: Pulmonary sequestration associated with unilateral pulmonary hypoplasia and massive pleural effusion. A case report and review of the literature. Pediatr Radiol 14:228, 1984.

193. Avishai V, Dolev E, Weissberg D, et al: Extralobar sequestration presenting as massive hemothorax. Chest 109:843, 1996.

194. Kirwan WO, Walbaum PR, McCormack RJM: Cystic intrathoracic derivatives of the foregut and their complications. Thorax 28:424, 1973.

195. Ward IM, Krahl JB: Enterogenous pulmonary cyst. Am J Dis Child 63:924, 1942.

196. Kellett HS, Lipphard D, Willis RA: Two unusual examples of heteroplasia in the lung. J Pathol Bacteriol 84:421, 1962.

197. Culiner MM: Intralobar bronchial cystic disease, the "sequestration complex," and cystic bronchiectasis. Dis Chest 53:462, 1968.

198. Wesley JR, Heidelberger KP, DiPietro MA, et al: Diagnosis and management of congenital cystic disease of the lung in children. J Pediatr Surg 21:202, 1986.

199. Reed JC, Sobonya RE: Morphologic analysis of foregut cysts in the thorax. Am J Roentgenol 120:851, 1974.

200. St. Georges R, Deslauriers J, Duranceau A: Clinical spectrum of bronchogenic cysts of the mediastinum and lung. Ann Thorac Surg 52:6, 1991.

201. DiLorenzo M, Collin PP, Vaillancourt R, et al: Bronchogenic cysts. J Pediatr Surg 24:988, 1989.

202. Suen HC, Mathisen DJ, Grillo HC, et al: Surgical management and radiological characteristics of bronchogenic cysts. Ann Thorac Surg 55:476, 1993.

203. Ramenofsky ML, Leape LI, McCauley RGK: Bronchogenic cysts. J Pediatr Surg 14:219, 1979.

204. Wilkinson N, Reid H, Hughes D: Intradural bronchogenic cysts. J Clin Pathol 45:1032, 1992.

205. Menke H, Roher HD, Gabbert H, et al: Bronchogenic cyst: A rare cause of a retroperitoneal mass. Eur J Surg 163:311, 1997.

206. Dagenais F, Nassif E, Dery R, et al: Bronchogenic cyst of the right hemidiaphragm. Ann Thorac Surg 59:1235, 1995.

207. Amendola MA, Shirazi KK, Brooks J, et al: Transdiaphragmatic bronchopulmonary foregut anomaly: "Dumbbell" bronchogenic cyst. Am J Radiol 138:1165, 1982.

208. Bergstrom JF, Yost RV, Ford KT, et al: Unusual roentgen manifestations of bronchogenic cysts. Radiology 107:49, 1973.

209. Bücheler E, Thurn P: The combination of arterial vascular hypoplasia and cystic lung changes. Radiologe 2:347, 1962.

210. Quinlan JJ, Holden HM, Schaffner VD, et al: Cystic disease of the lungs. Can Med Assoc J 79:1012, 1958.

211. Racz I, Baum GL: The relationship of ethnic origin to the prevalence of cystic lung disease in Israel: A preliminary report. Am Rev Respir Dis 91:552, 1965.

212. Baum GL, Racz I, Bubis J, et al: Cystic disease of the lung: Report of eighty-eight cases, with an ethnologic relationship. Am J Med 40:578, 1966.

213. Beecham JE: Fine needle aspiration biopsy of peripheral congenital bronchial cyst. Acta Cytol 32:663, 1987.

214. Okubo A, Sone E, Ogushi F, et al: A case of bronchogenic cyst with high production of antigen CA 19-9. Cancer 63:1994, 1989.

215. Salyer DC, Salyer WR, Eggleston JC: Benign developmental cysts of the mediastinum. Arch Pathol Lab Med 101:136, 1977.

216. Pryce DM: The lining of healed but persistent abscess cavities in the lung with epithelium of the ciliated columnar type. J Pathol Bacteriol 60:259, 1948.

217. Rogers LF, Osmer JC: Bronchogenic cyst: A review of 46 cases. Am J Roentgenol 91:273, 1964.

218. Houser WC, Dorff GJ, Rosenzweig DY, et al: Mycobacterial infection of a congenital bronchogenic cyst. Thorax 35:312, 1980.

219. Holden WE, Mulkey DD, Kessler S: Multiple peripheral lung cysts and hemoptysis in an otherwise asymptomatic adult. Am Rev Respir Dis 126:930, 1982.

220. Dahmash NS, Chen JT, Ravin CE, et al: Unusual radiologic manifestations of bronchogenic cyst. South Med J 77:762, 1984.

221. Dabbs CH, Berg R Jr, Peirce EC II: Intrapericardial bronchogenic cysts: Report of two cases and probable embryologic explanation. J Thorac Surg 34:718, 1957.

222. Cornell SH: Calcium in the fluid of mediastinal bronchogenic cyst: A new roentgenographic finding. Radiology 85:825, 1965.

223. Nakata H, Nakayama C, Kimoto T, et al: Computed tomography of mediastinal bronchogenic cysts. J Comput Assist Tomogr 6:733, 1982.

224. Mendelson DS, Rose JS, Efremidis SC, et al: Bronchogenic cysts with high CT numbers. Am J Radiol 140:463, 1983.

225. Naidich DP, Rumancik WM, Ettenger NA, et al: Congenital anomalies of the lungs in adults: MR diagnosis. Am J Roentgenol 151:13, 1988.

226. Nakata H, Egashira K, Watanabe H, et al: MR imaging of bronchogenic cysts. J Comput Assist Tomogr 17:267, 1993.

227. Aktogu S, Yuncu G, Halilcolar H, et al: Bronchogenic cysts: Clinicopathological presentation and treatment. Eur Respir J 9:2017, 1996.

228. Zaugg M, Kaplan V, Widmer URS, et al: Fatal air embolism in an airplane passenger with a giant intrapulmonary bronchogenic cyst. Am J Respir Crit Care Med 157:1686, 1998.

229. Kent DC: Bleeding into pulmonary cyst associated with anticoagulant therapy. Am Rev Respir Dis 92:108, 1965.

230. Brünner S, Poulsen PT, Vesterdal J: Cysts of the lung in infants and children. Acta Paediatr 49:39, 1960.

231. Golding F, Griffiths P, Hempleman HV, et al: Decompression sickness during construction of the Dartford Tunnel. Br J Industr Med 17:167, 1960.

232. Svennevig J-L, Bugge-Asperheim B, Boye NP: Carcinoma arising in a lung cyst. Scand J Thorac Cardiovasc Surg 13:153, 1979.

233. Tarpy SP, Kornfeld H, Moroz K, et al: Unusual presentation of a large tension bronchogenic cyst in an adult. Thorax 48:951, 1993.

234. Maier HC: Bronchiogenic cysts of the mediastinum. Ann Surg 127:476, 1948.

235. Steinberg I: Angiocardiography in the differential diagnosis of pericardial and mediastinal tumors. Am J Roentgenol 84:409, 1960.

236. Kwak DL, Stork WJ, Greenberg SD: Partial defect of the pericardium associated with a bronchogenic cyst. Radiology 101:287, 1971.
237. Agha FP, Master K, Kaplan S, et al: Multiple bronchogenic cysts in the mediastinum. Br J Radiol 48:54, 1975.
238. Nunzio MC, Evans AJ: Case report: The computed tomographic features of mediastinal bronchogenic cyst rupture into the bronchial tree. Br J Radiol 67:589, 1994.
239. Bier R, Ethier S: Quiz case. J Can Assoc Radiol 29:69, 1978.
240. Harris M, Woo-Ming MO, Miller CG: Acquired pulmonary stenosis due to compression by a bronchogenic cyst. Thorax 28:394, 1973.
241. Gill HS, Stetz J, Chong FK, et al: Nonresolving spontaneous pneumothorax in a 38-year-old woman. Chest 110:835, 1996.
242. Khalil A, Carette MF, Milleron B, et al: Bronchogenic cyst presenting as mediastinal mass with pleural effusion. Eur Respir J 8:2185, 1995.
243. Patel SR, Meeker DP, Biscotti CV, et al: Presentation and management of bronchogenic cysts in the adult. Chest 106:79, 1994.
244. Yernault J-C, Kuhn G, Dumortier P, et al: "Solid" mediastinal bronchogenic cyst: Mineralogic analysis. Am J Roentgenol 146:73, 1986.
244a. Coiffi U, Bonavina L, De Simone M, et al: Presentation and surgical management of bronchogenic and esophageal duplication cysts in adults. Chest 113:1492, 1998.
245. Patel SR, Meeker DP, Biscotti CV, et al: Presentation and management of bronchogenic cysts in the adult. Chest 106:79, 1994.
246. Ribet ME, Copin MC, Gosselin B: Bronchogenic cysts of the mediastinum. J Thorac Cardiovasc Surg 109:1003, 1995.
247. Storer J, Kiragus C: Considerations on an unrecognized mediastinal cyst. J Pediatr 51:194, 1957.
248. Cohen SR, Geller KA, Birns JW, et al: Foregut cysts in infants and children: Diagnosis and management. Ann Otol Rhinol Laryngol 91:622, 1982.
249. Davis JG, Simonton JH: Mediastinal carinal bronchogenic cysts. Radiology 7:391, 1956.
250. Johnston SRD, Adam A, Allison DJ, et al: Recurrent respiratory obstruction from a mediastinal bronchogenic cyst. Thorax 47:660, 1992.
251. Harris M, Woo-Ming MO, Miller CG: Acquired pulmonary stenosis due to compression by a bronchogenic cyst. Thorax 28:394, 1973.
252. Fratellone PM, Coplan N, Friedman M, et al: Hemodynamic compromise secondary to a mediastinal bronchogenic cyst. Chest 106:610, 1994.
253. Miller DC, Walter JP, Guthaner DF, et al: Recurrent mediastinal bronchogenic cyst: Cause of bronchial obstruction and compression of superior vena cava and pulmonary artery. Chest 74:218, 1978.
254. Gayet C, Villard J, Andre-Fouet X, et al: Superior vena caval thrombosis and recurrent pericarditis caused by a bronchogenic cyst. J Cardiovasc Surg (Torino) 25:86, 1984.
255. Metersky ML, Moskowitz H, Thayer JO: Recurrent mediastinal bronchogenic cyst. Respiration 62:234, 1995.
255a. Okada Y, Mori H, Maeda T, et al: Congenital mediastinal bronchogenic cyst with malignant transformation: An autopsy report. Pathol Int 46:594, 1996.
256. Kissane JM: Pathology of Infancy and Childhood. 2nd ed. St. Louis, CV Mosby, 1975, p 504.
257. Spencer H: Pathology of the Lung (Excluding Pulmonary Tuberculosis). Vol 1. 4th ed. New York, Pergamon Press, 1985.
258. Williams HE, Landau LI, Phelan PD: Generalized bronchiectasis due to extensive deficiency of bronchial cartilage. Arch Dis Child 47:423, 1972.
259. Williams H, Campbell P: Generalized bronchiectasis associated with deficiency of cartilage in the bronchial tree. Arch Dis Child 35:182, 1960.
260. Wayne KS, Taussig LM: Probable familial congenital bronchiectasis due to cartilage deficiency (Williams-Campbell syndrome). Ann Rev Respir Dis 114:15, 1976.
261. Jones VF, Eid NS, Franco SM, et al: Familial congenital bronchiectasis: Williams-Campbell syndrome. Pediatr Pulmonol 16:263, 1993.
262. Hutchin P, Friedman PJ, Saltzstein SL: Congenital cystic adenomatoid malformation with anomalous blood supply. J Thorac Cardiovasc Surg 62:220, 1971.
263. Rashad F, Grisoni E, Gaglione S: Aberrant arterial supply in congenital cystic adenomatoid malformation of the lung. J Pediatr Surg 23:1007, 1988.
264. Miller RK, Sieber WK, Yunis EJ: Congenital adenomatoid malformation of the lung: A report of 17 cases, and review of the literature. In Sommers SC, Rosen PP (eds): Pathology Annual, Part I. New York, Appleton-Century-Crofts, 1980, p 387.
265. Avitabile AM, Greco MA, Hulnick DH, et al: Congenital cystic adenomatoid malformation of the lung in adults. Am J Surg Pathol 8:193, 1984.
265a. Hulnick DH, Naidich DP, McCauley DI, et al: Late presentation of congenital cystic adenomatoid malformation of the lung. Radiology 151:569, 1984.
265b. Patz EF, Müller NL, Swensen SJ, Dodd LG. Congenital cystic adenomatoid malformation in adults: CT findings. J Comput Assist Tomogr 19:361, 1995.
266. van Dijk C, Wagenvoort CA: The various types of congenital adenomatoid malformation of the lung. J Pathol 110:131, 1973.
267. Bale PM: Congenital cystic malformation of the lung: A form of congenital bronchiolar ("adenomatoid") malformation. Am J Clin Pathol 71:411, 1979.
268. Cangiarella J, Greco MA, Askin F, et al: Congenital cystic adenomatoid malformation of the lung: Insights into the pathogenesis utilizing quantitative analysis of vascular marker CD34 (QBEND-10) and cell proliferation marker MIB-1. Mod Pathol 8:913, 1995.
269. Cachia R, Sobonya RE: Congenital cystic adenomatoid malformation of the lung with bronchial atresia. Hum Pathol 12:947, 1981.
270. Mendoza A, Wolf P, Edwards DK, et al: Prenatal ultrasonographic diagnosis

of congenital adenomatoid malformation of the lung. Arch Pathol Lab Med 110:402, 1986.
271. Stocker JT, Madewell JE, Drake RM: Congenital cystic adenomatoid malformation of the lung: Classification and morphologic spectrum. Hum Pathol 8:155, 1977.
272. Ostor AG, Fortune DW: Congenital cystic adenomatoid malformation of the lung. Am J Clin Pathol 70:595, 1978.
273. Daroca PJ Jr: Mucogenic cells of congenital adenomatoid malformation of lung. Arch Pathol Lab Med 103:258, 1979.
274. Hernanz-Schulman M: Cysts and cystlike lesions of the lung. Radiol Clin North Am 31:631, 1993.
275. Lackner RP, Thompson AB 3rd, Rikkers LF, et al: Cystic adenomatoid malformation involving an entire lung in a 22-year-old woman. Ann Thorac Surg 61:1827, 1996.
276. Fasanelli S, Bellussi A, Patti GL, et al: Congenital cystic adenomatoid malformation: Unusual presentation. Rays (Roma) 5:43, 1980.
277. Hulnick DH, Naidich DP, McCauley DI, et al: Late presentation of congenital cystic adenomatoid malformation of the lung. Radiology 151:569, 1984.
278. Patz EF, Müller NL, Swensen SJ, et al: Congenital cystic adenomatoid malformation in adults: CT findings. J Comput Assist Tomogr 19:361, 1995.
279. Kim WS, Lee KS, Kim IO, et al: Congenital cystic adenomatoid malformation of the lung: CT-pathologic correlation. Am J Roentgenol 168:47, 1997.
280. Sheffield EA, Addis BJ, Corrin B, et al: Epithelial hyperplasia and malignant change in congenital lung cysts. J Clin Pathol 40:612, 1987.
281. Benjamin DR, Cahill JL: Bronchioloalveolar carcinoma of the lung and congenital cystic adenomatoid malformation. Am J Clin Pathol 95:889, 1991.
282. Ribet ME, Copin MC, Soots JG, et al: Bronchioloalveolar carcinoma and congenital cystic adenomatoid malformation. Ann Thorac Surg 60:1126, 1995.
283. Landing BH, Wells TR: Tracheobronchial anomalies in children. In Rosenberg HS, Bolands RP (eds): Perspectives in Pediatric Pathology. Vol I. Chicago, Year Book Medical Publishers, 1973, p 1.
283a. Gupta TGCM, Goldberg SJ, Lewis E, et al: Congenital bronchomalacia. Am J Dis Child 115:88, 1968.
283b. MacMahon HE, Ruggieri J: Congenital segmental bronchomalacia: Report of a case. Am J Dis Child 118:923, 1969.
283c. Chang N, Hertzler JH, Gregg RH, et al: Congenital stenosis of the right mainstem bronchus: A case report. Pediatrics 41:739, 1968.
283d. Wallace JE: Two cases of congenital web of a bronchus. Arch Pathol 39:47, 1945.
284. Gupta TGCM, Goldberg SJ, Lewis E, et al: Congenital bronchomalacia. Am J Dis Child 115:88, 1968.
285. MacMahon HE, Ruggieri J: Congenital segmental bronchomalacia: Report of a case. Am J Dis Child 118:923, 1969.
286. Chang N, Hertzler JH, Gregg RH, et al: Congenital stenosis of the right mainstem bronchus: A case report. Pediatrics 41:739, 1968.
287. Chang N, Hertzler JH, Gregg RH, et al: Congenital stenosis of the right mainstem bronchus: A case report. Pediatrics 41:739, 1968.
288. Wallace JE: Two cases of congenital web of a bronchus. Arch Pathol 39:47, 1945.
289. Meng RL, Jensik RJ, Faber LP, et al: Bronchial atresia. Ann Thorac Surg 25:184, 1978.
290. Williams AJ, Schuster SR: Bronchial atresia associated with a bronchogenic cyst: Evidence of early appearance of atretic segments. Chest 87:396, 1985.
291. van Klaveren RJ, Morshuis WJ, Lacquet LK, et al: Congenital bronchial atresia with regional emphysema associated with pectus excavatum. Thorax 47:1082, 1992.
292. Van Renterghem D: Letter to the Editor. Embryology of bronchial atresia. Chest 89:619, 1986.
293. Schuster SR, Harris GB, Williams A, et al: Bronchial atresia: A recognizable entity in the pediatric age group. J Pediatr Surg 13:682, 1978.
294. Haller JA Jr, Tepas JJ, White JJ, et al: The natural history of bronchial atresia: Serial observations of a case from birth to operative correction. J Thorac Cardiovasc Surg 79:868, 1980.
295. Reid L: The Pathology of Emphysema. London, Lloyd-Luke (Medical Books) Ltd, 1967.
296. Culiner MM: Bronchial cysts and collateral ventilation. Dis Chest 45:627, 1964.
297. Culiner MM, Grimes OF: Localized emphysema in association with bronchial cysts or mucoceles. J Thorac Cardiovasc Surg 41:306, 1961.
298. Robotham JL, Menkes HA, Chipps B, et al: A physiologic assessment of segmental bronchial atresia. Am Rev Respir Dis 121:533, 1980.
299. Sedivy R, Bankl HC, Stimpfl T, et al: Sudden, unexpected death of a young marathon runner as a result of bronchial malformation. Mod Pathol 10:247, 1997.
300. Jederlinic PJ, Sicilian LS, Baigelman W, et al: Congenital bronchial atresia: A report of 4 cases and review of the literature. Medicine 66:73, 1986.
301. Cohen AM, Solomon EH, Alfidi RJ: Computed tomography in bronchial atresia. Am J Roentgenol 135:1097, 1980.
302. Pugatch RD, Gale ME: Obscure pulmonary masses: Bronchial impaction revealed by CT. Am J Roentgenol 141:909, 1983.
303. Finck S, Milne ENC: A case report of segmental bronchial atresia: Radiologic evaluation including computed tomography and magnetic resonance imaging. J Thorac Imaging 3:53, 1988.
304. Rossoff LJ, Steinberg H: Bronchial atresia and mucocele: A report of two cases. Respir Med 88:789, 1994.
305. Miller KE, Edwards DK, Hilton S, et al: Acquired lobar emphysema in premature

infants with bronchopulmonary dysplasia: An iatrogenic disease? Radiology 138:589, 1981.

306. Murray GF: Congenital lobar emphysema. Surg Gynecol Obstet 124:611, 1967.

307. Staple TW, Hudson HH, Hartman AF Jr, et al: The angiographic findings in four cases of infantile lobar emphysema. Am J Roentgenol 97:195, 1966.

308. Cottom DG, Myers NA: Congenital lobar emphysema. BMJ 1:1394, 1957.

309. Hendren W, McKee DM: Lobar emphysema of infancy. J Paediatr Surg 1:24, 1966.

310. Reid JM, Barclay RS, Stevenson JG, et al: Congenital obstructive lobar emphysema. Dis Chest 49:359, 1966.

311. May L, Meese EH, Timmes JJ: Congenital lobar emphysema: Case report of bilateral involvement. J Thorac Cardiovasc Surg 48:850, 1964.

312. Floyd FW, Repici AJ, Gibson ET, et al: Bilateral congenital lobar emphysema surgically corrected. Pediatrics 31:87, 1963.

313. Wall MA, Eisenberg JD, Campbell JR: Congenital lobar emphysema in a mother and daughter. Pediatrics 70:131, 1982.

314. Kruse RL, Lynn HB: Lobar emphysema in infants. Mayo Clin Proc 44:525, 1969.

315. Lewis JE, Potts WJ: Obstructive emphysema with a defect of the anterior mediastinum: Report of a case. J Thorac Surg 21:438, 1951.

316. Binet JP, Nezelof C, Fredet J: Five cases of lobar tension emphysema in infancy: Importance of bronchial malformation and value of postoperative steroid therapy. Dis Chest 41:126, 1962.

317. High RH, Arey JB: Lobar emphysema in infants. Am J Dis Child 92:498, 1956.

318. Campbell PE: Congenital lobar emphysema: Etiological studies. Aust Paediatr J 5:226, 1969.

319. Powell HC, Elliott ML: Congenital lobar emphysema. Virchows Arch Pathol Anat Histol 374:197, 1977.

320. Hislop A, Reid L: New pathological findings in emphysema of childhood: I. Polyalveolar lobe with emphysema. Thorax 25:682, 1970.

321. Hislop A, Reid L: New pathological findings in emphysema of childhood: II. Overinflation of a normal lobe. Thorax 26:190, 1971.

322. Henderson R, Hislop A, Reid L: New pathologic findings in emphysema of childhood: III. Unilateral congenital emphysema with hypoplasia—and compensatory emphysema of contralateral lung. Thorax 26:195, 1971.

323. Mandelbaum I, Heimburger I, Battersby JS: Congenital lobar obstructive emphysema: Report of eight cases and literature review. Ann Surg 162:1075, 1965.

324. Leape LL, Longino LA: Infantile lobar emphysema. Pediatrics 34:246, 1964.

325. Allen RP, Taylor RL, Reiquam CW: Congenital lobar emphysema with dilated septal lymphatics. Radiology 86:929, 1966.

326. Franken EA, Buehl I: Infantile lobar emphysema: Report of two cases with unusual roentgenographic manifestation. Am J Roentgenol 98:354, 1966.

327. Fagan CJ, Swischuk LE: The opaque lung in lobar emphysema. Am J Roentgenol 114:300, 1972.

328. Kennedy CD, Habibi P, Matthew DJ, et al: Lobar emphysema: Long-term imaging follow-up. Radiology 180:189, 1991.

329. Roghair GD: Nonoperative management of lobar emphysema. Radiology 102:125, 1972.

330. Landing BH: Congenital malformations and genetic disorders of the respiratory tract (larynx, trachea, bronchi, and lungs): State of the art. Am Rev Respir Dis 120:151, 1979.

331. Myers NA: Congenital lobar emphysema. Aust N Z J Surg 30:32, 1960.

332. Roghair GD: Nonoperative management of lobar emphysema: Long-term follow-up. Radiology 102:125, 1972.

333. Warkany J: The lung. In Warkany J (ed): Congenital Malformations. Chicago, Year Book Medical Publishers, 1971, p 604.

334. Warkany J: The trachea and bronchi. In Warkany J (ed): Congenital Malformations. Chicago, Year Book Medical Publishers, 1971, p 599.

335. Atwell SW: Major anomalies of the tracheobronchial tree with a list of the minor anomalies. Dis Chest 52:611, 1967.

336. Smith FR, Boyden EA: An analysis of variations of the segmental bronchi of the right lower lobe of fifty injected lungs. J Thorac Surg 18:195, 1949.

337. Bense L, Eklund G, Wiman LG: Bilateral bronchial anomaly: A pathogenetic factor in spontaneous pneumothorax. Am Rev Respir Dis 146:513, 1992.

338. Mangiulea VG, Stinghe RV: The accessory cardiac bronchus: Bronchologic aspect and review of the literature. Dis Chest 54:35, 1968.

339. McLaughlin FJ, Strieder DJ, Harris GBC, et al: Tracheal bronchus: Association with respiratory morbidity in childhood. J Pediatr 106:751, 1985.

340. Ritsema GH: Ectopic right bronchus: Indication for bronchography. Am J Roentgenol 140:671, 1983.

341. Jackson GD, Littleton JT: Simultaneous occurrence of anomalous cardiac and tracheal bronchi: A case study. J Thorac Imaging 3:59, 1988.

342. Shipley RT, McLoud TC, Dedrick CG, et al: Computed tomography of the tracheal bronchus. J Comput Assist Tomogr 9:53, 1985.

343. Ritsema GH: Ectopic right bronchus: Indication for bronchography. Am J Roentgenol 150:671, 1983.

344. McLaughlin FJ, Strieder DJ, Harris GBC, et al: Tracheal bronchus: Association with respiratory morbidity in childhood. J Pediatr 106:751, 1985.

345. Hosker HSR, Clague HW, Morritt GN: Ectopic right upper lobe bronchus as a cause of breathlessness. Thorax 42:473, 1987.

346. Rémy J, Smith M, Marache P, et al: La bronche-tracheale-gauche pathogene. [Pathogenetic left tracheal bronchus. A review of the literature in connection with four cases.] J Radiol Electrol 58:41, 1977.

347. Gonzalez-Crussi F, Padilla L-M, Miller JK, et al: Bridging bronchus: A previously undescribed airway anomaly. Am J Dis Child 130:1015, 1976.

348. Starshak RJ, Sty JR, Woods G, et al: Bridging bronchus: A rare airway anomaly. Radiology 140:95, 1981.

349. Landing BH, Lawrence TYK, Payne VC Jr, et al: Bronchial anatomy in syndromes with abnormal visceral situs, abnormal spleen and congenital heart disease. Am J Cardiol 28:456, 1971.

350. Soto B, Pacifico AD, Souza AS, et al: Identification of thoracic isomerism from the plain chest radiograph. Am J Roentgenol 131:995, 1978.

351. Landay MJ, Shaw C, Bordlee RP: Bilateral left lungs: Unusual variation of hilar anatomy. Am J Radiol 138:1162, 1982.

352. Shtasel P, Jordan L: The accessory cardiac bronchial stump: Case reports. J Am Osteopath Assoc 65:486, 1966.

353. Mangiula VG, Razvzn VS: The accessory cardiac bronchus: Bronchologic aspect and review of the literature. Chest 54:33, 1968.

354. McGuinness G, Naidich DP, Garay SM, et al: Accessory cardiac bronchus: CT features and clinical significance. Radiology 189:563, 1993.

355. Sotile SC, Brady MB, Brogdon BG: Accessory cardiac bronchus: Demonstration by computed tomography. J Comput Assist Tomogr 12:144, 1988.

356. Watanabe H, Aoki T, Nakata H, et al: A case of squamous cell lung cancer arising from the accessory cardiac bronchus. J Thorac Imaging 12:227, 1997.

357. Dabbs DJ, Duhaylongsod F, Schour L: Fine needle aspiration cytology of congenital tracheal diverticulum: A case report. Acta Cytol 38:98, 1994.

358. Moller GM, ten Berge EJ, Stassen CM: Tracheocele: A rare cause of difficult endotracheal intubation and subsequent pneumomediastinum. Eur Respir J 7:1376, 1994.

359. Infante M, Mattavelli F, Valente M, et al: Tracheal diverticulum: A rare cause and consequence of chronic cough. Eur J Surg 160:315, 1994.

360. Moller GM, ten Berge EJ, Stassen CM: Tracheocele: A rare cause of difficult endotracheal intubation and subsequent pneumomediastinum. Eur Respir J 7:1376, 1994.

361. Morgan CL, Grossman H, Leonidas J: Roentgenographic findings in a spectrum of uncommon tracheo-oesophageal anomalies. Clin Radiol 30:353, 1979.

362. Holden MP, Wooler GH: Tracheo-oesophageal fistula and oesophageal atresia: Results of 30 years' experience. Thorax 25:406, 1970.

363. Black RJ: Congenital tracheo-oesophageal fistula in the adult. Thorax 37:61, 1982.

364. Kluth D: Atlas of esophageal atresia. J Pediatr Surg 11:901, 1976.

365. Salzberg AM: Congenital malformations of the lower respiratory tract: Respiratory disorders in the newborn. In Kendig EL, Chernick V (eds): Disorders of the Respiratory Tract. Philadelphia, WB Saunders, 1983, p 183.

366. Holman WL, Vaezy A, Postlethwait RW, et al: Surgical treatment of H-type tracheoesophageal fistula diagnosed in an adult. Ann Thorac Surg 41:453, 1986.

367. Ramo OJ, Salo JA, Mattila SP: Congenital bronchoesophageal fistula in the adult. Ann Thorac Surg 59:887, 1995.

368. Blackburn WR, Amoury RA: Congenital esophago-pulmonary fistulas without esophageal atresia: An analysis of 260 fistulas in infants, children and adults. Rev Surg 23:153, 1966.

369. Moreno AM, Ruiz de Adana JC, Sanchez UL, et al: Congenital oesophagobronchial fistula in an adult involving left main bronchus. Thorax 49:835, 1994.

370. Osinowo O, Harley HRS, Janigan D: Congenital broncho-oesophageal fistula in the adult. Thorax 38:138, 1983.

371. Levi-Montalcini R: Nerve-growth factor in familial dysautonomia. N Engl J Med 95:671, 1976.

372. Kameya S, Umeda Y, Mizuno K, et al: Congenital esophagobronchial fistula in the adult. Am J Gastroenterol 79:589, 1984.

373. Lacina S, Townley R, Radecki L, et al: Esophageal lung with cardiac abnormalities. Chest 79:468, 1981.

374. Leithiser RE Jr, Capitanio MA, Macpherson RI, et al: "Communicating" bronchopulmonary foregut malformations. Am J Roentgenol 146:227, 1986.

375. Braimbridge MV, Keith HI: Oesophago-bronchial fistula in the adult. Thorax 20:226, 1965.

376. Olivet RT, Payne WS: Congenital H-type tracheoesophageal fistula complicated by achalasia in an adult: Report of a case. Mayo Clin Proc 50:464, 1975.

377. Bekoe S, Magoven GJ, Liebler GA, et al: Congenital bronchoesophageal fistula in the adult. Chest 66:201, 1974.

378. Hicks LM, Mansfield PB: Esophageal atresia and tracheoesophageal fistula: Review of 13 years' experience. J Thorac Cardiovasc Surg 81:358, 1981.

379. Shermeta DW, Whitington PF, Seto DS, et al: Lower esophageal sphincter dysfunction in esophageal atresia: Nocturnal regurgitation and aspiration pneumonia. J Pediatr Surg 12:871, 1977.

380. Nakazato Y, Wells TR, Landing BH: Abnormal tracheal innervation in patients with esophageal atresia and tracheoesophageal fistula: Study of the intrinsic tracheal nerve plexuses by a microdissection technique. J Pediatr Surg 21:838, 1986.

381. Gundry SR, Orringer MB: Esophageal motor dysfunction in an adult with a congenital tracheoesophageal fistula. Arch Surg 120:1082, 1985.

382. Levasseur P, Navajas M: Congenital tracheobiliary fistula. Ann Thorac Surg 44:318, 1987.

383. Sane SM, Sieber WK, Girdany BR: Congenital bronchobiliary fistula. Surgery 69:599, 1971.

384. Moreira VF, Arocena C, Cruz F, et al: Bronchobiliary fistula secondary to biliary lithiasis: Treatment by endoscopic sphincterotomy. Dig Dis Sci 39:1994, 1994.

385. Hennigar GR, Choy SH: Accessory lung with persistent left superior vena cava and duplication of intestine. J Thorac Surg 35:469, 1958.

386. Brownlee RT, Dafoe CS: Complete reduplication of the right lung. J Thorac Cardiovasc Surg 55:653, 1968.

386a. Singer G, Haag E, Anabitarte M: Cutaneous lung tissue heterotopia. Histopathology 32:60, 1998.

387. Chi JG, Shong Y-K: Diffuse striated muscle heteroplasia of the lung. Arch Pathol Lab Med 106:641, 1982.
388. Armin A, Castelli M: Congenital adrenal tissue in the lung with adrenal cytomegaly: Case report and review of the literature. Am J Clin Pathol 82:225, 1984.
389. Mendoza A, Voland J, Wolf P, et al: Supradiaphragmatic liver in the lung. Arch Pathol Lab Med 110:1085, 1986.
390. Warkany J: The lung. *In* Warkany J (ed): Congenital Malformations. Chicago, Year Book Medical Publishers, 1971, p 604.
391. Marchevsky AM: Lung tumors derived from ectopic tissues. Semin Diagn Pathol 12:172, 1995.
392. Gonzalez-Crussi F, Boggs JD, Raffensperger JG: Brain heterotopia in the lungs: A rare cause of respiratory distress in the newborn. Am J Clin Pathol 73:281, 1980.
393. Dupuis C, Remy J, Remy-Jardin M, et al: The "horseshoe" lung: Six new cases. Pediatr Pulmonol 17:124, 1994.
394. Ersöz A, Soncul H, Gökgöz L, et al: Horseshoe lung with left lung hypoplasia. Thorax 47:205, 1992.
395. Chen SJ, Li YW, Wu MH, et al: Crossed ectopic left lung with fusion to the right lung: A variant of horseshoe lung? Am J Roentgenol 168:1347, 1997.
396. Freedom RM, Burrows PE, Moes CAF: "Horseshoe" lung: Report of five new cases. Am J Roentgenol 146:211, 1986.
397. Frank JL, Poole CA, Rosas G: Horseshoe lung: Clinical, pathologic, and radiologic features and a new plain film finding. Am J Roentgenol 146:217, 1986.

CHAPTER 23

Developmental Anomalies Affecting the Pulmonary Vessels

ANOMALIES OF THE PULMONARY ARTERIES, 637
  Absence of the Main Pulmonary Artery, 637
  Proximal Interruption (Absence) of the Right or Left
    Pulmonary Artery, 637
  Anomalous Origin of the Left Pulmonary Artery from
    the Right, 638
  Pulmonary Artery Stenosis, 642
  Congenital Aneurysms of the Pulmonary Arteries, 642
  Direct Communication of the Right Pulmonary Artery
    with the Left Atrium, 642
ANOMALIES OF THE PULMONARY VEINS, 642
  Congenital Pulmonary Venous Obstruction, 642
  Varicosities of the Pulmonary Veins, 645
  Anomalous Pulmonary Venous Drainage, 647
    Partial Anomalous Venous Drainage, 647
    Total Anomalous Venous Drainage, 648
ANOMALIES OF BOTH ARTERIES AND VEINS, 653
  Hypogenetic Lung (Scimitar) Syndrome, 653
  Pulmonary Arteriovenous Malformation, 655
    Pathologic Characteristics, 657
    Radiologic Manifestations, 657
    Clinical Manifestations, 661
ANOMALIES OF PULMONARY LYMPHATICS, 662
  Lymphangioma, 662
  Diffuse Pulmonary Lymphangiomatosis, 662
  Congenital Pulmonary Lymphangiectasia, 663
MISCELLANEOUS VASCULAR ANOMALIES, 664
  Anomalies of the Heart and Great Vessels, 664
    *Anomalies Resulting in Increased Pulmonary Blood
      Flow, 664*
    *Anomalies Resulting in Decreased Pulmonary Blood
      Flow, 665*
  Systemic Arterial Supply to the Lung, 665
CONGENITAL DEFICIENCY OF THE LEFT SIDE OF THE
PARIETAL PERICARDIUM, 667

For convenience of discussion, developmental anomalies of pulmonary vessels have been grouped into those affecting the arteries and veins alone, those affecting both arteries and veins, and those affecting the lymphatics. This distinction is somewhat artificial, and precise categorization of every abnormality into one of these groups is not possible. Moreover, there is also overlap with developmental anomalies of the airways and pulmonary parenchyma.[1-3]

ANOMALIES OF THE PULMONARY ARTERIES

Absence of the Main Pulmonary Artery

Absence of the main pulmonary artery can be manifested by a variety of anatomic patterns.[4] In some cases, the artery is atretic, either in its proximal portion or over its entire length, and a residual fibrous cord marks its usual position. In this situation, the right and left main pulmonary arteries may persist in their normal sites and receive their blood supply from the aorta via a patent ductus.

In other cases, all morphologic evidence of a main pulmonary artery is lost, in which case a single great artery arises from a common semilunar heart valve, invariably in association with a ventricular septal defect (persistent truncus arteriosus). Independent pulmonary arteries thus are absent, and pulmonary blood supply is derived from branches of the single trunk vessel at systemic pressure. Several anatomic subtypes have been described.[5] Type I is characterized by partial septation of the truncus arteriosus with a short pulmonary trunk arising from it and dividing into the pulmonary arteries. In Type II, the right and left pulmonary arteries arise separately from the posterior wall of the truncus. In Type III, they arise from the lateral aspect. Type IV is believed to represent a complete failure of development of the sixth aortic arch, pulmonary blood supply being derived solely from bronchial arteries. Although complete absence of pulmonary arteries may occur in this form, dissection of pulmonary hila in some patients has revealed patent pulmonary arteries distally, atresia being limited to the mediastinal portion of the vessels.[6] Several other variations have been described in addition to these four main types.[4, 7]

Pulmonary atresia with ventricular septal defect is a relatively common form of congenital heart disease.[8] As indicated, pulmonary blood flow before and at birth is supplied by a patent ductus arteriosus or by collateral systemic arteries.[8] After birth, the patent ductus narrows or closes, and the infant becomes severely hypoxemic. In about 50% of patients, major aortopulmonary collateral arteries persist as the main source of pulmonary blood flow; usually, these are one to six in number and arise from the descending thoracic aorta.[8] The prognosis is poor: the majority of patients die in infancy unless they undergo successful corrective surgery.[8, 9] Some patients, however, survive into middle age without intervention with minimal or no dyspnea.[10, 11]

Proximal Interruption (Absence) of the Right or Left Pulmonary Artery

Although rare examples of complete absence of both intrapulmonary and extrapulmonary artery branches have been described,[12] this anomaly is better designated *proximal interruption* of the right or left pulmonary artery because the vessels in the lung are usually intact and patent.[13] The majority of cases are diagnosed in childhood; occasionally the abnormality is first recognized in an adult.[14-16] As with absence of the main pulmonary artery, blood supply to the pulmonary vasculature distal to the stenosis is provided by a systemic vessel, usually a patent ductus arteriosus or bronchial collaterals and, occasionally, by an artery arising directly from the ascending aorta.[8, 17]

Interruption of the right pulmonary artery is more common, with several hundred cases having been reported.[8] The vast majority of affected patients have a left aortic arch and develop substantial bronchial collateral circulation during childhood. Patients can be classified into four groups:[8] (1) proximal interruption without pulmonary arterial hypertension, in which case patients are usually asymptomatic and the diagnosis is made on the basis of the radiologic findings; (2) proximal interruption with pulmonary arterial hypertension, in the majority of cases associated with symptoms in early childhood; (3) proximal interruption with recurrent pulmonary infection or hemoptysis, often secondary to associated malformations of the lung parenchyma;[18] and (4) proximal interruption with left patent ductus arteriosus or congenital heart disease.

Careful inspection of the right-sided collateral vessels frequently reveals focal stenotic or atretic segments;[19, 20] histologic examination of these segments has shown an appearance similar to that of the ductus arteriosus, and it has been suggested that these vessels represent (in part) persistence of a right ductus, the stenosis being a normal attempt at duct closure.[19, 20] Anomalous collaterals that arise from the ascending aorta may show no narrowing and histologically resemble a normal pulmonary artery.[17, 19] In some cases, histologic examination of right-sided intrapulmonary vessels has shown decreased medial thickness and focal intimal sclerosis.[19-21]

The radiographic findings consist of a decreased size of the right lung associated with small right and enlarged left hila (Fig. 23–1).[8] Enlargement of the intercostal arteries may result in rib notching. Despite its reduced volume, the lung usually is hyperlucent; when taken in conjunction with the diminutive hilar shadow, this finding may lead to the erroneous diagnosis of Swyer-James syndrome. Differentiation is usually possible by radiography in full expiration: patients with Swyer-James syndrome show ipsilateral air trapping as a result of bronchiolar obstruction, a sign that is absent in cases of proximal pulmonary artery interruption. The diagnosis also may be confirmed by echocardiography and perfusion lung scans.[8] Perfusion is absent and ventilation normal in the affected lung in proximal interruption, whereas in Swyer-James syndrome there is substantial reduction in both perfusion and ventilation.[22, 23] Chronic thromboembolic occlusion of a pulmonary artery may mimic proximal interruption even on angiography.[24] Contrast-enhanced CT and MR imaging allow demonstration of the absent proximal artery and the patent intrapulmonary arteries, which are typically decreased in caliber.[25-27] They may also allow demonstration of bronchial collaterals or the less common transpleural intercostal collaterals.[16, 27]

Proximal interruption of the left pulmonary artery is less common than right-sided interruption and has a high incidence of associated congenital cardiovascular anomalies, particularly tetralogy of Fallot.[17] The distal left pulmonary artery may be supplied by a patent ductus arteriosus, by acquired bronchial artery collaterals, or by a vessel originating in the ascending aorta.[8] Although usually diagnosed in infancy, the abnormality occasionally is undetected until adulthood on the basis of an abnormal chest radiograph.[16, 28] The radiographic findings are similar to those of the right-sided anomaly and consist of decreased size of the left lung and hemithorax, absent left pulmonary artery shadow, elevation of the left hemidiaphragm, and ipsilateral shift of the mediastinum.[16, 28] The pulmonary vessels may be absent or markedly decreased in size. Ventilation-perfusion scans demonstrate absent perfusion and decreased ventilation without any evidence of air trapping;[16] definitive diagnosis can be made by MR, contrast-enhanced CT, or angiography.[16, 25, 28] One patient has been reported to have concomitant left lower lobe bronchiectasis.[16] Hemoptysis, sometimes massive, may occur.[29]

Anomalous Origin of the Left Pulmonary Artery from the Right

Of the many anomalous origins of the pulmonary arteries,[30] derivation of the left from the right is particularly interesting because of its effects on the lungs.[31, 32] From its point of origin, the aberrant left artery passes posteriorly and to the right to reach the right side of the distal trachea or right main bronchus; it then turns sharply to the left and passes between the esophagus and trachea in its course to the left hilum (thus the designation *pulmonary sling*). Its intimate relationship to the right main bronchus and trachea results in their compression and various obstructive effects on the right lung or both lungs.[30]

The pathogenesis of the anomaly has been hypothesized to be faulty development or reabsorption of the ventral portion of the left sixth aortic arch, leaving the developing left pulmonary plexus to connect with the right sixth aortic arch (subsequently the right pulmonary artery).[33] There is evidence that it may be related to a 22q11.2 chromosomal deletion.[33a]

Airway obstruction usually becomes manifest shortly after birth. The affected infant almost invariably presents with stridor and often with feeding problems and respiratory tract infections; the right lung is frequently overinflated.[34, 35] The abnormality is commonly associated with tracheobronchial anomalies, such as tracheal stenosis (*see* farther on) and anomalous origin of the right upper lobe bronchus from the trachea; cardiovascular malformations are also frequent. Occasional patients are asymptomatic, and the abnormality is detected as an incidental finding on the chest radiograph in adulthood.[36-38] One elderly patient presented with dysphagia.[39] Conventional chest radiographs may reveal an anterior impression on the distal trachea and an extraparatracheal opacity.[40] The demonstration of local posterior displacement of the barium-filled esophagus in the region of the lower trachea makes the diagnosis virtually certain. The diagnosis can be confirmed by CT (Fig. 23–2) or MR, both of which demonstrate the origin and course of the anomalous artery as well as the presence of associated airway abnormalities.[38, 41, 42]

The condition is usually fatal unless treated.[35] Early recognition is vital because surgical correction is feasible and usually results in abatement of respiratory symptoms and

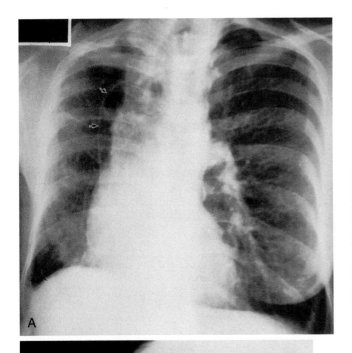

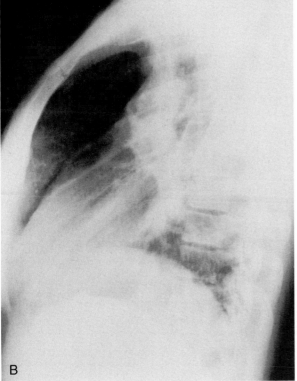

Figure 23–1. Proximal Interruption of the Right Pulmonary Artery. A posteroanterior radiograph *(A)* reveals moderate elevation of the right hemidiaphragm and shift of the mediastinum to the right, indicating considerable loss of volume of the right lung. A right hilar shadow cannot be identified, and the vascularity of the right lung is markedly reduced in amount and atypical in pattern. The overinflated left lung is displaced into the right hemithorax, as indicated by the anterior pleural junction line *(arrows)*; note the deep retrosternal air space in lateral projection *(B)*. A rectilinear lung scan (anterior view) *(C)* reveals no perfusion of the right lung; note the faint but definite activity extending into the right hemithorax from the overinflated left lung. (Courtesy of Dr. Richard Lesperance, Montreal Chest Hospital Center.)

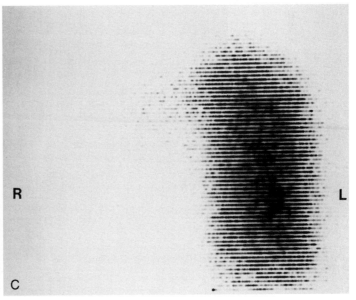

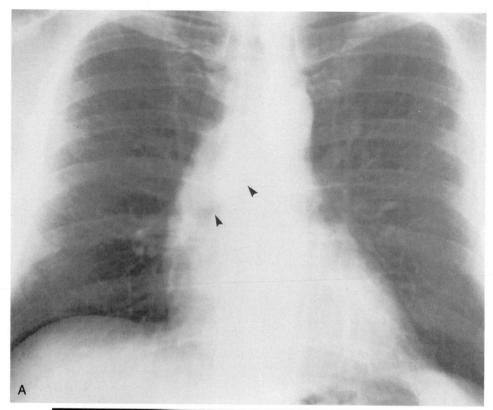

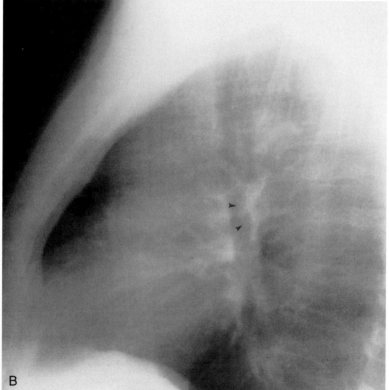

Figure 23–2. Anomalous Origin of the Left Pulmonary Artery from the Right. Posteroanterior (PA) *(A)* and lateral *(B)* chest radiographs reveal an abnormal mediastinal opacity on the PA view *(small arrowheads)* overlying the right side of the cardiac silhouette. On the lateral projection, the normal right hilar vascular shadow and the intermediate stem line are not seen; note also the impression on the posterior aspect of an airway *(small arrowheads)*.

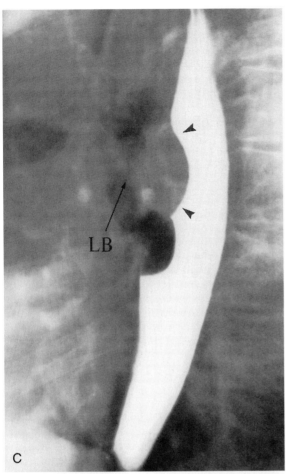

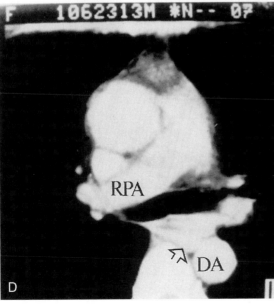

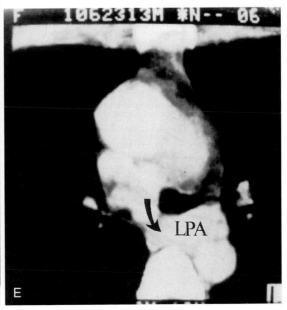

Figure 23–2 *Continued.* A lateral projection of the chest with barium in the esophagus *(C)* reveals the left pulmonary artery impressing the left main bronchus anteriorly (LB) and the esophagus posteriorly *(arrowheads).* CT scans through the right pulmonary artery (RPA) *(D)* and a level more cephalad *(E)* reveal the left pulmonary artery (LPA) arising from the right pulmonary artery from which it passes behind the left main bronchus before entering the left hilum *(curved arrow).* The esophagus *(open arrow)* lies anteromedial to the descending aorta (DA) behind the anomalous pulmonary artery. The patient was a 46-year-old man with essential hypertension. (From Stone DN, Bein ME, Garris JB: Anomalous left pulmonary artery: Two new adult cases. Am J Roentgenol 135:1259–1263, 1980.)

signs. Associated congenital defects, usually cardiovascular, are common and may be of greater prognostic significance.[40]

Tracheobronchial anomalies have been found in approximately 50% of cases studied at autopsy;[40] of particular importance is tracheal stenosis caused by incomplete septation of the cartilaginous rings (*napkin ring* or *funnel* trachea). Because of the frequency of this associated anomaly, bronchoscopy is recommended before surgery in any patient with anomalous left pulmonary artery origin to establish whether respiratory difficulty might be caused by such an intrinsic tracheal anomaly rather than by the vascular anomaly itself.[43] The term *ring/sling complex* has been suggested for this entity; in addition to the anomalous left pulmonary artery, radiographic findings include a low carina, horizontal equal-length right and left main bronchi, and a long segment of stenotic trachea.[44]

Pulmonary Artery Stenosis

Stenosis (coarctation) of the pulmonary artery may be single or multiple, short or long, unilateral or bilateral and may occur anywhere from the pulmonary valve to small pulmonary arteries.[45] Stenosis affecting the main branch or proximal branches of the pulmonary artery is often associated with cardiovascular anomalies, most frequently infundibular, valvular, or supravalvular pulmonic stenosis (60% of cases)[46, 47] and atrial septal defect.[48] In one review of 20 cases, pulmonary artery stenosis was present without other abnormalities in 5 cases, was associated with congenital cardiac anomalies in 9, and was part of the Williams-Beuren syndrome (pulmonary artery stenoses, supravalvular aortic stenosis, mental retardation, and peculiar facies) in 6.[52, 53]

The etiology of the abnormality is variable. In some cases, it is associated with pulmonary artery stenoses in other family members[50] or with Ehlers-Danlos syndrome,[51] Down's syndrome,[45] or Alagille syndrome (decreased intrahepatic bile ducts, cholestasis, and peculiar facies),[54] suggesting a genetic defect. Other cases occur after maternal rubella.[55]

Radiographically the pulmonary vasculature may appear normal, diminished, or increased, depending on the presence and nature of associated malformations (Figs. 23–3 and 23–4).[49] In those instances in which the pulmonary artery stenosis is the only or major anomaly, the chest radiograph may reveal poststenotic dilation of affected pulmonary artery branches, diffuse pulmonary oligemia, and signs of pulmonary arterial hypertension and cor pulmonale. Selective pulmonary angiography has been recommended in all cases of presumed pulmonary valvular stenosis to rule out associated peripheral pulmonary coarctation.[56]

In patients with peripheral pulmonary stenosis or coarctation, the pulmonic second sound is accentuated and a grade 2 to 4/6 murmur usually is audible bilaterally over the upper part of the chest anteriorly, radiating to the neck and back;[47] however, when stenosis is severe, flow may be so reduced that the lesions are acoustically silent.[57] A murmur also may not be heard at the site of the pulmonary arterial stenosis in patients with associated cardiac anomalies, presumably because flow is decreased by the valvular or infundibular stenosis.

Congenital Aneurysms of the Pulmonary Arteries

Congenital aneurysms of the pulmonary arteries are rare lesions that are usually seen with other pulmonary abnormalities, such as arteriovenous malformations or bronchopulmonary sequestration.[30] Approximately 40% to 50% are associated with congenital cardiac defects, such as pulmonic valve stenosis, tetralogy of Fallot, and ventricular septal defect.[58, 59] These aneurysms are usually present at birth and are often the result of turbulent blood flow created by pulmonary valvular stenosis. Such poststenotic dilation affects the left pulmonary artery much more commonly than the right; in fact, enlargement of the main pulmonary artery and its left branch in conjunction with a normal right hilum should strongly suggest the diagnosis of pulmonary valvular stenosis (Fig. 23–5). Dilation also may occur as an isolated anomaly unassociated with pulmonary stenosis, in which case it is usually (albeit not always [Fig. 23–6]) confined to the pulmonary trunk;[60] although often fusiform in shape, it may be saccular. The abnormality may be confused radiographically with a central or peripheral neoplasm.[61] Definitive diagnosis may be made with contrast-enhanced CT, MR, or angiography.[62]

Clinical manifestations include asymmetry of the thorax (the left side usually being more prominent), a systolic ejection murmur (attributable to the stenosis of the pulmonary valve orifice in relation to the increased caliber of the main pulmonary artery), and accentuation of the second pulmonic sound (possibly caused by the proximity of the dilated pulmonary artery to the anterior chest wall rather than by pulmonary hypertension[63]). The abnormality is compatible with a normal life span.[63]

Direct Communication of the Right Pulmonary Artery with the Left Atrium

This is a rare congenital malformation characterized by a direct communication between a branch of the right pulmonary artery and the left atrium without intervening lung parenchyma; 35 cases had been reported by 1989.[64] Aneurysmal dilation of the anomalous branch is common. In some cases, the right lung itself is normal, the anomalous artery behaving as a supernumerary vessel arising from an otherwise unremarkable right pulmonary artery. In others, there is aplasia or severe hypoplasia of the lower lobe,[65, 66] in which case the vessel appears to represent a residual interlobar or lower lobe artery that persists in the absence of peripheral portions of the pulmonary vascular bed.

Although the chest radiograph may be normal,[67] it most often reveals a round opacity 2 to 3 cm in diameter in the right hemithorax adjacent to the left atrium.[68] Definitive diagnosis may be made by angiography or MR;[67] with the latter, the communication is best seen on images obtained in the oblique sagittal plane.[67] The diagnosis is usually made in infancy or childhood; occasional examples have been reported in adults.[66, 67] Patients complain of dyspnea, and there may be cyanosis and clubbing. The condition can be corrected relatively easily in most cases by ligating or dividing the aberrant vessel.

ANOMALIES OF THE PULMONARY VEINS

Congenital Pulmonary Venous Obstruction

Congenital obstruction of the pulmonary veins can be caused by compression by an intrathoracic mass or by intrin-

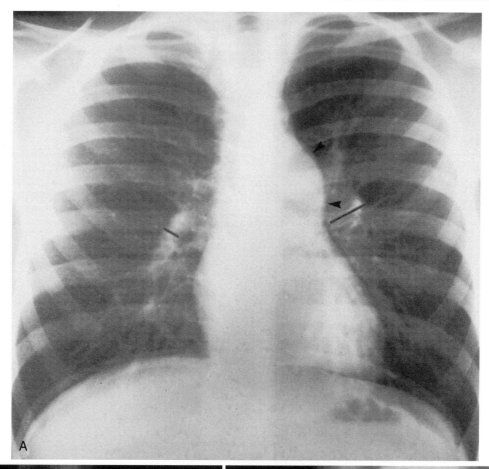

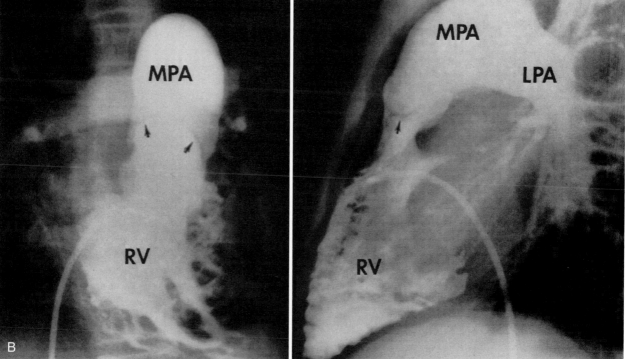

Figure 23–3. Valvular Pulmonary Stenosis with Poststenotic Arterial Dilation. A posteroanterior chest radiograph *(A)* demonstrates a prominent main pulmonary artery *(arrowheads)* and a sharp discrepancy between the size of the right and left interlobar arteries at comparable levels *(oblique bars)*. The midlung vasculature is normal on both sides. These features should suggest pulmonary valvular stenosis with poststenotic dilation of the main and proximal left interlobar pulmonary arteries. A right ventricular (RV) angiogram *(B)* in anteroposterior *(left)* and lateral *(right)* projection reveals dilation of the right ventricle. The pulmonic valves *(arrows)* are thickened and domed, indicating stenosis. Note the poststenotic dilation of the main pulmonary artery (MPA) and the proximal portion of the left interlobar artery (LPA). The patient was a 10-year-old boy with a loud precordial systolic murmur.

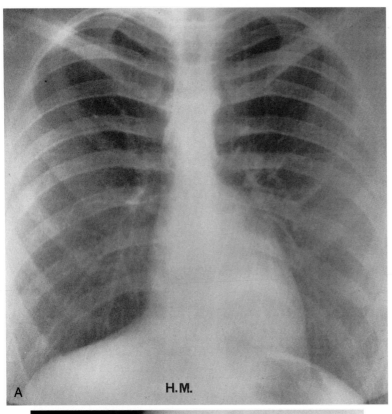

H.M.

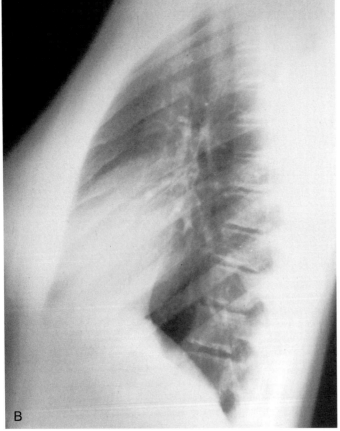

Figure 23–4. Combined Pulmonary Valvular and Arterial Stenosis. Conventional posteroanterior *(A)* and lateral *(B)* chest radiographs disclose right ventricular enlargement, absence of the main pulmonary artery segment on the left heart border, diminutive hilar arteries, and diffuse pulmonary oligemia.

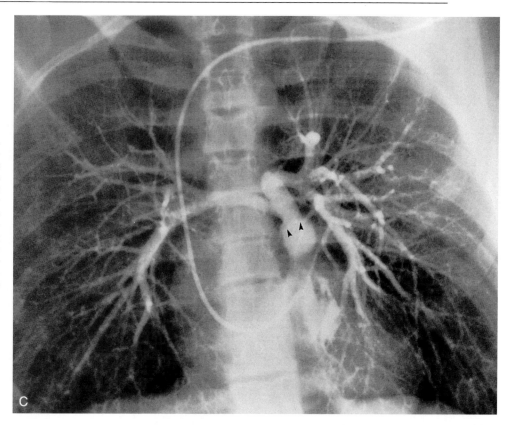

Figure 23–4 *Continued.* A right ventricular angiogram in anteroposterior projection *(C)* discloses severe generalized narrowing of the central and hilar pulmonary arteries consistent with diffuse pulmonary artery coarctation. Venous drainage (not shown) was through the pulmonary veins to the left atrium. Doming of the pulmonic valves *(arrowheads)* indicates valvular stenosis. The patient was a young woman with exertional dyspnea and loud systolic murmurs throughout the precordium.

sic abnormalities of the veins themselves. In addition, some cardiac anomalies, such as cor triatriatum, can result in venous obstruction that is clinically indistinguishable from the other two forms.

The intrinsic anomaly, characterized by stenosis or atresia of one or more pulmonary veins, is rare.[69, 70] Most cases of isolated stenosis are recognized in the first 3 years of life; occasional individuals have survived to 13 years of age before diagnosis.[69] As might be expected, common vein atresia is invariably identified in the neonatal period.[70] Many patients have an associated cardiovascular anomaly.

Morphologically the abnormality is localized to the venoatrial junction and consists of either stenosis or complete atresia.[71] The stenosis can be caused by a primary abnormality of either the atrium or the veins themselves, the former consisting of endocardial thickening at the mouth of the vein and the latter of medial muscular hypertrophy, intimal fibrosis, or a combination of the two. Stenotic vessels can become completely occluded by secondary thrombus formation.

In patients without associated cardiovascular anomalies, radiologic manifestations consist of signs of pulmonary venous hypertension, with or without arterial hypertension and right ventricular enlargement. In an infant presenting with hemoptysis, the presence of asymmetric vascularity and a unilateral reticular pattern in a lung of normal or small size should suggest the diagnosis of localized stenosis; confirmation can be obtained by a pulmonary arteriogram that reveals a small ipsilateral pulmonary artery, pruned peripheral branches, stasis of contrast medium, and nonopacification of draining pulmonary veins.[71–74]

Clinically the most common symptoms are failure to thrive, fatigue, dyspnea, recurrent respiratory infections, and hemoptysis.[72] Signs and symptoms of pulmonary venous and arterial hypertension are common but may be modified by associated cardiovascular anomalies.

Varicosities of the Pulmonary Veins

Varicosities of the pulmonary veins are a rare abnormality that may be either congenital or acquired and consist of abnormal tortuosity and dilation of one or more pulmonary veins just before their entrance into the left atrium. By 1984, 53 cases of the congenital form had been reported.[75] The abnormality usually is not recognized until the patient reaches adulthood, although cases have been reported in infants.[76] The defect is thought to occur during the period of transition from splanchnic to pulmonary venous drainage, although the reason for the localized dilation at that time is not understood.[77] One case has been reported in association with the Klippel-Trenaunay syndrome (varicosities of systemic veins, cutaneous and soft tissue hypertrophy, and hemangiomas).[78]

The majority of cases in which the vein has been studied have shown normal structure,[77] and an intrinsic defect of the vessel wall does not seem likely. In most cases, the lesion is apparent radiologically as one or more round or oval homogeneous opacities, somewhat lobulated but well defined, in the medial third of either lung (Fig. 23–7). On the left, the lingular vein is usually affected; on the right, it is most often a branch of the inferior pulmonary vein in the region of the medial basal segment of the right lower lobe.[80, 81]

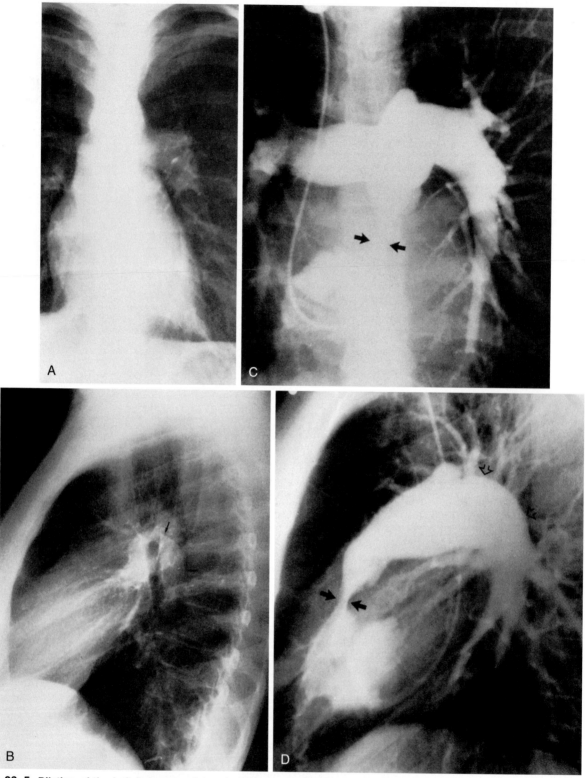

Figure 23–5. Dilation of the Left Pulmonary Artery in Infundibular Pulmonic Stenosis. In posteroanterior projection *(A)*, the left hilum is larger than the right, its configuration suggesting dilation of its vascular components; in lateral projection *(B)*, the dilated left interlobar artery can be identified *(arrows)* curving over the left upper lobe bronchus. A pulmonary angiogram *(C* and *D)* shows a severe degree of infundibular pulmonic stenosis *(solid arrows)* and selective dilation of the left pulmonary artery *(open arrows* in *D).*

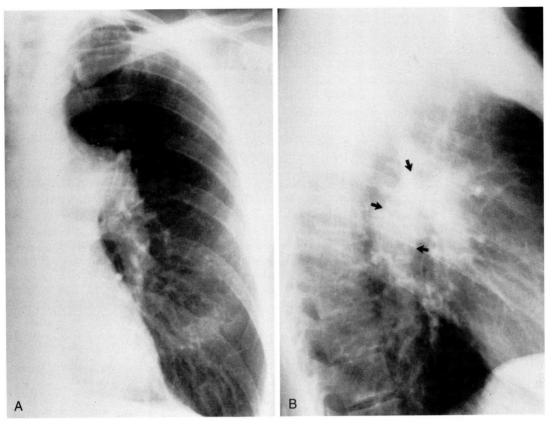

Figure 23–6. Idiopathic Dilation of the Pulmonary Artery. Posteroanterior *(A)* and lateral *(B)* radiographs of the left lung reveal marked dilation of the left main pulmonary artery and its interlobar branch. The increased diameter of the interlobar artery is well illustrated in lateral projection *(arrows in B)*. This 44-year-old man was asymptomatic and had no abnormal findings on physical examination.

Acquired varicosities of the pulmonary veins are invariably associated with disease of the mitral valve, most commonly regurgitation.[82] They usually occur on the right side, a striking unilaterality that can be attributed to the anatomy of the mitral valve, whose plane is directed posteriorly, superiorly, and to the right.

The radiographic differential diagnosis includes all masses in the lungs. The definitive diagnosis can be readily made with contrast-enhanced CT,[83] MR, or angiography[75, 84] (*see* Fig. 23–7). The varicosities may opacify more slowly than normal pulmonary veins and, because of sluggish flow, may clear more slowly.[84] Caution should be exercised in such circumstances, however, because a case has been described in which a bronchogenic cyst opacified during the venous phase of a pulmonary angiogram,[76] and two cases have been reported in which atresia of one pulmonary vein was accompanied by abnormal dilation of the remaining ipsilateral pulmonary vein, mimicking a pulmonary varix.[85, 86]

Pulmonary venous varicosities seldom give rise to symptoms; however, hemoptysis and death have been reported after rupture.[84, 87] In one case, chronic collapse of the right middle lobe was attributed to bronchial obstruction by the abnormal vessel.[88]

Anomalous Pulmonary Venous Drainage

Anomalous pulmonary venous drainage occurs when pulmonary venous blood flows directly into the right heart or systemic veins. It may be partial or total, both forms producing an extracardiac left-to-right shunt; in addition, a total anomalous connection is associated with a right-to-left shunt through an obligatory septal defect. The anatomy of the anomalous connections is highly variable. Although approximately 30 patterns have been described,[89] drainage may be considered in four groups:[90] (1) *supracardiac*, usually to a persistent left superior vena cava and thence to the left innominate vein (approximately 50% of cases); (2) *cardiac*, in which a direct connection is established with the right atrium or coronary sinus (30% of cases); (3) *infradiaphragmatic*, in which a common vein extends below the diaphragm to join the portal vein or one of its radicles (15% of cases); and (4) *mixed* (approximately 5% of cases). It is probable that there are several pathogenetic mechanisms to explain these anatomic variations;[90] the most important is likely a failure of connection between the primitive pulmonary splanchnic plexus and the common pulmonary vein derived from the atrium.[90]

Partial Anomalous Venous Drainage

The partial anomaly incorporates the venous drainage from part or all of one lung via one or more pulmonary veins. It is probably more common than clinical and routine postmortem examinations suggest; in two series of 550 consecutive autopsies, the incidence was 0.7%.[91] When symptoms are present, the abnormality is often associated with other cardiovascular anomalies, particularly atrial septal de-

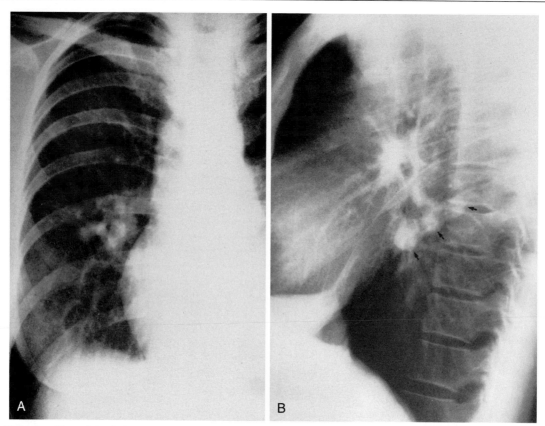

Figure 23–7. Varicosities of the Pulmonary Veins. Posteroanterior *(A)* and lateral *(B)* radiographs of this asymptomatic 39-year-old woman reveal a lobulated opacity projected in the plane of the right hilum and situated slightly posterior to it *(arrows in B)*.

fect. The special situation in which the anomalous vein drains the right lung and is associated with other right-sided anomalies is considered separately (hypogenetic lung syndrome, *see* page 653).

The anomalous vein may be visible on plain radiographs, although a more precise characterization of the anomaly can be achieved by CT.[92] The most common site identified on CT in adults is probably the left upper lobe (Fig. 23–8).[93] In this situation, the anomalous vein courses cephalad lateral to the aortic arch and usually drains into the left brachiocephalic vein, a course that is particularly well demonstrated with contrast-enhanced dynamic or spiral CT and multiplanar or three-dimensional reconstructions.[93] CT findings also may be diagnostic in cases involving the left lower lobe,[94] right lower lobe,[95] and partial right pulmonary venous drainage into the azygos vein.[96] MR or pulmonary angiography may be required to confirm the diagnosis (Fig. 23–9).[97, 98, 98a] In one study of 11 patients with a total of 14 anomalous pulmonary venous connections, MR allowed identification of all 14, whereas only 8 were identified by echocardiography.[98] MR also allows identification of associated cardiac abnormalities, the most common being atrial septal defect.[98]

When the venous drainage of an entire lung passes into the systemic venous system and the atrial septum is intact,[99] the hemodynamics of the two lungs obviously differ—as has been described in association with mitral stenosis[100] and mitral atresia[101]—indicating the possibility of differing degrees of pulmonary venous hypertension in the two lungs.

In this situation, the increased blood flow to the involved lung may be manifested by enlargement of the pulmonary artery and prominence of the vascular markings.[100]

Because there is usually no significant obstruction to blood flow, pulmonary vascular changes and congestive heart failure tend to develop late in the course of the disease; in fact, patients can survive into adulthood and old age without clinical evidence of cardiopulmonary abnormality.[90, 91, 102, 103] When present, symptoms and signs are identical to those of atrial septal defect: the second heart sound is often widely split, and there is usually an ejection systolic murmur and gallop rhythm. Because pulmonary venous blood mixes with systemic venous blood at or before the right atrium, oxygen saturation tends to be identical in all heart chambers and the two major vessels; in the absence of severe pulmonary hypertension, this may be a clue to the venous anomaly. Occasionally, the abnormality occurs in adults with an intact atrial septum who present with "unexplained" pulmonary arterial hypertension.[104]

Total Anomalous Venous Drainage

Total anomalous pulmonary venous drainage is a relatively uncommon abnormality,[90] in which an atrial septal defect or patent ductus arteriosus is necessary for survival. Other cardiovascular anomalies are present in approximately one third of cases;[102] syndromes of deranged bronchial anatomy and splenic abnormalities are also frequent.[105, 106] Typically the pulmonary veins join directly behind the heart to

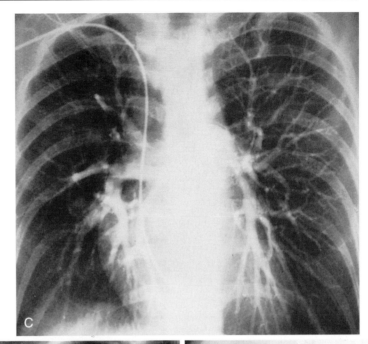

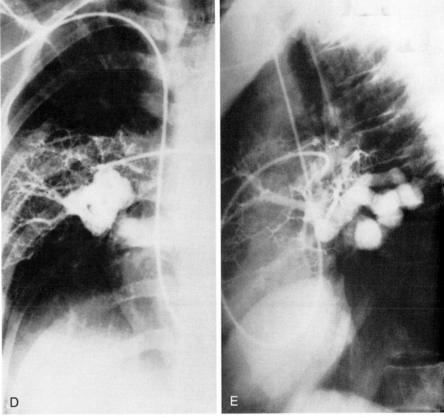

Figure 23–7 *Continued.* The arterial phase of a flood pulmonary angiogram *(C)* reveals no evidence of opacification of the mass. The anterior segmental artery of the right upper lobe was selectively catheterized, and contrast medium was injected; during the venous phase of the injection *(D and E)*, dense opacification of several spherical vascular spaces occurred, draining via large dilated veins into the left atrium. (Courtesy of Dr. W. E. Beamish, University of Alberta Hospital, Edmonton, Alberta.)

form a common, somewhat dilated sac before communicating with the systemic venous system.[90, 107] A case has been reported of a 55-year-old asymptomatic man who had a single pulmonary vein draining into the left atrium after collecting the total venous circulation from both lungs.[107a] The chest radiograph demonstrated a scimitar-like tubular structure caudad to the right hilum. Three-dimensional reconstructions from a spiral CT demonstrated progression of veins from both lungs toward a retrocardiac junction, at which they created a single vein that coursed cranially to enter the right side of the left atrium at the level of the right hilum.

The clinical and pathologic manifestations can result from the large left-to-right shunt (in which case there is frequently pulmonary arterial and right ventricular dilation[108]) or from obstruction to venous blood flow. The latter may occur by several mechanisms: (1) drainage of the entire pulmonary blood flow through the hepatic portal circulation,

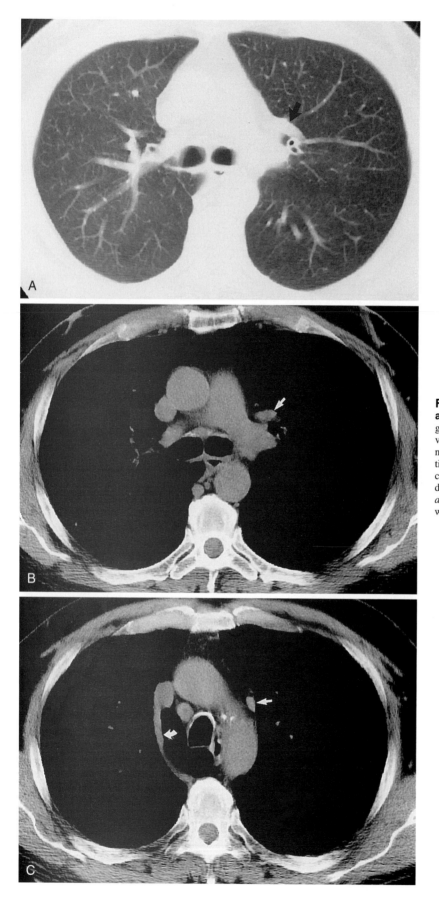

Figure 23–8. Partial Anomalous Venous Drainage of the Left Upper Lobe. CT scan *(A)* photographed at lung windows demonstrates an anomalous vein coursing from the left upper lobe into the mediastinum *(arrow)*. CT scans *(B* and *C)* photographed at soft tissue windows demonstrate the anomalous vein coursing cranially lateral to the aortic arch *(straight arrows)*. Incidental note is also made of the azygos vein *(curved arrow)* coursing within an azygos fissure. The patient was a 51-year-old man.

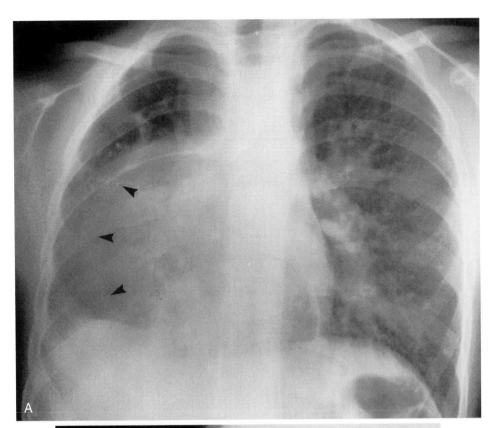

Figure 23–9. Anomalous Pulmonary Venous Return. Posteroanterior *(A)* and lateral *(B)* chest radiographs show a broad curvilinear vessel *(arrowheads)* in the right lung. The heart is displaced to the right, and the right lung is of small volume compared with the left.

Illustration continued on following page

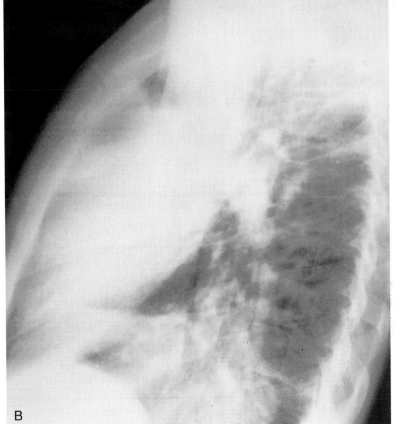

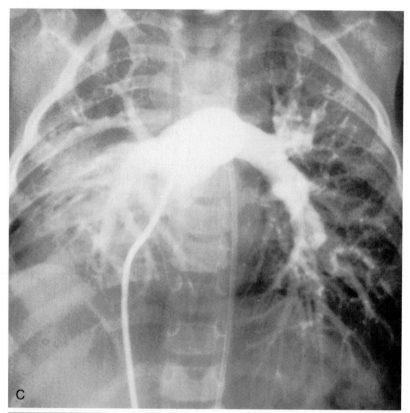

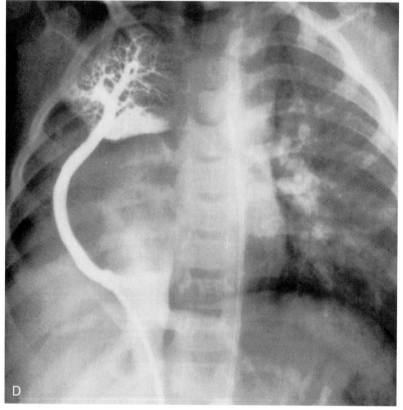

Figure 23–9 *Continued.* Pulmonary angiogram in anteroposterior projection *(C)* reveals a normal complement of pulmonary arteries on both sides. Selective catheterization of the anomalous vessel via the inferior vena cava *(D)* shows an anomalous vein that drains into the hepatic venous system. Although this vein possesses the typical configuration of a scimitar, the patient does not manifest all the anomalies usually associated with the hypogenetic lung (scimitar) syndrome (see Fig. 23–10).

in which case obstruction is invariable; (2) intrinsic stenosis of the abnormal common pulmonary vein;[109] (3) compression of the anomalous common vein between the left main pulmonary artery and the left main bronchus;[109, 110] and (4) a small atrial septal defect, especially when it is a simple patent foramen ovale.

Morphologic studies of autopsy specimens have shown medial hypertrophy of muscular arteries and veins, arteriolization of both small arterioles and veins, and parenchymal interstitial thickening, the last-named especially in cases with infradiaphragmatic connection.[106, 108]

The radiographic features are variable. Cases with communication at the supracardiac or cardiac level usually are characterized by severe pulmonary pleonemia.[107] Those with significant pulmonary venous obstruction and hypertension show a characteristic radiographic combination of interstitial pulmonary edema and a normal-sized heart. Definitive diagnosis can be made with echocardiography, MR, or angiography.[97, 111] In one investigation of 77 patients in which the three procedures were compared (including 56 patients with a variety of congenital cardiac abnormalities but normal pulmonary veins and 21 with various anomalous pulmonary venous connections), overall detection rates were 95% with MR imaging, 69% with cardiac angiography, and 38% with echocardiography.[97] In another prospective study of 13 patients, MR imaging demonstrated the anomalous connection in all cases, whereas the diagnostic accuracy of echocardiography was 57%.[112] Rarely a large vein may drain blood from one pulmonary lobe to an ipsilateral lobe, simulating the scimitar syndrome.[113]

The majority of patients with total anomalous pulmonary venous drainage die in infancy;[114, 115] even with surgical correction, the mortality rate is about 40%.[116] Patients who survive to adulthood characteristically have a large septal defect and a short anomalous pathway, drainage being directly into the superior vena cava or right atrium.[117] When total anomalous pulmonary venous drainage is associated with tetralogy of Fallot, any obstruction to pulmonary venous drainage causes severe pulmonary edema if the tetralogy is corrected by systemic-to–pulmonary artery shunt.

ANOMALIES OF BOTH ARTERIES AND VEINS

Hypogenetic Lung (Scimitar) Syndrome

Hypogenetic lung (scimitar) syndrome is a rare congenital anomaly characterized principally by hypoplasia of the right lung and anomalous pulmonary venous drainage from it to the inferior vena cava.[3, 118, 119] The incidence is estimated to be 1 to 3 per 100,000 births.[120] The anomalous pulmonary vein most commonly drains into the inferior vena cava below the level of the right hemidiaphragm,[118, 119] although it may also join with the suprahepatic portion of the inferior vena cava, hepatic veins, portal vein, azygos vein, coronary sinus, or right atrium.[3, 96, 118, 119] Hypoplasia of the right pulmonary artery and partial or complete arterial supply to the right lung by systemic arteries originating from the descending thoracic or upper abdominal aorta are also usually present.[118, 119, 121] The anomalous systemic artery runs most frequently to the lower lobe, although the entire right lung may be thus supplied.[118] Its vascular distribution does not overlap with

the territory of either pulmonary or bronchial arteries; however, its branching pattern is similar to that of the pulmonary arteries, and it acts as the sole vascular supply for the pulmonary parenchyma it subtends.[122] Other pulmonary abnormalities found in the syndrome include anomalies of the right bronchial tree (commonly mirror image), diverticula (possibly the cause of recurrent bronchopulmonary infections in later life[122]) and, occasionally, extension of a portion of the right lung across the midline into the left hemithorax.[123] Associated cardiovascular anomalies are also frequent, the most common being atrial septal defect (present in 25% of patients in one series[124]), ventricular septal defect, tetralogy of Fallot, patent ductus arteriosus, coarctation of the aorta, persistence of the left superior vena cava, cardiac dextroposition, and pulmonary stenosis.

The pathogenesis of the abnormality is unclear; however, the multiplicity of pulmonary anomalies suggests that it most likely represents a profound developmental derangement of the entire lung bud early in embryogenesis. Why the combination of changes is so consistently located on the right side is unknown. The syndrome has been reported in a father and daughter,[125] in a father and son,[120] and in two of four siblings born to parents who were first cousins,[120] suggesting a genetic influence; however, most cases are sporadic.

The anomalous vein is usually visible radiographically as a broad, gently curved shadow descending to the diaphragm just to the right of the heart; this shadow is shaped like a Turkish sword or scimitar, accounting for the designation *scimitar* syndrome (Fig. 23–10).[121, 126, 126a] Although the entire right lung is drained by the anomalous vein in most cases,[127] other patterns can occur; for example, one group has reported a long vein that pursued a circuitous course throughout the right lung before it drained into the inferior vena cava and the left atrium as well as into two large veins that joined before entering the inferior vena cava.[128]

The diagnosis can often be made on the chest radiograph: the characteristic findings consist of a small right lung with small hilum and diminished vascularity, a shift of the heart and mediastinum to the right, and a curved appearance of the anomalous draining vein next to the right atrium.[124] In one review of 122 patients, hypoplasia of the right lung (usually mild) and dextrocardia were each identified on the chest radiograph in 80% of cases and a scimitar vein in 70%;[120] hypervascularization of the left lung was visible in almost 20% of cases. Although highly suggestive of the diagnosis, the presence of a scimitar-like vein is not pathognomonic of the syndrome: a similar appearance is occasionally caused by a meandering right pulmonary vein draining normally into the right atrium[129, 130] or into the inferior vena cava and left atrium without associated pulmonary or cardiac anomalies.[130] In one case, a scimitar-shaped vein draining normally into the left atrium was associated with systemic arterial supply to the posterobasal segment of the right lower lobe.[131]

If radiographic findings are not definitive, the diagnosis can usually be made with CT.[120, 132–134] The procedure also allows identification of associated abnormalities, such as bilobed right lung with absence of the minor fissure and horseshoe lung.[120, 134] The diagnosis may also be made using MR imaging.[135] In some cases, angiography or echocardiog-

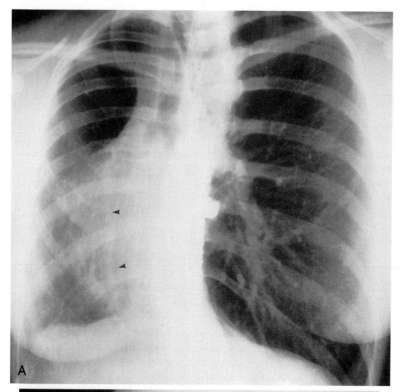

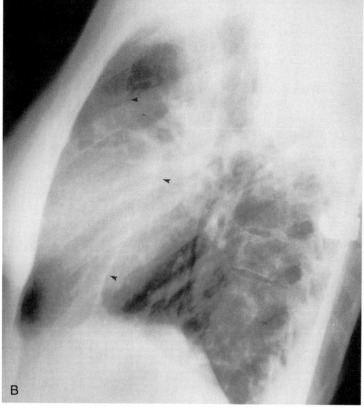

Figure 23–10. Hypogenetic Lung (Scimitar) Syndrome. Posteroanterior (PA) *(A)* and lateral *(B)* chest radiographs reveal a small right hemithorax. The pulmonary vasculature of the right lung is diminutive and disorganized, whereas that of the left lung is normal. A large vascular shadow *(arrowheads),* coursing caudally from the midlung zone toward the cardiophrenic angle, can be identified through a dextroposed cardiac silhouette. In lateral projection, note the serpentine interface *(arrowheads)* extending from a point behind the manubrium to the top of the right hemidiaphragm. This appearance, in conjunction with the obscured right cardiac border on the PA projection, is caused by an accumulation of adipose tissue anteriorly and should not be confused with right hemidiaphragmatic duplication, whose appearance is similar. A Harrington rod has been inserted for correction of dextroscoliosis.

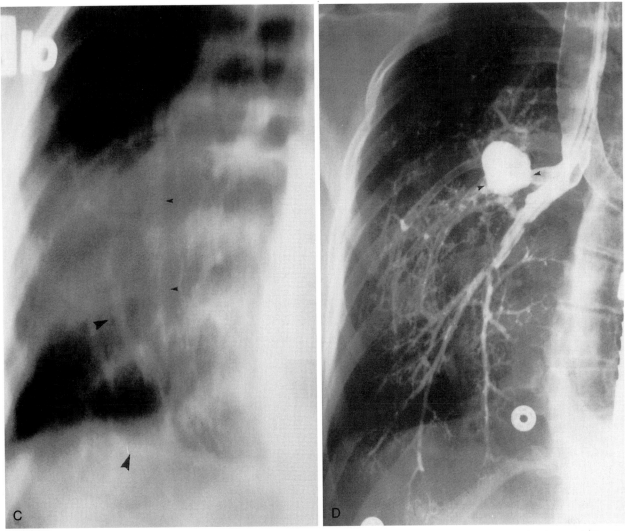

Figure 23–10 *Continued.* A conventional linear tomogram through the lower thorax in anteroposterior projection *(C)* reveals a vertically oriented, branching, broad linear opacity *(small arrowheads)* consistent with an anomalous vein (note the scimitar shape). Several other abnormal vessels *(large arrowheads)* can also be identified. A right tracheobronchogram *(D)* reveals a hypoplastic right bronchial tree. A large diverticulum *(arrowheads)* arises from the right upper lobe bronchus.

Illustration continued on following page

raphy may be required to make a definitive diagnosis or to assess the presence of associated cardiac anomalies.[131, 136, 137]

More than half of patients with hypogenetic lung syndrome have cardiorespiratory symptoms, similar in many respects to those of large left-to-right shunts with pulmonary arterial hypertension; in one study, 31 (60%) of the 53 patients whose clinical status was known were symptomatic.[118] Some patients have repeated bronchopulmonary infections or hemoptysis. A systolic murmur of moderate intensity usually is heard along the left sternal border. Patients without pulmonary arterial hypertension or symptoms in infancy have a good prognosis and often lead a normal life without surgical correction of the abnormalities.[120]

Pulmonary Arteriovenous Malformation

The term *pulmonary arteriovenous malformation* (arteriovenous fistula, arteriovenous aneurysm) is used here to describe a spectrum of abnormal vascular communications between pulmonary arteries and pulmonary veins.[138] This spectrum ranges from microscopic communications that are too small to be visualized radiologically to complex aneurysms with multiple feeding arteries and draining veins, which may involve the entire blood supply of a segment or lobe and may have arterial communication with the neighboring chest wall or adjacent lung segments.[138–141] Depending on their size and number, the lesions may be unassociated with symptoms or result in an anatomic right-to-left shunt that can be complicated by a reduction in the arterial oxygen saturation, cyanosis, polycythemia,[140, 141] or paradoxical emboli.[142, 143] Although pulmonary sequestration and hypogenetic lung syndrome also constitute forms of congenital arteriovenous communication in which a systemic vessel under high pressure connects with relatively thin-walled pulmonary vessels under low pressure, these are generally considered distinct entities and are discussed elsewhere.

The abnormality has been considered to be caused by a defect in the terminal capillary loops that allows dilation and the formation of thin-walled vascular sacs supplied by a

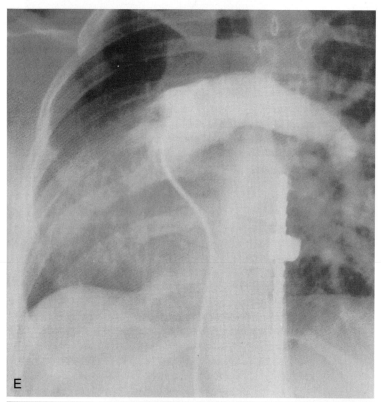

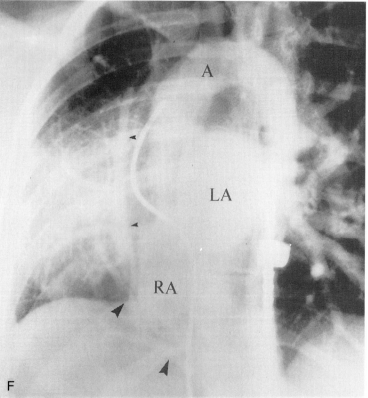

Figure 23–10 _Continued._ A pulmonary arteriogram performed with the catheter tip in the main pulmonary artery _(E)_ demonstrates an absent right pulmonary artery; the left is normal. During the levo phase of the study _(F)_, venous return from the right lung is entirely through the anomalous veins _(small arrowheads)_ to the inferior vena cava and right atrium (RA). Note the small vessels in the cardiophrenic angle _(large arrowheads)_ that were subsequently shown by aortography to represent aberrant arterial supply to the right lung from the aorta. (A, aorta; LA, left atrium.)

single distended afferent artery and drained by a single distended efferent vein (however, *see* farther on).[142, 143] It has also been proposed that the malformations result from incomplete degeneration of vascular septa connecting the primitive pulmonary arterial and venous plexuses.[144]

Approximately one third of patients have multiple lesions in the lungs, identifiable either radiologically or in resected specimens.[139, 145] It has also been estimated that approximately 60% of patients with pulmonary lesions have arteriovenous communications in the skin, mucous membranes, or other organs.[146] This situation, known as *hereditary hemorrhagic telangiectasia* (Rendu-Osler-Weber disease), has been shown to have an autosomal dominant pattern of inheritance.[147] Although it is assumed that the vascular defect is present at birth, it seldom becomes manifest clinically until adult life when the vessels have been subjected to pressure over several decades.[142] In one family of 91 individuals known to have hereditary hemorrhagic telangiectasia, 14 (15%) were found to have arteriovenous fistulas in the lungs.[142] Multiple pulmonary arteriovenous malformations have also been described in patients with Fanconi's syndrome[148] and polysplenia syndrome with multiple cardiac anomalies.[149]

Most lesions are not recognized until the twenties or thirties; approximately 10% are identified in infancy or childhood.[150] They occur twice as frequently in women as in men.

Pathologic Characteristics

Grossly, pulmonary arteriovenous malformations appear as red, more or less spherical, vascular masses ranging from 1 mm to several centimeters in diameter (Fig. 23–11). Some patients also have telangiectasia of the bronchial mucosa, which can be associated with hemoptysis and be seen bronchoscopically.[151] Although the malformations can be recognized microscopically (and, in fact, have occasionally been diagnosed by open-lung biopsy),[152] they are best studied by preparing corrosion casts of the pulmonary vasculature.[140, 153, 154] The few cases thus examined have shown the fistulas to be supplied and drained by several vessels, the draining veins usually being somewhat larger than the feeding arteries. The intervening vessels may be more or less uniform in diameter and show a complex branching mass resembling a Medusa's head; sometimes a markedly dilated arteriovenous communication is present without the intervening tortuous complex.[152]

Microscopic examination shows multiple endothelial-lined, blood-containing spaces interspersed throughout an architecturally normal pulmonary parenchyma. Vascular walls are typically thin, especially in the larger vessels, a characteristic that presumably explains the frequent presence of recent or remote parenchymal hemorrhage. Intramural elastic tissue and muscle are typically sparse.

Radiologic Manifestations

Pulmonary arteriovenous malformations are seen more commonly in the lower lobes than in the middle or upper lobes[143, 155] and are single in about two thirds of cases.[139, 156] The characteristic radiographic appearance is of a round or oval homogeneous mass of unit density, somewhat lobulated in contour but sharply defined, most often in the medial

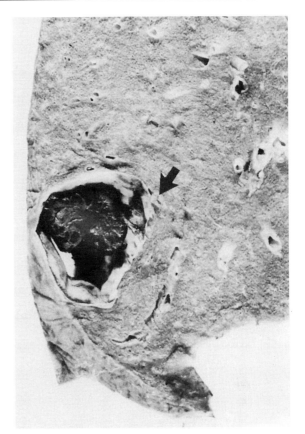

Figure 23–11. Pulmonary Arteriovenous Malformation. A magnified view of a lower lobe shows a well-circumscribed, subpleural cystic space filled with blood clot. A portion of the feeder pulmonary artery is evident at the right *(arrow).* Histologic sections showed the cyst wall to have a variable appearance, focally resembling pulmonary artery and focally pulmonary vein.

third of the lung, ranging from less than 1 cm to several centimeters in diameter (Fig. 23–12). A feeding artery and draining vein can often be identified, the artery relating to the hilum and the vein deviating from the course of the artery toward the left atrium (Fig. 23–13). In a minority of cases, a fairly extensive racemose opacity, somewhat ill-defined but homogeneous in density, occupies much of one bronchopulmonary segment;[156] this more complex angiomatous mass possesses several feeding and draining vessels.[139] In some cases, plain radiography does not reveal lesions because they are obscured by hemorrhage into contiguous parenchyma or (uncommonly) by hemothorax following spontaneous intrapleural rupture[156a] or atelectasis resulting from bronchial compression.[155] Calcification occurs occasionally, probably related to phleboliths.[142]

Although radiographic abnormalities have been described in many patients who have pulmonary arteriovenous malformations,[146, 157] further evaluation is necessary to confirm the diagnosis and to demonstrate the presence of smaller malformations that may not be initially apparent. A variety of imaging modalities can be used, including CT,[158–160] radionuclide scanning, echocardiography,[161, 162] Doppler ultrasound and amplitude ultrasound angiography,[162a] and angiography.[160, 163] Although arteriovenous malformations can also be readily diagnosed on MR,[164–166] it is seldom used in clinical practice. In patients undergoing surgery or embolo-

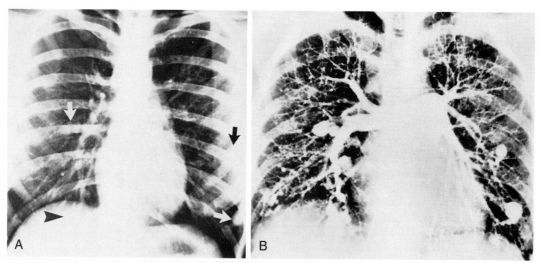

Figure 23–12. Multiple Arteriovenous Malformations. This young woman had had several small hemoptyses over the past couple of years and had noticed increasing shortness of breath on exertion. A posteroanterior chest radiograph *(A)* reveals several fairly sharply defined nodular opacities in both lungs *(arrows)*. Note that the opacity in the right lower lobe *(arrowhead)* appears to possess an intimate relationship to vessels. A pulmonary angiogram during the arterial phase *(B)* reveals many more large arteriovenous communications than are evident on the chest radiograph.

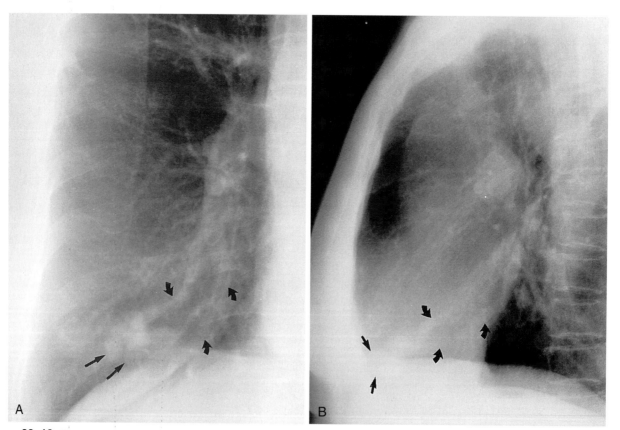

Figure 23–13. Pulmonary Arteriovenous Malformation. Views of the right lung from posteroanterior *(A)* and lateral chest radiographs *(B)* in a 71-year-old woman demonstrate a serpiginous soft tissue opacity in the right middle lobe *(straight arrows)*. The associated large feeding artery and draining vein *(curved arrows)* are diagnostic of arteriovenous malformation.

therapy, precise information regarding the number, location, and architecture of the lesions is essential;[167, 168] such assessment requires either angiography or three-dimensional spiral CT.[167, 168]

The characteristic CT finding of arteriovenous malformations consists of a homogeneous, circumscribed nodule or serpiginous mass connected with blood vessels.[158, 160] In one study, 40 patients with 109 malformations were separated into three groups to assess the usefulness of CT: (1) Group 1 (20 patients), to compare the CT diagnosis and pretherapeutic management with pulmonary angiography; (2) Group 2 (27 patients), to assess the follow-up of patients who received treatment; and (3) Group 3 (11 patients), to assess CT as an isolated diagnostic procedure in elderly patients or family members with hereditary hemorrhagic telangiectasia.[160] In Group 1, conventional and dynamic CT enabled identification of 107 lesions (98%) compared to 65 (60%) with angiography. Follow-up CT scans in patients with successful embolotherapy demonstrated progressive decrease in size of the malformations over time. Lack of change in size was related to unsuccessful treatment and was observed in only 4% of cases. In 67% of patients who had

follow-up CT scans several months to 10 years after successful embolotherapy, the arteriovenous malformations were no longer detectable. In elderly patients or family members with hereditary hemorrhagic telangiectasia (Group 3), CT demonstrated arteriovenous malformations in three of eight asymptomatic individuals, all of whom underwent subsequent angiography and embolotherapy.

Optimal investigation of arteriovenous malformations by CT requires the use of spiral volumetric CT. This allows assessment of the entire lung in one or two breath holds, thus minimizing the risk of missing small lesions. The procedure also enables image reconstruction of various levels within the lesion, thereby facilitating depiction of the center of the malformation (Fig. 23–14).[160, 168] Three-dimensional reconstruction using spiral CT also permits assessment of the architecture of the malformations (Fig. 23–15). One group of investigators compared the results of pulmonary angiography in 37 arteriovenous malformations with those of spiral CT using single-threshold, shaded-surface displays with 2- or 5-mm section thickness, a pitch of 1, and a 360-degree linear interpolation algorithm but without intravenous contrast material.[168] A reliable demonstration of the angioar-

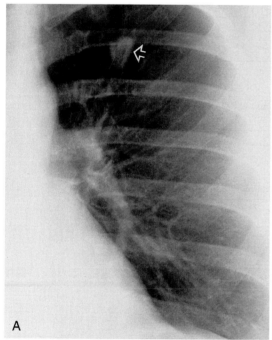

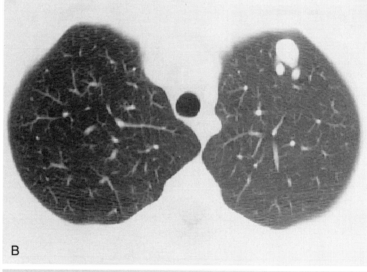

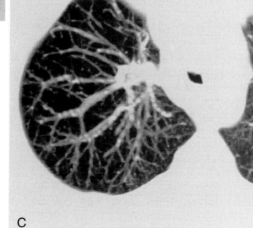

Figure 23–14. Arteriovenous Malformation. A view of the left lung from a posteroanterior chest radiograph *(A)* in a 33-year-old man with Rendu-Osler-Weber disease demonstrates slightly lobulated soft tissue opacity in the left upper lobe *(arrow)*. A 5-mm collimation spiral CT performed without intravenous contrast material *(B)* shows the soft tissue opacity with the associated feeding artery and draining vein. Maximal intensity projection (MIP) reconstruction obtained using the volumetric spiral CT data *(C)* allows better depiction of the vascular nature of the lesion with demonstration of the feeding artery and draining vein *(arrows)*.

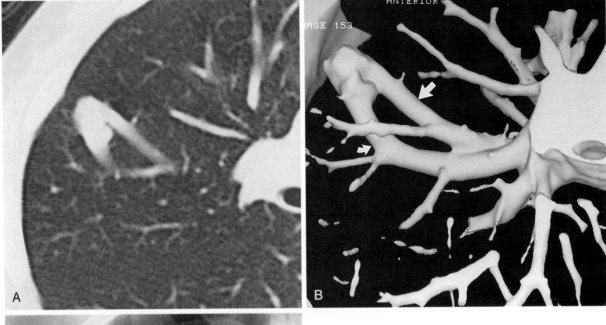

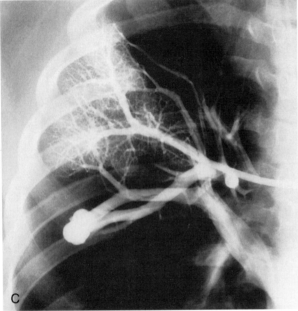

Figure 23–15. Arteriovenous Malformation. A 2-mm collimation spiral CT scan *(A)* in a 15-year-old boy demonstrates a pulmonary arteriovenous malformation in the right upper lobe. The angioarchitecture of the malformation is clearly depicted on the three-dimensional image *(B)*. The feeding artery *(straight arrow)* originates from the anterior segmental artery, and the draining vein *(curved arrow)* joins the apical segmental vein. The features are those of a simple pulmonary arteriovenous malformation. This CT image was obtained using an on-line single-threshold, three-dimensional–shaded-surface display of a stack of 20 spiral CT sections of 2-mm collimation. A selective pulmonary angiogram *(C)* confirms the CT findings. (Case courtesy of Professeur Jacques Remy, Centre Hospitalier Regional et Universitaire de Lille, Lille, France.)

chitecture was made with three-dimensional spiral CT in 28 (76%) cases, including 25 simple and 3 complex arteriovenous malformations. Combined interpretation of the three-dimensional images and transverse sections led to accurate evaluation of 35 (95%) malformations. Two of the malformations remained nonanalyzable on CT as a result of respiratory motion artifacts and incomplete reconstruction of the volume of interest. By comparison, selective unilateral pulmonary angiography allowed assessment of the anatomic features in only 9 (32%) malformations; the remaining 19 cases were considered nonanalyzable because of superimposition of the vessels (although documentation of the angioarchitecture was made in all cases with hyperselective angiography). On the basis of these observations, it is reasonable to conclude that spiral CT is the procedure of choice in the diagnosis of pulmonary arteriovenous malformations.

The presence of arteriovenous malformation–related shunt can be assessed with perfusion scintigraphy or echocardiography.[161, 169] In this situation, a fraction of the tagged albumen particles escapes into the systemic circulation, where the particles are detected by a gamma camera placed over the kidneys. Perfusion scanning allows quantification of the amount of shunt and shows good agreement with the 100% oxygen technique.[170] Contrast echocardiography also allows demonstration of the presence of intrapulmonary shunts,[171] although it is qualitative rather than quantitative.

Despite the value of spiral CT, pulmonary angiography is performed routinely before treatment of arteriovenous malformations for absolute confirmation of the presence of the malformation, analysis of the feeding arterial and draining venous structures, and detection of other malformations (Fig. 23–16).[143, 160, 171a] Care must be exercised in obtaining angiographic visualization of all portions of both lungs; it is not enough to perform selective angiography of the lung in

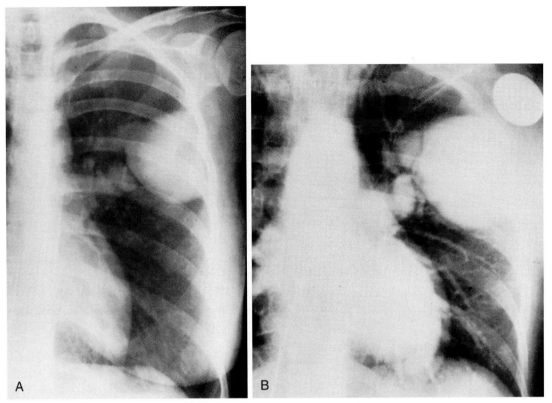

Figure 23–16. Pulmonary Arteriovenous Malformation. A view of the left hemithorax from a posteroanterior radiograph *(A)* reveals a large, sharply circumscribed, homogeneous mass in the midlung zone. A broad, serpentine shadow extends from the medial aspect of the mass to the left hilum. A late venous phase of a pulmonary angiogram *(B)* shows uniform opacification of the large mass as well as the broad serpentine structure extending medially. The markedly delayed circulation time is indicated by the fact that the arteriovenous malformation is uniformly opacified at a time when the right pulmonary veins, the left ventricle, and the aorta are already opacified. The patient was a 28-year-old woman with Rendu-Osler-Weber syndrome. (Courtesy of Dr. Harold Jacobson, Montefiore Hospital, Bronx, New York.)

question, because lesions may be present in the contralateral lung and may not be visible on the plain radiograph (*see* Fig. 23–12).[145, 156, 172] In fact, multiple tiny fistulas have been demonstrated in patients with normal plain radiographs,[142] notably in asymptomatic siblings of patients with known malformations and in patients in whom the diagnosis was suspected clinically because of polycythemia and cyanosis.[173, 174] Although typically stable in size, an increase in size of a malformation is sometimes seen; for example, in one patient, three lesions presented as nodules on a routine chest radiograph, despite the fact that the patient had had a completely normal radiograph 2 years earlier.[175]

Clinical Manifestations

The incidence of symptoms varies in different series.[141, 155, 156] In the family of 91 persons with hereditary hemorrhagic telangiectasia referred to previously, 8 of the 14 patients with pulmonary arteriovenous fistulas were asymptomatic.[142] By contrast, the authors of one study of 21 cases and a review of the literature found the majority of patients to be symptomatic;[155] however, most had multiple lesions, and symptoms may have been related to involvement of organs other than the lungs, including the upper respiratory tract (epistaxis), the gastrointestinal tract (hematemesis), and the brain (cerebrovascular hemorrhage).

As might be expected, hemoptysis is the most common presenting complaint of patients with pulmonary lesions. Dyspnea is present in 60% of cases.[155] Signs suggestive of

the abnormality include cyanosis, finger clubbing, and a continuous murmur or bruit audible over the lesion(s).[150, 155, 176] Rarely, hemothorax causes pleuritic pain, with the attendant signs of friction rub, decreased breath sounds, and dullness on percussion.[139, 142] Such pleural hemorrhage is a serious complication that can be fatal;[177] in one review of the literature, the authors found nine such episodes with five deaths.[178]

Involvement of extrathoracic sites is not uncommon and may be an important clue to the diagnosis. As indicated previously, telangiectasis in the skin or mucous membranes is present in many patients. Symptoms of central nervous system disease may be the result of metastatic abscess, hypoxemia, cerebral thromboemboli, cerebral thrombosis from secondary polycythemia, and cerebral hemorrhage from a concomitant intracerebral arteriovenous aneurysm.[155, 179] Cerebral symptoms are transitory in many cases and are not uncommon in patients with hereditary hemorrhagic telangiectasia, even in the absence of pulmonary arteriovenous fistulas; these episodes have never been satisfactorily explained.[142] Although some patients have polycythemia,[155] repeated hemorrhages from the nose or lungs may cause anemia.[180–182] An unusual combination of abnormalities, consisting of polyposis of the colon and duodenal bulb, pulmonary arteriovenous malformations, and hypertrophic osteoarthropathy, has been described in a 15-year-old girl.[183]

Arterial blood gas analysis and cardiac catheterization may provide useful data in confirming the diagnosis: Po_2 and arterial oxygen saturation are decreased, cardiac output

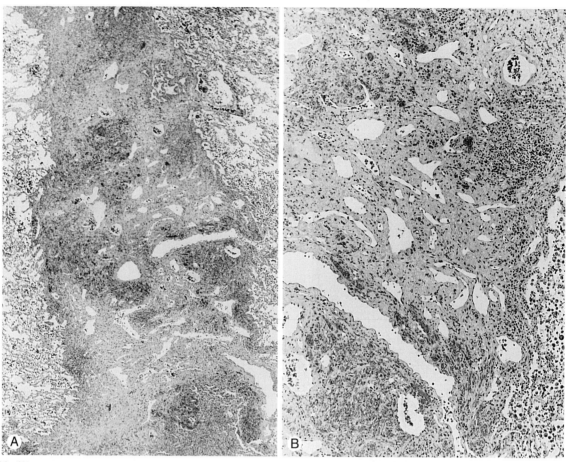

Figure 23–17. Diffuse Pulmonary Lymphangiomatosis. Sections (*A* and *B*) show marked thickening of an interlobular septum by a combination of fibrous tissue and numerous, irregularly shaped small vessels (magnified in *B*).

is increased, and the pulmonary artery pressure is normal.[155, 184] The electrocardiogram usually is normal, a useful sign in differentiation from congenital heart disease.[155] Blood volume studies reveal increased red blood cell mass in many cases, with normal or near-normal plasma volume.[155] An unusual case has been reported of a 35-year-old woman who had a single large arteriovenous malformation in her right lower lobe.[185] When she stood erect, a loud bruit was heard over the lesion and the Po_2 was low, indicating gravity-related increased flow through the shunt; when she lay on her right side, the Po_2 increased and the bruit disappeared, indicating reduced flow. Angiography performed while she was in the latter position showed kinking of the artery and vein, interfering with flow through the shunt.

Transcatheter embolization has become a safe, effective means of vascular occlusion[186–190] and is widely considered to be the procedure of choice for the treatment of arteriovenous malformations.[143, 189–191] Several different embolic materials have been employed, including polyvinyl alcohol (Ivalon), wool coils, stainless steel coils, and detachable silicone balloons.

ANOMALIES OF PULMONARY LYMPHATICS

Lymphangioma

Lymphangiomas probably represent developmental malformations in which there is a failure of communication between a peripheral portion of the lymphatic system and its draining vessels. The majority of intrathoracic lesions arise within the mediastinum; however, occasional examples apparently develop within the lung.[192, 193] Accumulation of lymph within the "sequestered" vessels results in their distention and the formation of a tumor-like mass that may be large enough to cause respiratory embarrassment.[193] Although probably most common in infancy, occasional cases have been reported in adults.[194, 195]

Diffuse Pulmonary Lymphangiomatosis

Lymphangiomatosis is a rare pulmonary abnormality that has sometimes been confused with lymphangiectasia (*see* farther on).[196] To obviate this confusion, it has been proposed that the latter term should be confined to lesions characterized by dilation of existing lymphatic vessels, without an increase in number or complexity;[196] by contrast, lymphangiomatosis is used to refer to lesions in which the primary abnormality is an increase in the number of lymphatics. The abnormality has also been referred to as *diffuse pulmonary angiomatosis* by some authors because of uncertainty as to the origin of the abnormal vascular channels.[197]

The condition is most common in infancy and childhood, during which time it has been estimated to account for approximately 5% of all chronic interstitial disease.[198] Recognition of the abnormality in older individuals also occurs—as in one report of individuals 16, 20, and 33 years of age[196]—although symptoms dating to childhood may be discovered on close questioning.

Pathologically, there is a proliferation of variably sized, anastomosing lymphatic vessels in pleural, interlobular septal, and peribronchovascular connective tissue (Fig. 23–17).[196, 199] Aggregates of spindle cells with clear cytoplasm and ultrastructural and immunohistochemical features of smooth muscle differentiation may be seen adjacent to the abnormal vessels.

Chest radiographs show bilateral interstitial disease, sometimes with a lower lobe predominance (Fig. 23–18).[196, 197] Pleural effusion (chylothorax), either unilateral or bilateral, is common;[200] chylopericardium is seen occasionally.[200] In one study of eight patients ranging in age from 3 to 35 years, the main CT abnormality (seen in all patients) was smooth thickening of the interlobular septa and bronchoarterial bundles.[201] Seven patients also had patchy bilateral areas of ground-glass attenuation, which were presumed to represent pulmonary edema; all had diffuse increased attenuation of mediastinal fat approximating that of water. Seven of the eight patients had bilateral pleural effusions or smooth thickening of the pleura, and two had regions of calcified pleural thickening.

Clinical manifestations of "asthma" have been noted in a number of patients.[196] Concomitant mediastinal, skeletal, and other visceral lymphangiomatous malformations are present in some individuals.[201–203] One case has been reported in a patient with the Klippel-Trenaunay syndrome (varicosities of systemic veins, cutaneous and soft tissue hypertrophy, and hemangiomas).[204] Pulmonary function tests often show combined restrictive and obstructive features.[196]

Congenital Pulmonary Lymphangiectasia

Congenital pulmonary lymphangiectasia is an almost invariably fatal abnormality that usually becomes manifest at birth. As discussed previously, the condition consists predominantly of dilation of the pulmonary lymphatics without evidence of an increase in number or complexity;[196] in its severest degree, this dilation can reach cystic proportions.

The abnormality has been classified into three subtypes

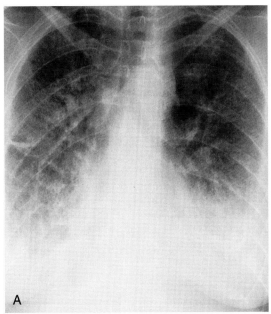

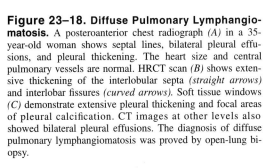

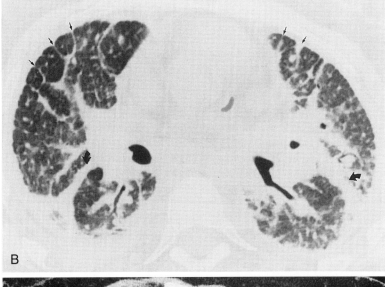

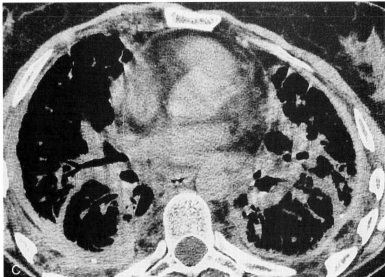

Figure 23–18. Diffuse Pulmonary Lymphangiomatosis. A posteroanterior chest radiograph *(A)* in a 35-year-old woman shows septal lines, bilateral pleural effusions, and pleural thickening. The heart size and central pulmonary vessels are normal. HRCT scan *(B)* shows extensive thickening of the interlobular septa *(straight arrows)* and interlobar fissures *(curved arrows)*. Soft tissue windows *(C)* demonstrate extensive pleural thickening and focal areas of pleural calcification. CT images at other levels also showed bilateral pleural effusions. The diagnosis of diffuse pulmonary lymphangiomatosis was proved by open-lung biopsy.

based on the presence or absence of congenital cardiac malformations, involvement of other viscera, and early or late presentation. In patients with a cardiac anomaly (Group I, comprising approximately one third of cases), there appears to be a close association with obstruction to pulmonary venous return: hemodynamic factors tend to keep pulmonary lymphatics dilated and probably play a major role in the pathogenesis of the lymphangiectasia.[204] An association with the asplenia syndrome[206] has been noted in some patients. The radiologic findings in this group are highly variable, ranging from clear evidence of pulmonary venous obstruction (interstitial edema), through patchy areas of pneumonia and atelectasis, to normal chest radiographs.

Group II comprises patients in whom the lymphangiectasia is not associated with cardiac anomalies (approximately two thirds of reported cases). This form is thought to result from abnormal development of the lung between the 14th and 20th weeks of gestation. During the early part of this phase, the pulmonary lymphatics are large in relation to the remainder of the lung, whereas by the 18th and 20th weeks the lung's connective tissue elements normally diminish, and the lymphatics become much narrower. It has been postulated that lymphangiectasia may represent a failure of the lymphatics to undergo regression while lung parenchyma continues to grow.[207] In contrast to Group I patients, many Group II patients have congenital abnormalities of other structures, most commonly polycystic or other renal disease[204] or congenital ichthyosis.[204, 208] The radiographic changes in this group are again highly variable. Most commonly, there is marked prominence of interstitial markings in the form of Kerley A and B lines simulating interstitial pulmonary edema; in some patients, however, the radiographic findings consist of no more than patchy areas of consolidation, atelectasis, and focal overinflation.

Patients in Group III have a combination of pulmonary disease and lymphangiectasia in other viscera, especially the intestine.[209] Retroperitoneal and mediastinal lymphatics may also be affected, and hemangiomas of bone and other sites may be present. Pulmonary involvement is less severe than in Groups I and II and is associated with a better prognosis.

In one unusual report of three patients between 13 and 19 years of age, each came to medical attention because of an abnormal chest radiograph, changes being limited to one or two lobes and the mediastinum.[210] All had morphologic findings characteristic of lymphangiectasia, but the late presentation, lack of symptoms, and lobar localization—features seen infrequently in the other subgroups—suggested a possible additional variant of the disease.

Pathologic findings are similar in all groups.[207, 211] Grossly the lungs are bulky and firm and show numerous small cystic spaces, which can measure up to 5 mm in diameter. Microscopically the elongated "cysts" are lined by a flattened endothelium and are located within interstitial connective tissue of the bronchovascular bundles, interlobular septa, and pleura. Infrequent smooth muscle cells may be seen in their walls, and their lumens contain hypocellular eosinophilic fluid characteristic of lymph.

MISCELLANEOUS VASCULAR ANOMALIES

Anomalies of the Heart and Great Vessels

Anomalies Resulting in Increased Pulmonary Blood Flow

Anomalies resulting in increased pulmonary blood flow include atrial and ventricular septal defect, patent ductus arteriosus, aorticopulmonary window, and anomalous pulmonary venous drainage. Rarely a congenital aneurysm of the aortic sinus of Valsalva ruptures into the right atrium, right ventricle, or pulmonary artery, immediately increasing pulmonary blood flow.[212] The left-to-right shunt results in some degree of increased pulmonary blood flow, which may be recognizable radiologically as increased size in the central and peripheral pulmonary arteries (Fig. 23–19). Pathologic findings are those of pulmonary hypertension, typically of plexogenic arteriopathy (*see* page 1882).[213]

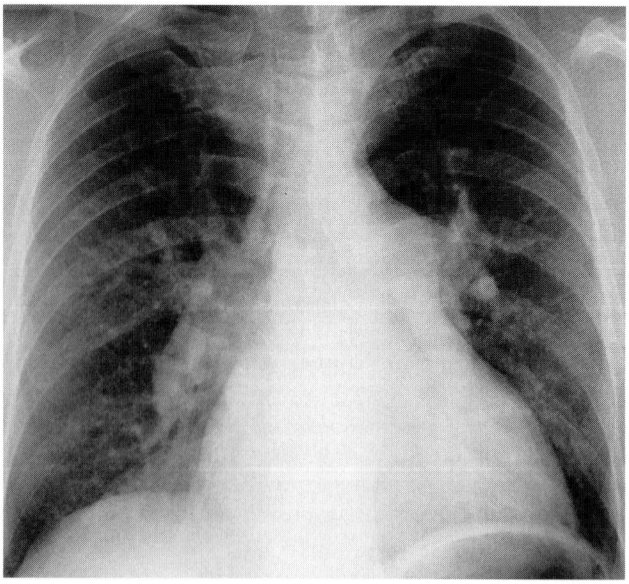

Figure 23–19. Increased Size of Pulmonary Vessels: Atrial Septal Defect (ASD). A posteroanterior chest radiograph in a 56-year-old man demonstrates enlargement of the central pulmonary arteries and increased size of the peripheral vessels. Also note mild cardiomegaly and decreased size of the aortic arch, findings frequently seen in patients with long-standing ASD. The patient had proven ASD with associated pulmonary arterial hypertension.

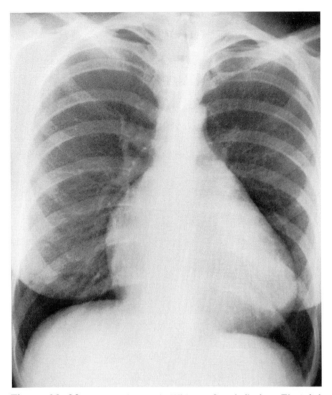

Figure 23–20. Diffuse Oligemia Without Overinflation: Ebstein's Anomaly. The peripheral pulmonary markings are diminished in caliber, and the hila are diminutive; the lungs are not overinflated. The contour of the markedly enlarged heart is consistent with Ebstein's anomaly.

Anomalies Resulting in Decreased Pulmonary Blood Flow

By far the most common cause of general pulmonary oligemia as a result of diminished flow is a congenital anomaly of the right ventricular outflow tract (isolated pulmonic stenosis, tetralogy of Fallot with pulmonary atresia, Type IV persistent truncus arteriosus, and Ebstein's anomaly) (Fig. 23–20). The caliber of the pulmonary vessels generally reflects the severity of the flow decrease, the hila usually being diminutive and the peripheral vessels correspondingly small (except with valvular pulmonic stenosis, in which poststenotic dilation may enlarge the main or left pulmonary artery). The reduction in flow throughout the lungs is more or less uniform, although both physiologic[214] and radiologic[215] studies have shown discrepant flow through the two upper zones in patients with isolated pulmonary stenosis or tetralogy of Fallot. It is not clear from these reports, however, on which side the greater flow usually occurs: flow was greater in the left lung during physiologic studies using carbon dioxide labeled with ^{15}O,[214] and in the right lung during angiographic investigation.[215] The mechanics producing asymmetric flow are not thoroughly understood.

Morphologic abnormalities of the pulmonary vasculature have been studied in cases of isolated pulmonary atresia and stenosis,[216–218] pulmonary stenosis associated with other cardiac malformations,[219] and tetralogy of Fallot.[217–221] In cases of pulmonary stenosis, studies of neonatal and infant lungs have shown a significant decrease in arterial medial thickness, primarily as a result of a decrease in the amount of muscle. It has been suggested that this decrease may be

related to the relatively low intrauterine pulmonary pressure.[216] Studies of arterial media in cases of tetralogy of Fallot have shown more variable results, some authors[221] finding an increase in arterial muscularization and others a decrease.[217, 218, 220] A variety of other quantitative and qualitative arterial abnormalities have also been reported.[220, 221] Alveoli have been found to be small and decreased in number in some patients.[220]

Because decreased pulmonary circulation always increases bronchial collateral flow,[222–225] the pulmonary vascular pattern throughout the lungs may be formed partly or wholly by a greatly hypertrophied bronchial arterial system. This extensive systemic arterial supply is particularly evident in tetralogy of Fallot and in Type IV pulmonary artery atresia. Although pulmonary arterial flow is negligible in these cases, the diminutive vascular markings throughout the lungs may represent the pulmonary arterial tree being filled through systemic–pulmonary artery anastomoses. Long-term follow-up of patients with surgically corrected tetralogy of Fallot has shown no evidence of pulmonary function abnormalities.[226]

Systemic Arterial Supply to the Lung

A portion of lung, which may be normal or abnormal, may be supplied by a systemic artery arising from the aorta or one of its branches. The abnormality may be congenital or acquired.[227] As indicated elsewhere in this chapter, the congenital form is seen in association with a variety of other anomalies, including bronchopulmonary sequestration, hypogenetic lung syndrome, congenital cystic adenomatoid malformation, absence of the main pulmonary artery, and proximal interruption of a pulmonary artery.[3, 8, 119]

A systemic artery may also enter the lung in the absence of these conditions, either in the form of a systemic–pulmonary vascular fistula[228, 229] or as a localized blood supply of otherwise normal lung.[230–235] In the latter situation, a large systemic artery supplies a portion of one lung, invariably the basal segments of one of the lower lobes, either partly or completely (Fig. 23–21). Examination of the bronchial tree shows normal architecture, by definition excluding sequestration. Additional pulmonary artery supply to the affected segments may or may not be present, but the main pulmonary artery and its branches to other lobes are normal. The anomalous artery is usually solitary and arises from the descending aorta; rare examples of multiple feeding vessels have been reported.[236] The cause and pathogenesis are unknown. Because of the frequent involvement of the basal lung segments, it is possible that abnormal development of one or more of the pulmonary ligament arteries may be implicated (*see* page 601).[237]

The chest radiograph shows normal or increased vascular markings.[235, 238] The increased blood flow from the systemic artery causes dilation of the draining inferior pulmonary vein, which may result in a tubular shadow visible radiographically in the left lower lobe.[233, 234] The dilated vein and the increased vascularity in the lower lobe are readily recognized on CT.[233, 234] Ipsilateral rib notching may be present.[236] Pulmonary angiography, CT, or MR imaging can be used to determine whether there is an absence of pulmonary arterial supply to the involved lung. Because of the high pressure, angiography may reveal absent or incomplete

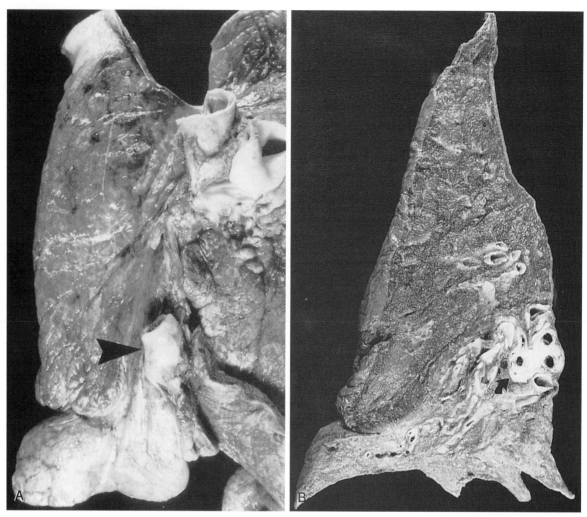

Figure 23–21. Systemic Arterial Supply of Normal Lung. The medial surface of a left lower lobe *(A)* shows a prominent 1-cm vessel entering the basal aspect *(arrowhead)*. This connected with the midthoracic aorta and showed marked atherosclerotic stenosis (seen on the cut section in *B [arrow]*). The basal parenchyma supplied by the abnormal vessel is atelectatic; histologic examination revealed marked interstitial fibrosis and nonspecific chronic inflammation. The pulmonary vessels and airways showed a normal anatomic distribution. Incidental finding in a 70-year-old woman with no respiratory complaints.

filling of the segments served by the systemic vessel.[236] Ventilation-perfusion scans show perfusion defects and normal ventilation of the affected lung.[235]

Patients may present in infancy or early childhood with a chest murmur or cardiac decompensation secondary to a left-to-left shunt.[231, 232] One 21-year-old patient presented with several episodes of hemoptysis.[233] The anomaly also may cause no symptoms and become evident on a screening chest radiograph or at autopsy.

Congenital systemic–pulmonary vascular fistulas may involve either normal or anomalous systemic arterial branches, and communication may be with either pulmonary veins or arteries, usually in the basal segment of one of the lower lobes.[228] Affected patients may be asymptomatic or may suffer from recurrent hemoptysis; a murmur may be audible over the defect.[228, 229] Morphologic and angiographic studies have shown a complex arrangement of intercommunicating vessels. When the communication exists with a pulmonary artery, catheterization of this vessel may reveal increased oxygen saturation, providing evidence of left-to-right shunt.

Similar systemic–pulmonary vascular fistulas may be secondary to infection, trauma, or surgery. Although the incidence of such acquired systemic arterialization of the lung is unknown, it is probably much higher than is commonly realized. The authors have seen several cases on radiographic examination in which obliteration of the pleural space by fibrous tissue as a result of pleuritis has been accompanied by extension of systemic vessels from the chest wall across the pleura into contiguous lung parenchyma; such transgression undoubtedly occurs frequently, especially if the underlying lung has been damaged by infection (e.g., in bronchiectasis) (Fig. 23–22). Occasionally, significant symptoms result from the subsequent shunt.[239] An unusual form of acquired systemic-pulmonary anastomosis has been described in patients with severe pulmonic stenosis.[240] In this situation, collateral vessels develop chiefly over the apices of the lungs and cause hemorrhage with secondary pleuritis and fibrosis. The radiographic appearance has been described as *pseudofibrosis of the cyanotic* and possesses a striking resemblance to tuberculosis.

Aortography is usually necessary to make a definitive

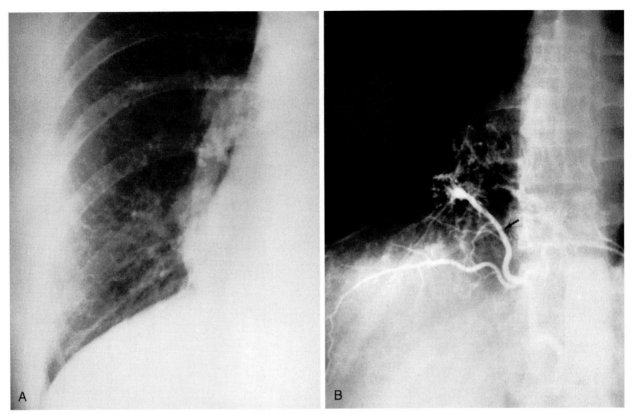

Figure 23–22. Systemic Arterial Supply of the Lung in Association with Chronic Bronchiectasis. A detail view of the lower half of the right lung from a posteroanterior radiograph *(A)* reveals loss of visibility of the right heart border caused by airlessness of contiguous right middle lobe parenchyma. The lateral view was noncontributory. This 25-year-old woman complained of chronic productive cough, and a bronchogram revealed severe bronchiectasis of the right middle lobe, the anterior basal segment of the right lower lobe, and probably of the anterior segment of the right upper lobe. An abdominal aortogram *(B)* revealed opacification of a large branch of the right phrenic artery *(arrow)*, which divided into a multitude of smaller radicals that entered the medial portion of the right lung. It is suggested that this represents systemic arterialization of the lung in response to chronic suppurative disease (severe bronchiectasis). There is no good evidence to suggest that the abnormality represents intrapulmonary sequestration. (Courtesy of Dr. W. E. Beamish, University Hospital, Edmonton, Alberta.)

diagnosis of all these conditions (Fig. 23–23). As with bronchopulmonary sequestration, preoperative recognition of the systemic vascular supply may prevent potentially fatal hemorrhage at thoracotomy.

CONGENITAL DEFICIENCY OF THE LEFT SIDE OF THE PARIETAL PERICARDIUM

Absence of the left side of the pericardium may be complete or partial and is accompanied by herniation of a portion of heart through the defect into the left hemithorax. Discussion of the anomaly is included here to familiarize the reader with the specific signs and to avoid confusion with the mediastinal displacement that may occur secondary to atelectasis of the left lower lobe.

In a review of six patients with complete absence of the left side of the pericardium, the radiographic findings were summarized as follows (Fig. 23–24):[241] (1) a shift of the heart to the left; (2) an unusual cardiac silhouette, with an elongated left heart border and three convexities (the aortic arch; a long, prominent, sharply demarcated pulmonary artery segment; and a left ventricular segment); (3) a band of radiolucency between the aortic arch and the main pulmonary artery; and (4) a band of radiolucency between

the left hemidiaphragm and the base of the heart, caused by interposed air-containing lung (radiographs exposed in the supine position may be necessary to reveal this last sign). Although some investigators have confirmed the diagnosis by demonstrating pneumopericardium after inducing diagnostic pneumothorax (Fig. 23–24), this procedure is not required for diagnosis and may, in fact, be hazardous.[241]

Patients complain of nonspecific anterior chest pain of short duration, often brought on by exercise or by lying on the left side, and of mild shortness of breath on exertion.[241] In the study of six patients cited earlier, the apical impulse was in the left axilla, and there was a sustained left ventricular thrust; all patients had systolic ejection murmurs of grade I to III/VI intensity, and two had diastolic murmurs along the left sternal border. Electrocardiography characteristically reveals right axis deviation and clockwise rotation of the QRS complex.[241, 242] The diagnosis can be confirmed if necessary by CT or MR.[243] Echocardiography can also be useful in excluding associated cardiovascular anomalies,[244] although it is not diagnostic of the pericardial deficiency itself.

Complete absence of the left side of the parietal pericardium is a benign condition quite compatible with a normal life span, as illustrated by the single case report of its presence in a 77-year-old asymptomatic man.[242] Although

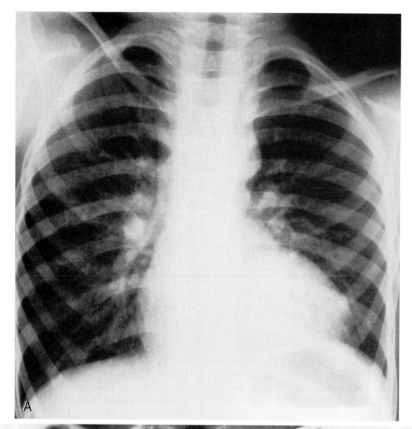

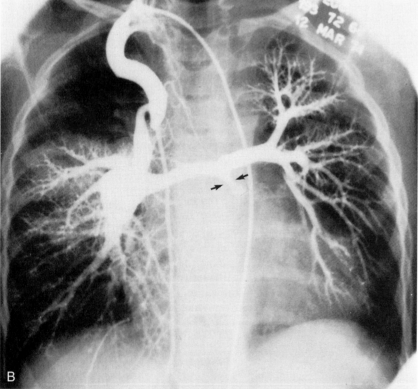

Figure 23–23. Systemic Arterial Supply to the Lung: Tetralogy of Fallot. A posteroanterior radiograph *(A)* reveals an abnormal cardiac configuration, there being a prominent concavity of the left border of the heart in the region of the main pulmonary artery. The hila are normal or slightly enlarged, and the pulmonary vasculature is generally within normal limits. Following selective injection of contrast medium into the right internal mammary artery *(B)*, at least 80% of the pulmonary arterial tree has been opacified via a large branch of this artery, which joins the pulmonary artery in the right hilum. Note the diminutive main pulmonary artery *(arrows in B)*. The patient was a 6-year-old boy with pulmonary atresia and ventricular septal defect; his course was excellent following establishment of a conduit between the right ventricle and main pulmonary artery and closure of the ventricular septal defect. (Courtesy of Dr. Kent Ellis, Columbia–Presbyterian Medical Center, New York.)

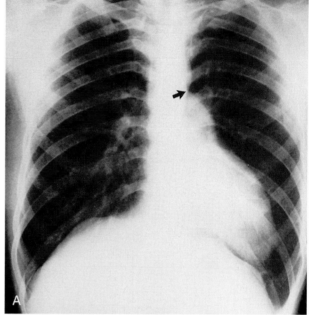

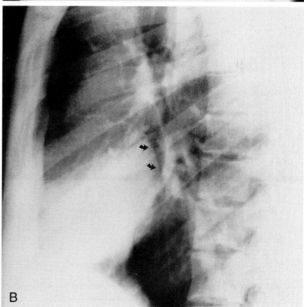

Figure 23–24. Congenital Deficiency of the Parietal Pericardium. A posteroanterior radiograph *(A)* shows a shift of the heart to the left and three convexities along the elongated left heart border—the aortic arch, the pulmonary artery segment, and the ventricular segment. The main pulmonary artery is unusually prominent, and a radiolucent cleft separates it from the aortic arch *(arrow)*. In lateral projection *(B)*, the anterior surface of the main pulmonary artery is exceptionally well seen, as is the posterior wall of the left atrium *(arrows)*.

Illustration continued on following page

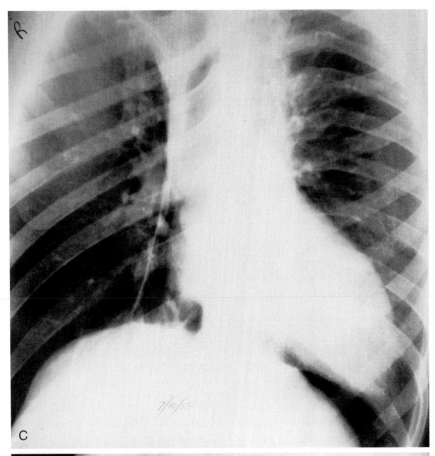

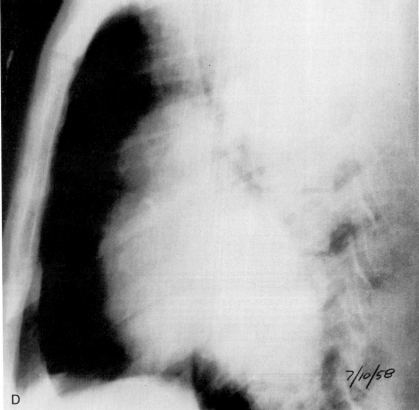

Figure 23–24 *Continued.* After introduction of 500 ml of air into the left pleural space, a lateral decubitus radiograph with the left side down and a horizontal x-ray beam *(C)* shows gas separating the heart from the diaphragm. In addition, gas has passed to the right side of the heart, creating a linear opacity that represents the combined thickness of the right side of the pericardium and adjacent mediastinal pleura separating the right pericardial space from the right lung. A lateral radiograph of the chest with the patient supine *(D)* shows the heart to have fallen away from the anterior chest wall and diaphragm owing to the lack of support of the left side of the pericardium. The patient was a 26-year-old man with a 6-year history of intermittent left precordial pain and tightness in the chest. (From Ellis K, Leeds NE, Himmelstein A: Am J Roentgenol 82:125, 1959.)

more rare, partial absence of the pericardium appears to be more serious: there have been at least three reported deaths from this condition as a result of herniation of the left ventricle; by contrast, herniation of the left atrium or atrial appendage alone is not a fatal condition.[241, 245] Focal absence of the left side of the parietal pericardium with herniation of the left atrium or left atrial appendage is recognized radiographically by the presence of a typical bulge along the left upper cardiac border.[137] The diagnosis can be easily confirmed by MR imaging.[137]

REFERENCES

1. Clements BS, Warner JO, Shinebourne EA: Congenital bronchopulmonary vascular malformations: Clinical application of a simple anatomical approach in 25 cases. Thorax 42:409, 1987.
2. Clements BS, Warner JO: Pulmonary sequestration and related congenital bronchopulmonary-vascular malformations: Nomenclature and classification based on anatomical and embryological considerations. Thorax 42:401, 1987.
3. Panicek DM, Heitzman ER, Randall PA, et al: The continuum of pulmonary developmental anomalies. RadioGraphics 7:747, 1987.
4. Edwards JE, McGoon DC: Clinicopathologic correlations: Absence of anatomic origin from heart of pulmonary arterial supply. Circulation 47:393, 1973.
5. Collett RW, Edwards JE: Persistent truncus arteriosus: A classification according to anatomic types. Surg Clin North Am 29:1245, 1949.
6. Sotomora RF, Edwards JE: Anatomic identification of so-called absent pulmonary artery. Circulation 57:624, 1978.
7. Davis GD, Fulton RE, Ritter DG, et al: Congenital pulmonary atresia with ventricular septal defect: Angiographic and surgical correlates. Radiology 128:133, 1978.
8. Ellis K: Developmental abnormalities in the systemic blood supply to the lungs. Am J Roentgenol 156:669, 1991.
9. Marcelletti C, McGoon DC, Mair DD: The natural history of truncus arteriosus. Circulation 54:108, 1976.
10. Hicken P, Evans D, Heath D: Persistent truncus arteriosus with survival to the age of 38 years. Br Heart J 28:284, 1966.
11. Carter JB, Blieden LC, Edwards JE: Persistent truncus arteriosus: Report of survival to age 52 years. Minn Med 56:280, 1973.
12. Spencer H: Pathology of the Lung (Excluding Pulmonary Tuberculosis). Vol. 1. 4th ed. New York, Pergamon Press, 1985.
13. Anderson RC, Char F, Adams P Jr: Proximal interruption of a pulmonary arch (absence of one pulmonary artery): Case report and a new embryologic interpretation. Dis Chest 34:73, 1958.
14. Ko T, Gatz MG, Reisz GR: Congenital unilateral absence of a pulmonary artery: A report of two adult cases. Am Rev Respir Dis 141:795, 1990.
15. Debatin JF, Moon RE, Spritzer CE, et al: MRI of absent left pulmonary artery. J Comput Assist Tomogr 16:641, 1992.
16. Bouros D, Paré P, Panagou P, et al: The varied manifestation of pulmonary artery agenesis in adulthood. Chest 108:670, 1995.
17. Pool PE, Vogel JHK, Blount SG Jr: Congenital unilateral absence of a pulmonary artery: The importance of flow in pulmonary hypertension. Am J Cardiol 1:706, 1962.
18. Cogswell TL, Singh S: Agenesis of the left pulmonary artery as a cause of hemoptysis. Angiology 73(3 pt 1):154, 1986.
19. Kauffman SL, Yao AC, Webber CB, et al: Origin of the right pulmonary artery from the aorta: A clinical-pathologic study of two types based on caliber of the pulmonary artery. Am J Cardiol 19:741, 1967.
20. Wagenvoort CA, Neufeld HN, Birge RF, et al: Origin of right pulmonary artery from ascending aorta. Circulation 23:84, 1961.
21. Yamaki S, Suzuki Y, Ishizawa E, et al: Isolated aortic origin of right pulmonary artery: Report of a case with special reference to pulmonary vascular disease in the left and right lungs. Chest 83:575, 1983.
22. Isawa T, Taplin GV: Unilateral pulmonary artery agenesis, stenosis, and hypoplasia. Radiology 99:605, 1971.
23. Gluck MC, Moser KM: Pulmonary artery agenesis: Diagnosis with ventilation and perfusion scintiphotography. Circulation 41:859, 1970.
24. Moser KM, Olson LK, Schlusselberg M, et al: Chronic thromboembolic occlusion in adult can mimic pulmonary artery agenesis. Chest 95:503, 1989.
25. Lynch DA, Higgins CB: MR imaging of unilateral pulmonary artery anomalies. J Comput Assist Tomogr 14:187, 1990.
26. Catala FJ, Marti-Bonatti L, Morales-Martin P: Proximal absence of right pulmonary artery in the adult: Computed tomography and magnetic resonance findings. J Thorac Imaging 8:244, 1993.
27. Morgan PW, Foley DW, Erickson SJ: Proximal interruption of a main pulmonary artery with transpleural collateral vessels: CT and MR appearances. J Comput Assist Tomogr 15:311, 1991.
28. Harris KM, Lloyd DCF, Morrissey B, et al: The computed tomographic appearances in pulmonary artery atresia. Clin Radiol 45:382, 1992.
29. Chiu RCJ, Herba MJ, Viloria J, et al: Thoracopulmonary hypogenesis with systemic artery-pulmonary vessel fistulae: Report of a case. Ann Thorac Surg 31:360, 1981.
30. Ellis K, Seaman WB, Griffiths SP, et al: Some congenital anomalies of the pulmonary arteries. Semin Roentgenol 2:325, 1967.
31. Philp T, Sumerling MD, Fleming J, et al: Aberrant left pulmonary artery. Clin Radiol 23:153, 1972.
32. Berdon WE, Baker DH: Vascular anomalies and the infant lung: Rings, slings and other things. Semin Roentgenol 7:39, 1972.
33. Gallo P, Fazzari F, La Magra C, et al: Facio-auriculo-vertebral anomalad and pulmonary artery sling: A hitherto undescribed but probably noncausal association. Pathol Res Pract 173:172, 1981.
33a. McDonald-McGinn DM, Driscoll DA, Bason L, et al: Autosomal dominant "Opitz" GBBB syndrome due to a 22q11.2 deletion. Am J Med Genet 59:103, 1995.
34. Lincoln JCR, Deverall PB, Stark J, et al: Vascular anomalies compressing the oesophagus and trachea. Thorax 24:295, 1969.
35. Capitanio MA, Ramos R, Kirkpatrick JA: Pulmonary sling: Roentgen observations. Am J Roentgenol 112:28, 1971.
36. Jue KL, Raghib G, Amplatz K, et al: Anomalous origin of the left pulmonary artery from the right pulmonary artery: Report of 2 cases and review of the literature. Am J Roentgenol 95:598, 1965.
37. Hatten HP, Forman JG, Rosenblum HD: Pulmonary sling in the adult. Am J Roentgenol 128:919, 1977.
38. Stone DN, Bein ME, Garris JB: Anomalous left pulmonary artery: Two new adult cases. Am J Roentgenol 135:1259, 1980.
39. Dumler MP: A rare cause of dysphagia: Anomalous left pulmonary artery. JAMA 197:233, 1966.
40. Gumbiner CH, Mullins CE, McNamara DG: Pulmonary artery sling. Am J Cardiol 45:311, 1980.
41. Malmgren N, Laurin S, Lundstrom N-R: Pulmonary artery sling. Acta Radiol 29:7, 1988.
42. Vogl TJ, Diebold T, Bergman C, et al: MRI in pre- and postoperative assessment of tracheal stenosis due to pulmonary artery sling. J Comput Assist Tomogr 17:878, 1993.
43. Landing BH: Syndromes of congenital heart disease with tracheobronchial anomalies. Edward BD Neuhauser Lecture, 1974. Am J Roentgenol 123:679, 1975.
44. Berdon WE, Baker DH, Wung J-T, et al: Complete cartilage-ring tracheal stenosis associated with anomalous left pulmonary artery: The ring-sling complex. Radiology 152:57, 1984.
45. McCue CM, Robertson LW, Lester RG, et al: Pulmonary artery coarctations: A report of 20 cases with review of 319 cases from the literature. J Pediatr 67:222, 1965.
46. Gay BB Jr, Franch RH, Shuford WH, et al: The roentgenologic features of single and multiple coarctations of the pulmonary artery and branches. Am J Roentgenol 90:599, 1963.
47. Baum D, Khoury GH, Ongley PA, et al: Congenital stenosis of the pulmonary artery branches. Circulation 29:680, 1964.
48. Bousvaros G, Palmer WH: Phonocardiographic features of the systolic murmur in pulmonary artery stenosis. Br Heart J 27:374, 1965.
49. Hoeffel JC, Henry M, Jimenez J, et al: Congenital stenosis of the pulmonary artery and its branches. Clin Radiol 25:481, 1974.
50. McDonald AH, Gerlis LM, Somerville J: Familial arteriopathy with associated pulmonary and systemic arterial stenoses. Br Heart J 31:375, 1969.
51. Lees MH, Menashe VD, Sunderland CO, et al: Ehlers-Danlos syndrome associated with multiple pulmonary artery stenoses and tortuous systemic arteries. J Pediatr 75:1031, 1969.
52. Pagon RA, Bennet FC, LaVeck B, et al: Williams syndrome: Features in late childhood and adolescence. Pediatrics 80:85, 1987.
53. Wessel A, Pankau R, Kececioglu D, et al: Three decades of follow-up of aortic and pulmonary vascular lesions in the Williams-Beuren syndrome. Am J Med Genet 52:297, 1994.
54. Alagille D, Estrada A, Hadchouel M, et al: Syndromic paucity of interlobular bile ducts, Alagille syndrome or arteriohepatic dysplasia: Review of 80 cases. J Pediatr 110:195, 1987.
55. Rowe RD: Maternal rubella and pulmonary artery stenosis. Pediatrics 32:180, 1963.
56. Winfield ME, McDonnel GM, Steckel RJ: Multiple coarctations of the pulmonary arteries with associated infundibular pulmonic stenosis: Case report with serial right-heart catheterization studies obtained at a three-year interval. Radiology 83:854, 1964.
57. Massumi R, Just G, Tawakkol A, et al: Acoustically silent stenosis of a branch of the pulmonary artery: A hemodynamic explanation. Am J Med 40:773, 1966.
58. Bartter T, Irwin RS, Nash G: Aneurysms of the pulmonary arteries. Chest 94:1065, 1988.
59. Bhandari AK, Nanda NC: Pulmonary artery aneurysms: Echocardiographic features in 5 patients. Am J Cardiol 53:1438, 1984.
60. Challis TW, Fay JE: Isolated dilatation of the main pulmonary artery: A report of three cases and a review of the literature. J Can Assoc Radiol 20:180, 1969.
61. Buckingham WB, Sutton GC, Meszaros WT: Abnormalities of the pulmonary artery resembling intrathoracic neoplasms. Dis Chest 40:698, 1961.
62. Silverman JM, Julien PJ, Herfkens RJ, et al: Magnetic resonance imaging evaluation of pulmonary vascular malformations. Chest 106:1333, 1994.
63. Trell E: Pulmonary arterial aneurysm. Thorax 28:644, 1973.
64. Jimenez M, Fournier A, Choussat A: Pulmonary artery to the left atrium fistula as an unusual cause of cyanosis in the newborn. Pediatr Cardiol 10:216, 1989.
65. Lucas RV Jr, Lund GW, Edwards JE: Direct communication of a pulmonary artery with the left atrium: An unusual variant of pulmonary arteriovenous fistula. Circulation 24:1409, 1961.
66. Ohara H, Ito K, Kohguchi N, et al: Direct communication between the right pulmonary artery and the left hilum: A case report. J Thorac Cardiovasc Surg 77:742, 1979.
67. Stuckey S: Direct communication between the right pulmonary artery and the left atrium: Magnetic resonance findings. Australas Radiol 37:216, 1993.
68. Krause DW, Kuehn HJ, Sellers RD, et al: Roentgen sign associated with an aberrant vessel connecting right main pulmonary artery to left atrium. Radiology 111:177, 1974.
69. Vogel M, Ash J, Rowe R, et al: Congenital unilateral pulmonary vein stenosis complicating transposition of the great arteries. Am J Cardiol 54:166, 1984.

70. Khonsari S, Saunders PW, Lees MH, et al: Common pulmonary vein atresia: Importance of immediate recognition and surgical intervention. J Thorac Cardiovasc Surg 83:443, 1982.

71. Mortensson W, Lundström N-R: Congenital obstruction of the pulmonary veins at their atrial junctions: Review of the literature and a case report. Am Heart J 87:359, 1974.

72. Swischuk LE, L'Heureux P: Unilateral pulmonary vein atresia. Am J Roentgenol 135:667, 1980.

73. Belcourt CL, Roy DL, Nanton MA, et al: Stenosis of individual pulmonary veins: Radiologic findings. Radiology 161:109, 1986.

74. Adey CK, Soto B, Shin MS: Congenital pulmonary vein stenosis: A radiographic study. Radiology 161:113, 1986.

75. Asayama J, Shiguma R, Katsume H, et al: Pulmonary varix. Angiology 35:735, 1984.

76. Chilton SJ, Campbell JB: Pulmonary varix in early infancy: Case report with 8-year follow up. Radiology 129:400, 1978.

77. Ben-Menachem Y, Kuroda K, Kyger ER III, et al: The various forms of pulmonary varices: Report of three new cases and review of the literature. Am J Roentgenol 125:881, 1975.

78. Owens DW, Garcia E, Pierce RR, et al: Klippel-Trenaunay syndrome with pulmonary vein varicosity. Arch Dermatol 108:111, 1973.

79. Hagen H, Heinz K: Varixknoten im Lingulaast der Vena pulmonalis. [Varicosities in the lingular branch of the pulmonary vein.] Fortschr Roentgenstr 93:151, 1960.

80. Bryk D, Levin EJ: Pulmonary varicosity. Radiology 85:834, 1965.

81. Steinberg I: Pulmonary varices mistaken for pulmonary and hilar disease. Am J Roentgenol 101:947, 1967.

82. Shida T, Ohashi H, Nakamura K, et al: Pulmonary varices associated with mitral valve disease: A case report and survey of the literature. Ann Thorac Surg 34:452, 1982.

83. Borkowski GP, O'Donovan PB, Troup BR: Pulmonary varix: CT findings. J Comput Assist Tomogr 5:827, 1981.

84. Poller S, Wholey MH: Pulmonary varix: Evaluation by selective pulmonary angiography. Radiology 86:1078, 1966.

85. Hasuo K, Numaguchi Y, Kishikawa T, et al: Anomalous unilateral single pulmonary vein mimicking pulmonary varices. Chest 79:602, 1981.

86. Benfield JR, Gots RE, Mills D: Anomalous single left pulmonary vein mimicking a parenchymal nodule. Chest 59:101, 1971.

87. Klinck GH Jr, Hunt HD: Pulmonary varix with spontaneous rupture and death: Report of a case. Arch Pathol 15:227, 1933.

88. Kozuka T, Nosaki T: A pulmonary vein anomaly: Unusual connection and tortuosity of the right lower lobe vein. Br J Radiol 41:232, 1968.

89. Blake HA, Hall RJ, Manion WC: Anomalous pulmonary venous return. Circulation 32:406, 1965.

90. Darling RC, Rothney WB, Craig JM: Total pulmonary venous drainage into the right side of the heart. Lab Invest 6:44, 1957.

91. Hughes CW, Rumore PC: Anomalous pulmonary veins. Arch Pathol 37:364, 1944.

92. Greene R, Miller SW: Cross-sectional imaging of silent pulmonary venous anomalies. Radiology 159:279, 1986.

93. Dillon EH, Camputaro C: Partial anomalous pulmonary venous drainage of the left upper lobe vs duplication of the superior vena cava: Distinction based on CT findings. Am J Roentgenol 160:375, 1993.

94. Pennes DR, Ellis JH: Anomalous pulmonary venous drainage of the left lower lobe shown by CT scans. Radiology 159:23, 1986.

95. Schatz SL, Ryvicker MJ, Deutsch AM, et al: Partial anomalous pulmonary venous drainage of the right lower lobe shown by CT scans. Radiology 159:21, 1986.

96. Thorsen MK, Erickson SJ, Mewissen MW, et al: CT and MR imaging of partial anomalous pulmonary venous return to the azygos vein. J Comput Assist Tomogr 14:1007, 1990.

97. Masui T, Seelos KC, Kersting-Sommerhoff BA, et al: Abnormalities of the pulmonary veins: Evaluation with MR imaging and comparison with cardiac angiography and echocardiography. Radiology 181:645, 1991.

98. Vesely TM, Julsrud PR, Brown JJ, et al: MR imaging of partial anomalous pulmonary venous connections. J Comput Assist Tomogr 15:752, 1991.

98a. White CS, Baffa JM, Haney PJ, et al: Anomalies of pulmonary veins: Usefulness of spin-echo and gradient-echo MR images. Am J Roentgenol 170:1365, 1998.

99. Miller SW, Dinsmore RE, Liberthson RR, et al: Anomalous pulmonary venous connection of entire left lung with intact atrial septum. Radiology 122:591, 1977.

100. Wolfe WG, Ebert PA: Total anomalous pulmonary venous return with intact atrial septum and associated mitral stenosis. Thorax 25:769, 1970.

101. Shone JD, Edwards JE: Mitral atresia associated with pulmonary venous anomalies. Br Heart J 26:241, 1964.

102. Brody H: Drainage of the pulmonary veins into the right side of the heart. Arch Pathol 33:221, 1942.

103. Kissner DG, Sorkin RP: Anomalous pulmonary venous connection: Medical therapy. Chest 89:752, 1986.

104. Babb JD, McGlynn TJ, Pierce WS, et al: Isolated partial anomalous venous connection: A congenital defect with late and serious complications. Ann Thorac Surg 31:540, 1981.

105. Landing BH, Lawrence TYK, Payne VC Jr, et al: Bronchial anatomy in syndromes with abnormal visceral situs, abnormal spleen and congenital heart disease. Am J Cardiol 28:456, 1971.

106. Petersen RC, Edwards WD: Pulmonary vascular disease in 57 necropsy cases of total anomalous pulmonary venous connection. Histopathology 7:487, 1983.

107. Elliott LP, Schiebler GL: A roentgenologic-electrocardiographic approach to cyanotic forms of heart disease. Pediatr Clin North Am 18:1133, 1971.

107a. Hidvegi RS, Lapin J: Anomalous bilateral single pulmonary vein demonstrated by three-dimensional reconstruction of helical computed tomographic angiography: Case report. Can Assoc Radiol J 49:262, 1998.

108. Haworth SG, Reid L: Structural study of pulmonary circulation and of heart in total anomalous pulmonary venous return in early infancy. Br Heart J 39:80, 1977.

109. Carey LS, Edwards JE: Severe pulmonary venous obstruction in total anomalous pulmonary venous connection to the left innominate vein. Am J Roentgenol 90:593, 1963.

110. Kauffman SL, Ores CN, Andersen DH: Two cases of total anomalous pulmonary venous return of the supracardiac type with stenosis simulating infradiaphragmatic drainage. Circulation 25:376, 1962.

111. Hsu YH, Chien CT, Hwang M, et al: Magnetic resonance imaging of total anomalous pulmonary venous drainage. Am Heart J 121:1560, 1991.

112. Choe YH, Lee HJ, Kim HS, et al: MRI of total anomalous pulmonary venous connections. J Comput Assist Tomogr 18:243, 1994.

113. Everhart FJ, Korns ME, Amplatz K, et al: Intrapulmonary segment in anomalous pulmonary venous connection: Resemblance to scimitar syndrome. Circulation 35:1163, 1967.

114. Carter REB, Capriles M, Noe Y: Total anomalous pulmonary venous drainage: A clinical and anatomical study of 75 children. Br Heart J 31:45, 1969.

115. Gathman GE, Nadas AS: Total anomalous pulmonary venous connection: Clinical and physiologic observations of 75 pediatric patients. Circulation 42:143, 1970.

116. Bove EL, DeLaval MR, Taylor JFN, et al: Infradiaphragmatic total anomalous pulmonary venous drainage: Surgical treatment and long-term results. Ann Thorac Surg 31:544, 1981.

117. Singh R, Weisinger B, Carpenter M, et al: Total anomalous pulmonary venous return, surgically corrected in two patients beyond 40 years of age. Chest 60:38, 1971.

118. Mathey J, Galey JJ, Logeais Y, et al: Anomalous pulmonary venous return into inferior vena cava and associated bronchovascular anomalies (the scimitar syndrome). Thorax 23:398, 1968.

119. Woodring JH, Howard TA, Kanga JF: Congenital pulmonary venolobar syndrome revisited. RadioGraphics 14:349, 1994.

120. Dupuis C, Charaf LAC, Brevię GM, et al: The "adult" form of the scimitar syndrome. Am J Cardiol 70:502, 1992.

121. Jue KL, Amplatz K, Adams P Jr, et al: Anomalies of great vessels associated with lung hypoplasia: The scimitar syndrome. Am J Dis Child 111:35, 1966.

122. Halasz NA, Halloran KH, Liebow AA: Bronchial and arterial anomalies with drainage of the right lung into the inferior vena cava. Circulation 14:826, 1956.

123. Clements BS, Warner JO: The crossover lung segment: Congenital malformation associated with a variant of scimitar syndrome. Thorax 42:417, 1987.

124. Kiely B, Filler J, Stone S, et al: Syndrome of anomalous venous drainage of the right lung to the inferior vena cava: A review of 67 reported cases and three new cases in children. Am J Cardiol 20:102, 1967.

125. Neil CA, Ferencz C, Sabiston DC, et al: The familial occurrence of hypoplastic right lung with systemic arterial supply and venous drainage: "Scimitar syndrome." Bull Johns Hopkins Hosp 107:1, 1960.

126. Roehm JOF Jr, Jue KL, Amplatz K: Radiographic features of the scimitar syndrome. Radiology 86:856, 1966.

126a. Cirillo RL: The scimitar sign. Radiology 206:623, 1998.

127. Bessolo RJ, Maddison FE: Scimitar syndrome: Report of a case with unusual variations. Am J Roentgenol 103:572, 1968.

128. Osborn AG, Silverman JF: Unusual venous drainage patterns in the scimitar syndrome. Radiology 113:601, 1974.

129. Goodman LR, Jamshidi A, Hipona FA: Meandering right pulmonary vein simulating the scimitar syndrome. Chest 62:510, 1972.

130. Takeda SI, Imachi T, Arimitsu K, et al: Two cases of scimitar variant. Chest 105:292, 1994.

131. Cukier A, Kavakama J, Teixeira LR, et al: Scimitar sign with normal pulmonary venous drainage and systemic arterial supply: Scimitar syndrome or bronchopulmonary sequestration? Chest 105:294, 1994.

132. Godwin JD, Tarver RD: Scimitar syndrome: Four new cases examined with CT. Radiology 159:15, 1986.

133. Olson MA, Becker GJ: The scimitar syndrome: CT findings in partial anomalous pulmonary venous return. Radiology 159:25, 1986.

134. Gilkeson RC, Basile V, Sands MJ, et al: Chest case of the day. Am J Roentgenol 169:266, 1997.

135. Baran R, Kir A, Tor MM, et al: Scimitar syndrome: Confirmation of diagnosis by a noninvasive technique (MRI). Eur Radiol 6:92, 1996.

136. Folger GM Jr: The scimitar syndrome: Anatomic, physiologic, developmental and therapeutic considerations. Angiology 23:373, 1976.

137. Crowley JJ, Oh KS, Newman B, et al: Telltale signs of congenital heart disease. Radiol Clin North Am 31:573, 1993.

138. Burke CM, Safai C, Nelson DP, et al: Pulmonary arteriovenous malformations: A critical update. Am Rev Respir Dis 134:334, 1986.

139. Abbott OA, Haebich AT, Van Flent WE: Changing patterns relative to the surgical treatment of pulmonary arteriovenous fistulas. Am Surg 25:674, 1959.

140. Steinberg I, Maisel B, Vogel FS: Pulmonary arteriovenous fistula associated with capillary telangiectasia (Rendu-Osler-Weber disease): Report of a case illustrating use of metal casting for demonstrating the lesion. J Thorac Surg 35:517, 1958.

141. Sammons BP: Arteriovenous fistula of the lung. Radiology 72:710, 1959.

142. Hodgson CH, Burchell HB, Good CA, et al: Hereditary hemorrhagic telangiectasia and pulmonary arteriovenous fistula: Survey of a large family. N Engl J Med 261:625, 1959.
143. Stork WJ: Pulmonary arteriovenous fistulas. Am J Roentgenol 74:441, 1955.
144. Prager RL, Laws KH, Bender HW Jr: Arteriovenous fistula of the lung. Ann Thorac Surg 36:231, 1983.
145. Ellman P, Hanson A: Pulmonary arteriovenous aneurysm. Br J Dis Chest 53:165, 1959.
146. Dines DE, Arms RA, Bernatz PE, et al: Pulmonary arteriovenous fistula. Mayo Clin Proc 49:460, 1974.
147. Guttmacher AE, Marchuk DA, White RI Jr: Hereditary hemorrhagic telangiectasia. N Engl J Med 333:918, 1995.
148. Taxman RM, Halloran MJ, Parker BM: Multiple pulmonary arteriovenous malformations in association with Fanconi's syndrome. Chest 64:118, 1973.
149. Papagiannis J, Kanter RJ, Effman EL, et al: Polysplenia with pulmonary arteriovenous malformations. Pediatr Cardiol 14:127, 1993.
150. Gomes MMR, Bernatz PE: Arteriovenous fistula: A review and ten-year experience at the Mayo Clinic. Mayo Clin Proc 45:81, 1970.
151. Masson RG, Altose MD, Maycock RL: Isolated bronchial telangiectasia. Chest 65:450, 1974.
152. Cooley DA, McNamara DG: Pulmonary telangiectasia: Report of a case proved by pulmonary biopsy. J Thorac Surg 27:614, 1954.
153. Lindskog GE, Liebow A, Kausel H, et al: Pulmonary arteriovenous aneurysm. Ann Surg 132:591, 1950.
154. Hales MR: Multiple small arteriovenous fistulae of the lungs. Am J Pathol 32:927, 1956.
155. Moyer JH, Glantz G, Brest AN: Pulmonary arteriovenous fistulas: Physiologic and clinical considerations. Am J Med 32:417, 1962.
156. Steinberg I, Finby N: Roentgen manifestations of pulmonary arteriovenous fistula: Diagnosis and treatment of four new cases. Am J Roentgenol 78:234, 1957.
156a. Edinburgh KJ, Chung MH, Webb WR: CT of spontaneous hemothorax from intrapleural rupture of a pulmonary arteriovenous malformation. Am J Roentgenol 170:1399, 1998.
157. Hodgson CH, Burchell HB, Good CA, et al: Hereditary hemorrhagic telangiectasia and pulmonary arteriovenous fistula: Survey of a large family. N Engl J Med 261:625, 1959.
158. Godwin JD, Webb WR: Dynamic computed tomography in the evaluation of vascular lung lesions. Radiology 138:629, 1981.
159. Rankin S, Faling J, Pugatch RD: CT diagnosis of pulmonary arteriovenous malformations. J Comput Assist Tomogr 6:746, 1982.
160. Remy J, Remy-Jardin M, Wattinne L, et al: Pulmonary arteriovenous malformations: Evaluation with CT of the chest before and after treatment. Radiology 182:809, 1992.
161. Moser RJ, Tenholder MF: Diagnostic imaging of pulmonary arteriovenous malformations: Evaluation with roentgenographic, sonographic and radionuclide imaging. Chest 89:586, 1986.
162. Hernandez A, Strauss AW, McKnight R, et al: Diagnosis of pulmonary arteriovenous fistula by contrast echocardiography. J Pediatr 93:258, 1978.
162a. Wang H-C, Kuo P-H, Liaw Y-S, et al: Diagnosis of pulmonary arteriovenous malformations by colour Doppler ultrasound and amplitude ultrasound angiography. Thorax 53:372, 1998.
163. Sagel SS, Greenspan RH: Minute pulmonary arteriovenous fistulas demonstrated by magnification pulmonary angiography—case report. Radiology 97:529, 1970.
164. Gutierrez FR, Glazer HS, Levitt RG, et al: NMR imaging of pulmonary arteriovenous fistulae. J Comput Assist Tomogr 8:750, 1984.
165. Webb WR, Gamsu G, Golden JA: Nuclear magnetic resonance of pulmonary arteriovenous fistula: Effects of flow. J Comput Assist Tomogr 8:155, 1984.
166. Dinsmore BJ, Gefter WB, Hatabu H, et al: Pulmonary arteriovenous malformations: Diagnosis by gradient refocused MR imaging. J Comput Assist Tomogr 14:918, 1990.
167. White RI, Mitchell SE, Barth KH, et al: Angioarchitecture of pulmonary arteriovenous malformations: An important consideration before embolotherapy. Am J Roentgenol 140:681, 1983.
168. Remy J, Remy-Jardin M, Giraud F, et al: Angioarchitecture of pulmonary arteriovenous malformations: Clinical utility of three-dimensional helical CT. Radiology 191:657, 1994.
169. Lewis AB, Gates G, Stanley P: Echocardiography and perfusion scintigraphy in the diagnosis of pulmonary arteriovenous fistula. Chest 73:675, 1978.
170. Whyte MKB, Peters AM, Hughes JMB, et al: Quantification of right to left shunt at rest and during exercise in patients with pulmonary arteriovenous malformations. Thorax 47:790, 1992.
171. Barzilai B, Waggoner AD, Spessert C, et al: Two-dimensional echocardiography in the detection and follow-up of congenital pulmonary arteriovenous malformations. Am J Cardiol 68:1507, 1991.
171a. Coley SC, Jackson JE: Pulmonary arteriovenous malformations. Clin Radiol 53:396, 1998.
172. van de Weyer KH: Zur Röntgendiagnostik arteriovenöser Lungenfisteln. [The roentgen diagnosis of pulmonary arteriovenous fistulas.] Fortschr Roentgenstr 102:393, 1965.
173. Apthorp GH, Bates DV: Report of a case of pulmonary telangiectasia. Thorax 12:65, 1957.
174. MacNee W, Buist TA, Finlayson ND, et al: Multiple microscopic pulmonary arteriovenous connections in the lungs presenting as cyanosis. Thorax 40:316, 1985.
175. Hoffman R, Rabens R: Evolving pulmonary nodules: Multiple pulmonary arteriovenous fistulas. Am J Roentgenol 120:861, 1974.
176. Dines DE: Diagnostic significance of pneumatocele of the lung. JAMA 204:1169, 1968.
177. Kintzer JS, Jones FL, Pharr WF: Intrapleural haemorrhage complicating pulmonary arteriovenous fistula. Br J Dis Chest 72:155, 1978.
178. Dalton ML Jr, Goodwin FC, Bronwell AW, et al: Intrapleural rupture of pulmonary arteriovenous aneurysm: Report of a case. Dis Chest 52:97, 1967.
179. Hunter DD: Pulmonary arteriovenous malformation: An unusual cause of cerebral embolism. Can Med Assoc J 93:662, 1965.
180. Steinberg I, McClenahan J: Pulmonary arteriovenous fistula. Angiocardiographic observations in nine cases. Am J Med 19:549, 1955.
181. Takeuchi A, Ise S, Morioka T, et al: Pulmonary arteriovenous fistula without signs of anoxemia: Report of a case and review of the literature. Jpn J Thorac Surg 121:557, 1959.
182. Standefer JE, Tabakin BS, Hanson JS: Pulmonary arteriovenous fistulas: Case report with cine-angiographic studies. Am Rev Respir Dis 89:95, 1964.
183. Baert AL, Casteels-Van Daele M, Broeckx J, et al: Generalized juvenile polyposis with pulmonary arteriovenous malformations and hypertrophic osteoarthropathy. Am J Roentgenol 141:661, 1983.
184. Sanders JS, Marth JM: Multiple small pulmonary arteriovenous fistulas: Diagnosis by cardiac catheterization. Circulation 25:383, 1962.
185. Hazlett DR, Medina J: Postural effects on the bruit and right-to-left shunt of pulmonary arteriovenous fistula. Chest 60:89, 1971.
186. Castaneda-Zuniga W, Epstein M, Zollikofer C, et al: Embolization of multiple pulmonary artery fistulas. Radiology 134:309, 1980.
187. Kaufman SL, Kumar AAJ, Roland JA, et al: Transcatheter embolization in the management of congenital arteriovenous malformations. Radiology 137:21, 1980.
188. Barth KH, White RI, Kaufman SL, et al: Embolotherapy of pulmonary arteriovenous malformations with detachable balloons. Radiology 142:599, 1982.
189. White RI, Lynch-Nyhan A, Terry P, et al: Pulmonary artery malformations: Techniques and long term outcome of embolotherapy. Radiology 169:663, 1988.
190. Dutton JAE, Jackson JE, Hughes JMB, et al: Pulmonary arteriovenous malformations: Results of treatment with coil embolization in 53 patients. Am J Roentgenol 165:1119, 1995.
191. Burke CM, Safai C, Nelson DP, et al: Pulmonary arteriovenous malformations: A critical update. Am Rev Respir Dis 134:334, 1986.
192. Redo SF, Williams JR, Bass R, et al: Respiratory obstruction secondary to lymphangioma of the trachea. J Thorac Cardiovasc Surg 49:1026, 1965.
193. Milovic I, Oluic D: Lymphangioma of the lung associated with respiratory distress in a neonate. Pediatr Radiol 22:156, 1992.
194. Wada A, Tateishi R, Terazawa T, et al: Lymphangioma of the lung. Arch Pathol 98:211, 1974.
195. Holden WE, Morris JF, Antonovic R, et al: Adult intrapulmonary and mediastinal lymphangioma causing haemoptysis. Thorax 42:635, 1987.
196. Tazelaar HD, Kerr D, Yousem SA, et al: Diffuse pulmonary lymphangiomatosis. Hum Pathol 24:1313, 1993.
197. Canny GJ, Cutz E, MacLusky IB, et al: Diffuse pulmonary angiomatosis. Thorax 46:851, 1991.
198. Fan LL, Muellen ALW, Brugman SM, et al: Clinical spectrum of chronic interstitial lung disease in children. J Pediatr 121:867, 1992.
199. Carlson KC, Parnassus WH, Klatt EC: Thoracic lymphangiomatosis. Arch Pathol Lab Med 111:475, 1987.
200. Ramani P, Shah A: Lymphangiomatosis: Histologic and immunohistochemical analysis of four cases. Am J Surg Pathol 17:329, 1993.
201. Swensen SJ, Hartman TE, Mayo JR, et al: Diffuse pulmonary lymphangiomatosis: CT findings. J Comput Assist Tomogr 19:348, 1995.
202. Bhatti MA, Ferrante JW, Gielchinsky I, et al: Pleuropulmonary and skeletal lymphangiomatosis with chylothorax and chylopericardium. Ann Thorac Surg 40:398, 1985.
203. Takahashi K, Takahashi H, Maeda K, et al: An adult case of lymphangiomatosis of the mediastinum, pulmonary interstitium and retroperitoneum complicated by chronic disseminated intravascular coagulation. Eur Respir J 8:1799, 1995.
204. Felman AH, Rhatigan RM, Pierson KK: Pulmonary lymphangiectasia: Observation in 17 patients and proposed classification. Am J Roentgenol 116:548, 1972.
205. Hernandez RJ, Stern AM, Rosenthal A: Pulmonary lymphangiectasis in Noonan syndrome. Am J Radiol 134:75, 1980.
206. Esterly JR, Oppenheimer EH: Lymphangiectasis and other pulmonary lesions in the asplenia syndrome. Arch Pathol 90:553, 1970.
207. Laurence KM: Congenital pulmonary cystic lymphangiectasis. J Pathol Bacteriol 70:325, 1955.
208. Rhatigan RM, Hobin FP: Congenital pulmonary lymphangiectasis and ichthyosis congenita: A case report. Am J Clin Pathol 53:95, 1970.
209. Noonan JA, Walters LR, Reeves JT: Congenital pulmonary lymphangiectasis. Am J Dis Child 120:314, 1970.
210. Wagenaar SJ, Swierenga J, Wagenvoort CA: Late presentation of primary pulmonary lymphangiectasis. Thorax 33:791, 1978.
211. Laurence KM: Congenital pulmonary lymphangiectasis. J Clin Pathol 12:62, 1959.
212. Sethi GK, Class RN, Scott SM, et al: Aortic sinus of Valsalva–pulmonary artery fistula: Diagnosis and management. Chest 65:568, 1974.
213. Haworth SG: Pulmonary vascular disease in ventricular septal defect: Structural and functional correlations in lung biopsies from 85 patients, with outcome of intracardiac repair. J Pathol 152:157, 1987.
214. Dollery CT, West JB, Wilcken DEL, et al: A comparison of the pulmonary blood flow between left and right lungs in normal subjects and patients with congenital heart disease. Circulation 24:617, 1961.

215. Wilson WJ, Amplatz K: Unequal vascularity in tetralogy of Fallot. Am J Roentgenol 100:318, 1967.
216. Haworth SG, Reid L: Quantitative structural study of pulmonary circulation in the newborn with pulmonary atresia. Thorax 32:129, 1977.
217. Wagenvoort CA, Edwards JE: The pulmonary arterial tree in pulmonic atresia. Arch Pathol 71:56, 1961.
218. Naeye RL: Perinatal changes in the pulmonary vascular bed with stenosis and atresia of the pulmonic valve. Am Heart J 61:586, 1961.
219. de Matteis A: The vascular pathology of the lung in congenital malformations of the heart with severe pulmonary stenosis or atresia and right-to-left shunt. Respiration 26:337, 1969.
220. Johnson RJ, Haworth SG: Pulmonary vascular and alveolar development in tetralogy of Fallot: A recommendation for early correction. Thorax 37:893, 1982.
221. Hislop A, Reid L: Structural changes in the pulmonary arteries and veins in tetralogy of Fallot. Br Heart J 35:1178, 1973.
222. Turner-Warwick M: Systemic arterial patterns in the lung and clubbing of the fingers. Thorax 18:238, 1963.
223. Felson B: Chest Roentgenology. Philadelphia, WB Saunders, 1973.
224. Liebow AA, Hales MR, Harrison W, et al: The genesis and functional implications of collateral circulation of the lungs. Yale J Biol Med 22:637, 1950.
225. Heimburg P: Bronchial collateral circulation in experimental stenosis of the pulmonary artery. Thorax 19:306, 1964.
226. Jonsson H, Wahlgren H, Ivert T: Pulmonary artery abnormalities in tetralogy of Fallot and relation to late physical performance. Scand J Thorac Cardiovasc Surg 30:21, 1996.
227. Tadavarthy SM, Klugman J, Castaneda-Zuniga WR, et al: Systemic-to-pulmonary collaterals in pathological states. Radiology 144:55, 1982.
228. Currarino G, Willis K, Miller W: Congenital fistula between an aberrant systemic artery and a pulmonary vein without sequestration: A report of three cases. Pediatrics 87:554, 1975.
229. Brundage BH, Gomez AC, Cheitlin MD, et al: Systemic artery to pulmonary vessel fistulas: Report of two cases and a review of the literature. Chest 62:19, 1972.
230. Flisak ME, Chandrasekar AJ, Marsan RE, et al: Systemic arterialization of lung without sequestration. Am J Roentgenol 138:751, 1982.
231. Litwin SB, Plauth WH Jr, Nadas AS: Anomalous systemic arterial supply to the lung causing pulmonary artery hypertension. N Engl J Med 283:1098, 1970.
232. Kirks DR, Kane PE, Free EA, et al: Systemic arterial supply to normal basilar segments of the left lower lobe. Am J Roentgenol 126:817, 1976.
233. Matzinger FR, Bhargava R, Peterson RA, et al: Systemic arterial supply to the lung without sequestration: An unusual cause of hemoptysis. Can Assoc Radiol J 45:44, 1994.
234. Hirai T, Ohtake Y, Mutoh S, et al: Anomalous systemic arterial supply to normal basal segments of the left lower lobe: A report of two cases. Chest 109:286, 1996.
235. Miyake H, Hori Y, Takeoka H, et al: Systemic arterial supply to normal basal segments of the left lung: Characteristic features on chest radiography and CT. Am J Roentgenol 171:387, 1998.
236. Piessens J, De Geest H, Kesteloot H, et al: Anomalous collateral systemic pulmonary circulation to a normal lung. Chest 59:222, 1971.
237. Stocker JT, Malczak HT: A study of pulmonary ligament arteries: Relationship to intralobar pulmonary sequestration. Chest 86:611, 1984.
238. Painter RL, Billig DM, Epstein I: Brief recordings: Anomalous systemic arterialization of the lung without sequestration. N Engl J Med 279:866, 1968.
239. Syme J: Systemic to pulmonary arterial fistula of the chest wall and lung following lobectomy. Australas Radiol 19:326, 1975.
240. Haroutunian LM, Neill CA, Dorst JP: Pulmonary pseudofibrosis in cyanotic heart disease: A clinical syndrome mimicking tuberculosis in patients with extreme pulmonic stenosis. Chest 62:587, 1972.
241. Morgan JR, Rogers AK, Forker AD: Congenital absence of the left pericardium: Clinical findings. Ann Intern Med 74:370, 1971.
242. Glancy DL, Sanders CV, Porta A: Posterior chest wall pulsation in congenital complete absence of the left pericardium. Chest 65:564, 1974.
243. Baim RS, MacDonald IL, Wise DJ, et al: Computed tomography of absent left pericardium. Radiology 135:127, 1980.
244. Nicolosi GL, Borgioni L, Alberti E, et al: M-Mode and two-dimensional echocardiography in congenital absence of the pericardium. Chest 81:610, 1982.
245. Robin E, Ganguly SN, Fowler MS: Strangulation of the left atrial appendage through a congenital partial pericardial defect. Chest 67:354, 1975.

CHAPTER 24

Hereditary Abnormalities of Pulmonary Connective Tissue

MARFAN'S SYNDROME, 676
EHLERS-DANLOS SYNDROME, 677
CUTIS LAXA, 677
PSEUDOXANTHOMA ELASTICUM, 677
ALKAPTONURIA (OCHRONOSIS), 677
LYMPHANGIOLEIOMYOMATOSIS, 679
    Etiology and Pathogenesis, 679
    Pathologic Characteristics, 679
    Radiologic Manifestations, 683
    Clinical Manifestations, 685
    Natural History and Prognosis, 686
TUBEROUS SCLEROSIS, 686
NEUROFIBROMATOSIS, 690

This chapter is concerned with a variety of conditions in which the principal pulmonary abnormality is related to a hereditary or developmental derangement of the lungs' mesenchymal tissue. The former group is perhaps the more easy to understand because it appears to be characterized by genetic deficiencies of connective tissue metabolism. The inclusion of the second group of diseases—lymphangioleiomyomatosis, tuberous sclerosis, and neurofibromatosis—under a developmental heading is more tenuous because their pathogenesis has not been clearly defined. Their association with a variety of mesenchymal abnormalities in different organs and the hereditary nature of the last two, however, argue that they can be considered appropriately at this point.

There are more than 100 distinct heritable disorders of connective tissue, each presumed to be caused by a mutation in a single gene that controls the structure or metabolism of one or more macromolecules.[1] In several of these disorders, specific enzyme deficiencies have been identified that are believed to be responsible for various manifestations of disease.[2, 3] An example is lysyl oxidase, the enzyme responsible for the initial deamination of lysine and hydroxylysine, which results in the formation of compounds that produce the characteristic cross-links of elastin and collagen. The molecule has cupric ion as a cofactor, and animals on copper-deficient diets show changes in certain tissues and organs that are considered to be the result of an interference with cross-linking of collagen and elastin.[4, 5] Defective binding between collagen and elastin also occurs in animals fed on the seed of the sweet pea (*Lathyrus odoratus*) and is believed to be the underlying mechanism for the inherited emphysema-like changes found in the lungs of the blotchy mouse.[4]

Even in young individuals, significant emphysema can develop in a variety of heritable disorders of connective tissue, such as cutis laxa, osteogenesis imperfecta, and Marfan's syndrome. In some of these patients, concomitant cigarette smoking or antiprotease deficiency may be important in the development of disease.[6]

MARFAN'S SYNDROME

Marfan's syndrome is characterized by abnormally long extremities (particularly the fingers and toes), subluxation of the lens, and cardiovascular abnormalities (particularly aortic dilation and dissection).[3, 7] Its incidence has been estimated to be about 5 per 100,000.[7] It shows an autosomal dominant pattern of inheritance with variable penetrance and has been shown to be related to mutation of the fibrillin 1 gene.[8]

The most common chest radiographic manifestations are a long thin body habitus, scoliosis, and pectus excavatum;[9] in one series of 50 patients, 34 (68%) had pectus deformity and 22 (44%) had scoliosis.[7] The most frequently reported pulmonary abnormality is spontaneous pneumothorax,[9–11] a complication that arises in about 5% to 10% of patients (values that are several hundred times greater than those of the general population).[9, 10] Other pulmonary manifestations include apical bullae (Fig. 24–1) and, less commonly, diffuse emphysema, bronchiectasis, or upper lobe fibrosis.[9–11]

Cardiovascular disease develops in the vast majority of patients who have Marfan's syndrome and is the cause of death in more than 90%.[12, 13] The most common abnormalities are aortic aneurysm, aortic dissection, and aortic and mitral valve regurgitation.[13] The first two of these usually involve the ascending aorta and thus may come to the attention of chest physicians (Fig. 24–2). Serial chest radiographs may show progressive aortic enlargement and commonly show cardiomegaly as a result of aortic regurgitation.[14] The diagnosis is usually confirmed by computed tomography (CT); diagnostic features include the presence of an intimal flap and a false lumen.[13, 14] Aortic aneurysms and dissection as well as the associated cardiovascular abnormalities can also be readily recognized on MR imaging and echocardiography.[15, 16] In one investigation of 49 symptomatic patients with clinically suspected thoracic aortic dissection of various causes, contrast-enhanced CT, multiplanar

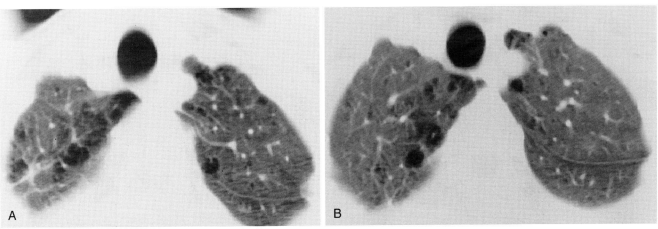

Figure 24–1. Marfan's Syndrome. CT scans (*A* and *B*) in a 29-year-old man with Marfan's syndrome demonstrate bilateral apical bullae. The bullae were found incidentally at CT during assessment of aortic dissection.

transesophageal echocardiography, and MR imaging all had a 100% sensitivity in the detection of dissection;[17] the specificity was 100% for spiral CT, 94% for echocardiography, and 94% for MR imaging.

Aortic dissection is often manifested by the sudden onset of chest pain; in a patient with Marfan's syndrome, this complaint should lead to its rapid diagnosis or exclusion (pneumothorax being the most likely differential diagnosis). The complication has been reported to be particularly frequent during pregnancy.[18] Isolated cystic medial "necrosis" of a pulmonary artery associated with a dissecting aneurysm also has been reported in the absence of other stigmata of Marfan's syndrome.[19] Another rare manifestation is aneurysm of the ductus arteriosus.[20, 21]

EHLERS-DANLOS SYNDROME

Ehlers-Danlos syndrome consists of a group of inherited disorders of connective tissue that can be divided into several different types on the basis of clinical, genetic, and biochemical features. In some types, specific deficiencies appear to play a role in the pathogenesis; for example, in Type IV (the variety predominantly associated with fragile skin and vessel rupture), there is a deficiency of Type III procollagen produced by fibroblasts.[22] Structural abnormalities of collagen are likely the cause of most apparent clinical findings.[23, 24]

Pleuropulmonary and thoracic skeletal abnormalities consist most commonly of emphysema, often associated with bullae (Fig. 24–3), pneumothorax, and scoliosis.[25] Easy bruisability is also a prominent feature of the disease, especially Type IV, and rupture of pulmonary vessels can be associated with significant pulmonary hemorrhage.[26] Irregularly arranged and quantitatively decreased collagen has been documented by some investigators.[27, 28] Some cases have also been reported in which weakness of airway walls appeared to result in tracheal and bronchial dilation (tracheobronchomegaly [Mounier-Kuhn syndrome]).[29, 30] Other pulmonary abnormalities include pulmonary artery stenoses,[31] bronchiectasis,[32] thin-walled cavitary lesions,[33] and fibrous pseudotumors and cysts.[34, 35] In one 18-year-old woman who presented with recurrent hemoptysis, solid and cavitated nodules as well as thin-walled cystic lesions were evident

on the chest radiograph and CT;[36] open lung biopsy revealed fibrous pseudotumors and blood-filled cysts, some of which appeared to arise from or to be part of pulmonary arterioles and venules.

CUTIS LAXA

Cutis laxa (generalized elastolysis) is a hereditary connective tissue disorder usually transmitted in an autosomal recessive fashion and characterized by loose skin and subcutaneous tissue that hangs in folds, resulting in an appearance of premature aging. Thoracic complications include panacinar emphysema with normal α_1-antiprotease levels,[3, 30, 37] tracheobronchomegaly (Mounier-Kuhn syndrome),[38] bronchiectasis,[30] and aortic aneurysms.[30]

PSEUDOXANTHOMA ELASTICUM

A single patient has been reported with pseudoxanthoma elasticum who had fragmented and swollen elastic fibers in pulmonary vessels and calcification of alveolar septa and vessel walls.[39] The authors considered these changes to be a manifestation of this disease, although they noted that other histologic studies of pulmonary tissue in this condition had failed to document similar changes.

ALKAPTONURIA (OCHRONOSIS)

Alkaptonuria is a rare hereditary disorder caused by a lack of homogentisic acid oxidase. The result is secretion of homogentisic acid in the urine and its accumulation in cartilage and other connective tissues; with time, this causes abnormal connective tissue pigmentation (ochronosis) and arthritis. A characteristic slate-gray or coal-black color of the tracheobronchial cartilage rings has been described at both autopsy and bronchoscopy.[40] The pigment accumulates predominantly in the peribronchial fibrous tissue but also can be seen in the cartilage matrix, fibrous tissue of the mucosa, and parenchymal scars. There are no clinical or functional abnormalities related to the lungs.

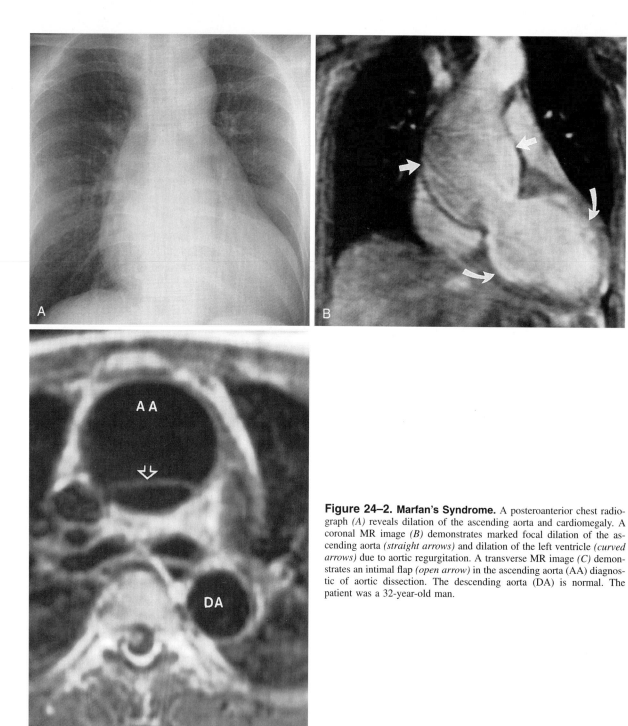

Figure 24–2. Marfan's Syndrome. A posteroanterior chest radiograph *(A)* reveals dilation of the ascending aorta and cardiomegaly. A coronal MR image *(B)* demonstrates marked focal dilation of the ascending aorta *(straight arrows)* and dilation of the left ventricle *(curved arrows)* due to aortic regurgitation. A transverse MR image *(C)* demonstrates an intimal flap *(open arrow)* in the ascending aorta (AA) diagnostic of aortic dissection. The descending aorta (DA) is normal. The patient was a 32-year-old man.

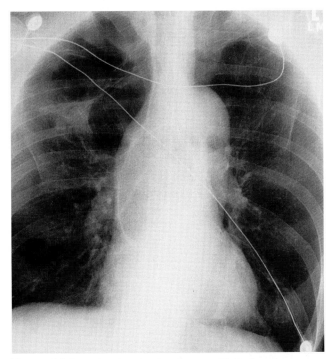

Figure 24–3. Ehlers-Danlos Syndrome with Bullae. A posteroanterior chest radiograph in a 43-year-old man with Ehlers-Danlos syndrome demonstrates large bullae involving mainly the upper lobes. Localized areas of scarring and a nodular opacity in the right upper lobe of unknown cause are also seen.

LYMPHANGIOLEIOMYOMATOSIS

Lymphangioleiomyomatosis (LAM) (lymphangiomyomatosis, myomatosis) is a rare condition characterized by a predominantly peribronchovascular proliferation of smooth muscle associated with airway and vascular obstruction and cyst formation. The condition should not be confused with pulmonary lymphangiomatosis,[41] an abnormality that most likely represents a developmental anomaly of pulmonary lymphatics (*see* page 662).

The condition is uncommon: by 1981, fewer than 100 cases had been documented in the literature;[42] in two relatively large series published in 1990[43] and 1995,[44] 32 and 46 patients were reviewed. The disease is confined to women and is by far most common during the childbearing years, the average age at presentation being 30 to 35.[43] It can also occur in postmenopausal women[45] and has been reported to present in a patient of 72 years.[46] In such individuals, it is possible that the onset of slowly progressive disease precedes clinical recognition.[46]

Etiology and Pathogenesis

The cause and pathogenesis of LAM are not known. The close similarity of its pathologic, clinical, and radiologic features to pulmonary disease in tuberous sclerosis, a condition considered to be a disease of disordered development, suggests that LAM is itself a developmental (hamartomatous) abnormality; in fact, some authorities consider LAM to represent a *forme fruste* of tuberous sclerosis.[47–49] Supporting this hypothesis are observations that patients with tuber-

ous sclerosis who have pulmonary disease are almost all female and experience the onset of disease at the same age as patients with LAM.[50, 51] In addition, some patients with LAM show abnormalities usually associated with tuberous sclerosis, such as renal angiomyolipoma.[47, 49, 52] Chromosomal abnormalities have also been identified in some patients,[53] and there is evidence that abnormal genes in both diseases may be located close together on chromosome 12.[54] One case has also been reported of a patient who had both LAM and cerebrotendinous xanthomatosis, a rare hereditary disorder.[55]

Despite these observations, the recurrence of LAM in some patients who have allograft lung transplants[56] suggests that factors other than an intrinsic tissue abnormality are important in the pathogenesis of the disease. The fact that LAM is almost always seen in women during the reproductive years raises the possibility of an effect of altered hormone secretion or tissue response to hormones. A variety of epidemiologic, clinical, and pathologic evidence supports this hypothesis. Although the use of the contraceptive pill has not been associated with the development of disease, patients have been found to have had fewer pregnancies than expected.[57] Exacerbations of disease have been documented during pregnancy[58, 59] and after the administration of exogenous estrogens.[60] Moreover, there is fairly convincing evidence that hormonal therapy—particularly with progesterone—can lead to improvement in some patients.[43] Receptors for estrogen and progesterone have also been identified in tissue from affected patients by both biochemical[61, 62] and immunohistochemical[63, 64] techniques, although their presence does not appear to predict response to hormonal therapy.[43]

Pathologic Characteristics

The earliest histologic abnormality in LAM appears to be a proliferation of abnormal muscle cells in the vicinity of small bronchioles, blood and lymphatic vessels, and pleura (Fig. 24–4). The abnormal cells are generally round or polygonal in shape; have large, somewhat pleomorphic nuclei; and sometimes show mitotic activity (Fig. 24–4).[65, 66] Focally, the cells may have a spindle shape reminiscent of more typical smooth muscle cells. In advanced disease, large portions of the lung parenchyma may be replaced by the abnormal muscle (Fig. 24–5). Immunohistochemical studies generally show strong reactivity of the proliferating cells for HMB45 (a monoclonal antibody directed toward a component of developing melanosomes) and muscle-specific actin.[67–69]

Gross slices of the lungs at autopsy or pneumonectomy typically show innumerable cystic spaces of variable size (usually 0.2 to 2.0 cm in diameter) separated by thickened interstitial tissue (Fig. 24–6).[65, 70] The pathogenesis of the development of the cysts is not clear; although some investigators have suggested that degradation of elastic fibers may be involved,[71] it is possible that obstruction of small airways by the proliferating smooth muscle cells is more important.[72] Histologic examination of the cyst walls may show only small foci of abnormal muscle or relatively thick, eccentric or concentric foci of proliferation (Fig. 24–7). Vascular obstruction has been implicated in the development of pulmo-

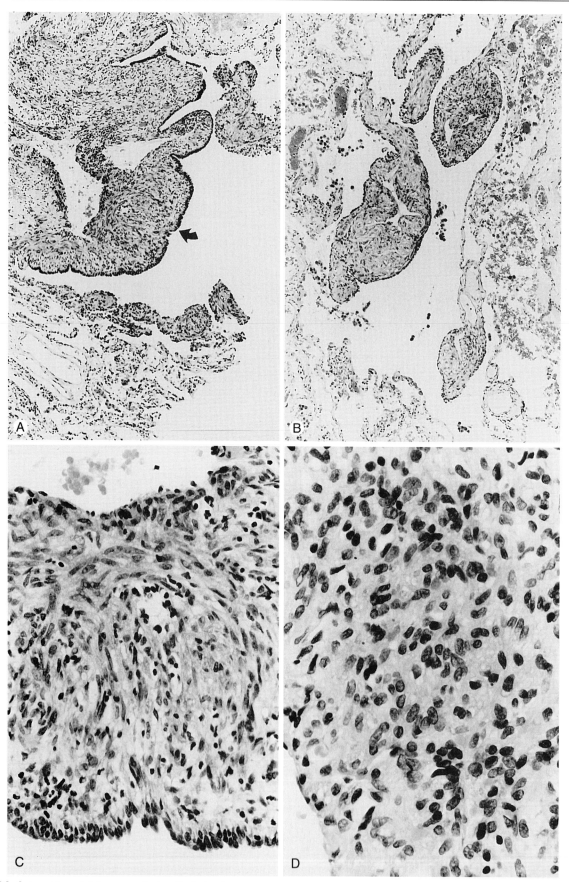

Figure 24–4. Lymphangioleiomyomatosis—Early Lesions. Sections of the walls of two small bronchioles (*A* and *B*) show thickening by a cellular proliferation, more marked on one side. A magnified view of the region indicated by the *arrow* in *A (C)* shows spindle-shaped nuclei suggestive of smooth muscle cells. A similar view of a deeper cut of *C (D)* shows cells with oval or round nuclei whose precise differentiation is difficult to ascertain.

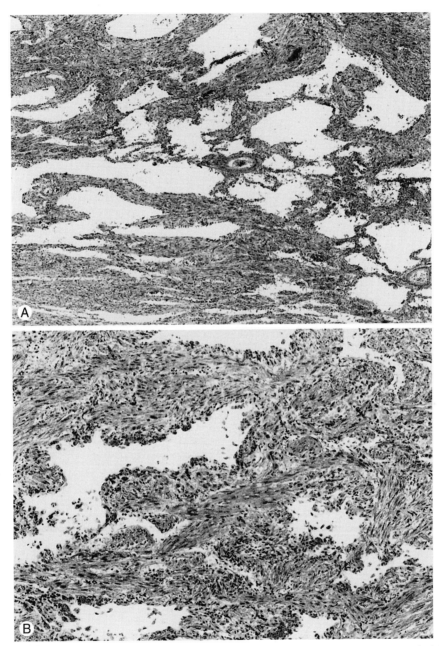

Figure 24–5. Lymphangioleiomyomatosis—Advanced Disease. A histologic section *(A)* reveals moderate-to-marked thickening of the parenchymal interstitium; only a few normal alveolar septa remain. A section at higher magnification *(B)* shows the thickening to be caused by a proliferation of uniform spindle cells with abundant cytoplasm consistent with smooth muscle. *(A,* ×30; *B,* ×100.)

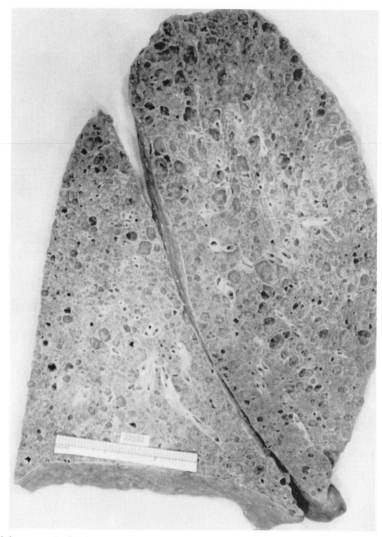

Figure 24–6. Lymphangioleiomyomatosis. A sagittal slice through the midportion of the left lung shows numerous cystic spaces of variable size throughout both lobes.

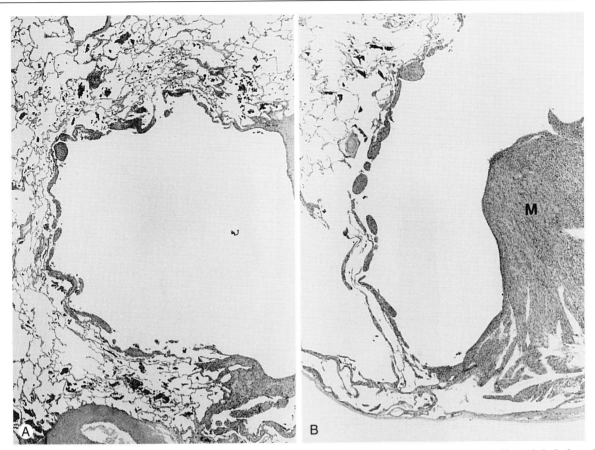

Figure 24–7. Lymphangioleiomyomatosis—Cystic Lesions. Sections (*A* and *B*) show two cystic spaces, one with a relatively large focus of muscle cell proliferation on one side (M) and the other with relatively mild wall thickening.

nary hemorrhage (manifested pathologically by hemosiderin-laden macrophages)[73] and dilation of both intrapulmonary and extrapulmonary lymphatics. Minute (1 to 3 mm) nodules composed of a benign (presumably hyperplastic) proliferation of Type II pneumocytes can be seen in some cases (*see* Fig. 24–10).[28]

An unusual case has been reported of a patient with severe pulmonary hypertension whose lung showed a more or less diffuse interstitial proliferation of smooth muscle in a pattern different from that of typical LAM;[74] the authors proposed that it may represent a hamartomatous abnormality distinct from both the latter condition and tuberous sclerosis.

Smooth muscle proliferation may also be seen in the thoracic duct, which may be totally obliterated, and in lymph nodes in the mediastinum and retroperitoneum. Involvement of all these structures causes some degree of disturbance in lymph flow and may result in the development of chylothorax, chyloperitoneum, or chylopericardium.

Radiologic Manifestations

The most common radiographic finding of LAM (seen in 80% to 90% of patients) is a bilateral reticular pattern (Fig. 24–8).[75–77] In approximately 80% of cases, it involves all lung zones to a similar degree; in the remainder, it is more marked in the lower lung zones.[75] Cysts can be identified in 50% to 60% of cases.[76, 77] Evidence of hyperinflation with

increase in the retrosternal air space or flattening of the diaphragm is seen at presentation in many patients.[75–77] Pneumothorax has been reported in 30% to 40% of cases[75, 77] and unilateral or bilateral pleural effusions in 10% to 20%.[75, 77] The pulmonary parenchymal abnormalities may precede, accompany, or follow the pleural manifestations.[75] In 2% to 20% of cases, the chest radiograph is normal.[75–77]

The characteristic HRCT finding consists of numerous air-filled cysts surrounded by normal lung parenchyma (Fig. 24–9).[75, 76] This abnormality is common: in 69 cases reported in four separate studies, it was identified in 68.[75–78] Cysts can be seen in patients who have normal radiographs[75] or who have radiographs showing only reticular opacities.[75, 76] They usually measure between 0.2 and 2 cm in diameter, although they may be as large as 6 cm.[75, 76] Their size varies with severity of disease, the majority of patients with relatively mild involvement having cysts less than 1 cm in diameter.[75] Most cysts are round and have smooth walls ranging from faintly perceptible to 4 mm in thickness.[75, 76] They are distributed diffusely throughout the lungs, without central, peripheral, or lower lung zone predominance.[75] In most cases, the parenchyma between the cysts appears normal; occasionally, there is a slight increase in interstitial markings,[79, 80] interlobular septal thickening,[76, 80] or patchy areas of ground-glass attenuation (presumably the result of pulmonary hemorrhage).[75] Rarely, a few small nodular opacities can be seen.[77]

The cysts can be easily distinguished from honey-

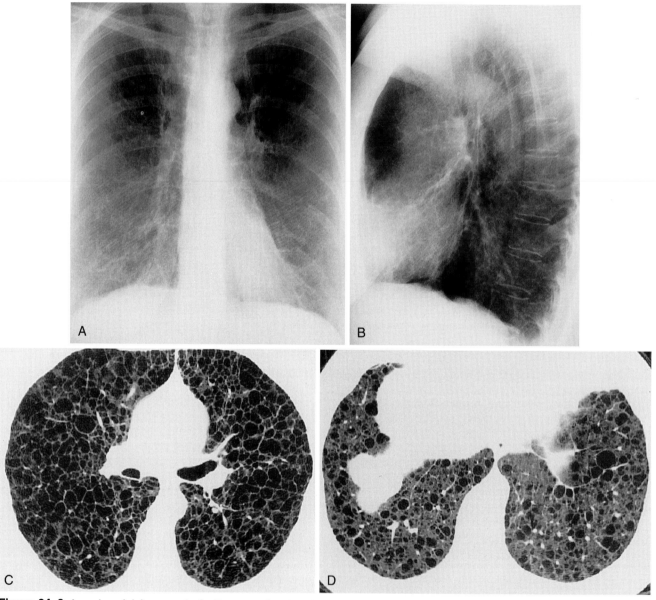

Figure 24–8. Lymphangioleiomyomatosis. Posteroanterior *(A)* and lateral *(B)* chest radiographs reveal a diffuse bilateral reticular pattern. A few individual cysts can be identified. The lung volumes are increased. HRCT scans *(C* and *D)* demonstrate that the reticular pattern seen on the radiograph is due to diffuse involvement of both lungs by air-filled cysts. The majority of cysts are round, measure 0.5 to 2 cm in diameter, and have well-defined smooth walls. The patient was a 40-year-old woman.

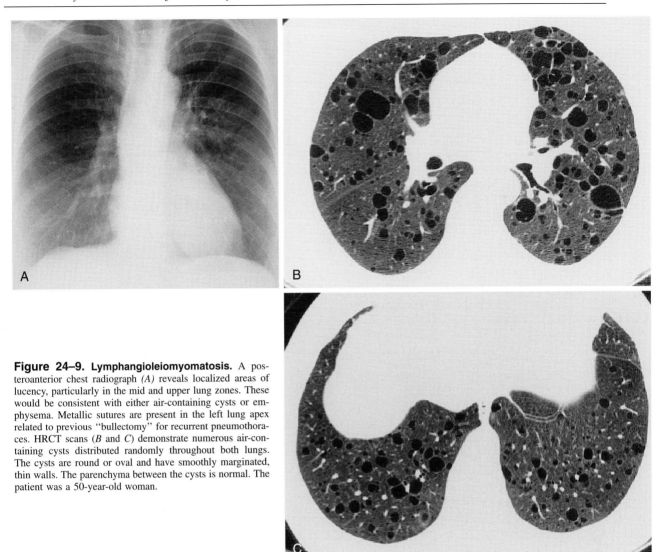

Figure 24–9. Lymphangioleiomyomatosis. A posteroanterior chest radiograph *(A)* reveals localized areas of lucency, particularly in the mid and upper lung zones. These would be consistent with either air-containing cysts or emphysema. Metallic sutures are present in the left lung apex related to previous "bullectomy" for recurrent pneumothoraces. HRCT scans *(B* and *C)* demonstrate numerous air-containing cysts distributed randomly throughout both lungs. The cysts are round or oval and have smoothly marginated, thin walls. The parenchyma between the cysts is normal. The patient was a 50-year-old woman.

combing related to idiopathic pulmonary fibrosis by their diffuse distribution and the presence of relatively normal intervening parenchyma.[75, 76] The main differential diagnosis on HRCT is with Langerhans' cell histiocytosis.[75, 81, 82] The latter is characterized by air-filled cysts involving the mid-lung and upper lung zones with relative sparing of the lung bases;[81, 82] in addition, the majority of patients with Langerhans' cell histiocytosis have pulmonary nodules, a finding that is rarely seen in LAM.[77, 82, 82a]

As with radiographs, pneumothorax and pleural effusions are commonly seen on CT.[75, 77] Lymphadenopathy is evident occasionally;[83, 84] for example, in one review of the CT findings in eight patients, anterior mediastinal, aortopulmonary window, and paratracheal lymphadenopathy was seen in three and retrocrural lymphadenopathy in one.[83] However, in another study of 38 patients, there was no evidence of either hilar or mediastinal lymphadenopathy.[77]

The extent of disease on HRCT correlates better with the severity of clinical and functional impairment than do the radiographic findings.[75, 76, 78] The best correlation is with impairment in gas transfer as assessed by the carbon monoxide diffusing capacity (DL_{CO});[75, 76, 78] however, significant associations have also been demonstrated between the extent

of cystic disease and the severity of air-flow obstruction[76, 85] and air trapping.[75, 85] Although the diagnosis may also be made using spin-echo MR imaging,[86] the procedure is inferior to HRCT in the assessment of the presence and extent of cysts and interstitial lung disease and is thus of limited value.[87]

Clinical Manifestations

The presenting complaint is usually shortness of breath, sometimes gradual and sometimes acute, in which case there is usually an associated pneumothorax.[43] The latter manifestation can be quite troublesome, because of either bilaterality or recurrence;[88, 89] for example, in one investigation of six patients, four had a total of 25 episodes.[70] Cough, hemoptysis, and chest pain are uncommon presenting symptoms but have been found to occur in 35% to 45% of patients at some time in the course of the disease.[43] Chylothorax is also a common manifestation;[73, 90, 91] occasionally, chyle is coughed up (chyloptysis) or passed in the urine (chyluria).

Extrapulmonary manifestations of disease are generally related to involvement of thoracic or abdominal lymph nodes and include mostly chyloperitoneum and chylopericardium.[91–94] When abnormalities such as renal angiomyolipoma[52] or other myomatous tumors[95] are identified, the possibility of tuberous sclerosis should be considered.

The pulmonary function pattern is generally one of obstruction,[43, 96] with the FEV_1/FVC ratio usually well below the predicted normal value.[70, 97] Lung volumes are usually normal or increased, except in patients with large chylous effusions.[54] The DLco is usually reduced, and hypoxemia is common and may be severe; however, Pco_2 is almost invariably decreased.[73, 97]

Although the classic picture of dyspnea and chylothorax, with or without pneumothorax, in a woman of childbearing age likely suggests the diagnosis to most pulmonary physicians, such a picture appears to be relatively uncommon. In one investigation of 32 patients, the most common presentations were isolated pneumothorax or exertional dyspnea, not uncommonly in association with a normal chest radiograph.[43] The diagnosis has been confirmed on tissue fragments obtained by needle aspiration;[97a] however, specimens obtained by transbronchial or lung biopsy are clearly likely to be more informative.[43, 68] Although not all authorities agree,[54] we believe the diagnosis can be reasonably made in the majority of patients on the basis of a combination of clinical and HRCT findings, precluding the need for biopsy.

Natural History and Prognosis

The prognosis of LAM is generally believed to be poor, some investigators having found that most patients die of the disease within 10 years of diagnosis.[73] The results of more recent studies of patients who have been treated with hormonal therapy, however, suggest that prognosis may be better; for example, in the study of 32 patients cited previously, 25 (78%) were alive 8.5 years after the onset of disease.[43]

TUBEROUS SCLEROSIS

Tuberous sclerosis is an autosomal dominant disorder of mesodermal development that affects males and females equally. Approximately 25% of patients give positive family histories.[66] The disease is characterized classically by the triad of mental retardation, epilepsy, and adenoma sebaceum; however, a variety of other abnormalities can also be seen, including retinal phacoma, angiomyolipomas of the kidneys, rhabdomyomas of the heart, sclerotic lesions of bones, and subungual fibromas. These various manifestations usually appear in infancy or early childhood, and 75% of patients so affected die before they reach age 20.[98]

Pulmonary involvement is uncommon, occurring in about 1% to 2.5% of patients.[51, 99, 100] In a review of the literature published in 1972, 28 well-documented cases were identified, 27 in women ranging in age from 21 to 50 years.[50] Other investigators have also noted a striking female predominance of the complication.[100] As discussed earlier, the pathologic characteristics of tuberous sclerosis and LAM are virtually identical in most cases.[66, 101] Some investigators, however, have found differences in the nature and distribution of the lesions (e.g., little evidence of smooth muscle proliferation in the cyst walls in tuberous sclerosis).[99, 102]

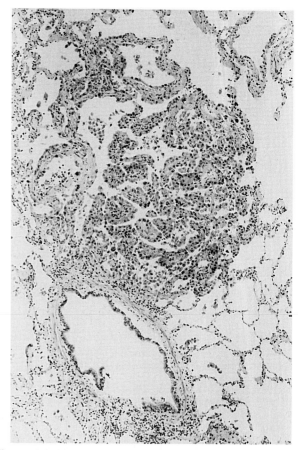

Figure 24–10. Tuberous Sclerosis—Type II Cell Hyperplasia. Section shows a discrete, somewhat nodular focus of alveolar interstitial thickening and alveolar Type II cell hyperplasia. (Courtesy of Dr. P. Russo, Hôpital St. Justine, Montreal, Canada.)

Nodular foci of Type II cell hyperplasia can be found in some patients (Fig. 24–10).[103, 104] A possible association with clear cell tumor has also been reported.[104a]

The radiographic and CT manifestations of thoracic involvement are similar to those of LAM (Fig. 24–11). The former consist of a diffuse reticular pattern with or without cystic or bullous changes.[76, 105] HRCT demonstrates thin-walled cysts throughout both lungs,[76, 105, 106] sometimes in patients with normal chest radiographs.[105] Similar to LAM, pneumothorax is common, having been reported in up to 50% of patients who have tuberous sclerosis and pulmonary involvement.[105, 107] Chylous pleural effusion is distinctly unusual.[90, 105, 108] The diagnosis of tuberous sclerosis should be considered when bilateral renal angiomyolipomas are seen on CT images through the upper abdomen. These tumors have a characteristic appearance of mixed fat and soft tissue attenuation on CT (Fig. 24–11). Although bilateral angiomyolipomas are characteristic of tuberous sclerosis, unilateral or bilateral renal angiomyolipomas are seen in 15% of patients with LAM.[105]

Clinical manifestations of pulmonary involvement are also similar to those of LAM. Respiratory symptoms are usually first noted between 20 and 45 years of age.[51, 100] Dyspnea is the most common complaint; hemoptysis and cough are seen occasionally.[51, 100] In one series of nine patients, pneumothorax complicated the course of disease in

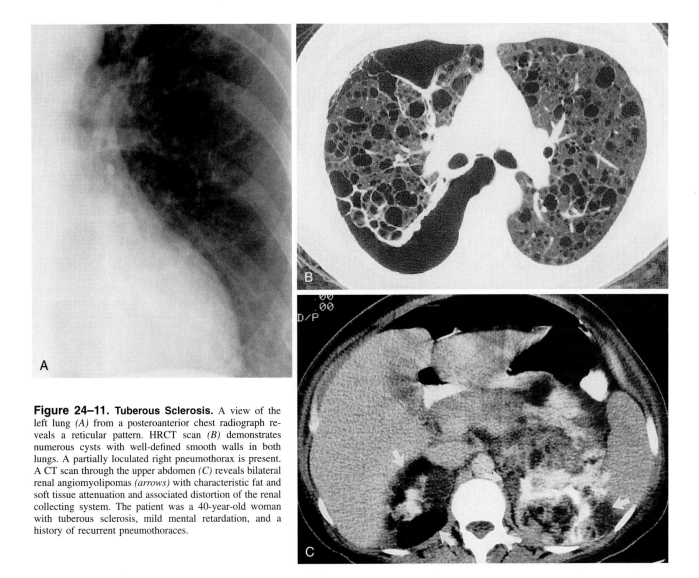

Figure 24–11. Tuberous Sclerosis. A view of the left lung *(A)* from a posteroanterior chest radiograph reveals a reticular pattern. HRCT scan *(B)* demonstrates numerous cysts with well-defined smooth walls in both lungs. A partially loculated right pneumothorax is present. A CT scan through the upper abdomen *(C)* reveals bilateral renal angiomyolipomas *(arrows)* with characteristic fat and soft tissue attenuation and associated distortion of the renal collecting system. The patient was a 40-year-old woman with tuberous sclerosis, mild mental retardation, and a history of recurrent pneumothoraces.

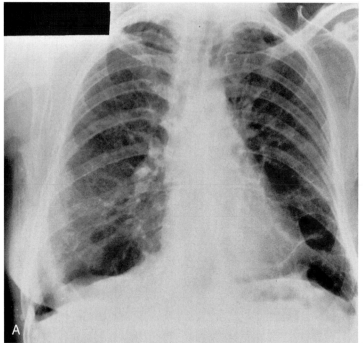

Figure 24–12. Neurofibromatosis—Pulmonary and Cutaneous Manifestations. Posteroanterior views of the chest in inspiration *(A)* and expiration *(B)* reveal numerous bullae in the lower portion of both lungs, most evident on the expiratory film because of air trapping. A background of diffuse reticulation is present, suggesting interstitial pulmonary fibrosis. Along the lateral chest wall *(A)* and on the anterior and posterior chest walls in lateral projection *(C)* are numerous nodular opacities representing cutaneous neurofibromas.

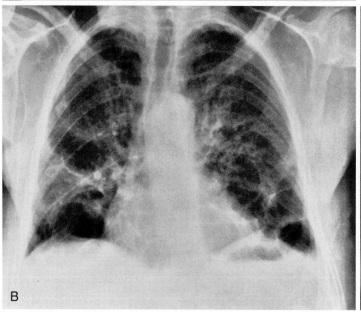

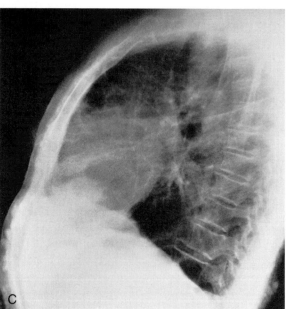

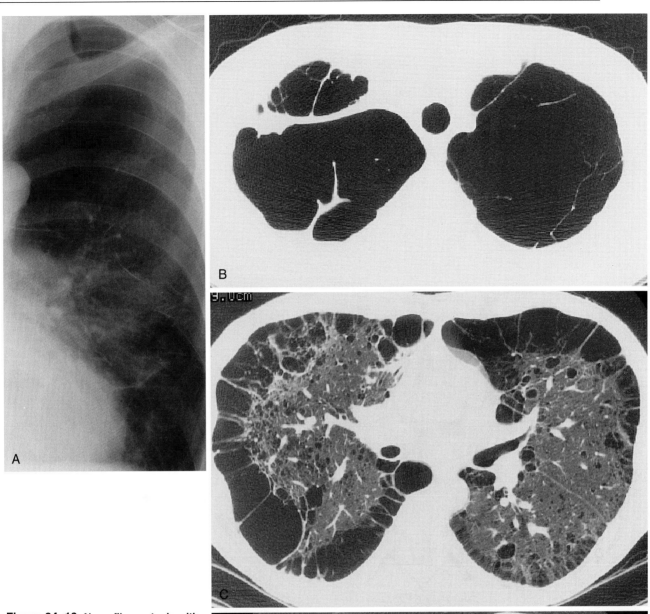

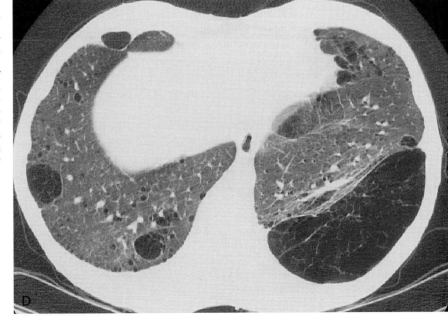

Figure 24–13. Neurofibromatosis with Bullae. A view of the left lung *(A)* from a posteroanterior chest radiograph reveals severe emphysema involving mainly the upper lobe. Similar findings were present in the right lung. HRCT scan through the lung apices *(B)* demonstrates almost complete replacement of the parenchyma by large bullae. HRCT scan through the midlung zones *(C)* reveals predominantly subpleural emphysema with relative sparing of the central lung regions. Only a few bullae are present in the lung bases *(D)*. The patient was a 34-year-old man with neurofibromatosis and a 15 pack-year smoking history.

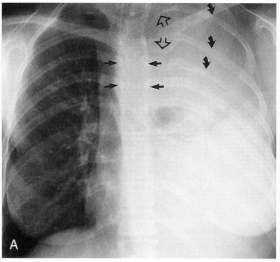
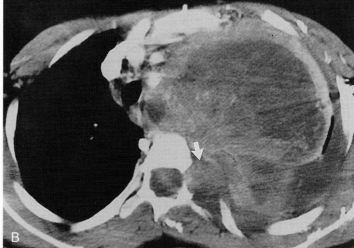
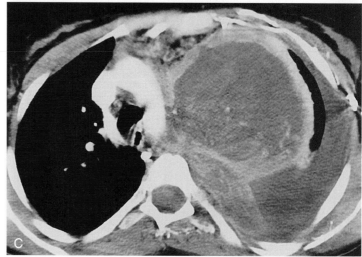

Figure 24–14. Neurofibromatosis with Neurofibro-sarcoma. A posteroanterior chest radiograph *(A)* reveals opacification of the left hemithorax, compression of the left main bronchus, and shift of the mediastinum to the right. Note scalloping of the vertebral bodies with increased distance between the pedicles *(straight arrows)* of several of the upper thoracic vertebrae. Also note twisted-ribbon deformity of several of the left ribs *(curved arrows)*. Widening of the space between the posterior left third and fourth ribs *(open arrows)* indicates the origin of the neurogenic tumor. Contrast-enhanced CT scans *(B and C)* demonstrate a large inhomogeneous mass occupying most of the left hemithorax associated with shift of the mediastinum to the right. Also present is a left pleural effusion. At surgery, the mass was shown to be a neurofibro-sarcoma arising from an intercostal nerve in the left paraspinal region *(white arrow in B)*. Widening of the spinal canal and erosion of the adjacent pedicle and rib can also be seen. The patient was an 18-year-old woman.

four.[100] Extrathoracic manifestations of tuberous sclerosis are seen in virtually all patients and include most commonly seizures, renal angiomyolipomas, cerebral calcification, skin lesions, and retinal hamartomas.[100] Pulmonary function tests show severe obstruction, hyperinflation, increased airway resistance, low DL_{CO}, hypoxemia, and hypocarbia.[98–100] The course of the pulmonary disease is variable: some patients experience slowly progressive dyspnea and eventual death from respiratory failure, and others remain stable, with or without hormonal therapy.[100]

NEUROFIBROMATOSIS

Neurofibromatosis (von Recklinghausen's disease) is a relatively common familial disorder with a frequency of about 1 in 3,000. Although it is inexorably progressive, only about 20% of affected patients develop disabling disease.[109] The most prominent manifestations are cutaneous café-au-lait spots and neurofibromas of the cutaneous and subcutaneous peripheral nerves, nerve roots, and viscera.[109] A variety of other neoplasms can also be seen, including central nervous system gliomas, meningiomas, peripheral nerve sarcomas and schwannomas, pheochromocytomas, and angiosarcomas.[109–113] Thoracic neoplasms are usually neurogenic.

They can arise in the intercostal nerves (in which case they may be associated with rib destruction, a chest wall mass, or, rarely, hemorrhage from an eroded intercostal vessel[114]), in the mediastinum,[115] and in the lungs themselves.[116] In one unusual case of a human immunodeficiency virus–positive man, multiple biopsy specimens showed extensive neurofibromas in the bronchial submucosa;[117] spinal root tumors were also present.

The most common pulmonary manifestations consist of diffuse interstitial fibrosis and bullae, either alone or in combination. The prevalence of interstitial fibrosis is about 5% to 10%;[110, 118, 119] bullae have been seen in almost 20% of patients in some series.[118] Pathologically, the interstitial disease is similar to that of interstitial pneumonitis of other causes, with variably severe fibrosis and chronic inflammation usually most prominent in the subpleural region. Increased numbers of intra-alveolar macrophages are common and can be sufficiently numerous to suggest a diagnosis of desquamative interstitial pneumonitis.[120] Immunofluorescence studies in one case failed to show specific immunofluorescence to IgG, IgM, IgA, complement, or fibrinogen.[121]

Radiologically the interstitial disease is characterized by a reticular pattern that involves both lungs symmetrically with some basal predominance (Fig. 24–12). Bullae usually are asymmetric and tend to develop in the upper lobes,[118] seldom the lower.[110] In some cases, bullae are unassociated with radiographic evidence of interstitial fibrosis,[118] although this has been seen in virtually all patients with bullae whose lungs have been examined histologically.[119, 122] In one study of the conventional CT findings in two patients, a reticular pattern involving mainly the lower lung zones without peripheral or central predominance was found;[123] extensive apical bullous disease was apparent, although it was not readily appreciated on the radiograph. We have seen three patients who had extensive paraseptal emphysema involving mainly the upper lobes and in whom there was no evidence of fibrosis on the radiograph or HRCT (Fig. 24–13).

Cutaneous neurofibromas are seen as nodular opacities on the chest radiograph and may mimic intrapulmonary nodules such as might be found with metastases from neurofibrosarcomas; in these cases, CT may be helpful.[124, 125] Other relatively common chest wall abnormalities include scoliosis and twisted-ribbon deformity of the ribs.[126, 127] Although scoliosis itself is a nonspecific finding, the presence of acute-angle lower thoracic scoliosis involving five or fewer vertebrae is characteristic of neurofibromatosis.[127] Additional characteristic findings include scalloping of vertebral bodies because of dural ectasia[128] and lateral thoracic meningoceles.[129] Paraspinal masses may also be caused by neural tumors. When the latter arise from the intercostal nerves, they may be seen as extrapleural soft tissue masses running parallel to and occasionally eroding a rib;[129] occasionally, such tumors become large (Fig. 24–14). Tumors of the vagus or phrenic nerves may result in mediastinal masses. Rarely, plexiform neurofibromas originating from the sympathetic chain or phrenic or vagus nerves may be seen as masses infiltrating contiguous mediastinal structures;[130, 131] these tumors have a lower attenuation than chest wall muscle, with CT attenuation values ranging from 15 to 30 HU.[130, 131]

Clinically, the diagnosis is readily made by the presence on the skin of multiple sessile or pedunculated neurofibromas. Pulmonary disease typically does not become evident until the patient reaches adulthood. Respiratory symptoms are usually mild, the most common complaint being dyspnea on exertion.[119] Pulmonary hypertension has been reported in some patients.[132] Pulmonary function tests usually reveal evidence of obstruction, although a restrictive pattern may be dominant; DLco is often decreased.[119] As in interstitial fibrosis associated with other conditions, the disease occasionally is complicated by the development of carcinoma.[119, 120]

REFERENCES

1. Prockop DJ, Kivirikko KL: Heritable diseases of collagen. N Engl J Med 311:376, 1984.
2. Pyeritz RE: Connective tissue in the lung: Lessons from the Marfan syndrome. Ann Intern Med 103:289, 1985.
3. Mainardi CL, Kang AH: Collagen disease: A new perspective. Am J Med 71:913, 1981.
4. Fisk DE, Kuhn C: Emphysema-like changes in the lungs of the blotchy mouse. Am Rev Respir Dis 113:787, 1976.
5. Pyeritz RE, McKusick VA: Basic defects in the Marfan syndrome. N Engl J Med 305:1011, 1981.
6. Corbett E, Glaisyer H, Chan C, et al: Congenital cutis laxa with a dominant inheritance and early onset emphysema. Thorax 49:836, 1994.
7. Pyeritz RE, McKusick VA: The Marfan syndrome: Diagnosis and management. N Engl J Med 300:772, 1979.
8. Ramirez F: Fibrillin mutations in Marfan syndrome and related phenotypes. Curr Opin Genet Dev 6:309, 1996.
9. Tanoue LT: Pulmonary involvement in collagen vascular disease: A review of the pulmonary manifestations of the Marfan syndrome, ankylosing spondylitis, Sjögren's syndrome, and relapsing polychondritis. J Thorac Imaging 7:62, 1992.
10. Hall JR, Pyeritz RE, Dudgeon DL, et al: Pneumothorax in the Marfan syndrome: Prevalence and therapy. Ann Thorac Surg 37:500, 1984.
11. Wood JR, Bellamy D, Child AH, et al: Pulmonary disease in patients with Marfan syndrome. Thorax 39:780, 1984.
12. Murdoch JL, Walker BA, Halpern BL, et al: Life expectancy and causes of death in the Marfan syndrome. N Engl J Med 286:804, 1972.
13. Posniak HV, Olson MC, Demos TC, et al: CT of thoracic aortic aneurysms. RadioGraphics 10:839, 1990.
14. Fisher ER, Stern EJ, Godwin JD, et al: Acute aortic dissection: Typical and atypical imaging features. RadioGraphics 14:1263, 1994.
15. Kersting-Sommerhoff BA, Higgins CB, White RD, et al: Aortic dissection: Sensitivity and specificity of MR imaging. Radiology 166:651, 1988.
16. Mayo JR: Magnetic resonance imaging of the chest: Where we stand. Radiol Clin North Am 32:795, 1994.
17. Sommer T, Fehske W, Holzknecht N, et al: Aortic dissection: A comparative study of diagnosis with spiral CT, multiplanar transesophageal echocardiography, and MR imaging. Radiology 199:347, 1996.
18. Pyeritz RE: Maternal and fetal complications of pregnancy in the Marfan syndrome. Am J Med 71:784, 1981.
19. Shilkin KB, Low LP, Chen BTM: Dissecting aneurysm of the pulmonary artery. J Pathol 98:25, 1969.
20. Crisfield RJ: Spontaneous aneurysm of the ductus arteriosus in a patient with Marfan's syndrome. J Thorac Cardiovasc Surg 62:243, 1971.
21. Müller NL, Mayo J, Culham JAG, et al: Ductus arteriosus aneurysm in Marfan syndrome. Can Assoc Radiol J 37:195, 1986.
22. Clark JG, Kuhn C III, Uitto J: Lung collagen in type IV Ehlers-Danlos syndrome: Ultrastructural and biochemical studies. Am Rev Respir Dis 122:971, 1980.
23. Barabas AP: Heterogeneity of the Ehlers-Danlos syndrome: Description of three clinical types and a hypothesis to explain the basic defect(s). BMJ 2:612, 1967.
24. Robitaille GA: Ehlers-Danlos syndrome and recurrent hemoptysis. Ann Intern Med 61:716, 1964.
25. Smit J, Alberts C, Balk AG: Pneumothorax in the Ehlers-Danlos syndrome: Consequence or coincidence? Scand J Respir Dis 59:239, 1978.
26. Yost BA, Vogelsang JP, Lie JT: Fatal hemoptysis in Ehlers-Danlos syndrome: Old malady with a new curse. Chest 107:1465, 1995.
27. Nerlich AG, Stoss H, Lehmann H, et al: Pathomorphological and biochemical alterations in Ehlers-Danlos-syndrome type IV. Pathol Res Pract 190:697, 1994.
28. Muir TE, Leslie KO, Popper H, et al: Micronodular pneumocyte hyperplasia. Am J Surg Pathol 22:465, 1998.
29. Aaby GV, Blake HA: Tracheobronchomegaly. Ann Thorac Surg 2:64, 1966.
30. Franquet T, Giménez A, Cáceres J, et al: Imaging of pulmonary-cutaneous disorders: Matching the radiologic and dermatologic findings. RadioGraphics 16:855, 1996.
31. Lees MH, Menashe VD, Sunderland CO, et al: Ehlers-Danlos syndrome associated with multiple pulmonary artery stenoses and tortuous systemic arteries. J Pediatr 75:1031, 1969.
32. Robitaille GA: Ehlers Danlos syndrome and recurrent hemoptysis. Ann Intern Med 61:716, 1964.
33. Herman TE, McAlister WH: Cavitary pulmonary lesions in type IV Ehlers-Danlos syndrome. Pediatr Radiol 24:263, 1994.
34. Corrin B, Simpson CG, Fisher C: Fibrous pseudotumours and cyst formation in the lungs in Ehlers-Danlos syndrome. Histopathology 17:478, 1990.
35. Murray RA, Poulton TB, Saltarelli MG, et al: Rare pulmonary manifestation of Ehlers-Danlos syndrome. J Thorac Imaging 10:138, 1995.
36. Murray RA, Poulton TB, Saltarelli MG, et al: Rare pulmonary manifestation of Ehlers-Danlos syndrome. J Thorac Imaging 10:138, 1995.
37. Turner-Stokes L, Turton C, Pope FM, et al: Emphysema and cutis laxa. Thorax 38:790, 1983.
38. Wanderer AA, Ellis EF, Goltz RW, et al: Tracheobronchomegaly and acquired cutis laxa in a child. Pediatrics 44:709, 1969.
39. Jackson A, Loh C-L: Pulmonary calcification and elastic tissue damage in pseudoxanthoma elasticum. Histopathology 4:607, 1980.
40. Gaines JJ Jr: The pathology of alkaptonuric ochronosis. Hum Pathol 20:40, 1989.
41. Tazelaar HD, Kerr D, Yousem SA, et al: Diffuse pulmonary lymphangiomatosis. Hum Pathol 24:1313, 1993.
42. Berger JL, Shaff MI: Pulmonary lymphangioleiomyomatosis. J Comput Assist Tomogr 5:565, 1981.
43. Taylor JR, Ryu J, Colby TV, et al: Lymphangioleiomyomatosis: Clinical course in 32 patients. N Engl J Med 323:1254, 1990.
44. Kitaichi M, Nishimura K, Itoh H, et al: Pulmonary lymphangioleiomyomatosis: A report of 46 patients including a clinicopathologic study of prognostic factors. Am J Respir Crit Care Med 151:527, 1995.
45. Baldi S, Papotti M, Valente ML, et al: Pulmonary lymphangioleiomyomatosis in postmenopausal women: Report of two cases and review of the literature. Eur Respir J 7:1013, 1994.
46. Sinclair W, Wright JL, Churg A: Lymphangioleiomyomatosis presenting in a postmenopausal woman. Thorax 40:475, 1985.
47. Capron F, Ameille J, Leclerc P, et al: Pulmonary lymphangioleiomyomatosis and Bourneville's tuberous sclerosis with pulmonary involvement: The same disease? Cancer 52:851, 1983.
48. Valensi QJ: Pulmonary lymphangiomyoma, a probable *forme fruste* of tuberous sclerosis: A case report and survey of the literature. Am Rev Respir Dis 108:1411, 1973.
49. Maziak DE, Kesten S, Rappaport DC, et al: Extrathoracic angiomyolipomas in lymphangioleiomyomatosis. Eur Respir J 9:402, 1996.
50. Jao J, Gilbert S, Messer R: Lymphangiomyoma and tuberous sclerosis. Cancer 29:1188, 1972.
51. Dwyer JM, Hickie JB, Garvan J: Pulmonary tuberous sclerosis: Report of three patients and a review of the literature. QJM 40:115, 1971.
52. Kerr LA, Blute ML, Ryu JH, et al: Renal angiomyolipoma in association with pulmonary lymphangioleiomyomatosis: Forme fruste of tuberous sclerosis? Urology 41:440, 1993.
53. Popper HH, Gamperl R, Pongratz MG, et al: Chromosome typing in lymphangioleiomyomatosis of the lung with and without tuberous sclerosis. Eur Respir J 6:753, 1993.
54. Kalassian KG, Doyle R, Kao P, et al: Lymphangioleiomyomatosis: New insights. Am J Respir Crit Care Med 155:1183, 1997.
55. Dormans TP, Verrips A, Bulten J, et al: Pulmonary lymphangioleiomyomatosis and cerebrotendinous xanthomatosis: Is there a link? Chest 112:273, 1997.
56. Nine JS, Yousem SA, Paradis IL, et al: Lymphangioleiomyomatosis: Recurrence after lung transplantation. J Heart Lung Transplant 13:714, 1994.
57. Wahedna I, Cooper S, Williams J, et al: Relation of pulmonary lymphangioleiomyomatosis to use of the oral contraceptive pill and fertility in the UK: A national case control study. Thorax 49:910, 1994.
58. Kitzsteiner KA, Mallen RG: Pulmonary lymphangiomyomatosis: Treatment with castration. Cancer 46:2248, 1980.
59. Hughes E, Hodder RV: Pulmonary lymphangiomyomatosis complicating pregnancy: A case report. J Reprod Med 32:553, 1987.
60. Shen A, Iseman MD, Waldron JA, et al: Exacerbation of pulmonary lymphangioleiomyomatosis by exogenous estrogens. Chest 91:782, 1987.
61. Graham ML II, Spelsberg TC, Dines DE, et al: Pulmonary lymphangiomyomatosis: With particular reference to steroid-receptor assay studies and pathologic correlation. Mayo Clin Proc 59:3, 1984.
62. Brentani MM, Carvalho CR, Saldiva PH, et al: Steroid receptors in pulmonary lymphangiomyomatosis. Chest 85:96, 1984.
63. Colley MH, Geppert E, Franklin WA: Immunohistochemical detection of steroid receptors in a case of pulmonary lymphangioleiomyomatosis. Am J Surg Pathol 13:803, 1989.
64. Berger U, Khaghani A, Pomerance A, et al: Pulmonary lymphangioleiomyomatosis: An immunocytochemical study. Am J Clin Pathol 903:609, 1990.
65. Corrin B, Liebow AA, Friedman PJ: Pulmonary lymphangiomyomatosis. Am J Pathol 79:348, 1975.
66. Valensi QJ: Pulmonary lymphangiomyoma, a probable *forme fruste* of tuberous sclerosis: A case report and survey of the literature. Am Rev Respir Dis 108:1411, 1973.
67. Tanaka H, Imada A, Morikawa T, et al: Diagnosis of pulmonary lymphangioleiomyomatosis by HMB45 in surgically treated spontaneous pneumothorax. Eur Respir J 8:1879, 1995.
68. Guinee DG Jr, Feuerstein I, Koss MN, et al: Pulmonary lymphangioleiomyomatosis: Diagnosis based on results of transbronchial biopsy and immunohistochemical studies and correlation with high-resolution computed tomography findings. Arch Pathol Lab Med 118:846, 1994.
69. Matthews TJ, Hornall D, Sheppard MN: Comparison of the use of antibodies to alpha smooth muscle actin and desmin in pulmonary lymphangioleiomyomatosis. J Clin Pathol 46:479, 1993.
70. Carrington CB, Cugell DW, Gaensler EA, et al: Lymphangioleiomyomatosis: Physiologic-pathologic-radiologic correlations. Am Rev Respir Dis 116:977, 1977.
71. Fukuda Y, Kawamoto M, Yamamoto A, et al: Role of elastic fiber degradation in emphysema-like lesions of pulmonary lymphangiomyomatosis. Hum Pathol 21:1252, 1990.
72. Sobonya RE, Quan SF, Fleishman JS: Pulmonary lymphangioleiomyomatosis: Quantitative analysis of lesions producing airflow limitation. Hum Pathol 16:1122, 1985.

73. Corrin B, Liebow AA, Friedman PJ: Pulmonary lymphangiomyomatosis. Am J Pathol 79:347, 1975.
74. Kay JM, Kahana LM, Rihal C: Diffuse smooth muscle proliferation of the lungs with severe pulmonary hypertension. Hum Pathol 27:969, 1996.
75. Müller NL, Chiles C, Kullnig P: Pulmonary lymphangiomyomatosis: Correlation of CT with radiographic and functional findings. Radiology 175:335, 1990.
76. Lenoir S, Grenier P, Brauner MW, et al: Pulmonary lymphangiomyomatosis and tuberous sclerosis: Comparison of radiographic and thin-section CT findings. Radiology 175:329, 1990.
77. Kitaichi M, Nishimura K, Itoh H, et al: Pulmonary lymphangioleiomyomatosis: A report of 46 patients including a clinicopathologic study of prognostic factors. Am J Respir Crit Care Med 151:527, 1995.
78. Aberle DR, Hansell DM, Brown K, et al: Lymphangiomyomatosis: CT, chest radiographic, and functional correlations. Radiology 176:381, 1990.
79. Rappaport DC, Weisbrod GL, Herman SJ, et al: Pulmonary lymphangioleiomyomatosis: High-resolution CT findings in four cases. Am J Roentgenol 152:961, 1989.
80. Templeton PA, McLoud TC, Müller NL, et al: Pulmonary lymphangioleiomyomatosis: CT and pathologic findings. J Comput Assist Tomogr 13:54, 1989.
81. Moore ADA, Godwin JD, Müller NL, et al: Pulmonary histiocytosis X: Comparison of radiographic and CT findings. Radiology 172:249, 1989.
82. Brauner MW, Grenier P, Mouelhi MM, et al: Pulmonary histiocytosis X: Evaluation with high-resolution CT. Radiology 172:255, 1989.
82a. Bonelli FS, Hartman TE, Swensen SJ, et al: Accuracy of high-resolution CT in diagnosing lung diseases. Am J Roentgenol 170:1507, 1998.
83. Sherrier RH, Chiles C, Roggli V: Pulmonary lymphangioleiomyomatosis: CT findings. Am J Roentgenol 153:937, 1989.
84. Woodring JH, Howard RS II, Johnson MV: Massive low-attenuation mediastinal, retroperitoneal, and pelvic lymphadenopathy on CT from lymphangioleiomyomatosis: Case report. Clin Imaging 18:7, 1994.
85. Crausman RS, Lynch DA, Mortenson RL, et al: Quantitative CT predicts the severity of physiologic dysfunction in patients with lymphangioleiomyomatosis. Chest 109:131, 1996.
86. King MA: MR diagnosis of lymphangioleiomyomatosis: Visibility of pulmonary cysts on spin-echo images. Magn Reson Imaging 14:361, 1996.
87. Müller NL, Mayo JR, Zwirewich CV: Value of MR imaging in the evaluation of chronic infiltrative lung diseases: Comparison with CT. Am J Roentgenol 158:1205, 1992.
88. Graf-Deuel E, Knoblauch A: Simultaneous bilateral spontaneous pneumothorax. Chest 105:1142, 1994.
89. Berkman N, Bloom A, Cohen P, et al: Bilateral spontaneous pneumothorax as the presenting feature in lymphangioleiomyomatosis. Respir Med 89:381, 1995.
90. Stovin PGI, Lum LC, Flower CDR, et al: The lungs in lymphangiomyomatosis and in tuberous sclerosis. Thorax 30:497, 1975.
91. Chew QT, Nouri MS: Pulmonary and retroperitoneal lymphangiomyomatosis: Clinical and radiographic features. N Y State J Med 79:250, 1979.
92. Kanbe A, Hajiro K, Adachi Y, et al: Lymphangiomyomatosis associated with chylous ascites and high serum CA-125 levels: A case report. Jpn J Med 26:237, 1987.
93. Sheth RA, Greenberg SD, Jenkins DE, et al: Lymphangiomyomatosis with chylous effusions. South Med J 77:1032, 1984.
94. Jenner RE, Oo HLA: Isolated chylopericardium due to mediastinal lymphangiomatous hamartoma. Thorax 30:113, 1975.
95. Ernst JC, Sohaey R, Cary JM: Pelvic lymphangioleiomyomatosis: Atypical precursor to pulmonary disease. Chest 106:1267, 1994.
96. Crausman RS, Jennings CA, Mortenson RL, et al: Lymphangioleiomyomatosis: The pathophysiology of diminished exercise capacity. Am J Respir Crit Care Med 153:1368, 1996.
97. McCarty KS Jr, Mossler JA, McLelland R, et al: Pulmonary lymphangiomyomatosis responsive to progesterone. N Engl J Med 303:1461, 1980.
97a. Berner A, Franzen S, Heilo A: Fine-needle aspiration cytology as a diagnostic approach to lymphangioleiomyomatosis: A case report. Acta Cytol 41:877, 1997.
98. Harris JO, Waltuck BL, Swenson EW: The pathophysiology of the lungs in tuberous sclerosis: A case report and literature review. Am Rev Respir Dis 100:379, 1969.
99. Lie JT, Miller RD, Williams DE: Cystic disease of the lungs in tuberous sclerosis: Clinicopathologic correlation, including body plethysmographic lung function tests. Mayo Clin Proc 55:547, 1980.
100. Castro M, Shepherd CW, Gomez MR, et al: Pulmonary tuberous sclerosis. Chest 107:189, 1995.
101. Capron F, Ameille J, Leclerc P, et al: Pulmonary lymphangioleiomyomatosis and Bourneville's tuberous sclerosis with pulmonary involvement: The same disease? Cancer 52:851, 1983.
102. Stovin PGI, Lum LC, Flower CDR, et al: The lungs in lymphangiomyomatosis and in tuberous sclerosis. Thorax 30:497, 1975.
103. Popper HH, Juettner-Smolle FM, Pongratz MG: Micronodular hyperplasia of type II pneumocytes—a new lung lesion associated with tuberous sclerosis. Histopathology 18:347, 1991.
104. Guinee D, Singh R, Azumi N, et al: Multifocal micronodular pneumocyte hyperplasia: A distinctive pulmonary manifestation of tuberous sclerosis. Mod Pathol 8:902, 1995.
104a. Flieder DB, Travis WD: Clear cell "sugar" tumor of the lung: Association with lymphangioleiomyomatosis and multifocal micronodular pneumocyte hyperplasia in a patient with tuberous sclerosis. Am J Surg Pathol 21:1242, 1997.
105. Castro M, Shepherd CW, Gomez MR, et al: Pulmonary tuberous sclerosis. Chest 107:189, 1995.
106. Kullnig P, Melzer G, Smolle-Jüttner FM: High-resolution-computertomographie des thorax bei lymphangioleiomyomatose and tuberöser sklerose. ROFO 151:32, 1989.
107. Dwyer JM, Hickie JB, Garvan J: Pulmonary tuberous sclerosis: Report of three patients and a review of the literature. QJM 40:115, 1971.
108. Broughton RBK: Pulmonary tuberous sclerosis presenting with pleural effusion. BMJ 1:477, 1970.
109. Riccardi VM: von Recklinghausen neurofibromatosis. N Engl J Med 305:1617, 1981.
110. Burkhalter JL, Morano JU, McCay MB: Diffuse interstitial lung disease in neurofibromatosis. South Med J 79:944, 1986.
111. Larrieu AJ, Hashimoto SA, Allen P: Spontaneous massive haemothorax in von Recklinghausen's disease. Thorax 37:151, 1982.
112. Riccardi VM, Wheeler TM, Pickard LR, et al: The pathophysiology of neurofibromatosis: II. Angiosarcoma as a complication. Cancer Genet Cytogenet 12:275, 1984.
113. Arpornchayanon O, Hirota T, Itabashi M, et al: Malignant peripheral nerve tumors: A clinicopathological and electron microscopic study. Jpn J Clin Oncol 14:57, 1984.
114. Larrieu AJ, Hashimoto SA, Allen P: Spontaneous massive haemothorax in von Recklinghausen's disease. Thorax 37:151, 1982.
115. Bourgouin PM, Shepard JO, Moore EH, et al: Plexiform neurofibromatosis of the mediastinum: CT appearance. Am J Roentgenol 151:461, 1988.
116. Unger PD, Geller SA, Anderson PJ: Pulmonary lesions in a patient with neurofibromatosis. Arch Pathol Lab Med 108:654, 1984.
117. Gillissen A, Kotterba S, Rasche K, et al: A rare manifestation of von Recklinghausen neurofibromatosis: Advanced neurofibromatous infiltration in lung of an HIV-positive patient. Respiration 61:292, 1994.
118. Massaro D, Katz S: Fibrosing alveolitis: Its occurrence, roentgenographic and pathologic features in von Recklinghausen's neurofibromatosis. Am Rev Respir Dis 93:934, 1966.
119. Webb WR, Goodman PC: Fibrosing alveolitis in patients with neurofibromatosis. Radiology 122:289, 1977.
120. De Scheerder I, Elinck W, Van Renterghem D, et al: Desquamative interstitial pneumonia and scar cancer of the lung complicating generalized neurofibromatosis. Eur J Respir Dis 65:623, 1984.
121. Patchefsky AS, Atkinson WG, Hoch WS, et al: Interstitial pulmonary fibrosis and von Recklinghausen's disease: An ultrastructural and immunofluorescent study. Chest 64:459, 1973.
122. Klatte EC, Franken EA, Smith JA: The radiographic spectrum in neurofibromatosis. Semin Roentgenol 11:17, 1976.
123. Bergin CJ, Müller NL: CT in the diagnosis of interstitial lung disease. Am J Roentgenol 145:505, 1985.
124. Patel YD, Moorhouse HT: Neurofibrosarcomas in neurofibromatosis: Role of CT scanning and angiography. Clin Radiol 33:555, 1982.
125. Schabel SI, Schmidt GE, Vujic I: Overlooked pulmonary malignancy in neurofibromatosis. Can Assoc Radiol J 31:135, 1980.
126. Casselman ES, Miller WT, Lin SR, et al: Von Recklinghausen's disease: Incidence of roentgenographic findings with a clinical review of the literature. CRC Crit Rev Diagn Imaging 9:387, 1978.
127. Hunt JC, Pugh DG: Skeletal lesions in neurofibromatosis. Radiology 76:1, 1961.
128. Casselman ES, Mandell GA: Vertebral scalloping in neurofibromatosis. Radiology 131:89, 1979.
129. Klatte EC, Franken EA, Smith JA: The radiographic spectrum in neurofibromatosis. Semin Roentgenol 11:17, 1976.
130. Bourgouin PM, Shepard JAO, Moore EH, et al: Plexiform neurofibromatosis of the mediastinum: CT appearance. Am J Roentgenol 151:461, 1988.
131. Gossios KJ, Guy RL: Case report: Imaging of widespread plexiform neurofibromatosis. Clin Radiol 47:211, 1993.
132. Porterfield JK, Pyeritz RE, Traill TA: Pulmonary hypertension and interstitial fibrosis in von Recklinghausen neurofibromatosis. Am J Med Genet 25:531, 1986.

Index

Note: Page numbers in *italics* refer to illustrations; numbers followed by t indicate tables; numbers followed by n indicate notes.

Abdomen, pleural effusion related to disease within, 2763–2766
  sarcoidosis involving, 1563, 1565
  surgery on, pleural effusion after, 2763–2765, 2766
    pulmonary complications in, 2672, 2674
  upper, mechanoreceptors in, in ventilatory control, 238
Abdominal drainage tubes, complications of, 2677
Abdominal muscles, in ventilation, 247, 255, 256, 3056
  recruitment of, in diaphragmatic paralysis, 3059, *3060*
Abscess, cavity vs., 462
  hepatic, in amebiasis, 1034, 1035, *1035,* 2753
  intrabdominal, pleural effusion due to, 2765
  lung. See *Lung abscess.*
  mediastinal, radiologic features of, 2852, *2854, 2855*
    retropharyngeal abscess with, upper airway obstruction due to, 2022, *2023*
  retropharyngeal, acute, upper airway obstruction due to, 2021, 2022, *2023*
    mediastinitis due to, *2852*
  retrosternal, after sternotomy, 2660, *2660, 3019, 3019*
  subphrenic, in amebiasis, 1034
    pleural effusion with, 2766
    postoperative, 2672–2674
  with skeletal tuberculosis, 837–838, *838*
Acanthosis nigricans, in pulmonary carcinoma, 1174
Acariasis, 1061
Accessory cardiac bronchus, 626–627, *627*
Accessory diaphragm, 3006
Accessory fissures, imaging of, 160–165, *163–166*
Accessory lobe, inferior, 164–165, *165*
Accessory lung, 628
  bronchopulmonary sequestration vs., 601
Acetaldehyde, defect in metabolism of, alcohol-induced asthma and, 2116
Acetylation, slow, drug-induced lupus and, 1424–1425
Acetylcholine, endothelial response to, 148
  pulmonary vascular response to, 106
Acetylcysteine, mucus viscosity and, 63
Acetylsalicylic acid. See also *Salicylates.*
  asthma provoked by, 2112–2113
    leukotrienes in, 2091, 2113
  mucociliary clearance and, 129
  thoracic disease due to, 2539t, 2565

Achalasia, 2967, *2967, 3183*
  esophageal involvement in progressive systemic sclerosis vs., 1457
Acid, daily production of, 115
Acid maltase deficiency, 2727, 3064
Acid-base balance, 115–119
  disorders of. See also *Acidosis; Alkalosis.*
    classification of, 115
    compensatory mechanisms in, 115–116
    mixed, 115
    nomogram for, 119, *120*
    renal response to, 116
    in COPD, 2228
Acidemia, acidosis vs., 115n
Acidosis, carotid body response to, 235–237
  defined, 115n
  metabolic, 117–118, 118t
    central ventilatory response to, 237
    hyperventilation in, 3067
    in asthma, 2139
    pulmonary vascular response to, 106
  pleural fluid, 2743
  respiratory, 116–117
    in COPD, 2228
Acinar adenocarcinoma, pulmonary, 1101, *1102.*
    See also *Adenocarcinoma, pulmonary.*
Acinar nodule, 438
Acinetobacter infection, 764
Acinic cell carcinoma, tracheobronchial gland, 1258
Acino-nodose lesions, in tuberculosis, problems with term, 828
Acinus(i), 26–31, *31, 32, 2190*
  channels of airway communication with, 31–33, *32*
  development and growth of, 137, *139*
    postnatal, 138–139
  gas composition in, 53, *54*
  gas diffusion in, 107
  perfusion of, 104
    matching acinar ventilation to, 108–111, *109.* See also *Ventilation/perfusion* entries.
  ventilation of, 53–60
    matching capillary blood flow to, 108–111, *109.* See also *Ventilation/perfusion* entries.
Acquired immunodeficiency syndrome (AIDS).
    See also *Human immunodeficiency virus (HIV) infection.*
  bronchoalveolar lavage in infection diagnosis in, 343
  epidemiology of, 1641–1643, *1642*

Acquired immunodeficiency syndrome (AIDS) (Continued)
  Kaposi's sarcoma in. See *Kaposi's sarcoma, in HIV infection.*
  Mycobacterium avium complex infection in, 1654–1655, *1654–1656*
    histologic features of, 853, *854*
  Pneumocystis carinii pneumonia in. See Pneumocystis carinii *pneumonia, in HIV infection.*
  spontaneous pneumothorax in, 2787
Acrocyanosis, 398
Acrodermatitis enteropathica, 726
Acromegaly, 2729
  with carcinoid tumor, 1241, 1242
Acrylate glue embolism, 1865, *1867*
ACTH, intraoperative measurement of, during carcinoid tumor excision, 1242
Actinobacillus actinomycetemcomitans infection, 776
Actinomycosis, 952–957
  cavities or cysts in, 3102t
  clinical features of, 956–957
  endobronchial, 957
  epidemiology of, 953
  homogeneous nonsegmental opacity in, 3080t
  pathogenesis of, 953–954
  pathologic features of, 954, *954*
  pleural boundary crossing by, 460
  pleural effusion in, 2751
  radiologic features of, 954–956, *955, 956*
Acute lung injury. See also *Adult respiratory distress syndrome (ARDS); Pulmonary edema, permeability.*
  diagnostic criteria for, 1995, 1995t
Acute respiratory disease syndrome, adenovirus infection and, 995
Acute-phase reactants, in tuberculosis, 847
Acyclovir, thoracic disease due to, 2572
Addison's disease, due to tuberculosis, 840
Adenocarcinoid tumor, 1232
Adenocarcinoma. See also *Carcinoma.*
  cervical, metastatic to lung, 1408
  colorectal, metastatic to lung, *1385, 1387, 1396, 1400*
  endometrial, metastatic to lung, 1407
  mesothelioma vs., 1165, *1165,* 2818–2820, *2819, 2826*
  metastatic to lung, calcification in, 467
    from cervical primary, 1408
    from colorectal primary, *1385, 1387, 1396, 1400*
    from endometrial primary, 1407

Adenocarcinoma *(Continued)*
　from unknown primary, *1389*
　pulmonary, 1098–1110
　　acinar, 1101, *1102*
　　anatomic location of, 1121
　　bronchioloalveolar, 1101–1106, *1103–1108.*
　　　See also *Bronchioloalveolar carci-
　　　noma.*
　　classification of, 1098–1100
　　epidemiology of, 1072
　　gross and histologic features of, *1086,*
　　　1100–1108, *1100–1109, 1120*
　　histogenesis of, 1100
　　immunohistochemical features of, *1086,*
　　　1108–1110
　　metastases from, 1172
　　mucin-secreting, calcification in, 467
　　nonbronchioloalveolar, 1100–1101, *1100–
　　　1102*
　　papillary, 1101, *1102*
　　　calcification in, 467
　　paraneoplastic vascular disorders with,
　　　1177, 1178
　　pleural tags with, 1139, *1140–1141*
　　prognosis in, 1196
　　solitary nodule due to, *3114*
　　ultrastructural features of, 1108, *1110*
　　well-differentiated fetal, 1368–1369, *1369*
Adenoid(s), hypertrophy of, upper airway
　　obstruction due to, 2030
Adenoid cystic carcinoma, submaxillary gland,
　　metastatic to lung, *1388*
　tracheal, 2036, *2039, 3180*
　tracheobronchial gland, 1253–1256, *1253–
　　1256*
Adenoma, adrenal, metastasis vs., 1192
　alveolar, 1267
　bronchial, 1229, 1251
　mediastinal, pleomorphic, 2929
　mucous gland, 1259
　papillary, 1266–1267
　parathyroid, 2913–2914, *2914*
　pulmonary, 1265–1267
　tracheobronchial gland, 1258–1259
Adenomatoid tumor of pleura, 2838
Adenosine deaminase, in tuberculous pleural
　　effusion, 2746
Adenosine-5′-monophosphate, airway narrowing
　　in response to, in asthma, 422
Adenosquamous carcinoma, pulmonary,
　　1113–1114, *1115.* See also *Carcinoma,
　　pulmonary.*
　　mucoepidermoid carcinoma and, 1256–1257
　　prognosis in, 1196
Adenovirus infection, 994–996, *995, 996*
　acute bronchiolitis due to, 2333, *2334*
　in childhood, COPD and, 2176
　inhomogeneous segmental opacity in, 3097t
Adhesive atelectasis, 522, *525.* See also
　　Atelectasis.
　after radiation therapy, 2596
　defined, 513, 525
　postoperative, *2670,* 2671
　　homogeneous segmental opacity in, 3088t
Adiaspiromycosis, 950–951
Adipose tissue. See *Fat.*
Adrenal glands, adenoma of, metastasis vs.,
　　1192
　carcinoma of, metastatic, enlarged azygos
　　　node with, *2939*
　pulmonary carcinoma metastatic to, 1173
　　detection of, 1191–1192, *1192*
　tuberculosis involving, 840
β-Adrenergic agonists, mucociliary clearance
　　and, 129
　pulmonary vascular response to, 106

β$_2$-Adrenergic agonists, for asthma, mortality
　　and, 2142
β-Adrenergic blockers, asthma provoked by,
　　2116
　thoracic disease due to, 2539t, 2571
Adrenergic nervous system, cholinergic system
　　interaction with, 145, 148
　in lung innervation, 148
α-Adrenergic receptors, bronchial hyper-
　　responsiveness and, 2099–2100
β-Adrenergic receptors, bronchial hyper-
　　responsiveness and, 2099
β$_2$-Adrenergic receptors, in lung, 148
　variations in, in asthma, 2082
Adult respiratory distress syndrome (ARDS).
　　See also *Pulmonary edema, permeability.*
　acute interstitial pneumonitis and, 1619–1621
　after trauma, 2005, *2005*
　causes of, 1978t
　clinical features of, 1994–1995
　diagnosis of, 1995–1997
　　criteria for, 1995, 1995t
　diffuse air-space pattern in, 3130t
　epidemiology of, 1977
　herpes simplex virus type I and, 999
　in pancreatitis, 2003–2005, *2004*
　pathogenesis of, 1977–1983
　pathologic features of, 1983–1986, *1984, 1985*
　prognosis in, 1997–1999
　pulmonary function tests in, 1997
　pulmonary hypertension in, endothelial dys-
　　function and, 1882
　radiologic features of, 1986–1994, *1986–1993*
　with amniotic fluid embolism, 1852
　with fat embolism, 2005, *2005*
Advanced Multiple-Beam Equalization
　　Radiography (AMBER), 302–303
Aeromonas infection, 758–759
Aerosols, cough threshold measurement using,
　　2136
　inhalation of, for bronchial reactivity assess-
　　ment, 421t, 422
　technetium-labeled, for ventilation imaging,
　　329–330
　water-mist, mucus mobility and, 63
African tick typhus, 1022
Agammaglobulinemia, X-linked, 724–725
Age, pulmonary function and, 405, 2171–2172,
　　2172
　Streptococcus pneumoniae infection risk and,
　　736
　tuberculosis risk and, 801–802
Agenesis, corpus callosum, 726
　pulmonary, 598, 599–601, *600, 601*
　pulmonary artery, 637–638, *639*
　　Swyer-James syndrome vs., 504, 638, 2337
Agranulocytosis, pneumonia patterns in, 700
AIDS. See *Acquired immunodeficiency syndrome
　　(AIDS); Human immunodeficiency virus
　　(HIV) infection.*
Air, partial pressures of gases in, 53
Air alveologram, 438, *439*
Air bronchiologram, 438
Air bronchogram, *435,* 437–438, *437*
　in atelectasis, 526, *529,* 533–534
　in pneumothorax, 519, *519*
　with solitary nodule, 1142, *1142*
Air embolism, 1854–1857
　due to bulla enlargement, 2240
　pulmonary (venous), 1855–1856, 1856t
　systemic (arterial), 1854–1855, 1854t
　with central venous catheter, 2685, *2685*
Air gap technique, for conventional radiographs,
　　302
Air pollution, asthma provoked by, 2114–2115
　COPD and, 2173–2175

Air pollution *(Continued)*
　cough and, 380
Air trapping, esophageal, 2967
　in asthma, 2130–2132, *2133*
　in healthy persons, 291, *292,* 2331
　in Swyer-James syndrome, 2337, *2340*
　inspiratory-expiratory radiography for detec-
　　tion of, 303, *304*
　local overinflation with, 497–498, *497,* 499,
　　500, 501
　with airway obstruction, 514, *515*
　with bulla, 508, *508*
　with congenital bronchial atresia, 620
　with metastatic neoplasm, *1401*
Air-blood barrier, development and growth of,
　　137
　oxygen diffusion across, 107
　structure of, 17–21, *18, 20, 23–24, 23, 24*
　pulmonary edema and, 1947–1949, *1948*
Air-crescent sign, in angioinvasive aspergillosis,
　　940–941, *944, 946*
　in echinococcosis, 1056
　with aspergilloma, 923, 925, *925, 926*
Air-drying, for lung specimen preparation, 350,
　　352–353
Airflow obstruction, chronic. See *Chronic
　　obstructive pulmonary disease (COPD).*
Air-space nodule, 438, *439*
Air-space pattern, diffuse lung disease with,
　　differential diagnosis of, 3130, 3130t, *3131,
　　3132*
　in bronchioloalveolar carcinoma, 1149–1156,
　　1150–1155
　increased density with, 434–439, *434–439*
　　due to interstitial disease, *440*
　　interstitial pattern combined with, 454–455,
　　　456, 457
Airway(s). See also *Bronchial tree;
　　Bronchiole(s); Bronchus(i); Trachea.*
　adventitious sounds originating in, 394–395
　anatomy of, 3–51
　　nomenclature of wall in, 12
　central, expiratory collapse of, in COPD,
　　2222, *2222, 2223*
　channels of acinar communication with, 31–
　　33, *32*
　closure of, at low lung volumes, 111
　congenital stenosis of, 618–620
　decreased starting caliber of, bronchial hyper-
　　responsiveness and, 2096–2097
　development and growth of, 136–139, *137–
　　139*
　　anomalies affecting, 597–629
　disease of, 2019–2353. See also specific disor-
　　ders.
　　with normal chest radiograph, 3047
　displacement of, in atelectasis, 533, *534*
　diverticula of, 626–627, *627*
　epithelium of. See *Bronchial epithelium; Epi-
　　thelium.*
　esophageal carcinoma invading, 2965
　fibrosarcoma of, 1349, *1349*
　function of, 51–63
　imaging of, 33–51
　infection of, 701, *701, 702.* See also *Bronchio-
　　litis; Bronchitis; Tracheitis.*
　lipoma of, 1347
　melanoma of, 1267
　metastasis via, 1383
　morphologic investigation techniques for, 351
　obstruction of. See *Airway obstruction.*
　papillomas of, 1262–1265, *1262–1266*
　pulmonary infection via, 698–713
　quantitative assessment of wall dimensions of,
　　2085, *2087*
　rupture of, homogeneous segmental opacity
　　due to, 3088t

Airway(s) *(Continued)*
 pneumomediastinum and, 2618, *2621,* 2865
  with blunt trauma, 2618–2622, *2621, 2622*
 small. See also *Bronchiole(s).*
 tests of function of, 414, 2220–2221
 smooth muscle of. See *Airway smooth muscle.*
 structural changes in, in asthma, 2083–2087,
   2086, 2087
  bronchial hyper-responsiveness and,
    2096–2097
  in COPD, 2189–2190
 upper, carcinoma of, pulmonary carcinoma
   and, 1201–1202
  compliance of, in obstructive sleep apnea,
    2060–2061
  muscles of, 246. See also specific muscles.
   control of, 242–243
   dysfunction of, in obstructive sleep ap-
     nea, 2061–2062
   in ventilation, *236,* 239
  obstruction of. See *Airway obstruction,*
    upper.
  radiologic measurement of, in obstructive
    sleep apnea, 2063, *2064, 2065*
  receptors in, in ventilatory control, *236,*
    237, 241
  structural narrowing of, obstructive sleep
    apnea and, 2059–2060
Airway conductance, 412
Airway ganglia, 145, *147*
Airway hyper-responsiveness. See *Bronchial*
  hyper-responsiveness.
Airway obstruction, bronchiectasis due to, 2269,
  2270
 due to endotracheal intubation, 2680
 due to metastasis, 1397–1399, *1400–1403*
 dynamic compliance in, 412
 in asthma, mechanisms of, 2087–2088
 in fibrosing mediastinitis, 2857–2860, *2859*
 in mediastinal histoplasmosis, 886
 in obstructive sleep apnea, site of, 2059, 2061
 in sarcoidosis, mechanisms of, 1567
 intralobar sequestration and, 602
 neonatal lobar hyperinflation and, 623, *625*
 partial, by endobronchial lesion, lung volume
   and, 497, 498, 499, *499–501*
  normal chest radiograph with, 3047
  oligemia due to, 503–504, *506*
  Swyer-James syndrome vs., 2340, *2343*
 pulmonary carcinoma and, 1081
 resorption atelectasis and, 513–517, *514–518*
 spontaneous pneumothorax and, 2783
 total atelectasis due to, 539, *540*
 upper, 2021–2048
  acute, 2021–2025, *2023–2025*
   causes of, 2021, 2022t
  chronic, 2025–2048
   causes of, 2025–2027, 2026t
   clinical features of, 2030
   due to laryngeal dysfunction, 2032–2033
   due to relapsing polychondritis, 2040–
     2042, *2044*
   due to saber-sheath trachea, 2036–2040,
     2042, 2043
   due to thyroid disorders, 2030–2032,
     2031, 2032
   due to tonsil and adenoid hypertrophy,
     2030
   due to tracheal neoplasms, 2035–2036,
     2037–2041
   due to tracheal stenosis, 2033–2035,
     2034–2036
   due to tracheobronchomegaly, 2046–
     2048, *2047*
   due to tracheobronchopathia osteochon-
     droplastica, 2042, *2045*

Airway obstruction *(Continued)*
   due to tracheomalacia, 2042–2046
   general features of, 2025–2030
   physiologic features of, 2027–2029, *2027*
   radiologic features of, 2029, *2030*
   fixed vs. variable, 2027–2028, *2027*
   in rheumatoid disease, 1449
   in systemic lupus erythematosus, 1431
   phrenic nerve pacing and, 246
   pulmonary function tests in diagnosis of,
     2028
   severe, pulmonary edema with, 2002–2003,
     2003
   VisoV in determining site of, 409–410
Airway resistance, density dependence of, in
  COPD, 2224
 frictional, in work of breathing, 58–59
 measurement of, 412–413
 upper, during sleep, 2055
Airway smooth muscle, 13–14, *14*
 biochemistry and mechanics of contraction of,
   2100, 2101–2102
 hyperplasia of, 14
 in asthma, 2087
  bronchial hyper-responsiveness and, 2097,
    2100–2102
  myogenic response of, to stretch, 2116
 tumors of, 1332, 1333–1334
Airway stents, complications of, 2674
Airway wall remodeling, in asthma, 2085–2087,
  2086, 2087
 bronchial hyper-responsiveness and, 2096–
   2097
 in COPD, 2189–2190
Alagille syndrome, 642
Alariasis, 1052
Albinism, partial, 726
Albumin, technetium-labeled, for perfusion
  scanning, 326–327, 1800
Alcaligenes infection, 764
Alcohol, aspiration of, 2512
 consumption of, asthma provoked by, 2116
  chest wall pain due to, in Hodgkin's dis-
    ease, 387
  obstructive sleep apnea and, 2057, 2062
  tuberculosis risk and, 801
  ventilatory response and, 240
Algae, sea, airborne toxins from, 2124
 hypoventilation due to poisoning from,
   3062
Alkalemia, alkalosis vs., 115n
Alkalosis, defined, 115n
 metabolic, 118–119
  hypoventilation due to, 3054
 respiratory, 117
  lactic acidosis development in, 3067
Alkaptonuria, 677
Alkylating agents. See also *Chemotherapy;*
  specific drugs.
 thoracic disease due to, 2538t, 2544–2551
Allergens, asthma provocation by, 2104–2106,
  2105
Allergic alveolitis, extrinsic. See *Extrinsic*
  allergic alveolitis.
Allergic bronchopulmonary aspergillosis. See
  under *Aspergillosis.*
Allergic granulomatosis and angiitis. See *Churg-*
  Strauss syndrome.
Allergy. See also *Atopy.*
 angioneurotic edema and, 2022
 Churg-Strauss syndrome and, 1507, 1509
 genetic considerations in, 2080–2082, 2081t
 occupational asthma and, possible causes of,
   2119t, 2121–2122
  proven causes of, 2117–2121, 2118t–2119t
Allescheria boydii infection, 951

Almitrine, ventilatory response and, 240
Alpha chain disease. See also *Heavy chain*
   disease.
 pleural effusion due to, 2760
Alpha₁-protease inhibitor. See α_1-*Protease*
  inhibitor.
ALPS (mnemonic), 742
Altered measles syndrome, 988, 990, 2752
Alternans, respiratory, 258
Alternaria infection, 952
Altitude, bronchoarterial diameter ratio and,
  2275
 hypoxemia due to, 115. See also *Mountain*
   sickness.
 diffusion defect and, 114
Aluminum, occupational COPD due to, 2122
 pneumoconiosis due to, 2460–2463, *2461,*
   2462
Alveolar adenoma, 1267
Alveolar air equation, 112
Alveolar capillaries. See *Pulmonary*
  capillary(ies); Pulmonary vasculature.
Alveolar damage, diffuse. See *Diffuse alveolar*
  damage.
Alveolar ducts, 17
Alveolar epithelial cells. See also *Alveolar*
  epithelium.
 type I, 18–19, *18*
  development and growth of, 137
  replacement of, 19
 type II, 19–20, *19*
  development and growth of, 137
  in defense against oxidant damage, 2521
  lipid metabolism in, 131
Alveolar epithelium, 17, 18–20, *18, 19*
 cells of. See *Alveolar epithelial cells.*
 damage to, in idiopathic pulmonary fibrosis
   pathogenesis, 1587–1590, *1590*
 fluid transport across, 1955
  in pulmonary edema, 1958
 focal hyperplasia of, *1009,* 1108
 in adult respiratory distress syndrome, 1978
 permeability of, 1951
 structure of, 17, 18–20, *18, 19*
  pulmonary edema and, 1949, *1949*
Alveolar fenestrae, 32
 in emphysema, 2191, *2192*
 collateral resistance and, 60
Alveolar fibrosis, diffuse. See *Pulmonary*
  fibrosis, idiopathic.
Alveolar hemorrhage. See also *Hemorrhage,*
  pulmonary.
 diffuse, after bone marrow transplantation,
   1726–1727, *1727*
  differential diagnosis of, 1764
  diffuse air-space pattern in, 3130t
  in systemic lupus erythematosus, 1426–
    1427, *1428,* 1430
Alveolar hypersensitivity. See *Extrinsic allergic*
  alveolitis.
Alveolar hyperventilation, 3065–3067. See also
  Hyperventilation.
Alveolar hypoventilation, 3048–3065
 causes of, 416–417
  nonpulmonary, 3048–3049, 3049t
  pulmonary, 3048t
 chronic, sequelae of, 3049
 daytime, in obesity hypoventilation syndrome,
   2066
 due to respiratory pump disorders, 3049t,
   3056–3065
 due to ventilatory control disorders, 3049–
   3056, 3049t
 during sleep in COPD, 2227
 hypoxemia due to, 115
 in kyphoscoliosis, 3022

Alveolar hypoventilation *(Continued)*
  primary. See *Sleep apnea, central.*
  pulmonary hypertension in, 1918, *1918*
  respiratory acidosis due to, 116
  with normal arterial carbon dioxide tension,
    3048
Alveolar lipoproteinosis. See *Alveolar
  proteinosis.*
Alveolar macrophages, 21–23, *22*
  in adult respiratory distress syndrome, 1978–
    1979
  in alveolar proteinosis, 2703
  in asbestosis, 2422, *2423*
  in asthmatic airway inflammation, 2090
  in clearance of alveolar air space, 22, 130
  in extrinsic allergic alveolitis, 2363
  in host response to neoplasia, 1084
  in progressive systemic sclerosis, 1452–1453
  in sarcoidosis, 1536–1537
  in silicosis, 2391
  Langerhans' cells vs., 1630
  surfactant's protective functions for, 58
Alveolar microlithiasis, 2719–2722, *2720*
  radiologic features of, *278*, 2721, *2722, 2723*
Alveolar period of lung development, 138
Alveolar phospholipidosis. See *Alveolar
  proteinosis.*
Alveolar pores, 31–32, *32*
Alveolar proteinosis, 2700–2708
  after bone marrow transplantation, 1732
  bronchial cast formation in, *2291*, 2292
  clinical features of, 2706, *2709*
  diagnosis of, 2706
  in HIV infection, 1687, 2701
  pathogenesis of, 2701–2703
  pathologic features of, 2703, *2704, 2705*
  prognosis in, 2706–2708, *2710*
  radiologic features of, 454, 457, 2704–2706,
    2706–2708
  recurrent, after lung transplantation, 1720
  tuberculosis risk and, 803
Alveolar sacs, 17
Alveolar septum. See *Air-blood barrier.*
Alveolar soft part sarcoma, 1357, 2929
Alveolar ventilation, 53–60
  determinants of, 53
  matching alveolar perfusion to, 108–111, *109.*
    See also *Ventilation/perfusion* entries.
Alveolar-arterial oxygen gradient, in ventilation/
  perfusion mismatch assessment, 112, 113
Alveolar-capillary gas exchange, acinar gas
  partial pressures and, 53, *54*
Alveolitis, cryptogenic fibrosing, 1585. See also
  Pulmonary fibrosis, idiopathic.
  extrinsic allergic. See *Extrinsic allergic alveo-
    litis.*
  lymphocytic, in HIV infection, 1674, 1686
  in response to asbestos exposure, 2423
Alveolocapillary membrane. See *Air-blood
  barrier.*
Alveologram, air, 438, *439*
Alveolus(i), 17–24, *18*
  development and growth of, *139*
    factors influencing, 142
    postnatal, 139
  epithelium of. See *Alveolar epithelial cells;
    Alveolar epithelium.*
  fluid lining of, 1951
  geometry and dimensions of, 23–24, *23, 24*
  interstitium of, 17–18, 20–21
  particle clearance from, 130
  perfusion of, 104
    matching alveolar ventilation to, 108–111,
      109. See also *Ventilation/perfusion*
      entries.
  rupture of, pneumomediastinum and, 2863–
    2865

Alveolus(i) *(Continued)*
  ventilation of, 53–60
    determinants of, 53
    matching alveolar perfusion to, 108–111,
      109. See also *Ventilation/perfusion*
      entries.
AMBER (Advanced Multiple-Beam Equalization
  Radiography), 302–303
Amebiasis, 1034–1036, *1035*, 3080t
  pleural effusion in, 2753
American Joint Committee on Cancer, lymph
  node classification of, for lung cancer
  staging, 180–184, *185*, 188t, 1186, *1186,*
  1187t
American Thoracic Society, regional nodal
  stations of, 180–184, 184t, *185–187*, 1186
Amiloride, for cystic fibrosis, mechanism of
  action of, 2300
Aminoaciduria, renal, familial retardation of
  growth and cor pulmonale with, 2728
γ-Aminobutyric acid, in respiratory rhythm
  generation, 240
Aminoglycosides, myasthenia-like syndromes
  due to, 3063
Aminophylline, ventilatory response and, 240
β-Aminopropionitrile, experimental emphysema
  induced by, 2185–2186
Aminorex fumarate, pulmonary hypertension due
  to, 1903
Amiodarone, thoracic disease due to, 2538t,
  2559–2564
    clinical features of, 2563
    diffuse reticular pattern in, 3136t
    laboratory findings in, 2563–2564
    pathogenesis of, 2559
    pathologic features of, 2559–2560, *2560–
      2561*
    prognosis in, 2564
    radiologic features of, 2560–2563, *2562,
      2563*
Amitriptyline, thoracic disease due to, 2539t,
  2569
Amitrole-containing herbicide, 2587
Ammonia inhalation, 2524–2525
Amniotic fluid, cystic adenomatoid malformation
  and, 618
    embolization of, 1850–1853
    pulmonary hypoplasia and, 142, 598, 599
Amoxicillin resistance, in *Haemophilus
  influenzae*, 770
Amphoric breathing, 394
Amphotericin B, thoracic disease due to, 2538t,
  2558
Ampicillin, thoracic disease due to, 2538t, 2558
Amputation neuroma, presenting in lung, 1346
Amylase, in pleural fluid, in pancreatitis, 2743,
  2765
Amyloidosis, 2708–2718
    classification of, 2708–2709
    clinical features of, 2718
    diagnosis of, 2718
    in cystic fibrosis, 2312
    in multiple myeloma, 1297
    in rheumatoid disease, 1451
    pathogenesis of, 2709–2711
    pathologic features of, 2711, *2711–2715*
    pleural, 2840
    pleuropulmonary diseases resulting in, 2709
    prognosis in, 2718
    radiologic features of, 2711–2718, *2715–2719*
    tracheobronchial, airway narrowing due to,
      2042, *2045*, 2718
    radiologic features of, 2711, *2715, 2716*
Amyotrophic lateral sclerosis, 3061
Anabolic steroids, pulmonary peliosis due to,
  2571

Anaerobic bacteria, classification and
  nomenclature of, 735t
    empyema and, 2747
    pneumonia due to, 778–783
      cavities or cysts in, 3102t
      clinical features of, 781–782
      community-acquired, 721
      diagnosis of, 782–783
      epidemiology of, 778–779
      homogeneous opacity in, nonsegmental,
        3079t
        segmental, 3087t
      hospital-acquired, 723
      laboratory findings in, 782
      pathogenesis of, 779
      pathologic features of, 779, *780*
      prognosis in, 783
      radiologic features of, 779–781, *781, 782*
Anaerobic threshold, 241
Analgesics. See also *Acetylsalicylic acid;
  Salicylates.*
    asthma provoked by, 2112–2113
    thoracic disease due to, 2539t, 2565
Anaphylatoxin, in adult respiratory distress
  syndrome, 1981
Anaphylaxis, 2106
    exercise-induced, 2109
    mast cell mediators in, 2109
Anasarca, neonatal, cystic adenomatoid
  malformation and, 618
Anatase, pneumoconiosis due to, 2465–2466,
  2467
Anchovy paste sputum, in amebiasis, 1035
Ancylostomiasis, 1043, 1047, 1752
Androgens, obstructive sleep apnea and, 2059,
  2067
Anemia, Fanconi's, 726
    in pulmonary carcinoma, 1178
    iron-deficiency, in idiopathic pulmonary hem-
      orrhage, 1762–1763
    sickle cell, pulmonary complications of, 1832–
      1834
Anergy, in HIV infection, 1653
    tuberculin testing and, 842–843, 843t
Aneurysm, aortic. See *Aortic aneurysm.*
    false, defined, 2951
    of aorta, *2634*, 2952
    inferior vena cava, 2947
    innominate artery, 2961, 3178t
    pulmonary arteriovenous, 655–662
      clinical features of, 395, 661–662
      pathologic features of, 657, *657*
      radiologic features of, 657–661, *658–661*
    pulmonary artery, 1935–1937, 1935t, *1936,
      1937*
      congenital, 642, *643*, 646, *647*
      in Behçet's disease, 1519, *1519, 1520*
    Rasmussen's, 817–818, 1935
    superior vena cava, 2947, *2948*
Angiitis. See also *Vasculitis.*
    cutaneous leukocytoclastic, 1490t
Angina pectoris, 388
Angiocentric immunoproliferative lesion,
  1280–1281, *1282–1285*
Angioendotheliomatosis, 1291
Angiofibroma, endobronchial, 1351
Angiofollicular lymph node hyperplasia, 2760,
  2938–2940, *2940–2942*
Angiography, 322–326, *323–326*. See also
  Pulmonary angiography.
    selective, with parathyroid hormone measure-
      ment, in parathyroid adenoma assess-
      ment, 2914
Angioimmunoblastic lymphadenopathy,
  1312–1313, *1314*
Angioimmunoproliferative lesion, 1280–1281,
  1282–1285

Angiokeratoma corporis diffusum universale, 2724

Angiomatoid lesions, in pulmonary hypertension, 1884, *1888*

Angiomatosis, bacillary, 1647, *1647*
  diffuse pulmonary, 662–663, *662, 663*

Angiomyolipoma, renal, bilateral, in tuberous sclerosis, 686, *687*

Angioneurotic edema, upper airway obstruction due to, 2022–2023

Angiosarcoma, mediastinal, 2920–2921
  metastatic to lung, 1409–1410
  pulmonary, 1343
  sclerosing epithelioid. See *Epithelioid hemangioendothelioma.*

Angiostrongyloides costaricensis, 1040

Angiotensin, plasma levels of, in asthma, 2093
  pulmonary metabolism of, 131

Angiotensin-converting enzyme, actions of, in lung, 131
  elevated, diseases associated with, 1569t
  in serum or BAL fluid in sarcoidosis, 1568–1569
    prognosis and, 1573
  in silicosis, 2407

Angiotensin-converting enzyme inhibitors, angioneurotic edema due to, 2022
  asthma and, 2116–2117
  cough due to, 382
  thoracic disease due to, 2539t, 2570–2571

Angiotropic lymphoma, 1291

Anhydrides, lung disease due to, 2362t. See also *Extrinsic allergic alveolitis.*
  occupational asthma due to, 2121

Animal confinement buildings, 2379
  COPD and, 2175

Animal exposure, asthma and, 2106
  in patient's history, 390

Animal lipids, aspiration of, 2501, 2506, *2508*

Animal products, occupational asthma due to, 2118t, 2120

Anion gap, calculation of, 117

Anisakiasis, 1047

Ankylosing spondylitis, 3022–3023

Anomalous pulmonary venous drainage. See under *Pulmonary venous drainage.*

Anorectic drugs, pulmonary hypertension due to, 1903

Anterior axillary fold, on radiographs, 259

Anterior diaphragmatic lymph nodes, 176, *178*
  enlargement of, 2929

Anterior horn cell disorders, 3061

Anterior junction line (anterior mediastinal line), 201–204, *204, 205*

Anterior mediastinal lymph nodes, in ATS classification, 184t, *186*
  in Hodgkin's disease, 1299–1302, *1300, 1301, 1304*

Anterior mediastinal triangle, 202, *204*

Anterior mediastinum. See *Mediastinum, anterior.*

Anterior parietal lymph nodes, 175–176, *176*

Anteroposterior chest diameter, lung volume and, 496–497

Anterosuperior mediastinal lymph nodes, 176–179, *179*

Anthracosis, 2409

Anthrax, 749

Antiarrhythmic drugs, thoracic disease due to, 2538t, 2559–2564
  myasthenia-like syndromes due to, 3063

Anti–basement membrane antibody, in Goodpasture's syndrome, 1757–1758
  detection of, 1764

Antibiotics, cytotoxic, thoracic disease due to, 2538t, 2540–2544

Antibiotics *(Continued)*
  thoracic disease due to, 2538t, 2558–2559

Anticardiolipin antibodies, in systemic lupus erythematosus, 1430

Anticentromere antibodies, in CREST syndrome, 1453, 1460

α_1-Antichymotrypsin, deficiency of, COPD and, 2178
  in tracheobronchial secretions, 61

Anticonvulsant drugs, thoracic disease due to, 2539t, 2564–2565

Antidepressants, thoracic disease due to, 2539t, 2569

Antidiuretic hormone, elevated, in asthma, 2136–2137
  inappropriate secretion of, paraneoplastic, in pulmonary carcinoma, 1176–1177

Anti–endothelial cell antibodies, in systemic lupus erythematosus, 1431
  Wegener's granulomatosis and, 1493

Antigenic drift, in influenza virus, 981

Antigenic shift, in influenza virus, 981

Anti-Hu antibodies, in small cell carcinoma–associated neuropathy, 1174

Anti-Jo-1 antibodies, in dermatomyositis/polymyositis, 1463

Antikeratin antibodies, in adenocarcinoma vs. mesothelioma, 2819

Antileukoproteinase, in emphysema pathogenesis, 2182–2183, *2183*

Antilung antibodies, in coal workers' pneumoconiosis, 2410–2411

Antimetabolites, thoracic disease due to, 2538t, 2551–2555

Antimicrobials. See also *Antibiotics.*
  thoracic disease due to, 2538t, 2556–2559

Antimony, pneumoconiosis due to, 2456

Antineutrophil cytoplasmic antibodies (ANCA), disease associations of, 1492
  genetic assocation with, 1492
  in Churg-Strauss syndrome, 1507, 1511
  in microscopic polyangiitis, 1513
  in rheumatoid disease, pulmonary vasculitis and, 1450–1451
  in systemic lupus erythematosus, 1423
  Wegener's granulomatosis and, 1492–1493, 1505

Antinuclear antibodies (ANA), in coal workers' pneumoconiosis, 2410–2411
  in CREST syndrome, 1453, 1460
  in mixed connective tissue disease, 1470
  in progressive systemic sclerosis, 1422, 1453
  in rheumatoid disease, 1434
  in systemic lupus erythematosus, 1422–1423
  in pleural fluid, 2753

Antioxidants, in pulmonary defense, 2521
  pulmonary carcinoma and, 1081–1082

Antiphospholipid antibodies, disease associations with, 1423
  in systemic lupus erythematosus, 1430

Antiphospholipid syndrome, pulmonary hypertension with, 1912–1914
  venous thrombosis and, 1779

α_1-Antiprotease. See α_1-*Protease inhibitor.*

Antiproteases, in tracheobronchial secretions, 61

Antipsychotic drugs, thoracic disease due to, 2539t, 2569

Antirheumatic drugs, thoracic disease due to, 2539t, 2565–2566

Antisynthetase antibodies, in dermatomyositis/polymyositis, 1463

Antithrombin III deficiency, venous thrombosis and, 1779

α_1-Antitrypsin. See α_1-*Protease inhibitor.*

Anxiety, chronic cough and, 382
  dyspnea due to, 387, 388

Aorta, aneurysm of. See *Aortic aneurysm.*
  coarctation of, rib notching with, *3014,* 3015
  congenital anomalies of, 2961, *2962–2965*
    aortography in evaluation of, 325
  esophageal carcinoma invading, 2965
  MR evaluation of, 321
  penetrating trauma to, 2648–2652, *2652, 2653*
  rupture of, 2626–2633
    aortography in, *2627–2629, 2633*
    clinical features of, 2633
    CT imaging of, 2629–2632, *2630, 2631*
    hemothorax due to, 2761
    mediastinal hemorrhage with, 2627, *2627, 2630–2631, 2630, 2870–2871, 2870*
    radiographic features of, 2627–2629, *2627–2629*
    transesophageal echocardiography in, 2632–2633

Aortic aneurysm, 2951–2955, *2954–2956*
  chest pain due to, 386
  false, *2634,* 2952
  hemothorax due to, 2761
  in Marfan's syndrome, 676
  mediastinal mass due to, in anterior compartment, 3172t
    in middle-posterior compartment, 3178t, *3181, 3182*
  mycotic, 2952, *2954, 3181*
  traumatic, *2627,* 2633, *2635*

Aortic aperture of diaphragm, 2987, *2988*

Aortic body, in respiratory control, *3050,* 3051

Aortic dissection, 2955–2957, *2958–2960, 3180*
  in Marfan's syndrome, 676–677, *678*

Aortic line, 215, *216, 217*

Aortic nipple, 209, *210, 211,* 2951

Aorticopulmonary paraganglioma, 2942–2943, *2943*

Aorticosympathetic paraganglioma, 2977–2978

Aortitis, syphilitic, 2943

Aortobronchial fistula, 2290t, 2291
  postoperative, 2674

Aortography, 324–325, *325*
  in aortic rupture, *2627–2629,* 2633
  in bronchopulmonary sequestration, 604, *605*

Aortopulmonary line, 211–212, *213–214*

Aortopulmonary lymph nodes, in ATS classification, 184t, *185, 186*

Aortopulmonary window, 211–212, *212–214*

Aortopulmonary window lymph nodes, 179, *183*
  in classification for lung cancer staging, *185,* 188t, *1186,* 1187t

APACHE II score, adult respiratory distress syndrome prognosis and, 1998

Apical cap, 582, *583,* 2795–2796, *2796–2798*
  with aortic rupture, *2627,* 2629
  with pleural effusion, 572

Apical carcinoma, pulmonary, 1156–1165, *1162–1164.* See also *Carcinoma, pulmonary.*
  apical cap vs., 2796, *2798*
  extrapulmonary features of, 1171–1172

Aplasia, pulmonary, 598, *599–601*

Apnea, sleep. See *Sleep apnea.*

Apnea index, 2056

Apnea-hypopnea index, 2056

Apneustic center, *236,* 238, 3050–3051, *3050*

Appetite suppressants, pulmonary hypertension due to, 1903

Arachidonic acid, metabolites of. See also *Leukotrienes; Prostaglandins.*
  in adult respiratory distress syndrome pathogenesis, 1983
  in pulmonary hypertension pathogenesis, 1881
  pulmonary metabolism of, 131

Arachnia propionica infection, 952

Arcuate ligaments, 253–254, *253*
ARDS. See *Adult respiratory distress syndrome (ARDS); Pulmonary edema, permeability.*
Arenaviruses, 994
Argon inhalation, closing volume measurement using, 413–414
Argyrophilia, in pulmonary neuroendocrine cells, 10
Argyrosiderosis, 2454–2455
Armillifer infestation, 1059–1061
Arnold-Chiari malformation, 3056
Aromatic hydrocarbons, polycyclic, pulmonary carcinoma and, 1077–1078
Arousal, defined, 2055
  in obstructive sleep apnea, 2062
Arrhythmias, in COPD, 2218–2219
  obstructive sleep apnea and, 2067
Arsenic, pulmonary carcinoma and, 1076
Arterialization, in pulmonary hypertension, of pulmonary arterioles, 1883
  of pulmonary veins, 1919, *1919*
Arteriography. See *Angiography; Aortography; Pulmonary angiography.*
Arteriovenous anastomoses, bronchial, 77
  pulmonary, 77
Arteriovenous fistula, pulmonary, developmental. See *Arteriovenous malformation, pulmonary.*
  with penetrating wound, 2648, *2653*
Arteriovenous malformation, pulmonary, 655–662
  clinical features of, 395, 661–662
  multiple masses or nodules due to, 3123t
  pathologic features of, 657, *657*
  radiologic features of, 657–661, *658–661*
  solitary nodule due to, 3111t, *3113*
Arteritis, giant cell (temporal), 1517–1518, *1518*
  defined, 1490t
  Takayasu's, 1513–1517, 1515t, *1516, 1517*
  defined, 1490t
  rib notching in, 3015
Artery-bronchus ratios, 78–80, 284–286
  altitude and, 2275
  in asthma, 2130
  in bronchiectasis diagnosis, 2274, *2274*, 2275–2276
  in hydrostatic pulmonary edema, 1959–1961, *1960*
Arthralgia, in *Mycoplasma pneumoniae* infection, 1014
Arthritis, in *Mycoplasma pneumoniae* infection, 1014
  in sarcoidosis, 1565
  rheumatoid. See also *Rheumatoid disease.*
    juvenile, 1451–1452
  septic, of sternoclavicular and sternochondral joints, in heroin addict, 3020
Arthropathy, in cystic fibrosis, 2312
Arthropods, 1059–1061
Aryl hydrocarbon hydroxylase, pulmonary activity of, pulmonary carcinoma and, 1082
ASA. See *Acetylsalicylic acid.*
Asbestos, 2419–2448
  benign pleural effusion due to, 2754–2756
  bronchiolitis due to, *2327*
  COPD and, 2175
  disease related to. See also *Asbestosis.*
    clinical features of, 2443–2445
    diagnosis of, 2446–2448
    epidemiology of, 2420–2422, 2421t
    pathogenesis of, 2422–2423
    pathologic features of, 2423–2430, *2425–2433*
    prognosis in, 2448
    pulmonary function tests in, 2445–2446
    radiologic features of, 2430–2443, *2433–2448*

Asbestos *(Continued)*
  with normal radiograph, 2448, 3048
  lymphoproliferative disease and, 1275
  mesothelioma and, 2448, 2807–2809. See also *Mesothelioma.*
  pleural calcification and, 583, *585*
  pleural disease related to, pathologic features of, 2424–2425, *2425–2427*
    pulmonary function tests in, 2446
    radiologic features of, 2431–2437, *2433–2443*
  pleural fibrosis due to, diffuse, 582, *582*, 2804, *2804*, 2805
    pathologic features of, 2424, *2429*
    focal visceral, 2424, *2427*
  pleural plaques associated with, 2796
    normal chest radiograph with, 3048
  pulmonary carcinoma and, 1074–1076, 2448
  pulmonary disease related to, pathologic features of, 2425–2430, *2428–2433*
    radiologic features of, 2437–2443, *2438–2440, 2444–2448*
  round atelectasis due to, 522, 3118t, *3121*
    pathologic features of, 2430, *2432, 2433*
    pulmonary carcinoma vs., 2443, 2448
    radiologic features of, *2438–2440*, 2441–2443, *2447, 2448*
  sources of exposure to, 2420–2422, 2421t, 2808–2809, 2808t
  types of, 2419–2420, *2420*
    mesothelioma risk and, 2809, 2810
Asbestos bodies, 2425–2429, *2428*
Asbestosis, clinical features of, 2443–2445
  defined, 2429
  diagnosis of, 2448
    waveform analysis of crackles in, 394, 2443
  diffuse reticular pattern in, 3136t, *3143*
  pathogenesis of, 2422–2423
  pathologic features of, 2429–2430, *2429–2431*
  prognosis in, 2448
  pulmonary carcinoma and, 1075–1076
  radiologic features of, 2437–2441, *2444–2446*
  screening for, 2441
  with normal chest radiograph, 2448
Ascariasis, 1039–1040, *1040*, 1752, 3080t
Ascites, pleural effusion vs., on CT, 572–574, *573–576*
  pleural effusion with, mechanisms of, 2763, 2764
Askin tumor, in paravertebral region, 2974
  of chest wall, 3028–3029
L-Asparaginase, thoracic disease due to, 2538t, 2555
Aspergilloma, 923–927, *924–927*
  at bronchial stump after pneumonectomy, 2672
  in HIV disease, 1673
  in tuberculosis, *3106*
  progressing to invasive aspergillosis, *922*
  solitary nodule due to, 3111t
Aspergillosis, 919–945
  acute bronchopneumonia due to, 437, *437*, 936–937, *937–940*
    after bone marrow transplantation, 1730
  acute tracheobronchitis due to, *701*, 944, *946*
    in HIV disease, 1673
  after bone marrow transplantation, 1730, *1731*
  after heart-lung or lung transplantation, 1717, *1718*
  allergic, in HIV disease, 1673
  allergic bronchopulmonary, 927–936
    aspergilloma and, 923
    clinical features of, 935
    diagnosis of, 927–928
    eosinophilia with, 1753
    in cystic fibrosis, 928, 2308, 2309–2310

Aspergillosis *(Continued)*
  marijuana and, 2569
  pathogenesis of, 928
  pathologic features of, 928–929, *929, 930*
  prognosis in, 935–936
  radiologic features of, 483, 929–935, *931–935*
  angioinvasive, *436*, 940–942, *941–946*
    after transplantation, *1718, 1731*
    in HIV disease, *1672, 1673*
    multiple masses or nodules in, *3126*
  bronchiolitis with, *2331*
  cavities or cysts in, 3103t
  chronic necrotizing, 944–945
    in HIV disease, 1672, 1673
  due to hypersensitivity, 927. See also *Aspergillosis, allergic bronchopulmonary.*
  homogeneous segmental opacity in, 3087t
  in HIV disease, 1672–1673, *1672, 1673*
  invasive, 936–945
    diagnosis of, 945, 947
    epidemiology of, 936
    fungus ball progressing to, *922*
    homogeneous nonsegmental opacity in, 3080t
    in HIV disease, 1672–1673, *1672, 1673*
    multiple masses or nodules in, 3123t, *3126*
    pathogenesis of, 936
    prognosis in, 947
  pathogenesis of, 921
  pleural effusion in, 2751–2752
  saprophytic, 921–927
    airway colonization in, 921–923
    fungus ball in, 923–927. See also *Aspergilloma.*
    invasion of necrotic tissue in, 927
    solitary nodule due to. See *Aspergilloma.*
Aspergillus species, 919–921, *920*. See also *Aspergillosis.*
  Mucor species vs., 946
Asphyxia, traumatic, 2645
Asphyxiating thoracic dystrophy of the newborn, 3015
Aspiration (event), 2485–2513. See also *Aspiration pneumonia.*
  anaerobic pneumonia and, 778, 779
  bronchiolitis due to, *2326*
  of alcohol, 2512
  of barium, *2512*, 2513
  of carbohydrate solutions, 2512
  of corrosive fluids, 2512
  of esophageal contents, in gastroesophageal reflux, asthma and, 2113
  of gastric or oropharyngeal secretions, 2491–2500
    clinical features of, 2500
    conditions predisposing to, 2491
    pathogenesis of pulmonary damage due to, 2491–2492
    pathologic features of, 2492–2494, *2492–2496*
    prognosis in, 2500
    radiologic features of, 2494, *2497–2499*
  of kerosine, 2512
  of lipids, 2500–2507
    causes and pathogenesis of, 2500–2501
    clinical features of, 2506
    diagnosis of, 2506–2507
    pathologic features of, 2501, *2502–2504*
    prognosis in, 2506
    radiologic features of, *1139*, 2501–2506, *2504–2508*
    segmental opacity due to, homogeneous, 3088t
    inhomogeneous, 3098t
    solitary mass due to, 3118t

Aspiration (event) *(Continued)*
  of metallic mercury, 2513
  of solid foreign bodies, 2485–2490
    clinical features of, 2487–2490
    pathologic features of, 2486, *2487, 2490*
    pulmonary oligemia with, 3157t
    radiologic features of, 2486–2487, *2488–2490*
    segmental opacity due to, homogeneous, 3088t
      inhomogeneous, 3098t, *3100*
    upper airway obstruction due to, 2024, *2024*
  of water, 2507–2512
    clinical features of, 2510–2511
    diffuse air-space pattern in, 3130t
    pathogenesis of pulmonary reaction to, 2508–2509
    pathologic features of, 2509
    prognosis in, 2511–2512
    radiologic features of, 2509–2510, *2509–2511*
  of water-soluble contrast agents, 2512
  pneumatocele due to, in HIV infection, *1662, 1664*
  pulmonary infection acquisition by, 698, 699
  recurrent, inhomogeneous segmental opacity in, 3098t
Aspiration (procedure). See also *Fine-needle aspiration.*
  endotracheal, in pneumonia diagnosis, 719
  gastric, specimen collection by, in tuberculosis diagnosis, 844
Aspiration pneumonia. See also *Aspiration (event).*
  acute, pathologic features of, *2493*
    radiologic features of, *2494, 2497, 2498*
  anatomic bias of, *436,* 476
  chronic, pathologic features of, *2492, 2492*
    radiologic features of, *2494, 2499*
  consolidation in, 436, *436*
  defined, 778
  in polymyositis, 1465
  pathogenesis of, 699
  usage of term, 698, 2491
Aspirin. See *Acetylsalicylic acid.*
Asteroid bodies, in *Sporothrix schenckii* smear, 950
Asthma, 2077–2143
  ACE inhibitors and, 2570–2571
  acute episodes of, predicting recovery from, 2140
  adult-onset, obstructing tracheal tumor and, 1251, *5024*
  allergic, 2078
  allergic bronchopulmonary aspergillosis vs., 928
  atopic, 2078
  atopy and, 2078, 2079
  chronic bronchitis vs., 2170
  classification of, 2078–2079
  clinical features of, 2132–2136, 2135t
  complications of, 2140
  control of breathing in, 2139–2140
  corticosteroid therapy for, hypoventilation due to, 3065
  cough due to, 381, 2136
  cryptogenic, 2078
  cystic fibrosis and, 2309, 2310
  defined, 2077–2078
  diagnosis of, chest radiograph in, 2126–2127
    history in, 2132–2133
    in elderly persons, 2135
    nonspecific bronchial responsiveness measurement in, 2103–2104, *2103.* See also *Inhalation challenge tests.*
    physical examination in, 2133–2135

Asthma *(Continued)*
    diaphragmatic contour in, 496
    emphysema vs., *2027, 2221*
    environmental factors in, 2081
    epidemiology of, 2079–2080
    exercise-induced, 2078, 2106–2111
      delayed response in, 2111
      pathogenesis of, 2108–2110
      refractory period in, 2110–2111
    extrinsic, 2078
    extrinsic allergic alveolitis and, 2374
    extrinsic nonatopic, 2078
    flow-volume loop of, *2027, 2221*
    genetic considerations in, 2080–2082, 2081t
    heroin abuse and, 2567
    intrinsic, 2078
    laboratory findings in, 2136–2137
    laryngeal narrowing in, 2033
    meat-wrapper's, 2122
    mortality due to, 2141–2143
    nocturnal, 2078, 2135–2136
    nonatopic, 2078
    nonspecific occupational bronchoconstriction in, 2123
    normal chest radiographs in, 3047
    occupational, 2117–2124
      acquired airway hyper-responsiveness in, 2102
      causes of, possibly allergic, 2119t, 2121–2122
        proven allergic, 2117–2121, 2118t–2119t
      diagnosis of, 2122–2123
        nonspecific bronchial responsiveness measurement in, 2104
      organic dust toxic syndrome vs., 2124
      reactive airways dysfunction syndrome vs., 2124
    pathogenesis of, 2087–2124, *2088*
      bronchial hyper-responsivness in, 2094–2104, *2096.* See also under *Bronchial hyper-responsiveness.*
      inflammation in, 2088–2093, *2088*
      mucus and mucociliary clearance in, 2093–2094
      provoking factors in, 2104–2117
    pathologic features of, 2082–2087, *2083–2087*
    Pneumocystis carinii pneumonia and, 1668
    potroom, 2122
    prognosis in, 2140–2143
    pulmonary carcinoma and, 1081
    pulmonary function tests in, 2137–2140
    radiologic features of, 2124–2132
      on high-resolution CT, 2127–2132, *2131–2133*
      on plain radiographs, 2125–2127, *2125–2130*
    remissions in, 2140–2141
    respiratory syncytial virus infection and, 987, 2079–2080, 2111–2112
    rhinovirus infection and, 991, 2111–2112
    risk factors for, 2079–2080
    severity of, clinical grading scheme for, 2135, 2135t
    steroid-resistant, 2135
    strongyloidiasis and, 1041
    swine confinement areas and, 2379
    Tokyo-Yokohama, 2114
    tracheobronchial polyps and, 1371
    ventilation-perfusion abnormalities in, 2130–2132, *2134,* 2138–2139
Asthmatic bronchitis, defined, 2170
Ataxia-telangiectasia, 728
Atelectasis, 513–560
  adhesive, 522, *525*
    after radiation therapy, 2596
    defined, 513, 525

Atelectasis *(Continued)*
    postoperative, *2670, 2671,* 3088t
    after radiation therapy, 2596, *2600, 2602*
    air bronchogram in, 437–438
    cicatrization, 522–525, *526–528.* See also *Pulmonary fibrosis.*
      after radiation therapy, *2602*
      defined, 513, 525
      compensatory mechanisms in, 526–533, *531–536*
    compression, 513, 519, *520, 521*
      defined, 513
    discoid, 554–560, *558*
    due to metastatic neoplasm, *1402*
    due to pulmonary carcinoma, 1121–1128, *1122–1126, 1128, 1129*
    due to pulmonary thromboembolism, 1781
    gravity-dependent, 287, *291,* 513, 519–521, *521*
    in asthma, 2140
    in bronchiectasis, 2272, *2274*
    in bullous disease, 2237, *2240, 2241*
    in sarcoidosis, 1562
    in tuberculosis, 810–811
    interlobar fissure displacement in, 459
    linear, 554–560, *558*
    lobar, 539–554
      combined, 552–554, *555, 556*
      of left upper lobe, 543–549, *545–548*
      of lingula, 549
      of lower lobes, *536,* 552, *552, 553*
      of right middle lobe, 549–551, *549–551*
      of right upper lobe, 539–543, *542–544*
      subpulmonary effusion vs., 554, 568
    local overinflation with, 498, *498*
    loculated interlobar effusion vs., 581
    lung density in, 517–519, *519,* 539, *541*
    mechanisms of, 513–525
    nonobstructive, 513
    passive, 517–522, *519–521, 523, 524*
      defined, 513, 525
      dependent opacity on CT due to, 287, *291,* 513, 519–521, *521*
    patterns of, 534–560
    platelike, 554–560, *558*
    pleural effusion vs., 533, 554, 568, 581
    pleural relationships in, 534–539, *538*
    pneumothorax *ex vacuo* with, 2787
    postoperative, 2670–2671, *2670,* 3088t
      with nonthoracic surgery, 2672
    post-traumatic, 2623
    radiologic signs of, 525–534, *529–537,* 529t
    relaxation (passive), 517–522, *519–521, 523, 524*
      defined, 513, 525
      dependent opacity on CT due to, 287, *291,* 513, 519–521, *521*
    resorption, 513–517, *514–518*
      air bronchogram and, 533
      defined, 513, 525
    round, 521–522, *523, 524*
      asbestos-related, 522
        pathologic features of, *2430, 2432, 2433*
        pulmonary carcinoma vs., 2443, 2448
        radiologic features of, *523, 2438–2440, 2441–2443, 2447, 2448*
        solitary mass due to, 3118t, *3121*
    segmental, 554, *557*
    surfactant disruption in, 58
    total pulmonary, 539, *540*
    with endotracheal intubation, 2680
    with suspected lung cancer, investigation of, 1194
    with tracheobronchial fracture, 2621, *2621*
Atherosclerosis, pulmonary arterial, *13,* 72–74
    pulmonary hypertension with, 1882–1883, *1883*

Athletes, exercise-induced asthma in, 2107
ventilatory response of, genetic factors and, 240–241
Atopy, 2078. See also *Allergy.*
angioneurotic edema in, 2022
asthma and, 2078, 2079
bronchial hyper-responsiveness in, mechanisms of, 2094
childhood respiratory infection and, 2080
COPD and, 2180–2181
cystic fibrosis and, 2309, 2310
eosinophilic lung disease and, 1744, 1748
genetic considerations in, 2080–2082, 2081t
idiopathic pulmonary fibrosis and, 1586
occupational asthma and, 2117–2120
Atrial myxoma, pulmonary hypertension with, *1927–1928,* 1928
Atrial septal defect, increased pulmonary blood flow with, 664, *664*
pulmonary hypertension due to, *1892, 1894, 1895, 1895, 1896, 1896–1897*
Atrium, left, direct communication of right pulmonary artery with, 642
Atropine, before bronchoscopy, 367
mucociliary clearance and, 129
Attenuation, 291–292
ground-glass, in bronchiolitis, *2330,* 2331–2333, *2331, 2334*
in interstitial disease, 453–454, *455*
on high-resolution CT, 453, *455,* 456
mosaic, in bronchiolitis, 2330–2331, *2332*
in chronic pulmonary thromboembolism, 1811, 1813, *1815*
in healthy subjects, 290, 2331
in thromboembolic pulmonary hypertension, 1908, *1910*
of lung parenchyma, 287–291, *290, 291,* 292–294, *292, 293*
clinical significance of measurements of, 294
normal gradient of, 287–290, *290, 291*
structure identification and, 313
tissue density and, 269–270, 291–292
Augmentation mammoplasty, oil injection for, pulmonary embolism due to, 1871
silicone implants for, systemic lupus erythematosus and, 1425
silicone injection for, pulmonary embolism due to, 1870
Auscultation, in chest examination, 392–395
Autoantibodies. See also specific types of antibodies.
HLA antigens and, 1423–1424
in asbestos-exposed persons, 2423
in coal workers' pneumoconiosis, 2410–2411
in dermatomyositis/polymyositis, 1462–1463
in pulmonary vasculitis, 1489–1490
in Sjögren's syndrome, 1466
in systemic lupus erythematosus, 1422–1423, 1425
Autoimmune disease. See also *Connective tissue disease;* specific diseases.
focal lymphoid hyperplasia and, 1271
follicular bronchitis or bronchiolitis and, 1273, *1274*
idiopathic pulmonary fibrosis and, 1586, 1587
thymoma and, 2894–2896
Autonomic dysfunction syndromes, hypoventilation in, 3056
Autonomic nervous system, bronchial hyper-responsiveness and, 2098
Autonomic neuropathy, paraneoplastic, in pulmonary carcinoma, 1174
Auto-PEEP, 407, 495
in COPD, 2224
Axillary fold, anterior, on radiographs, 259

Axon reflex, in inflammation, 145
Axoneme, of airway cilium, 7, *8*
Azathioprine, for rheumatoid disease, malignancy and, 1451
thoracic disease due to, 2538t, 2555
Azoospermia, obstructive, 2283–2284
Azygoesophageal recess, 228–229, *232*
Azygos arch, 223–227, *226*
Azygos continuation of inferior vena cava, 2950, *2951–2953*
Azygos fissure, 162–164, *163, 164*
Azygos lobe, 162–164, *163, 164*
Azygos lymph node, 179
enlarged, dilated azygos vein vs., 2950, *2951*
in metastatic carcinoma, *2939*
in classification for lung cancer staging, *185, 1186*
Azygos vein, 218, *218*
azygos fissure and, 162–164, *163, 164*
dilation of, 2946, *2948,* 2950–2951, 2950t, *2951,* 3178t
measurement of, 223
size variation in, 223–227, *227–229*

Babesiosis, 1038
Bacillary angiomatosis, 1647, *1647*
Bacille Calmette-Guérin, 799, 848–849
tuberculin test response and, 842
Bacillus infection, 749–750
BACTEC method, for tuberculosis diagnosis, 845
Bacteremia, abscesses associated with, 3123t, *3125*
Bacteria. See also specific genera and species.
classification and nomenclature of, 735t
infection due to, 734–861
after bone marrow transplantation, 1730
after lung transplantation, 1713–1716, *1716*
cavities or cysts in, 3102t, *3105, 3106*
COPD exacerbations and, 2176–2177
diffuse nodular pattern in, 3145t, *3146, 3147*
due to aerobic and facultative organisms, 736–778
due to anaerobes, 778–783. See also *Anaerobic bacteria.*
homogeneous consolidation in, nonsegmental, 3079t–3080t
segmental, 3087t, *3089*
in HIV disease, 1643–1656
in sterile pulmonary infarct, 1829, *1829*
in systemic lupus erythematosus, 1432
inhomogeneous consolidation in, nonsegmental, 3093t, *3094*
segmental, 3097t, *3099*
lymph node enlargement in, 3164t, *3166*
pleural infusion due to, 2743–2751, 2744t
solitary mass due to, 3117t
solitary nodule due to, 3111t, *3113*
superimposed on viral infection, 980
Bacterial pseudomycosis, 958–960
Bacteroides infection, 779, 781
clinical features of, 782
diagnosis of, 783
pyopneumothorax due to, 2749
Bagassosis, 2362t, 2377–2378. See also *Extrinsic allergic alveolitis.*
Ball clay, pneumoconiosis due to, 2451–2452
BALT (bronchus-associated lymphoid tissue), 16, *16*
primary pulmonary lymphoma and, 1275
Bare area sign, 573, *575*
Barium, aspiration of, *2497, 2512,* 2513
embolization of, 1865–1868

Barium *(Continued)*
pneumoconiosis due to, 2456
Barium swallow, in esophageal obstruction diagnosis, 2861
in suspected esophageal perforation, 2852
Baroreceptors, in pulmonary arteries, 149
Barotrauma, air embolism due to, 1855
pneumomediastinum and, 2863–2865
to pulmonary capillary endothelium, in neurogenic pulmonary edema, 1976
Bartonella henselae infection, bacillary angiomatosis due to, 1647, *1647*
cat-scratch disease due to, 765
Bartonella quintana infection, in HIV disease, 1647, *1647*
Basal cells, of tracheobronchial epithelium, 6, 7, 8, 9
Basaloid carcinoma, pulmonary, 1113, *1114.* See also *Carcinoma, pulmonary.*
Basophils, in asthmatic airway inflammation, 2089
Bat's wing pattern, 437, 3130
in cardiogenic pulmonary edema, *435,* 1969–1970, *1972*
clinical features associated with, 1971
Bauxite, pneumoconiosis due to, 2460–2461, *2461*
Bayou virus, 992
Bazex's syndrome, 1174
Bcl-2 gene, 1083
BCNU (carmustine), thoracic disease due to, 2538t, 2548–2550, *2551*
Beclomethasone dipropionate, inhaled, thoracic disease due to, 2539t, 2571
Bedside radiography, 305–306
Behçet's disease, 1518–1521, *1519, 1520*
pulmonary artery aneurysm in, 1936, *1936, 1937*
Beryllium, pneumoconiosis due to, 2456–2460, *2458, 2459*
pulmonary carcinoma and, 1077, 2460
Besnier-Boeck-Schaumann disease. See *Sarcoidosis.*
Bicalutamide, thoracic disease due to, 2538t, 2551
Bicarbonate, as buffer, 116
carbon dioxide transport as, 114
Bifidobacterium eriksonii infection, 952
Biliary cirrhosis, in cystic fibrosis, 2312
primary, pulmonary involvement in, 1475
sarcoidosis vs., 1565
Biliary disease, pleural effusion with, 2764
Biliary-pleural fistula, 2764
Biliptysis, 380
Biologic response modifiers, thoracic disease due to, 2538t, 2555–2556
Biopsy, 369–374
after lung transplantation, in acute rejection diagnosis, 1703, 1705, 1706
in obliterative bronchiolitis diagnosis, 1710
bronchial, 369
in sarcoidosis diagnosis, 1570–1571
in idopathic pulmonary fibrosis diagnosis, 1611
in pleural effusion diagnosis, 2743
in tuberculosis, 2746
in sarcoidosis diagnosis, 1570–1571
in tuberculosis diagnosis, 844, 2746
mediastinal, 373–374
open lung, by thoracotomy, 372
pleural, closed, 372–373
scalene node, 374
in sarcoidosis diagnosis, 1571
surveillance, after lung transplantation, 1705
thoracoscopic, 371–372
transbronchial, 369–370

Biopsy (*Continued*)
  in carcinoid tumor diagnosis, 1242
  in extrinsic allergic alveolitis, 2375
  in sarcoidosis diagnosis, 1571
  in tuberculosis diagnosis, 844
  transthoracic needle, 370–371
    CT-guided, 315, 370
    of pleura, 372–373
    ultrasound-guided, 334, 370
Biotin-dependent carboxylase deficiency, 726
Biot's breathing, 2054n
Bipolaris infection, 952
Birbeck granules, 11, 1630, *1632*
    transmission electron microscopy for identification of, 354, *355*
Bird-fancier's lung, 2362t, 2377. See also
    Extrinsic allergic alveolitis.
  diffuse nodular pattern in, *3148*
  radiologic features of, *2370, 2372, 2374*
Bis(chloromethyl)ether, pulmonary carcinoma
    and, 1077
Black blood signal, 317
Black Creek virus, 992
Black Death, 758
Black lung. See *Coal workers' pneumoconiosis.*
Black pleural line, in alveolar microlithiasis,
    2721
Black-fat smoking, 2500
Blastoma, pleuropulmonary, 2840
  pulmonary, 1367–1369, *1369, 1370*
Blastomycosis, North American, 899–902,
    899–902
    cavities or cysts in, 3103t
    in HIV disease, 1672
    nonsegmental opacity in, homogeneous,
      3080t
      inhomogeneous, 3093t
    pleural effusion in, 2751
    solitary mass due to, 3117t
  South American, 902–904, *904*
Blebs, 508
  spontaneous pneumothorax and, 2781–2784,
    2782, 2790
Bleeding. See *Hemorrhage.*
Bleomycin, thoracic disease due to, 2538t,
    2540–2543, *2542, 2543*
Blood flow, pulmonary. See *Pulmonary blood
    flow.*
  systemic, alterations in, in venous thrombosis
    development, 1778
Blood fluke. See *Schistosomiasis.*
Blood gases, 114–115
  in COPD, 2225–2229
  renal function and, 2216–2217
Blood groups, COPD and, 2179
  venous thrombosis risk and, 1780
Blood pressure, systemic arterial, 395–396
  obstructive sleep apnea and, 2066–2067
Blood volume, pulmonary, defined, 104
  lung density and, 270, *271*
Blood-air barrier, development and growth of,
    137
  oxygen diffusion across, 107
  structure of, 17–21, *18, 20, 23–24, 23, 24*
  pulmonary edema and, 1947–1949, *1948*
Bloom's syndrome, 726
Blue bloaters, 2215. See also *Chronic
    obstructive pulmonary disease (COPD).*
  arterial desaturation during sleep in, 2227
  ventilation/perfusion mismatch in, 2225
Blue bodies, in desquamative interstitial
    pneumonia, 1611, *1613*
Bochdalek's foramen(ina), *248, 2987, 2988*
  hernia through, 2997–3001, *2998, 3002*
    middle-posterior mediastinal mass due to,
      3178t

Bochdalek's foramen(ina) (*Continued*)
    paravertebral mass due to, 3185t, *3189*
Body box, for airway resistance measurement,
    412
  for lung volume measurement, 407–408
    in COPD, 2225
Boeck's sarcoid. See *Sarcoidosis.*
Boerhaave's syndrome, pleural effusion with,
    2761
Bone, carcinoid tumor metastatic to, 1237
  in lung parenchyma, in pulmonary hyperten-
    sion, 1919, *1920, 1923, 1930*
  neoplasms of. See also specific neoplasms.
    in chest wall, 3029–3032, *3031–3038*
    in lung, 1345–1346
    paravertebral mass due to, 3185t
  pulmonary carcinoma invading, 1166, *1166*
  pulmonary carcinoma metastatic to, 1166,
    1167, 1173
    detection of, 1192
  radiation therapy's effects on, 2597
  sarcoidosis involving, 1562, 1565
  tuberculosis involving, 837–838, *838, 839*
  Wegener's granulomatosis involving, 1504
Bone marrow, embolization of, 1850, *1851*
  fat embolism from, 1846
    in sickle cell disease, 1833
Bone marrow transplantation, 1726–1732
  bronchiolitis after, 1728–1729, *1728, 1729,
    2332, 2336–2337*
  complications of, 1726–1732
  diffuse alveolar hemorrhage after, 1726–1727,
    1727
  graft-versus-host disease after, 1729
    obliterative bronchiolitis and, 1729
  idiopathic pneumonia syndrome after, 1727–
    1728
  infection after, 1730–1731, *1731*
  lymphocytic bronchitis after, 1729–1730
  pleural disease after, 1731–1732
  pulmonary edema after, 1726
  pulmonary function after, 1732
  tuberculosis risk and, 803–804
Booster phenomenon, in tuberculin testing, 843
Bordetella infection, 765. See also *Pertussis.*
Borrelia burgdorferi, sarcoidosis and, 1535
Botryomycosis, 958–960
Botulism, 3064
Boutonneuse fever, 1022
Boyden nomenclature of bronchial segments, 33,
    33t
Boyle's law, 407
Brachiocephalic vascular syndrome, due to
    cervical rib, 3013
Brachytherapy, complications of, 2592, 2604,
    2674–2675
Bradykinin, airway narrowing in response to, in
    asthma, 422
  in adult respiratory distress syndrome patho-
    genesis, 1983
  in asthmatic airway inflammation, 2093
  pulmonary metabolism of, 131
Brain. See *Central nervous system.*
Brainstem, in ventilatory control, *236*, 238–239,
    3050–3051, *3050*
Branhamella catarrhalis (*Moraxella catarrhalis*),
    bronchiectasis and, 2267
  pneumonia due to, 722, 748
Brasfield scoring system, for cystic fibrosis,
    2306
Breast augmentation, oil injection for, pulmonary
    embolism due to, 1871
  silicone implants for, systemic lupus erythema-
    tosus and, 1425
  silicone injection for, pulmonary embolism
    due to, 1870

Breast cancer, metastatic to lung, *1389*, 1405
  lymphangitic pattern of, *1391–1393*
  pleural effusion due to, 2759
  radiation therapy for, pulmonary carcinoma
    and, 1079, 1201
Breath sounds, adventitious, 394–395
  normal, 393–394
Breathing. See *Respiration; Ventilation.*
Brevetoxin, 3062
Bridging bronchus, 626
Bromocarbamide, thoracic disease due to, 2539t,
    2567
Bromocriptine, thoracic disease due to, 2571,
    2756
Bronchial adenoma, as term, problems with,
    1229, 1251
Bronchial arteriography, 325–326, *326*
Bronchial arteriovenous anastomoses, 77
Bronchial artery(ies), 119–120. See also
    Bronchial circulation.
  increased flow in, with decreased pulmonary
    circulation, 665
  innervation of, 149
  metastasis via, 1382
  pulmonary artery anastomoses with, 77
    in bronchiectasis, 395
Bronchial artery embolism, *1870*, 1871, *1871*
Bronchial artery embolization therapy, bronchial
    artery angiography before, 325–326, *326*
  for massive hemoptysis, 384
  pathologic findings after, *1870*, 1871
  radiologic findings after, 1871, *1871*
Bronchial atresia, congenital, 620–621, *621–624*
    hyperinflation with air trapping in, 497, *497*
    pulmonary oligemia in, 3157t, *3158*
Bronchial biopsy, 369
  in sarcoidosis diagnosis, 1570–1571
Bronchial breath sound, 394
Bronchial brushings, cytologic examination of,
    339–342, *342*, 367
    specimen processing for, 340
    in pneumonia diagnosis, 719–720
    in tuberculosis diagnosis, 843
Bronchial capillaries, 120
Bronchial challenge testing. See *Inhalation
    challenge tests.*
Bronchial circulation. See also *Bronchial
    artery(ies).*
  anatomy of, 119–120
  blood flow in, 120–121
  function of, 121
  in asthma, 2087, 2110
  in pulmonary fluid exchange, 1950
  innervation of, 120–121
  pulmonary circulation anastomoses with, 77
    in bronchiectasis, 395
Bronchial cuff sign, in pulmonary carcinoma,
    1129–1133, *1132–1134*
Bronchial cystadenoma, 1259
Bronchial epithelium, 5–12, *6, 7*
  damage to, in asthma, 2083, *2086*
    airway hyper-responsiveness and, 2097–
      2098
  development and growth of, 136, *138*
  fluid transport across, in pulmonary edema,
    1958
  in asthmatic airway inflammation, 2090
  response of, to injury, 9
Bronchial fistulas, 2289–2291, 2290t, *2291*
Bronchial glands. See *Tracheobronchial glands.*
Bronchial hyper-responsiveness, acquired, in
    occupational asthma, 2102
  defined, 2094
  genetic factors in, 2081
  in chronic pulmonary edema, 1972
  nonspecific, COPD and, 2180–2181

Bronchial hyper-responsiveness *(Continued)*
  genetic factors in, 2081
  in asthma, 2094–2104, *2096*
    airway smooth muscle alterations and,
        2100–2102
    altered aerosol deposition and, 2097
    increased mucosal permeability and,
        2097–2098
    inflammation and, 2102–2103
    neurohumoral control abnormalities and,
        2098–2100
    pathogenesis of, 2096–2103, *2096*
    starting airway caliber and, 2096–2097
  tests for. See *Inhalation challenge tests.*
Bronchial isomerism, 626
Bronchial mucus proteinase inhibitor, in
    emphysema pathogenesis, 2182–2183, *2183*
Bronchial nerves, 145, *147, 148*
Bronchial provocation testing. See *Inhalation
    challenge tests.*
Bronchial responsiveness. See also *Bronchial
    hyper-responsiveness.*
  nonspecific, defined, 2094
  tests for. See *Inhalation challenge tests.*
Bronchial stenosis, after transplantation,
        1722–1723, *1723*
  breath and voice sound changes with, 394
  congenital, 620
  in relapsing polychondritis, 1471, *1472*
  tuberculous, radiologic features of, 830–831,
        836
Bronchial tree. See also *Airway(s);
    Bronchiole(s); Bronchus(i); Trachea.*
  branching of, anomalous, 625–627, *627*
    factors influencing, 142
  cast preparation from, 351
  left, anteroposterior view of, *40–41*
    lateral view of, *42–43*
  right, anteroposterior view of, *36–37*
    lateral view of, *38–39*
Bronchial veins, 120
  pulmonary vein anastomoses with, 77
Bronchial wall thickening, in asthma,
        2125–2126, *2129, 2130*
    CT assessment of, 2127–2128, *2129–2130,
        2131*
  in chronic bronchitis, 2199–2203, *2202, 2203*
  in hydrostatic pulmonary edema, 1962–1963,
        1964
  in pulmonary carcinoma, 1129–1133, *1132–
        1134*
  visualization of, on high-resolution CT, 2127–
        2128, 2276
    on plain radiographs, 483, *485–487*
Bronchial washings, cytologic examination of,
        339–342, *342*
    specimen processing for, 340
  in pulmonary metastasis diagnosis, 1412
Bronchial–pulmonary artery fistula, 2290t, *2291,
        2291*
Bronchial-to-arterial diameter ratio. See *Artery-
    bronchus ratios.*
Bronchiectasis, 2265–2292
  after transplantation, 1723
  causes of, 2266t
  chronic, systemic arterial supply to the lung
        in, 666, *667*
  chronic bronchiolitis due to, 2269, *2271, 2326*
  classification of, 2266t
  clinical features of, 395, 2278
  congenital, 615
  cylindrical, *2268, 2268, 2270, 2271*
    bronchography in, *2278*
    CT findings in, 2275
  cystic (saccular), *2268, 2269, 2269, 2270*
    bronchography in, *2280*

Bronchiectasis *(Continued)*
    CT findings in, 2275, *2275, 2277*
    radiologic findings in, 2272, *2273,* 3104t,
        3109
  diagnosis of, bronchography in, 322
    CT in, *312, 385*
  heroin abuse and, 2567
  in allergic bronchopulmonary aspergillosis,
        929–935, *932–934*
  in chronic pulmonary thromboembolism, 1812
  in cystic fibrosis, 2304, *2309, 2310*
    lymphadenopathy with, 2277
    pathogenesis of, 2267
  in dyskinetic cilia syndrome, 2267, 2281,
        2283, *2284*
  in idiopathic pulmonary fibrosis, 1591, 1599,
        1600
  in Mounier-Kuhn syndrome, 2285–2287, *2286*
  in *Mycobacterium avium* complex infection,
        853, 855, *857–859*
  in panlobular emphysema, 2212
  in rheumatoid disease, 1448–1449, *1449*
  in tuberculosis, pathologic features of, *815,
        816,* 817, *823, 824,* 2269, *2270*
    radiologic features of, 830, *836*
  in Williams-Campbell syndrome, 2285
  in yellow nail syndrome, 2284–2285, *2285*
  in Young's syndrome, 2283–2284
  inhomogeneous segmental opacity due to,
        3098t
  normal chest radiographs in, 3047
  pathogenesis of, 2265–2268
  pathologic features of, 2268–2269, *2268–2271*
  prognosis in, 2281
  pulmonary function tests in, 2278–2281
  radiologic features of, *482, 483, 484,* 2272–
        2277, *2272–2280*
  traction, 525, *526,* 2267
    in pulmonary fibrosis, 1591, 1599, *1600,
        2271*
  varicose, 2268–2269
    bronchography in, *2279*
    CT findings in, 2275, *2275*
Bronchiectasis sicca, in tuberculosis, 817
Bronchiolar epithelium, 17, *17*
  development and growth of, 137
Bronchiole(s), lobular (preterminal), 26
  membranous, grading of inflammatory reac-
        tion in, 2189
    morphology and cell function of, 5–17, *8,
        11, 14, 16*
    smooth muscle of, 14, *14*
  respiratory, 17, *17*
    grading of inflammatory reaction in, 2189
Bronchiolectasis, traction, 525, *526*
Bronchiolitis, 701, *702,* 2321–2353
  acute, 2322, 2323t, 2333–2336
    due to infection, *2325, 2330,* 2333–2335,
        2335, 2336
    due to toxin inhalation, 2335–2336
    pathologic features of, *2325*
  causes of, 2322t
  chronic, 2336–2353
    histologic classification of, 2322–2327,
        2323t
    nonspecific, pathologic features of, 2324,
        2325–2327
    transmural, 2324–2327
  classification of, 2321–2327, 2322t–2324t
  constrictive. See also *Bronchiolitis, oblitera-
    tive.*
    cryptogenic, 2324
  diffuse, 2323t, 2349–2353, *2351, 2352*
  follicular, 1273, *1274,* 2323t, 2349, *2349,
        2350*
    in rheumatoid disease, 1273, *1274,* 1446–
        1448, *1447, 1448,* 2349, *2349, 2350*

Bronchiolitis *(Continued)*
  in bronchiectasis, 2269, *2271, 2326*
  in connective tissue disease, 2336
  in extrinsic allergic alveolitis, 2365, *2368*
  in invasive aspergillosis, *940*
  in Swyer-James syndrome pathogenesis, 2337,
        2338
  obliterative, 2324t
    after bone marrow transplantation, 1728–
        1729, *1728, 1729, 2332,* 2336–2337
    after lung transplantation, 1707–1711,
        1708–1710, 2336
      parainfluenza virus and, 1717
    due to aspiration of gastric contents, 2494,
        2496
    in rheumatoid disease, 1445–1446, *1446,
        1447*
    in systemic lupus erythematosus, 1431
    oligemia in, 3150t, *3155*
    pathologic features of, 2327, *2328*
    radiologic features of, *2329,* 2330–2331,
        2332
  pathologic features of, 2321–2327, 2323t–
        2324t, *2325–2328*
  radiologic features of, *30, 31,* 2327–2333,
        2329–2334
  respiratory, 2323t, 2348–2349, *2348*
    radiologic features of, 2331, *2331*
  viral, in infancy, asthma risk and, 2079–2080,
        2112
Bronchiolitis obliterans organizing pneumonia
    (BOOP), 2324t, 2344–2348
  after lung transplantation, 1711
  asbestos exposure and, 2430
  clinical features of, 2347
  defined, 1584
  homogeneous nonsegmental opacity in, 3081t
  in dermatomyositis/polymyositis, 1463, *1464*
  in rheumatoid disease, 1446
  in systemic lupus erythematosus, 1426, *1427,*
        1431
  pathologic features of, 2327, *2328,* 2344,
        2344, 2345
  prognosis in, 2347–2348
  radiologic features of, *2330,* 2331, *2333,*
        2344–2347, *2346, 2347*
    prognosis and, 2347–2348
Bronchioloalveolar carcinoma. See also
    Adenocarcinoma, pulmonary.
  air-space pattern in, 1149–1156, *1150–1155*
  bronchorrhea in, 1169–1170
  bubble lucencies in, 463, *470,* 1142, *1142*
  gross and histologic features of, 1101–1106,
        1103–1108
  homogeneous nonsegmental opacity in, 3081t,
        3085
  inflammatory reaction to, *1106,* 1120
  lymphangitic spread of, *1392*
  mucinous subtype of, *1008,* 1106
  nodular pattern in, 447, *452,* 3145t
  prognosis in, 1196
  pulmonary metastasis from, 1399
  sclerosing subtype of, 1106, *1107*
  ultrastructural features of, *1110*
  unusual presentations of, 1156
Bronchiologram, air, 438
Bronchitis, 701
  asthmatic, 2170
  chronic, 2170. See also *Chronic obstructive
    pulmonary disease (COPD).*
    asthma vs., 2170
    COPD and, 2168–2170, *2169*
    extrinsic allergic alveolitis and, 2374–2375
    mucociliary clearance in, 2181–2182
    pulmonary carcinoma and, 1081
    radiologic features of, 2199–2203, *2202,
        2203*

Bronchitis *(Continued)*
  swine confinement areas and, 2379
  follicular, 1273, *1274*
    in rheumatoid disease, 1446–1448
  in childhood, COPD and, 2176
  lymphocytic, after bone marrow transplanta-
    tion, 1729–1730
  obliterative, 2292
  plastic, *2291,* 2292
    in allergic bronchopulmonary aspergillosis,
      928
  tuberculous, 830
Bronchoalveolar lavage, 343
  in adult respiratory distress syndrome, 1996
  in alveolar proteinosis, 2706
    for treatment, 2708, *2709*
  in *Pneumocystis carinii* pneumonia, 1668
  in pneumonia, 720
  in pulmonary carcinoma, 1179
  in rejection, 1707
  in sarcoidosis, 1536, 1568
    prognosis and, 1573, 1573t
  in tuberculosis, 843–844
  indications for, 343, 367
Bronchoarterial diameter ratio. See *Artery-
  bronchus ratios.*
Bronchoarterial fistula, in coccidioidomycosis,
  894, *896*
Bronchobiliary fistula, 628, 2290t, *2291*
Bronchocele formation, in pulmonary carcinoma,
  1124–1125, 1131
Bronchocentric granulomatosis, in allergic
  bronchopulmonary aspergillosis, 928, *930*
  in tuberculosis, 817, *823*
Bronchoconstriction, due to pulmonary
  thromboembolism, 1781
  exercise-induced, 423–424
  nonspecific occupational, 2123
  reflex, bronchial hyper-responsiveness and,
    2098
Bronchodilator, response to, in COPD,
  2222–2223
  in cystic fibrosis, 2313
  testing for, 409
Bronchoesophageal fistula, 628, 2290–2291,
  2290t, 2967
  due to esophageal rupture, 2634
Bronchogenic carcinoma. See *Carcinoma,
  pulmonary.*
Bronchogenic cyst, 609–615
  anatomic bias of, 478
  mediastinal, *610,* 612–615, *613–617*
    middle-posterior mass due to, *2943, 2945,*
      3177t, *3179*
  on MRI, 614, *616*
  pathologic features of, 610–611, *610, 611*
  pulmonary, 611–612, *611–613*
    solitary nodule due to, 3111t
  rupture of, 614, *617*
Bronchogram, air, *435,* 437–438, *437*
  in atelectasis, 526, *529,* 533–534
  in pneumothorax, 519, *519*
  with solitary nodule, 1142, *1142*
Bronchography, 322
  in bronchiectasis, 2277, *2278–2280*
  specimen, 351
Bronchohepatic fistula, in amebiasis, 1035
  in echinococcosis, 1055
Broncholithiasis, 2287–2288, *2287–2289*
  in histoplasmosis, 881, *882,* 2287, *2288*
Bronchomycosis feniseciorum. See *Extrinsic
  allergic alveolitis; Farmer's lung.*
Bronchopancreatic fistula, with diaphragmatic
  rupture, 2643
Bronchophony, 394
Bronchopleural fistula, 2289–2290, 2290t

Bronchopleural fistula *(Continued)*
  after lung resection, 2663, 2762
Bronchopneumonia, 702–707, *706–711.* See also
  Pneumonia.
  acute, in invasive aspergillosis, 936–937, *937–
    940*
  combined air-space and interstitial pattern of
    increased density in, 454, *456*
  consolidation in, 437, *437*
  healing pattern in, 703, *707*
  pathologic features of, 702–703, *706, 707*
  pathophysiology of, 703–707, *709–711*
Bronchopulmonary lymph nodes, 180, *183, 184*
Bronchopulmonary sequestration, 601–609
  anatomic bias of, 477–478
  extralobar, 609
  intralobar, 602–609
    clinical features of, 609
    homogeneous nonsegmental opacity in,
      3079t
    pathologic features of, 602–604, *603*
    radiologic features of, 604–609, *605–608*
    solitary mass due to, 3117t
  pathogenesis of, 601–602
Bronchorrhea, in bronchioloalveolar carcinoma,
  1169–1170
Bronchoscopy, 367–369
  biopsy using, 369–370. See also *Biopsy, trans-
    bronchial.*
  complications of, 367
  cytologic examination of specimen collected
    by, 339–342, *342,* 367
  guidelines for, in adults, 368t
  in pneumonia diagnosis, 719–720
  in pulmonary metastasis diagnosis, 1412
  in tuberculosis diagnosis, 843–844
  in Wegener's granulomatosis diagnosis, 1505
  indications for, 367–369
  rigid, 369
  technical considerations in, 367
  therapeutic applications of, 369
  virtual, 311
Bronchospasm, wheezing and, 395
Bronchostenosis. See *Bronchial stenosis.*
Bronchovascular resistance, gas tension changes
  and, 121
Bronchus(i). See also *Airway(s); Bronchial tree.*
  abnormal number of, 626
  accessory cardiac, 626–627, *627*
  bridging, 626
  cartilage plates of, 12–13, *12, 13*
    calcification of, 474, *476*
    development and growth of, 136, *138*
    in COPD, 2187
  dehiscence of, after transplantation, 1721–
    1722, *1722*
  deviation of, in aortic rupture, 2628
  dilatation of, in asthma, 2130, *2132*
  displacement of, in atelectasis, 533, *534*
    in pulmonary venous hypertension, 533,
      535
  diverticula of, in COPD, 2187, *2188*
  epithelium of. See *Bronchial epithelium.*
  expiratory collapse of, in COPD, 2222, *2222,
    2223*
  fracture of, homogeneous segmental opacity
    in, 3088t
    with blunt trauma, 2618–2622, *2621, 2622*
  intermediate, 35
    defined, 33
    on CT, 50, *51*
  left lower lobe, *40–43,* 46, *49,* 50
    on CT, 50–51, *51–52*
  left upper lobe, *40–43,* 46, *48*
    on CT, 50, *51*
    on lateral radiograph, 84, *88–89*

Bronchus(i) *(Continued)*
  lingular, *40–43,* 46, *48, 49*
    on CT, 50, *51–52*
  lobar, abnormal origin of, 626, *627*
    development and growth of, 136, *137*
    imaging of, 35–36, *36–50*
  lower lobe, defined, 33
  main, defined, 33
    imaging of, 35
    measurement of, 35
  metastasis to, 1397–1398, *1400–1402*
  middle lobe, defined, 33
  morphology and cell function of, 5–17, *5–7,
    12, 13, 15*
  mucosa of, increased permeability of, airway
    hyper-responsiveness and, 2097–2098
  on CT, 46–51, *51–52,* 281–286, *282*
  pig, 35, 626, *627*
  right lower lobe, 35–46, *36–39, 45–47*
    on CT, 50–51, *51–52*
  right middle lobe, 35, *36–39, 45*
    on CT, 50, *51–52*
  right upper lobe, 35, *36–39, 44*
    on CT, 46–50, *51*
    on lateral radiograph, 84–87, *88–89*
  segmental, abnormal origin of, 626, *627*
    imaging of, 35–36, *36–50*
    nomenclature of, 33, 33t
  smooth muscle of, 14. See also *Airway
    smooth muscle.*
  tracheal, 35, 626, *627*
  transplantation complications involving, 1721–
    1724, *1722, 1723*
  upper lobe, defined, 33
  wall of, in asthma, 2083–2087, *2086, 2087*
    radiographic visualization of, 483, *486, 487*
    thickening of. See *Bronchial wall thick-
      ening.*
Bronchus suis, 35, 626, *627*
Bronchus-associated lymphoid tissue (BALT),
  16, *16*
  primary pulmonary lymphoma and, 1275
Brown induration, in postcapillary pulmonary
  hypertension, 1919
Brownian movement, in particle deposition, 127
Brucella species, *Francisella tularensis* cross-
  reactivity with, 767
  pulmonary infection due to, 765
Brucellosis, 765
Brugia malayi infestation. See *Eosinophilia,
  tropical.*
Brush cell, in tracheobronchial epithelium, 9
Brushings, bronchial. See *Bronchial brushings.*
Bruton's agammaglobulinemia, 724–725
Bubble lucencies, 463, *470*
  in solitary nodules, 1142, *1142*
Buffers, in acid-base balance maintenance, 116
Building-associated allergic alveolitis, 2362t,
  2378. See also *Extrinsic allergic alveolitis.*
Bulging fissure sign, in nonsegmental air-space
  pneumonia, 702, *705*
Bulla(e), 504–508, *507–509.* See also *Bullous
  disease.*
  apical, in Marfan's syndrome, 676, *677*
  collapsed lung adjacent to, 519, *521*
  defined, 2234
  in ankylosing spondylitis, 3022
  in Ehlers-Danlos syndrome, 677, *679*
  in emphysema, 2204, *2204–2206,* 2234–2235,
    2235, 2236, 2238–2239
  in neurofibromatosis, *688, 689,* 690–691
  infected, 2237, *2242*
  pathologic features of, 2234–2236, *2235, 2236*
  primary spontaneous pneumothorax and,
    2781–2784, *2782, 2783*
  radiologic definition of, 461

Bulla(e) *(Continued)*
    radiologic features of, 2236–2240, *2237–2243,* 3104t, *3109*
    secondary spontaneous pneumothorax and, 2784, 2785–2787, *2785*
Bullectomy, 2242, 2243
Bullet fragment embolism, 1868, *1868,* 2652
Bullet wound, 2647–2648, 2648–2652, *2648, 2649, 2651*
Bullous disease, 2234–2243. See also *Bulla(e).*
    clinical features of, 2240
    pathologic features of, 2234–2236, *2235, 2236*
    pulmonary function tests in, 2240–2243
    radiologic features of, 2236–2240, *2237–2243*
Bumetanide, thoracic disease due to, 2572
Bupivacaine, thoracic disease due to, 2572
Buprenorphine, thoracic disease due to, 2539t, 2567
Burkholderia cepacia infection, in cystic fibrosis, 761
    lung transplantation and, 1700
    pathogenetic role of, 2301, 2302
    prognosis and, 2315
Burkholderia gladioli infection, 761
Burkholderia mallei infection, 760–761
Burkholderia picketti (Ralstonia picketti) infection, 765
Burkholderia pseudomallei infection, 759–760
Burkitt's lymphoma, 1291
    in HIV infection, 1681–1682
Burns, bronchopulmonary disease associated with, 2528–2531, *2529, 2530*
    upper airway obstruction due to, 2023–2024
Busulfan, thoracic disease due to, 2538t, 2544–2545, *2546–2548*
Butterfly pattern, 437
    in cardiogenic pulmonary edema, *435,* 1969–1970, *1972*
    clinical features associated with, 1971
Byssinosis, 2124

C receptors. See *J receptors.*
C1 esterase inhibitor, in angioneurotic edema, 2023
C5a (complement component), in adult respiratory distress syndrome, 1981
Cabergoline, pleural effusion due to, 2756
Cadmium exposure, 2527–2528
    COPD and, 2175
    experimental emphysema induced by, 2186
    pulmonary carcinoma and, 1078
Café-coronary syndrome, 2487–2490, *2490*
Calcification, benign patterns of, 467, *472*
    due to remote *Varicellavirus* pneumonia, 1001, *1003*
    eggshell, *452, 474, 476*
        in sarcoidosis, 1545, 1547
        in silicosis, *452,* 474, 2402, *2403*
    in airway cartilage plates, 13, *13,* 474, *476*
    in bronchogenic cyst, 611, *613,* 614
    in carcinoid tumor, 1237
    in coal workers' pneumoconiosis, 2414, 2416–2418
    in costal cartilage, 261–262, *261*
    in diffuse pleural fibrosis, *2803, 2804, 2804, 2805*
    in focal fibrosing mediastinitis, 2857, 2861, *2863*
    in histoplasmosis, 880, 881, *881–884*
    in pleural plaques, 583, *585,* 2435, *2436,* 2801, *2803*
    in pulmonary hamartoma, 467, *472,* 1352–1354, *1354–1357*
    in pulmonary metastasis, 1389, *1391*

Calcification *(Continued)*
    in silicosis, *452,* 474, 2394, *2398,* 2402, *2403*
    in solitary mass, 1148, *1148*
    in solitary nodule, *315,* 1135–1139, *1136–1138,* 1193
    in thymoma, 2886, *2893*
    in tuberculoma, 827, *832*
    in tuberculosis, 463–467, *476,* 805, 811, *812,* 827, *833*
    intra-arterial, after fat embolism, 1848
    metastatic, 2699–2700, *2700, 2701*
        after liver transplantation, 1732–1734
    nodular, 467–474, *475*
    of lymph nodes, *452,* 467, *471,* 474, *476*
        after radiation therapy in Hodgkin's disease, 1302, *1305*
        in sarcoidosis, 1545, 1547, *1550*
        in silicosis, 2402, *2403*
    on radiographs and CT, 463–474, *471–476*
    parenchymal, diffuse, 467–474, *474, 475*
        local, 463–467, *471*
    pericardial, after radiation therapy, 2597, *2605*
    pleural, 583, *584, 585*
        in pancreatitis, 2765
    popcorn, in pulmonary hamartoma, 467, *472,* 1354, *1354*
    pulmonary artery, in pulmonary hypertension, 1886, *1890*
    punctate, 467, *474*
Calcifying fibrous pseudotumor of pleura, 2840
Calcitonin, pulmonary carcinoma secreting, 1177
Calcitriol, in sarcoidosis pathogenesis, 1566
Calcium, in airway smooth muscle contraction, 2100
Calcium oxalate crystals, in aspergillosis, *920, 921*
Calcofluor white, in fungal infection diagnosis, 876
Canalicular period of lung development, 137, *139*
Canal(s) of Lambert, 32
Candidiasis, 916–919, *917–919*
    after transplantation, 1717, *1719*
    chronic mucocutaneous, 725–726
Cantharidin poisoning, 3062
Capillariasis, 1047
Capillaritis, *1426, 1498*
    in microscopic polyangiitis, 1513
    in systemic lupus erythematosus, 1426
    in Wegener's granulomatosis, 1496
Caplan's syndrome, 1438–1443, 2416, *2417*
    in silicosis, 2402–2404
Capnocytophaga infection, 776
Capsaicin, afferent nerve effects of, 145
    cough evaluation using, 381
Carbachol inhalation, for bronchial reactivity assessment, 421, 421t
Carbamate insecticides, 2587
Carbamazepine, thoracic disease due to, 2539t, 2564–2565
Carbohydrate, aspiration of solutions of, 2512
    dietary, exercise capacity and, in COPD, 2227–2228
Carbon black, pneumoconiosis due to, 2409–2410, 2413
Carbon dioxide. See also *Hypercapnia.*
    daily production of, 115
    diffusion of, from blood to acinar gas, 107
    receptors for, in upper airway and lung, in control of ventilation, 241
    transport of, in blood, 114
Carbon dioxide dissociation curve of blood, *110*
    ventilation/perfusion mismatch and, 110
Carbon dioxide partial pressure, acinar, 53, *54*
    arterial, determinants of, 115
Carbon monoxide, diffusing capacity measurement using, 108, 414–416

Carbon monoxide *(Continued)*
    in COPD, 2229
    poisoning by, 3068–3069
Carbon oxychloride inhalation, 2526
Carbonic anhydrase, in red blood cells, 114
Carborundum, pneumoconiosis due to, 2463–2465, *2465, 2466*
Carboxylase deficiency, biotin-dependent, 726
Carcinoembryonic antigen, in adenocarcinoma vs. mesothelioma, 2818–2819, 2826
    in carcinoid tumors, 1233
Carcinoid syndrome, 1241–1242
    diagnosis of, 1242
    paraneoplastic, in pulmonary carcinoma, 1176
Carcinoid tumor, 1229–1243
    atypical, pathologic features of, 1234, *1236*
        prognosis in, 1243
        radiologic features of, 1237–1241, *1241, 1242*
        usage of term, 1246
    clinical features of, 1241–1242
    diagnosis of, 1242–1243
    metastases from, 1237, 1243
    oligemia with, 3157t, *3160*
    pathologic features of, 1230–1234, *1230–1236*
    prognosis in, 1243
    pulmonary tumorlets/neuroendocrine cell hyperplasia and, 1243–1245, *1244–1246*
    radiologic features of, 467, 1234–1241, *1237–1242*
    segmental opacity due to, homogeneous, 3087t
        inhomogeneous, 3097t
    small cell carcinoma vs., 1234, 1242
    solitary nodule due to, 3112t
    thymic, 2900–2901, *2900, 2901*
    ultrastructure of, 1233–1234, *1235*
Carcinoma. See also *specific types.*
    acinic cell, tracheobronchial gland, 1258
    adenoid cystic, submaxillary gland, metastatic to lung, *1388*
        tracheal, 2036, *2039, 3180*
        tracheobronchial gland, 1253–1256, *1253–1256*
    adrenal, metastatic, enlarged azygos node with, *2939*
    at site of foreign body, 2653
    breast, metastatic to lung, *1389,* 1405
        lymphangitic pattern of, *1391–1393*
        pleural effusion due to, 2759
        radiation therapy for, pulmonary carcinoma and, 1079, 1201
    bronchioloalveolar. See *Bronchioloalveolar carcinoma.*
    cervical, metastatic, in lung, 1407–1408
        in thoracic skeleton, *3038*
    colorectal, metastatic to lung, *1385, 1387, 1396, 1400,* 1404–1405
    dermatomyositis/polymyositis and, 1465
    esophageal, 2961–2965, *2966*
        radiation therapy for, airway-esophageal fistula due to, 2967
        with perforation, mediastinitis with, *2855*
    head and neck, metastatic to lung, 1405
        cavitation in, 1389, *1390*
        pulmonary carcinoma and, 1201–1202
    hepatocellular, metastatic to lung, 1405
    laryngeal, pulmonary carcinoma and, 1202
    metastatic. See *Metastasis(es); specific primary tumors and sites.*
    mucoepidermoid, tracheobronchial, *1252,* 1256–1258, *1257, 1258*
    oropharyngeal, metastatic to trachea, *2041*
    ovarian, metastatic, in diaphragm, 3006
        in lung, 1408
    pleural, 2838
    pleural effusion due to, 2756–2759, *2758*

Carcinoma *(Continued)*
   prostatic, metastatic to lung, 1408
   pulmonary, 1069–1202. See also *Adenocarcinoma, pulmonary.*
      adenosquamous, 1113–1114, *1115*
         mucoepidermoid carcinoma and, 1256–1257
         prognosis in, 1196
      air bronchogram with, 1142, *1142*
      anatomic bias of, 477, 1120–1121
      apical, 1156–1165, *1162–1164*
         apical cap vs., 2796, *2798*
         extrapulmonary features of, 1171–1172
      asbestos exposure and, 1074–1076, 2448
      atelectasis due to, 1121–1128, *1122–1126, 1128, 1129*
      basaloid, 1113, *1114*
      beryllium and, 1077, 2460
      bone involvement in, 1166, *1166, 1167*
      bronchial wall thickening in, 1129–1133, *1132–1134*
      bronchioloalveolar. See *Bronchioloalveolar carcinoma.*
      bronchogenic cyst and, 612, 615
      bubble lucencies in, 463, *470*
      calcification in, 1135, *1137, 1138,* 1148, *1148*
      causes of, 1072–1082
      cavitation in, 462, *465, 1091,* 1148–1149, *1149,* 3104t, *3108*
      chest wall involvement in, *1164,* 1165–1166, *1166*
      classification of, 1071t, 1084–1085
      clear cell, 1112–1113, *1113*
      clinical features of, 1169–1178
         bronchopulmonary, 1169–1170
         extrapulmonary intrathoracic, 1170–1172, *1170*
         extrathoracic, 1172–1178
         prognosis and, 1199–1200
      coal workers' pneumoconiosis vs., 2416
      constitutional symptoms in, 1173
      contrast enhancement of, 1143–1146, *1146, 1147*
      cystic lesion due to, 510, 3104t
      diagnosis of, 1179–1181
         bronchial brushings and washings in, 341, *342,* 1179
         bronchoscopy in, 369
         CT in, *384,* 1180
         sputum cytology in, 340–341, *342,* 1179
         transthoracic needle aspiration in, 346, *347*
      doubling time of, 1142–1143, *1144, 1145*
      epidemiology of, 1070–1072
      genetic factors in, 1082
      giant cell, 1117, *1118*
         autonomic neuropathy in, 1174
         doubling time of, 1143, *1145*
         prognosis in, 1196
      hepatoid, 1113
      hilar enlargement in, 1156, *1157, 1158*
      idiopathic pulmonary fibrosis and, 1608
      in HIV infection, 1683
      in Hodgkin's disease, 1312
      in progressive systemic sclerosis, 1460, *1461*
      in rheumatoid disease, 1451
      infection in, 1121–1128, *1128*
      inflammatory reaction to, *1106,* 1120, *1120*
      interlobar fissure displacement in, 459–460, *461*
      investigation of patient with, 1178–1194
         with specific radiographic patterns, 1193–1194
      iron dust exposure and, 2454

Carcinoma *(Continued)*
      large cell, 1110–1113. See also *Large cell carcinoma, pulmonary.*
      local spread of, 1117, *1119*
      lung volume change in, 1128–1129, *1129*
      lymph node enlargement in, 3165t, *3168*
      lymphoepithelioma-like, 1113, *1115*
         Epstein-Barr virus and, 1079
         prognosis in, 1196
      mediastinal involvement in, 1156, *1158–1161*
         clinical features of, 1170–1171, *1170*
      metastases from, clinical features of, 1172–1173
         detection of, 1181, 1191–1193, *1192*
         pulmonary, 1399
         thromboembolism vs., *1821*
      metastatic pulmonary nodule vs., 1387–1388
      mucoid impaction in, *1124–1125,* 1129, *1130, 1131*
      multiple primary, 1201
      neoplasms associated with, 1201–1202
      nodule-lung interface in, 1139, *1139–1141*
      oat cell, 1091–1096, *1096.* See also *Small cell carcinoma, pulmonary.*
      obstructive pneumonitis due to, 1121–1128, *1122–1127, 1129*
      oligemia with, 3157t
      paraneoplastic syndromes with, 1173–1178
      pathogenesis of, 1082–1084
      pathologic features of, 1084–1120
         heterogeneity of, 1085, *1086*
      pleomorphic, 1114–1117, *1116*
         prognosis in, 1196
      pleural effusion due to, 2758
      pleural involvement in, 1165, *1165*
         clinical features of, 1170
         mesothelioma vs., 1165, *1165,* 2818–2820, *2819,* 2826
      prognosis in, 1195–1201, 1198t, *1199*
      pulmonary artery compression by, unilateral oligemia due to, *506*
      radiologic features of, 1120–1169
         time of appearance of, 3046
      round atelectasis vs., 2443, 2448
      sarcomatoid, 1116
      scar, 1080, *1080*
      screening for, 1194–1195
      second primary, 1201
         after small cell carcinoma treatment, 1196
      segmental opacity in, homogeneous, 3087t–3088, *3090*
         inhomogeneous, 3097t
      silicosis and, 1077, 2408
      small cell, 1091–1098. See also *Small cell carcinoma, pulmonary.*
      solitary mass due to, 3117t, *3120*
      solitary nodule due to, 3112t, *3114*
      spindle cell, 1114
      spontaneous regression of, 1201
      squamous cell, 1085–1091. See also *Squamous cell carcinoma, pulmonary.*
      staging of, 1181–1193
         clinical-severity, 1200
         M assessment in, 1191–1193, *1192*
         methods of, 1181
         N assessment in, 1183–1191, *1186,* 1187t, *1188, 1189*
         prognosis and, 1198–1199, 1198t, *1199*
         regional lymph node classification for, 180–184, *185,* 188t, 1186, *1186,* 1187t
         schemes for, 1181, 1182t
         T assessment in, 1182–1183, *1183–1185*

Carcinoma *(Continued)*
      thoracoscopic biopsy in, 371–372
      superior vena cava syndrome due to, 1171, 2949, 2950, *2950*
      three-dimensional morphology of, 1120, *1121*
      tuberculosis and, 848, 1080–1081
      tumor markers for, 1179
         prognosis and, 1200–1201
      vascular invasion and proliferation by, 1118–1120
      vascular supply of, 1117–1118
      small cell. See *Small cell carcinoma.*
      squamous cell. See *Squamous cell carcinoma.*
      thymic, 2897–2899, *2898, 2899,* 3171t
      thyroid, 2913
         metastatic, calcification in, 467
            to chest wall, *3035*
            to lung, 1405–1407
         upper airway obstruction due to, 2031–2032, *2032*
      tracheal, 2942
         upper airway obstruction due to, 2035–2036, *2037, 2039*
      tracheobronchial gland, 1251–1258
         acinic cell, 1258
         adenoid cystic, 1253–1256, *1253–1256*
         mucoepidermoid, *1252,* 1256–1258, *1257, 1258*
      upper airway, pulmonary carcinoma and, 1201–1202
Carcinomatosis, lymphangitic. See *Lymphangitic carcinomatosis.*
Carcinosarcoma, pleural, 2835
   pulmonary, 1114–1117, *1116, 1117*
      prognosis in, 1196
      pulmonary blastoma and, 1367–1368
Cardiac. See also *Heart* entries.
Cardiac bronchus, accessory, 626–627, *627*
Cardiac catheterization, in pulmonary hypertension, complications of, 1891
Cardiac incisura, 204–205, *206*
Cardiac output, pulmonary artery pressure and, 104, *105*
Cardiac tamponade, with pulmonary carcinoma, 1171
Cardiomyopathy, congestive, after radiation therapy, *2605*
Cardiophrenic angle, fat in, enlargement of, *2916, 2918,* 2925–2927
   radiographic interpretation of, 233
   tumors in, 2925–2929
Cardioplegia, cold, unilateral diaphragmatic paralysis due to, 2989
Cardiothoracic ratio, 229
Carinal angle, measurement of, 35
Carinal lymph nodes, 179, *182*
Carmustine (BCNU), thoracic disease due to, 2538t, 2548–2550, *2551*
Carney's triad, 1344, *1344, 1345*
Carnitine deficiency, rhabdomyolysis due to, 3065
Carotenoids, mesothelioma and, 2810
   pulmonary carcinoma and, 1081–1082
Carotid artery, buckling of, 2961
Carotid body, excision of, hypoventilation due to, 3056
   in respiratory control, 235–237, *236, 3050, 3051*
   in ventilatory response to exercise, 241
Carotid endarterectomy, hypoventilation due to, 3052, 3056
Cartilage, costal, calcification of, 261–262, *261*
   in conducting airways, 12–13, *12, 13*
      calcification of, 474, *476*
      development and growth of, 136, *138*

Cartilage (Continued)
in COPD, 2187
neoplasms of, 1343–1345. See also specific
neoplasms.
paravertebral mass due to, 3185t
Cartilage hypoplasia, immunodeficiency with,
726
Carvallo's sign, in cor pulmonale, 1934
Caseation necrosis, in tuberculosis, 805,
807–809
Cast formation, bronchial, 2291, 2292
Castleman's disease, 2760, 2938–2940,
2940–2942
Cat dander, asthma and, 2106
Catalase, in defense against oxidant damage,
2521
Catecholamines, endogenous release of, in
asthma, 2099
Catheter(s), central venous, complications of,
2682–2685, 2682–2687
pleural effusion due to, 2762
superior vena cava syndrome due to, 2949
complications of, 2681–2690
for empyema drainage, ultrasound-guided,
334, 334
for pulmonary angiography, improvements in,
1818
intravascular, cytologic examination of material aspirated from, 348
embolization of, 1868, 1869
pulmonary arterial, indwelling balloon-tipped,
complications of, 2685–2690, 2688,
2689
cytologic examination of material aspirated from, 348
pleural effusion due to, 2762
transtracheal, complications of, 2681
Cat-scratch disease, 765
Caveolae intracellulares, in pulmonary
endothelium, 75, 75
Cavitation, 461–463, 463–470
benign vs. malignant, 1148–1149
differential diagnosis of, 3101, 3102t–3104t,
3105–3109
in coccidioidomycosis, 894, 894, 895, 897,
3103t
in Hodgkin's disease, 1302–1306, 1308
in pulmonary carcinoma, 1091, 1148–1149,
1149, 3104t, 3108
anatomic bias and, 477
in pulmonary metastasis, 1389, 1390, 3104t
in sarcoidosis, 1561, 1561, 1562, 3104t
in tuberculosis, disease transmission and, 800
pathologic features of, 813–814, 813, 814,
817–819
radiologic features of, 463, 824, 829, 3106
in Wegener's granulomatosis, 462, 466, 1499,
1500, 3104t, 3108
Cavity. See also Cavitation.
radiologic definition of, 461–462
CCNU (lomustine), thoracic disease due to,
2538t, 2548
CD11/CD18 protein, in leukocyte–endothelial
cell adherence in adult respiratory distress
syndrome, 1979
Cedar, occupational asthma due to, 2121
Celiac disease, extrinsic allergic alveolitis and,
2375
idiopathic pulmonary hemorrhage and, 1758,
1763
Cell-mediated immunity, in dermatomyositis/
polymyositis, 1463
in host response to neoplasia, 1083–1084
in pulmonary vasculitis, 1490
in rheumatoid disease, 1434
in Wegener's granulomatosis, 1493–1494

Cell-mediated immunity (Continued)
pulmonary, 131
Cellulose embolism, 1857–1861
pathologic features of, 1858
Cement dust, pneumoconiosis due to, 2468
Central nervous system, Churg-Strauss syndrome
involving, 1510
coccidioidomycosis involving, 895
disorders of, alveolar hypoventilation due to,
3049t, 3051–3055
hyperventilation due to, 3066
Mycoplasma pneumoniae infection involving,
1014
neoplasms of, metastatic to lung, 1411–1412
pulmonary carcinoma metastatic to, 1172–
1173
sarcoidosis involving, 1566
tuberculosis involving, 838–839
Wegener's granulomatosis involving, 1504
Central sleep apnea. See Sleep apnea, central.
Central tendon of diaphragm, 248, 248, 249
Central venous catheter(s), complications of,
2682–2685, 2682–2687
pleural effusion due to, 2762
superior vena cava syndrome due to, 2949
Cepacia syndrome, 2302
Cephalometry, lateral, in obstructive sleep apnea,
2063, 2064
Cephalosporins, thoracic disease due to, 2538t,
2558
Cephradine, thoracic disease due to, 2558
c-erbB-2 gene, 1083
Cerebellar degeneration, subacute, paraneo-
plastic, in pulmonary carcinoma, 1174
Cerebral dysfunction, alveolar hypoventilation
due to, 3051–3052
Cerebral venous thrombosis, in pulmonary
carcinoma, 1177
Cerebrospinal fluid, hydrogen ion concentration
in, ventilatory response and, 237
in tuberculosis diagnosis, 844
Cerebrotendinous xanthomatosis, 2727
Cerebrovascular accident, alveolar
hypoventilation due to, 3051
central apnea after, 3053
obstructive sleep apnea and, 2067
Cerium, pneumoconiosis due to, 2456
Ceroidosis, 2727
Cervical aortic arch, 2961
Cervical carcinoma, metastatic, in lung,
1407–1408
in thoracic skeleton, 3038
Cervical fascia, deep, 198
Cervical lymph nodes, in metastatic upper
airway cancer vs. primary lung cancer
distinction, 1202
Cervical rib, 262, 263, 3012–3013, 3013
Cervicomediastinal continuum, 197–198,
197–199
Cervicothoracic continuum, 198
Cervicothoracic sign, 97, 197
Cestodes, 1053–1059. See also specific diseases.
CFTR (cystic fibrosis transmembrane regulator),
62, 2300
COPD and, 2178
Chaetomium species infection, 952
Challenge testing. See Inhalation challenge tests.
Charcot-Leyden crystals, in asthma, 2083, 2084
Chédiak-Higashi syndrome, 727
Cheese-worker's lung, 2362t. See also Extrinsic
allergic alveolitis.
Chemicals, inhaled. See Inhaled substances;
specific substances.
Chemodectomas, 1363–1364
aorticopulmonary, 2942–2943, 2943
aorticosympathetic, 2977–2978

Chemodectomas (Continued)
minute pulmonary, 74, 1364, 1374–1375, 1376
pulmonary chondroma with, 1344
Chemokines, in adult respiratory distress
syndrome, 1979
in asthmatic airway inflammation, 2092
Chemoreceptors, in pulmonary veins, 149
in respiratory control, 3050, 3051
peripheral, hypoventilation due to disorders of,
3056
Chemotactic factors, in asthmatic airway
inflammation, 2092
Chemotherapy. See also specific drugs and
classes of drugs.
for Hodgkin's disease, long-term effects of,
1312
for small cell pulmonary carcinoma, acute leukemia after, 1202
Pneumocystis carinii pneumonia and, 909
radiation effect enhancement by, 2593
thoracic disease due to, 2538t, 2540–2551
thymic rebound hyperplasia after, 2877, 2879
Chest. See also Chest wall.
anteroposterior diameter of, lung volume and,
496–497
deformity of, pulmonary hypertension with,
1918
injury to, pneumothorax due to, 2790
physical examination of, 391–395
Chest drainage tubes, complications of,
2676–2677, 2677–2679
Chest pain, 385–387
Chest syndrome, acute, in sickle cell disease,
1832–1834
Chest wall, 3011–3032
actinomycosis involving, 955, 2751
bones of, imaging of, 260–264, 261–264
edema of, after thoracentesis, 2741, 2742
MR evaluation of, 321, 322
neoplasms of, 3023–3032, 3026–3038
nocardiosis involving, 2751
nonpenetrating trauma's effects on, 2644–2647
pressure-volume relationships of, 53–54, 55,
56
pulmonary carcinoma involving, 1164, 1165–
1166, 1166
radiographic anatomy of, 259–264, 259–264
soft tissues of, imaging of, 259–260, 259–261
surgical complications involving, 2659–
2660
Chest wall pain, 386–387
pleural pain vs., 385–386, 387
Cheyne-Stokes respiration, 2054n, 3066
Chickenpox, clinical features of, 1001–1003
epidemiology of, 999–1000
laboratory findings in, 1003
pathogenesis of, 1000–1001
pneumonia due to. See under Varicellavirus infection.
Child(ren). See also Infant(s); Neonate(s).
empyema in, 2747–2749
hoarseness in, 389
pneumonia in, bronchiectasis and, 2267, 2278
respiratory tract infection in, asthma and, 987,
991, 2080, 2111–2112
atopy and, 2080
COPD and, 2176
China clay, pneumoconiosis due to, 2451–2452
Chlamydia(e), 1015–1019
Chlamydia pneumoniae, 722, 1016–1017, 3097t
Chlamydia psittaci, 1017–1019, 1019, 3097t
Chlamydia trachomatis, 1017
Chlorambucil, thoracic disease due to, 2538t,
2547–2548
Chlordiazepoxide, thoracic disease due to, 2539t,
2567

Chloride transport, in airway epithelium, 62
    in cystic fibrosis, 2300
Chlorine gas inhalation, 2525–2526, *2526*
Chloromethyl methyl ether, pulmonary
    carcinoma and, 1077
Chlorpromazine, thoracic disease due to, 2569
Chocolate sauce sputum, in amebiasis, 1035,
    2753
Chokes, 1856
Cholecystectomy, pulmonary complications of,
    2672, 2674
Cholesterol, dietary, pulmonary carcinoma and,
    1082
Cholinergic nervous system, adrenergic system
    interaction with, 145, 148
    bronchial hyper-responsiveness and, 2098
    in efferent lung innervation, 147–148
    in exercise-induced asthma, 2110
    in pulmonary artery innervation, 149
Cholinergic receptors, in lung, 148, 2098
Cholinergic urticaria, 2109
Chondritis, tuberculous, of rib, 3017, *3017*
Chondrodynia, costosternal, 3017
Chondroitin sulfate, in mesothelioma, 2820
    in pulmonary interstitial connective tissue,
        1950
Chondroma, mediastinal, 2925
    pulmonary, *1342,* 1343–1344, *1343–1345*
        hamartoma and, 1343, 1350–1351, *1350*
Chondrosarcoma, 3032, *3033*
    mediastinal, 2925
    metastatic, calcification in, 467
    pulmonary, 1344–1345
Chordoma, 2979
Choriocarcinoma, mediastinal, 2910–2911
    metastatic to lung, *1384*
        from gestational primary, 1408–1409
        from testicular primary, *1383, 1406,* 1407
    pulmonary, primary, 1367
Choroiditis, tuberculous, 840
Chromium, pulmonary carcinoma and,
    1076–1077
Chromobacterium violaceum infection, 759
Chronic granulomatous disease of childhood,
    726–727, *727*
Chronic obstructive pulmonary disease (COPD),
    2168–2243. See also *Bronchitis, chronic;*
    Emphysema.
    adenovirus infection and, 996, 2176
    causes of, 2171–2181, *2172,* 2178t
    clinical features of, 2215–2216
    cystic fibrosis and, 2313
    definitions in, 2168–2170
    dyspnea in, 388
    epidemiology of, 2171
    genetic factors in, 2177–2180, 2178t
    in smokers, pulmonary carcinoma and, 1081
    increased tracheal compliance in, 2048
    laboratory findings in, 2216–2217
    laryngeal narrowing in, 2033
    lung transplantation for, pulmonary function
        after, 1724
    mucociliary clearance in, 2181–2182
    occupational, 2174–2175
        aluminum-related, 2122
    panic disorder and, 388
    pathogenesis of, 2181–2186, *2183*
        sequence of events in, 2199
    pathologic features of, 2186–2199
        in bronchioles, 2187–2190, *2189*
        in large airways, 2186–2187, *2187, 2188*
        in lung parenchyma, 2190–2198, *2190–2200*
    prognosis in, 2229–2231
        cardiovascular abnormalities and, 2219
    pulmonary function in, 2220–2229, *2221–2223*

Chronic obstructive pulmonary disease (COPD)
    (Continued)
    effects of smoking cessation on, 2229, *2229*
    pulmonary hemodynamics and cardiac func-
        tion in, 2217–2219
    pulmonary hypertension in, 1915, *1917*
        thromboembolism-induced hypertension vs.,
            1782
    pulmonary thromboembolism in, ventilation/
        perfusion scans in diagnosis of, 1806–
        1807
    radiologic features of, 2199–2215
    respiratory muscle function in, 2219–2220
    risk factors for, *2169*
    saber-sheath trachea and, 2040
    small airway tests in, 414, 2220–2221
    surgical complication risk and, 2672
    ventilatory response in, genetic influences on,
        240
Chryseobacterium infection, 764–765
Chrysosporium parvum infection, 950–951
Churg-Strauss syndrome, 1506–1511
    clinical features of, 1509–1511
    defined, 1490t
    diagnostic criteria for, 1506–1507, 1507t
    epidemiology of, 1507
    laboratory findings in, 1511
    limited form of, 1507
    pathogenesis of, 1507
    pathologic features of, 1507–1509, *1508*
    prognosis in, 1511
    radiologic features of, 1509, *1509–1511*
Chyliform effusion, 2745t, 2768. See also
    Pseudochylous effusion.
    in rheumatoid disease, 2754
Chyloma, 2769
Chylomicrons, fat embolism from, 1846–1847
Chylopericardium, in lymphangioleio-
    myomatosis, 683, 685
Chyloperitoneum, in lymphangioleiomyomatosis,
    683, 685
Chyloptysis, in lymphangioleiomyomatosis,
    685
Chylothorax, 2745t, 2768–2769, 2768t, *2769*
    CT identification of, 574
    in chronic lymphocytic leukemia, 2760
    in lymphangioleiomyomatosis, 683, 685
    in lymphoma, 2759
    pleural fluid characteristics in, 2743
    rheumatoid pleural effusion vs., 2754
    traumatic, 2634–2636
Chyluria, in lymphangioleiomyomatosis, 685
Cicatricial emphysema, 2190. See also *Chronic*
    obstructive pulmonary disease (COPD);
    Emphysema.
    COPD and, 2170
    pathologic features of, 2196–2198, *2199, 2200*
Cicatrization atelectasis, 522–525, *526–528.* See
    also *Pulmonary fibrosis.*
    after radiation therapy, *2602*
    defined, 513, 525
Cigarette smoking. See *Smoking.*
Ciguatera fish poisoning, 3062
Cilia of tracheobronchial epithelium, 6–7, *6, 7.*
    See also *Mucociliary clearance.*
    acquired abnormalities of, 7, *8*
        dyskinetic cilia syndrome vs., 2283
    congenital dysfunction of. See *Dyskinetic cilia*
        syndrome.
    normal function of, 127–129, *128*
Ciliary dyskinesia, primary. See *Dyskinetic cilia*
    syndrome.
Ciliated cells of tracheobronchial epithelium,
    6–7, *6–8*
Circulation, bronchial. See *Bronchial artery(ies);*
    Bronchial circulation.

Circulation *(Continued)*
    pulmonary. See *Pulmonary artery(ies); Pulmo-*
        nary capillary(ies); Pulmonary vascula-
        ture; Pulmonary vein(s).
    systemic, physical examination of, 395–396
Cirrhosis, biliary, in cystic fibrosis, 2312
        primary, pulmonary involvement in, 1475
            sarcoidosis vs., 1565
    extrapulmonary venoarterial shunts in, 3067–
        3068
    in α₁-protease inhibitor deficiency, 2232
    intrapulmonary shunting in, normal chest
        radiographs with, 3047–3048
    pleural effusion with, 2764
    pulmonary edema in, 1974
    pulmonary hypertension with, 1903–1904,
        1904
Cisterna chyli, 175
Citric acid aerosol, cough threshold
    measurement with, 2136
Citrobacter species infection, 758
Clara cell(s), 9–10, *9*
    foreign chemical metabolism in, 132
    in lung development, 136
Clara cell–specific protein, 10
Classification of organisms, defined, 735
Clavicle, anatomic variants of, on radiographs,
    263, *264*
    companion shadow of, 259
    congenital anomalies of, 3011
    dislocation of, 2645–2646
    neoplasms of, 3030
Clay, pneumoconiosis due to, 2451–2452
Clear cell carcinoma, pulmonary, 1112–1113,
    1113. See also *Carcinoma, pulmonary.*
Clear cell tumor, benign, 1363, *1364*
Cleidocranial dysostosis, 3011
Climate, asthma and, 2117
    COPD and, 2177
Clinical history. See *History.*
Clomipramine, thoracic disease due to, 2539t,
    2569
Clonorchis sinensis, 1052
Closing capacity measurement, 413–414, *413*
    in COPD, 2121
Closing volume, 111
    measurement of, 413–414, *413*
    in COPD, 2121
Clostridium botulinum poisoning, 3064
Clostridium infection, 779, 781
    pyopneumothorax due to, 2749
Clubbing, 396
    in asbestosis, 2445
Cluster-of-grapes appearance, in allergic
    bronchopulmonary aspergillosis, 929
Coagulation factors, in reperfusion injury, 1701
Coagulation system, abnormalities of, in venous
    thrombosis development, acquired,
    1779–1780
        inherited, 1778–1779
    in adult respiratory distress syndrome patho-
        genesis, 1981–1982
Coal macule, 2411–2412, *2411*
Coal miners, COPD in, 2174–2175
Coal workers' pneumoconiosis, 2409–2419
    clinical features of, 2418–2419
    epidemiology of, 2409–2410
    laboratory findings in, 2419
    multiple masses or nodules due to, 3124t
    nodular pattern in, 447, 453, 2413–2414,
        2415, 3145t, *3149*
    pathogenesis of, 2410–2411
    pathologic features of, 2411–2413, *2411–2414*
    prognosis in, 2419
    pulmonary fibrosis in. See under *Progressive*
        massive fibrosis.

Coal workers' pneumoconiosis *(Continued)*
  pulmonary function tests in, 2419
  radiologic features of, 2413–2418, *2415–2418*
  rheumatoid disease and, 1438–1443, 2411,
    2416, *2417*
  solitary mass due to, 3118t
Coarctation of the aorta, rib notching with, *3014,*
  3015
Coarctation of the pulmonary artery, 642,
  644–645
  in congenital rubella, 993
  pulmonary hypertension with, 1915
Cobb method, for scoliosis assessment, 3020
Cocaine, thoracic disease due to, 2539t,
  2567–2569
Coccidioidomas, 893, *894*
Coccidioidomycosis, 890–899
  cavities or cysts in, 3103t
  chronic progressive, 894–895
  disseminated, 895–897, *898*
  eosinophilia with, 1753
  epidemiology of, 890–891
  in HIV disease, 1671–1672
  laboratory findings in, 897–899
  lymph node enlargement in, 3164t
  miliary, 895–897, *898*
  nonsegmental opacity in, homogeneous, 3080t
    inhomogeneous, 3093t
  pleural effusion in, 2751
  primary, 891–893, *892, 893*
    persistent, 893–894, *894–897*
  solitary nodule due to, 3111t
Cockroaches, asthma and, 2106
Codeine, thoracic disease due to, 2539t, 2567
Coefficient of variation, 406
Coffee-worker's lung, 2362t. See also *Extrinsic
  allergic alveolitis.*
Cold, common, cough due to, 380
Cold agglutinins, pneumonia with, 1014, 2752
Cold air, airway response to, exercise-induced
  asthma and, 2107–2109
  inhibition of ventilation in response to, 237
  sensitivity to, in COPD, 2177
Cold cardioplegia, unilateral diaphragmatic
  paralysis due to, 2989
Collagen, in alveolar interstitium, 20–21, *20,* 24
  in fetal pulmonary arteries, 140
  in visceral pleura, 151
Collapse therapy, for tuberculosis, 814
  complications of, 818, *824*
Collar sign, with visceral diaphragmatic
  herniation, 2638, *2641*
Collateral ventilation, anatomic pathways of,
  31–33, *32*
  factors determining effectiveness of, 59–60
  resistance in, 59–60
  with airway obstruction, resorption atelectasis
    and, 514, *515*
Collecting duct of tracheobronchial gland, 14
Collimation, in CT, 309, *312, 314*
Colobronchial fistula, 2290t, 2291
Colon, carcinoma of, metastatic to lung, *1385,
  1387, 1400,* 1404–1405
  volvulus of, with diaphragmatic paralysis,
    2992
Colonic aganglionosis, 3052–3053
Colonization, by inhaled or aspirated
  microorganisms, factors facilitating, 699
Colophony, occupational asthma due to, 2122
Colorectal carcinoma, metastatic to lung, *1385,
  1387, 1396, 1400,* 1404–1405
Coma, as symptom of respiratory disease, 389
Comet-tail sign, in round atelectasis, 521, 522,
  523, 524, 2440, 2441, *2447, 2448*
Common cold, cough due to, 380
Common variable immunodeficiency, 725

Complement, deficiency of, 726
  systemic lupus erythematosus and, 1424
  in adult respiratory distress syndrome, 1981
  in angioneurotic edema, 2023
  in pleural fluid in rheumatoid disease, 2754
Compliance, lung. See *Lung compliance.*
  respiratory system, 54, *56*
  surfactant and, 58
  upper airway, in obstructive sleep apnea,
    2060–2061
Composter's lung, 2362t. See also *Extrinsic
  allergic alveolitis.*
Compression atelectasis, 513, 519, *520, 521.* See
  also *Atelectasis.*
Computed radiography, dual-energy, calcification
  detection on, in solitary nodule, 1138–1139
Computed tomography (CT), 309–315
  bronchial anatomy on, 46–51, *51–52*
  chest wall bones on, 263, *264, 264*
  chest wall soft tissue on, 259–260, *260, 261*
  conventional, 310
    high-resolution CT vs., 281, *282,* 312
  diaphragm on, 251–254, *252–256*
  display parameters in, 281–283, *285, 286*
  electron beam, 309
  emphysema quantification using, 2212–2215,
    2213, 2214
  expiratory scans, 290–291, *291, 292*
  high-resolution (HRCT), 312, *314*
    chest radiography vs., 456–457
    conventional CT vs., 281, *282,* 312
    ground-glass attenuation on, 453, *455,* 456
    indications for, 315, *316*
    pleural anatomy on, 154, *156*
    radiation dose in, 313–314
    secondary lobule abnormalities on, 26,
      28–31
  hilar anatomy on, 87–96, *96–100*
  hilar lymph node assessment on, 191–192,
    192
  indications for, 314–315, *315, 316*
  lung density on, 269–270, 291–294. See also
    Attenuation.
  lymph node measurement on, 187–188, *189,
    1186*
  mediastinal lymph node assessment on, MRI
    vs., *181–184,* 189–191, *190*
  MRI vs., 320, *321*
  normal interlobar fissures on, *157,* 158–160,
    159–163
  normal lung on, 281–294
  pleural effusion on, 572–577, *573–578*
  radiation dose in, 313–314
  scan orientation in, 281, *282*
  single-photon emission. See *Single-photon
    emission computed tomography (SPECT).*
  spiral (helical), 310–311, *310, 311*
    emphysema quantification using, 2214,
      2214
    with minimum intensity projection, in em-
      physema, 2211, *2211*
  technical parameters in, 311–313, *312–314*
  thoracic inlet on, *199*
  transthoracic needle aspiration guided by,
    345–346
  transthoracic needle biopsy guided by, 370
  upper airway dimension assessment using,
    2063, *2065*
  venography using, in deep vein thrombosis,
    1820–1823
Conductance, airway, 412
Conducting zone of lungs, 3–17
  geometry and dimensions of, 3–5
  morphology and cell function of, 5–17
Conduit lymphatics, 172–174
Confusion, as symptom of respiratory disease,
  389

Congestion, in *Streptococcus pneumoniae*
  pneumonia, 737, *738*
Congestive cardiomyopathy, after radiation
  therapy, 2605
Congestive heart failure. See *Heart failure.*
Connective tissue, abnormalities of proteins of,
  COPD and, 2180
  hereditary abnormalities of, 676–691
  of alveolar interstitium, 20–21, *20,* 23–24
  of conducting airways, 14
Connective tissue disease, 1421–1475. See also
  specific diseases.
  bronchiolitis in, 2336
  eosinophilia with, 1753
  idiopathic pulmonary fibrosis vs., 1611
  mixed, 1469–1470, *1471.* See also *Overlap
    syndrome(s).*
  myopathy in, hypoventilation due to, 3065
  pleural effusion in, 2744t–2745t, 2753–2754
  pulmonary hypertension with, 1912, *1913*
    oligemia in, 3151t
  pulmonary lymphoma and, 1275, 1277
  rib notching in, 3015–3016
  sarcoidosis and, 1563
  silicosis and, 2408–2409
Consolidation, 434–435, *434, 435*
  border characteristics of, *435,* 457
  breath and voice sound changes with, 394
  homogeneous, nonsegmental, differential diag-
    nosis of, 3078, 3079t–3081t, *3082–3085*
    segmental, differential diagnosis of, 3086,
      3087t–3088t, *3089–3091*
  in nonsegmental air-space pneumonia, 701–
    702, *703–705*
  inhomogeneous, nonsegmental, differential di-
    agnosis of, 3092, 3093t, *3094, 3095*
    segmental, differential diagnosis of, 3096,
      3097t–3098t, *3099, 3100*
  interstitial thickening with, 454–455, *456, 457*
  on high-resolution CT, 437, *437, 438*
  radiologic features of, 435–439, *435–439*
  spread of, across incomplete fissure, 462
Constrictive bronchiolitis. See also *Bronchiolitis,
  obliterative.*
  cryptogenic, 2324
Consumption, galloping, 814
Contarini's condition, 2740, *2740*
Continuous diaphragm sign, 2865, *2868*
Contraceptives, oral, pulmonary veno-occlusive
  disease and, 1930–1931
  venous thrombosis and, 1780
Contractile interstitial cell. See *Myofibroblast(s).*
Contrast medium(a), asthma provoked by, 2117
  for esophagography, in suspected esophageal
    perforation, 2852
  for venography, venous thrombosis due to,
    1778
  iodized oil, pulmonary edema due to, 2005
    pulmonary embolism due to, 1861–1863,
      1865, 2569
  ionic, adverse reactions to, 2570
    thoracic disease due to, 2539t, 2569–2570
  water-soluble, aspiration of, 2512–2513
    pulmonary edema due to, 2006, 2539t,
      2569–2570
Contusion, pulmonary, 2611–2613, *2612, 2613*
  fat embolism vs., 1848, 2612
  hematoma with, *2616, 2617*
  homogeneous nonsegmental opacity in,
    3081t
Copper, deficiency of, lysyl oxidase deficiency
  due to, 676
  lung function and, 2186
Cor pulmonale, acute, 1934
  chronic, 1934
    chronic pulmonary thromboembolism with,
      1822–1823

Cor pulmonale *(Continued)*
    familial retardation of growth and renal amino-
        aciduria with, 2728
    in coal workers' pneumoconiosis, 2413
    in COPD, 2218–2219
        prognosis and, 2230
    in upper airway obstruction, 2029
Coracoclavicular joint, 263
Cord factor, 804
Cordotomy, ventilatory failure after, 3051, 3052,
    3055
Corner vessels, 106, 1947, *1947*
Corona radiata, in solitary nodule, 1139, *1139*
Coronary artery bypass surgery, atelectasis after,
    522
Coronaviruses, 994
Corpora amylacea, 2721, *2721*
Corpus callosum, agenesis of, 726
Corrosive fluids, aspiration of, 2512
Corticosteroids, for asthma, bronchial narrowing
        in response to, 2113
    hypoventilation due to, 3065
    muscle weakness due to, 2140
    for fetal lung maturation stimulation, 57, 58
    for Wegener's granulomatosis, complications
        of, 1506
    lung development and, 142
    Pneumocystis carinii pneumonia and, 909–910
    tuberculosis risk and, 803
Corticotropin (ACTH), intraoperative
        measurement of, during carcinoid tumor
        excision, 1242
Corynebacterium equi (*Rhodococcus equi*)
        infection, 750
    in HIV disease, 1645–1647, *1646*
Corynebacterium infection, 750
Costal cartilage, calcification of, 261–262, *261*
Costal fibers of diaphragm, 248–249, *248, 249,*
    2987
    on CT, 252, *252, 253*
Costochondral osteochondritis. See *Tietze's
    syndrome.*
Costophrenic muscle slips, from diaphragm to
        ribs, clinical significance of, 495
Costosternal chondrodynia, 3017
Cotton dust exposure, 2124. See also *Organic
    dust toxic syndrome.*
Cotton fiber embolism, 1865, *1867*
Cotton-candy lung, 2196
Cough, 380–382
    chest wall pain due to, 387
    in asthma, 2136
        exercise-induced, 2107–2108
    in respiratory defense, 129–130
Cough fracture, of ribs, 2645
Cough receptors. See *Irritant receptors.*
Cough threshold measurement, 2136
Counterpulsation balloons, intra-aortic,
        complications of, 2690
Cowden's disease, 1351
Coxiella burnetii infection, 722, 1019–1020,
    1021, 3087t
Coxsackievirus, 990
Crack cocaine, thoracic disease due to, 2539t,
    2567–2569
Crackles, 394
Craniofacial structure, obstructive sleep apnea
        and, 2058, 2059
Crazy-paving pattern, in alveolar proteinosis,
    2706, *2708*
Creola bodies, 2083
Crescent sign, in angioinvasive aspergillosis,
        940–941, *944, 946*
    in echinococcosis, 1056
    with aspergilloma, 923, 925, *925, 926*
CREST syndrome, 1460

CREST syndrome *(Continued)*
    antinuclear antibodies in, 1453, 1460
    pulmonary hypertension in, 1460
        pathogenesis of, 1453–1454
        pathologic features of, *1454,* 1455
    systemic lupus erythematosus with, pathologic
        features of pulmonary hypertension in,
        1454
Cricoarytenoid joint, rheumatoid disease
        involving, 1449
Cricothyroid joint, rheumatoid disease involving,
    1449
Crohn's disease, 1473–1475
    pleural effusion in, 2766
Crotalaria species, pulmonary hypertension and,
    1902
Croup, upper airway obstruction due to, 2021
Crural fibers of diaphragm, 248–249, *248, 249,*
    2987
    on CT, 252–253, *253, 254*
Cryoglobulinemia, mixed, 1521
Cryoglobulinemic vasculitis, essential, 1490t.
    See also *Vasculitis.*
Cryptococcosis, 904–909
    cavities or cysts in, 3103t
    clinical features of, 907–908
    disseminated, 907, 908
    epidemiology of, 905
    homogeneous nonsegmental opacity in, 3080t
    in HIV disease, 1670–1671, *1671*
    laboratory findings in, 908–909
    pathogenesis of, 905
    pathologic features of, 905–907, *906, 907*
    pleural effusion in, 2751
    radiologic features of, 907, *907, 908*
Cryptogenic bilateral fibrosing pleuritis, 2804
Cryptogenic constrictive bronchiolitis, 2324. See
    also *Bronchiolitis.*
Cryptogenic fibrosing alveolitis, 1585. See also
    Pulmonary fibrosis, idiopathic.
Cryptogenic organizing pneumonia. See
    *Bronchiolitis obliterans organizing
    pneumonia (BOOP).*
Cryptosporidiosis, 1039
    in HIV infection, 1676, *1676*
CT angiogram sign, 1153–1156, *1156*
CT quotient, 292
Cultures, cytomegalovirus, 1007
    in histoplasmosis, 888–889
    in pneumonia diagnosis, 719, 720, 721
    influenza virus, 984–985
    lung, 351
    mycobacterial, 798–799
        in tuberculosis diagnosis, 845
        nontuberculous, 860
    Mycoplasma pneumoniae, 1014–1015
    viral, 981
Currant jelly sputum, in *Klebsiella pneumoniae*
        infection, 753
Curschmann spirals, in asthma, 2083, *2084*
Curvularia lunata infection, 952
Cushing's syndrome, mediastinal lipomatosis
        and, 2915, *2916*
    paraneoplastic, in pulmonary carcinoma,
        1175–1176
    with carcinoid tumor, 1241, 2900
Cutaneous leukocytoclastic angiitis, 1490t. See
    also *Vasculitis.*
Cutis laxa, 677
Cutis verticis gyrata, in pachydermoperiostosis,
    397
Cyanide, inhalation of smoke containing,
    2528–2529
Cyanosis, 397–398
    pseudofibrosis with, 666
Cyclic adenosine monophosphate, in regulation
        of airway smooth muscle contraction, 2100

Cyclooxygenase, in prostaglandin production,
    2091
Cyclophosphamide, for Wegener's
        granulomatosis, complications of, 1506
    thoracic disease due to, 2538t, 2545–2547,
        2549, 2550
Cyclosporin A, thoracic disease due to, 2538t,
    2551
Cylindrical bronchiectasis, 2268, *2268, 2270,*
    2271. See also *Bronchiectasis.*
    bronchography in, *2278*
    CT findings in, 2275
Cylindroma. See *Adenoid cystic carcinoma.*
Cyst(s), bronchogenic. See *Bronchogenic cyst.*
    diaphragmatic, 3006, *3006, 3007*
    differential diagnosis of, 3101, 3102t–3104t,
        3105–3109
    enteric, 2979
    esophageal, 2943–2944, *2944*
    gastroenteric, 2979–2980
    hydatid. See *Echinococcosis.*
    in bronchiectasis, 2272, *2273*
    in bronchopulmonary sequestration, 602–604,
        607, 608, 608
    in lymphangioleiomyomatosis, 679, *682,* 683–
        685, *683–685*
    lung, traumatic, 3104t
    mediastinal, bronchial vs. esophageal origin
        of, 611, 2943
        bronchogenic, *610,* 612–615, *613–617*
        in middle-posterior compartment, 2943–
            2945, *2944–2946*
    mesothelial, 2927–2928, *2927, 2928,* 3171t,
        3173
    neurenteric, 2979–2980
    paravertebral, 2979–2980, *2980*
    radiologic definition of, 461, 510
    thoracic duct, 2945
    thymic, 2882, *2883–2885,* 3169t
        after radiation therapy for Hodgkin's dis-
            ease, 2604
Cystadenoma, bronchial, 1259
    mucinous, 1101, 1265–1266
Cystic adenomatoid malformation, 615–618,
    618–620
    spontaneous pneumothorax with, *2787*
Cystic bronchiectasis, 2268, 2269, *2269, 2270.*
    See also *Bronchiectasis.*
    bronchography in, *2280*
    CT findings in, 2275, *2275, 2277*
    radiologic findings in, 2272, *2273,* 3104t,
        3109
Cystic fibrosis, 2298–2315
    allergic bronchopulmonary aspergillosis in,
        928, 2308, 2309–2310
    Aspergillus colonization of airways in, 921–
        923
    bronchiectasis in, 2304, *2309, 2310*
        lymphadenopathy with, 2277
        pathogenesis of, 2267
    bronchitis in, 701
    Burkholderia cepacia infection in, 761
        lung transplantation and, 1700
        pathogenetic role of, 2301, 2302
        prognosis and, 2315
    clinical features of, 2308–2312
        in gastrointestinal tract, 2311–2312
        in genitourinary tract, 2310–2311
    diagnosis of, 2312–2313
    diffuse reticular pattern in, 3136t
    epidemiology of, 2298
    genetic factors in, 2298–2299
    heterozygosity for, asthma and, 2082
        population screening for, 2313
    laboratory findings in, 2312–2314

Cystic fibrosis (Continued)
  nontuberculous mycobacterial infection in,
    850
  pathogenesis of, 2299–2303
    infection in, 2301–2303
  pathologic features of, 2303–2304, 2303–2306
  pneumothorax in, mechanism of, 2790
  prognosis in, 2314–2315
  pulmonary function tests in, 2313–2314
  radiologic features of, 484, 2304–2308, 2307–2311
    pulmonary function correlation with, 2314
  Young's syndrome and, 2283–2284
Cystic fibrosis transmembrane regulator (CFTR),
    62, 2300
  COPD and, 2178
Cystic hamartoma, mesenchymal, 1373–1374
Cystic hygroma, 2921
Cystic medial degeneration, of aorta, 2951–2952,
    2955
Cystic teratoma, 2903–2906, 2907–2909. See
    also Teratoma.
  mature, anterior mediastinal mass due to, 3174
  of diaphragm, 3005
  rupture of, 2906–2907
Cysticercosis, 1059, 1060
Cytochrome P-450 enzymes, COPD and, 2179
  in lung, 132
Cytogenetics, 356
Cytokines, in adult respiratory distress
    syndrome, 1983
  in sarcoidosis, 1536–1537
Cytology, 339–348
Cytomegalovirus infection, 1004–1008
  after bone marrow transplantation, 1730
  after lung transplantation, 1716–1717
    obliterative bronchiolitis risk and, 1707–
      1708
  clinical features of, 1007
  diffuse air-space pattern in, 3130t
  epidemiology of, 1004
  in HIV disease, 1674–1675, 1674, 1675
  laboratory findings in, 1007–1008
  mesothelioma and, 2810
  pathogenesis of, 1004
  pathologic features of, 1004–1006, 1005, 1006
  pleural effusion in, 2752
  Pneumocystis carinii pneumonia and, 1006,
    1670
  radiologic features of, 712, 1006–1007, 1007,
    1008
Cytosine arabinoside, thoracic disease due to,
    2538t, 2555
Cytotoxic therapy. See Chemotherapy; specific
    drugs.

Dantrolene, thoracic disease due to, 2572, 2756
Dead space, alveolar, ventilation/perfusion ratio
    and, 109, 109
  physiologic, in ventilation/perfusion mismatch
    assessment, 111–112
Decompression syndrome, pulmonary air
    embolism due to, 1855–1856
Deep cervical fascia, 198
Deep sulcus sign, in pneumothorax, 589, 591
Deep vein thrombosis. See under Thrombosis.
Dehydration, mucociliary clearance and, 129
Dendriform pulmonary ossification, 474, 2700,
    2702, 2703
Dendritic cells of tracheobronchial epithelium,
    11–12, 11
  in asthmatic airway inflammation, 2090
Density, of lung. See Lung density.
  optical, 302

Density (Continued)
  radiopacity vs., 269n
Density mask, emphysema quantification using,
    2213–2214, 2213
Dental technicians, dust exposure in, 2468
Deoxyribonucleic acid. See DNA entries.
Dermatitis, in cystic fibrosis, 2312
Dermatomyositis, 1462–1465. See also
    Polymyositis.
  hypoventilation in, 3065
Desferrioxamine, thoracic disease due to, 2539t
Desmoid tumors, of chest wall, 3025
Desmoplastic small round cell tumor of pleura,
    2838–2840
Desquamative interstitial pneumonitis. See under
    Interstitial pneumonitis.
Destructive index, in emphysema, 2192
Detergent-worker's lung, 2362t, 2379. See also
    Extrinsic allergic alveolitis.
Developmental lung disease, 595–691. See also
    specific disorders.
  affecting airways and parenchyma, 597–629
  affecting connective tissue, 676–691
  affecting pulmonary vessels, 637–671
Dexfenfluramine, pulmonary hypertension due
    to, 1903
Diabetes mellitus, autonomic neuropathy in,
    hypoventilation due to, 3056
  in cystic fibrosis, 2312
  insulin-dependent, progressive systemic sclero-
    sis–like syndrome with, 1459
  ketoacidosis in, pulmonary edema with, 2005
  pulmonary abnormalities in, 2728–2729
  tuberculosis risk and, 803
Dialysis. See also Hemodialysis patients.
  peritoneal, pleural effusion with, 2764
Diaphragm, 247–255, 2987–3007
  accessory, 3006
  age-related changes in, 254, 255
  anatomy of, 248–251, 248, 250, 2987, 2988
  CT scan at level of, 573
  cysts of, 3006, 3006, 3007
  defects in, 3006. See also Diaphragmatic
    hernia.
    catamenial pneumothorax and, 2787
    fluid passage via, 2763
    focal, 254, 255
      in healthy persons, 2638
    thoracic endometriosis and, 2767
  development of, 247–248, 247
  dysfunction of, in systemic lupus erythemato-
    sus, 1431
  electromyography of, in respiratory fatigue
    detection, 258
    in ventilatory control assessment, 419, 420
  elevation of, in atelectasis, 528–529, 530
    in response to inflammation, 2995
    with pulmonary thromboembolism, 1796,
      1796, 1797
  energy sources of, 257
  eventration of, 251, 2994–2995
    diaphragmatic hernia vs., 2990, 2995
  fatigue of, assessment of, 258, 420
  fenestrations of. See Diaphragmatic fenestra-
    tions.
  flattened, in emphysema, 2207, 2207, 2209
    with hyperinflation, 495–496, 496
  function of, 249, 255–259
  hematoma of, 3006, 3006
  hernia of. See Diaphragmatic hernia.
  imaging of, 251–254, 251–256
  in ventilation, 3056
    during sleep, 243
  innervation of, 250–251
    spinal levels of, 3055
  inversion of, pleural effusion mimicking intra-
    peritoneal fluid with, 573–574, 576

Diaphragm (Continued)
  motion of, 254–255
    abnormalities of, 2989–2995
    assessment of, 2988–2989
    normal, 2987–2988
    restriction of, 2995
  muscle slips from, clinical significance of,
    251, 252
  neoplasms of, 3004–3006, 3005
  normal radiographic appearance of, 2987
  paralysis of, bilateral, 2993–2994, 2994t,
    2996–2997
    clinical manifestations of, 3057–3059,
      3058–3060
    in pulmonary carcinoma, 1166, 1168
    pulmonary function tests in, 3059–3061
    unilateral, 2989–2993, 2989t, 2990–2992
  position of, abnormalities of, 2989–2995
  receptors in, in ventilatory control, 238
  rupture of, 2636–2644
    clinical features of, 2638–2644
    injuries associated with, 2636–2637
    pneumatocele vs., 2614
    radiologic features of, 2637–2638, 2637–2645
  scalloping of, 251, 251
  strength estimate for, 419–420
  surgical complications involving, 2669
  tension-time index of, 257, 420, 3057
    in COPD, 2220
  tonic contraction of, 2995
  trauma to, nonpenetrating, 2636–2644
    penetrating, 2648, 2652
  ultrasonography in assessment of, 334
  weakness of, bilateral, 2993, 2994
    clinical manifestations of, 3057–3059,
      3058–3060
    pulmonary function tests in, 3059–3061
Diaphragm sign, 572, 574
Diaphragmatic fenestrations, air migration
    through, catamenial pneumothorax and,
    2787
  tissue migration through, pleural endometrio-
    sis and, 2788–2789
Diaphragmatic flutter, 2995
Diaphragmatic hernia, 2995–3004
  anterior mediastinal mass due to, 3172t
  Bochdalek's, 2997–3001, 2998, 3002
    middle-posterior mediastinal mass due to,
      3178t
    paravertebral mass due to, 3185t, 3189
  congenital, pulmonary hypertension with,
    1918
  diaphragmatic paralysis vs., 2990
  hiatus, 2996–2997, 2998–3001, 3178t
    middle-posterior mediastinal mass due to,
      3178t
  Morgagni's (retrosternal, parasternal), 2926,
    2998, 3001–3004, 3003, 3004, 3172t
  multiple acquired, 2998
  omental fat protrusion with, 254, 255
  paravertebral mass due to, 3185t, 3189
  pulmonary hypoplasia and, 598
  Streptococcus agalactiae infection and, 748
  traumatic, 2637
    clinical features of, 2643
    pleural effusion with, 2762
    radiologic features of, 2637–2638, 2637–2644
Diaphragmatic lymph nodes, 176, 178
  enlargement of, 2929
  in ATS classification, 184t, 187
Diaphragmatic pacing, obstructive sleep apnea
    during, 2062
  upper airway obstruction and, 246
Diaphragmatic sinuses, tissue migration through,
    pleural endometriosis and, 2788

Diatomaceous earth, silicosis due to, 2390
Diclofenac, thoracic disease due to, 2539t, 2565
Diesel fumes, pulmonary carcinoma and, 1078
Diet, asthma and, 2081
    COPD and, 2180, 2227–2228
    mesothelioma and, 2810
    pulmonary carcinoma and, 1081–1082
Diethylenetriamine pentaacetic acid, technetium-labeled, for ventilation imaging, 330
Diffuse alveolar damage, in adult respiratory distress syndrome, 1984–1986, *1984, 1985*
    in idiopathic pulmonary fibrosis, *1619,* 1621
    in influenza, 982
    in interstitial pneumonia, 707, *713,* 1619–1621
    in *Pneumocystis carinii* pneumonia, 911
Diffuse alveolar fibrosis. See *Pulmonary fibrosis, idiopathic.*
Diffuse alveolar hemorrhage. See *Hemorrhage, pulmonary.*
Diffuse fasciitis with eosinophilia, 1459
Diffuse lung disease. See also *Interstitial disease, diffuse.*
    high-resolution CT in assessment of, 315, *316*
    with air-space pattern predominant, differential diagnosis of, 3130, 3130t, *3131, 3132*
    with reticular pattern predominant, differential diagnosis of, 3133, 3134t–3136t, *3137–3143*
    with small nodular pattern predominant, differential diagnosis of, 3144, 3145t, *3146–3149*
Diffuse pulmonary angiomatosis, 662–663, *662, 663*
Diffusing capacity, in asthma, 2138
    in COPD, 107, 2229
    measurement of, 107–108
        in *Pneumocystis carinii* pneumonia diagnosis, 1668
    reduction of, with heavy exercise, 107
    tests of, 414–416, 415t
Diffusion, in particle deposition, 127
    of gases, from acinus to red blood cell, 107–108, *108*
        impairment of, hypoxemia due to, 114
        mechanisms of, 107, *108*
        ventilation/perfusion mismatch assessment and, 113
    intravascular, 107
Diffusive pendelluft, 413
Diflunisal, thoracic disease due to, 2539t, 2565
DiGeorge's syndrome, 728
Digital radiography, 306–308, *308*
Digital subtraction angiography, 322–323, *323*
    in pulmonary thromboembolism diagnosis, 1815–1816, *1818*
Dilation lesions, in pulmonary hypertension, 1884, *1888*
Diltiazem, thoracic disease due to, 2539t, 2572
D-Dimers, plasma, in pulmonary thromboembolism diagnosis, 1826
Dimorphism, defined, 876
Dinoflagellates, airborne toxins from, 2124
    hypoventilation due to poisoning by, 3062
Dipalmitoyl phosphatidylcholine, in surfactant, 56, 57
Diphenylhydantoin, thoracic disease due to, 2539t, 2564
Diphenylmethane diisocyanate, allergic alveolitis associated with, 2362t, 2378–2379. See also *Extrinsic allergic alveolitis.*
Diphtheria, 750
Diplococcus pneumoniae. See Streptococcus pneumoniae *pneumonia.*
Direct smear technique for sputum processing, 340
Dirofilariasis, 1045, *1046*

Dirofilariasis *(Continued)*
    pulmonary embolism in, 1853
Dirty chest, in chronic bronchitis, 2203
Discoid atelectasis, 554–560, *558.* See also *Atelectasis.*
Diskitis, staphylococcal, *3024*
Dislocation, of clavicle, 2645–2646
Displaced crus sign, 573, *574*
Disseminated intravascular coagulation, adult respiratory distress syndrome and, 1982
    due to amniotic fluid embolism, 1852
    in acute promyelocytic leukemia, 1320
    pulmonary microvascular thrombosis in, 1774, *1775*
    venous thrombosis and, 1780
Distal intestinal obstruction syndrome, in cystic fibrosis, 2311
Diverticulosis, tracheal, 2047
Diverticulum(a), airway, 626–627, *627*
    bronchial wall, in COPD, 2187, *2188*
    ductus, aortic injury vs., 2633
    esophageal, 2966–2967, 3177t
    Kommerell's, 2961, *2964, 2965*
    pharyngeal, 3177t
    Zenker's, 2966–2967
        aspiration pneumonia secondary to, *2499*
Diving, air embolism due to, 1855–1856
    radiologic features of, 1857
Diving reflex, nasal receptors in, 237
DNA, in sputum, viscosity and, in cystic fibrosis, 2301
DNA content analysis, flow cytometry for, 357, *357*
DNA hybridization techniques, for tuberculosis diagnosis, 845
DNA viruses, 994–1010. See also specific viruses.
DNAse I, recombinant, aerosolized therapy with, in cystic fibrosis, 2301
Dobbhoff feeding tube, faulty insertion of, *2679*
Docosahexaenoic acid, dietary, COPD and, 2180
Doege-Potter syndrome, with solitary fibrous tumor of pleura, 2833
Dorsal lobe of Nelson, 165
Dorsal respiratory group, in medullary control of ventilation, *236,* 238–239, *3050,* 3051
Double density of cardiac silhouette, with pericardiophrenic lymph node enlargement, 1302, *1303, 1304*
Double indicator dilution technique, extra-vascular lung water volume assessment using, 1996–1997
Double-fissure artefact, 286, *287*
Doubling time, of pulmonary nodule, 479, *480,* 1142–1143, *1144, 1145*
Down's syndrome, immunodeficiency in, 726
    obstructive sleep apnea in, 2058
    pulmonary artery stenosis in, 642
    pulmonary hyperplasia in, 599
Drain cleaners, potassium hydroxide, aspiration of, 2512
Dressler's syndrome, pleural effusion in, 2766
Drowned lung, 517, *517*
Drowning, 2507. See also *Aspiration (event), of water.*
    mortality due to, 2508
Drug(s). See also specific drugs and classes of drugs.
    adverse reactions to, types of, 2537–2540
    anaphylaxis due to, 2106
    asthma provoked by, 2116–2117
    bronchiolitis due to, 2322t
    eosinophilic lung disease due to, 1744t, 1751–1752
    illicit, thoracic disease due to, 2539t, 2567–2569, *2568*

Drug(s) *(Continued)*
    methemoglobinemia due to, 3068
    myasthenia-like syndromes due to, 3063–3064
    pleural effusion due to, 2756, 2756t
    pulmonary hypertension due to, 1902–1903
    respiratory depression due to, 3051
    systemic lupus erythematosus due to, 1424–1425
        clinical features of, 1432
    thoracic disease due to, 2537–2572, 2538t–2539t
        diffuse reticular pattern in, 3136t
        homogeneous nonsegmental opacities in, 3081t
Drug abuse, emboli of filler material in, 1857–1861. See also *Talcosis, intravenous.*
    pneumothorax in, 2790
    thoracic disease due to, 2539t, 2567–2569, *2568*
    tuberculosis risk and, 801
Drug history, 389
Drug resistance, in *Burkholderia cepacia,* 2302
    in *Haemophilus influenzae,* 770
    in *Staphylococcus aureus,* 744
    in *Streptococcus pneumoniae,* 736
    in tuberculosis, 804, 1654
Dry cold air. See also *Cold air.*
    airway response to, exercise-induced asthma and, 2107–2109
Dry-drowning, 2508
Dual-energy computed radiography, calcification detection on, in solitary nodule, 1138–1139
Duchenne type muscular dystrophy, 3064
Ductus diverticulum, aortic injury vs., 2633
Dung lung, 2524
Duodenal ulcer, pleural effusion with, 2766
Dust exposure, idiopathic pulmonary fibrosis and, 1586
    inert radiopaque, 2452–2456
    inorganic, 2386–2468. See also *Pneumoconiosis;* specific materials.
        establishing causal relationship of, to biologic effect, 2387
    occupational, airway macrophages in, 16
        COPD and, 2174–2175
    organic, 2361–2380. See also *Extrinsic allergic alveolitis; Organic dust toxic syndrome.*
        in animal confinement areas, 2379
        COPD and, 2175
    volcanic, 2466
Dust mites, asthma and, 2106
Dutch hypothesis of COPD, 2180–2181
Dwarfism, short-limbed, 726
Dynamic compliance, frequency dependence of, 412
    in COPD, 2220–2221
    measurement of, 411–412
Dysautonomia, familial, 3056
Dyskinesia, respiratory, 3051–3052
Dyskinetic cilia syndrome, 2281–2283, *2282, 2284*
    bronchiectasis in, 2267, 2281, 2283, *2284*
    transmission electron microscopy in diagnosis of, 354
Dyspnea, 242, 387–389
    during pregnancy, 388
    functional, 387–388
    in COPD, 2215
        during exercise, 2228
    in pulmonary thromboembolism, 1825

Eaton-Lambert syndrome, 1173–1174, 3063
Ebstein's anomaly, 500–501, *501,* 665, *665,* 3151t, *3152*

Echinococcosis, 1053–1059
  cavities or cysts in, 3103t
  diaphragmatic involvement in, 3006, *3007*
  due to *E. granulosus,* 1053–1056, *1054–1058*
  due to *E. multilocularis,* 1056–1059
  due to *E. vogeli,* 1059
  hepatic, pulmonary embolism in, 1854
  in middle mediastinum, 2943
  in paravertebral region, 2980, *2980*
  of rib, 3017
  of sternum, 3020
  pastoral, 1053
  pleural effusion in, 2753, *2754*
  solitary mass due to, 3117t, *3119*
  solitary nodule due to, 3111t
  sylvatic, 1053
  water-lily sign in, 463, *467,* 1056, *1056,* 2753,
    2754
ECHO virus, 991
Echocardiography, contrast, for intrapulmonary
    shunt detection, 3047
  for pulmonary artery pressure estimation,
    2218
  in pulmonary hypertension diagnosis, 1889–
    1891
  transesophageal, in aortic rupture, 2632–2633
Ecthyma gangrenosum, in *Pseudomonas
    aeruginosa* pneumonia, 762
Edema, chest wall, after thoracentesis, 2741,
    2742
  peripheral, in COPD, 2217
  pulmonary. See *Pulmonary edema.*
  upper airway obstruction due to, 2022–2024
EDRF (endothelium-derived relaxant factor). See
    Nitric oxide.
Eggshell calcification, *452, 474, 476*
  in sarcoidosis, 1545, *1547*
  in silicosis, *452, 474,* 2402, *2403*
Egophony, 394
Ehlers-Danlos syndrome, 677, *679*
  pulmonary artery stenosis in, 642
Eicosapentaenoic acid, dietary, COPD and, 2180
Eikenella corrodens infection, 776
Eisenmenger's syndrome, 1892–1894, *1895,*
    1896
Ejection fraction, in COPD, 2218
Elastance, respiratory system, 54
Elastase, experimental emphysema induced by,
    2185
  neutrophil, in adult respiratory distress syn-
    drome, 1980, 1981, 1983
    in cystic fibrosis, 2302–2303
    in emphysema, 2182, *2183,* 2185
    smoking and, 2184
Elastic recoil, of lung and thoracic cage, 53–54,
    55, 56
  loss of, emphysema and, 2198–2199, *2201*
    hyperinflation and, 494
  maximal expiratory flow and, 410, *410*
  measurement of, 410–411, *411*
  pleural cavity pressure and, 168
  surface tension and, 54–58
Elastic tissue, in conducting airways, *6, 13, 13*
Elasticity, in respiratory mucus, 62–63
Elastin, degradation of, in emphysema,
    2184–2185
  in alveolar development, 142
  in alveolar interstitium, 20
Elastolysis, generalized, 677
Electrocardiography, in right ventricular
    hypertrophy detection, in COPD, 2218
Electroencephalography, in obstructive sleep
    apnea diagnosis, 2068
Electromyography, in respiratory fatigue
    detection, 258
  in ventilatory control assessment, 419, *420*

Electron beam computed tomography, 309
Electron microscopy, 351–355
  scanning, 354–355, *355*
  transmission, 351–354, *355*
Elementary bodies, 1016
Embolism. See also *Thromboembolism.*
  acrylate glue, 1865, *1867*
  air, 1854–1857
    due to bulla enlargement, 2240
    pulmonary (venous), 1855–1856, 1856t
    systemic (arterial), 1854–1855, 1854t
    with central venous catheter, 2685, *2685*
  amniotic fluid, 1850–1853
  barium, 1865–1868
  bone marrow, 1850, *1851*
  bronchial artery, *1870,* 1871, *1871*
  bullet, 1868, *1868,* 2652
  cellulose, 1857–1861
    pathologic features of, 1858
  cotton fiber, 1865, *1867*
  fat, 1845–1850. See also *Fat embolism.*
  in parasitic infestation, 1853–1854
  iodized oil, 1861–1863, *1865,* 2569
    pulmonary edema and, 2005
  metallic mercury, 1863–1865, *1866*
  of drug filler material, 1857–1861. See also
    Talcosis, intravenous.
  of microscopic particulates in IV fluid, 1868
  of neoplastic tissue, 1854
    with pulmonary metastasis, 1382, 1388–
      1389, *1389, 1397, 1398, 1399*
  of plastic intravenous catheter, 1868, *1869*
  of radiopaque foreign bodies, 1868
  of tissue and tissue secretions, 1845–1846,
    1846t
  pleural effusion due to, 2745t
  polytef (Teflon), 1870
  septic. See *Septic embolism.*
  shrapnel, 1868, *1868*
  silicone, 1868–1870
  talc, 1857–1861. See also *Talcosis, intrave-
    nous.*
  to lungs, without clinical significance, 132
  vegetable oil, 1871
Embolization therapy, bronchial artery. See
    Bronchial artery embolization therapy.
  for pulmonary arteriovenous malformation,
    662
  for vascular malformations, pulmonary acry-
    late glue embolism due to, 1865, *1867*
  with oil, for hepatocellular carcinoma, thoracic
    disease due to, 2570
Embryonic period of lung development, 136,
    137
Emotional distress. See also *Psychogenic* entries.
  asthma provoked by, 2114
Emotional laryngeal wheezing, 2032
Emphysema, 2170. See also *Chronic obstructive
    pulmonary disease (COPD).*
  asbestos-related disease and, 2445
  asthma vs., *2027,* 2221
  bullae in, 2204, *2204–2206,* 2234–2235, *2235,
    2236, 2238–2239*
  cadmium and, 2527–2528
  centrilobular (proximal acinar), 2190
    bulla in, *2236*
    oligemia in, *3153*
    panlobular emphysema vs., 2192
    pathologic features of, 2191–2192, *2191–
      2195, 2197*
    radiologic features of, *2207, 2210,* 2211,
      2211
  coal workers' pneumoconiosis and, 2418–
    2419
  collateral resistance in, 60
  cor pulmonale in, 1934

Emphysema *(Continued)*
  experimental, 2185–2186
  extrinsic allergic alveolitis and, 2375
  flow-volume loop of, *2027,* 2221
  focal, in coal workers' pneumoconiosis, *2411,*
    2412
    primary spontaneous pneumothorax and,
      2781–2784, *2782*
  hyperinflation in, radiologic signs of, 495–
    496, *496*
  in silicosis, 2405–2406, *2408*
  interstitial, in primary spontaneous pneumotho-
    rax, 2790, *2790*
    with pneumomediastinum, 2868, *2869*
  irregular (scar, cicatricial), 2190
    COPD and, 2170
    pathologic features of, 2196–2198, *2199,
      2200*
  lobar. See also *Swyer-James syndrome.*
    congenital, 621–625, *625, 626*
    oligemia in, 3157t, *3159*
  lung transplantation for, 1699
  mediastinal. See *Pneumomediastinum.*
  miscellaneous causes of, 2243
  normal chest radiographs in, 3047
  objective quantification of, 2212–2215, *2213,
    2214*
  oligemia in, diffuse, 502–503, *502, 503,*
    3151t, *3152–3154*
    local, 504, *507,* 3157t
  panlobular (panacinar), 2190
    centrilobular emphysema vs., 2192
    oligemia in, *3153*
    pathologic features of, 2192–2196, *2196–
      2198*
    radiologic features of, 2211–2212, *2212*
  paraseptal (distal acinar), 2190
    bullae in, 2234, *2238–2239*
    COPD and, 2170
    pathologic features of, 2196, *2198*
    radiologic features of, 2212, *2212*
  pathogenesis of, 2182–2186, *2183*
    sequence of events in, 2199
  pathologic assessment of severity of, 2190–
    2191
  pathologic features of, 2190–2198, *2190–2200*
  pneumonia with, 700, *700,* 739
  α_1-protease inhibitor and, 2182, *2183,* 2231–
    2232
  pulmonary carcinoma and, 1081
  pulmonary diffusing capacity in, 107
  pulmonary hypertension in, 1915, *1917,* 2209,
    2209
  radiologic features of, 270, *271,* 2204–2209,
    2204–2209
    on CT, 2209–2212, *2210–2213*
  senile, 2190n
  spontaneous pneumothorax and, primary,
    2790, *2790*
    secondary, 2784, 2785–2787, *2785, 2787*
  structure-function correlation in, 2198–2199,
    2201
  subcutaneous, after thoracic surgery, 2659–
    2660
    in blunt chest trauma, 2625, *2625*
  unilateral. See *Swyer-James syndrome.*
  vascular and cardiac anomalies in, 2199
Empyema. See also *Pleural effusion.*
  after lung resection, 2665, *2666, 2668,* 2762
  after lung transplantation, 1720
  bacterial, 2747–2751
  causes of, 2747
  chest tube position in, 2677
  CT identification of, 575–576, *577, 579, 579,
    580*
  identification of causative organism of, 2749

Empyema (Continued)
in anaerobic pneumonia, 779, 781
in rheumatoid disease, 2754
incidence of, 2747
parapneumonic effusion vs., 2747n
pathologic features of, 2747, 2750, 2751
pleural calcification due to, 583
prognosis in, 2749–2751
radiologic features of, 2749
squamous cell carcinoma of pleura and, 2838
ultrasonography in assessment of, 334, 334
with esophageal rupture, 2634, 2636
with hemothorax, 2761
with lung abscess, 2749
Empyema necessitatis, 2747
after pneumonectomy, 2668
Encephalitis, tuberculous, 838–839
Encephalitozoon infection, 1039
Encephalomyelopathy, paraneoplastic, in
pulmonary carcinoma, 1174
subacute necrotizing, central apnea with, 3052
Endarteritis obliterans, of pulmonary arteries, in
tuberculosis, 817
Endocarditis, cancer-associated nonbacterial
thrombotic, 1172, 1177
Loeffler's, 1748–1751, 1751, 1752
pulmonary hypertension with, 1933
of tricuspid valve, septic pulmonary embolism
with, 1829, 1831–1832
Endocrine tumors, atypical, 1229, 1246
Endodermal sinus tumor, mediastinal,
2909–2910, 2910
Endometrial malignancy, metastatic to lung,
1407
Endometriosis, pleural, 2767–2768
catamenial pneumothorax and, 2788–2789
pulmonary parenchymal involvement in,
1375–1376
Endopleura, 151
Endoscopy, 366–369. See also specific
procedures.
Endothelial tumor, sclerosing. See Epithelioid
hemangioendothelioma.
Endotheliitis, in acute rejection, 1703, 1704
Endothelin(s), pulmonary synthesis of, 132
Endothelin-1, in adult respiratory distress
syndrome, 1983
in asthmatic airway inflammation, 2093
in progressive systemic sclerosis, 1453
in pulmonary hypertension, 1881
Endothelium, acetylcholine's effects on, 148
bronchial vascular, fluid transport across, 1955
in asthmatic airway inflammation, 2090
in pulmonary fluid exchange, 1950
damage to, in adult respiratory distress syndrome, 1977–1978
markers of, 1998
tests for, 1996
in idiopathic pulmonary fibrosis, 1587,
1590, 1590
in venous thrombosis development, 1778
lymphatic capillary, 174
permeability of, 1951
products of, in pulmonary hypertension, 1881–
1882
pulmonary capillary, anatomy of, 74–76, 75,
76
in fluid exchange, 1947–1949, 1949
permeability of, 1949
Endothelium-derived relaxant factor. See Nitric
oxide.
Endothoracic fascia, on high-resolution CT, 154,
156
Endotoxin, experimental emphysema induced by,
2185
in adult respiratory distress syndrome, alveolar
macrophage response to, 1978–1979

Endotoxin (Continued)
endothelial response to, 1977–1978
neutrophil response to, 1980
in organic dust toxic syndrome, 2124, 2175
Endotracheal aspiration, in pneumonia diagnosis,
719
Endotracheal intubation, complications of,
2680–2681, 2681
upper airway obstruction due to, 2024–
2025, 2025
optimal tube placement for, 2025
tracheal stenosis due to, 2033–2035, 2034,
2035
Entamoeba histolytica infection, 1034–1036,
1035, 3080t
pleural effusion in, 2753
Enteric cysts, intrapulmonary, 610
Enterobacter infection, 751–753
cavitary or cystic disease in, 3102t
homogeneous opacity in, nonsegmental, 3079t
segmental, 3087t
inhomogeneous opacity in, nonsegmental,
3093t
segmental, 3097t
Enterobacteriaceae. See also specific organisms.
pneumonia due to, 751–758
Enterobiasis, 1047
Enterococci, group D (Enterococcus faecalis), 748
Enterocytozoon infection, 1039
Enteroviruses, 990–991
Environmental factors, asthma and, 2081,
2114–2115
COPD and, 2173–2175
cough and, 380
systemic lupus erythematosus and, 1424–1425
Environmental tobacco smoke. See Smoking,
passive.
Eosinophil(s), function of, 1743–1744
in asthmatic airway inflammation, 2089–2090
in pleural fluid specimen, 344
Eosinophil cationic protein, in asthmatic airway
inflammation, 2090
in sputum, in asthma diagnosis, 2136
Eosinophilia, diffuse fasciitis with, 1459
in pulmonary carcinoma, 1178
in sputum, in asthma diagnosis, 2136
simple pulmonary, 1744–1746, 1745, 1746
nonsegmental opacity in, homogeneous,
3081t, 3083
inhomogeneous, 3093t
tropical, 1043–1045, 1044, 1752–1753
Eosinophilia-myalgia syndrome, 1752, 3065
pulmonary hypertension in, 1902
Eosinophilic collagen disease, disseminated. See
Loeffler's endocarditis.
Eosinophilic granuloma, 1627. See also
Langerhans' cell histiocytosis.
Eosinophilic leukemia. See Loeffler's
endocarditis.
Eosinophilic lung disease, 1743–1753
classification of, 1744t
connective tissue disease and, 1753
drug-induced, 1744t, 1751–1752
due to parasitic infestation, 1744t, 1752–1753
fungal, 1744t, 1753
idiopathic, 1744–1751
acute eosinophilic pneumonia and, 1746
chronic eosinophilic pneumonia and, 1747
hypereosinophilic syndrome and, 1748
simple pulmonary eosinophilia and, 1744
vasculitis and, 1753
Eosinophilic pleuritis, with pneumothorax, 2790,
2790
Eosinophilic pneumonia, acute, 1746, 1746,
1747
chronic, 1747–1748, 1748–1750, 3081t, 3084

Eotaxin, in asthmatic airway inflammation, 2092
Ependymoma, pulmonary, 1370
Epiglottitis, 769, 2021–2022
Epinephrine, pulmonary vascular response to,
106
Episodic paroxysmal laryngospasm, 2032–2033
Epithelial-mesenchyme interaction, in lung
development, 141–142
Epithelioid angiosarcoma, sclerosing. See
Epithelioid hemangioendothelioma.
Epithelioid hemangioendothelioma, mediastinal,
2920, 2920, 2921
pulmonary, 1339–1343, 1340, 1341
Epithelium, alveolar. See Alveolar epithelial
cells; Alveolar epithelium.
bronchial. See Bronchial epithelium.
bronchiolar, 17, 17
development and growth of, 137
tracheal, 5–12, 7, 11
response of, to injury, 9
Epoxy resins, 2528
Epstein-Barr virus infection, 1008–1009, 1009
after transplantation, 1717
lymphoproliferative disorder and, 1711–
1712
angiocentric immunoproliferative lesion and,
1281
hereditarily determined susceptibility to, 726
idiopathic pulmonary fibrosis and, 1585
lymph node enlargement in, 3164t
pleural lymphoma and, 2838
pulmonary carcinoma and, 1079
Erdheim-Chester disease, 2727
Ergometrine, asthma provoked by, 2117
Ergotamine, thoracic disease due to, 2539t, 2571
Erionite, mesothelioma and, 2809
pneumoconiosis due to, 2452
Erythema gyratum repens, in pulmonary
carcinoma, 1174
Erythema multiforme, in Mycoplasma
pneumoniae infection, 1014
Erythema nodosum, in sarcoidosis, 1563, 1564
Erythrocytes, in carbon dioxide transport, 114
in pleural fluid specimen, 344
Erythromycin, for diffuse panbronchiolitis, 2353
Escherichia coli infection, 753–755, 756, 757
cavities or cysts in, 3102t
homogeneous nonsegmental opacity in, 3080t
Esophageal atresia, tracheoesophageal fistula
with, 628
Esophageal cyst, 2943–2944, 2944
Esophageal hiatus, 2987, 2988
hernia through, 2996–2997, 2998–3001, 3178t
Esophageal lung, 628
Esophageal sphincter, lower, incompetent, with
tracheobronchial-esophageal fistula, 628
Esophageal stripes, superior, 211, 223, 226
Esophageal varices, 2967–2968, 2968
sclerotherapy for, complications of, 2761,
2968
Esophagobronchial fistula, 628, 2290–2291,
2290t, 2967
due to esophageal rupture, 2634
Esophagography, in esophageal obstruction
diagnosis, 2861
in suspected esophageal perforation, 2852
Esophagopleural fistula, due to esophageal
perforation, 2634, 2856
due to sclerotherapy for esophageal varices,
2968
postoperative, 2663
Esophagopleural stripes, inferior, 218, 229, 232
superior, 211, 223, 226
Esophagoscopy, 367
Esophagus, air trapping in, 2967
carcinoma of, 2961–2965, 2966

Esophagus *(Continued)*
　radiation therapy for, airway-esophageal fistula due to, 2967
　　with perforation, mediastinitis with, *2855*
　cystic fibrosis involving, 2311
　disease of, chest pain due to, 386
　　presenting as middle-posterior mediastinal mass, 2961–2968, *2966–2968*
　diverticula of, 2966–2967, 3177t
　endotracheal tube inserted into, 2681, *2681*
　foreign body in, airway obstruction due to, 2024, 2486
　neoplasms of, mesenchymal, 2965–2966
　　middle-posterior mediastinal mass due to, 3178t
　obstruction of, by mediastinal histoplasmosis, 886–888
　　in fibrosing mediastinitis, 2861
　on PA chest radiograph, 211
　penetrating trauma to, 2648, *2651*
　perforation of, causes of, 2851
　　clinical features of, 2856
　　complicating therapeutic procedures, 2675, *2676*
　　mediastinitis due to, radiologic features of, 2852, *2853–2855*
　　pleural effusion with, 2761
　　pneumomediastinum and, 2865, 2868
　　pneumonia with abscess secondary to, *718*
　　with closed chest trauma, 2633–2634, *2636*
　progressive systemic sclerosis involving, 1457, *1458*
　pulmonary carcinoma involving, 1156, *1160–1161*, 1171
Essential cryoglobulinemic vasculitis. See also *Vasculitis.*
　defined, 1490t
Estrogens, lymphangioleiomyomatosis and, 679
　systemic lupus erythematosus and, 1425
Ethambutol, thoracic disease due to, 2538t, 2558
Ethanol. See *Alcohol.*
Ethchlorvynol, thoracic disease due to, 2539t, 2567
Ethiodized oil, embolization of, 1861–1863, *1865*, 2569
　pulmonary edema and, 2005
Etoposide, thoracic disease due to, 2538t, 2551
Eventration of diaphragm, 251, 2994–2995
　diaphragmatic hernia vs., 2990, 2995
Exanthem subitum, 999
Excluded volume of interstitial fluid, 1950
Exercise, anaphylaxis due to, 2109
　asthma provoked by, 2078, 2106–2111
　　delayed response in, 2111
　　pathogenesis of, 2108–2110
　　refractory period in, 2110–2111
　blood gases during, in COPD, 2227–2228
　bronchoconstriction due to, assessment of, 423–424
　diffusing capacity and, 107, 416
　hypoxemia due to, diffusion defect and, 114
　pulmonary function testing with, in *Pneumocystis carinii* pneumonia diagnosis, 1667–1668
　ventilation/perfusion heterogeneity and, 111
　ventilatory response to, 241
　　genetic factors in, 240–241
Exercise lability index, 2107
Exercise testing, in asbestos-related disease, 2446
Expectoration, 380
Expiratory muscles, 247. See also *Respiratory muscles; specific muscles.*
Expiratory reserve volume (ERV), 406, *406*
Exserohilum infection, 952
External intercostal muscles, 260, *260*

External intercostal muscles *(Continued)*
　in inspiration, 246–247
　spinal levels of innervation of, 3055
External oblique muscle, in expiration, 247
　spinal levels of innervation of, 3055
Extramedullary hematopoiesis, 1320, 2980–2981, *2981*, 3185t, *3190*
Extrapulmonary sign, 459, *459*
Extrinsic allergic alveolitis, 2361–2379
　acute, *2368, 2369,* 2372
　building-associated, 2362t, 2378
　chronic, *2371, 2372*
　clinical features of, 2373–2375
　diagnosis of, 2375
　　criteria for, 2361
　differential diagnosis of, 2373, 2375
　diffuse air-space pattern in, 3130t
　diffuse nodular pattern in, 3145t, *3148*
　diffuse reticular pattern in, 3136t, *3142*
　due to *Aspergillus* hypersensitivity, 927
　high-resolution CT findings in, 454, *455,* 2331–2333, *2334*
　idiopathic pulmonary fibrosis vs., 1611, 2373
　isocyanate-associated, 2362t, 2378–2379
　Japanese summer-type, 2362t, 2378
　pathogenesis of, 2361–2364
　pathologic features of, 2364–2365, *2366–2368*
　prognosis in, 2375–2376
　pulmonary function tests in, 2375
　radiologic features of, 2365–2373, *2368–2374*
　　time of appearance of, 3046
　subacute, 454, *455,* 2365–2372, *2369, 2373, 2374*
　varieties of, 2362t–2363t, 2376–2379
Eye, sarcoidosis involving, 1564
　tuberculosis involving, 840
　Wegener's granulomatosis involving, 1504

Fabry's disease, 2724
Facioscapulohumeral dystrophy, 3064
Fallen lung sign, with tracheobronchial fracture, 2621, *2621*
Familial Mediterranean fever, 2766–2767
Family history, 390
Fanconi's syndrome, immunodeficiency in, 726
　pulmonary arteriovenous malformations in, 657
Farmer's lung, 2362t, 2376–2377. See also *Extrinsic allergic alveolitis.*
　radiologic features of, *2368, 2369*
Fasciitis, diffuse, with eosinophilia, 1459
Fasciola hepatica, 1052
Fast-twitch glycolytic fatigable fibers, in diaphragm, 249
Fast-twitch oxidative glycolytic fatigue-resistant fibers, in diaphragm, 249
Fat, dietary, pulmonary carcinoma and, 1082
　extrapleural, pleural plaques vs., 2800, *2801*
　in bronchial tree, 14
　in cardiophrenic angle, enlargement of, *2916, 2918,* 2925–2927
　　radiographic interpretation of, 233
　in neck, obstructive sleep apnea and, 2059–2060
　mediastinal, normal distribution of, 212–214, *215, 216*
　neoplasms of, 1347. See also specific neoplasms.
　omental, herniation of, through diaphragmatic defect, 254, *255*
　pleuropericardial, enlargement of, *2916, 2918,* 2925–2927
　　radiographic interpretation of, 233
Fat embolism, 1845–1850

Fat embolism *(Continued)*
　adult respiratory distress syndrome with, 2005, *2005*
　causes of, 1846, 1847t
　clinical features of, 1848–1849
　diagnosis of, 1849–1850
　epidemiology of, 1846
　from bone infarcts, in sickle cell disease, 1833
　laboratory findings in, 1849
　pathogenesis of clinical syndrome of, 1846–1848
　pathologic features of, 1848, *1848*
　prognosis in, 1850
　pulmonary contusion vs., 1848, 2612
　radiologic features of, 1848, *1849*
Fatigue, reader, in radiographic interpretation, 279
　respiratory muscle. See under *Respiratory muscles.*
FDG. See ^{18}F-*Fludeoxyglucose* entries.
Febarbamate, thoracic disease due to, 2539t, 2567
Feeding tube, faulty insertion of, 2679–2680, *2679*
Feeding vessel sign, in pulmonary metastasis, 1389
　in *Staphylococcus aureus* pneumonia, 746
　in Wegener's granulomatosis, 1499, *1501*
　with septic emboli, 716
Fenestrae, alveolar, 32
　in emphysema, 2191, *2192*
　　collateral resistance and, 60
Fenestrations, diaphragmatic, air migration through, catamenial pneumothorax and, 2787
　tissue migration through, pleural endometriosis and, 2788–2789
Fenfluramine, pulmonary hypertension due to, 1903
Fenoterol, asthma deaths and, 2142
Ferruginous bodies, asbestos-related, 2425–2429, *2428*
　in coal workers' pneumoconiosis, 2412, *2412*
　particles forming, 2428
　talc-associated, 2449
Fetal adenocarcinoma, well-differentiated, 1368–1369, *1369*
Fever, 389
Fiber(s), inhaled, deposition of, 127
Fiberglass, pneumoconiosis due to, 2467–2468
Fibrin bodies, pleural, *2839,* 2840
Fibrinoid necrosis, in pulmonary hypertension, 1884–1885, *1888*
Fibroblasts, in asthmatic airway inflammation, 2090
Fibrobullous disease, upper lobe, in rheumatoid disease, 1438, *1439–1440*
Fibrocystic pulmonary dysplasia, familial, 1586, *1587–1589*
Fibrodysplasia ossificans progressiva, 3015
Fibroleiomyoma, pulmonary, 1409
Fibroma, esophageal, 2965, 2966
　mediastinal, 2925
　pleural (subpleural, submesothelial). See *Fibrous tumor of pleura, solitary.*
　pulmonary, 1347, 1371
　　hamartoma and, 1347, 1350–1351
Fibronectin, alveolar macrophage secretion of, 23
　in alveolar interstitium, 21
Fibrosarcoma, chest wall, *3026–3027*
　mediastinal, 2925
　pleural. See *Fibrous tumor of pleura, solitary.*
　pulmonary, 1349–1350, *1349*
Fibrosclerosis, multifocal, 2857

Fibrosing alveolitis, cryptogenic, 1585. See also *Pulmonary fibrosis, idiopathic.*
Fibrosing mediastinitis, 2856–2863
  causes of, 2856
  clinical features of, 2863
  diffuse, 2857
  focal, 2857, *2859, 2862, 2863*
  in Riedel's thyroiditis, upper airway obstruction with, 2031, *2031*
  in silicosis, 2402, *2404*
  pathogenesis of, 2856–2857
  pathologic features of, 2857, *2857, 2858*
  radiologic features of, 2857–2861, *2859–2864,* 3177t
  tuberculous, 835, 2856
Fibrosing pleuritis, cryptogenic bilateral, 2804
Fibrothorax, *2803,* 2804–2805, *2804, 2805*
  after penetrating wound, 2648, *2650*
  calcific, *584*
  in sarcoidosis, 1562
  pulmonary hypertension and, 1917
  radiologic differential diagnosis of, 582
Fibrous dysplasia, 3031, *3031*
Fibrous histiocytoma, benign, mediastinal, 2925
  pulmonary, 1371–1373
  borderline, 1347
  malignant, mediastinal, 2925
    of rib, *3033*
  pulmonary, 1347–1349
Fibrous pseudotumor of pleura, calcifying, 2840
Fibrous tumor of pleura, solitary, 2828–2835
  calcifying fibrous pseudotumor and, 2840
  clinical features of, 2833
  pathologic features of, 2829, *2830–2833*
  prognosis in, 2833–2835
  radiologic features of, *583, 586,* 2829–2833, *2834–2837*
Fibroxanthoma, pulmonary, 1371
Filariasis, 1043–1045, *1044,* 1752–1753
  pleural effusion in, 2752
Film digitization, 307–308
Film latitude, 302, 305
Filtration, wedge, for conventional radiographs, 302
Filtration coefficient, in pulmonary fluid and solute exchange, 1954
Fine-needle aspiration, 345–348
  transbronchial, 347–348
    in sarcoidosis diagnosis, 1571
  transthoracic, 345–347
    in pneumonia diagnosis, 721
    in pulmonary metastasis diagnosis, 1412
    in tuberculosis diagnosis, 846
  ultrasound-guided, 334, *334*
Fire clay, pneumoconiosis due to, 2451–2452
Firefighters, lung function in, 2531
Fish poisoning, 3062–3063
Fishmeal-worker's lung, 2362t. See also *Extrinsic allergic alveolitis.*
Fissures, 153–154, *155*
  accessory, imaging of, 160–165, *163–166*
  imaging of, 154–165
  incomplete, 153–154, *155*
    identification of, on high-resolution CT, 159–160, *162*
    pleural effusion configuration with, 564–565, *566*
    spread of pathologic process and, 461, *462*
  interlobar, bulging, in pneumonia, 702, *705,* 752, *754*
  displacement of, 459–461, *460, 461*
    in atelectasis, 525–526, *529, 530*
  on conventional CT, *157,* 158–159, *159, 161,* 286–287, *287, 288*
  on high-resolution CT, 159–160, *160, 162, 163,* 286, 287, *287, 289*

Fissures *(Continued)*
  on radiographs, 155–158, *157, 158, 160, 161*
  thickening of, in asbestos-exposed persons, 2433
Fistula(s), aortobronchial, 2290t, 2291
  postoperative, 2674
  biliary-pleural, 2764
  bronchial, 2289–2291, 2290t, *2291*
  bronchial–pulmonary artery, 2290t, 2291, *2291*
  bronchoarterial, in coccidioidomycosis, 894, *896*
  bronchobiliary, 628, 2290t, 2291
  bronchoesophageal, 628, 2290–2291, 2290t, 2967
    due to esophageal rupture, 2634
  bronchopancreatic, with diaphragmatic rupture, 2643
  bronchopleural, 2289–2290, 2290t
    after lung resection, 2663, 2762
  colobronchial, 2290t, 2291
  esophagopleural, due to esophageal perforation, 2634, 2856
    due to sclerotherapy for esophageal varices, 2968
    postoperative, 2663
  gastrobronchial, postoperative, 2674
  hepatobronchial, in amebiasis, 1035
    in echinococcosis, 1055
  pancreaticopleural, in chronic pancreatitis, 2765
  pulmonary arteriovenous, developmental. See *Arteriovenous malformation, pulmonary.*
    with penetrating wound, 2648, *2653*
  subarachnoid-pleural, pleural effusion due to, 2762
  systemic–pulmonary vascular, 666–667, *667, 668*
    with chest tube, 2677
  thoracobiliary, with diaphragmatic rupture, 2643
  tracheoesophageal, acquired, 2967
    congenital, 627–628, 2500
Flatworms, 1047–1052. See also specific diseases.
Fleischner lines, 554–560, *558*
Fleischner's sign, in pulmonary thromboembolism, 504, 1788, *1794*
Flow cytometry, 356–358, *357*
Flow interruption technique, for airway resistance measurement, 412
Flow-void phenomenon, in magnetic resonance imaging, 101, *101*
Flow-volume curves, in COPD, 2221–2222, *2221*
  in forced expiration, 408, *408*
  in obstructive conditions, 2027–2028, *2027*
  in obstructive sleep apnea, 2060, *2060*
Fludarabine, thoracic disease due to, 2538t, 2555
^{18}F-Fludeoxyglucose positron emission tomography (FDG-PET), 332–333
  in lymphoma staging, 1293
  in mesothelioma diagnosis, 2824
  in pulmonary carcinoma, for diagnosis, 1181
    for staging, 1191, 1192
  lymph node assessment on, 190
    in pulmonary carcinoma staging, 1191
  round atelectasis vs. pulmonary carcinoma on, 2443
  solitary nodule assessment on, 1146
^{18}F-Fludeoxyglucose single-photon emission computed tomography (FDG-SPECT), 332
  solitary nodule assessment on, 1146, *1147*
Fluid exchange, pulmonary, 1947–1956, *1947–1949, 1952*
  safety factors in, 1955–1956

Fluid transport equation, pulmonary fluid and solute exchange and, 1952–1955, *1952*
Flukes, blood. See *Schistosomiasis.*
  liver, 1052, 1753
  lung, 1047–1048, *1048–1051*
2-(^{18}F)-Fluoro-2-deoxy-D-glucose. See ^{18}F-*Fludeoxyglucose* entries.
Fluoroscopy, for diaphragmatic motion assessment, 2988, 2994
5-Fluorouracil, thoracic disease due to, 2538t, 2555
Fluoxetine, thoracic disease due to, 2539t, 2569
Fly ash, pneumoconiosis and, 2409
Focal-film distance, 302
Folded lung. See *Round atelectasis.*
Follicular bronchiolitis, 1273, *1274,* 2323t, 2349, *2349, 2350.* See also *Bronchiolitis.*
  in rheumatoid disease, 1446–1448, *1447, 1448*
Follicular bronchitis, 1273, *1274*
  in rheumatoid disease, 1446–1448
Follicular hyperplasia of thymus, in myasthenia gravis, 2877–2880, *2880*
Food additives, asthma provoked by, 2116
Food allergens, asthma and, 2106
Foramen(ina) of Bochdalek, 248, 2987, *2988*
  hernia through, 2997–3001, *2998, 3002*
    middle-posterior mediastinal mass due to, 3178t
    paravertebral mass due to, 3185t, *3189*
Foramen(ina) of Morgagni, 248, 2987, *2988*
  hernia through, *2926,* 2998, 3001–3004, *3003, 3004,* 3172t
Forced expiratory volume, in one second (FEV$_1$), age-related decline in, 2171–2172, *2172*
  forced vital capacity and, 406
  in COPD, 2121–2224, *2221–2223*
  measurement of, 408–410, *408*
  signal-to-noise ratio for, 410
Forced oscillation technique, for total respiratory system resistance measurement, 412
Forced vital capacity (FVC), measurement of, 406
  95% confidence limits for, 409
  signal-to-noise ratio for, 410
Foreign body(ies), aspiration of, 2485–2490. See also *Aspiration (event), of solid foreign bodies.*
  carcinoma at site of, 2653
  esophageal, airway obstruction due to, 2024, 2486
  from spinal stabilization, migration of, 2652
  in pleural cavity, with penetrating wound, 2648, *2650*
  radiopaque, embolization of, 1868
Form elasticity of lung, 564
Formaldehyde, 2526–2527
  occupational asthma due to, 2122
  pulmonary carcinoma and, 1078
Formalin inflation, for lung specimen fixation, 348–350, *350*
Fracture(s), after radiation therapy, 2597
  airway, homogeneous segmental opacity due to, 3088t
    pneumomediastinum and, 2618, *2621,* 2865
    with blunt trauma, 2618–2622, *2621, 2622*
  rib. See *Rib(s), fracture of.*
  vertebral, 2646, *2646,* 3023
    paravertebral mass due to, 3185t
    signs resembling aortic rupture in, 2626–2627
Francisella tularensis infection, 766–767, *768,* 2749
Fremitus, 392
Friction rub, pleural, 395
α-L-Fucosidase deficiency, mucus abnormality in, 63

Fryns syndrome, 599
Fuller's earth, pneumoconiosis due to, 2451
Fumes, metal, inhalation of, 2527–2528
    occupational exposure to, COPD and, 2174–2175
Functional residual capacity (FRC), 406, *406*
    in COPD, 2224
    measurement of, 407–408
Fungal infection, 875–952. See also *Fungus ball*; specific diseases.
    after bone marrow transplantation, 1730, *1731*
    after heart-lung or lung transplantation, 1717–1720, *1718–1721*
    cavities or cysts in, 3103t, *3107*
    diagnosis of, 876
    diffuse nodular pattern in, 3145t
    eosinophilic lung disease due to, 1744t, 1753
    homogeneous consolidation in, nonsegmental, 3080t
        segmental, 3087t
    in HIV disease, 1656–1673
    inhomogeneous consolidation in, nonsegmental, 3093t
        segmental, 3097t
    lymph node enlargement in, 3164t
    pleural effusion due to, 2745t, 2751–2752
    solitary mass due to, 3117t
    solitary nodule due to, 3111t
    types of, 876
Fungus(i). See also *Fungal infection; Fungus ball*; specific fungal diseases.
    asthma and, 2106
Fungus ball. See also *Aspergilloma*.
    in pseudallescheriasis, 951
    in sarcoidosis, 923, 1542, 1561, *1562*
    in tuberculosis, 814, 817, *824, 922, 923, 925, 926, 3106*
    intracavitary, 463, *466*
    non-*Aspergillus* species causing, 923
Funnel chest, 3018–3019, *3018*
Funnel trachea, anomalous origin of left pulmonary artery with, 642
Fusarium species infection, 952
Fusobacterium infection, 779, 782

α-Galactosidase A deficiency, in Fabry's disease, 2724
β-Galactosidase deficiency, in G$_{M1}$ gangliosidosis, 2724–2725
Gallium scintigraphy, 331–332, *331, 332*
    in Kaposi's sarcoma diagnosis, 332, 1679
    in lymphoma, 1293
    in sarcoidosis, 331, *331*, 1568, *1568*
        prognosis and, 1573
Galloping consumption, 814
Ganglioneuroblastoma, 2976–2977
Ganglioneuroma, 2976–2977, *2977, 2978*
    of chest wall, 3028
Gangrene, pulmonary, 463, *468–469*, 707, *710*
    in tuberculosis, 817
    with *Klebsiella pneumoniae* infection, 752, 753
Gap junctions, in alveolar epithelium, 18
Gardener's lung, 2362t. See also *Extrinsic allergic alveolitis*.
Gas(es). See also specific gases.
    inhaled, 2519–2527
        oxidant, 2519–2524
Gas embolism. See *Air embolism*.
Gastrectomy, partial, tuberculosis risk after, 803
Gastric aspiration, specimen collection by, in tuberculosis diagnosis, 844
Gastric pressure, abnormal swings in, in diaphragmatic paralysis, 2993, 2994

Gastric secretions, aspiration of. See under *Aspiration (event)*.
Gastric ulcer, pleural effusion with, 2766
Gastrobronchial fistula, postoperative, 2674
Gastroenteric cyst, 2979–2980
Gastroesophageal reflux, after tracheoesophageal fistula repair, 628
    aspiration and, 2491
    asthma and, 2113–2114
    chest pain due to, 386
    cough due to, 381
    in cystic fibrosis, 2311
    in progressive systemic sclerosis, 1453
Gastrointestinal tract. See also *Colon; Stomach*.
    Churg-Strauss syndrome involving, 1509
    cystic fibrosis involving, 2311–2312
    disease of, pleural effusion in, 2765–2766
    pulmonary carcinoma metastatic to, 1173
    sarcoidosis involving, 1565
    tuberculosis involving, 840
    upper, hemorrhage from, hemoptysis vs., 382
    Wegener's granulomatosis involving, 1504
Gaucher's disease, 2722–2724, *2725*
Gemcitabine, thoracic disease due to, 2555
Genetic fingerprinting, in epidemiologic investigation of tuberculosis, 846
Genioglossal muscles, in maintenance of airway patency, 242–243
    in ventilation, 246
Geniohyoid muscle, in ventilation, 246
Genitourinary tract, cystic fibrosis involving, 2310–2311
    disease of, pleural effusion with, 2764
    tuberculosis involving, 835–837
    Wegener's granulomatosis involving, 1504
Geotrichosis, 949
Germ cell neoplasm(s). See also specific neoplasms.
    malignant, 2902, *2902*, 2903t
    of anterior mediastinum, 2901–2911, 3171t, *3174*
    pulmonary, 1365–1367, *1368*
    sarcoidosis and, 1572
    testicular, metastatic to lung, *1383, 1406, 1407, 1407*
    thymic cyst and, 2882
Germinoma, mediastinal, 2908–2909, *2910*
    testicular, metastatic to lung, 1407
Gestational trophoblastic neoplasms. See also *Choriocarcinoma*.
    metastatic to lung, 1408–1409
Ghon focus, 463–467, *471*, 805, *809*
Giant cell arteritis, 1490t, 1517–1518, *1518*
Giant cell carcinoma, pulmonary, 1117, *1118*.
    See also *Carcinoma, pulmonary*.
    autonomic neuropathy in, 1174
    doubling time of, 1143, *1145*
    prognosis in, 1196
Giant cell interstitial pneumonia, 1584
Giant cell pneumonia, in measles, 988, *988, 989*, 990
Giant cell reaction, to aspirated gastric contents, 2492, *2494, 2495*
Giant cell tumor of bone, metastatic to lung, 1410–1411
Giant lymph node hyperplasia, 2760, 2938–2940, *2940–2942*
Giardiasis, 1039
Gibson's sign, in diaphragmatic rupture, 2643
Glanders, 760–761
Glial fibrillary acidic protein, in carcinoid tumors, 1233
Globoid leukodystrophy, 2727
Glomangioma, pulmonary, 1335–1336
Glomerulonephritis, acute, pleural effusion in, 2764

Glomerulonephritis *(Continued)*
    paraneoplastic, in pulmonary carcinoma, 1178
Glomus body, 1335
Glomus cells, 1335
Glomus pulmonale, 149
Glomus tumor, pulmonary, 1335–1336
Glossopharyngeal breathing, with spinal cord injury, 3055
Gloved-finger appearance, 483, *484*
    in allergic bronchopulmonary aspergillosis, 483, 929, *934*
Glucose, in pleural fluid, 2743, 2746
    in rheumatoid disease, 2754
β-Glucosidase deficiency, in Gaucher's disease, 2722–2724
Glutamate, in respiratory rhythm generation, 240
Glutaraldehyde, occupational asthma due to, 2122
Glutathione, in defense against oxidant damage, 2521
Glutathione-*S*-transferase deficiency, pulmonary carcinoma and, 1082
Glutathione-*S*-transferase gene, COPD and, 2179
Glycine, in respiratory rhythm generation, 240
Glycogen storage disease, 2727, 3064
Glycolipids, in tracheobronchial secretions, 61
G$_{M1}$ gangliosidosis, 2724–2725
Gnathostomiasis, 1046–1047
Goblet cells of tracheobronchial epithelium, 6, 7–8, *8, 9*
    hyperplasia of, in asthma, 2083, *2085*
Goiter, mediastinal, 198, 2912, *2912*, 2913, *2913*
    in anterior compartment, 3171t
    in middle-posterior compartment, 3175t
    upper airway obstruction due to, 2030–2031
Gold miners, COPD in, 2175
Gold therapy, obliterative bronchiolitis in rheumatoid disease and, 1445
    thoracic disease due to, 2539t, 2566
Golden's sign, 460, 543, *544, 548, 549*
    in pulmonary carcinoma, 1121, *1126*
Golgi tendon apparatus, of diaphragm, in ventilatory control, 238
Goodpasture's syndrome, 1757–1765
    clinical features of, 1763
    diagnosis of, 1764
    diffuse air-space pattern in, 3130t
    epidemiology of, 1757
    pathogenesis of, 1757–1758
    pathologic features of, 1758–1759, *1759*
    prognosis in, 1765
    pulmonary function tests in, 1763
    radiologic features of, 1759–1762, *1760, 1762*
Gorham's syndrome, 3031
Gossypiboma, 1371
Gottron's papules, 1462
Graft-versus-host disease, after bone marrow transplantation, 1729
    bronchiolitis and, 1729, *2332*, 2336–2337
    chronic, progressive systemic sclerosis and, 1459
    idiopathic pneumonia syndrome and, 1727, 1728
Grain dust, COPD and, 2175
    occupational asthma due to, 2120
    Wegener's granulomatosis and, 1492
Grain fever, 2175. See also *Organic dust toxic syndrome*.
Gram stain, for pneumonia diagnosis, 719
Gram-negative bacilli. See also specific genera and species.
    classification and nomenclature of, 735t
    pulmonary infection due to, 751–765
Gram-negative cocci. See also specific genera and species.
    classification and nomenclature of, 735t

Gram-negative cocci *(Continued)*
pulmonary infection due to, 748
Gram-negative coccobacilli. See also specific
genera and species.
classification and nomenclature of, 735t
pulmonary infection due to, 765–776
Gram-positive bacilli. See also specific genera
and species.
classification and nomenclature of, 735t
pulmonary infection due to, 749–750
Gram-positive cocci. See also specific genera
and species.
classification and nomenclature of, 735t
pulmonary infection due to, 736–748
Granular cell tumor, pulmonary, 1346
Granular pneumocyte. See *Alveolar epithelial
cells, type II.*
Granulocyte-macrophage colony-stimulating
factor, thoracic disease due to, 2538t, 2556
Granulocytic sarcoma, 1317, 1319, *1319*
Granuloma(s), calcified, CT detection of, *315*
in extrinsic allergic alveolitis, 2365, *2366–
2368*
in sarcoidosis, 1537, *1538–1540*
in tuberculosis, 805, *806–807*
mediastinal, problems with term, 2856
non-necrotizing, differential diagnosis of,
1537–1541, 1565
plasma cell, 1371–1373, *1372*
pulmonary hyalinizing, 1373, *1374, 1375*
shifting, in atelectasis, 534
Granulomatosis, bronchocentric, in allergic
bronchopulmonary aspergillosis, 928, *930*
in tuberculosis, 817, *823*
Langerhans' cell. See *Langerhans' cell histiocytosis.*
lymphomatoid, 1280–1281, *1282–1285*
necrotizing sarcoid, 1521–1523, *1522–1524*
Wegener's. See *Wegener's granulomatosis.*
Granulomatous hepatitis, 1565
Granulomatous interstitial nephritis, in
sarcoidosis, 1566
Granulomatous lymphadenitis, 2940–2942
necrotizing, broncholithiasis with, 2287
Granulomatous mediastinitis, 2856–2863. See
also *Fibrosing mediastinitis.*
Graphite, pneumoconiosis due to, 2409, 2413
Graves' disease. See also *Hyperthyroidism.*
thymic hyperplasia in, 2877
Gravitational shift test, in pneumonia vs.
pulmonary edema, 1969
Gravity, pulmonary circulation and, 104–106,
105, 110
pulmonary diffusing capacity and, 108
ventilation/perfusion ratio variation and, 110–
111
Gray hepatization, in *Streptococcus pneumoniae*
pneumonia, 737, *738*
Great white plague, 799
Grid technique, for bedside radiography, 305
for conventional radiography, 302
Ground-glass pattern, in bronchiolitis, *2330,
2331–2333, 2331, 2334*
in interstitial disease, 453–454, *455*
on high-resolution CT, 453, *455, 456*
Growing teratoma syndrome, 2902
Growth factors, in pulmonary carcinoma, 1083
Growth retardation, familial, renal aminoaciduria
and cor pulmonale with, 2728
Guaifenesin, mucus mobility and, 63
Guillain-Barré syndrome, 3061–3062
influenza and, 984
Gunshot wound, 2647–2648, 2648–2652, *2648,
2649, 2651*
bullet fragment embolism after, 1868, *1868,*
2652

Gynecomastia, pulmonary carcinoma and, 1177

Haemophilus influenzae infection, 767–770
community-acquired, 721
homogeneous opacity in, nonsegmental, 3079t
segmental, 3087t
in HIV disease, 1645
in influenza, 983–984
inhomogeneous segmental opacity in, 3097t,
3099
parapneumonic effusion in, 2749
radiologic features of, 769–770, *769*
Haemophilus parainfluenzae infection, 770
Hafnia alvei infection, 758
Hair spray, granulomatous pneumonitis
associated with, 2531
Hairy cell leukemia, nontuberculous
mycobacterial infection in, 853, 855
Halitosis, 389
Halo sign, in angioinvasive aspergillosis, 941,
945
in zygomycosis, 946
Halothane, ventilatory response and, 240
Hamartoma, calcification with, 467, 472
endobronchial, *1353*
atelectasis due to, *536*
epidemiology of, 1351
pathologic features of, 1352, *1353*
radiologic features of, 1355, *1357*
mesenchymal cystic, 1373–1374
pulmonary, 1350–1355
chondroma and, 1343, 1350–1351, *1350*
clinical features of, 1355
epidemiology of, 1351
fibroma and, 1347, 1350–1351
lipoma and, 1347, 1350–1351, *1353*
pathologic features of, *1350,* 1351–1352,
1351–1353
prognosis in, 1355
radiologic features of, 1352–1355, *1354–
1357*
solitary nodule due to, 3112t, *3115*
Hamazaki-Wesenberg bodies, in sarcoidosis,
1537
Hamman-Rich disease. See *Pulmonary fibrosis,
idiopathic.*
Hamman's sign, 2140, 2870
pneumothorax and, 2791
with esophageal rupture, 2634, 2856
Hampton's hump, 1796, *1798–1800,* 3088t, *3091*
Hand-Schüller-Christian disease, 1627. See also
Langerhans' cell histiocytosis.
Hansenula polymorpha infection, 952
Hantaviruses, 992–993, *992, 993*
Hard metal lung disease, 2463, *2463, 2464*
Harvester's lung. See *Extrinsic allergic
alveolitis; Farmer's lung.*
Hassall's corpuscles, 198
Head and neck cancer, metastatic to lung, 1405
cavitation in, 1389, *1390*
pulmonary carcinoma and, 1201–1202
Head trauma, hypoxemia with, 2647
pulmonary edema due to, 1974–1976
Headache, "benign" cough, 382
morning, in obstructive sleep apnea, 2067
Heaf and Disk tine test, 841–842
Heart. See also *Cardiac; Cardio-* entries.
Churg-Strauss syndrome involving, 1510
developmental anomalies of, 664–665, *664,
665*
herniation of, after pneumonectomy, 2665
with parietal pericardium deficiency, 667–
671, *669–670*
MR evaluation of, 320–321

Heart *(Continued)*
normal radiographic appearance of, 229–233
paradoxical change in size of, in upper airway
obstruction, 2029
perforation of, in pulmonary angiography,
1818, *1818*
with central venous catheter, 2685
physical examination of, 395–396
progressive systemic sclerosis involving,
1457–1458
pulmonary carcinoma involving, 1170–1171
sarcoidosis involving, 1562–1563, *1563–1564*
prognosis in, 1572
Wegener's granulomatosis involving, 1504
Heart disease, congenital, pulmonary
arteriovenous malformation vs., 662
pulmonary artery aneurysm in, 1935
pulmonary oligemia in, 500–501, *501,*
3151t, *3152*
pulmonary vascular changes in, grading of,
1885–1886
sternal abnormalities and, 3019
with increased flow, pulmonary hypertension due to, 1891–1896, *1892, 1894–
1897*
ischemic. See also *Myocardial infarction.*
asbestos exposure and, 2448
chest pain due to, 386
Heart failure, left-sided, pulmonary hypertension
due to, 1918–1919
obstructive sleep apnea and, 2067
pleural effusion due to, 579–581, *580,* 2760–
2761, *2762*
pulmonary infarction and, 1781
right-sided, due to pulmonary thromboembolism, 1782, 1825
in COPD, blood gas tensions and, 2226
prognosis and, 2230
Heart surgery, atelectasis after, 522, *2670,* 2671
chylothorax after, 2769
pleural effusion after, 2762, 2766
pulmonary edema after, 2671
Heart-lung transplantation, 1698–1726
bronchiolitis after, 2336
complications of, 1700–1724
pleural, 1720–1721
indications for, 1699
infection after, bacterial, 1713–1715
fungal, 1717, *1718, 1720*
lung diseases treated by, 1699t
prognosis after, 1726
pulmonary function tests after, 1724–1726
in obliterative bronchiolitis diagnosis, 1711
rejection after. See *Lung transplantation,
rejection after.*
reperfusion edema after, 1702
Heartworm (dirofilariasis), 1045, *1046*
pulmonary embolism in, 1853
Heat loss, respiratory, bronchoconstriction in
response to, 2108
Heat shock proteins, connective tissue disease
and, 1424
in *Legionella* infection, 772
Heath-Edwards system, for grading pulmonary
vascular changes in congenital heart
disease, 1885–1886
Heavy chain disease, 1297–1298
pleural effusion due to, 2760
Heerfordt's syndrome, 1565
Helical computed tomography, 310–311, *310,
311.* See also *Computed tomography (CT).*
emphysema quantification using, 2214, *2214*
with minimum intensity projection, in emphysema, 2211, *2211*
Helium inhalation, change in maximal expiratory
flow with, in airway obstruction diagnosis,
409–410

Helium inhalation (*Continued*)
  closing volume measurement using, 413–414
  functional residual capacity determination using, 407
  inspired gas distribution assessment using, in COPD, 2225
  total lung capacity estimation from, in COPD, 2225
Helminths, 1039–1059. See also specific diseases.
Hemangioendothelioma, epithelioid, mediastinal, 2920, *2920, 2921*
  pulmonary, 1339–1343, *1340, 1341*
Hemangioma, histiocytoid. See *Hemangio-endothelioma.*
  mediastinal, 2917–2920
  pulmonary, 1376–1377
  sclerosing, 1364–1365, *1366, 1367*
Hemangiomatosis, pulmonary capillary, 1914–1915, *1914*
Hemangiopericytoma, mediastinal, 2921
  pulmonary, 1336–1337, *1337*
Hematologic malignancy. See also specific disorders.
  mediastinal germ cell neoplasms and, 2902
Hematoma, chronic expanding, 2614
  diaphragmatic, 3006, *3006*
  extrapleural, postsurgical, 2661, *2662*
  mediastinal, anterior mass due to, 3172t
    middle-posterior mass due to, 3178t
  pulmonary, 2613–2618, *2614–2617, 2619–2620*
    multiple masses or nodules due to, 3124t
    postoperative, 2669–2670, *2669*
    solitary mass due to, 3118t
    solitary nodule due to, 3112t
  with penetrating wound, 2648, *2651*
  with vertebral fracture, paravertebral mass due to, 3185t
Hematopoiesis, extramedullary, 1320, 2980–2981, *2981*
Hemiazygos vein, 218
  dilation of, 2950–2951, 2950t, 3178t
Hemodialysis patients, asthma in, 2106
  granulomatous pneumonitis with foreign material in, 1868–1870, *1870*
  hypoventilation with normal arterial carbon dioxide tension in, 3048
  metastatic pulmonary calcification in, 2699
  pleural effusion in, 2764
  pulmonary edema in, 1973–1974
Hemoglobin concentration, diffusing capacity measurement and, 416
Hemolytic-uremic syndrome, mitomycin-induced, 2544
Hemopneumothorax, spontaneous, 2791
Hemoptysis, 382–385, 383t
  in systemic lupus erythematosus, differential diagnosis of, 1430
  in tuberculosis, 831
Hemorrhage, mediastinal, 2625–2626, *2626, 2870–2871, 2870*
  after sternotomy, 2664
  anterior mass due to, 3172t
  in aortic rupture, 2627, *2627,* 2630–2631, *2630*
  middle-posterior mass due to, 3178t
  pulmonary, after bone marrow transplantation, 1726–1727, *1727*
    differential diagnosis of, 1764
    diffuse air-space pattern in, 3130t
    due to thromboembolism, 1780–1781
      pathologic features of, 1783
    idiopathic, 1757–1765
      clinical features of, 1762–1763
      diagnosis of, 1764

Hemorrhage (*Continued*)
      epidemiology of, 1757
      pathogenesis of, 1758
      pathologic features of, 1758–1759
      prognosis in, 1764–1765
      pulmonary function tests in, 1763
      radiologic features of, 1759–1762, *1761, 1763*
    in coccidioidomycosis, *896*
    in systemic lupus erythematosus, 1426–1427, *1428,* 1430
    on high-resolution CT, *438*
    usage of term, 1780n
  retropharyngeal, upper airway obstruction due to, 2024
  with transthoracic needle biopsy, 370
Hemorrhagic fever with renal syndrome, 992, 993
Hemosiderosis, pulmonary, idiopathic. See *Hemorrhage, pulmonary, idiopathic.*
  in pulmonary hypertension, 1919, *1920, 1923, 1929*
Hemothorax. See also *Pleural effusion.*
  after thoracotomy, 2661, *2661*
  CT identification of, 574, *576*
  defined, 2763
  due to malignancy, 2763
  due to trauma, 2761
    blunt, 2623
    penetrating, 2648, *2648,* 2651, *2652*
  in thoracic endometriosis, 2767
  pleural calcification due to, 583
  rare causes of, 2763
Henderson equation, 116
Henoch-Schönlein purpura, 1490t, 1521
Heparin, functions of, in lung, 17
Hepatitis, granulomatous, 1565
  viral, pleural effusion in, 2752
Hepatitis C virus, idiopathic pulmonary fibrosis and, 1585–1586
Hepatization, in *Streptococcus pneumoniae* pneumonia, 737, *738*
Hepatobronchial fistula, in amebiasis, 1035
  in echinococcosis, 1055
Hepatocellular carcinoma, metastatic to lung, 1405
Hepatoid carcinoma, pulmonary, 1113
Hepatopulmonary syndrome, liver transplantation's effects on, 1734
HER2/*neu* gene, 1083
Herbicide poisoning, 2584, 2585–2587, *2586, 2587*
Hereditary hemorrhagic telangiectasia, pulmonary arteriovenous malformations in, 657, *659,* 661, *661, 3113*
Hering-Breuer reflex, stretch receptors in, 237
Hermansky-Pudlak syndrome, 2727
Herniation, cardiac, after pneumonectomy, 2665
  with parietal pericardium deficiency, 667–671, *669–670*
  diaphragmatic. See *Diaphragmatic hernia.*
  mediastinal, 531–532, *532*
  pulmonary, 3012, *3013*
    postoperative, 2671, *2672*
    post-traumatic, 2646–2647, *2647*
Heroin, septic arthritis of sternoclavicular and sternochondral joints in addicts of, 3020
  thoracic disease due to, 2539t, 2567
Herpes simplex infection, after bone marrow transplantation, 1730
  pleural effusion in, 2752
  type I, 996–999, *997–999*
  type II, 999
Herpes zoster. See *Zoster.*
Herpes varicella. See *Varicellavirus infection.*
Herpesvirus(es), 996–1009. See also specific viruses.

Herpesvirus 6, 999
Herpesvirus 8, 999
  Kaposi's sarcoma and, 1677, 1681
  primary effusion lymphoma and, 1682, 2838
Herpesvirus simiae, 996
Hexamethylene diisocyanate, allergic alveolitis associated with, 2362t, 2378. See also *Extrinsic allergic alveolitis.*
Hiatus hernia, 2996–2997, *2998–3001,* 3178t
Hiccups, persistent, 2995
High-altitude pulmonary edema, 1999–2001
Highest mediastinal lymph nodes, in classification for lung cancer staging, *185,* 188t, *1186,* 1187t
High-resolution computed tomography. See under *Computed tomography (CT).*
Hilar lymph nodes, 180, *183, 184,* 191–192, *192.* See also *Lymph nodes.*
  CT assessment of, in pulmonary carcinoma staging, 1187, *1188*
  enlarged, differential diagnosis of, 3163, 3164t–3165t, *3166–3169*
    in cystic fibrosis, 2277, 2304, *2307*
    in suspected lung cancer, investigation of, 1194
    in angioimmunoblastic lymphadenopathy, 1313, *1314*
    in classification for lung cancer staging, *185,* 188t, *1186,* 1187t
    in Hodgkin's disease, 1299, *1301*
      symptoms due to, 1311–1312
    in sarcoidosis, 1545–1547, *1546–1549,* 1547t, 1550, *1550, 1551*
    Hodgkin's disease vs., 1311–1312, 1545
  silicosis involving, 2394, 2402, *2403*
Hilum(a), defined, 81
  displacement of, in atelectasis, 532–533, *533*
  enlargement of, in pulmonary carcinoma, 1156, *1157, 1158*
  imaging of, 81–104
  line shadows connecting peripheral mass to, 483
  lymph nodes of. See *Hilar lymph nodes; Lymph nodes.*
  on conventional radiographs, on lateral projection, 84–87, *88–95*
    on posteroanterior projection, 81–84, *82–86*
  on CT, 87–96, *96–100*
  on MRI, 96–104, *101–103,* 321
  vascular pseudotumors of, on lateral projection, 87, *92*
    on posteroanterior projection, 84, *85, 86*
  vasculature of, nomenclature of, 87
Hilum overlay sign, in mediastinal lymphoma, *1294*
Hirschsprung's disease, 3052–3053
Hirudiniasis, 1061
Histamine, in asthmatic airway inflammation, 2090–2091
  in exercise-induced asthma, 2109
  inhalation of, for bronchial responsiveness measurement, 420–423, 421t, *423,* 2095, *2095*
  irritant receptor response to, 237
  pulmonary vascular response to, 106
Histamine receptors, bronchial hyper-responsiveness and, 2100
  in asthma, 2091
Histiocytes, sea-blue, in Niemann-Pick disease, 2724
Histiocytoid hemangioma. See *Epithelioid hemangioendothelioma.*
Histiocytoma, fibrous. See *Fibrous histiocytoma.*
  pulmonary, 1371
Histiocytosis, malignant, 1291
Histiocytosis X. See *Langerhans' cell histiocytosis.*

Histoplasmoma, 878, *879*, 881, *883–885*
Histoplasmosis, 876–890
  acute, *878,* 880–881, *880–882*
  asymptomatic, 880
  broncholithiasis in, 881, *882,* 2287, *2288*
  cavities or cysts in, 3103t
  chronic, 881–888
    inactive, *879*
    mediastinal, 884–888, *887*
    pulmonary, 881–884, *886*
  clinical categories of, 879–880
  disseminated, 888, *889*
  due to *H. duboisii,* 890
  epidemiology of, 877
  fibrosing mediastinitis due to, 2856, *2861, 2863*
  homogeneous nonsegmental opacity in, 3080t
  in HIV disease, 1671
  inhomogeneous opacity in, nonsegmental, 3093t
    segmental, 3097t
  laboratory findings in, 888–890
  local parenchymal calcification in, 463–467
  lymph node enlargement in, 3164t
  multiple masses or nodules in, 3123t
  pathogenesis of, 877–878, *878, 879*
  pathologic features of, 877–880, *878, 879*
  pleural effusion in, 2751
  simulating necrotizing sarcoid granulomatosis, *1522*
  solitary nodule due to, 3111t
  tuberculosis vs., 811, 879
History, 379–391
  family, 390
  in asthma diagnosis, 2132–2133
  occupational, 390
    in asthma diagnosis, 2122
  past medical, 389
  residence and travel, 390
  respiratory disease symptoms in, 380–389
HIV. See *Acquired immunodeficiency syndrome (AIDS); Human immunodeficiency virus (HIV) infection.*
HLA antigens, allergy and, 2082
  anhydride-related occupational asthma and, 2121
  animal-related occupational asthma and, 2120
  ankylosing spondylitis and, 3022
  anti–Jo-1 antibodies and, 1463
  aspirin-induced asthma and, 2113
  Behçet's disease and, 1518
  berylliosis and, 2458
  Caplan's syndrome and, 1441
  coal workers' pneumoconiosis and, 2411
  COPD and, 2179
  CREST syndrome and, 1460
  cryptogenic bilateral fibrosing pleuritis and, 2804
  diffuse panbronchiolitis and, 2349–2352
  echinococcosis and, 1058
  extrinsic allergic alveolitis and, 2364
  Goodpasture's syndrome and, 1757
  HIV-associated pulmonary hypertension and, 1914
  idiopathic pulmonary fibrosis and, 1586
  idiopathic pulmonary hemorrhage and, 1758
  isocyanate sensitivity and, 2122
  lymphocytic interstitial pneumonitis in HIV infection and, 1686
  mismatched, acute rejection and, 1702
  obliterative bronchiolitis in rheumatoid disease and, 1445
  obstructive sleep apnea and, 2059
  pleural effusion in rheumatoid disease and, 2754
  pleuropulmonary disease in juvenile rheumatoid arthritis and, 1451–1452

HLA antigens *(Continued)*
  pneumothorax and, 2781
  primary pulmonary hypertension and, 1898
  relapsing polychondritis and, 1471
  rheumatoid disease and, 1434
  sarcoidosis and, 1535–1536
  silicosis and, 2392
  Sjögren's syndrome and, 1466
  systemic lupus erythematosus and, 1423–1424
  Takayasu's arteritis and, 1515
  tuberculosis risk and, 802
  Wegener's granulomatosis and, 1492
Hoarseness, 389
Hodgkin's disease, 1298–1312
  anterior mediastinal mass in, 1302, 2911, *2911, 3172t*
  bronchoalveolar lavage in, 343
  chemotherapy for, long-term effects of, 1312
  chest wall involvement in, 1306, 3025, 3031
  chest wall pain due to alcohol consumption in, 387
  clinical features of, 1311–1312
  differential diagnosis of, 1299
  endobronchial, 1306, *1308, 1309*
  gallium lung scanning in, 332
  laboratory findings in, 1312
  lymph node enlargement in, 3165t
    diaphragmatic, 2929
    mediastinal, 1299–1302, *1300–1305*
    sarcoidosis vs., 1311–1312, 1545
  middle-posterior mediastinal mass in, 3176t
  pathologic features of, 1298–1299, *1298, 1299*
  pleural effusion due to, 2759
  pleuropulmonary involvement in, radiologic features of, 1302–1306, *1305–1309*
  prognosis in, 1312
  pulmonary consolidation in, 1302, *1306, 1307*
    homogeneous nonsegmental, 3081t, *3084*
  radiation therapy for, abnormalities after, 2604
    long-term effects of, 1312
    pulmonary carcinoma and, 1201
  radiologic features of, 1299–1311, *1300–1311*
    after therapy, 1306–1310
  recurrent, 1310–1311
    rebound thymic hyperplasia vs., 2877
    residual, rebound thymic hyperplasia vs., 2877
  skeletal involvement in, 1306, *1310, 1311,* 3031–3032
  thymic cyst and, 2882
  thymic involvement in, 1302
Homogentisic acid oxidase deficiency, in alkaptonuria, 677
Honeycombing, 446–447, *447, 449*
  cystic lesions of lymphangioleiomyomatosis vs., 685
  diffuse lung disease with, 3133
  in idiopathic pulmonary fibrosis, *1594, 1598, 1599, 1599, 1601–1602, 3139*
    bronchiectasis vs., 2269, *2271*
    on CT, 1604, *1605, 1606*
  in Langerhans' cell histiocytosis, 446–447, 1630, *1634, 1635*
  in rheumatoid disease, 1434, *1435, 1437, 1437*
  in sarcoidosis, 446–447, 1542, *1543,* 1551–1554, *1555,* 1558, *1561*
Hookworm disease, 1043, 1047
  eosinophilic lung disease in, 1752
Hoover's sign, 391, 2216
Hormones. See also *specific hormones.*
  exogenous, thoracic disease due to, 2538t, 2551
  lung development and, 142
  tumor secretion of, in pulmonary carcinoma, 1175–1177
Horse race effect, in FEV₁ decline, 2172, *2172,* 2173

Horseshoe lung, 628–629
Horsfield-Cumming system, for describing airway geometry, 3–4, *4*
Hot-tub-bather's lung, 2362t. See also *Extrinsic allergic alveolitis.*
Hounsfield units, 269–270, 291–292
House dust mites, asthma and, 2106
Hughes-Stovin syndrome, 1518, 1936, 1937
Human albumin microspheres, technetium-labeled, for perfusion scanning, 326–327, 1800
Human chorionic gonadotropin, pulmonary carcinoma secreting, 1177
  α-subunit of, in carcinoid tumors, 1233
Human immunodeficiency virus (HIV) infection. See also *Acquired immunodeficiency syndrome (AIDS).*
  alveolar proteinosis in, 1687, 2701
  aspergillosis in, 1672–1673, *1672, 1673*
  Bartonella infection in, 1647, *1647*
  blastomycosis in, 1672
  coccidioidomycosis in, 1671–1672
  community-acquired pneumonia in, organisms causing, 722
  cryptococcosis in, 1670–1671, *1671*
    pleural effusion in, 2751
  emphysema in, 2243
  epidemiology of, 1642–1643
  gallium scintigraphy in, 331–332, *332*
  Haemophilus influenzae infection in, 1645
  histoplasmosis in, 1671
  Kaposi's sarcoma in, 1337, 1676–1681. See also under *Kaposi's sarcoma.*
  Legionella infection in, 1645
  mesothelioma and, 2810
  Nocardia asteroides infection in, 1648
  nontuberculous mycobacterial infection in, 853, *854,* 1654–1655, *1654–1656*
  parapneumonic pleural effusion in, 2747
  Pneumocystis carinii pneumonia in, 722, 1656–1670. See also under *Pneumocystis carinii* pneumonia.
  Pseudomonas aeruginosa infection in, 1645
  pulmonary, 991–992, 1673–1674
    lymphocytic interstitial pneumonitis and, 1674, 1685–1686
    pulmonary hypertension with, 1686, 1914
    pulmonary manifestations of, 1641–1687, 1644t
      epidemiology of, 1643
      infectious, 1643–1676, 1644t
      neoplastic, 1644t, 1676–1683
  Rhodococcus equi infection in, 1645–1647, *1646*
  risk factors for, 1642
  Staphylococcus aureus infection in, 1645
  Streptococcus pneumoniae infection in, 742, 1645
  tuberculosis in, 1648–1654. See also under *Tuberculosis.*
Human neurofilament subunits, in carcinoid tumors, 1233
Human papillomavirus. See *Papillomavirus(es).*
Human T-cell leukemia virus, 991
Humidification of inspired air, bronchial circulation in, 121
Humidifier fever. See *Organic dust toxic syndrome.*
Humidifier lung, 2362t. See also *Extrinsic allergic alveolitis.*
Humoral immunity, in host response to neoplasia, 1084
  in rheumatoid disease, 1434
  pulmonary, 130–131
Hyaline membranes, in adult respiratory distress syndrome, 1984, *1984*

Hyalinizing granuloma, pulmonary, 1373, *1374, 1375*
Hyaluronic acid, in mesothelioma, 2818, 2820, 2826
  in pleural fluid, 2743
  in pulmonary interstitial connective tissue, 1950
Hydatid disease. See *Echinococcosis.*
Hydramnios, cystic adenomatoid malformation and, 618
Hydrocarbons, ingestion of, pulmonary disease due to, 2588–2589
  polycyclic aromatic, pulmonary carcinoma and, 1077–1078
Hydrochloric acid, in polyvinyl chloride fires, 2529
Hydrochlorothiazide, thoracic disease due to, 2539t, 2571, *2571*
Hydrocortisone, systemic, bronchial narrowing in response to, in asthma, 2113
Hydrogen sulfide, acute exposure to, 2524
Hydronephrosis, pleural effusion with, 2764
Hydropneumothorax, 589, *591*
Hydrostatic pressure, in pulmonary fluid and solute exchange, 1953–1954
Hydrothorax. See also *Pleural effusion.*
  due to heart failure, 2761, *2762*
  hepatic, 2764
  tension, 592
    due to malignancy, 2757, *2758*
  typical configuration of, 564
5-Hydroxyindoleacetic acid, urinary, in carcinoid syndrome diagnosis, 1242
Hygroma, cystic, 2921
Hymenoptera sting, anaphylaxis due to, 2106
Hypercalcemia, in sarcoidosis, 1566, 1570
  in tuberculosis, 847
  metastatic pulmonary calcification in, 2699
  paraneoplastic, in pulmonary carcinoma, 1176
Hypercapnia, carotid body response to, 235–237
  in asthma, 2139
  in COPD, 2226–2227
  pattern of central response to, 239
  pulmonary vascular response to, 106
  ventilatory failure with. See *Alveolar hypoventilation.*
  ventilatory response to, 240–241, 417–418, *417*
    during sleep, 243, 2055
    genetic influences on, 240–241
    upper airway muscle control in, 242, 246
Hypercatabolism of immunoglobulins, 726
Hypercortisolism. See also *Cushing's syndrome.*
  mediastinal lipomatosis and, 2915, *2916*
Hypereosinophilic syndrome. See *Loeffler's syndrome.*
Hyperhomocystinemia, venous thrombosis and, 1779
Hyperimmunoglobulin E syndrome, 725
Hyperinfection syndrome, in strongyloidiasis, 1041, 1042, *1042,* 1043
Hyperinflation, 494–495
  compensatory, 498, *498*
    in atelectasis, 529–532, *531, 532*
  dynamic signs of, 499, *501*
  general, radiologic signs of, 495–497, *496*
  in asthma, 2125, *2125, 2126*
    consequences of, 2138
    mechanisms of, 2138
    radiographic detection of, 3047
  in emphysema, radiologic signs of, 2207–2209, *2207–2209*
  local, radiologic signs of, 497–499, *497–501*
  neonatal lobar, 621–625, *625, 626*
  oligemia with, 3156, *3158, 3159*
  static signs of, 498–499, *499, 500*

Hyperlucent lung, after radiation therapy, 2596, *2599*
  unilateral. See also *Swyer-James syndrome.*
    differential diagnosis of, 2340–2343
Hypermagnesemia, hypoventilation due to, 3065
  in salt-water near-drowning, 2510–2511
Hyperparathyroidism, 2729
  paraneoplastic syndrome resembling, in pulmonary carcinoma, 1176
Hyper-reactivity, airway. See also *Bronchial hyper-responsiveness.*
  defined, 422
  of smooth muscle cells, prejunctional vs. postjunctional, 2100
Hyper-responsiveness, airway. See also *Bronchial hyper-responsiveness.*
  defined, 422
Hypersensitivity, alveolar. See *Extrinsic allergic alveolitis.*
  delayed, in tuberculosis, 805, 813
  in inhalation challenge tests, 422
  in irradiation-induced lung damage, 2593–2594
  in respiratory syncytial virus infection, 986
  to *Aspergillus* organisms, 927. See also *Aspergillosis, allergic bronchopulmonary.*
Hypersensitivity pneumonitis. See *Extrinsic allergic alveolitis.*
Hypersomnolence, daytime, in obstructive sleep apnea, 2065–2066
Hypertension, obstructive sleep apnea and, 2066–2067
  pulmonary. See *Pulmonary hypertension.*
Hyperthyroidism, 2729
  hyperventilation due to, 3067
  hypoventilation in, 3065
  thymic hyperplasia in, 2877
Hypertrichosis lanuginosa, in pulmonary carcinoma, 1174
Hypertrophic osteoarthropathy, 396–397, 397t
  in cystic fibrosis, 2310
  in pulmonary carcinoma, 1175
  solitary fibrous tumor of pleura and, 2833
  with pulmonary metastasis, 1389
Hyperventilation, defined, 3065
  due to extrapulmonary disorders, 3066–3067
  due to pulmonary disease, 3065–3066
  in compensation in metabolic acidosis, 118
  isocapnic, in bronchial reactivity assessment, 423–424
  prolonged, overcompensation in, 3067
  psychogenic, 3066–3067
  respiratory alkalosis due to, 117
Hyperviscosity syndrome, in rheumatoid disease, 1451
Hypervolemia, pulmonary edema associated with, 1973–1974, *1973*
Hypnotics, obstructive sleep apnea and, 2062
  thoracic disease due to, 2539t, 2567
Hypocomplementemic urticarial vasculitis, 1432–1433
  emphysema in, 2243
Hypogenetic lung syndrome, 653–655, *654–656,* 3157t
Hypoglycemia, with pulmonary carcinoma, 1177
  with solitary fibrous tumor of pleura, 2833
Hypokalemia, hypoventilation due to, 3065
  in paraneoplastic Cushing's syndrome, 1176
Hyponatremia, in tuberculosis, 847
  with inappropriate antidiuretic hormone secretion, in pulmonary carcinoma, 1177
Hypopharynx, receptors in, in ventilatory control, 246
  systemic lupus erythematosus involving, 1431
Hypophosphatemia, hypoventilation due to, 3065
Hypopituitarism, 2729

Hypoplasia, pulmonary, 598–601
  pulmonary artery, parenchymal hypoplasia and, 598
Hypopnea, sleep, defined, 2054, 2056
Hypoproteinemia, pulmonary edema associated with, 1973–1974, *1973*
Hypothyroidism, 2729
  hypoventilation in, 3054
  pleural effusion in, 2766
  progressive systemic sclerosis with, 1459
Hypoventilation. See *Alveolar hypoventilation.*
Hypoxemia, arterial, mechanisms causing, 114–115
  due to pulmonary thromboembolism, 1783
  in asthma, 2138–2139
  in COPD, 2226
    during sleep, 2227
  in cystic fibrosis, 2313–2314
  in drug-induced pulmonary edema, 2567
  in hepatopulmonary syndrome, liver transplantation's effects on, 1734
  in pulmonary hypertension pathogenesis, 1915
  ventilatory response to, 418, *418*
  with nonthoracic trauma, 2647
Hypoxia, carotid body response to, 235–237
  pattern of central response to, 239
  pulmonary vascular effects of, 106
  ventilatory response to, 240–241
    during sleep, 243, 2055
    genetic influences on, 240–241
    upper airway muscle control in, 242, 246

Iceberg tumor, *1230,* 1231
Identification of organisms, defined, 735
Idiopathic pulmonary fibrosis. See *Pulmonary fibrosis, idiopathic.*
Ifosfamide, thoracic disease due to, 2538t, 2545
Imaging, 299–334. See also specific imaging modalities.
Imipramine, thoracic disease due to, 2569
Immotile cilia syndrome. See *Dyskinetic cilia syndrome.*
Immune complexes, in idiopathic pulmonary fibrosis, 1587
  in pulmonary vasculitis, 1489
  in Wegener's granulomatosis, 1493
Immune mediators, alveolar macrophage production of, 23
Immunity, cell-mediated. See *Cell-mediated immunity.*
  humoral, in host response to neoplasia, 1084
  in rheumatoid disease, 1434
  pulmonary, 130–131
Immunoblastic lymphadenopathy, 1312–1313, *1314*
Immunochemistry, 355–356
Immunocompromised host. See also *Immunodeficiency(ies);* specific immunodeficiency conditions.
  bronchoalveolar lavage in infection diagnosis in, 343
  inflammatory disease detection in, gallium scintigraphy in, 331–332, *332*
  nontuberculous mycobacterial infection in, histologic features of, 853, *854, 855*
  pneumonia in, 724–728
    patterns of, 700
  tuberculosis risk for, 803–804
Immunodeficiency(ies). See also *Immunocompromised host;* specific immunodeficiency conditions.
  alveolar proteinosis in, 2701
  associated with other diseases, 725–726
  bronchiectasis in, 2267

Immunodeficiency(ies) *(Continued)*
 combined, 724
 common variable, 725
 inherited, classification of, 724
 with defective phagocytic function, 726–728
 with predominant antibody deficiency, 724–725
Immunoenzymatic techniques, 356
Immunofluorescence tests, 356
Immunoglobulin(s). See also specific immunoglobulins.
 hypercatabolism of, 726
Immunoglobulin A, in tracheobronchial secretions, 61, 130
 selective deficiency of, 725
 COPD and, 2180
Immunoglobulin E, COPD and, 2181
 deficiency of, 725
 in allergic airway response, 2105
 serum, in allergic bronchopulmonary aspergillosis, 928
 smoking and, 2181
Immunoglobulin G, in tracheobronchial secretions, 130–131
 subclass deficiency of, 725
Impedance plethysmography, in deep vein thrombosis, 1824
Inciters of airway hyper-responsiveness, 2102
India ink test, for cryptococcosis, 908
Indian tick typhus, 1022
Inducers of airway hyper-responsiveness, 2102
Inert gas inhalation. See also *Helium inhalation.*
 for closing volume measurement, 413–414
 for functional residual capacity determination, 407
Inertial impaction, in particle deposition, 126
Infant(s). See also *Child(ren); Neonate(s).*
 acute infectious bronchiolitis in, 2333, 2334
 pulmonary function testing in, in cystic fibrosis, 2313
Infantile sex-linked agammaglobulinemia, 724–725
Infarction, bone, in sickle cell disease, fat embolism from, 1833
 myocardial. See *Myocardial infarction.*
 pulmonary, anatomic bias of, 477
 as term, usage of, 1780n
 clinical features of, 1825
 consolidation in, 436, *436*
 homogeneous segmental, 3088t, *3091*
 due to intravascular metastasis, 1397
 due to thromboembolism, 1780–1781
 CT findings with, 1811, *1814, 1815*
 pathologic features of, 1783, *1784–1787*
 radiologic features of, 1794–1799, *1795–1801*
 healed, linear shadow with, 483, *559*
 hemorrhagic, in aspergillosis, consolidation due to, *436*, 437
 in pulmonary carcinoma, 1166–1169, *1169*
 pleural effusion with, 2760
 with bacterial superinfection, 1829, *1829*
 with Swan-Ganz catheter, 2688–2689, *2688*
Infection, 695–1061. See also *Pneumonia;* specific infections.
 actinomycetous, 952–958. See also *Actinomycosis; Nocardiosis.*
 acute bronchiolitis due to, *2325, 2330,* 2333–2335, *2335, 2336*
 after bone marrow transplantation, 1730–1731, *1731*
 after lung transplantation, 1713–1720, *1716, 1718–1721*
 airway, 701, *701, 702.* See also *Bronchiolitis; Bronchitis; Tracheitis.*
 alveolar proteinosis and, 2702

Infection *(Continued)*
 asthma provoked by, 2111–2112
 bacterial. See *Bacteria, infection due to;* specific genera and species.
 by direct spread from extrapulmonary site, 716, *718*
 cavities or cysts due to, 3102t–3103t, *3105–3107*
 COPD and, 2175–2177
 diagnosis of, cytologic, 341–342
 general considerations in, 716–721
 transmission electron microscopy in, 353–354
 transthoracic needle aspiration in, 347
 diffuse air-space pattern in, 3130t, *3131*
 diffuse nodular pattern in, 3145t, *3146, 3147*
 diffuse reticular pattern in, 3134t
 fungal, 875–972. See also *Fungal infection; Fungus ball;* specific diseases.
 general features of, 697–728
 homogeneous consolidation in, nonsegmental, 3079t–3080t, *3082*
 segmental, 3087t, *3089*
 in bullous disease, 2237, *2242*
 in cystic fibrosis, 2308
 pathogenetic role of, 2301–2303
 in diabetes mellitus, 2728
 in fibrosing mediastinitis, 2856–2857
 in HIV disease, 1643–1676, 1644t
 in Hodgkin's disease, 1312
 in rheumatoid disease, 1451
 in systemic lupus erythematosus, 1432
 pathogenetic role of, 1424
 inhalational transmission of, 698–699
 inhomogeneous consolidation in, nonsegmental, 3093t, *3094*
 segmental, 3097t, *3099*
 localized, of middle mediastinum, 2943
 lymph node enlargement in, 3164t, *3166*
 mesothelioma and, 2810
 middle-posterior mediastinal mass due to, 3177t
 multiple masses or nodules due to, 3123t, *3125, 3126*
 mycobacterial, 798–861. See also *Mycobacterial infection; Tuberculosis.*
 paravertebral mass due to, 3185t, *3186*
 pathogenesis of, 698–716
 patterns of, 698–716
 pleural effusion due to, 2743–2753
 pulmonary artery aneurysm due to, 1935
 sarcoidosis and, 1534–1555
 solitary mass due to, 3117t, *3119*
 solitary nodule due to, 3111t, *3113*
 upper airway obstruction due to, 2021–2022, *2023*
 via pulmonary vasculature, 713–716
 via tracheobronchial tree, 698–713
 viral, 979–1010. See also *Viral infection;* specific viruses and groups.
 Wegener's granulomatosis and, 1492
 with central venous catheter, 2683
Infectious mononucleosis, 1008–1009, *1009*
 pleural effusion in, 2752
Inferior accessory fissure, 164–165, *165*
Inferior accessory lobe, 164–165, *165*
Inferior esophagopleural stripes, 218, 229, *232*
Inferior hemiazygos vein, 218
Inferior phrenic artery, 254, *256*
Inferior phrenic vein, 254, *256*
Inferior recess(es), of anterior mediastinum, 204
 of posterior mediastinum, 223, *224–225*
Inferior vena cava, azygos continuation of, 2950, *2951–2953*
 dilation of, 2947
Inferior vena cava aperture of diaphragm, 2987, *2988*

Inflammation, in asthma, bronchial hyper-responsiveness and, 2102–2103
 mechanisms of, 2088–2093, *2088*
 in bronchiectasis, 2265–2267
 in cystic fibrosis, 2302–2303
 in pulmonary defense, 130
 mediators of, alveolar macrophage production of, 23
 in adult respiratory distress syndrome, 1983
 in asthma, 2090–2093
 in response to exercise, 2109–2110
Inflammatory bowel disease, 1473–1475, *1474*
 pleural effusion in, 2766
Inflammatory myofibroblastic tumor, pulmonary, 1371–1373
Inflammatory pseudotumor, pulmonary, 1371–1373, *1372, 1373*
Influenza, 981–985, *983, 984*
 diffuse air-space pattern in, 3130t
 hospital-acquired pneumonia due to, 723
 inhomogeneous segmental opacity in, 3097t
 pleural effusion in, 2752
 Staphylococcus aureus pneumonia and, 744
Infra-aortic area, 197, 211–218, *212–217*
Infra-azygos area, 197, 228–229, *232*
Inhalation, injury due to. See also *Dust exposure; Inhaled substances;* specific substances.
 bronchiolitis in, 2335–2336
 pulmonary infection acquired by, 698–699
 smoke, 2335–2336, 2528–2531, *2529, 2530*
 upper airway obstruction due to, 2023
Inhalation challenge tests, 420–424, 421t, *423*
 nonspecific, 420–423, 421t, 423–424, *423,* 2095–2096, *2095*
 in asthma diagnosis, 2103–2104, *2103*
 in occupational asthma diagnosis, 2104, 2123
 specific, 423, 2137
Inhaled substances. See also *Dust exposure;* specific substances.
 altered deposition of, bronchial hyper-responsiveness and, 2097
 idiopathic pulmonary fibrosis and, 1586
 occupational asthma due to, 2119t, 2121–2122
 pulmonary carcinoma and, 1074–1078
 pulmonary metabolism of, 132
 reactive airways dysfunction syndrome due to, 2123, 2123t
 toxic, 2519–2531
 pulmonary edema due to, 2519, *2520*
 Wegener's granulomatosis and, 1492
Injury Severity Score, adult respiratory distress syndrome prognosis and, 1998
Innermost intercostal muscles, 260
Innominate artery, aneurysm of, 2961, 3178t
 avulsion of, 2626
 buckling of, 2957–2961, *2961,* 3178t
Insect allergens, asthma and, 2106
Insect sting, anaphylaxis due to, 2106
Insecticide poisoning, 2584–2585, *2585,* 2587
Inspiration, deep, airway caliber change in response to, in asthma, 2101, 2115–2116, *2115*
Inspiratory capacity (IC), 406, *406*
Inspiratory muscles, 246–247. See also *Respiratory muscles;* specific muscles.
 fatigue of, in COPD, 2219–2220
 mechanical model of, 249, *249*
Inspiratory reserve volume (IRV), 406, *406*
β_2-Integrins, in leukocyte–endothelial cell adherence in adult respiratory distress syndrome, 1979
Intensive care units, indications for daily chest radiographs in, 305–306
Interbronchial angle, 35

Intercellular adhesion molecule 1 (ICAM-1), in asthmatic airway inflammation, 2090
Intercellular clefts, in pulmonary endothelium,, 75, 76
Interception, in particle deposition, 127
Intercostal arteries, in blood supply to diaphragm, 249
Intercostal lymph nodes, 176, *177*
Intercostal muscles, electromyography of, in ventilatory control assessment, 419
  external, 260, *260*
    in inspiration, 246–247
    spinal levels of innervation of, 3055
  in ventilation, 3056
  innermost, 260
  internal, 260, *260*
    in expiration, 247
    spinal levels of innervation of, 3055
  pain originating in, 387
  parasternal, spinal levels of innervation of, 3055
  receptors in, in ventilatory control, 238
Intercostal nerve, radicular pain originating from, 387
Intercostal vein(s), left superior, 209–211, *209–211*
  dilation of, 2951, *2953*
  on high-resolution CT, 154, *156*
Interface sign, 572–573, *574*
Interferon, atopy and, 2081
  in tuberculous pleural effusion, 2746
  thoracic disease due to, 2538t, 2556
Interleukins, in adult respiratory distress syndrome, 1983
  in asthmatic airway inflammation, 2089
  thoracic disease due to, 2538t, 2555–2556
Interlobar artery(ies), enlargement of, in pulmonary hypertension, 1886, 1915
  in pulmonary thromboembolism, 1788–1791, *1792, 1793*
  left, 79, 80
  loss of visibility of, in atelectasis, 533, *534, 536*
  right, 78, *78, 79*
    measurement of, 78, 80
Interlobar fissures. See *Fissures.*
Interlobar lymph nodes, in classification for lung cancer staging, *185,* 188t, *1186,* 1187t
Interlobular septum(a), 25–26, *25, 27, 28*
  functional significance of, 26, *28*
  on CT, *283, 287, 290*
  radiographic identification of, 26, *29*
Intermediate cells, of pulmonary arteriolar wall, 74
  of tracheobronchial epithelium, *6, 8–9*
Intermediate stem line, 87, *88–91*
Internal bronchial diameter–to–pulmonary artery diameter ratio. See *Artery-bronchus ratios.*
Internal intercostal muscles, 260, *260*
  in expiration, 247
  spinal levels of innervation of, 3055
Internal mammary artery, in blood supply to diaphragm, 249
Internal mammary lymph nodes, 175–176, *176*
Internal oblique muscle, in expiration, 247
  spinal levels of innervation of, 3055
International Labor Office system, for pneumoconiosis radiograph interpretation, 441, 2387–2390
Intersegmental septum, 165, 166, *167*
  on CT, 254, *256*
Interstitial disease. See also specific disorders.
  air bronchogram in, 438
  air-space pattern of lung density in, *440*
  diffuse, conventional radiographs in, problems in interpretation of, 441

Interstitial disease (*Continued*)
  crackles in, 394
  increased lung density in, radiographic patterns of, 439–454
  pulmonary hypertension in, 1915–1917
  thoracoscopic biopsy in, 371
  respiratory bronchiolitis–associated, 2348–2349
Interstitial fibrosis. See *Pulmonary fibrosis.*
Interstitial nephritis, granulomatous, in sarcoidosis, 1566
Interstitial pattern, increased density with, 439–454
  air-space pattern combined with, 454–455, *456, 457*
Interstitial plasma cell pneumonitis, 909, 911, 913. See also Pneumocystis carinii *pneumonia.*
Interstitial pneumonia, 707–713, *712–715.* See also *Interstitial pneumonitis; Pulmonary fibrosis, idiopathic.*
Interstitial pneumonitis. See also *Interstitial pneumonia; Pulmonary fibrosis, idiopathic.*
  acute, 1619–1621, *1620*
  after bone marrow transplantation, 1727–1728
  desquamative, 1584, 1611–1617
    clinical features of, 1617
    diffuse reticular pattern in, 3135t
    pathogenesis of, 1611
    pathologic features of, 1611, *1612, 1613*
    prognosis in, *1616,* 1617
    radiologic features of, 454, 1611–1617, *1614–1616*
    usual interstitial pneumonia and, 1584–1585
  diffuse, in rheumatoid disease, 1434–1438, *1435–1437*
    in systemic lupus erythematosus, 1429–1430
  due to cytomegalovirus, 1005, *1005*
  giant cell, 1584
  in congenital rubella, 993–994
  in neurofibromatosis, 690
  in progressive systemic sclerosis, pathogenesis of, 1452–1453
    radiologic features of, 1456–1457, *1456*
  in sarcoidosis, 1541, *1541*
  lymphoid, 1271–1273, *1271–1273,* 1584
    in HIV infection, 1674, 1685–1686, *1685, 1686*
    in Sjögren's syndrome, 1466, 1468, *1468*
  nonspecific, 1617–1619, *1617, 1618*
    diffuse reticular pattern in, 3135t
    in HIV infection, 1674, 1684–1685, *1684*
  usual, 1584. See also *Pulmonary fibrosis, idiopathic.*
    desquamative interstitial pneumonia and, 1584–1585
Interstitial pressure, in pulmonary fluid and solute exchange, 1953–1954
Interstitial vascular sarcoma, sclerosing. See *Epithelioid hemangioendothelioma.*
Interstitium, alveolar, 17–18, 20–21
  pulmonary, fluid accumulation in, interstitial pressure and, 1956
    in pulmonary edema development, 1951, *1951*
    in pulmonary fluid exchange, 1950
    radiologic anatomy of, 439–441
Intersublobar septum, 165, 166, *167*
  on CT, 254, *256*
Intervascular anastomoses, 77
Intestinal tract. See *Colon; Gastrointestinal tract.*
Intimal fibrosis, in pulmonary arteries, 74
  in pulmonary hypertension, 1883–1884, *1883, 1884, 1886, 1887*

Intimal fibrosis (*Continued*)
  in pulmonary veins, in pulmonary hypertension, 1919, *1919*
Intra-aortic counterpulsation balloons, complications of, 2690
Intracranial pressure, elevated, pulmonary edema with, 1974–1976
Intrapulmonary lymph nodes, in ATS classification, 184t, *185,* 187
Intrathoracic rib, 262–263, 3013–3014
Intravascular bronchioloalveolar tumor. See *Epithelioid hemangioendothelioma.*
Intravascular lymphomatosis, 1291
Intubation. See also *Endotracheal intubation.*
  complications of, 2675–2681
Inversion recovery sequence, 317–319
Inverted V appearance, in allergic bronchopulmonary aspergillosis, 929
Inverted Y appearance, in allergic bronchopulmonary aspergillosis, 929, *931, 932*
Iodized oil embolism, 1861–1863, *1865,* 2569
  pulmonary edema and, 2005
Ion transport, in airway epithelium, 62, 2299–2300
  in cystic fibrosis, 2300
  in pulmonary edema prevention, 1956
Iron, pneumoconiosis due to, 2452–2455, *2453–2455*
Iron overload. See also *Hemosiderosis.*
  tuberculosis risk and, 803
Iron-deficiency anemia, in idiopathic pulmonary hemorrhage, 1762–1763
Irradiation. See *Radiation* entries.
Irrationality, as symptom of respiratory disease, 389
Irritant receptors, 146, *146*
  bronchial hyper-responsiveness and, 2098
  in ventilatory control, *236,* 237
Ischemic heart disease. See also *Myocardial infarction.*
  asbestos exposure and, 2448
  chest pain due to, 386
Isocapnic hyperventilation, in bronchial reactivity assessment, 423–424
Isocyanates, allergic alveolitis associated with, 2362t, 2378–2379. See also *Extrinsic allergic alveolitis.*
  occupational asthma due to, 2119t, 2121–2122, 2124
  reactive airways dysfunction syndrome due to, 2123
Isomerism, bronchial, 626
Isoniazid (INH), thoracic disease due to, 2539t
Isoxsuprine, thoracic disease due to, 2566
IVBAT (intravascular bronchioloalveolar tumor). See *Epithelioid hemangioendothelioma.*
Ivory vertebra, in Hodgkin's disease, 1306, *1310, 1311*

J receptors, 147
  in ventilatory control, *236,* 238
Jaagsiekte, 1079
"Jack and the Beanstalk," 2057
Jackson-Humber nomenclature of bronchial segments, 33, 33t
Japanese summer-type allergic alveolitis, 2362t, 2378. See also *Extrinsic allergic alveolitis.*
Jaundice, in *Streptococcus pneumoniae* pneumonia, 741
Jejunoileal bypass, tuberculosis risk after, 803
Job's syndrome, 725
Joints, sarcoidosis involving, 1565
  tuberculosis involving, 837–838

Joints *(Continued)*
  Wegener's granulomatosis involving, 1504
Juxta-alveolar lymphatics, 172, *174*
Juxtacapillary receptors, 147
  in ventilatory control, *236,* 238
Juxtaphrenic lymph nodes, 176, *178*
  enlargement of, 2929
Juxtaphrenic peak, with right upper lobe
  atelectasis, 539, *543*
Juxtavertebral lymph nodes, 176, *177*

K cells. See *Neuroendocrine cells.*
K complexes, in non-REM sleep, 2054, 2068
Kala-azar, 1039
Kaolin, pneumoconiosis due to, 2451–2452
Kaolinite, in secondary lysosomes in alveolar
  macrophages, 21
Kaposi's sarcoma, 1337–1339, *1338, 1339*
  in HIV infection, 1337, 1676–1681
    cause of, 1676–1677
    clinical features of, 1680
    diagnosis of, 1680–1681
    pathologic features of, 1677, *1678, 1679*
    prognosis in, 1681
    radiologic features of, 1677–1679, *1679–
      1681*
  lung scintigraphy in, 332, 1679
Kaposi's sarcoma–associated herpesvirus, 999
  Kaposi's sarcoma and, 1677, 1681
  primary effusion lymphoma and, 1682, 2838
Kartagener's syndrome. See *Dyskinetic cilia
  syndrome.*
Kawasaki disease, 1490t
Kerley lines, 172
  in pulmonary edema, *442,* 444, *444, 446,* 480,
    *481, 482, 1961, 1961, 1962, 1964, 1965,
    1967,* 1994
Kerosene, aspiration of, 2512
Kidneys. See also *Renal* entries.
  Churg-Strauss syndrome involving, 1510–1511
  ectopic, in mediastinum, 2981
  progressive systemic sclerosis involving,
    1458–1459
  sarcoidosis involving, 1566
  Wegener's granulomatosis involving, 1499
Killer cells, lymphokine-activated, in host
  response to neoplasia, 1083–1084
  natural (NK), in host response to neoplasia,
    1083
Klebsiella infection, *705,* 751–753, *752–755.* See
  also Klebsiella pneumoniae *infection.*
  cavities or cysts in, 3102t
  homogeneous opacity in, nonsegmental, 3079t
    segmental, 3087t
  inhomogeneous opacity in, nonsegmental,
    3093t
    segmental, 3097t
  pleural effusion with, 2749
Klebsiella pneumoniae infection, 751
  clinical features of, 753
  pathologic features of, 752, *752, 753*
  pulmonary gangrene in, 707, *710*
  radiologic features of, 459, 752–753, *754, 755*
Klinefelter's syndrome, 2729
  mediastinal germ cell neoplasms in, 2902
Klippel-Feil syndrome, 599, 3011
Kluyveromyces fragilis infection, 952
Knife wound, 2648, *2651, 2653*
Knuckle sign, in pulmonary thromboembolism,
  1791–1792, *1792, 1794, 1795*
Kommerell's diverticulum, 2961, *2964, 2965*
Koplik's spots, in measles, 988
Krabbe's disease, 2727
Krypton 81m, for ventilation imaging, 329

Kugelberg-Welander syndrome, 3061
Kuhn, pores of, 31–32, *32*
Kulchitsky cell carcinoma. See *Carcinoid tumor,
  atypical.*
Kveim test, in sarcoidosis diagnosis, 1571
Kyphoscoliosis, 3020–3022, *3021*
  pulmonary hypertension with, 1918

Laboratory-worker's lung, 2362t. See also
  Extrinsic allergic alveolitis.
Laceration, pulmonary, 2613–2618
  cavities or cysts with, 3104t
  classification of, 2614
  with contusion, 2612
Lacrimal glands, in sarcoidosis, 1565
  in Sjögren's syndrome, 1468, 1469
Lactate dehydrogenase, in pleural fluid,
  2741–2742
  serum, in *Pneumocystis carinii* pneumonia,
    915, 1667
Lactic acidosis, 117
Lactobacillus casei ss *rhamnosus,* 750
Lactoferrin, in tracheobronchial secretions, 61
Lambda pattern, on gallium scintigraphy in
  sarcoidosis, 1568, *1568*
Lambert, canals of, 32
Lambert-Eaton myasthenic syndrome,
  1173–1174, 3063
Lamina propria, of conducting airways, *6,* 12–17
Landry-Guillain-Barré syndrome, 3061–3062
  influenza and, 984
Langerhans' cell(s), in tracheobronchial
  epithelium, 11–12
Langerhans' cell histiocytosis, 1627–1638
  clinical features of, 1636
  desquamative interstitial pneumonitis–like pat-
    tern in, 1611, *1613*
  diagnosis of, 1636–1637
    transmission electron microscopy in, 354,
      355
  diffuse reticular pattern in, 3135t, *3140*
  etiology of, 1627
  honeycombing in, 446–447, 1630, *1634, 1635*
  idiopathic pulmonary fibrosis vs., 1611, 1628,
    1631
  lymphangioleiomyomatosis vs., 685, 1631
  pathogenesis of, 1627–1628
  pathologic features of, 1628–1630, *1628–1632*
  pneumothorax-associated pleuritis vs., 2790,
    2790
  prognosis in, 1637–1638
  pulmonary function in, 1636
  radiologic features of, 1630–1636, *1633–1638*
Lanthanum, pneumoconiosis due to, 2456
Large cell carcinoma, pulmonary, 1110–1113.
  See also *Carcinoma, pulmonary.*
  basaloid subtype of, 1113, *1114*
  clear cell subtype of, 1112–1113, *1113*
  epidemiology of, 1072
  gonadotropin secretion by, 1177
  hematologic disorders with, 1178
  incidence of, 1110
  lymphoepithelioma-like, 1113, *1115*
    Epstein-Barr virus and, 1079
    prognosis in, 1196
  pathologic features of, 1110–1113, *1111–
    1115*
  prognosis in, 1196
  with neuroendocrine differentiation, 1229,
    1246
Larmor frequency, 317
Larva currens, in strongyloidiasis, 1043
Larva migrans, cutaneous, 1047, 1752
  visceral, 1045–1046, 1753

Laryngeal nerve, recurrent, hoarseness due to
  dysfunction of, 389
    in pulmonary innervation, 145
    pulmonary carcinoma invading, 1171
Laryngeal stenosis, in tuberculosis, 2022
Laryngitis, acute infectious, hoarseness due to,
  389
  tuberculous, 800, 840
Laryngocele, infected, upper airway obstruction
  due to, 2022
Laryngomalacia, upper airway obstruction due
  to, 2046
Laryngoscopy, 366
Laryngospasm, episodic paroxysmal, 2032–2033
Laryngotracheitis, acute, upper airway
  obstruction due to, 2021
Larynx, carcinoma of, pulmonary carcinoma
  and, 1202
  dysfunction of, upper airway obstruction due
    to, 2032–2033
  edema of, upper airway obstruction due to,
    2022–2023
  muscles of, in ventilation, 239
  papillomatosis of, 1262–1263
  receptors in, in ventilatory control, *236,* 237,
    246
  relapsing polychondritis involving, 1472
  rheumatoid disease involving, 1449
  systemic lupus erythematosus involving, 1431
Laser film scanners, film digitization using, 307
Laser therapy, complications of, 2675
Lassa fever, pleural effusion in, 2752
Latch bridge state, in asthma, 2101
Lateral arcuate ligament, 253–254
Lateral cephalometry, in obstructive sleep apnea,
  2063, *2064*
Lateral decubitus projection, for conventional
  radiography, 300–301, *301*
Lateral pericardiac lymph nodes, 176, *178*
  enlargement of, 2929
Latex allergy, 2106
  occupational asthma due to, 2120
Lathyrus odoratus seed, collagen-elastin binding
  defect due to, 676
Latissimus dorsi, in inspiration, 246
  on CT, 260
Latitude, of film, 302, 305
Leber's disease, 3052
Leeches, 1061
Left-handedness, obstructive sleep apnea and,
  2057
Legionella infection, 770–775
  clinical features of, 700, 773–775
  community-acquired, 722
  diagnosis of, 775
  epidemiology of, 770–772
  homogeneous nonsegmental opacity in, 3079t
  hospital-acquired, 723
  in HIV disease, 1645
  laboratory findings in, 775
  pathogenesis of, 772
  pathologic features of, 772, *773*
  pleural effusion in, 2749
  prognosis in, 775
  radiologic features of, 772–773, *774–776*
Legionnaires' disease, 770–775. See also
  Legionella *infection.*
Leigh's disease, 3052
Leiomyoma, benign metastasizing, 1409
  esophageal, 2965–2966
  mediastinal, 2925
  pulmonary, 1331–1334
Leiomyosarcoma, esophageal, 2965
  gastric, pulmonary chondroma with, 1344
  mediastinal, 2925
  metastatic to lung, *1387,* 1409, *1410, 1411*

Leiomyosarcoma *(Continued)*
  pulmonary, 1331–1334, *1334–1336*
Leiperia cincinnalais, 1059
Leishmaniasis, 1039
Lemierre's syndrome, 779, 1829, 1831
Length-tension relationship of muscle, 2102, 3057
Leptospira interrogans infection, 776–777
Leser-Trélat sign, in pulmonary carcinoma, 1174
Letterer-Siwe disease, 1627. See also *Langerhans' cell histiocytosis.*
Leukemia, 1313–1323
  acute, after small cell carcinoma treatment, 1202
  adult T-cell, 1321, 1323
  chronic lymphocytic, *1320,* 1321–1323, *1321, 1322*
    pleural effusion due to, 2760
    pulmonary carcinoma and, 1201
  eosinophilic. See *Loeffler's endocarditis.*
  hairy cell, nontuberculous mycobacterial infection in, 853, *855*
  lymph node enlargement in, 3165t
  lymphoblastic, mediastinal involvement in, 1292
  megakaryocytic, megakaryocytic capillary stasis in, 1317–1318, *1317*
  myelogenous, clinical features of, 1319–1320
    invasive aspergillosis in, 936, *944–946*
    pathologic features of, 1313–1318, *1315–1318*
    radiologic features of, 1318–1319, *1319*
    Sweet's syndrome and, 1320
  parenchymal infiltration in, time of appearance of radiologic features of, 3046
  pleural effusion due to, 2760
  promyelocytic, disseminated intravascular coagulation in, 1320
Leukocyte(s). See also specific classes of leukocytes.
  marginated pool of, in lungs, 132–133
  polymorphonuclear. See *Neutrophil(s).*
Leukocyte adhesion deficiency syndrome, 727
Leukocyte count, lung function and, 2183
Leukocytoclastic angiitis, cutaneous, 1490t. See also *Vasculitis.*
Leukocytosis, in pulmonary carcinoma, 1178
Leukoencephalopathy, progressive multifocal, sarcoidosis and, 1566
Leukostasis, pulmonary, in leukemia, *1316,* 1317, 1319
Leukotrienes, in adult respiratory distress syndrome, 1983
  in aspirin-induced asthma, 2091, 2113
  in asthmatic airway inflammation, 2090, 2091
  in exercise-induced asthma, 2109, 2110
  mucociliary clearance and, in asthma, 2093–2094
Leu-M1, in adenocarcinoma vs. mesothelioma, 2819
Levator palatini, in ventilation, 246
Levator scapulae, on CT, 260
Levodopa, thoracic disease due to, 2572
Lidocaine, antibacterial activity of, 367
  for bronchoscopy, 367
  thoracic disease due to, 2538t, 2564
Light, systemic lupus erythematosus and, 1424
Light chain deposition, amyloidosis vs., 2711
Light chain disease, 1298
Ligneous perityphlitis, fibrosing mediastinitis with, 2857
Line shadows, 479–483, *481, 482, 484–488*
Linear atelectasis, 554–560, *558.* See also *Atelectasis.*
Linguatula serrata infestation, 1059–1061

Lingula, atelectasis of, 549
  nonspecific vascular changes and fibrosis in, 372
Lipid(s). See also *Fat.*
  aspiration of. See under *Aspiration (event).*
  metabolism of, in lung, 131
  neutral, in surfactant, 56
  in tracheobronchial secretions, 61
Lipid pneumonia. See *Aspiration (event), of lipids.*
Lipid storage disease, 2722–2727, *2725, 2726*
Lipid-containing interstitial cell, in alveolar development, 142
Lipoid pneumonia. See *Aspiration (event), of lipids.*
Lipoid proteinosis, 2728
Lipoma, chest wall, 3025–3028, *3028*
  diaphragmatic, 3004, *3005*
  esophageal, 2965, 2966
  mediastinal, 2914–2915, *2915*
  pleural, 583, *586,* 2835, *2837*
  pulmonary, 1347
    hamartoma and, 1347, 1350–1351, *1353*
Lipomatosis, mediastinal, 2915, *2916–2919,* 3177t
Lipoprotein(s), altered, fat embolism from, 1846–1847
Lipoprotein lipases, in capillary endothelial cells, 131
Lipoproteinosis, alveolar. See *Alveolar proteinosis.*
Liposarcoma, chest wall, 3028, *3029*
  mediastinal, *1348,* 2917
  pleural, 2835, *2838*
  pulmonary, 1347, *1348*
Liquid ventilation, with perflubron, in adult respiratory distress syndrome, 1987, *1990, 1991*
Listeria monocytogenes infection, 750
Lithoptysis, in broncholithiasis, 2288
Liver, abscess of, in amebiasis, 1034, 1035, *1035,* 2753
  carcinoma of, metastatic to lung, 1405
  disease of. See also specific disorders.
    cystic, diaphragmatic involvement in, 3006, *3007*
    in α$_1$-protease inhibitor deficiency, 2232
    pleural effusion with, 2764
    pulmonary hypertension with, 1903–1904, *1904*
  pulmonary carcinoma metastatic to, 1173
    detection of, 1192
  sarcoidosis involving, 1563, 1564–1565
  transplantation of, 1732–1734, *1734*
    pleural effusion after, 2764
    pulmonary edema after, 1974
  tuberculosis involving, 840
Liver failure, pulmonary edema in, 1974
Liver flukes, 1052, 1753
Liver scan, in diaphragmatic rupture diagnosis, 2637
Livestock confinement buildings, 2379
  COPD and, 2175
Lobar atelectasis. See under *Atelectasis.*
Lobar emphysema. See also *Swyer-James syndrome.*
  congenital, 621–625, *625, 626*
  oligemia in, 3157t, *3159*
Lobar fusion, 153–154, *155*
  identification of, on high-resolution CT, 159–160, *162*
  pleural effusion configuration with, 564–565, *566*
  spread of pathologic process and, 461, *462*
Lobar lymph nodes, in classification for lung cancer staging, *185,* 188t, *1186,* 1187t

Lobar torsion, 2622–2623, *2624*
  after transplantation, 1724, *1725*
  postoperative, 2671–2672, *2673*
Lobectomy, atelectasis after, 2670
  bronchopleural fistula after, 2289–2290
  empyema after, 2762
  examination of specimen from, 348–351, *349, 350, 352–353*
  mediastinal displacement after, 2665
  pulmonary function after, prediction of, 331, 1181
  reorientation of lobes and fissures after, 2669
Lobular artery, 26
Lobular bronchioles, 26
Lobule, primary, 24, *25,* 31
  secondary, 24–26, *25, 27, 28*
    abnormalities of, on high-resolution CT, 26, *28–31*
Loeffler's endocarditis, 1748–1751, *1751, 1752*
  pulmonary hypertension with, 1933
Loeffler's syndrome, 1744–1746, *1745, 1746*
  nonsegmental opacity in, homogeneous, 3081t, *3083*
  inhomogeneous, 3093t
Löfgren's syndrome, 1563
Lomustine (CCNU), thoracic disease due to, 2538t, 2548
Lordotic projection, for radiography, 300
Lower esophageal sphincter, incompetent, with tracheobronchial-esophageal fistula, 628
Lower paratracheal lymph nodes, in ATS classification, 184t, *185,* 186
  in classification for lung cancer staging, *185,* 188t, *1186,* 1187t
L-selectin, in leukocyte–endothelial cell adherence, in adult respiratory distress syndrome, 1979
Luftsichel sign, left-sided, 543, *545, 547*
  right-sided, *542*
Lung(s). See also *Pulmonary* entries.
  abscess of. See *Lung abscess.*
  accessory, 628
    bronchopulmonary sequestration vs., 601
  agenesis of, 598, 599–601, *600, 601*
  anatomy of, on CT, 281–291
  aplasia of, 598, 599–601
  biopsy of, open, by thoracotomy, 372
    transbronchial. See under *Biopsy.*
    transthoracic, 370–371
      CT-guided, 315, 370
      ultrasound-guided, 334, 370
  collapse of, 539, *540.* See also *Atelectasis.*
  conducting zone of, 3–17
    geometry and dimensions of, 3–5
    morphology and cell function of, 5–17
  defense mechanisms of, 126–131
    immune, 130–131
    inflammation in, 130
    particle clearance in, 127–130, *128*
  density of. See *Lung density.*
  development of, 136–142
    anomalies of, 597–629
    factors influencing, 141–142
    periods of, 136
  diagrammatic representation of, for radiology discussion, *434*
  disease distribution within, 474–478, *477*
  esophageal, 628
  fetal, maturation of, 57, 58
  filtering function of, 132–133
  fluid and solute exchange in, 1947–1956, *1947–1949, 1952*
  fundamental "unit" of, 24–31
  growth of, after pneumonectomy, 139
  herniation of, 3012, *3013*
    postoperative, 2671, *2672*

Lung(s) (Continued)
post-traumatic, 2646–2647, 2647
heterotopic tissue within, 628
horseshoe, 628–629
innervation of, 145–149, 146
lymphatics of, 172–174, 173, 174, 192–193
masses in, multiple, differential diagnosis of, 3122, 3123t–3124t, 3125–3129
solitary, 1146–1148, 1148
differential diagnosis of, 3116, 3117t–3118t, 3119–3121
metabolism in, 131–132
neoplasms of, 1067–1412. See also specific neoplasms.
histologic classification of, 1071t
nonrespiratory functions of, 126–133
perforation of, with chest tube, 2677, 2677–2679
pressure-volume relationships of, 53–54, 55, 56
resection of. See Lobectomy; Pneumonectomy.
respiratory zone of, 3, 17–24
geometry and dimensions of, 23–24
morphology and cell function of, 17–23
surgical complications involving, 2669–2672, 2669, 2670, 2672–2674
systemic arterial supply to, 665–667, 666–668
transitional zone of, 3, 17
transplantation of. See Heart-lung transplantation; Lung transplantation.
trauma's effects on, nonpenetrating, 2611–2623
nonthoracic, 2647
penetrating, 2647–2653
zones of, 3
Lung abscess, 703–707, 709
acute, interlobar fissure displacement in, 459, 460
after transplantation, 1716
empyema vs., 579, 580
empyema with, 2749
healed cavity from, bronchogenic cyst vs., 611–612
in actinomycosis, 954, 956
in anaerobic pneumonia, 781, 781, 782
mortality with, 783
in Klebsiella pneumonia, 705, 752–753, 753–755
in Legionella infection, 773, 774
in melioidosis, 760
in Pseudomonas aeruginosa pneumonia, 762, 764
in pulmonary carcinoma, 1121, 1128
in Salmonella infection, 755, 758
in Staphylococcus aureus infection, 744, 745, 746, 747, 3105
infected bulla vs., 2237
multiple masses or nodules due to, 3123t, 3125
nonspecific, problems with term, 778
primary, problems with term, 778
radiographic features of, 460, 462, 464
solitary mass due to, 3117t
Lung cancer. See Carcinoma, pulmonary; specific types.
Lung capacities, 406–408, 406. See also Total lung capacity (TLC).
in COPD, 2224–2225
Lung compliance, dynamic, frequency dependence of, 412
in COPD, 2220–2221
measurement of, 411–412
increase in, hyperinflation and, 494–495
measurement of, 410–411, 411
Lung cultures, 351
Lung density, alterations in, 270–272, 271–273

Lung density (Continued)
due to perfusion abnormalities, 270, 271
decreased, 493–511
classification of abnormalities with, 494, 494–496
due to pulmonary vasculature change, 499–504, 501–507
due to pulmonary volume change, 494–499, 494–501
extrapulmonary abnormalities causing, 493, 493
in atelectasis, 517–519, 519, 539, 541
increased, 433–488
classification of, 433–434
general signs with, 457–479
limitations of pattern approach to, 455–457
with combined air-space and interstitial pattern, 454–455, 456, 457
with predominant air-space pattern, 434–439, 434–439
with predominant interstitial pattern, 439–454
normal, 269–270
on CT, 269–270, 291–294. See also Attenuation.
on MRI, 270
radiopacity vs., 269n
with pneumothorax, 587, 589
Lung extravascular water, estimation of volume of, 1964–1965, 1996–1997
Lung fluke. See Paragonimiasis.
Lung markings, prominent, in chronic bronchitis, 2203
Lung scanning. See Gallium scintigraphy; Ventilation/perfusion scanning.
Lung sounds, adventitious, 394–395
normal, 393–394
Lung transplantation, 1698–1726
bronchiolitis obliterans organizing pneumonia after, 1711
complications of, 1700–1724
bronchial, 1721–1724, 1722, 1723
pleural, 1720–1721, 1722
pulmonary vascular, 1724, 1725
double, 1698–1699
in cystic fibrosis, survival after, 2315
infection after, 1713–1720
bacterial, 1713–1716, 1716
fungal, 1717–1720, 1718–1721
viral, 1716–1717
lung diseases treated by, 1699t
lymphoproliferative disorder after, 1711–1713, 1712–1715
obliterative bronchiolitis after, 1707–1711, 1708–1710, 2336
parainfluenza virus and, 1717
operative procedures for, 1698–1699
patient selection for, 1699–1700, 1700t
prognosis after, 1726
pulmonary function tests after, 1724–1726
in obliterative bronchiolitis, 1711
in rejection, 1705–1707
recurrence of primary disease after, 1720
rejection after, acute, 1702–1707
biopsy in, 1703, 1705, 1706
bronchoalveolar lavage in, 1707
classification and grading of, 1703t
clinical features of, 1705
cytomegalovirus infection vs., 1716–1717
pathogenesis of, 1702
pathologic features of, 1703, 1703–1705
pulmonary function tests in, 1705–1707
radiologic features of, 1703–1705, 1706
chronic, 1707
bronchial involvement in, 1723–1724
vascular involvement in, 1724

Lung transplantation (Continued)
hyperacute, 1702
reperfusion edema after, 1700–1702, 1701, 1702
single, bilateral sequential, 1699
Lung volume, 406–408, 406
alterations in lung density with, 270, 272
attenuation and, 290–291, 291, 292–294, 292, 293
in COPD, 2224–2225
low, airway closure at, 111
pulmonary vascular resistance and, 106
radiologic methods for determination of, 308–309
Lung worm, 1047
Lupus anticoagulant, chronic thromboembolic pulmonary hypertension and, 1782
venous thrombosis and, 1779
Lupus erythematosus, subacute cutaneous, paraneoplastic, in pulmonary carcinoma, 1174
systemic. See Systemic lupus erythematosus (SLE).
Lupus pernio, in sarcoidosis, 1564
Lupus pneumonitis, acute, 1426, 1426, 1427, 1429
Lycoperdonosis, 2362t. See also Extrinsic allergic alveolitis.
Lymph nodes, calcification of, 452, 467, 471, 474, 476
after radiation therapy in Hodgkin's disease, 1302, 1305
in sarcoidosis, 1545, 1547, 1550
in silicosis, 2302, 2403
cervical, in metastatic upper airway cancer vs. primary lung cancer distinction, 1202
diaphragmatic, 176, 178
enlargement of, 2929
in ATS classification, 184t, 187
hilar. See Hilar lymph nodes.
histoplasmosis involving, 877–878, 879, 881, 882
in pulmonary defense, 130
mediastinal. See Mediastinal lymph nodes; specific nodal groups.
nontuberculous mycobacterial infection involving, 858
parietal, 175–176, 176–178
pulmonary carcinoma involving, assessment of, 1183–1191, 1186, 1187t, 1188, 1189
pulmonary carcinoma metastatic to, 1172
monoclonal antibody in detection of, 1181
sarcoidosis involving, clinical features of, 1564
diffuse pulmonary disease and, 1558, 1558, 1559
pathologic features of, 1542, 1546
radiologic features of, 1545–1550, 1546–1551, 1547t
tuberculosis involving, 805–806, 808, 809, 834–835
in HIV infection, 1649–1651, 1650, 1652
radiologic features of, 807–810, 810–812
visceral, 176–180, 179–184
Lymphadenitis, granulomatous, 2940–2942
necrotizing, bronchiolithiasis with, 2287
Lymphangiectasia, congenital pulmonary, 663–664
lymphangiomatosis vs., 662
Lymphangiography, in chylothorax diagnosis, 2769
oil embolism complicating, 1861–1863, 1865, 2539t, 2569
Lymphangioleiomyomatosis, 679–686
clinical features of, 685–686
diffuse reticular pattern in, 3134t

Lymphangioleiomyomatosis *(Continued)*
  Langerhans' cell histiocytosis vs., 685, 1631
  natural history and prognosis in, 686
  pathogenesis of, 679
  pathologic features of, 679–683, *680–683*
  radiologic features of, 446, 447, *449*, 683–685, *684, 685*
  renal angiomyolipoma in, 686
  spontaneous pneumothorax with, 2785
  tuberous sclerosis and, 679, 686
Lymphangioma, mediastinal, 2921–2924, *2922–2924*
  pulmonary, 662, 1377
Lymphangiomatosis, diffuse pulmonary, 662–663, *662, 663*
  mediastinal, 2924–2925
Lymphangiomyomatosis. See *Lymphangioleiomyomatosis.*
Lymphangitic carcinomatosis, 1390–1397
  clinical features of, 1397
  diagnosis of, 1397, 1412
  diffuse reticular pattern in, 3135t
  Kaposi's sarcoma vs., 1677
  pathogenesis of, 1382–1383
  pathologic features of, 1390, *1391, 1392*
  radiologic features of, 444, *446*, 1390–1397, *1393–1397*
Lymphatic capillaries, 174
  permeability of endothelium of, 1951
Lymphatic duct, right, 175
Lymphatic system, 172–193
  function of, 174–175
  hypoplasia of, pleural effusion in, 2766
  in particle clearance from interstitial tissue, 130
  in pleural fluid drainage, 169, 172
  in pulmonary fluid and solute exchange, 1951–1952, 1955–1956
  of lungs, 172–174, *173, 174*
    developmental anomalies of, 662–664
    metastasis via, 1382–1383
  of pleura, 172, *173*
    in clearance of pulmonary edema fluid, 1958
    metastasis via, 1382–1383
Lymphedema, congenital, chylothorax in, 2769
  pleural effusion in, 2766
  in yellow nail syndrome, 2284–2285, *2285, 2766*
Lymphocele, mediastinal, due to thoracic duct rupture, 2636
Lymphocytes, cytokine-activated, in host response to neoplasia, 1083–1084
  flow cytometry for subset analysis of, 358
  in conducting airways, 12, 16, *16*
  in extrinsic allergic alveolitis, 2364
  in pleural fluid specimen, 344
  T. See *T lymphocytes.*
Lymphocytic alveolitis, in HIV infection, 1674, 1686
  in response to asbestos exposure, 2423
Lymphocytic angiitis and granulomatosis, benign, 1281
Lymphocytic bronchitis, after bone marrow transplantation, 1729–1730
Lymphocytic interstitial pneumonitis, 1271–1273, *1271–1273*, 1584
  in HIV infection, 1674, 1685–1686, *1685, 1686*
  in Sjögren's syndrome, 1466, 1468, *1468*
Lymphocytic proliferation, small (well-differentiated), 1269–1271, *1270*, 1277
Lymphocytopenia, in pulmonary carcinoma, 1178
Lymphoepithelial lesion, 1276, *1276*

Lymphoepithelioma-like carcinoma, pulmonary, 1113, *1115*. See also *Carcinoma, pulmonary.*
  Epstein-Barr virus and, 1079
  prognosis in, 1196
Lymphoid aggregates, in airways. See *Bronchus-associated lymphoid tissue (BALT).*
Lymphoid hyperplasia, of thymus, 2877–2880, *2880*
  pulmonary, 1269–1273
    diffuse, 1271–1273, *1271–1274*. See also *Follicular bronchiolitis; Lymphoid interstitial pneumonia.*
    focal (nodular), 1269–1271, *1270*, 1277
  Lymphoid interstitial pneumonia, 1271–1273, *1271–1273*
    in HIV infection, 1674, 1685–1686, *1685, 1686*
    in Sjögren's syndrome, 1466, 1468, *1468*
Lymphoid tissue, intraparenchymal, 180
  of conducting airways. See *Bronchus-associated lymphoid tissue (BALT).*
Lymphokine-activated killer cells, in host response to neoplasia, 1083–1084
Lymphoma, 1273–1293
  after transplantation, 1711
  AILD-like T-cell, 1313
  angiotropic, 1291
  bronchoalveolar lavage in diagnosis of, 343
  Burkitt's, 1291
    in HIV infection, 1681–1682
  diffuse large cell (immunoblastic), in HIV infection, 1682
  mediastinal, 1292, *1293, 1294*, 2912, *3175*
  diffuse reticular pattern in, 3135t
  gallium lung scanning in, 332, 1293
  Hodgkin's. See *Hodgkin's disease.*
  in HIV infection, 1681–1683, *1682, 1683*
  in Sjögren's syndrome, 1469
  lymph node enlargement in, 3165t
  lymphoblastic, mediastinal, 1292, *1295*, 2911–2912
  mediastinal, 1291–1293, *1293–1295*, 2911–2912
    in anterior compartment, 3172t, *3175*
    in middle-posterior compartment, 3178t
  of thoracic spine, 3031–3032
  pleural, 1288, 1290, *1290*, 2838
  pleural effusion due to, 2759–2760
  primary effusion, 2759, 2838
    in HIV infection, 1682
  pulmonary, *443*, 1274–1281
    high-grade, 1278–1280
    homogeneous nonsegmental opacity in, 3081t
    low-grade B-cell (small lymphocytic), 1275–1278, *1275–1280*
    multiple masses or nodules due to, 3123t
    secondary, 1281–1291, *1286–1290*
      clinical features of, 1288
      laboratory findings in, 1288–1290
      pathologic features of, *1286*, 1287, *1287*
      radiologic features of, 1287–1288, *1288–1290*
      specific forms of, 1290–1291
  residual or recurrent tumor in, rebound thymic hyperplasia vs., 2877
  T-cell–rich B-cell, 1278
Lymphomatoid granulomatosis, 1280–1281, *1282–1285*
Lymphomatosis, intravascular, 1291
Lymphoproliferative disorders, 1269–1313. See also specific disorders.
  after bone marrow transplantation, 1732, *1733*
  after heart-lung or lung transplantation, 1711–1713, *1712–1715*

Lymphoproliferative disorders *(Continued)*
  sarcoidosis and, 1572
  with immunosuppressive therapy for rheumatoid disease, 1451
  with leukemia, 1321–1323
Lymphoreticular cells, in alveolar interstitium, 21
  in tracheobronchial epithelium, 11–12, *11*
Lymphoreticular malignancies. See also specific disorders.
  invasive aspergillosis in, 936
Lysozyme, in pleural fluid, 2743, 2746
  in tracheobronchial secretions, 61
  serum level of, in sarcoidosis diagnosis, 1569t
Lysyl oxidase, deficiency of, copper deficiency and, 676
  in emphysema, 2183, *2183*, 2185–2186

Mach bands, 215, *216, 217*
Machine-operator's lung, 2362t. See also *Extrinsic allergic alveolitis.*
Macleod's syndrome. See *Swyer-James syndrome.*
Macroaggregated albumin, technetium-labeled, for perfusion scanning, 326–327, 1800
α_2-Macroglobulin, COPD and, 2179
Macrophages, flow cytometry for subset analysis of, 358
  in airways, 16, *16*
  in asthmatic airway inflammation, 2090
  in idiopathic pulmonary fibrosis pathogenesis, 1590
  pulmonary. See also *Alveolar macrophages.*
    classification of, 21
Maduromycosis, 957
Magnetic resonance angiography, in pulmonary thromboembolism diagnosis, 1813
Magnetic resonance imaging (MRI), 315–322
  CT vs., 320, *321*
  diaphragm assessment on, 2989
  emphysema quantification using, 2215
  hilar anatomy on, 96–104, *101–103*
  indications for, 320–322, *321, 322*
  lung density on, 270
  mediastinal lymph node assessment on, CT vs., *181–184*, 189–191, *190*
  of postpneumonectomy space, 2661
  physical principles of, 315–320, *318–321*
  upper airway dimension assessment using, 2063, *2065*
Major basic protein (MBP), in asthmatic airway inflammation, 2090
Major fissures. See *Fissures, interlobar.*
Malakoplakia, 724
Malaria, 1039
Malassezia furfur, 952
Malathion, 2584
Malignancy. See *Neoplasm(s), malignant;* specific types and sites.
Malignant fibrous histiocytoma, of lung, 1347–1349
  of mediastinum, 2925
  of rib, *3033*
Malignant neuroleptic syndrome, 2569
Malignant small cell tumor of thoracopulmonary region, 2974, 3028
Mallory's hyaline inclusions, in type II cells in asbestosis, 2429, *2431*
Maloprim, thoracic disease due to, 2538t, 2558
Maltoma, 1275
Malt-worker's lung, 2362t, 2378. See also *Extrinsic allergic alveolitis.*
Mammary artery, internal, in blood supply to diaphragm, 249

Mammary lymph nodes, internal, 175–176, *176*
Mammomanogamus laryngeus infestation, 1046
Mammoplasty, augmentation, oil injection for, pulmonary embolism due to, 1871
 silicone implants for, systemic lupus erythematosus and, 1425
 silicone injection for, pulmonary embolism due to, 1870
Manganese, inhalation of fumes from, 2527
Mantoux test, 841, 842
Manubrium, imaging of, 264
Maple bark–worker's lung, 2362t, 2378. See also *Extrinsic allergic alveolitis.*
Marenostrin, in familial paroxysmal polyserositis, 2766
Marfan's syndrome, 676–677, *677, 678*
 obstructive sleep apnea in, 2061
Marijuana, aspergillosis and, 920–921
 chronic airflow obstruction due to smoking of, 2175
 thoracic disease due to, 2569
Mass(es), mediastinal. See *Mediastinum, masses in.*
 paravertebral, 2974–2981
  differential diagnosis of, 3184, 3185t, *3186–3190*
 pulmonary, multiple, differential diagnosis of, 3122, 3123t–3124t, *3125–3129*
  solitary, 1146–1148, *1148*
   differential diagnosis of, 3116, 3117t–3118t, *3119–3121*
Mast cells, adjacent to pulmonary vessels, 74
 in alveoli, 21
 in conducting airways, 16–17
 in asthma, 2087, 2089, 2109
 in extrinsic allergic alveolitis, 2364
 in idiopathic pulmonary fibrosis, 1590
Mastitis, tuberculous, 840
Mastoiditis, septic pulmonary embolism with, 1829
 tuberculous, 840
Matthew-Wood syndrome, 599
Maximal expiratory flow, density dependence of, 409–410
 in asthma assessment, 2137
 in COPD, 2121
 in COPD, 2121–2224, *2221–2223*
Maximal expiratory flow–elastic recoil curve, 410, *410*
Maximal expiratory pressure, measurement of, in respiratory muscle performance assessment, 419
Maximal inspiratory pressure, measurement of, in respiratory muscle performance assessment, 419
Maximal transdiaphragmatic pressure, measurement of, in respiratory muscle performance assessment, 419–420
Maximal voluntary ventilation (MVV), 410
Measles, 987–990, *988, 989*
 atypical, 988, 990, 2752
 bacterial superinfection in, 987, 990
 pneumonia due to, bronchiectasis and, 2267
Meat-wrapper's asthma, 2122
Mechanical ventilation, dependence on, lung transplantation and, 1700
 high-frequency oscillatory, mucociliary clearance and, 129
 in adult respiratory distress syndrome, radiographic changes with, 1987, *1988–1990,* 1993
 in asthma, 2140
 in Guillain-Barré syndrome, 3062
 intermittent, in neuromuscular disease, 3061
 partial liquid, in adult respiratory distress syndrome, 1987, *1990, 1991*

Mechanical ventilation *(Continued)*
 pneumomediastinum and, 2865
 pneumonia associated with. See *Pneumonia, ventilator-associated.*
 pneumothorax with, 2789–2790
Mechanic's hands, in dermatomyositis/polymyositis, 1463
Meconium ileus, in cystic fibrosis, 2311
Meconium ileus equivalent, in cystic fibrosis, 2311
Medial arcuate ligament, 253, *253,* 254
Medial hypertrophy, of pulmonary vessels, in pulmonary hypertension, 1883, *1885,* 1919, *1919*
Mediastinal emphysema. See *Pneumomediastinum.*
Mediastinal fibrosis, idiopathic, 2856–2863. See also *Fibrosing mediastinitis.*
Mediastinal granuloma, problems with term, 2856
Mediastinal hemorrhage, 2625–2626, *2626,* 2870–2871, *2870*
 after sternotomy, 2664
 anterior mass due to, 3172t
 in aortic rupture, 2627, *2627,* 2630–2631, *2630*
 middle-posterior mass due to, 3178t
Mediastinal herniation, 531–532, *532*
Mediastinal line, anterior, 201–204, *204, 205*
Mediastinal lymph nodes, 175–191. See also *Lymph nodes; specific nodal groups.*
 classification of, American Thoracic Society system of, 180–184, 184t, *185–187,* 186
  for lung cancer staging, 180–184, *185,* 188t, *1186,* *1186,* 1187t
 CT vs. MRI for assessment of, *181–184,* 189–191, *190*
 enlarged, 2938–2942, *2939–2942*
  differential diagnosis of, 3163, 3164t–3165t, *3166–3169*
  in cystic fibrosis, 2277, 2304–2306
  in extrinsic allergic alveolitis, 2365
  in progressive systemic sclerosis, 1456–1457
  in suspected lung cancer, investigation of, 1194
 imaging of, 175
 in angioimmunoblastic lymphadenopathy, 1313
 in Hodgkin's disease, 1299–1302, *1300–1305*
 in mediastinal lymphoma, 1292, *1293–1295*
 measurement of, on CT, 187–188, *189,* 1186
 metastasis to, FDG-PET imaging for detection of, 333
  pleural effusion due to, 2757
 silicosis involving, 2394, 2402, *2403*
 size of, 184–189, *189,* 189t
  criteria for, in pulmonary carcinoma staging, 1188
 thoracoscopic assessment of, 371–372
Mediastinal pain, 386
Mediastinal pleura, defined, 587n
Mediastinal triangle, anterior, 202, *204*
 posterior, 223, *225*
Mediastinal veins, dilation of, 2946–2951, *2947, 2948, 2950–2953,* 2950t
Mediastinitis, 2851–2863
 acute, 2851–2856
  causes of, 2851
  clinical features of, 2856
  prognosis in, 2856
  radiologic features of, 2852–2856, *2852–2855,* 3177t
 localized infectious, 2943
 postoperative, risk factors for, 2851–2852

Mediastinitis *(Continued)*
 sclerosing, chronic (fibrosing, granulomatous), 2856–2863. See also *Fibrosing mediastinitis.*
  in rheumatoid disease, 1433
 tuberculous, 835
Mediastinoscopy, 373–374
 fine-needle aspiration during, 348
Mediastinotomy, anterior, 374
Mediastinum, abscess in, radiologic features of, 2852, *2854, 2855*
  retropharyngeal abscess with, upper airway obstruction due to, 2022, *2023*
 adipose tumors of, *1348,* 2914–2917, *2915–2919*
 anatomy of, 196–233
 anterior, in Heitzman classification, 197
  anatomy of, 198–205, *200–207*
  masses predominantly in, 2875–2929
   differential diagnosis of, 3170, 3171t–3172t, *3173–3175*
   in Hodgkin's disease, 1302
 biopsy techniques in, 373–374
 cartilaginous tumors of, 2925
 chronic histoplasmosis of, 884–888, *887*
 compartments of, 196–197, 2875–2876, *2876*
 CT assessment of, indications for, 314
 cysts of, bronchial vs. esophageal origin of, 611, 2943
  bronchogenic, *610,* 612–615, *613–617*
  in middle-posterior compartment, 2943–2945, *2944–2946*
 displacement of, in atelectasis, 529, *530,* 531–532, *532*
 fat distribution in, 212–214, *215, 216*
 fibrohistiocytic tumors of, 2925
 fibrous tumors of, 2925
 germ cell tumors of, 2901–2911, *2902, 2904–2910*
  staging of, 2903t
 Heitzman's regions of, 197
 hematoma in, anterior mass due to, 3172t
  middle-posterior mass due to, 3178t
 lymph nodes of. See *Lymph nodes; Mediastinal lymph nodes; specific nodal groups.*
 lymphocele of, due to thoracic duct rupture, 2636
 lymphoma of, 1291–1293, *1293–1295,* 2911–2912
 masses in, anatomic classification of, 2875–2876, *2876*
  in anterior cardiophrenic angle, 2925–2929
  in anterior compartment, 2875–2929
   differential diagnosis of, 3170, 3171t–3172t, *3173–3175*
   in Hodgkin's disease, 1302
  in middle-posterior compartment, 2938–2968
   differential diagnosis of, 3176, 3177t–3178t, *3179–3183*
   types of, frequency of, 2876
 metastasis to, anterior mass due to, 3172t
  from gonadal tumor, 2902
  middle-posterior mass due to, 3178t
 middle-posterior, masses predominantly in, 2938–2968
  differential diagnosis of, 3176, 3177t–3178t, *3179–3183*
 MR evaluation of, 321, *321*
 muscle tumors of, 2925
 osteogenic tumors of, 2925
 pleomorphic adenoma of, 2929
 pulmonary carcinoma involving, 1156, *1158–1161*
  clinical features of, 1170–1171, *1170*
 surgical complications involving, 2663–2669, *2664, 2666–2668*

Mediastinum *(Continued)*
  trauma to, aortography in evaluation of, 324–325
    CT in, 325, *325*
    nonpenetrating, 2625–2636
    vascular tumors of, 2917–2925, *2920–2924*
    widening of, in aortic rupture, 2627–2628, *2627, 2630*
Medical history, 389
Medication(s). See *Drug(s);* specific drugs and classes of drugs.
Mediterranean spotted fever, 1022
Medulla, in respiratory control, *236,* 238–239, *3050,* 3051
Megaesophagus, 2967, *2967,* 3178t, *3183*
Megakaryocytes, in lungs, 132, *133*
Megakaryocytic capillary stasis, in leukemia, 1317–1318, *1317*
Meigs-Salmon syndrome, 2765
Melanocytic schwannoma, 2976
Melanoma, metastatic, in lung, *1401, 1403,* 1407
  in trachea, *2040*
  pleural, 2838
  tracheobronchial, 1267
Melanoptysis, in coal workers' pneumoconiosis, 2418
Melioidosis, 759–760
Melphalan, thoracic disease due to, 2538t, 2548
Melting sign, with pulmonary infarct resolution, 1797, *1801*
Membranous bronchioles, grading of inflammatory reaction in, 2189
  morphology of, 5–17, *8, 11, 14, 16*
  smooth muscle of, 14, *14*
Membranous pneumocyte. See *Alveolar epithelial cells, type I.*
Meningioma, metastatic to lung, 1411–1412
  pulmonary, 1370
Meningitis, in coccidioidomycosis, 895
  tuberculous, 838–839
Meningocele, 2978–2979, *2979,* 3185t, *3186*
Meningomyelocele, 2978–2979, 3185t
Meningothelial-like nodules, pulmonary, 74, 1364, 1374–1375, *1376*
Meniscus sign. See *Air-crescent sign.*
Menstruation, asthma and, 2117
  pneumothorax and, 2767–2768, 2787–2789
6-Mercaptopurine, thoracic disease due to, 2538t, 2555
Mercurous chloride, Young's syndrome and, 2284
Mercury, metallic, aspiration of, 2513
  embolism of, 1863–1865, *1866*
  inhalation of fumes from, 2527
Mesalamine, thoracic disease due to, 2539t, 2565
Mesenchymal cystic hamartoma, 1373–1374
Mesenchymal neoplasms. See also specific neoplasms.
  esophageal, 2965–2966
  pleural, 2828–2835
  pulmonary, 1331–1357, 3088t
Mesenchymoma, mediastinal, 2929
  pulmonary, 1350. See also *Hamartoma.*
    malignant, 1357
Mesothelial cells, of pleura, 151–153, *152, 154, 155*
Mesothelial cysts, 2927–2928, *2927, 2928,* 3171t, *3173*
Mesothelial hyperplasia, mesothelioma vs., 2816–2818, *2817, 2818*
Mesothelioma, 2807–2828
  benign (local, fibrous). See *Fibrous tumor of pleura, solitary.*
  benign pleural thickening vs., 587, *588,* 2435, 2437, *2443,* 2824, *2825*

Mesothelioma *(Continued)*
  causes of, 2807–2810
  clinical features of, 2824–2825
  diagnosis of, pleural fluid cytology in, 345
    thoracoscopic biopsy in, 371
  epidemiology of, 2807
  histologic classification of, 2811, *2814–2816*
    prognosis and, 2826
  laboratory findings in, 2825–2826
  latent period for, 2825
  metastasis from, 2824, 2826
  multicystic, 2840
  pathogenesis of, 2810–2811
  pathologic features of, 2811–2820, *2812–2816,* 2820t, *2821*
  pleural effusion and, 2435
  polio vaccine and, 990, 2810
  prognosis in, 2448, 2826–2828, *2827*
  pulmonary carcinoma with pleural involvement vs., 1165, *1165,* 2818–2820, *2819,* 2826
  radiologic features of, 583–587, *587,* 2437, *2441–2443,* 2820–2824, *2822–2825*
  spontaneous pneumothorax with, 2786
  staging of, 2826, 2828t
  synthetic mineral fibers and, 2468
  ultrastructural features of, 2819–2820, *2821*
  well-differentiated papillary, 2838
Mesulergine, thoracic disease due to, 2571
Metabisulfite, asthma provoked by, 2116
Metabolic acidosis, 117–118, 118t
  central ventilatory response to, 237
  hyperventilation in, 3067
  in asthma, 2139
  pulmonary vascular response to, 106
Metabolic alkalosis, 118–119
  hypoventilation due to, 3054
Metabolic disease, 2699–2729. See also specific disorders.
  inherited, immunodeficiency with, 726
Metal(s). See also specific metals.
  exposure to dust of, idiopathic pulmonary fibrosis and, 1586
  hard, pneumoconiosis due to, 2463, *2463, 2464*
  inhalation of fumes from, 2527–2528
  occupational asthma due to, 2119t, 2122
Metalloproteinases, in emphysema pathogenesis, 2182
Metastasectomy, for pulmonary metastasis, 1387
  from osteosarcoma, 1411
  from renal cell carcinoma, 1404
  from soft tissue sarcoma, 1410
Metastasis(es), airway obstruction due to, 1397–1399, *1400–1403*
  CT in detection of, 314
  cytologic findings in, 1412
  defined, 1382
  from adenocarcinoma, *1389*
  from adenoid cystic carcinoma of submaxillary gland, *1388*
  from adrenal carcinoma, enlarged azygos node in, *2939*
  from angiosarcoma, 1409–1410
  from bone tumors, 1410–1411
  from breast cancer, *1389,* 1405
    lymphangitic pattern of, *1391–1393*
    pleural effusion due to, 2759
  from bronchioloalveolar carcinoma, 1399
    lymphangitic pattern of, *1392*
  from carcinoid tumors, 1237, 1243
  from carcinoma, mediastinal germ cell neoplasm vs., 2902
  from central nervous system tumors, 1411–1412
  from cervical carcinoma, 1407–1408, *3038*

Metastasis(es) *(Continued)*
  from chondrosarcoma, calcification in, 467
  from choriocarcinoma, *1383, 1384, 1406,* 1407, 1408–1409
  from colorectal cancer, *1385, 1387, 1396, 1400,* 1404–1405
  from endometrial malignancy, 1407
  from extrapulmonary lymphoma. See *Lymphoma, pulmonary, secondary.*
  from gestational trophoblastic neoplasms, 1408–1409
  from giant cell tumor of bone, 1410–1411
  from head and neck cancer, 1405
    cavitation in, 1389, *1390*
  from hepatocellular carcinoma, 1405
  from leiomyosarcoma, 1332, *1387,* 1409, *1410, 1411*
  from malignant fibrous histiocytoma, 1349
  from melanoma, *1401, 1403,* 1407, *2040*
  from mesothelioma, 2824, 2826
  from oropharyngeal carcinoma, *2041*
  from osteosarcoma, 1410, 1411
    calcification in, 467, *473, 1391*
  from ovarian cancer, in diaphragm, 3006
    in lung, 1408
  from prostatic carcinoma, 1408
  from pulmonary carcinoma, clinical features of, 1172–1173
    detection of, 1181, 1191–1193, *1192*
    pulmonary, 1399
    thromboembolism vs., *1821*
  from renal cell carcinoma, 1399–1404, *1399, 1402, 1404*
    lymph node enlargement in, *3169*
  from soft tissue sarcomas, 1409–1410
  from testicular germ cell tumor, *1383, 1406,* 1407, *1407*
  from thymoma, 2896
  from thyroid cancer, calcification in, 467
    in chest wall, *3035*
    in lung, 1405–1407
  from upper airway cancer, pulmonary carcinoma vs., 1202
  from Wilms' tumor, *1386*
  intravascular, pulmonary hypertension and infarction due to, 1397, *1398, 1399*
  lymph node enlargement in, 3165t, *3169*
  pathogenesis of, 1381, 1382–1383
  patterns of, 1383–1399
  pleural effusion due to, 2756–2757, 2758–2759
  pulmonary function tests in, 1412
  spontaneous regression of, 1412
  to adrenals, 1173
    detection of, 1191–1192, *1192*
  to bone, from carcinoid tumor, 1237
    from pulmonary carcinoma, 1166, *1167,* 1173
    detection of, 1192
  to bronchus, 1397–1398, *1400–1402*
  to central nervous system, 1172–1173
  to chest wall, 3032, *3035, 3038*
  to diaphragm, 3004–3006
  to gastrointestinal tract, 1173
  to lung, 1381–1412
    anatomic bias of, 477, *477*
    calcification in, 467, *473*
    cavities or cysts due to, 510, *511,* 3104t
    diagnosis of, bronchoalveolar lavage in, 343
    cytologic, 341
    transthoracic needle aspiration in, 347
    diffuse nodular pattern in, 3145t
    from primary pulmonary carcinoma, 1399
    from specific sites, 1399–1412
    hematogenous, nodular interstitial pattern in, 447–453

Metastasis(es) (Continued)
    laboratory findings in, 1412
    multiple masses or nodules due to, 3123t,
        3128
    nodular. See Nodule(s), metastatic parenchy-
        mal.
    solitary mass due to, 3117t
    solitary nodule due to, 3112t
    spontaneous regression of, 1412
    vascular supply of, 1384
    with interstitial thickening. See Lymphan-
        gitic carcinomatosis.
    to mediastinal lymph nodes, FDG-PET im-
        aging for detection of, 333
    pleural effusion due to, 2757
    to mediastinum, anterior mass due to, 3172t
        from gonadal tumor, 2902
        middle-posterior mass due to, 3178t
    to pleura, mesothelioma vs., 2818–2820, 2819,
        2820t
    to rib, chest wall pain due to, 387
    to sternum, 3031, 3037
    to thymus, 2898
    to trachea, 1398–1399, 1403, 2036, 2040,
        2041
    via airways, 1383
    via pleural space, 1383
    via pulmonary or bronchial arteries, 1382
    via pulmonary or pleural lymphatics, 1382–
        1383
Metastrongyloidiasis, 1047
Methacholine inhalation, for bronchial
    responsiveness measurement, 420–423,
    421t, 2095
Methadone, thoracic disease due to, 2539t, 2567,
    2568
Methemoglobinemia, 398, 3068
Methicillin resistance, in Staphylococcus aureus,
    744
Methotrexate, for rheumatoid disease,
    opportunistic infection with, 1451
    thoracic disease due to, 2538t, 2551–2555,
        2553, 2554
Methyl CCNU (semustine), thoracic disease due
    to, 2548
Methyldopa, thoracic disease due to, 2572
Methylphenidate (Ritalin), intravenous abuse of,
    1860
Methysergide, multifocal fibrosclerosis and,
    2857
    pleural effusion due to, 2756
Mica, pneumoconiosis due to, 2450–2451
Microangiitis, 1513. See also Capillaritis.
Microatelectasis. See Atelectasis, adhesive.
Microfilaria, pleural effusion due to, 2752
    pulmonary disease due to, 1043–1045, 1044,
        1752–1753
β2-Microglobulin, in amyloidosis, 2709
Microlithiasis, alveolar, 2719–2722, 2720
    radiologic features of, 278, 2721, 2722,
        2723
Micronodules, interstitial, problems with term,
    447
Microscopic polyangiitis, 1490t, 1511, 1513,
    1514
Microsomal epoxide hydrolase enzyme, COPD
    and, 2179
Microsporidiosis, 1039
Microthromboembolism, 1828–1829
Microvascular pressure, in pulmonary fluid and
    solute exchange, 1953
Microvilli, in adenocarcinoma vs. mesothelioma,
    2819–2820, 2821
    of mesothelial cells, 152, 154, 155
Midazolam, before bronchoscopy, 367
Middle diaphragmatic lymph nodes, 176, 178

Middle diaphragmatic lymph nodes (Continued)
    enlargement of, 2929
Middle lobe syndrome, in bronchiectasis, 2268
Midsternal stripe, after sternotomy, 2661
Migratory polyarthritis, in Churg-Strauss
    syndrome, 1511
Migratory thrombophlebitis, in pulmonary
    carcinoma, 1177
Miliary infection, 713–715. See also
    Tuberculosis, miliary.
Mineral dust airway disease, asbestosis and,
    2429–2430, 2431
Mineral fibers, synthetic, pneumoconiosis due to,
    2467–2468
Mineral oil aspiration, 2500
    clinical features of, 2506
    diagnosis of, 2506–2507
    pathologic features of, 2501, 2502–2504
    prognosis in, 2507
    radiologic features of, 2505, 2506, 2506, 2507
Minimal change nephropathy, paraneoplastic, in
    pulmonary carcinoma, 1178
Minocycline, thoracic disease due to, 2538t,
    2558
Minor fissure, left, 165, 166
    right. See Fissures, interlobar.
Minute pulmonary chemodectomas, 74, 1364,
    1374–1375, 1376
Mitomycin, thoracic disease due to, 2538t,
    2543–2544, 2544
Mitral insufficiency, pulmonary hypertension in,
    1923, 1928
Mitral stenosis, pulmonary hypertension in,
    1919, 1919, 1920, 1923, 1923, 1930
    clinical features of, 1928
    pulmonary function tests in, 1928
    pulmonary ossification in, 474, 475
    pulmonary veno-occlusive disease vs., 1931
    surgical correction of, hemodynamic assess-
        ment after, 1923–1926
    pulmonary function improvement after,
        1928–1930
Mitral valve prolapse, pulmonary hypertension
    in, 1924–1925
Mixed connective tissue disease, 1469–1470,
    1471. See also Overlap syndrome(s).
Moebius' syndrome, 3052
Molecular biology, 358
Mollusk shell–worker's lung, 2362t. See also
    Extrinsic allergic alveolitis.
Monge's disease, 3053–3054
Moraxella catarrhalis (Branhamella catarrhalis),
    bronchiectasis and, 2267
    pneumonia due to, 722, 748
Morgagni's foramen(ina), 248, 2987, 2988
    hernia through, 2926, 2998, 3001–3004, 3003,
        3004, 3172t
Morganella infections, 755–756
Morphometry, 356
Mosaic perfusion, in bronchiolitis, 2330–2331,
    2332
    in chronic pulmonary thromboembolism, 1811,
        1813, 1815
    in healthy subjects, 290, 2331
    in thromboembolic pulmonary hypertension,
        1908, 1910
Mounier-Kuhn syndrome, 2285–2287, 2286
    in cutis laxa, 677
    in Ehlers-Danlos syndrome, 677
    upper airway obstruction due to, 2046–2048,
        2047
Mountain sickness, acute, 1999–2001
    chronic, 3053–3054
Mouth breathing, obstructive sleep apnea and,
    2059
Mouth occlusion pressure, measurement of,
    418–419

Mucinous cystic tumor, 1101, 1265–1266
Mucin-secreting adenocarcinoma. See also
    Adenocarcinoma, pulmonary.
    calcification in, 467
Mucocele, 1253, 2269, 2269
Mucociliary clearance, 127–129, 128
    bronchiectasis and, 2267
    in asthma, 2093–2094
    in chronic bronchitis, 2181–2182
    in COPD, 2181–2182
    in cystic fibrosis, 2301
    in dyskinetic cilia syndrome, 2283
    smoking and, 2181–2182
Mucoepidermoid carcinoma, tracheobronchial,
    1252, 1256–1258, 1257, 1258
Mucoid impaction, 483, 484
    in allergic bronchopulmonary aspergillosis,
        928, 929
    radiologic features of, 483, 929, 931–935
    in pulmonary carcinoma, 1124–1125, 1129,
        1130, 1131
    with congenital bronchial atresia, 621, 622,
        623
Mucoid pseudotumor, tracheobronchial gland
    tumor vs., 1253
Mucopolysaccharide storage diseases, 2727–2728
Mucormycosis, 947–949, 948, 2752
Mucosa, bronchial, increased permeability of,
    airway hyper-responsiveness and,
    2097–2098
Mucosa-associated lymphoid tissue (MALT),
    pulmonary lymphoma and, 1275
Mucous cells, in tracheobronchial glands, 14, 15,
    15
Mucous gland adenoma, 1259
Mucous plugs, in asthma, 2083, 2083
Mucoviscidosis. See Cystic fibrosis.
Mucus, 60–63
    in asthma, 2093–2094
Müller maneuver, 275n
    chest radiographs with, 305
    clinical utility of, 275, 276
Müller-Hermelink classification of thymoma,
    2886, 2887–2891
Mullite, pneumoconiosis due to, 2452
Multicentric reticulohistiocytosis, 1313
Multifocal leukoencephalopathy, progressive,
    sarcoidosis and, 1566
Multiple endocrine neoplasia syndrome, with
    thymic carcinoid, 2900
Multiple hamartoma syndrome, 1351
Multiple myeloma, 1293–1297, 1296
    after transplantation, 1711
    of chest wall, 3032, 3034, 3036, 3037
    pain due to, 387
    pleural effusion due to, 2760
    with immunosuppressive therapy for rheuma-
        toid disease, 1451
Multiple organ dysfunction syndrome, 1977n
    adult respiratory distress syndrome and, 1977,
        1998
Multiple sclerosis, 3053
Multiple sleep latency test, 2066
Multiple system organ failure, 1977n
    adult respiratory distress syndrome and, 1977,
        1998
Muscarinic receptors, in lung, 148
Muscle, length-tension relationship of, 2102,
    3057
    skeletal, sarcoidosis involving, 1565
        tuberculosis involving, 840
        Wegener's granulomatosis involving, 1504
    smooth, in airways. See Airway smooth mus-
        cle.
    multi-unit, 2101
    neoplasms of, 1331–1335. See also specific
        neoplasms.

Muscle (*Continued*)
  single-unit, 2100–2101
  weakness of, in asthma, 2140
Muscle fibers, types of, in diaphragm, 249–250
Muscle hypertrophy-hyperplasia, of pulmonary
    vessels, in pulmonary hypertension, 1883,
    1885
Muscle spindles, in respiratory muscles, in
    compensation for increased ventilatory
    load, 242
  in ventilatory control, 238
Muscovite, pneumoconiosis due to, 2450
Muscular dystrophy, dermatomyositis/
    polymyositis vs., 1462
  hypoventilation in, 3064
Musculophrenic artery, in blood supply to
    diaphragm, 249
Mushroom-worker's lung, 2362t, 2377. See also
    Extrinsic allergic alveolitis.
Mustard gas, pulmonary carcinoma and, 1077
Myasthenia gravis, CT in assessment of,
    2891–2894
  hypoventilation in, 3063–3064
  Lambert-Eaton myasthenic syndrome vs., 1173
  thymic lymphoid hyperplasia in, 2877–2880,
    2880
  thymoma and, 2894, 2897
  upper airway obstruction in, 2033
myc genes, 1082
Mycetoma. See *Fungus ball.*
Mycobacteria. See also *Mycobacterial infection;*
    Tuberculosis; specific organisms.
  characteristics of, 798–799
  identification of, 844–846
  nontuberculous, classification of, 849
    cystic fibrosis and, 850
    sarcoidosis and, 803, 1534–1535
Mycobacterial infection, 798–861. See also
    Tuberculosis; specific organisms.
  cavities or cysts in, 3102t
  in HIV disease, 1648–1655
  nontuberculous, 849–861
    clinical features of, 857–860
    diagnosis of, 853, 860–861, 861t
    disseminated, 858–860
    epidemiology of, 849–852
    in HIV disease, 853, *854,* 1654–1655,
      1654–1656
    pathologic features of, 852–853, *852–855*
    prognosis in, 861
    radiologic features of, *852,* 853–857, *856–*
      860
Mycobacterium abscessus infection, 851–852
Mycobacterium africanum, 799
Mycobacterium asiaticum, 849
Mycobacterium avium complex infection, 850
  bronchiectasis with, *853*
  disseminated, 858
  in AIDS, 853, *854,* 1654–1655, *1654–1656*
  radiologic features of, 853–855, *856–859*
Mycobacterium bovis infection, 799
Mycobacterium chelonae infection, 851–852
  clinical features of, 858
  disseminated, 858–860
Mycobacterium fortuitum infection, 851–852
  clinical features of, 858
Mycobacterium genavense infection, 851
Mycobacterium gordonae, 849
Mycobacterium haemophilum infection, 851
Mycobacterium intracellulare, 849. See also
    Mycobacterium avium *complex infection.*
Mycobacterium kansasii infection, 850–851
  disseminated, 858–860
  in hairy cell leukemia, 853, *855*
  in HIV disease, 1655
  radiologic features of, 855–857, *860*

Mycobacterium malmoense infection, 851
  radiologic features of, 857
Mycobacterium marinum infection, 851
  clinical features of, 858
Mycobacterium microti, 799
Mycobacterium scrofulaceum infection, 851
Mycobacterium simiae infection, 851
Mycobacterium szulgai infection, 851
Mycobacterium tuberculosis. See also
    Tuberculosis.
  sarcoidosis and, 803, 1534–1535
  skin test response to, atopy and, 2080
  transmission of, 800–801
Mycobacterium ulcerans infection, clinical
    features of, 858
Mycobacterium xenopi infection, 851
  idiopathic pulmonary fibrosis with, *852*
Mycolic acid profile analysis, in mycobacteria
    identification, 845, 860
Mycoplasma fermentans, 1010
Mycoplasma genitalium, 1010
Mycoplasma hominis, 1010
Mycoplasma pneumoniae infection, asthma
    provoked by, 2111–2112
  bronchiolitis due to, *702*
  bronchiolitis in, *2325, 2330,* 2333, *2335, 2336*
  clinical features of, 1011–1014
  community-acquired, 722
  diffuse reticular pattern in, 3134t
  epidemiology of, 1010
  inhomogeneous consolidation in, nonsegmen-
    tal, 3093t
    segmental, 3097t
  laboratory findings in, 1014–1015
  pathogenesis of, 1010–1011
  pathologic features of, 1011, *1012*
  pleural effusion in, 2752
  prognosis in, 1015
  radiologic features of, 455, *714,* 1011, *1013–*
    1016
Mycosis fungoides, 1291
Mycotoxicosis, 876. See also *Organic dust toxic*
    syndrome.
Myeloma. See *Multiple myeloma;*
    Plasmacytoma.
Myelopathy, necrotizing, paraneoplastic, in
    pulmonary carcinoma, 1174
Myeloproliferative disorders, 1313–1320. See
    also specific disorders.
Myiasis, 1061
Myoblastoma, granular cell, pulmonary, 1346
Myocardial infarction, acute pulmonary
    thromboembolism vs., 1819
  obstructive sleep apnea and, 2067
  pleural effusion after, 2766
Myoclonus, respiratory, 2995
Myoepithelial cells, in tracheobronchial glands,
    14
Myoepithelioma, peripheral lung, 1251–1253
Myofibroblast(s), in alveolar interstitium, 20, 21,
    23, *23, 24*
  in idiopathic pulmonary fibrosis pathogenesis,
    1590
Myofibroblastic tumor, inflammatory, 1371–1373
Myoglobinuria, 3065
Myomatosis. See *Lymphangioleiomyomatosis.*
Myoneural junction disorders, hypoventilation
    due to, 3063–3064
Myopathy, paraneoplastic, in pulmonary
    carcinoma, 1173–1174
Myopericarditis, in *Mycoplasma pneumoniae*
    infection, 1014
Myositis, after influenza, 984
Myotonic dystrophy, 3064
Myxedema, 2729
  hypoventilation in, 3054

Myxedema (*Continued*)
  pleural effusion in, 2766
  progressive systemic sclerosis with, 1459
Myxoma, atrial, pulmonary hypertension with,
    1927–1928, 1928
  mediastinal, 2929
  pulmonary, 1347
Myxoviruses, 981–990

Naclerio's sign, 2865
Nailfold capillary microscopy, abnormal pattern
    on, in CREST syndrome, 1460
  in progressive systemic sclerosis, 1459
Naloxone, thoracic disease due to, 2539t, 2567
Napkin ring trachea, anomalous origin of left
    pulmonary artery with, 642
Naproxen, thoracic disease due to, 2539t, 2565
Narcotics, thoracic disease due to, 2539t, 2567,
    2568
Nasal dilatory muscles, in ventilation, 246
Nasal obstruction, obstructive sleep apnea and,
    2059
Nasogastric tube(s), complications of,
    2677–2680, *2679, 2680*
  deviation of, in aortic rupture, 2628, *2629*
Nasopharynx, receptors in, in ventilatory control,
    236, 237
Nasu-Hakola disease, 2728
Natural killer (NK) cells, in host response to
    neoplasia, 1083
Near-drowning, 2507–2508. See also *Aspiration*
    (event), of water.
Necator americanus, 1043, 1752
Neck circumference, obstructive sleep apnea
    and, 2059–2060
Neck dissection, radical, chest radiograph
    appearance after, 3012
Necrobiotic nodules, in rheumatoid disease,
    1438, *1441–1443*
  Caplan's syndrome vs., 1442
Necrosis, in cavity formation, mechanisms of,
    462
Necrotizing encephalomyelopathy, subacute,
    central apnea with, 3052
Necrotizing granulomatous lymphadenitis,
    broncholithiasis with, 2287
Necrotizing myelopathy, paraneoplastic, in
    pulmonary carcinoma, 1174
Necrotizing pneumonia, bronchiectasis and, 2267
  Klebsiella, 705
Necrotizing pseudomembranous tracheo-
    bronchitis, acute, 701, *701,* 942, *947,* 2022
Necrotizing sarcoid granulomatosis, 1521–1523,
    1522–1524
Needle(s), for closed pleural biopsy, 372–373
  for transthoracic aspiration, 345
Needle aspiration. See *Fine-needle aspiration.*
Needle biopsy. See under *Biopsy.*
Neisseria catarrhalis. See Moraxella catarrhalis
    (Branhamella catarrhalis).
Neisseria gonorrhoeae infection, pulmonary, 748
Neisseria meningitidis infection, in influenza,
    982
  pulmonary, 748
Neisseria species, commensal, pulmonary
    infection due to, in immunocompromised
    persons, 748
Nelson, dorsal lobe of, 165
Nemaline myopathy, 3064–3065
Nematodes, 1039–1047. See also specific
    diseases.
Neocarzinostatin, thoracic disease due to, 2544
Neonatal respiratory distress syndrome, adhesive
    atelectasis in, 522

Neonatal respiratory distress syndrome
  (*Continued*)
    surfactant in, 58
Neonate(s). See also *Child(ren); Infant(s).*
  airway morphology in, 138–139
  anasarca in, cystic adenomatoid malformation
      and, 618
  asphyxiating thoracic dystrophy of, 3015
  central apnea in, 3052
  hoarseness in, 389
  lobar hyperinflation in, 621–625, *625, 626*
  persistent pulmonary hypertension in, 1882
Neoplasm(s). See also specific types and sites.
  chest wall, 3023–3032, *3026–3038*
  diagnosis of, CT in, 314
    positron emission tomography in, 332–333
    transmission electron microscopy in, 354
  diaphragmatic, 3004–3006, *3005*
  endobronchial, partial airway obstruction by,
      lung volume and, 497, 498, 499, *499–
      501*
    normal chest radiograph with, 3047
    oligemia due to, 503–504, *506*
    Swyer-James syndrome vs., 2340, *2343*
  endocrine gland, 2912–2914
  host response to, cell-mediated immunity in,
      1083–1084
  in anterior cardiophrenic angle, 2925–2929
  in HIV infection, 1644t, 1676–1683
  lymph node enlargement due to, 3165t, *3168–
      3169*
  malignant, after bone marrow transplantation,
      1732, *1733*
    calcification and, 467, *472, 473*
    chylothorax due to, 2768, *2769*
    diagnosis of, bronchoalveolar lavage in, 343
      pleural fluid cytology in, 344–345
      sputum or bronchial washing cytology in,
        340–341, *342*
    doubling time and, 479
    hemothorax due to, 2763
    Langerhans' cell histiocytosis and, 1637–
      1638
    pleural effusion due to, 2744t, 2756–2760,
      2758
      rheumatoid effusion vs., 2754
    tuberculoma vs., 825
    venous thrombosis and, 1779–1780
  mediastinal, in anterior compartment, 3171t,
      3174, 3175
    in middle-posterior compartment, 2942–
      2943, 3177t–3178t, *3180*
  mesenchymal, esophageal, 2965–2966
    pleural, 2828–2835
    pulmonary, 1331–1357
      homogeneous segmental opacity in, 3088t
  MR evaluation of, 321, *322*
  oligemia with, 3157t, *3160*
  ovarian, pleural effusion with, 2765
  parathyroid, 2913–2914, *2914*
  paravertebral, 2974–2979, 3185t, *3188*
  phantom, due to interlobar effusion, 579–581,
      580
  pleural, 583–587, *586, 587,* 2807–2840
    histologic classification of, 1071t
    of uncertain nature, 2840
  pulmonary, 1067–1412
    airway and alveolar epithelial, 1069–1202.
      See also *Carcinoma, pulmonary.*
    bronchiectasis due to, 2269, *2270*
    cavities or cysts due to, 3104t, *3108*
    diffuse nodular pattern in, 3145t
    diffuse reticular pattern in, 3135t
    histologic classification of, 1071t
    homogeneous consolidation due to, nonseg-
      mental, 3081t, *3084, 3085*

Neoplasm(s) (*Continued*)
    segmental, 3087t–3088, *3090*
    inhomogeneous consolidation due to, seg-
      mental, 3097t
    lymphoproliferative, 1269–1323
    mesenchymal, 1331–1357
    miscellaneous epithelial, 1262–1267
    multiple masses or nodules due to, 3123t,
      3128
    neuroendocrine, 1229–1246
    of uncertain histogenesis, 1363–1377
    secondary, 1381–1412. See also *Metastas-
      is(es).*
    solitary mass due to, 3117t, *3120*
    solitary nodule due to, 3112t, *3114, 3115*
    tracheobronchial gland, 1251–1259
  pulmonary embolism from, 1854
  recurrent, after pneumonectomy, 2665, *2667*
    in irradiated field, radiation fibrosis vs.,
      2597–2604
  sarcoidosis and, 1572
  secondary. See also *Metastasis(es).*
    in lung, 1381–1412
      occurring by direct extension, 1381–
        1382, *1382*
    soft tissue, of anterior mediastinum, 2914–
      2925
      of chest wall, 3025–3029, *3028–3030*
    thymic, 2880–2882, 2884–2901
    vanishing, due to interlobar effusion, 579–581,
      580
Nepheline, pneumoconiosis due to, 2452
Nephritis, granulomatous interstitial, in
    sarcoidosis, 1566
Nephrotic syndrome, in pulmonary carcinoma,
    1178
  pleural effusion in, 2764
Neuhauser's sign, in X-linked agamma-
    globulinemia, 725
Neuraminidase, in influenza virus, 981
Neurenteric cyst, 2979–2980
Neurilemoma. See also *Schwannoma.*
  chest wall, 3028, *3029*
  paravertebral, 2974–2975, *2975, 2976, 3188*
  tracheal, 2036, *2038*
Neuroblastoma, 2976–2977
Neuroectodermal tumor, peripheral primitive, in
    paravertebral region, 2974
  of chest wall, 3028–3029
Neuroendocrine carcinoma, large cell, 1229,
    1246
  well-differentiated. See *Carcinoid tumor, atypi-
    cal.*
Neuroendocrine cells, hyperplasia of,
    1243–1245, *1244–1246*
  in tracheobronchial epithelium, 10–11, *11*
  lung development and, 142
  in tracheobronchial glands, 14
Neuroendocrine neoplasms, pulmonary,
    1229–1246
  terminology of, 1229, 1246
  thymic, 2899–2901, *2900, 2901*
  tumor markers for, 1232–1233
Neuroepithelial bodies, in airway epithelium, 11,
    11
Neurofibroma, chest wall, 3028, *3030*
  paravertebral, 2974–2975, *2976*
  pulmonary, 1346
Neurofibromatosis, *688, 689,* 690–691, *690*
Neurofibrosarcoma, in neurofibromatosis, *690*
Neurogenic neoplasms. See also specific
    neoplasms.
  chest wall, 3028, *3029, 3030*
  paravertebral, 2974–2979, 3185t, *3188*
    from peripheral nerves, 2974–2976, *2975,
      2976*

Neurogenic neoplasms (*Continued*)
    from sympathetic ganglia, 2976–2978,
      2977, 2978
  pulmonary, 1346
Neurogenic sarcoma, paravertebral, 2974, *2975*
  pulmonary, 1346
Neurokinins, actions of, in lung, 131
  in asthmatic airway inflammation, 2092
Neuroleptic malignant syndrome, 2569
Neurologic syndromes, in pulmonary carcinoma,
    1172–1173
  paraneoplastic, 1173, 1174
Neuroma, amputation, presenting in lung, 1346
Neuromodulators, in respiratory rhythm
    generation, 240
Neuromuscular blockers, muscle weakness due
    to, in asthma, 2140
  myasthenia-like syndrome due to, 3063–3064
Neuromuscular disease, respiratory failure due
    to, clinical manifestations of, 3057–3059,
    3058–3060
  pulmonary function tests in, 3059–3061
Neuron-specific enolase, in carcinoid tumors,
    1233
Neurosecretory granules, in carcinoid tumors, in
    atypical tumors, 1234
  in typical tumors, 1231, 1233, *1233, 1235*
Neurotoxic shellfish poisoning, 3062
Neurotransmitters. See also specific
    neurotransmitters.
  in respiratory rhythm generation, 239–240
  noninnervated receptors for, on lung cells, 148
Neutral endopeptidases, actions of, in lung, 131
  in asthmatic airway inflammation, 2092
Neutrophil(s), in adult respiratory distress
    syndrome, 1979–1980
  in airways, 130
  in asbestosis, 2422
  in extrinsic allergic alveolitis, 2363–2364
  in pleural fluid specimen, 344
  in progressive systemic sclerosis, 1452–1453
  transit of, through pulmonary circulation, em-
    physema and, 2183–2184
Neutrophil chemotactic factor of anaphylaxis, in
    exercise-induced asthma, 2109
Neutrophil elastase, in adult respiratory distress
    syndrome, 1980, 1981, 1983
  in cystic fibrosis, 2302–2303
  in emphysema, 2182, *2183,* 2185
    smoking and, 2184
New Guinea lung, 2363t. See also *Extrinsic
    allergic alveolitis.*
Newborn. See *Neonate(s).*
Nickel, pulmonary carcinoma and, 1076
Niemann-Pick disease, 2724, *2726*
Nilutamide, thoracic disease due to, 2538t, 2551
Nitrates, methemoglobinemia due to, 3068
Nitric oxide, actions of, in lung, 131
  in asthmatic airway inflammation, 2092–2093
  in cigarette smoke, 2184
  in nonadrenergic noncholinergic inhibitory sys-
    tem, 148
  in pulmonary hypertension pathogenesis,
    1881–1882
  inhaled, response to, in COPD, 2228–2229
  pulmonary endothelial synthesis of, hypoxic
    vasoconstriction and, 106
Nitric oxide synthetase, in airway nerves, 148
Nitrofurantoin, pleural effusion due to, 2756
  thoracic disease due to, 2538t, 2556–2557,
    2557, 2558
    diffuse reticular pattern in, 3136t
Nitrogen dioxide, acute exposure to, 2522–2524,
    2523
  atmospheric, asthma and, 2115
  experimental emphysema induced by, 2186

Nitrogen washout test, multiple-breath method for, for assessment of distribution of inspired gas, 414
    for functional residual capacity determination, 407
    single-breath method for, 413–414, *413*
    in COPD, 2121
Nitrosoureas, thoracic disease due to, 2538t, 2548–2550, *2551*
NK cells, in host response to neoplasia, 1083
Nocardiosis, 957–958, *958–960*
    cavities or cysts in, 3102t
    homogeneous nonsegmental opacity in, 3080t
    in HIV disease, 1648
    pleural effusion in, 2751
Nocturnal dyspnea, paroxysmal, 388
Nodule(s), air-space, 438, *439*
    border characteristics of, 457–459, *458*
    centrilobular, in bronchiolitis, *30*
      in tuberculosis, *30,* 827–828, *833*
    disappearing or shifting, in atelectasis, 534, *537*
    doubling time of, 479, *480,* 1142–1143, *1144, 1145*
    in tuberculosis, *30,* 824–830, *830–835.* See also *Tuberculoma.*
    interstitial, 447–453, *450–453*
    metastatic parenchymal, 1383–1390
      clinical features of, 1389–1390
      detection of, 1384–1386
      multiple, *1383–1385,* 1388–1390, *1388–1391*
      primary pulmonary carcinoma vs., 1387–1388
      size and distribution of, 1383–1384
      solitary, 1386–1388, *1386, 1387,* 3112t
      with miliary pattern, *1384,* 1388
    multiple, differential diagnosis of, 3122, 3123t–3124t, *3125–3129*
    overlooked on radiograph, 3046
    solitary, air bronchogram with, 1142, *1142*
      benign vs. malignant, 1133–1146, 1135t, *1136–1142, 1144–1147*
      calcification in, *315,* 1135–1139, *1136–1138*
      character of lung interface with, 1139, *1139–1141*
      contrast enhancement of, 1143–1146, *1146, 1147*
      defined, 1133
      differential diagnosis of, 3110, 3111t–3112t, *3113–3115*
      doubling time of, 479, *480,* 1142–1143, *1144, 1145*
      investigation of, in suspected lung cancer, 1193–1194
      metastatic, 1386–1388, *1386, 1387,* 3112t
      size of, 1135
Nomenclature of organisms, defined, 735
Nonadrenergic noncholinergic inhibitory system, 145, 148–149
    bronchial hyper-responsiveness and, 2098–2099
Non-Hodgkin's lymphoma. See *Lymphoma.*
Nonsteroidal anti-inflammatory drugs, asthma provoked by, 2112–2113
    thoracic disease due to, 2539t, 2565
Noonan's syndrome, chylothorax in, 2769
Norepinephrine, pulmonary metabolism of, 131
    pulmonary vascular response to, 106
Norwegian hemp disease. See *Extrinsic allergic alveolitis; Farmer's lung.*
Nucleolar organizer regions, quantification of, in mesothelioma diagnosis, 2816
Nutrition, lung development and, 142
Nylon flock, pneumoconiosis due to, 2468

Oat cell carcinoma, pulmonary, 1091–1096, *1096.* See also *Small cell carcinoma, pulmonary.*
Obesity, genetic factors in, 2058
    hypoventilation in myxedema and, 3054
    obstructive sleep apnea and, 2056–2057, 2059–2060
Obesity hypoventilation syndrome, 2057, 2066, 3053. See also *Sleep apnea.*
Oblique fissures. See *Fissures, interlobar.*
Oblique projection, for conventional radiography, 301
Obliterative bronchiolitis. See under *Bronchiolitis.*
Obliterative bronchitis, 2292
Obstructive azoospermia, 2283–2284
Obstructive pneumonitis, atelectasis and, 514–517, *516, 517,* 554, *557*
    due to pulmonary carcinoma, 1121–1128, *1122–1127, 1129*
Obstructive sleep apnea. See *Sleep apnea, obstructive.*
Occluding junctions, in alveolar epithelium, 18, *18, 76,* 1949, *1949*
    in pulmonary capillary endothelium, 76, *76,* 1949, *1949*
Occupational airway disorders, 2123–2124. See also *Asthma, occupational.*
Occupational exposure. See also *Dust exposure; specific materials.*
    COPD and, 2122, 2174–2175
    in patient history, 390
      in asthma diagnosis, 2122
    nonspecific bronchoconstriction due to, 2123
    pulmonary carcinoma and, 1074–1078
Ochronosis, 677
Oil embolism, 1861–1863, *1865,* 1871, 2569
    pulmonary edema and, 2005
Oleothorax therapy, for tuberculosis, lipid pneumonia due to, 818
    pleural mass from, 2840
Oligemia, pulmonary, cardiovascular anomalies with, 665, *665*
    diffuse, 500–503, *501–503*
      differential diagnosis of, 3150, 3151t, *3152–3155*
    local, 503–504, *504–507*
      differential diagnosis of, 3156, 3157t, *3158–3160*
      with pulmonary thromboembolism, 501–502, *501, 502,* 504, *506,* 1787–1788, *1792, 1793*
    subpleural, in asthma, 2125, *2128*
Oligohydramnios, pulmonary hypoplasia and, 142, 598, *599*
Omental fat, herniation of, through diaphragmatic defect, 254, *255*
Omovertebral bones, 262, *263*
Onchocerciasis, 1047
Oncocytes, in tracheobronchial glands, 14, *15*
Oncocytoma, tracheobronchial, 1259
Oncogenes, in pulmonary carcinoma, 1082–1083
    prognosis and, 1200
Ondine's curse. See *Sleep apnea, central.*
1-2-3 sign, in sarcoidosis, 1545, *1546*
Opacity. See also *Consolidation.*
    density vs., 269n
    local increase in, in atelectasis, 528
    subpleural dependent, 287–290, *291,* 519–521, *521*
    on expiratory scans, 291, *291, 292*
Opisthorchis felineus, 1052
Opisthorchis sinensis, 1753
Opisthorchis viverrini, 1052, 1753
Opium, chronic airflow obstruction due to smoking of, 2175

Optical density, 302
Orbital pseudotumor, fibrosing mediastinitis with, 2857
Orchid-grower's lung, 2363t. See also *Extrinsic allergic alveolitis.*
Organic dust inhalation, 2361–2380. See also *Extrinsic allergic alveolitis; Organic dust toxic syndrome.*
    in animal confinement areas, 2379
    COPD and, 2175
Organic dust toxic syndrome, 876, 2124, 2336, 2379–2380
    occupational asthma vs., 2124
Organophosphates, occupational airway disorder due to, 2124
    poisoning by, 2584–2585, *2585*
    ventilatory failure due to, 3063, 3064
Ornithosis, 1017–1019, *1019,* 3097t
Oropharyngeal secretions, aspiration of. See under *Aspiration (event).*
Oropharynx, carcinoma of, metastatic to trachea, *2041*
    ulcer of, in histoplasmosis, 888
Oroticaciduria, type I, 726
Orthopnea, 388
    in COPD, 2215
Ortner's syndrome, with chronic thromboembolic pulmonary hypertension, 1825
Osler-Charcot disease. See *Pulmonary fibrosis, idiopathic.*
Osmotic pressure, in pulmonary fluid and solute exchange, 1954
Osmotic reflection coefficient, in pulmonary fluid and solute exchange, 1954–1955
Ossification. See also *Calcification.*
    dendriform pulmonary, 474, 2700, *2702, 2703*
    in amyloidosis, 2711
    in bronchial cartilage, 13, *13*
    in carcinoid tumors, 1233, *1234,* 1237, *1241*
    on radiographs and CT scans, 463, 467–474, *475*
Osteitis, tuberculous, of rib, 3017, *3017*
Osteochondritis, costochondral. See *Tietze's syndrome.*
Osteochondroma, 3031
Osteogenic sarcoma. See *Osteosarcoma.*
Osteomyelitis, of rib, 3016–3017, *3017*
    of spine, 3023, *3024, 3025*
    of sternum, after sternotomy, 2661, 3019–3020
    septic pulmonary embolism with, 1830
Osteoporosis, in cystic fibrosis, 2312
    lung transplantation and, 1700
Osteosarcoma, mediastinal, 2925
    metastatic, 1410, *1411*
      calcification in, 467, *473, 1391*
    of rib, chest wall pain due to, 387
    pulmonary, 1345–1346
Otitis media, tuberculous, 840
Outer bronchial diameter–to–pulmonary artery diameter ratio. See *Artery-bronchus ratios.*
Ovarian hyperstimulation syndrome, 2765, *2765*
Ovaries, cancer of, metastatic, in diaphragm, 3006
    in lung, 1408
    tumors of, pleural effusion with, 2765
Overflowing bathtub theory, 1958
Overinflation. See *Hyperinflation.*
Overlap syndrome(s), 1459, 1469–1470, *1471*
    polyangiitis, 1506, 1524
    pulmonary hypertension in, *1454*
Oxalic acid, *Aspergillus* production of, 921
Oxidant gases, inhaled, 2519–2524. See also specific gases.
Oximetry, in carbon monoxide poisoning diagnosis, 3069

Oximetry *(Continued)*
in obstructive sleep apnea diagnosis, 2068, 2069
Oxygen, alveolar-arterial gradient of, in ventilation/perfusion mismatch assessment, 112, 113
diffusion of, from acinus to red blood cell, 107–108, *108*
Oxygen dissociation curve of blood, *110*
ventilation/perfusion mismatch and, 110
Oxygen free radicals. See *Reactive oxygen species.*
Oxygen partial pressure, determination of, 114
in acinus, 53, *54*
in inhaled air, 53
Oxygen saturation, arterial, 114
Oxygen therapy, in COPD, effects of, 2228
for inspiratory muscle fatigue, 2220
for pulmonary hypertension, 2217
nocturnal, 2227
prognosis and, 2230
nocturnal, for central apnea, 3053
in COPD, 2227
Oxygen toxicity, 2521
surfactant disruption in, 58
Oxyphilic adenoma, tracheobronchial, 1259
Ozone, asthma and, 2114, 2115
collateral resistance and, 60
nonspecific airway responsiveness and, 2115
pulmonary injury due to, 2521–2522

p53 gene, 1083
p53 protein, in mesothelioma diagnosis, 2816
Pacemaker(s), complications of, 2690–2691, *2690*
superior vena cava syndrome due to, *2948*, 2949
Pachydermoperiostosis, 396, *397*
Pacing, diaphragmatic, obstructive sleep apnea during, 2062
upper airway obstruction and, 246
Paget's disease of bone, 3031, *3032*
Pain, chest, 385–387
chest wall, 386–387
pleural pain vs., 385–386, *387*
with Pancoast tumor, 1171–1172
with pleural effusion, 2740
Paint remover, carbon monoxide poisoning due to, 3068
Palatoglossus, in ventilation, 246
Palpation of chest, 392
Panbronchiolitis, diffuse, 2323t, 2349–2353, *2351, 2352*
Pancoast tumor, 1156–1165, *1162–1164*
apical cap vs., 2796, *2798*
extrapulmonary features of, 1171–1172
Pancreas, pseudocyst of, 2944–2945, *2946*
pulmonary carcinoma metastatic to, 1173
secretions of, in cystic fibrosis, 2300
tuberculosis involving, 840
Pancreatic extracts, occupational asthma due to, 2121
Pancreatic insufficiency, in cystic fibrosis, 2312, 2313
Pancreatic tissue, in mediastinal teratoma, 2903, 2907
Pancreaticopleural fistula, in chronic pancreatitis, 2765
Pancreatitis, adult respiratory distress syndrome in, 2003–2005, *2004*
pleural effusion in, 2743, 2764–2765
Panda pattern, on gallium scintigraphy in sarcoidosis, 1568
Panic disorder, chest pain in, 386

Panic disorder *(Continued)*
dyspnea and, 388
psychogenic hyperventilation and, 3066
Papain, experimental emphysema induced by, 2185
Papillary adenocarcinoma, metastatic to lung, calcification in, 467
pulmonary, 1101, *1102.* See also *Adenocarcinoma, pulmonary.*
calcification in, 467
Papillary adenoma, 1266–1267
Papillary mesothelioma, well-differentiated, 2838
Papilloma, tracheobronchial, 1262–1265, *1262–1266*
Papillomavirus(es), 1009–1010
pulmonary carcinoma and, 1079
tracheobronchial papillomas and, 1262, 1264, 1265
Papovaviruses, 1009–1010
Para-aminosalicylic acid, thoracic disease due to, 2538t, 2558
Para-aortic line, 215, *216, 217*
Para-aortic lymph nodes, in classification for lung cancer staging, *185*, 188t, *1186*, 1187t
Paracoccidioidomycosis, 902–904, *904*
Paradoxical chest wall motion, with spinal cord injury, 3055
Paraesophageal lymph nodes, in ATS classification, 184t, *186*
in classification for lung cancer staging, *185*, 188t, *1186*, 1187t
Paraesophageal varices, 2967–2968, *2968*
sclerotherapy for, complications of, 2761, 2968
Paraffinoma, 2501, *2504*
Paragangliomas, 1363–1364
aorticopulmonary, 2942–2943, *2943*
aorticosympathetic, 2977–2978
minute pulmonary, 74, 1364, 1374–1375, *1376*
pulmonary chondroma with, 1344
Paragonimiasis, 1047–1049, *1048–1051*
cavities or cysts in, 3103t
homogeneous nonsegmental opacity in, 3080t
multiple masses or nodules in, 3123t
pleural effusion in, 2753
Parainfluenza virus, 985–986
post-transplantation obliterative bronchiolitis and, 1717
Paraldehyde, thoracic disease due to, 2539t, 2567
Parallel inhomogeneity, 53
Paralytic shellfish poisoning, 3062
Paranasal sinuses, cystic fibrosis involving, 2312
Paraneoplastic syndromes, with pulmonary carcinoma, 1173–1178
with thymoma, 2887, 2894–2896
Paraquat poisoning, 2585–2587, *2586, 2587*
Parasitic disease, 1033–1061. See also specific parasites and groups.
asthma and, 2079
cavities or cysts in, 3103t
diagnosis of, 1033–1034
embolic manifestations of, 1853–1854
eosinophilic lung disease due to, 1744t, 1752–1753
homogeneous nonsegmental consolidation in, 3080t
in HIV infection, 1675–1676
pleural effusion in, 2752–2753
solitary mass due to, 3117t, *3119*
solitary nodule due to, 3111t
Paraspinal lines, 211, 212–215, *215–217*
Parasternal stripe, 204–205, *206*
Parasternal muscles, in inspiration, 246–247
Parasympathetic nervous system, in pulmonary innervation, 145, *146*

Parathion, 2584
Parathyroid hormone, selective arteriography with measurement of, in parathyroid adenoma assessment, 2914
Parathyroid tumors, 2913–2914, *2914*
Paratracheal lymph nodes, 179, *181*
enlarged, in pulmonary carcinoma, *3168*
in tuberculosis, *3166*
in ATS classification, 184t, *185, 186*
in classification for lung cancer staging, *185*, 188t, *1186*, 1187t
in Hodgkin's disease, 1299–1302, *1300, 1301*
in sarcoidosis, 1545, *1546*, 1547t, *1548, 1549, 1550, 1550, 1551*
Paratracheal stripe, left, 220
right, 219–220, *219–220*
widening of, in aortic rupture, *2627*, 2628–2629
Paravertebral lymph nodes, in Hodgkin's disease, 1302, *1302*
Paravertebral mass(es), 2974–2981
differential diagnosis of, 3184, 3185t, *3186–3190*
Paravertebral pleura, defined, 587n
Parenchymal bands, in asbestosis, 2440
Parietal lymph nodes, 175–176, *176–178*
Parkinsonism. See also *Parkinson's disease.*
with autonomic disturbance, hypoventilation in, 3054
Parkinson's disease. See also *Parkinsonism.*
respiratory insufficiency in, 3054
upper airway obstruction in, 2033
Paroxysmal laryngospasm, episodic, 2032–2033
Paroxysmal nocturnal dyspnea, 388
Paroxysmal polyserositis, familial, 2766
Particles, in intravenous fluid, embolization of, 1868
inhaled, alveolar macrophages and, 22, 130
clearance of, 127–130, *128*
deposition of, 126–127
Parvoviruses, 1010
Passive atelectasis, 517–522, *519–521, 523, 524.* See also *Atelectasis.*
defined, 513, 525
dependent opacity on CT due to, 287, *291*, 513, 519–521, *521*
Pasteurella multocida infection, 759
Pasteurella pestis. See *Yersinia pestis* infection.
Pasteurella tularensis. See *Francisella tularensis* infection.
Patent ductus arteriosus, 1896
Pathologic investigation methods, 339–358. See also specific techniques.
special techniques in, 351–358
Peak expiratory flow (PEF), measurement of, 409
signal-to-noise ratio for, 410
Peat moss–worker's lung, 2363t. See also *Extrinsic allergic alveolitis.*
Pectoral girdle, abnormalities of, 3011–3012, *3012, 3013*
Pectoral muscles, congenital absence of, 259, *259, 493*, 3011–3012, *3012*
in inspiration, 246
on CT, 259–260, *260*
on radiographs, 259
Pectoriloquy, wheezing, 394
Pectus carinatum, 3019
Pectus excavatum, 3018–3019, *3018*
Pectus index, 3018
Pel-Ebstein relapsing fever, in Hodgkin's disease, 1311
Pelvic rib, 263, 3015
Pendelluft, 53
diffusive, 413
Penicillamine, immunologic disorders associated with, 1424

Penicillamine *(Continued)*
  myasthenia-like syndrome due to, 3063
  obliterative bronchiolitis in rheumatoid disease
    and, 1445, 1446
  systemic lupus erythematosus and, 1424
  thoracic disease due to, 2539t, 2565–2566
Penicillin, anaphylaxis due to, 2106
  resistance to, in *Streptococcus pneumoniae,*
    736
  thoracic disease due to, 2538t, 2558–2559
Penicilliosis, 951–952
Pentasomiasis, 1059–1061
Peplomycin, thoracic disease due to, 2538t, 2544
Percentage fall index, in exercise-induced
  asthma, 2107
Percentage rise index, in exercise-induced
  asthma, 2107
Percussion, chest wall, in physiotherapy,
  atelectasis due to, 2623
  in chest examination, 392
Perflubron, partial liquid ventilation using, in
  adult respiratory distress syndrome, 1987,
  1990, 1991
Perfluorochemicals, thoracic disease due to, 2571
Perfumes, asthma provoked by, 2117
Perfusion. See also *Ventilation/perfusion* entries.
  alterations in, lung density alterations due to,
    270, *271,* 499–504, *501–507*
  alveolar, matching alveolar ventilation to,
    108–111, *109*
  intrauterine, pulmonary hypoplasia due to
    decrease in, 598
  of acinus, 104
  pulmonary artery, conditions associated with
    nonuniformity of, 1820t
  regional, exercise and, 111
    gravity and, 110, 111
Perfusion lung scanning, 326–327, *327, 329,*
  1800. See also *Ventilation/perfusion*
  scanning.
  in pulmonary arteriovenous malformation as-
    sessment, 660
  in pulmonary carcinoma diagnosis, 1180–1181
  in pulmonary thromboembolism diagnosis,
    1806
Periaortic lymph nodes, 179, *180*
Peribronchial lymph nodes, in ATS
  classification, 184t, *185, 187*
Peribronchial lymphatics, 172, *174*
Peribronchiolar fibrosis, in asbestosis,
  2429–2430, *2431*
Pericardiac lymph nodes, lateral, 176, *178*
  enlargement of, 2929
Pericardial calcification, after radiation therapy,
  2597, *2605*
Pericardial cysts, 2927–2928, *2927, 2928,* 3171t,
  3173
Pericardial fluid, in tuberculosis diagnosis, 844
Pericardioperitoneal canals, 247, *247*
Pericardiophrenic artery, in blood supply to
  diaphragm, 249
Pericardiophrenic lymph nodes, in Hodgkin's
  disease, 1302, *1303, 1304*
Pericarditis, acute, chest pain due to, 386
  due to radiation therapy, 2597
  in histoplasmosis, 888
  in *Mycoplasma pneumoniae* infection, 1014
  in rheumatoid disease, 1433
  tuberculous, 839–840
Pericardium, parietal, congenital deficiency of
  left side of, 667–671, *669–670*
  progressive systemic sclerosis involving, 1458
  pulmonary carcinoma involving, 1171
Perichondritis, chest wall pain due to, 387
Pericytes, in pulmonary arteriolar wall, 74
Periesophageal lymph nodes, 179, *180*

Peripheral nervous system, Churg-Strauss
  syndrome involving, 1509–1510
  hypoventilation due to disorders of, 3061–
    3063
  sarcoidosis involving, 1566
  tumors arising from, in paravertebral region,
    2974–2976, *2975, 2976*
  Wegener's granulomatosis involving, 1504
Peripheral neuropathy, paraneoplastic, in
  pulmonary carcinoma, 1174
Peripheral primitive neuroectodermal tumor, in
  paravertebral region, 2974
  of chest wall, 3028–3029
Peritoneal dialysis, pleural effusion with, 2764
Peritonitis, tuberculous, 840
Perityphlitis, ligneous, fibrosing mediastinitis
  with, 2857
Persistent pulmonary hypertension of the
  newborn, 1882
Persistent truncus arteriosus, 637, 3151t
Personality change, in obstructive sleep apnea,
  2067
Pertechnegas, for ventilation imaging, 330
Pertussis, 765–766
  cough due to, in adults, 381–382
  pneumonia due to, bronchiectasis and, 2267
Pesticide poisoning, 2584–2587, *2585–2587*
PET. See *Positron emission tomography (PET).*
Petit's eventration, 2995
Petriellidium boydii infection, 951
Petroleum products, ingestion of, pulmonary
  disease due to, 2588–2589
Phagocytic deficiency syndromes, 726–728
Phagocytosis, by alveolar macrophages, in
  clearance of alveolar air space, 22, 130
Phantom tumor, due to interlobar effusion,
  579–581, *580*
  in hydrothorax due to heart failure, 2761,
  2762
Pharyngitis, acute, upper airway obstruction due
  to, 2021
  septic pulmonary embolism with, 1829, 1831
Pharynx, dermatomyositis/polymyositis
  involving, 1465
  diverticulum of, middle-posterior mediastinal
    mass due to, 3177t
Phenytoin, thoracic disease due to, 2539t, 2564
Pheochromocytoma, pulmonary edema with,
  2005
Phleboliths, in mediastinal hemangioma, 2917,
  2920
Phlebothrombosis, with central venous
  catheterization, 2682–2683
Phlogopite, pneumoconiosis due to, 2450
Phonomyogram, in diaphragmatic strength
  assessment, 420
Phonopneumography, 393
Phosgene inhalation, 2526
Phosphate, occupational exposure to, pulmonary
  carcinoma and, 1078
Phosphate wasting, renal, in pulmonary
  carcinoma, 1178
Phosphatidylethanolamine, in surfactant, 56
Phosphatidylglycerol, in surfactant, 56
Phospholipase A$_2$, in adult respiratory distress
  syndrome, 1983
Phospholipid(s), in tracheobronchial secretions,
  61
Phospholipidosis, pulmonary alveolar. See
  Alveolar proteinosis.
Photodynamic therapy, complications of, 2675
Phrenic artery, in blood supply to diaphragm,
  249
  inferior, on CT, 254, *256*
Phrenic nerve, 250–251
  electrical pacing of, obstructive sleep apnea
    due to, 2062

Phrenic nerve *(Continued)*
  upper airway obstruction and, 246
  pulmonary carcinoma invading, 1166, 1171
  stimulation frequency of, diaphragmatic force
    and, 257
  stimulation of, in diaphragmatic paralysis diag-
    nosis, 2993
  in diaphragmatic strength assessment, 420
Phrenic vein, inferior, 254, *256*
Phycomycosis, 947–949, *948,* 2752
Physical examination, 391–398
  for extrathoracic manifestations of pulmonary
    disease, 396–398
  of chest, 391–395
  of heart and systemic vasculature, 395–396
Physiotherapy, chest wall percussion in,
  atelectasis due to, 2623
Pick-and-smear method for sputum processing,
  340
Pickwickian syndrome, 2057, 2066, 3053. See
  also *Sleep apnea.*
Picornaviruses, 990–991
Pig bronchus, 35, 626, *627*
Pig fever. See *Organic dust toxic syndrome.*
Pigeon breast, 3019
Pigeon-breeder's lung, 2362t, 2377. See also
  Extrinsic allergic alveolitis.
  diffuse nodular pattern in, *3148*
  radiologic features of, *2370, 2372, 2374*
Pink puffers, 2215. See also *Chronic obstructive
  pulmonary disease (COPD).*
  ventilation/perfusion mismatch in, 2225
PIOPED criteria, for interpretation of ventilation/
  perfusion scans, 1804, 1805t
Piperacillin, thoracic disease due to, 2558
Piroxicam, thoracic disease due to, 2539t, 2565
Pituitary snuff-taker's lung, 2363t, 2378. See
  also *Extrinsic allergic alveolitis.*
Pityrosporum orbiculare, 952
Pityrosporum ovale, 952
Pixel, defined, 309
Placentoid bullous lesion, 2235–2236
Plague, 756–758
  great white, 799
Plant lectins, inhaled, Wegener's granulomatosis
  and, 1492
Plasma cell(s), in airways, *15, 16*
  in amyloidosis, 2709–2711
Plasma cell granuloma, 1371–1373, *1372*
Plasma cell neoplasms, 1293–1298. See also
  specific disorders.
Plasma cell pneumonitis, interstitial, 909, 911,
  913. See also Pneumocystis carinii
  pneumonia.
Plasmacytic hyperplasia, after transplantation,
  1711
Plasmacytoma, 1297, *1298*
  of chest wall, 3032
  pleural effusion due to, 2760
Plasminogen activator inhibitor, type I, in
  venous thrombosis development, 1778
Plastic bronchitis, *2291, 2292*
  in allergic bronchopulmonary aspergillosis,
    928
Platelet(s), production of, in lungs, 132
Platelet aggregation, pulmonary, after liver
  transplantation, 1734, *1734*
Platelet-activating factor, in asthmatic airway
  inflammation, 2092
Platinum, occupational asthma due to, 2122
Platypnea, 388
  in COPD, 2215
Pleomorphic adenoma, mediastinal, 2929
  tracheobronchial gland, 1258–1259
Pleomorphic carcinoma, pulmonary, 1114–1117,
  1116. See also *Carcinoma, pulmonary.*

Pleomorphic carcinoma *(Continued)*
prognosis in, 1196
Plethysmography, body, for airway resistance
measurement, 412
for lung volume measurement, 407–408
in COPD, 2225
impedance, in deep vein thrombosis, 1824
respiratory inductive, 408
Pleura, 151–169
abnormalities of, radiologic signs of, 563–592
adventitious sounds originating in, 395
anatomy of, 151–154, *152–155*
calcification of, 583, *584, 585*
closed biopsy of, 372–373
disease of, 2737–2840. See also specific diseases.
parenchymal disease vs., contrast-enhanced CT for distinction of, 577, *578*
imaging of, 154–166
invagination of, linear atelectasis and, 559
lymphatics of, 172, *173*
in clearance of pulmonary edema fluid, 1958
mediastinal, defined, 587n
neoplasms of, 2807–2840. See also specific neoplasms.
histologic classification of, 1071t
of uncertain nature, 2840
radiologic features of, 583–587, *586, 587*
pain originating from, 385–386
chest wall pain vs., 385–386, *387*
paravertebral, defined, 587n
parietal, 151, *153*
capillary pressure in, 168
imaging of, 154, *156*
visceral pleura's relationship to, in atelectasis, 534–539, *538*
physiology of, 168–169, *169*
pulmonary carcinoma involving, 1165, *1165*
clinical features of, 1170
mesothelioma vs., 1165, *1165*, 2818–2820, *2819*, 2826
surgical complications involving, 2661–2663, *2661, 2663*
thickening of, benign vs. malignant, 587, *588*, 2435, 2437, *2443*, 2824, *2825*
diffuse, asbestos-related, 2435, *2437, 2443*
pleural plaque vs., 582
in mesothelioma, 2820, *2822, 2823, 2823–2825*
in progressive systemic sclerosis, 1457
radiologic signs of, 582–587, *582–588*
with effusion, 574–576, *577*
trauma to, nonpenetrating, 2623–2625
pleural fluid eosinophilia with, 344
visceral, 151, *152*
capillary pressure in, 168–169
imaging of, 154, *156*
line shadows connecting peripheral mass to, 483, *487*
parietal pleura's relationship to, in atelectasis, 534–539, *538*
Pleural cavity, metastasis via, 1383
pressures within, 168
gravity and, 110–111
pleural fluid formation and absorption and, 168–169, *169*
Pleural effusion, 2739–2769. See also *Empyema.*
after bone marrow transplantation, 1731–1732
after lung transplantation, 1720
after pneumonectomy, 2661, *2664*, 2665
asbestos-related, benign, 2754–2756
clinical features of, 2443
pathologic features of, 2424–2425
radiologic features of, 2435, *2438–2440*
ascites vs., on CT, 572–574, *573–576*

Pleural effusion *(Continued)*
asymptomatic, causes of, 2740
atelectasis vs., 533, 554, 568, 581
atelectasis with, 519, *520*
atypical distribution of, 577–579
biochemical findings in, 2741–2743
causes of, 2741t
miscellaneous, 2766–2768
chyliform, 2745t, 2768
in rheumatoid disease, 2754
chylous. See *Chylothorax.*
clinical features of, 2740–2741
CT findings with, 572–577, *573–578*
diagnosis of, thoracoscopic biopsy in, 371
ultrasonography in, 333–334, *333, 334*, 563, *564*, 568, 579
differential diagnosis of, 2739–2740
drug-related, 2756, 2756t
due to abdominal disease, 2763–2766
due to malignancy, 2744t, 2756–2760, *2758*
cytogenetic analysis in diagnosis of, 356
metastatic, 1399
rheumatoid effusion vs., 2754
due to trauma, 2745t, 2761–2763, *2763*
exudative, 2739
transudate vs., 574–575, 2742
general features of, 2739–2743
hemorrhagic. See *Hemothorax.*
in healthy adult, 563
in infection, 2743–2753
in rheumatoid disease, 1443–1444, *1444, 1445*, 2744t, 2753–2754
in sarcoidosis, 1562
in *Streptococcus pneumoniae* pneumonia, 740–741
in systemic lupus erythematosus, 1425, 1426, *1426, 1428*, 2745t, 2753
in tuberculosis, asbestos-related effusion vs., 2435
in HIV infection, 1652
in yellow nail syndrome, 2284–2285, *2285*, 2766
loculated, 579–581, *579–581*
adjacent to empyema, 2750
atelectasis vs., 581
massive, total collapse vs., 532, *532*
normal chest radiograph with, 3048
parapneumonic, 2744t, 2747–2751
classification of, 2750
defined, 2747n
incidence of, 2747
indications for surgical drainage of, 2750–2751
lateral decubitus radiographs for detection of, 2747, *2748*
prognosis in, 2749–2751
pseudochylous, 2743, 2768. See also *Pleural effusion, chyliform.*
pulmonary function tests in, 2741
radiologic signs of, 563–581
on lateral radiograph, 564, *565*, 2747, *2748*
on posteroanterior radiograph, 563, 564, *564, 565*
on supine radiograph, 572, *572*, 577
small, radiographic detection of, 300, 301, *301*, 3048
subpulmonary, 566–568, *568–571*
lobar atelectasis vs., 554, 568
terminology of, 2739n
thoracentesis for. See *Thoracentesis.*
transudative, 2739, 2744t
exudate vs., 574–575, 2742
typical configuration of, 564–566, *565–567*
with heart failure, 2760–2761, *2762*
with mesothelioma, *2823, 2824*, 2825–2826, *2825*

Pleural effusion *(Continued)*
with pneumothorax, 2791
with pulmonary carcinoma, 1165, 1170, 1194
with pulmonary thromboembolism, 1799, 1826–1827, 2745t, 2760
Pleural fibrosis, 2795–2805
asbestos-related, diffuse, 2424, *2429*, 2804, *2804*, 2805
focal visceral, 2424, *2427*
diffuse, *2803*, 2804–2805, *2804, 2805*. See also *Fibrothorax.*
asbestos-related, 2424, *2429*, 2804, *2804*, 2805
due to collapse therapy for tuberculosis, 818, *824*
in sarcoidosis, 1542, *1545*, 1562
local, 2795–2804
lung transplantation and, 1700
radiologic signs of, 582, *582*
round atelectasis and, 522, *523, 524*
systemic-pulmonary vascular fistula and, 666
Pleural fluid, analysis of, in pleural effusion diagnosis, 2741–2743
composition of, 168, 169
CT in determining, 574–577, *576, 577*
cytologic examination of, 343–345
in pulmonary carcinoma diagnosis, 1179
in pulmonary metastasis diagnosis, 1412
formation and absorption of, 168–169, *169*
free. See *Pleural effusion.*
in tuberculosis diagnosis, 844
loculated, 579–581, *579–581*
lymphatic absorption of, 169, 172
quantification of, ultrasonography for, 563
terminology of, 2739n
Pleural friction rub, 395
Pleural line, black, in alveolar microlithiasis, 2721
in pneumothorax, 587, *588*
Pleural pain, 2740
Pleural plaques, 2796–2804
calcified, 583, *585*, 2435, *2436*, 2801, *2803*
cause of, 2796
clinical features of, 2801–2804
diffuse pleural thickening vs., 582
normal chest radiograph with, 3048
pathologic features of, 2424, *2425, 2426*, 2796, *2799*
pulmonary carcinoma and, 1076
radiologic features of, 2431–2435, *2433–2436, 2438–2440*, 2796–2801, *2800–2803*
talc-associated, 2449
Pleural reflections, posterior, 212–215, *215–217*
Pleural space. See *Pleural cavity.*
Pleural tag, 483, *487*
with solitary nodule, 1139, *1140–1141*
Pleuritis, acute, normal chest radiograph with, 3048
cryptogenic bilateral fibrosing, 2804
due to radiation therapy, 2597, *2603*
eosinophilic, with pneumothorax, 2790, *2790*
healed, 2795
in rheumatoid disease, 1443–1444
Pleurodesis, for pneumothorax, long-term effects of, 2791
Pleurodynia, epidemic, 990
Pleuropericardial cysts, 2927–2928, *2927, 2928*, 3171t
Pleuropericardial fat, enlargement of, *2916, 2918*, 2925–2927
radiographic interpretation of, 233
Pleuroperitoneal membranes, 247, *247*, 248
Pleuropulmonary blastoma, 2840
Plexogenic pulmonary arteriopathy, in pulmonary hypertension, 1882–1886, *1883–1889*

Plicatic acid, occupational asthma due to, 2121
Ploidy determination, flow cytometry for, 357–358, *357*
Plombage, complications of, 2675
Pneumatocele, 508–510, *509, 510,* 707, *711*
　bulla vs., 2234
　in HIV infection, due to aspiration, *1662, 1664*
　　due to *Pneumocystis carinii* pneumonia, 1660, *1663*
　in *Staphylococcus aureus* pneumonia, 744, 746
　in *Streptococcus pneumoniae* pneumonia, 739, *740*
　traumatic, 2613–2618, *2615, 2618, 2620*
Pneumococcal pneumonia. See Streptococcus pneumoniae *pneumonia.*
Pneumoconiosis, 2386–2468
　Caplan's syndrome and, 1438–1441
　defined, 2386–2387
　due to aluminum, 2460–2463, *2461, 2462*
　due to asbestos, 2419–2448. See also *Asbestos; Asbestosis.*
　due to beryllium, 2456–2460, *2458, 2459*
　due to cement dust, 2468
　due to coal and carbon, 2409–2419. See also *Coal workers' pneumoconiosis.*
　due to cobalt, 2463
　due to inert radiopaque dusts, 2452–2456
　due to nylon flock, 2468
　due to polyvinyl chloride, 2465
　due to silica, 2390–2409. See also *Silicosis.*
　due to silicates, 2449–2452, *2450, 2451.* See also *Asbestosis.*
　due to silicon carbide, 2463–2465, *2465, 2466*
　due to synthetic mineral fibers, 2467–2468
　due to talc, 2449–2450, *2450, 2451*
　　cicatrization atelectasis due to, *528*
　　emphysema in, 2243
　due to titanium dioxide, 2465–2466, *2467*
　due to tungsten carbide, 2463
　due to volcanic dust, 2466
　due to zirconium, 2468
　establishing cause of, 2387
　idiopathic pulmonary fibrosis vs., 1611
　in dental technicians, 2468
　international classification of radiographs of, 441, 2387–2390
　mixed dust, 2387, *2388,* 2453–2454, *2453– 2455*
　para-occupational, 2387
　pulmonary fibrosis in. See *Progressive massive fibrosis.*
　scanning electron microscopy in, 355
　welder's, 2453–2454, *2453–2455*
Pneumocystis carinii, 909, *909.* See also Pneumocystis carinii *pneumonia.*
　extrapulmonary infection with, 1667
Pneumocystis carinii pneumonia, 909–916
　after bone marrow transplantation, 1730
　after heart-lung or lung transplantation, 1717– 1720, *1720, 1721*
　clinical features of, 913–915
　cyst formation in, 3103t, *3107*
　cytomegalovirus infection and, 1006, 1670
　diagnosis of, 915–916
　　bronchoalveolar lavage in, 343
　　cyst identification in, 912–913
　diffuse air-space pattern in, 3130t, *3131*
　diffuse reticular pattern in, 3134t
　epidemiology of, 909–910
　gallium scintigraphy in, 331, 332, *332*
　homogeneous nonsegmental opacity in, 3080t
　in HIV infection, 722, 1656–1670
　　clinical features of, 1667
　　cyst formation in, *3107*

Pneumocystis carinii pneumonia *(Continued)*
　diagnosis of, 1668–1669
　diffuse air-space pattern in, *3131*
　empiric therapy for, 1668–1669
　epidemiology of, 1656–1657
　ground-glass pattern in, 1660, 1663, *1663, 1666*
　Kaposi's sarcoma concurrent with, *1681*
　laboratory findings in, 1667
　pathogenesis of, 1657
　pathologic features of, 1657–1660, *1657– 1661*
　pneumatocele in, 1660, *1663, 1664*
　prognosis in, 1669–1670
　pulmonary function tests in, 1667–1668
　radiologic features of, *914,* 1660–1667, *1663–1666*
　infantile, 909, 911, 913
　laboratory findings in, 915–916
　pathogenesis of, 910–911, *911*
　pathologic features of, 911–913, *911, 912*
　pneumatocele in, 510, *510*
　prognosis in, 916
　prophylactic therapy for, 916
　radiologic features of, 454, *455,* 713, *715, 913, 914, 915*
Pneumocyte, granular. See *Alveolar epithelial cells, type II.*
　membranous. See *Alveolar epithelial cells, type I.*
Pneumocytoma, sclerosing, 1364–1365, *1366, 1367*
Pneumomediastinum, 2863–2870
　clinical features of, 2868–2870
　in asthma, 2140
　pathogenesis of, 2863–2865
　pathologic features of, 2865
　postoperative, 2663–2664
　radiologic features of, 2865–2868, *2866–2869*
　traumatic, 2625
　with tracheobronchial fracture, 2618, *2621,* 2865
Pneumonectomy, bronchopleural fistula after, 2289–2290, 2663
　complications of, 2665–2669, *2666–2668*
　empyema after, 2762
　examination of specimen from, 348–351, *349, 350,* 352–353
　lung growth after, 139
　MR imaging after, 2661
　normal radiographic changes after, *2664,* 2665
　pleural fluid accumulation after, 2661, *2664,* 2665
　pulmonary edema after, 2001, 2671
　pulmonary function after, prediction of, 331, 1181
　pulmonary hypertension in remaining lung after, 1917
　pulmonary wedge pressure measurement after, 1995
Pneumonia. See also *Infection;* specific infections.
　acute, interlobar fissure displacement in, 459
　　pulmonary infarction vs., 1796–1797
　anaerobic, 778–783. See also under *Anaerobic bacteria.*
　anatomic bias of, 476
　aspiration. See *Aspiration (event); Aspiration pneumonia.*
　bacterial, in HIV disease, 1643–1644
　　spontaneous pneumothorax with, *2786*
　　viral infection and, 713, 980
　bronchioloalveolar carcinoma vs., 1153–1156, *1154–1156*
　childhood, bronchiectasis and, 2267, 2278
　chronic destructive, 779

Pneumonia *(Continued)*
　community-acquired, 721–723
　　atypical, organisms causing, 722
　　enteric gram-negative infection in, 751
　　epidemiologic features of, 697–698
　　microbiologic diagnosis in, clinical significance of, 718
　　risk factors for complications or mortality in, 722–723
　consolidation in, *435,* 436, 437, 457
　　spread of, across incomplete fissure, *462*
　crackles in, 394
　cryptogenic organizing. See *Bronchiolitis obliterans organizing pneumonia (BOOP).*
　diagnosis of, clinical considerations in, 700– 701
　　general considerations in, 716–721
　　in specific patient groups, 721–728
　　techniques for, 719–721
　empiric therapy for, problems with, 718
　eosinophilic, acute, 1746, *1746, 1747*
　　chronic, 1747–1748, *1748–1750,* 3081t, *3084*
　epidemiologic features of, 697–698
　giant cell, in measles, 988, *988, 989,* 990
　herpes simplex, 998, *998, 999, 999*
　　after bone marrow transplantation, 1730
　hospital-acquired, 698, 723–724
　in bronchopulmonary sequestration, 604, *608,* 609
　in compromised host, 724–728
　　patterns of, 700
　in influenza, 982–983, *983, 984*
　inappropriate antibiotic treatment for, clinical significance of, 718
　interstitial. See *Interstitial pneumonia; Interstitial pneumonitis; Pulmonary fibrosis, idiopathic.*
　lipid. See *Aspiration (event), of lipids.*
　lobar (nonsegmental), 701–702, *703–705*
　　as term, usage of, 699n
　　causes of, 436
　　in tuberculosis, 822, *826*
　lobular. See also *Bronchopneumonia.*
　　as term, usage of, 699n
　　on high-resolution CT, 437
　necrotizing, bronchiectasis and, 2267
　　Klebsiella, 705
　pathogenesis of, 698–716
　pleural effusion with. See *Empyema; Pleural effusion, parapneumonic.*
　pneumatocele in, 508–510, *509, 510*
　pneumococcal. See Streptococcus pneumoniae *pneumonia.*
　primary atypical, 980n
　pulmonary carcinoma and, 1081
　pulmonary thromboembolism vs., 1825
　radiologic assessment of, limitations of, 699– 700
　recurrent, defined, 723
　round, in *Legionella* infection, 773, *775*
　　in *Streptococcus pneumoniae* infection, 737, *739*
　severe, defined, 722
　unilateral pulmonary edema vs., 1969
　ventilator-associated, diagnostic problems in, 716–717
　　diagnostic techniques for, 719–721
　　epidemiologic features of, 698
　　microbiologic diagnosis in, clinical significance of, 718
　　mortality due to, underlying illness and, 718–719
Pneumonia alba, 777
Pneumonia syndrome, idiopathic, after bone marrow transplantation, 1727–1728

Pneumonitis, acute, in systemic lupus
  erythematosus, 1426, *1426, 1427,* 1429
  hypersensitivity. See *Extrinsic allergic alveo-
    litis.*
  interstitial. See *Interstitial pneumonia; Intersti-
    tial pneumonitis; Pulmonary fibrosis, idio-
    pathic.*
  interstitial plasma cell, 909, 911, 913. See also
    Pneumocystis carinii *pneumonia.*
  obstructive, atelectasis and, 514–517, *516,
    517,* 554, *557*
    due to pulmonary carcinoma, 1121–1128,
      1122–1127, 1129
  ossifying, 474, 2700, *2702, 2703*
  radiation. See *Radiation pneumonitis.*
  rheumatic, 1470
Pneumopericardium, pneumomediastinum vs.,
  2865–2868
Pneumoperitoneum, catamenial pneumothorax
  and, 2787
  pneumomediastinum and, 2865
Pneumorrhachis, with pneumomediastinum,
  2868, *2868*
Pneumotaxic center, *236,* 238, 3050, *3050,* 3051
Pneumothorax, 2781–2791
  after lung transplantation, 1720–1721, *1722*
  after thoracentesis, 2743
  atelectasis with, 517–519, *519*
  bulla simulating, 2240, *2243*
  catamenial, 2767–2768, 2787–2789
  clinical features of, 2791
  epidemiology of, 2781
  ex vacuo, 2787
  expiratory radiography for detection of, 303–
    305, *304*
  in coccidioidomycosis, 894, *897*
  in lymphangioleiomyomatosis, 685, *685*
  in Pneumocystis carinii pneumonia, 915,
    1660, *1665*
  in pulmonary carcinoma, 1165
  in rheumatoid disease, 1444
  pathogenesis of, 2781–2790
  pathologic features of, 2790, *2790*
  pleural pain in, 386
  pneumomediastinum vs., 2865
  postsurgical, 2662–2663, *2663*
  prognosis in, 2791
  pulmonary function tests with, 2791
  radiologic signs of, 587–592, *588–592*
    pulmonary ligament and, 166, *168*
  sounds associated with, 394, 395
  spontaneous, bilateral, 2787, *2788*
    in bullous disease, 2237–2240
    in Marfan's syndrome, 676
    primary, pathogenesis of, 2781–2784, *2782,
      2783*
      pathologic features of, 2790, *2790*
    secondary, pathogenesis of, 2784–2787,
      2784–2787, 2784t
      pathologic features of, 2790
  tension, 589–592, *592,* 2791
  traumatic, pathogenesis of, 2789–2790, 2789t
    with penetrating wound, 2648, *2648, 2651*
    with pleural trauma, 2625
    with tracheobronchial fracture, 2618, *2621*
  typical configuration of, 564
  Valsalva maneuver and, 2789
  with pneumomediastinum, 2863
  with pulmonary carcinoma, 1170
  with pulmonary metastasis, 1389–1390
  with transthoracic needle aspiration, 346
  with transthoracic needle biopsy, 370
Poisons. See *Toxins;* specific toxins.
Poland's syndrome, 3011–3012
Polio vaccine, simian virus 40 in, mesothelioma
  and, 990, 2810

Poliomyelitis, 990, 3061
  chronic paralytic, rib notching in, 3015
  kyphoscoliosis after, *3021*
Pollens, asthma and, 2105–2106
Pollution, air, asthma provoked by, 2114–2115
  COPD and, 2173–2175
  cough and, 380
Polyangiitis, microscopic, 1490t, 1511, 1513,
  1514
Polyangiitis overlap syndrome, 1506, 1524
Polyarteritis nodosa, classic, 1490t, 1511–1513,
  1512
  microscopic, 1490t, 1511, 1513, *1514*
Polyarthritis, migratory, in Churg-Strauss
  syndrome, 1511
Polychondritis, relapsing, 1470–1473, *1472,
  1473*
  upper airway obstruction due to, 2040–
    2042, *2044*
Polycyclic aromatic hydrocarbons, pulmonary
  carcinoma and, 1077–1078
Polycythemia, in COPD, 2216
  in obstructive sleep apnea, 2067
Polyester powder lung, 2363t. See also *Extrinsic
  allergic alveolitis.*
Polyhydramnios, cystic adenomatoid
  malformation and, 618
Polymer fume fever, 2528
Polymerase chain reaction, 358
  for tuberculosis diagnosis, 845–846
Polymorphonuclear leukocytes. See
  Neutrophil(s).
Polymyositis, 1462–1465, *1464*
  hypoventilation in, 3065
  idiopathic pulmonary fibrosis vs., 1611
  paraneoplastic, in pulmonary carcinoma, 1174
  systemic lupus erythematosus with, *1464*
Polymyxins, myasthenia-like syndromes due to,
  3063
Polyneuritis, acute, 3061–3062
  influenza and, 984
Polyps, tracheobronchial, inflammatory, 1371
Polyserositis, familial paroxysmal (recurrent
  hereditary), 2766
Polysomnography, in obstructive sleep apnea
  diagnosis, 2068, 2069
Polysplenia syndrome, pulmonary arteriovenous
  malformations in, 657
Polytetrafluoroethylene (Teflon), embolization of,
  1870
  poisoning by, 2528
Polyurethane foam injection–worker's lung,
  2363t. See also *Extrinsic allergic alveolitis.*
Polyvinyl alcohol, bronchial artery embolization
  with, *1870,* 1871, *1871*
Polyvinyl chloride, inhalation of smoke from,
  2529
  pneumoconiosis due to, 2465
Pompe's disease (acid maltase deficiency), 2727,
  3064
Pons, in respiratory control, *236,* 238,
  3050–3051, *3050*
Pontiac fever, 770
Popcorn calcification, in pulmonary hamartoma,
  467, *472,* 1354, *1354*
Pores, of alveolar epithelium, in fluid and solute
  exchange, 1951
  of pulmonary capillary endothelium, in fluid
    and solute exchange, 1949–1950
Pores of Kuhn, 31–32, *32*
Porphyria, 3062
Positive end-expiratory pressure (PEEP), for
  pulmonary edema, mechanism of action of,
  1951
  in adult respiratory distress syndrome, 1987,
    1988–1990, 1993

Positive end-expiratory pressure (PEEP)
    (Continued)
  intrinsic, 407, 495
    in COPD, 2224
  left atrial pressure measurement during, 1995,
    2690
Positron emission tomography (PET), 332–333
  in lymphoma staging, 1293
  in pulmonary carcinoma, for diagnosis, 1181
    for staging, 1191, 1192–1193
  lymph node assessment on, 190
    in pulmonary carcinoma staging, 1191
  round atelectasis vs. pulmonary carcinoma on,
    2443
  solitary nodule assessment on, 1146
Postanginal sepsis, 779, 1829, 1831
Posterior diaphragmatic lymph nodes, 176, *178*
  enlargement of, 2929
Posterior junction line, 223, *224–225*
Posterior mediastinal lymph nodes, 179, *180*
Posterior mediastinal triangle, 223, *225*
Posterior parietal lymph nodes, 176, *177*
Posterior pleural reflections, 212–215, *215–217*
Posterior tracheal stripe, 220–223, *221–222*
Posteroinferior junction line, 229
Postinspiratory inspiratory activity, 239
Postnasal drip, cough due to, 381
Postpericardiectomy syndrome, pleural effusion
  in, 2766
Postpneumonectomy syndrome, 2665–2669
Potassium, depletion of, in COPD, 2217
  transport of, in airway epithelium, 62
Potassium hydroxide drain cleaners, aspiration
  of, 2512
Potroom asthma, 2122
Potter's syndrome, 598
Pott's disease, 837, *838,* 3023, *3025*
Pouch defects, on angiography, in chronic
  thromboembolic disease, 1911
Poxviruses, 1009
Prawn-worker's lung, 2363t. See also *Extrinsic
  allergic alveolitis.*
Prealbumin, in amyloidosis, 2709
Preaortic line, 216
Preaortic recess, 216–218
Precordial catch, 387
Pregnancy, aspiration risk during, 2491–2492
  azygos vein size in, 227
  cellular pulmonary emboli in, without clinical
    significance, 132
  chickenpox pneumonia during, 1000
  dyspnea during, 388
  influenza during, 985
  tuberculosis risk and, 802
Prekallikrein, in adult respiratory distress
  syndrome, 1983
Prepericardiac lymph nodes, 176, *178*
  enlargement of, 2929
Pressure-volume curves, 410–411, *411*
  average size of air spaces and, 2198–2199
  in COPD, 2225
Preterminal bronchioles, 26
Pretracheal fascia, 198
Prevascular lymph nodes, 176–179, *179*
  in classification for lung cancer staging, *185,*
    188t, *1186,* 1187t
Prevertebral fascia, 198
Prevertebral space, 198
Primitive neuroectodermal tumor, peripheral, in
    paravertebral region, 2974
  of chest wall, 3028–3029
Procainamide, myasthenia-like syndrome due to,
  3063
  thoracic disease due to, 2538t, 2564
Procarbazine, thoracic disease due to, 2538t,
  2551

Progesterone, obstructive sleep apnea and, 2059
Progressive massive fibrosis, in coal workers'
  pneumoconiosis, clinical features of,
  2418
    multiple masses or nodules due to, 3124t
    pathogenesis of, 2410
    pathologic features of, 2411, 2413, 2414
    prognosis in, 2419
    pulmonary function tests in, 2419
    radiologic features of, 2414–2416, 2416,
      2418
    solitary mass due to, 3118t
  in silicosis, 2391, 2392
    multiple masses or nodules due to, 3124t,
      3129
    pathologic features of, 2392–2394, 2393,
      2394, 2396
    radiologic features of, 2394, 2399–2402,
      2405
    sarcoidosis vs., 1558
    solitary mass due to, 3118t
Progressive multifocal leukoencephalopathy,
  sarcoidosis and, 1566
Progressive systemic sclerosis (PSS), 1452–1460
  antinuclear antibodies in, 1422, 1453
  clinical features of, 1457–1459
  diffuse reticular pattern in, 3134t
  follicular bronchiolitis in, 1274
  pathogenesis of, 1452–1454
  pathologic features of, 1454–1455, 1454
  prognosis in, 1460
  pulmonary carcinoma in, 1460, 1461
  pulmonary fibrosis in, pulmonary carcinoma
    associated with, 1460, 1461
  pulmonary function tests in, 1459
  radiologic features of, 1455–1457, 1455, 1456,
    1458
    time of appearance of, 3046
  silicosis and, 2408–2409
  variants of, 1459. See also CREST syndrome.
Prolactin, pulmonary carcinoma secreting, 1177
Proliferating cell nuclear antigen, quantification
    of, in mesothelioma, for diagnosis,
    2818
    for staging, 2826–2828
Proliferative index, 357–358
Prominent lung markings, in chronic bronchitis,
    2203
Propionibacterium acnes, sarcoidosis and, 1535
Propoxur, 2587
Propoxyphene, thoracic disease due to, 2539t,
    2567
Propranolol, thoracic disease due to, 2571
Propylthiouracil, thoracic disease due to, 2572
Prostaglandins, alterations in, pulmonary veno-
    occlusive disease and, 1930–1931
  in adult respiratory distress syndrome patho-
    genesis, 1983
  in asthmatic airway inflammation, 2091–2092
  in pulmonary hypertension pathogenesis, 1881
  pulmonary metabolism of, 131
  pulmonary vascular response to, 106
Prostatic carcinoma, metastatic to lung, 1408
α_1-Protease inhibitor, alveolar macrophage
    secretion of, 23
  circumstances affecting level of, 2231
  deficiency of, 2231–2234
    COPD and, 2177–2178
    emphysema and, 2231–2232
    hepatic disease in, 2232
    intermediate, COPD in, 2234
    severe, clinical and functional features of,
      2233–2234, 2233
  genetic variants affecting, 2231–2233
  in cystic fibrosis, 2302–2303
  in emphysema, 2182, 2183

α_1-Protease inhibitor (Continued)
  in tracheobronchial secretions, 61
  inhibition of, by cigarette smoke, 2184
  quantitative analysis of, 2231
Protein, in edema fluid, in adult respiratory
    distress syndrome diagnosis, 1996
  in pleural fluid, 2741–2742
Protein C, activated, resistance to, venous
    thrombosis and, 1778–1779
Protein S deficiency, venous thrombosis and,
    1779
Proteinase 3, antineutrophil cytoplasmic antibody
    and, 1492
  in Wegener's granulomatosis, 1493
Proteinosis, alveolar. See Alveolar proteinosis.
  lipoid, 2728
Proteoglycans, in pulmonary interstitial
    connective tissue, 1950–1951
Proteus infection, 755–756
  pleural effusion with, 2749
Proton density sequence, 320
Proto-oncogenes, 1082
Protozoal disease, 1034–1039. See also specific
    diseases.
Provocation testing. See Inhalation challenge
    tests.
Pruning, vascular, in pulmonary hypertension,
    1886–1887, 1890
Pseudallescheriasis, 951
Pseudoaneurysm, aortic, 2634, 2952
  defined, 2951
Pseudocavitation, 463, 470
  in solitary nodules, 1142, 1142
Pseudochylous effusion, 2743, 2768. See also
    Chyliform effusion.
Pseudocoarctation of the aorta, 2961, 2962
Pseudocyst, pancreatic, in middle-posterior
    mediastinum, 2944–2945, 2946
Pseudodiaphragmatic contour, with
    subpulmonary effusion, 566–568, 569–571
Pseudofibrosis of the cyanotic, 666
Pseudo-Gaucher cells, 2724
  in tuberculosis, 812
Pseudoglandular period of lung development,
    136–137, 137, 138
Pseudohemoptysis, in Serratia marcescens
    infection, 752
Pseudolymphoma, in Sjögren's syndrome, 1466,
    1468
  pulmonary, 1269–1271, 1270, 1277
Pseudomembrane formation, in tracheobronchial
    Aspergillus infection, 701, 701, 942, 947,
    2022
Pseudomeningocele, 2979
Pseudomonas aeruginosa. See also Pseudomonas
    aeruginosa infection.
  altered airway binding to, in cystic fibrosis,
    2300
  bronchiectasis and, 2267
  chronic colonization with, shift in IgG sub-
    classes in, 2302
Pseudomonas aeruginosa infection, 706,
    761–764, 763, 764
  cavities or cysts in, 3102t
  homogeneous opacity in, nonsegmental, 3079t
    segmental, 3087t
  hospital-acquired, 723
  in cystic fibrosis, pathogenetic role of, 2301–
    2302
    prognosis and, 2315
  in diffuse panbronchiolitis, 2353
  in HIV disease, 1645
Pseudomonas cepacia. See Burkholderia cepacia
    infection.
Pseudomonas mallei (Burkholderia mallei)
    infection, 760–761

Pseudomonas maltophilia (Stenotrophomonas
    maltophilia) infection, 764
Pseudomonas picketti (Ralstonia picketti)
    infection, 765
Pseudomonas pseudoalcaligenes infection, 765
Pseudomonas pseudomallei (Burkholderia
    pseudomallei) infection, 759–760
Pseudomycosis, bacterial, 958–960
Pseudoplaques, in coal workers'
    pneumoconiosis, 2416, 2418
  in silicosis, 2404, 2406, 2407
Pseudotumor(s), calcifying fibrous, of pleura,
    2840
  diaphragmatic, 254
  due to interlobar effusion, 579–581, 580
  hilar, on lateral projection, 87, 92
    on posteroanterior projection, 84, 85, 86
  in hydrothorax due to heart failure, 2761,
    2762
  inflammatory, pulmonary, 1371–1373, 1372,
    1373
  mucoid, tracheobronchial gland tumor vs.,
    1253
  orbital, fibrosing mediastinitis with, 2857
  spindle cell, in tuberculosis, 812
Pseudoxanthoma elasticum, 677
Psittacosis, 1017–1019, 1019, 3097t
Psychogenic hyperventilation, 3066–3067
Psychogenic stridor, 2032–2033
Psychosocial disruption, in obstructive sleep
    apnea, 2067
Psyllium, occupational asthma due to,
    2120–2121
Puffer fish poisoning, 3063
Pulmonary. See also Lung entries.
Pulmonary adenoma, 1265–1267
Pulmonary agenesis, 598, 599–601, 600, 601
Pulmonary alveolar fibrosis, diffuse. See
    Pulmonary fibrosis, idiopathic.
Pulmonary alveolar microlithiasis. See Alveolar
    microlithiasis.
Pulmonary alveolar proteinosis. See Alveolar
    proteinosis.
Pulmonary angiography, 322–324, 323, 324
  digital subtraction, 322–323, 323
    in pulmonary thromboembolism diagnosis,
      1815–1816, 1818
  in pulmonary arteriovenous malformation as-
    sessment, 658, 660–661, 661
  in pulmonary thromboembolism diagnosis,
    324, 324, 1814–1819
    complications of, 1816–1818, 1818
    criteria for, 1818–1819, 1819t, 1823
    technique for, 1814–1816, 1817, 1818
  in thromboembolic pulmonary hypertension
    diagnosis, 1910–1911, 1912
  magnetic resonance, in pulmonary thromboem-
    bolism diagnosis, 1813
  nonuniform perfusion on, conditions associ-
    ated with, 1820t
  specimen, 351, 354
Pulmonary angiomatosis, diffuse, 662–663, 662,
    663
Pulmonary aplasia, 598, 599–601
Pulmonary arterial catheter(s), indwelling
    balloon-tipped, complications of,
    2685–2690, 2688, 2689
  cytologic examination of material aspirated
    from, 348
  pleural effusion due to, 2762
Pulmonary arterial wedge pressure, 104, 1880
  in pulmonary edema diagnosis, 1995–1996
Pulmonary arterioles, 72
  in situ thrombosis of, 1774–1775, 1775
Pulmonary arteriopathy, plexogenic, in
    pulmonary hypertension, 1882–1886,
    1883–1889

Pulmonary arteriovenous anastomoses, 77
Pulmonary arteriovenous malformation, 655–662
  clinical features of, 395, 661–662
  pathologic features of, 657, *657*
  radiologic features of, 657–661, *658–661*
Pulmonary artery(ies). See also *Pulmonary vasculature.*
  agenesis of, 637–638, *639*
    Swyer-James syndrome vs., 504, 638, 2337
  age-related changes in intima of, 72–74
  anatomy of, 71–74, *72, 72t, 73*
  aneurysm of, 1935–1937, 1935t, *1936, 1937*
    congenital, 642, *643, 646, 647*
    in Behçet's disease, 1519, *1519, 1520*
    in tuberculosis, 817–818, 1935
  atresia of, with ventricular septal defect, 637
  bronchial artery anastomoses with, 77
    in bronchiectasis, 395
  calcification of walls of, 474
  compression of, by pulmonary carcinoma, 1171
    pulmonary hypertension with, 1915
  development and growth of, 139–140, *140*
    anomalies of, 637–642
      pulmonary angiography for detection of, 323–324
  dilation of, middle-posterior mediastinal mass due to, 2945, 3178t
  elastic, 71–72, *73*
  enlargement of, with pulmonary thromboembolism, 1788–1792, *1792–1795*
  fibrosing mediastinitis involving, *2860, 2860,* 2863
  hypoplasia of, parenchymal hypoplasia and, 598
  imaging of, 77–80, *78, 79*
    on conventional radiographs, 273, *274*
    on CT, 281–286, *282, 284*
    on MRI, 321
  innervation of, 149
  left, anomalous origin of, 638–642, *640–641*
  main, absence of, 637, 3151t
    dilation of, 2945–2946, *2947*
    measurement of, in pulmonary hypertension diagnosis, 1887–1889
  metastasis via, 1382
  muscular, 72, *73*
    development and growth of, 140
  obstruction of, by mediastinal histoplasmosis, 886
    by neoplasm, 504, *506*
  occlusion of, with Swan-Ganz catheter, 2688–2689, *2688*
  perforation of, with Swan-Ganz catheter, 2689–2690, *2689*
  proximal interruption of, 637–638, *639*
    Swyer-James syndrome vs., 504, 638, 2337
  pulmonary carcinoma invading, 1166–1169, *1169*
  right, direct communication of, with left atrium, 642
  sarcomas of, 1332–1333, *1333,* 1334, *1334–1336*
  stenosis of, 642, *644–645*
    in congenital rubella, 993
    multiple, pulmonary hypertension with, 1915, *1916*
  supernumerary, *13,* 71, 72
  syphilis involving, 777–778
  Takayasu's arteritis involving, 1517
  thrombosis of, *in situ,* 1773–1774, *1774*
  thrombosis of stump of, after pneumonectomy, 2672, *2674*
  wall changes in, with pulmonary thromboembolism, 1785, *1789*
Pulmonary artery pressure, cardiac output and, 104, *105*

Pulmonary artery pressure *(Continued)*
  in COPD, prognosis and, 2230
  in pulmonary thromboembolism diagnosis, 1819
  noninvasive estimation of, 2218
Pulmonary artery–to–outer bronchial diameter ratio. See *Artery-bronchus ratios.*
Pulmonary blastoma, 1367–1369, *1369, 1370*
Pulmonary blood flow, decreased. See *Oligemia, pulmonary.*
  distribution of, 273–275
  increased, cardiovascular anomalies with, 664, *664*
    pulmonary hypertension due to, 1891–1896
      clinical features of, 1895–1896
      pathologic features of, 1894
      prognosis in, 1896
      radiologic features of, 1894–1895, *1894–1897*
    leukocyte retention in microvasculature and, 1979
    redistribution of, in hydrostatic pulmonary edema, 1959–1961, *1959, 1960*
    in pulmonary venous hypertension, 1919–1923, *1921–1926*
    transthoracic pressure and, 275, *276*
Pulmonary blood volume, defined, 104
  lung density and, 270, *271*
Pulmonary capillaritis. See *Capillaritis.*
Pulmonary capillary(ies). See also *Pulmonary vasculature.*
  as corner vessels, 106, 1947, *1947*
  endothelium of, in fluid exchange, 1947–1949, *1949*
  permeability of, 1949
  filtering function of, 132–133
  geometry and dimensions of network of, 76–77, *77*
  in situ thrombosis of, 1774–1775
Pulmonary capillary blood volume, diffusing capacity measurement and, 415, 416
Pulmonary capillary hemangiomatosis, 1914–1915, *1914*
Pulmonary capillary pressure, 104
Pulmonary capillary wedge pressure, 104, 1880
  in pulmonary edema diagnosis, 1995–1996
Pulmonary carcinoma. See *Carcinoma, pulmonary.*
Pulmonary edema, 1946–2006
  after bone marrow transplantation, 1726
  after lung transplantation, 1700–1702, *1701, 1702*
  cardiogenic, 1958–1973
    air-space, 1966–1969, *1967–1971*
    alveolar proteinosis vs., 2704
    bat's wing or butterfly pattern of, *435,* 1969–1970, *1972*
      clinical features of, 1971
    clinical features of, 1970–1972
    combined air-space and interstitial pattern in, 454–455, *457*
    contralateral, 1966–1967, *1970*
    differential diagnosis of, 1971
    diffuse air-space pattern in, 3130t, *3132*
    diffuse reticular pattern in, 3136t, *3141*
    interstitial, 1959–1965, *1961–1967*
    permeability edema vs., 1963, 1993–1994
    pulmonary function tests in, 1972–1973
    radiologic features of, 1959–1970, *1959–1972*
    unilateral, 1966–1969, *1968–1971*
  classification of, 1958, 1958t
  development and clearance of, 1956–1958, *1957*
  diffuse, due to pulmonary thromboembolism, 1782–1783

Pulmonary edema *(Continued)*
  due to aspiration of gastric contents, cardiogenic pulmonary edema vs., 2494
  due to contrast media, 2005–2006
  due to inhaled toxins, 2519, *2520*
  due to narcotics, 2567, *2568*
  due to pulmonary vein abnormalities, 1974, *1975*
  estimation of volume of, 1964–1965, 1993, 1996–1997
  fat embolism and, 2005
  high-altitude, 1999–2001
  hydrostatic, 1958–1976, 1958t. See also *Pulmonary edema, cardiogenic.*
    diffuse air-space pattern in, 3130t, *3132*
    diffuse reticular pattern in, 3136t, *3141*
    in diabetic ketoacidosis, 2005
    in pulmonary hypertension, 454–455, *457,* 1923, *1924, 1929*
    in pulmonary veno-occlusive disease, 1931, *1932, 1933*
    in upper airway obstruction, 2029
    interlobular septal thickening in, *29,* 445, 446, 1956, *1957, 1963, 1966*
    interstitial, alveolar septum ultrastructure in, 1947, *1948*
    Kerley (septal) lines in, 441, *442,* 444, *444, 446,* 480, *481, 482,* 1961, *1961, 1962, 1964, 1965, 1967,* 1994
    lung lymph flow during, 1955–1956
    neurogenic, 1974–1976
    pancreatitis and, 2003
    pathogenesis of, 1947–1958
      anatomic aspects of, 1947–1952, *1947–1949, 1951*
      physiologic aspects of, 1952–1956, *1952*
      safety factors in, 1955–1956
    permeability, 1958t, 1976–2006. See also *Adult respiratory distress syndrome (ARDS).*
      cardiogenic edema vs., 1963, 1993–1994
      causes of, 1978t
      diffuse air-space pattern in, 3130t
      microvascular pressure and, 1996, *1996*
      specific forms of, 1999–2006
    postoperative, 2671
    postpneumonectomy, 2001
    re-expansion, *1968,* 2001–2002, *2002*
    reticular pattern in, 446
    sequence of fluid accumulation in, 441, *441, 442,* 1950, 1951, *1951,* 1956–1957
    surfactant and, 58, 1980–1981
    unilateral, 1966–1969, *1968–1971*
    with air embolism, 1855
    with hypervolemia, 1973–1974, *1973*
    with hypoproteinemia, 1973–1974, *1973*
    with pheochromocytoma, 2005
    with renal disease, 1973–1974, *1973*
    with severe upper airway obstruction, 2002–2003, *2003*
    with transfusion, 2003
Pulmonary fibrosis, autoantibodies associated with, 1423
  bronchiectasis with, 2269, *2271*
  crackles in, 394
  idiopathic, 1585–1611. See also *Interstitial pneumonia; Interstitial pneumonitis.*
    asbestosis vs., 2430
    bronchiectasis with, 2269, *2271*
    bronchoalveolar lavage in, prognosis and, 1609
    clinical features of, 1606–1607
      prognosis and, 1608
    dendriform ossification with, 2700, *2703*
    diagnosis of, 1610–1611
    diffuse alveolar damage in, *1619,* 1621

Pulmonary fibrosis *(Continued)*
  epidemiology of, 1585
  etiology of, 1585
  extrinsic allergic alveolitis vs., 1611, 2373
  familial form of, 1586, *1587–1589*
  Langerhans' cell histiocytosis vs., 1611,
    1628, 1631
  lymphangioleiomyomatosis vs., 685
  Mycobacterium xenopi pneumonia with,
    852
  pathogenesis of, 1585–1590, *1587–1590*
  pathologic features of, 1591–1599, *1591–
    1600*
    prognosis and, 1609
  prognosis in, 1608–1610, *1610*
  pulmonary carcinoma and, 1608
  pulmonary function tests in, 1607–1608
    prognosis and, 1608
  radiologic features of, 1599–1606, *1600–
    1603*
    on CT, 1604–1606, *1604–1607,* 1609–
      1610, *1610*
    prognosis and, 1609–1610, *1610*
    time of appearance of, 3046
  reticular pattern in, 446, 447, *447–449,*
    1599, *1600–1604,* 3135t, *3138, 3139*
  in adult respiratory distress syndrome, 1984,
    1985, 1987–1992, *1991,* 1997
  in extrinsic allergic alveolitis, pathogenesis of,
    2364
    pathologic features of, 2365
    radiologic features of, 2367, *2370, 2371,*
      2372
  in intravenous talcosis, 1858, *1863, 1864*
  in pneumoconiosis. See *Progressive massive fi-
    brosis.*
  in progressive systemic sclerosis, pathogenesis
    of, 1452–1453
    pathologic features of, 1455
    pulmonary carcinoma associated with, 1460,
      1461
    radiologic features of, 1455–1457, *1455,
      1456*
  in pulmonary hypertension, 1923, *1929*
    postcapillary, 1919, *1920*
  in rheumatoid disease, 1434–1438, *1435–
    1437, 3137*
  in sarcoidosis, 1542, *1543, 1555,* 1558, *1560*
  in systemic lupus erythematosus, 1427, *1428,*
    1429–1430
  lung volume loss in, 525, *527, 528*
  pulmonary carcinoma and, 1080, *1080*
  radiation-induced. See *Radiation fibrosis.*
Pulmonary function, postoperative, prediction of,
  331, 1180–1181
Pulmonary function tests, 404–424. See also
    specific parameters.
  in COPD, 2220–2229, *2221–2223*
  in infants, in cystic fibrosis, 2313
  indications for, 404
  levels of, 404–405
  predicted normal values on, 405–408
Pulmonary hyalinizing granuloma, 1373, *1374,
  1375*
  pulmonary hyperplasia and, 599
Pulmonary hypertension, 1879–1937
  arterial. See also *Pulmonary hypertension, pre-
    capillary.*
    defined, 1880
  causes of, 1881t, 1934t
  combined precapillary and postcapillary, 1919
  drug-related, 1902–1903
  due to intravascular metastasis, 1397, *1398,
    1399*
  general features of, 1879–1891
  in antiphospholipid syndrome, 1912–1914

Pulmonary hypertension *(Continued)*
  in connective tissue disease, pulmonary olige-
    mia in, 3151t
  in COPD, 1915, *1917,* 2217–2218
  in CREST syndrome, 1460
    pathogenesis of, 1453–1454
    pathologic features of, *1454,* 1455
  in emphysema, 1915, *1917,* 2209, *2209*
  in hepatic disease, 1903–1904, *1904*
  in HIV infection, 1686, 1914
  in intravenous talcosis, *1862*
  in obstructive sleep apnea, 1918, 2066
  in progressive systemic sclerosis, pathogenesis
    of, 1453–1454
    pathologic features of, *1454,* 1455
  in pulmonary capillary hemangiomatosis,
    1914–1915, *1914*
  in rheumatoid disease, 1449–1451, *1450*
  in Spanish toxic oil syndrome, 2587–2588
  in systemic immunologic disorders, 1912,
    1913
  in systemic lupus erythematosus, 1431
  oligemia due to, 501–502, *501, 502,* 504, *506,*
    1787–1788, *1792, 1793*
  pathogenesis of, 1880–1882
  pathologic features of, 1882–1886, *1883–1889*
  persistent, in newborn, 1882
  postcapillary, 1881t, 1918–1930
    blood flow redistribution in, 1919–1923,
      1921–1926, 1959–1961, *1959, 1960*
    bronchial displacement with, 533, *535*
    clinical and radiographic correlation in,
      1963
    clinical features of, 1928
    electrocardiographic findings in, 1928
    pathologic features of, 1919, *1919, 1920*
    pulmonary function tests in, 1928–1930
    radiologic features of, 1919–1926, *1921–
      1930*
  precapillary, 1881t, 1891–1918
    due to pleuropulmonary disease, 1881t,
      1915–1918
    due to vascular disease, 1881t, 1891–1915
    in asthma, 2125, *2127*
  primary, 1896–1902
    clinical features of, 1899–1902
    hemodynamic findings in, 1902
    lung transplantation for, 1699
    pathogenesis of, 1896–1898
    pathologic features of, 1898–1899
    prognosis in, 1902
    pulmonary function tests in, 1902
    pulmonary oligemia in, 3151t
    radiologic features of, 1899, *1899–1901*
  pulmonary artery aneurysm due to, 1936
  radiologic features of, 1886–1891, *1890, 1892,
    1893*
  toxin-related, 1902–1903
  venous. See also *Pulmonary hypertension,
    postcapillary.*
    defined, 1880
  with increased flow, 1891–1896
    clinical features of, 1895–1896
    pathologic features of, 1894
    prognosis in, 1896
    radiologic features of, 1894–1895, *1894–
      1897*
  with thrombosis and thromboembolism, 1904–
    1912
    acute, 1781–1782
    chronic, 1782, 1904–1906, *1905–1906*
      clinical features of, 1825–1826, 1912
      pathologic features of, 1907
      prognosis in, 1912
      radiologic features of, 1908, *1909–1911*
    clinical features of, 1911–1912

Pulmonary hypertension *(Continued)*
  diagnosis of, 1891, *1893*
  pathogenesis of, 1898
  pathologic features of, 1907, *1907*
  prognosis in, 1912
  pulmonary oligemia in, 3151t
  radiologic features of, 1907–1911, *1908–
    1912*
Pulmonary hypoplasia, 598–601
Pulmonary infarct. See *Infarction, pulmonary.*
Pulmonary ligament(s), imaging of, 165–166,
  167, 168
  on CT, 254, *256*
  lower lobe atelectasis pattern and, 552
Pulmonary ligament lymph nodes, in ATS
    classification, 184t
  in classification for lung cancer staging, *185,*
    188t, *1186,* 1187t
Pulmonary lymphangiomatosis, diffuse,
  662–663, *662, 663*
Pulmonary meningothelial-like nodules, 74,
  1364, 1374–1375, *1376*
Pulmonary mycotoxicosis. See *Organic dust
  toxic syndrome.*
Pulmonary overpressurization syndrome,
  systemic air embolism due to, 1855
Pulmonary reimplantation response, 1700–1702,
  1701, 1702
Pulmonary resistance, measurement of, 412
Pulmonary sequestration. See *Bronchopulmonary
  sequestration.*
Pulmonary sling, 638–642, *640–641*
Pulmonary tissue, accessory, 628
  intralobar sequestration vs., 601
  heterotopic, 628
Pulmonary trunk, 71
Pulmonary tumorlets, 1243–1245, *1244–1246*
Pulmonary vascular pressure-flow curves, 104,
  105
Pulmonary vascular resistance, calculation of,
  104, *105,* 1880
  gravity and, 105, *105,* 110
  lung volume and, 106
  regulation of, 1879–1880
Pulmonary vasculature, 71–119. See also
    *Pulmonary artery(ies); Pulmonary
    capillary(ies); Pulmonary vein(s).*
  adventitious sounds originating in, 395
  anatomy of, 71–77, 1879, *1880*
  compartments of, 1947
  crowded, in atelectasis, 526
  development and growth of, 139–141, *140,
    141*
    anomalies affecting, 637–671
  function of, 104–119
    factors influencing, 104–106, *105,* 110
    gravity and, 111
  imaging of, 77–104
  in fluid and solute exchange, 1947–1950,
    1947–1949
  infection acquired via, 713–716, *715–717*
  innervation of, 149
  morphologic investigation techniques for, 351,
    354
  sarcomas of, 1332–1333, *1333,* 1334, *1334–
    1336*
  systemic vessel anastomoses with, 77
  transplantation complications involving, 1724,
    1725
Pulmonary vein(s). See also *Pulmonary
  vasculature.*
  abnormalities of, pulmonary edema due to,
    1974, *1975*
  anatomy of, *73,* 74, 75t
  bronchial vein anastomoses with, 77
  changes in, in postcapillary pulmonary hyper-
    tension, 1919, *1919*

Pulmonary vein(s) *(Continued)*
   development and growth of, 140–141, *141*
     anomalies of, 642–653
   diameter of, as indicator of pulmonary venous
     hypertension, 1921–1923, *1926*
   imaging of, *78, 79, 80, 81*
     on conventional radiographs, 273, *274, 275*
     on CT scans, 281–286, *282–284*
   in plexogenic arteriopathy, 1885
   in situ thrombosis of, 1775
   innervation of, 149
   obstruction of, by mediastinal histoplasmosis,
     886
     congenital, 642–645
     supernumerary, 74
   varicosities of, 645–647, *648–649*
Pulmonary venous drainage, anomalous,
     647–653
   in hypogenetic lung syndrome, 653, *656*
   partial, 647–648, *650–652*
   pulmonary angiography for detection of,
     324
   pulmonary wedge pressure measurement in
     presence of, 1995
   total, 648–653
Pulmonary venous pressure, pulmonary wedge
     pressure as reflection of, 1995–1996
Pulmonary venules, 74
Pulmonary wedge pressure, 104, 1880
   in pulmonary edema diagnosis, 1995–1996
Pulmonary-renal syndromes, differential
     diagnosis of, 1764
Pulmonic stenosis, decreased pulmonary blood
     flow with, 665, 3151t
   infundibular, 642, *646*
   supravalvular, 642
   systemic-pulmonary vascular fistula and, 666
   valvular, 642, *643–645*
Pulse oximetry, in carbon monoxide poisoning
     diagnosis, 3069
   in obstructive sleep apnea diagnosis, 2068,
     2069
Pulsion diverticulum, 2966, 2967
Pulsus paradoxus, 395
   in asthma, 2134
   reversed, 395–396
Punctate calcification, 467, *474*
Pure red blood cell aplasia, thymoma and, 2894,
     2897
Purified protein derivative (PPD), T lymphocytes
     sensitized to, in tuberculous pleural
     effusion, 2745
   tuberculin test using, 841
     in HIV infection, 1652–1653
Purpura, in pulmonary carcinoma, 1178
Pyopneumothorax, in anaerobic pneumonia, 779,
     781
   organisms causing, 2749
Pyothorax. See *Empyema; Pleural effusion.*
Pyrimethamine, thoracic disease due to, 2538t,
     2558
Pyrin, in familial paroxysmal polyserositis, 2766
Pyrophosphate, technetium-labeled, for
     ventilation imaging, 330
Pyrrolizidine alkaloids, pulmonary hypertension
     and, 1902

Q fever, 722, 1019–1020, *1021*
   homogeneous segmental opacity in, 3087t
   pleural effusion in, 2752
Quadriplegia, due to cervical cord injury, rib
     notching in, 3015
Quantum efficiency, 307
Quantum mottle, 313

Radiation, 2592–2606. See also *Radiation
     therapy.*
   dose of, in CT, 313–314
   mesothelioma and, 2809–2810
   pulmonary carcinoma and, 1078–1079
Radiation fibrosis, cicatrization atelectasis due
     to, *526*
   clinical manifestations of, 2605
   pathogenesis of, 2593
   pathologic features of, 2595, *2595*
   radiologic features of, 2597, *2602–2604*
   recurrent tumor vs., 2597–2604
Radiation pneumonitis, adhesive atelectasis in,
     522, *525*
   as term, problems with, 2592
   clinical manifestations of, 2605
   epidemiology of, 2592
   nonsegmental opacity in, homogeneous, 3081t
     inhomogeneous, 3093t, *3095*
   pathogenesis of, 2592–2594
   pathologic features of, 2594–2595, *2594, 2595*
   radiologic features of, 2595–2604, *2596–2604*
Radiation recall, 2593
Radiation therapy, apical pleural cap after, 2795
   chest wall neoplasms due to, 3023–3025,
     3026–3027
   endobronchial, complications of, 2592, 2604,
     2674–2675
   for breast cancer, pulmonary carcinoma and,
     1201
   for esophageal carcinoma, airway-esophageal
     fistula due to, 2967
   for Hodgkin's disease, long-term effects of,
     1312
     lymph node calcification after, 1302, *1305*
     pulmonary carcinoma and, 1201
   late complications of, 2597, *2604, 2605*
   peripheral primitive neuroectodermal tumor
     after, 3028
   pleural effusion after, 2763
   pulmonary carcinoma and, 1079
   pulmonary damage due to. See *Radiation
     fibrosis; Radiation pneumonitis.*
   pulmonary function studies after, 2605–2606
   tangential ports for, reduction of damage with,
     2592
Radioallergosorbent test, in allergen
     identification, 2104
Radiography. See also *Computed tomography
     (CT).*
   bedside, 305–306
   conventional, 299–309
     basic techniques for, 301–303, *303*
     factors affecting interpretation in, 275–279,
       278
     high-resolution CT vs., 456–457
     indications for, 299–300, 300t
       in ICU patients, 305–306
     lung density in, technical mechanisms affect-
       ing, 271, *273*
     of chest wall, 259, *259, 261–264*
     of diaphragm, 251, *251, 252*
     of hila, 81–87, *82–86, 88–95*
     of interlobar fissures, 155–158, *157, 158,
       160, 161*
     of normal lung, 269–279
     postmortem, 351
     projections for, 299–301, *301*
     pulmonary markings in, 272–275, *274–276*
     respiration and, 302, 303–305, *304*
     special techniques for, 303–309, *304, 308*
     superimposition of abnormalities in, 441
   digital, 306–308, *308*
   dual-energy computed, calcification detection
     on, in solitary nodule, 1138–1139
   in pneumoconiosis diagnosis, international
     classification system for, 441, 2387–2390

Radiography *(Continued)*
   inspiratory-expiratory, 303–305, *304*
   lung density in. See also *Lung density.*
     decreased, 493–511
     increased, 433–488
     technical mechanisms affecting, 271, *273*
   normal findings on, pulmonary disease associ-
     ated with, 3043–3069
   scanning equalization systems for, 302–303
   selenium detector, 307
   signs of chest disease on, 431–592
   storage phosphor, 306–307, *308*
   time factor in diagnosis using, 438–439, 479,
     480
Radiometric techiques, for tuberculosis
     diagnosis, 845
Radionuclide imaging, 326–332. See also
     *Gallium scintigraphy; Ventilation/perfusion
     scanning.*
   in deep vein thrombosis, 1824
   in goiter diagnosis, 2913
   in Kaposi's sarcoma diagnosis, 332, 1679
   in pulmonary carcinoma, 1180–1181
     in distant metastasis detection, 1192
   of liver, in diaphragmatic rupture diagnosis,
     2637
   of mediastinal parathyroid glands, 2914
Radiopacity, density vs., 269n
Radiopaque foreign bodies, embolization of,
     1868
Radon, pulmonary carcinoma and, 1078–1079
Ralstonia picketti infection, 765
Ranke complex, 463–467, *471,* 805, 811, *812*
RANTES, in asthmatic airway inflammation,
     2092
Rapeseed oil, contaminated, 1459, 2587–2588
Rapidly adapting stretch receptors. See *Irritant
     receptors.*
Rapid-occlusion technique, for measuring
     pulmonary capillary pressure, 104
Rare earths, pneumoconiosis due to, 2456
ras genes, 1082–1083
Rasmussen's aneurysm, 817–818, 1935
Raynaud's disease, 398
Raynaud's phenomenon, 1462
   in CREST syndrome, 1460
   in overlap syndromes, 1459
   in progressive systemic sclerosis, 1453–1454
   in systemic lupus erythematosus, pulmonary
     hypertension and, 1431
Rb gene, 1083
Reactive airways dysfunction syndrome,
     2123–2124, 2123t
Reactive oxygen species, in adult respiratory
     distress syndrome, 1979–1980, 1982–1983
   in asbestosis, 2423
   in emphysema, 2184
   in oxidant gas–induced pulmonary injury,
     2519–2520
   in reperfusion injury, 1700
   smoking and, 2184
Reactivity, in inhalation challenge tests,
     421–422. See also *Bronchial hyper-
     responsiveness; Inhalation challenge tests.*
Reader fatigue, in radiographic interpretation,
     279
Rebreathing method, for assessment of
     ventilatory response, to carbon dioxide,
     417–418, *417*
   to hypoxemia, 418, *418*
   for diffusing capacity measurement, 415
Rectal prolapse, in cystic fibrosis, 2311
Rectum, adenocarcinoma of. See *Colorectal
     carcinoma.*
Rectus abdominis, in expiration, 247
   spinal levels of innervation of, 3055

Recurrent hereditary polyserositis, 2766
Recurrent laryngeal nerve, hoarseness due to
    dysfunction of, 389
    in pulmonary innervation, 145
    pulmonary carcinoma invading, 1171
Red blood cell(s), in carbon dioxide transport,
    114
    in pleural fluid specimen, 344
Red blood cell aplasia, thymoma and, 2894,
    2897
Red hepatization, in *Streptococcus pneumoniae*
    pneumonia, 737, *738*
Red tide, 2124, 3062
Reed-Sternberg cells, *1299*
Reflex bronchoconstriction, bronchial hyper-
    responsiveness and, 2098
Regional time constant, gravity and, 111
Reid index, 2186, *2187*
Rejection. See *Lung transplantation, rejection
    after.*
Relapsing polychondritis, 1470–1473, *1472,
    1473*
    upper airway obstruction due to, 2040–2042,
    2044
Relaxation atelectasis, 517–522, *519–521, 523,
    524.* See also *Atelectasis.*
    defined, 513, 525
    dependent opacity on CT due to, 287, *291,*
    513, 519–521, *521*
Relaxation times, in MRI, 317, *318, 319*
Renal. See also *Kidneys.*
Renal aminoaciduria, familial retardation of
    growth and cor pulmonale with, 2728
Renal angiomyolipoma, bilateral, in tuberous
    sclerosis, 686, *687*
Renal cell carcinoma, metastatic, 1399–1404,
    1399, 1402, 1404
    lymph node enlargement in, *3169*
Renal disease, pleural effusion with, 2764
    in systemic lupus erythematosus, 2753
    pulmonary edema with, 1973–1974, *1973*
Renal failure, chronic, tuberculosis risk and, 803
    venous thrombosis risk and, 1780
    in pulmonary carcinoma, 1178
Renal function, blood gases and, 2216–2217
Renal transplantation, tuberculosis risk and, 804
Renal tubular acidosis, in Sjögren's syndrome,
    1469
Rendu-Osler-Weber disease, pulmonary
    arteriovenous malformations in, 657, *659,*
    661, *661, 3113*
Renin, plasma levels of, in asthma, 2093
Reoviruses, 993
Reperfusion injury, after lung transplantation,
    1700–1702, *1701, 1702*
    pulmonary edema after lung re-expansion and,
    1902
Reservoir lymphatics, 172
Residual volume (RV), 406, *406*
    in COPD, 2224
    measurement of, 407–408
Resistance, airway, density dependence of, in
    COPD, 2224
    frictional, in work of breathing, 58–59
    measurement of, 412–413
    upper, during sleep, 2055
    bronchovascular, gas tension changes and, 121
    in work of breathing, 58–60
    measurement of, 412–413
    pulmonary vascular. See *Pulmonary vascular
    resistance.*
    regional, exercise and, 111
Resolution, spatial, defined, 307
Resorption atelectasis, 513–517, *514–518.* See
    also *Atelectasis.*
    air bronchogram and, 533

Resorption atelectasis *(Continued)*
    defined, 513, 525
Respiration. See also *Ventilation.*
    assessment of, during sleep, 2068
    conventional radiographs and, 302, 303–305,
    304
    fetal, lung development and, 142
Respiratory acidosis, 116–117
    in COPD, 2228
Respiratory alkalosis, 117
    lactic acidosis development in, 3067
Respiratory alternans, 258
Respiratory bronchioles, 17, *17*
    grading of inflammatory reaction in, 2189
Respiratory bronchiolitis, 2323t, 2348–2349,
    2348. See also *Bronchiolitis.*
    radiologic features of, 2331, *2331*
Respiratory bronchiolitis–associated interstitial
    disease, 2348–2349
Respiratory control system, 235–243, *236,
    3049–3051, 3050*
    assessment of, 240, 416–419, *417, 418*
    central controller in, 238–240
    factors affecting, 240–241
    input to, 235–238
    output from, 240–241
Respiratory cycle, neurologic phases of, 239
Respiratory distress syndrome, adult. See *Adult
    respiratory distress syndrome (ARDS);
    Pulmonary edema, permeability.*
    neonatal, adhesive atelectasis in, 522
    surfactant in, 58
Respiratory disturbance index, 2056
Respiratory drive, assessment of, 2226
    hypercapnia in COPD and, 2226
Respiratory dyskinesia, 3051–3052
Respiratory failure. See also *Alveolar
    hypoventilation.*
    acute-on-chronic, in COPD, prognosis and,
    2230
Respiratory heat loss, bronchoconstriction in
    response to, 2108
Respiratory inductive plethysmography, 408
Respiratory movements, fetal, decreased,
    pulmonary hypoplasia and, 598
Respiratory mucus, 60–63
    in asthma, 2093–2094
Respiratory muscles, 246–259. See also specific
    muscles and muscle groups.
    characteristics of, 3056
    energy sources of, 257
    fatigue and weakness of, 257–259, 3056–3057
    assessment of, 258, 420
    clinical features of, 3057–3059, *3058–3060*
    in COPD, 2219–2220
    in rheumatoid disease, 1451
    prediction of, 3057
    pulmonary function tests in, 3059–3061
    function of, *249,* 255–259
    hypoventilation due to disorders of, 3064–
    3065
    increased load on, compensatory mechanisms
    with, 241–242
    receptors in, in ventilatory control, 238
    spinal levels of innervation of, 3055
    strength of, determinants of, 3057
    tests of performance of, 419–420
    training of, to increase strength and endur-
    ance, 259
Respiratory myoclonus, 2995
Respiratory pump, *249,* 255–259
    hypoventilation due to disorders of, 3049t,
    3056–3065
Respiratory secretions. See *Tracheobronchial
    secretions.*
Respiratory syncytial virus, 986–987

Respiratory syncytial virus *(Continued)*
    acute bronchiolitis due to, 2333
    in infancy, asthma and, 987, 2079–2080,
    2112
    asthma exacerbations and, 2111, 2112
Respiratory system, compliance of, 54, *56.* See
    also *Lung compliance.*
    surfactant and, 58
    resistance of, total, measurement of, 412
Respiratory zone of lungs, 3, 17–24
    geometry and dimensions of, 23–24
    morphology and cell function of, 17–23
Restriction fragment length polymorphism
    analysis, in epidemiologic investigation of
    tuberculosis, 846
Reticular pattern, in interstitial disease, 444–447,
    447–449
    differential diagnosis of, 3133, 3134t–3136t,
    3137–3143
Reticulate bodies, 1016
Reticulohistiocytosis, multicentric, 1313
Reticulonodular pattern, in interstitial disease,
    453, *454*
    on conventional radiographs, problems in inter-
    pretation of, 441
Retinoblastoma gene, 1083
Retinoic acid, experimental emphysema reversed
    by, 2185
Retrobronchial line, left, 87, *88–89*
Retrobronchial stripe, left, 87, *89*
Retrocardiac lobe, 164–165, *165*
Retrocrural lymph nodes, 176, *178*
    enlargement of, 2929
Retroperitoneal fibrosis, fibrosing mediastinitis
    with, 2857, 2863
Retropharyngeal abscess, acute, upper airway
    obstruction due to, 2021, 2022, *2023*
    mediastinitis due to, *2852*
Retropharyngeal hemorrhage, upper airway
    obstruction due to, 2024
Retrosternal abscess, after sternotomy, 2660,
    2660, 3019, 3019
Retrosternal air space, increase in, in
    emphysema, 2209, *2209*
    with hyperinflation, 496, *496*
Retrosternal pain, 386
Retrosternal stripe, 204–205, *206*
Retrotracheal lymph nodes, in classification for
    lung cancer staging, *185,* 188t, *1186,* 1187t
Retroviruses, 991–992. See also *Human
    immunodeficiency virus (HIV).*
Rett's syndrome, 3052
Reversed pulmonary edema pattern, in chronic
    eosinophilic pneumonia, 1747–1748, *1749*
Rhabdomyolysis, 3065
Rhabdomyoma, mediastinal, 2925
Rhabdomyosarcoma, mediastinal, 2925
    pulmonary, 1334–1335
Rheumatic pneumonitis, 1470
Rheumatoid arthritis. See also *Rheumatoid
    disease.*
    juvenile, 1451–1452
Rheumatoid disease, 1433–1452, 1433t
    airway involvement in, 1444–1449, *1446–
    1449*
    bronchiectasis in, 1448–1449, *1449,* 2267–
    2268
    bronchiolitis in, 2336
    follicular, 1273, *1274,* 1446–1448, *1447,
    1448,* 2349, *2349,* 2350
    obliterative, 1445–1446, *1446, 1447*
    coal workers' pneumoconiosis and, 1438–
    1443, 2411, 2416, *2417*
    complications of drug therapy for, 1451
    diffuse reticular pattern in, 3134t, *3137*
    lymphoid interstitial pneumonia in, *1272*

Rheumatoid disease *(Continued)*
  parenchymal, 1434–1443, *1435–1437, 1439–1443*
  pathogenesis of, 1433–1434
  pleural, 1443–1444, *1444, 1445*
  pleural effusion in, 2744t, 2753–2754, *2755*
  prognosis in, 1451
  pulmonary vascular, 1449–1451, *1450*
  radiologic features of, time of appearance of, 3046
  silicosis and, 2402–2404
Rheumatoid factor, in coal workers'
    pneumoconiosis, 2410–2411
  in rheumatoid disease, 1434
Rheumatoid nodules, 1438, *1441–1443*
  Caplan's syndrome vs., 1442
Rhinocerebral mucormycosis, 949
Rhinovirus, 991
  asthma exacerbations and, 991, 2111–2112
Rhizopus infection, 945
Rhodococcus equi infection, 750
  in HIV disease, 1645–1647, *1646*
Rhomboid fossae, 263, *264*
Rhomboid muscles, on CT, 260, *260*
Rhonchi, 394, 395
  pleural friction rub vs., 395
Rib(s), abnormalities of, 3012–3017
    acquired, *3014*, 3015–3017, 3015t, *3016, 3017*
    congenital, 262–263, *263,* 3012–3015, *3013*
  actinomycosis involving, 955
  approximation of, in atelectasis, *530,* 533
  cervical, 262, *263,* 3012–3013, *3013*
  companion shadows of, 262, *262*
  fracture of, after sternotomy, 2661
    chest wall pain due to, 387
    pneumothorax with, 2790
    subcutaneous emphysema with, *2625*
    with blunt trauma, 2644–2645
  imaging of, 260–263, *261–264*
  intrathoracic, 262–263, 3013–3014
  multiple myeloma involving, 1294, *1296*
  neoplasms of, 3030, 3032, *3033–3036*
    chest wall pain due to, 387
  notching and erosion of, *3014,* 3015–3016, 3015t, *3016*
    in progressive systemic sclerosis, 1457
  pain originating in, 387
  pelvic, 263, 3015
  pulmonary carcinoma involving, 1166, *1166, 1167*
  surgical complications involving, 2660
  tuberculosis involving, 837–838, *839,* 3017, *3017*
Ribonucleic acid (RNA) viruses, 981–984. See
    also specific viruses.
Richter's syndrome, 1321
Rickettsial infection, 1019–1022
  homogeneous segmental consolidation in, 3087t
  pleural effusion in, 2752
Riedel's thyroiditis, fibrosing mediastinitis with, 2857, 2861, *2864*
  upper airway obstruction due to, 2031, *2031*
Right aortic arch, 2961, *2963*
Riley-Day syndrome, 3056
Ring-around-the-artery sign, in pneumo-
    mediastinum, 2865, *2866, 2867*
Ring/sling complex, 642
Ritalin (methylphenidate), intravenous abuse of, 1860
Ritodrine, thoracic disease due to, 2566
RNA viruses, 981–994. See also specific viruses.
Rochalimaea henselae. See *Bartonella henselae
    infection.*
Rocky Mountain spotted fever, 1020–1022

Roentgenography. See *Radiography.*
Roseola, 999
Round atelectasis, 521–522, *523, 524*
  asbestos-related, 522
    pathologic features of, 2430, *2432, 2433*
    pulmonary carcinoma vs., 2443, 2448
    radiologic features of, *523, 2438–2440, 2441–2443, 2447, 2448*
    solitary mass due to, 3118t, *3121*
Round pneumonia, in *Legionella* infection, 773, *775*
  in *Streptococcus pneumoniae* infection, 737, *739*
Roundup (herbicide), 2587
Roundworms, 1039–1047. See also specific
    diseases.
Rubella, 993–994
Rubeola. See *Measles.*
Runyon classification of nontuberculous
    mycobacteria, 849
Rutile, pneumoconiosis due to, 2465–2466, *2467*

S sign of Golden, 460, 543, *544, 548,* 549
  in pulmonary carcinoma, 1121, *1126*
Saber-sheath trachea, 2036–2040, *2042, 2043*
Sabin-Feldman dye test, for toxoplasmosis, 1038
Saccomanno method for sputum processing, 340
Saccular bronchiectasis, *2268,* 2269, *2269, 2270.*
    See also *Bronchiectasis.*
  bronchography in, *2280*
  CT findings in, 2275, *2275, 2277*
  radiologic findings in, 2272, *2273*
Saccular period of lung development, 137, *139*
Saculotubular lymphatics, 174
Sail sign, 200, *202*
Salicylates. See also *Acetylsalicylic acid.*
  hyperventilation due to, 3067
Saline aerosol inhalation, for bronchial reactivity
    assessment, 421t, 422
Saliva, in cystic fibrosis, 2300
  sputum vs., 380
Salivary glands, in sarcoidosis, 1565
  in Sjögren's syndrome, 1468, 1469
Salla disease, emphysema in, 2232
Salmonella infection, 755, *758*
  systemic lupus erythematosus and, 1424
Sandstorm appearance, in alveolar microlithiasis, 2721, *2723*
SAPHO syndrome, 3031
Sarcoid granulomatosis, necrotizing, 1521–1523, *1522–1524*
Sarcoidosis, 1533–1573
  angiotensin-converting enzyme in, 1568
  berylliosis vs., 2460
  cardiac, 1562–1563, *1563–1564*
    prognosis and, 1572
  clinical features of, 1563–1566
  CNS involvement in, 1566
  defined, 1533
  diagnosis of, 1570–1571
  differential diagnosis of, 1570–1571
  diffuse pulmonary disease in, 1550–1558, *1551–1561*
    air-space consolidation in, 1554, *1556, 1557*
    cavities or cysts in, 3104t
    ground-glass opacities in, 1554–1558, *1557*
    nodular pattern of, 453, 1551, *1551–1553,* 3145t, *3148*
    reticular pattern of, 1551–1554, *1555, 1556,* 3134t, *3138*
    reticulonodular pattern of, 453, *454,* 1551, *1554*
  epidemiology of, 1533–1534
  etiology of, 1534

Sarcoidosis *(Continued)*
  fungus ball in, 923, 1542, 1561, *1562*
  gallium scintigraphy in, 331, *331,* 1568, *1568*
    prognosis and, 1573
  gastrointestinal involvement in, 1564
  hematologic abnormalities in, 1570
  hepatic involvement in, 1564
  honeycombing in, 446–447, 1542, *1543, 1551–1554, 1555,* 1558, *1561*
  idiopathic pulmonary fibrosis vs., 1611
  Kiem test in, 1571
  laboratory findings in, 1567–1570
  lymphadenopathy in, 1545–1550, *1546–1551,* 1547t, 3164t, *3167*
    clinical features of, 1564
    diffuse pulmonary disease and, 1558, *1558, 1559*
    Hodgkin's disease vs., 1311–1312, 1545
  metastatic renal cell carcinoma mimicking, *1404*
  multiple masses or nodules in, 3123t
  musculoskeletal involvement in, 1564
  mycobacteria and, 1534
  necrotizing sarcoid granulomatosis and, 1523
  neoplasm with, 1572
  nodular, 1541
  ocular, 1564
  pathogenesis of, 1534–1537
  pathologic features of, 1537–1542, *1538–1546*
  prognosis in, 1571–1573, 1573t
  pulmonary fibrosis in, 1542, *1543, 1555,* 1558, *1560*
  pulmonary function tests in, 1566–1567
  radiologic features of, 1542–1563
    stage classification of, 1542–1545
    time of appearance of, 3046
    unusual, 1558–1563, *1561, 1562*
  recurrent, after lung transplantation, 1720
  renal involvement in, 1566
  salivary gland involvement in, 1564
  skin involvement in, 1564
  spontaneous pneumothorax with, *2784*
  tuberculosis and, 803, 1534–1535
  upper respiratory tract involvement in, 1566
Sarcoma. See also specific types and sites.
  alveolar soft part, 1357, 2929
  endometrial stromal, metastatic to lung, 1407
  granulocytic, 1317, 1319, *1319*
  neurogenic, paravertebral, 2974, 2975
  pulmonary, 1346
  osteogenic. See *Osteosarcoma.*
  pulmonary artery, 1332–1333, *1333,* 1334, *1334–1336*
  sclerosing interstitial vascular. See *Epithelioid
    hemangioendothelioma.*
  soft tissue, metastatic to lung, 1409–1410
  synovial, 1355
Sarcomatoid carcinoma, pulmonary, 1116. See
    also *Carcinoma, pulmonary.*
Satellite lesions, 459
  with solitary nodule, 1139
  with tuberculoma, 825
Saturation recovery sequence, 317
Sawmill-worker's lung, 2363t. See also *Extrinsic
    allergic alveolitis.*
Saw-toothing of flow-volume curve, in
    obstructive sleep apnea, 2060, *2060*
Saxitoxin, 3062
Scalded skin syndrome, 2291–2292
Scalene lymph node, biopsy of, 374
  in sarcoidosis diagnosis, 1571
  pulmonary carcinoma metastatic to, 1172
Scalene muscles, in inspiration, 246
  spinal levels of innervation of, 3055
Scandium, pneumoconiosis due to, 2456
Scanning electron microscopy, 354–355, *355*

Scanning equalization radiography, 302–303
Scapula, anatomic variants of, 263
  congenital anomalies of, 3011, *3012*
  neoplasms of, 3030
Scar carcinoma, 1080, *1080*
Scar emphysema, 2190. See also *Chronic obstructive pulmonary disease (COPD); Emphysema.*
  COPD and, 2170
  pathologic features of, 2196–2198, *2199, 2200*
Scarring, bullae with, 508, *508*
  parenchymal, 483, *488*
  pleural, mesothelioma and, 2810
Schaumann bodies, in berylliosis, 2458
  in sarcoid granuloma, 1537, *1539*
Schistosomiasis, 1049–1052
  eosinophilic lung disease due to, 1753
  pulmonary embolism in, 1853
Schlesinger mass, for specimen angiography or bronchography, 351
Schwannoma. See also *Neurilemoma.*
  cellular form of, neurogenic sarcoma vs., 2974
  malignant, 2976
  melanocytic, 2976
  pulmonary, 1346
Scimitar syndrome. See *Hypogenetic lung syndrome.*
Scintigraphy. See *Gallium scintigraphy; Radionuclide imaging; Ventilation/perfusion scanning.*
Scleroderma, 1452, 1452t. See also *Progressive systemic sclerosis (PSS).*
Sclerosing endothelial tumor. See *Epithelioid hemangioendothelioma.*
Sclerosing epithelioid angiosarcoma. See *Epithelioid hemangioendothelioma.*
Sclerosing hemangioma, 1364–1365, *1366, 1367*
Sclerosing interstitial vascular sarcoma. See *Epithelioid hemangioendothelioma.*
Sclerosing mediastinitis, chronic, 2856–2863.
  See also *Fibrosing mediastinitis.*
  in rheumatoid disease, 1433
Sclerosing pneumocytoma, 1364–1365, *1366, 1367*
Sclerosis, diseases associated with, 1452t, 1459
  limited systemic. See *CREST syndrome.*
  progressive systemic. See *Progressive systemic sclerosis (PSS).*
Sclerotherapy, for esophageal varices, complications of, 2761, 2968
Scoliosis, 3020–3022, *3021*
  in neurofibromatosis, 691
Scrub typhus, 1020
Sea algae, airborne toxins from, 2124
  hypoventilation due to poisoning from, 3062
Sea-blue histiocytes, in Niemann-Pick disease, 2724
Secretory component, in tracheobronchial secretions, 61, 130
Secretory leukocyte proteinase inhibitor, in emphysema pathogenesis, 2182–2183, *2183*
Sedatives, obstructive sleep apnea and, 2062
  thoracic disease due to, 2539t, 2567
Sedimentation, in particle deposition, 126–127
Segmental lymph nodes, in classification for lung cancer staging, *185*, 188t, *1186*, 1187t
Seizures, pulmonary edema due to, 1974–1976
Selectin, in leukocyte–endothelial cell adherence, in adult respiratory distress syndrome, 1979
Selenium detector digital radiography, 307
Seminoma, mediastinal, 2908–2909, *2910*
  testicular, metastatic to lung, 1407
Semistarvation, ventilatory response and, 240
Semustine (methyl CCNU), thoracic disease due to, 2548
Senecio jacobae, pulmonary hypertension and, 1902

Senile emphysema, 2190n
Sensitivity, in inhalation challenge tests, 421, 422, 2095. See also *Bronchial hyperresponsiveness; Inhalation challenge tests.*
Sepsis, 1977n
  adult respiratory distress syndrome and, 1998
  pattern of pulmonary infection associated with, 713, *715*
  postanginal, 779, 1829, 1831
Sepsis syndrome, 1977n
Septal pattern. See also *Kerley lines.*
  in interstitial disease, 441–444, *442, 444–446*
Septic arthritis, of sternoclavicular and sternochondral joints in heroin addict, 3020
Septic embolism, 1829–1832
  cavities or cysts with, 3104t
  clinical features of, 1831–1832
  multiple masses or nodules due to, 3124t
  pulmonary artery aneurysm due to, 1935
  pulmonary infection due to, 716, *717*
  radiologic features of, 1830–1831, *1830–1832, 1834*
  Staphylococcus aureus pneumonia due to, 746, *747*
Septic shock, 1977n
Septic thrombophlebitis, septic pulmonary embolism with, 1830
Septum transversum, of developing diaphragm, 247–248, *247*
Sequestration, pulmonary. See *Bronchopulmonary sequestration.*
Sequestrum formation, 707, *710*. See also *Gangrene, pulmonary.*
  in angioinvasive aspergillosis, 940, *943, 944*
Sequoiosis, 2363t. See also *Extrinsic allergic alveolitis.*
Series inhomogeneity, 53
Serotonin, asthma and, 2093
  drug-induced pulmonary hypertension and, 1903
  in pulmonary hypertension pathogenesis, 1881
  pulmonary metabolism of, 131
  pulmonary vascular response to, 106
  urinary, in carcinoid syndrome diagnosis, 1242
Serous cells, in tracheobronchial glands, 14, 15, *15*
Serratia infection, 751–753
  cavitary or cystic disease in, 3102t
  homogeneous opacity in, nonsegmental, 3079t
    segmental, 3087t
  inhomogeneous opacity in, nonsegmental, 3093t
    segmental, 3097t
Serratus anterior, in inspiration, 246
  on CT, 260, *260*
Serratus posterior, on CT, 260
Sex differences, in costal cartilage calcification patterns, 261–262, *261*
Sex-linked agammaglobulinemia, infantile, 724–725
Sézary's syndrome, 1291
Shaggy heart sign, in asbestosis, 2437
Shellfish poisoning, 3062–3063
Shifting granuloma, in atelectasis, 534
Shock, adult respiratory distress syndrome and, 1979
  septic, 1977n
Shrapnel embolism, 1868
Shrinking lung syndrome, 1431, 3065
Shunt. See also *Shunting.*
  ventriculoperitoneal, pleural effusion due to migration of, 2762
Shunting, bronchial circulation and, 121
  extrapulmonary, 3067–3068
  hypoxemia due to, 114–115
  intrapulmonary, 111

Shunting *(Continued)*
  alveolar-arterial oxygen gradient and, 112
  calculation of, in ventilation/perfusion mismatch assessment, 112–113
  in adult respiratory distress syndrome, 1997
  normal chest radiographs with, 3047–3048
  ventilation/perfusion ratio and, 109, *109*
  left-to-right, alteration in lung density with, 270, *271*
    pulmonary artery aneurysm with, 1936
    pulmonary blood flow redistribution in, *1960*
    pulmonary hypertension due to, 1891–1896, *1892, 1894–1897*
  right-to-left, due to increased pulmonary vascular resistance, 398
    in cirrhosis, normal chest radiograph with, 3047–3048
Shwachman-Diamond syndrome, 727, 2312
Shwachman-Kulczycki score, 2301n
  cystic fibrosis prognosis and, 2315
Shwachman's disease, 727, 2312
Sicca syndrome, 1466
Sickle cell disease, 1832–1834
Siderosilicosis, 2453, 2454, *2454*
Siderosis, 2452–2454, *2453, 2455*
Sign of the camalote, in echinococcosis, 463, *467*, 1056, *1056*, 2753, *2754*
Signal-to-noise ratio, for pulmonary function tests, 410
Signet-ring sign, in bronchiectasis, *2274, 2275*
Silhouette sign, 478, *478, 479*
  in left upper lobe atelectasis, 543
  in right middle lobe atelectasis, 551
  with large pleural effusion, 565
Silica. See also *Silicoproteinosis; Silicosis.*
  coal workers' pneumoconiosis and, 2410
  lymph node enlargement due to, 3165t
  pulmonary carcinoma and, 1077
  silicates vs., 2449
  systemic lupus erythematosus and, 1425
  Wegener's granulomatosis and, 1492
Silicates, pneumonoconiosis due to, 2449–2452.
  See also *Asbestosis.*
  silica vs., 2449
Silicon carbide, pneumoconiosis due to, 2463–2465, *2465, 2466*
Silicon dioxide, alveolar proteinosis and, 2702
  effects of, on alveolar macrophages, 22
Silicone, embolization of, 1868–1870
  implanted, systemic lupus erythematosus and, 1425
  injected, thoracic disease due to, 2539t, 2571
Silicoproteinosis, 2391, 2392
  clinical features of, 2407
  pathologic features of, 2394, *2396*
  radiologic features of, 2402
Silicosiderosis, 2453, 2454, *2454*
Silicosis, 2390–2409
  accelerated, 2402, *2405,* 2406–2407
  clinical features of, 2406–2407
  connective tissue disease and, 2408–2409
  diagnosis of, 2407
  diffuse nodular pattern in, 3145t, *3149*
  eggshell calcification in, *452,* 474, 2402, *2403*
  emphysema in, 2405–2406, 2408
  epidemiology of, 2390–2391
  in coal miners, 2390, 2409
  laboratory findings in, 2407–2408
  multiple masses or nodules due to, 3124t, *3129*
  pathogenesis of, 2391–2392
  pathologic features of, 2392–2394, *2393–2396*
  prognosis in, 2408–2409
  pulmonary carcinoma and, 1077, 2408
  pulmonary fibrosis in. See under *Progressive massive fibrosis.*

Silicosis (Continued)
  pulmonary function tests in, 2408
  radiologic features of, 447, *452,* 453, *453,*
      2394–2406, *2397–2407*
  solitary mass due to, 3118t
  tuberculosis and, 803, 2408
Silicotic nodule, 2391
  pathologic features of, 2392, *2393, 2395*
  radiologic features of, 2394, *2397, 2398, 2400*
Silo-filler's disease, 2523, 2524
Silver, pneumoconiosis due to, 2454–2455
Simian virus 40, in polio vaccine, mesothelioma
      and, 990, 2810
Simplified bacterial index, in quantitative
      bronchoalveolar lavage, 720
Sin Nombre virus, 992
Single-breath diffusing capacity measurement,
      414–415
  in COPD, 2229
Single-breath nitrogen washout test, 413–414,
      413
  in COPD, 2121
Single-photon emission computed tomography
      (SPECT), 332
  ^{18}F-fludeoxyglucose, 332
    solitary nodule assessment on, 1146, *1147*
  in parathyroid adenoma assessment, 2914
  thallium, in pulmonary carcinoma diagnosis,
      1181
Sjögren's syndrome, 1465–1469
  bronchiolitis in, 2336, 2349
  clinical features of, 1468–1469
  laboratory findings in, 1469
  lymphoid interstitial pneumonia in, *1273*
  pathogenesis of, 1466
  pathologic features of, 1466
  primary biliary cirrhosis and, 1475
  prognosis in, 1469
  pulmonary function tests in, 1469
  radiologic features of, 1466–1468, *1467, 1468*
Skeletal muscle, sarcoidosis involving, 1565
  tuberculosis involving, 840
  Wegener's granulomatosis involving, 1504
Skin, Churg-Strauss syndrome involving, 1510
  paraneoplastic lesions of, in pulmonary carci-
      noma, 1174
  progressive systemic sclerosis involving, 1457
  sarcoidosis involving, 1564
  tuberculosis involving, 839
  Wegener's granulomatosis involving, 1504
Skin fold, pneumothorax vs., 587, *588*
Skin tests, for coccidioidomycosis, 898–899
  for histoplasmosis, 889
  for nontuberculous mycobacterial infection,
      861
  for North American blastomycosis, 902
  for South American blastomycosis, 904
  for tuberculosis, 841–843, 841t–843t
    in HIV infection, 1652–1653
  in asthma diagnosis, 2137
  in occupational asthma diagnosis, 2122
Skodaic resonance, 392
Sleep, blood gases during, in COPD, 2227
  electrical activity during, 2068
  hypoxemia during, in cystic fibrosis, 2313–
      2314
  nocturnal asthma and, 2136
  non-REM, breathing during, 2054–2055
    electrical activity during, 2068
    normal, physiologic characteristics of, 2054–
      2055
  REM, breathing during, 2055
    electrical activity during, 2068
    hypoventilation during, in COPD, 2227
  ventilatory control during, 243, 243t
Sleep apnea, central, 3052–3053

Sleep apnea (Continued)
  after cordotomy, 3051, 3052
  defined, 2054
  in rheumatoid disease, 1449
  pulmonary hypertension in, 1918, *1918*
mixed, 2054
obstructive, 2054–2070
  cause of, 2057
  central sleep apnea vs., 3052
  clinical features of, 2063–2067
  conditions associated with, 2056–2057,
      2056t
  defined, 2054
  diagnosis of, 2068–2069
  epidemiology of, 2055–2057
  genetic factors in, 2058–2059
  hormonal factors in, 2059, 2067
  in rheumatoid disease, 1449
  increased airway compliance in, 2060–2061
  neuromuscular dysfunction in, 2061–2062
  obesity hypoventilation syndrome and,
      2057, 2066, 3053
  pathogenesis of, 2057–2062, *2058*
  prognosis in, 2069–2070
  pulmonary function tests in, 2069
  pulmonary hypertension in, 1918, 2066
  radiologic features of, 2062–2063, *2064,
      2065*
  structural airway narrowing in, 2059–2060
Sleep deprivation, ventilatory control and, 243
Sleep hypopnea, 2054, 2056
Sleep spindles, 2054, 2068
Sleepiness, daytime, in obstructive sleep apnea,
      2065–2066
Slendore-Hoeppli phenomenon, 950
Sliding microtubule hypothesis of ciliary
      beating, 127
Slow acetylation, drug-induced lupus and,
      1424–1425
Slowly adapting stretch receptors, *146,* 147
  in ventilatory control, *236,* 237–238, 241
Slow-twitch oxidative fatigue-resistant fibers, in
      diaphragm, 249, 250
Small airways disease, 2188n, 2324–2327
Small airways tests, 414, 2220–2221
Small cell carcinoma. See also *Carcinoma.*
  carcinoid tumor vs., 1234, 1242
  neuroendocrine tumors and, 1229
  pulmonary, 1091–1098
    anatomic location of, 1120–1121
    combined subtype of, 1096–1097, *1097,
        1098*
    endocrinopathy with, 1175–1176, 1176–
        1177
    epidemiology of, 1072
    gross and histologic features of, 1091–1097,
        1095–1098
    hilar enlargement with, 1156, *1157*
    immunohistochemical features of, 1098
    mediastinal involvement by, 1156, *1158*
    metastases from, pulmonary, 1399
      sites of, 1172
    neuromuscular syndromes with, 1173, 1174
    paraneoplastic syndromes with, 1173
    post-therapy neurologic syndrome with,
        1172–1173
    prognosis in, 1195–1196, 1199
    small cell variant of squamous cell carci-
        noma vs., 1090
    spontaneous regression of, 1201
    staging of, 1181
      prognosis and, 1199
    superior vena cava syndrome due to, 2949,
        2950
    ultrastructural features of, 1097–1098, *1099*
  thymic, 2900, 2901

Small cell tumor of thoracopulmonary region,
      malignant, 2974, 3028
Small mucous granule cell, 8
Small nodular pattern, diffuse lung disease with,
      differential diagnosis of, 3144, 3145t,
      3146–3149
Smear, for tuberculosis diagnosis, 844–845
Smoke inhalation, 2335–2336, 2528–2531, *2529,
      2530*
  upper airway obstruction due to, 2023
Smoking, allergic occupational asthma and, 2120
  asbestosis and, 2423
  black-fat, 2500
  carboxyhemoglobin levels and, 3069
  cessation of, in COPD, 2229, *2229*
  chronic bronchiolitis associated with, *2325*
  chronic bronchitis and, pulmonary carcinoma
      risk and, 1081
  ciliary abnormalities and, 7, *8*
  COPD and, 2172–2173, *2172*
  cough and, 380
  diffusing capacity and, 416, 2229
  effects of, on alveolar macrophages, 21, 22
  emphysema and, 2183–2184, *2183*
  extrinsic allergic alveolitis and, 2364
  herpetic tracheobronchitis and, 997
  idiopathic pulmonary fibrosis and, 1586
  immunoglobulin E levels and, 2181
  in patient's history, 389
  Langerhans' cell histiocytosis and, 1627
  mortality due to, 1072
  mucociliary clearance and, 2181–2182
  mucous cell hyperplasia and, *8*
  obesity hypoventilation syndrome and, 3053
  obstructive sleep apnea and, 2057
  oxidant stress and, 2184
  passive, asthma provoked by, 2117
    asthma risk and, 2079
    COPD and, 2173
    pulmonary carcinoma and, 1073–1074
  pulmonary carcinoma and, 1072–1074
    asbestos and, 1075
    genetic factors in, 1082
  pulmonary neutrophils and, 2183–2184
  sarcoidosis and, 1537
  silicosis and, 2392
Smooth muscle, in airways. See *Airway smooth
      muscle.*
  multi-unit, 2101
  neoplasms of, 1331–1335. See also specific
      neoplasms.
  single-unit, 2100–2101
Smudge cell, in adenovirus infection, 994
Snakebite, 3063
Sniff test, in diaphragmatic motion assessment,
      2988
  in diaphragmatic paralysis diagnosis, 2992,
      2993–2994
Snoring, in obstructive sleep apnea, 2063–2065
Sodium metabisulfite, airway narrowing in
      response to, in asthma, 422
Sodium transport, in airway epithelium, 62
  in pulmonary edema prevention, 1956
Soft tissue neoplasms. See also specific
      neoplasms.
  of anterior mediastinum, 2914–2925
  of chest wall, 3025–3029, *3028–3030*
  of middle-posterior mediastinum, 3177t–3178t
Soft tissue sarcomas, metastatic to lung,
      1409–1410
Solder flux, occupational asthma due to, 2122
Solids, aspiration of, 2485–2490. See also
      Aspiration (event), of solid foreign bodies.
Solute exchange, pulmonary, 1947–1956,
      1947–1949, 1952
Solute transport equation, pulmonary fluid and
      solute exchange and, 1952–1955, *1952*

Somatostatin, pulmonary carcinoma secreting, 1177

Somatostatin receptor scintigraphy, in carcinoid tumor diagnosis, 1243

Soot, pulmonary carcinoma and, 1078

Sotalol, thoracic disease due to, 2538t, 2564

South African tick bite fever, 1022

Soy sauce–brewer's lung, 2363t. See also *Extrinsic allergic alveolitis.*

Spanish toxic oil syndrome, 1459, 2587–2588

Sparganosis, 1059

Spastic paraparesis, tropical, 991

Spatial resolution, defined, 307

SPECT. See *Single-photon emission computed tomography (SPECT).*

Speech, ventilatory control during, 239

Sphingomyelinase deficiency, in Niemann-Pick disease, 2724

Spiculation, in pulmonary nodule margin, 457–459, *458*

Spinal cord, injury to, cervical, rib notching in, 3015

ischemic, with bronchial arteriography, 325

lesions of, hypoventilation due to, 3055

pulmonary carcinoma metastatic to, 1172

Spindle cell carcinoma, pulmonary, 1114. See also *Carcinoma, pulmonary.*

Spindle cell pseudotumor, in postprimary tuberculosis, 812

Spine, cervical, rheumatoid disease involving, 1449

chest wall pain due to disease of, 387

pulmonary carcinoma involving, 1166, *1167*

stabilization of, metallic implant migration after, 2652

thoracic, abnormalities of, 3020–3023, *3021, 3024, 3025*

fractures of, 2646, *2646,* 3023

paravertebral mass due to, 3185t

signs resembling aortic rupture in, 2626–2627

imaging of, 263–264

neoplasms of, 3031–3032

tuberculosis of, 837, *838,* 3023, *3025*

Spin-echo sequence, 319, *320*

Spin-lattice (T1) relaxation time, 317, *318, 319*

Spinnability, in respiratory mucus, 62

Spin-spin (T2) relaxation time, 317, *318–320*

Spiral computed tomography, 310–311, *310, 311.* See also *Computed tomography (CT).*

emphysema quantification using, 2214, *2214*

with minimum intensity projection, in emphysema, 2211, *2211*

Spirometry. See also *Pulmonary function tests; specific parameters.*

electronic, 409

Spleen, calcifications in, in histoplasmosis vs. tuberculosis distinction, 811

rupture of, pleural effusion with, 2762, *2763*

sarcoidosis involving, 1563, 1565

tuberculosis involving, 811, 840

Splenomegaly, in infectious mononucleosis, 1008

Splenosis, thoracic, 2840

with diaphragmatic rupture, 2643–2644, *2645*

Split pleura sign, 579, *579*

Spokewheel nodule, 438

Spoligotyping, in tuberculosis epidemiologic investigation, 846

Spondylitis, ankylosing, 3022–3023

infectious, 3023, *3024, 3025*

suppurative, paravertebral mass due to, 3185t

tuberculous, 837, *838,* 3023, *3025*

paravertebral mass due to, 3185t, *3186*

Sponge, retained, 2664, 2672, *2674*

Sporotrichosis, 949–950

Spotted fever, Mediterranean, 1022

Rocky Mountain, 1020–1022

Sprengel's deformity, 3011, *3012*

omovertebral bones with, 262, *263*

Sputum, collection of, 339–340, 843

culture of, for pneumonia diagnosis, 719

for tuberculosis diagnosis, 845

in HIV infection, 1653

cytologic examination of, 339–342, *342*

in *Pneumocystis carinii* pneumonia diagnosis, 1668

in pulmonary carcinoma diagnosis, 1179

in pulmonary metastasis diagnosis, 1412

in tuberculosis diagnosis, 844, 846

in HIV infection, 1653

specimen processing for, 340

defined, 60

in amebiasis, 1035, 2753

in asthma, 2093, 2136

ciliary inhibitory compound in, 2094

in *Klebsiella pneumoniae* infection, 753

malignant cells in, primary lung cancer vs. upper airway cancer metastasis as source of, 1202

purulent, physical characteristics of, 63

saliva vs., 380

viscosity of, in cystic fibrosis, 2301

Squames, intravascular, with amniotic fluid embolism, 1852, 1853

Squamous cell carcinoma. See also *Carcinoma.*

cervical, metastatic to thoracic skeleton, *3038*

oropharyngeal, metastatic to trachea, *2041*

pleural, 2838

pulmonary, 1085–1091

anatomic location of, 1120–1121

calcification in, 467

cavitation in, *1091, 1148, 1149, 3108*

epidemiology of, 1072

gross and histologic features of, 1085–1091, *1087–1093*

homogeneous segmental opacity in, *3090*

immunohistochemical features of, 1091

metastases from, sites of, 1172

multiple primary, 1201

prognosis in, 1195

small cell variant of, 1090

ultrastructural features of, 1091, *1094*

tracheal, 2036, *2037*

Stab wound, 2648, *2651, 2653*

Stannosis, 2455–2456

Staphylococcus aureus infection, 743–748

cavities or cysts in, 3102t, *3105*

clinical features of, 746

community-acquired, 721–722

diagnosis of, 746

empyema with hemothorax due to, 2761

epidemiology of, 743–744

extrapulmonary, septic pulmonary embolism with, *717*

hospital-acquired, 723

in HIV disease, 1645

in influenza, 982, 983–984

methicillin-resistant, 744

multiple bacteremic abscesses in, *3125*

of thoracic spine, *3024*

parapneumonic effusion with, 2747–2748, *2751*

pathogenesis of, 744

pathologic findings in, 744–745, *745*

prognosis in, 746–748

radiologic features of, *708, 709,* 745–746, *745–747*

segmental opacity in, homogeneous, 3087t, *3089*

inhomogeneous, 3097t

Staphylococcus cohnii pneumonia, 748

Starch embolism, 1857–1861

pathologic features of, 1858

Starch-spray lung, 2363t. See also *Extrinsic allergic alveolitis.*

Starling equation, pulmonary fluid and solute exchange and, 1952–1955, *1952*

Starvation, ventilatory response and, 240

Static maneuvers, in pulmonary function testing, 410–411

Steady-state method, for diffusing capacity measurement, 415

for ventilatory response assessment, 418, *418*

Stenotrophomonas maltophilia infection, 764

Stents, airway, complications of, 2674

vascular, complications of, 2674

Sternochondral joints, septic arthritis of, in heroin addict, 3020

Sternoclavicular joints, dislocation of, 2645–2646

septic arthritis of, in heroin addict, 3020

tuberculosis involving, 837–838

Sternocleidomastoid muscle, in inspiration, 246

on radiographs, 259

spinal levels of innervation of, 3055

Sternocostoclavicular hyperostosis, 3020

Sternotomy, complications of, 2660–2661, *2660*

infection after, 3019–3020, *3019*

Sternum, abnormalities of, 3018–3020, *3018, 3019*

imaging of, 264

metastasis to, 3031, *3037*

multiple myeloma involving, *3037*

neoplasms of, 3030, 3031

tuberculosis involving, 837–838

Steroids. See also *Corticosteroids.*

anabolic, pulmonary peliosis due to, 2571

Stevens-Johnson syndrome, 1014

Stipatosis, 2363t. See also *Extrinsic allergic alveolitis.*

Stoma(ta), of parietal pleura, 172, *173*

Stomach. See also *Gastric* entries; *Gastrointestinal tract.*

leiomyosarcoma of, with pulmonary chondroma, 1344

volvulus of, with diaphragmatic paralysis, 2990

with hiatus hernia, 2996, *3001*

Stomatococcus mucilaginosus pneumonia, 748

Storage phosphor radiography, 306–307, *308*

Strahler system for describing airway geometry, 3–4, *4*

Straight back syndrome, 3023

Streptococcal pneumonia, 736–743, 748. See also *Streptococcus pneumoniae pneumonia.*

in influenza, 982, 983–984

Streptococcus agalactiae infection, 748

Streptococcus faecalis (Enterococcus faecalis) infection, 748

Streptococcus milleri infection, 748

Streptococcus pneumoniae pneumonia, 736–742

cavities or cysts in, 3102t

clinical diagnosis of, 702

clinical features of, 741

community-acquired, 721

in HIV-infected persons, 722

complications of, 739–741

consolidation in, *435, 436, 437, 457, 703*

homogeneous nonsegmental, 3079t, *3082*

homogeneous segmental, 3087t

inhomogeneous segmental, 3097t

diagnosis of, 741

drug-resistant, 736

epidemiology of, 736

healing pattern in, 703

in HIV infection, 742, 1645

laboratory findings in, 741

Streptococcus pneumoniae pneumonia
(Continued)
pathogenesis of, 736–737
pathologic features of, 737, *738*
pleural effusion with, 2747
prognosis in, 741–742
radiologic features of, 459, *704*, 737–741,
739, 740
Streptococcus pyogenes pneumonia, 742–743,
743
segmental opacity in, homogeneous, 3087t
inhomogeneous, 3097t
Streptococcus viridans infection, 748
Streptokinase, intrapleural instillation of, adverse
reaction to, 2571
Stress failure, in pulmonary capillaries, high-
altitude pulmonary edema and, 2000
Stretch receptors, in compensation for increased
ventilatory load, 242
rapidly adapting. See *Irritant receptors.*
slowly adapting, *146,* 147
in ventilatory control, *236,* 237–238, 241
Stretched pore theory, 1949–1950
Stridor, 395
psychogenic, 2032–2033
Stroke, alveolar hypoventilation due to, 3051
central sleep apnea after, 3053
obstructive sleep apnea and, 2067
Strongyloidiasis, 1040–1043, *1041, 1042,* 1752
homogeneous nonsegmental opacity in, 3080t
in HIV infection, 1675
Subacinar nodule, 438
Subacute cerebellar degeneration, paraneoplastic,
in pulmonary carcinoma, 1174
Subacute necrotizing encephalomyelopathy,
central apnea with, 3052
Subaortic lymph nodes, in classification for lung
cancer staging, *185,* 188t, *1186,* 1187t
Subarachnoid-pleural fistula, pleural effusion due
to, 2762
Subcarinal angle, measurement of, 35
Subcarinal lymph nodes, in ATS classification,
184t, *185, 186*
in classification for lung cancer staging, *185,*
188t, *1186,* 1187t
in Hodgkin's disease, 1299, *1301*
Subclavian artery, left, 208–209, *208*
aberrant, 2961
right, aberrant, 209, *209,* 2961, *2963–2965*
Subclavian catheter, complications of,
2682–2684, 2686
Subclavian vein, compression of, with upper arm
abduction, 3013
Subcostal muscles, on CT, 260, *261*
Suberosis, 2363t, 2378. See also *Extrinsic
allergic alveolitis.*
Submaxillary gland, adenoid cystic carcinoma
of, metastatic to lung, *1388*
Submesothelial fibroma. See *Fibrous tumor of
pleura, solitary.*
Submucosa, of conducting airways, 12–17
Subphrenic abscess, in amebiasis, 1034
pleural effusion with, 2766
postoperative, 2672–2674
Subpleural curvilinear opacities, in dependent
atelectasis, 519
Subpleural dependent density, 287–290, *291*
on expiratory scans, 291, *291, 292*
Subpleural fibroma. See *Fibrous tumor of
pleura, solitary.*
Subpleural lines, in dependent atelectasis, 519
Subpulmonic effusion. See *Pleural effusion,
subpulmonary.*
Subsegmental lymph nodes, in classification for
lung cancer staging, *185,* 188t, *1186,* 1187t
Substance P, actions of, in lung, 131

Substance P *(Continued)*
in asthmatic airway inflammation, 2092
Sucralfate, aspiration of, 2512
Sudden infant death syndrome, obstructive sleep
apnea and, 2067
Sulfadoxine-pyrimethamine, thoracic disease due
to, 2558
Sulfasalazine, thoracic disease due to, 2538t,
2557
Sulfhemoglobinemia, cyanosis in, 398
Sulfonamides, thoracic disease due to, 2538t,
2558
Sulfur colloid, technetium-labeled, for ventilation
imaging, 330
Sulfur dioxide, acute exposure to, 2524, *2525*
atmospheric, asthma and, 2114–2115
from metabisulfite, asthma provoked by, 2116
Sulfur granules, in actinomycosis, 952–953, *953*
Sulfuric acid, acute exposure to, 2524, *2525*
Sulindac, thoracic disease due to, 2539t, 2565
Superior accessory fissure, 165, *166*
Superior esophageal stripes, 211, 223, *226*
Superior hemiazygos vein, 218
Superior intercostal vein, left, 209–211, *209–211*
dilation of, 2951, *2953*
Superior pulmonary sulcus tumor. See *Pancoast
tumor.*
Superior recess(es), of anterior mediastinum,
202, *204*
of posterior mediastinum, 223, *225*
Superior vena cava, dilation of, 2946–2949,
2947, 2948, 3178t
left, 2947–2949
obstruction of, by mediastinal histoplasmosis,
886, *887*
by mediastinal lymphoma, 1292, *1295*
Superior vena cava syndrome, *2948,* 2949–2950,
2949t, *2950*
in fibrosing mediastinitis, 2860, 2863, *2863*
with pulmonary carcinoma, 1171, 2949, 2950,
2950
Superoxide dismutase, in defense against oxidant
damage, 2521
Supersensitivity of smooth muscle cells,
prejunctional vs. postjunctional, 2100
Supra-aortic area, 197, 205–211, *208–211*
Supra-aortic triangle, 207
Supra-azygos area, 197, 218–228, *218–222,
224–231*
Supraclavicular fossa, 259
Supraclavicular lymph nodes, in ATS
classification, 184t
Suprasternal fossa, 259
Suprasternal space, 198
Surface tension, elastic recoil of lung and, 54–58
Surfactant, *20,* 56–58, *57*
adhesive atelectasis and, 522
disorders of metabolism of, 58
in adult respiratory distress syndrome, 1980–
1981
in alveolar proteinosis, 2702–2703
in extrinsic allergic alveolitis, 2364
in mucus, mucociliary clearance and, 129
in neonatal lungs, 57, 58
in reperfusion injury, 1701
Surfactant protein B, 56–57
inherited deficiency of, alveolar proteinosis in,
2701–2702
Surgery. See also specific procedures.
abdominal, pleural effusion after, 2763–2764,
2766
pulmonary complications in, 2672, 2674
adhesive atelectasis after, homogeneous segmental opacity in, 3088t
cardiac, atelectasis after, 522, *2670,* 2671
chylothorax after, 2769

Surgery *(Continued)*
pleural effusion after, 2762, 2766
pulmonary edema after, 2671
chylothorax due to, 2768–2769
diaphragmatic dysfunction after, 2995
nonthoracic, complications of, 2672–2674
pleural effusion after, 2761–2762
thoracic, complications of, 2659–2672
involving diaphragm, 2669
involving lungs, 2669–2672, *2669, 2670,
2672–2674*
involving mediastinum, 2663–2669,
2664, 2666–2668
involving pleura, 2661–2663, *2661, 2663*
involving soft tissues of chest wall,
2659–2660
involving thoracic cage, 2660–2661, *2660*
nonresectional, risk factors for pulmonary
complications in, 2672
thoracoscopic, 371–372
Surgical flaps, CT appearance of, 2665
Swan-Ganz catheter, complications of,
2685–2690, *2688, 2689*
cytologic examination of material aspirated
from, 348
pleural effusion due to, 2762
Sweat, in cystic fibrosis, 2300
Sweat test, 2312–2313
Sweet's syndrome, 1320
Swine confinement areas, 2379
COPD and, 2175
Swyer-James syndrome, 2337–2343
bronchiectasis in, 2267
clinical features of, 2343
oligemia with, 3157t, *3161*
pathogenesis of, 2337
pathologic features of, 2337
proximal interruption of pulmonary artery vs.,
504, 638, 2337
pulmonary hypoplasia vs., 601
radiologic features of, *271,* 503, *504, 505,*
2337–2343, *2338–2342*
Sympathetic nervous system, defined, 145
in pulmonary innervation, 145, *146*
tumors arising in ganglia of, in paravertebral
region, 2976–2978, *2977, 2978*
Sympathomimetic drugs. See also specific drugs.
thoracic disease due to, 2539t, 2566
Syncope, cough, 382
Syndrome of inappropriate secretion of
antidiuretic hormone, paraneoplastic, in
pulmonary carcinoma, 1176–1177
Syngamosis, 1046
Synovial sarcoma, 1355, 2929
Syphilis, 777–778
aortic involvement in, 2943
pulmonary artery aneurysm in, 1935
Syringomyelia, 3056
Systemic disease, in patient's history, 390–391
Systemic inflammatory response syndrome,
1977n
adult respiratory distress syndrome and, 1977
Systemic lupus erythematosus (SLE), 1422–1432
autoantibodies in, 1422–1423
clinical features of, 1422t, 1429–1432, 1429t
CREST syndrome with, pulmonary hypertension in, pathologic features of, *1454*
drug-induced, 1424–1425
clinical features of, 1432
pleural effusion in, 2756t
epidemiology of, 1422
hypoventilation in, 3065
pathogenesis of, 1423–1425
pathologic features of, 1425–1426, *1426*
pleural effusion in, 2745t, 2753
polymyositis with, pathologic features of,
1464

Systemic lupus erythematosus (SLE) *(Continued)*
  prognosis in, 1432
  pulmonary function tests in, 1432
  pulmonary hypertension in, 1912, *1913*
  radiologic features of, 1426–1429, *1426–1428*
    time of appearance of, 1427–1429, 3046
  tuberculosis and, 803, 1432
Systemic–pulmonary vascular fistula, 666–667,
    667, 668
  with chest tube, 2677

T lymphocytes, CD4+, *Pneumocystis carinii*
    pneumonia and, 910
  in asthmatic airway inflammation, 2089
  in host response to neoplasia, 1084
  in idiopathic pulmonary fibrosis, 1590
  in pulmonary defense, 131
  in sarcoidosis, 1536–1537
  sensitized to PPD, in tuberculous pleural effu-
    sion, 2745
T lymphocytopenia, CD4+, idiopathic, 727–728
T1 relaxation time, 317, *318, 319*
T1-weighted sequences, 319, *320, 321*
T2 relaxation time, 317, *318–320*
T2-weighted images, 319–320, *321*
Tachykinins, 145–146
Taconite, pneumoconiosis due to, 2452
Tactile fremitus, 392
Taenia solium infestation, 1059, *1060*
Tail sign, 483, *487*
  with solitary nodule, 1139, *1140–1141*
Takayasu's arteritis, 1513–1517, 1515t, *1516,*
    1517
  defined, 1490t
  rib notching in, 3015
Talc. See also *Talcosis.*
  intrapleural instillation of, adverse reaction to,
    2571
  pleural calcification and, 583
Talcosis, 2449–2450, *2450, 2451*
  cicatrization atelectasis due to, *528*
  emphysema in, 2243
  intravenous, 1857–1861
    clinical features of, 1860–1861
    multiple masses or nodules due to, 3124t
    nodular pattern in, 447, *451,* 1858, *1861,*
      1863, 3145t
    pathogenesis of, 1858
    pathologic features of, 1858, *1859, 1860*
    radiologic features of, 1858–1860, *1861–*
      1864
  solitary mass due to, 3118t
Tamoxifen, thoracic disease due to, 2538t, 2551
Tapeworms, 1053–1059. See also specific
    diseases.
Tardive dyskinesia, respiratory dyskinesia in,
    3052
Target lesion, in histoplasmosis, 881, *883*
Target sign, with septic embolism, 1830
Tartrazine, asthma provoked by, 2116
Technetium 99m, in parathyroid adenoma
    assessment, 2914
  in perfusion scanning, 326–327, 1800
  in ventilation imaging, 329–330
Teflon (polytetrafluoroethylene), embolization of,
    1870
  poisoning by, 2528
Telangiectasia, hereditary hemorrhagic,
    pulmonary arteriovenous malformations in,
    657, *659,* 661, *661, 3113*
Temporal arteritis, 1517–1518, *1518*
  defined, 1490t
Temporomandibular joint, rheumatoid disease
    involving, 1449

Tension-time index, in respiratory muscle fatigue
    prediction, 257, 257n, 420, 2219–2220,
    3057
Teratoma, 2903–2908
  clinical features of, 2906–2907
  complications of, 2906
  cystic, 2903–2906, *2907–2909*
    anterior mediastinal mass due to, *3174*
    of diaphragm, *3005*
    rupture of, 2906–2907
  growing, 2902
  immature, 2903, *2905*
    prognosis with, 2907
  mature, anterior mediastinal mass due to, *3174*
    clinical features of, 2906–2907
    pathologic features of, 2903, *2904*
    prognosis with, 2907
    radiologic features of, 2903–2906, *2906,*
      2907
  pathologic features of, 2903, *2904, 2905*
  prognosis with, 2907–2908
  pulmonary, 1365–1367, *1368*
  radiologic features of, 2903–2906, *2906–2909*
  with malignant transformation, pathologic fea-
    tures of, 2903, *2905*
    prognosis with, 2908
Terbutaline, thoracic disease due to, 2566
Testicular germ cell tumor, metastatic to lung,
    1383, 1406, 1407, *1407*
Testosterone, obstructive sleep apnea and, 2059,
    2067
Tetanus, 3054–3055, *3056*
Tetracaine, antibacterial activity of, 367
Tetracycline, thoracic disease due to, 2538t,
    2558
Tetralogy of Fallot, decreased pulmonary blood
    flow with, 500, 665, 3151t
  rib notching with, 3015, *3016*
  systemic arterial supply to the lung in, *668*
  total anomalous pulmonary venous drainage
    with, 653
Tetrodotoxin, 3063
Thallium poisoning, 2587
Thallium scintigraphy, in HIV-infected patient,
    332
  in Kaposi's sarcoma diagnosis, 1679
  with SPECT technique, in pulmonary carci-
    noma, 1181
Thermistor, respiratory air flow measurement
    using, 2068
Thesaurosis, 2531
Thixotropy, in respiratory mucus, 62
Thoracentesis, 373
  chest wall swelling after, 2741, *2742*
  complications of, 2743
  diagnostic, 2743
  pulmonary edema after, *1968,* 2001–2002,
    2002
  pulmonary function after, 2741
Thoracic duct, 175
  neoplasm involving, chylothorax due to, 2768,
    2769
  rupture of, 2634–2636
    chylothorax due to, 2768–2769
  smooth muscle proliferation in, in lymphangio-
    leiomyomatosis, 683
Thoracic duct cyst, 2945
Thoracic inlet, 197–198, *197–199*
Thoracic inlet tumor. See *Pancoast tumor.*
Thoracic outlet syndrome, 3013, *3013*
Thoracic spine. See under *Spine.*
Thoracic surgery. See *Surgery;* specific
    procedures.
Thoracoabdominal paradox, in bilateral
    diaphragmatic paralysis, 2994, *2996–2997*
Thoracobiliary fistula, with diaphragmatic
    rupture, 2643

Thoracoplasty, complications of, 2675
  for tuberculosis, 814
    complications of, 818, *824*
  pulmonary hypertension with, 1918
Thoracoscopy, 371–372
Thoracostomy, tube, complications of,
    2676–2677, *2677–2679*
Thoracotomy, fine-needle aspiration during, 348
  in pleural effusion diagnosis, 2743
  open lung biopsy using, 372
  pleural fluid accumulation after, 2661, *2661,*
    2761–2762
  rib abnormalities after, 2660
Thresher's lung. See *Extrinsic allergic alveolitis;*
    Farmer's lung.
Thrombocytopenia, autoantibodies associated
    with, 1423
  in adult respiratory distress syndrome, 1982
  in pulmonary carcinoma, 1178
Thrombocytosis, in pulmonary carcinoma, 1178
  venous thrombosis risk in, 1780
Thromboembolism, pulmonary, 1775–1828
  acute, CT findings in, 1808–1811, *1809,*
    1810, 1813–1815
  autoantibodies associated with, 1423
  chronic, angiographic findings in, 1819,
    1823
    cor pulmonale with, *1822–1823*
    CT findings in, 1811–1813, *1812, 1815*
    proximal interruption of pulmonary artery
      vs., 638
  clinical features of, 1824–1826
  consequences of, 1780–1783
  CT in, 1807–1813
    parenchymal findings on, 1811–1813,
      1813–1815
    technique for, 1808
    vascular findings on, 1808–1811, *1809,*
      1810, 1812
  diagnosis of, recommendations for, 1824
  electrocardiographic changes in, 1827–1828
  embolus degradation in, 1783–1785, *1787–*
    1789
  epidemiology of, 1775, 1776–1777
  in pulmonary carcinoma, 1177–1178
  intracavitary loose body with, 1830, *1833*
  laboratory findings in, 1826–1827
  linear opacities on postoperative radiograph
    and, *559,* 560
  massive, clinical features of, 1825
  metastatic pulmonary carcinoma mimicking,
    1821
  microscopic, 1828–1829
  MRI in, 1813–1814, *1816*
  oligemia due to, diffuse, 501–502, *501,*
    502, 1788, *1793*
    local, 504, *506,* 1787–1788, *1792,* 3157t
  pathogenesis of, 1777–1783
  pathologic features of, 1783–1786, *1784–*
    1791
  pleural effusion due to, 2745t, 2760
  postmortem identification of, 1785, *1790,*
    1791
  prognosis in, 1828
  pulmonary angiography in, 324, *324,* 1814–
    1819
    complications of, 1816–1818, *1818*
    criteria for, 1818–1819, 1819t, *1823*
    technique for, 1814–1816, *1817, 1818*
  pulmonary artery pressure measurement in,
    1819
  pulmonary function tests in, 1827
  pulmonary hypertension with. See *Pulmo-*
    nary hypertension, with thrombosis and
    thromboembolism.
  radiologic features of, 1786–1799, *1792–*
    1801

Thromboembolism *(Continued)*
  diagnostic accuracy of, 1799
    time of appearance of, 3046
  segmental opacity in, homogeneous, 3088t, *3091*
    inhomogeneous, 3098t
  septic. See *Septic embolism.*
  ventilation/perfusion scanning in, *328–329,* 330–331, 1800–1807
    diagnostic accuracy of, 330t, 1804–1807, 1806t
    diagnostic criteria for, 1802–1804, *1802–1804,* 1805t
    technique for, 1800–1802
  with infarction or hemorrhage, radiologic features of, 1794–1799, *1795–1801*
  without infarction or hemorrhage, radiologic features of, 1787–1794, *1792–1795*
  pulmonary filtering in, 132
Thrombomodulin, in venous thrombosis development, 1778
Thrombophlebitis, migratory, in pulmonary carcinoma, 1177
  septic, septic pulmonary embolism with, 1830
Thrombosis, calf vein, clinical value of assessment of, 1820
  cerebral venous, in pulmonary carcinoma, 1177
  deep vein, clinical features of, 1826
    diagnosis of, 1819–1824
    epidemiology of, 1775–1776
    in pulmonary carcinoma, 1177–1178
    pathogenesis of, 1777–1780
  in situ pulmonary, 1773–1775
    after liver transplantation, 1734, *1734*
    in Behçet's disease, 1519–1520, *1520*
    in sickle cell disease, 1833–1834
    pulmonary hypertension with. See *Pulmonary hypertension, with thrombosis and thromboembolism.*
  of pulmonary artery stump after pneumonectomy, 2672, *2674*
  paraneoplastic, in pulmonary carcinoma, 1177–1178
  recurrent, 1779
  venous, autoantibodies associated with, 1423
    in Behçet's disease, 1520, *1520*
    with cardiac pacemaker, 2690, *2690*
    with central venous catheter, 2682–2683
Thromboxane, in adult respiratory distress syndrome pathogenesis, 1983
  in pulmonary hypertension pathogenesis, 1881
Thunderstorms, asthma provoked by, 2105–2106, 2117
Thymic cyst, 2882, *2883–2885,* 3171t
  after radiation therapy for Hodgkin's disease, 2604
Thymic notch sign, 200
Thymic wave sign, 200, *202*
Thymolipoma, 2880–2882, *2881, 2882,* 3171t
Thymoma, 2884–2897
  anterior mediastinal mass due to, 3171t, *3176*
  atypical, 2897
  classification of, 2886, *2887–2891*
  clinical features of, 2894–2896
  immunodeficiency with, 726
  paraneoplastic syndromes with, 2894–2896, 2897
  pathologic features of, 2884–2886, *2885, 2887–2891*
  pleural involvement by, 2886–2891, *2894*
  pleural tumors resembling, 2838
  prognosis in, 2896–2897
  pulmonary, 1369–1370
  radiologic features of, 2886–2894, *2892–2895*
  staging of, 2896, 2896t

Thymoma *(Continued)*
  thymic carcinoma vs., 2898
  thymic cyst and, 2882
Thymus, anatomy of, 198–200, *200, 201*
  carcinoma of, 2897–2899, *2898, 2899*
    anterior mediastinal mass due to, 3171t
  Hodgkin's disease of, 1302
  hyperplasia of, 2877, *2878, 2879*
    follicular (lymphoid), 2877–2880, *2880*
    rebound, 2877, *2879*
  imaging of, 200–201, *200, 202–204*
  indications for CT assessment of, 314
  inflammatory conditions causing enlargement of, 2884
  measurement of, on CT scan, 2877, *2879*
  neuroendocrine neoplasms of, 2899–2901, *2900, 2901*
  size variation in, stress and, 201
  tumors and tumor-like conditions of, 2877–2901. See also specific tumors and conditions.
    anterior mediastinal mass due to, 3171t, *3174*
Thyroid, carcinoma of, 2913
  metastatic, calcification in, 467
    in chest wall, *3035*
    in lung, 1405–1407
  upper airway obstruction due to, 2031–2032, *2032*
  tuberculosis involving, 840
  tumors of, 2912–2913, *2912, 2913*
    anterior mediastinal mass due to, 3171t
    middle-posterior mediastinal mass due to, 3177t
Thyroid acropachy, 396
Thyroid scintigraphy, in goiter diagnosis, 2913
Thyroiditis, Riedel's, fibrosing mediastinitis with, 2857, 2861, *2864*
  upper airway obstruction due to, 2031, *2031*
Tick bite, 3063
Tick typhus, African, 1022
Tidal volume (V_T), 406, *406*
  clinical use of, 406–407
Tietze's syndrome, 387, 3017
Tight junctions, in alveolar epithelium, 18, *18, 76,* 1949, *1949*
  in pulmonary capillary endothelium, 76, *76,* 1949, *1949*
Time constant of lung unit, 412n
  regional, gravity and, 111
Tin, pneumoconiosis due to, 2455–2456
Tissue resistance, in work of breathing, 59
Titanium dioxide, pneumoconiosis due to, 2465–2466, *2467*
Titanium dust exposure, alveolar proteinosis and, 2702
TNM classification system, for pulmonary carcinoma staging, 1181, 1182t
  M assessment in, 1191–1193, *1192*
  N assessment in, 1183–1191, *1186,* 1187t, *1188, 1189*
  prognosis and, 1198–1199, 1198t, *1199*
  T assessment in, 1182–1183, *1183–1185*
Tobacco. See *Smoking.*
Tobacco-worker's lung, 2363t. See also *Extrinsic allergic alveolitis.*
Tocainide, thoracic disease due to, 2538t, 2564
Togaviruses, 993–994
Tokyo-Yokohama asthma, 2114
Tolfenamic acid, thoracic disease due to, 2539t, 2565
Toluene diisocyanate, allergic alveolitis associated with, 2362t, 2378. See also *Extrinsic allergic alveolitis.*
  occupational asthma due to, 2121–2122
Tomography, computed. See *Computed tomography (CT).*

Tomography *(Continued)*
  conventional, 309
  positron emission. See *Positron emission tomography (PET).*
Tonsil(s), hypertrophy of, upper airway obstruction due to, 2030
Tonsillitis, acute, upper airway obstruction due to, 2021
Torsion, of lung or lobe, 2622–2623, *2624*
  after transplantation, 1724, *1725*
  postoperative, 2671–2672, *2673*
Total lung capacity (TLC), 406, *406*
  in COPD, 2224–2225
  measurement of, 407–408
  radiologic estimation of, 308–309
Toxaphene, 2587
Toxic epidermal necrolysis, 2291–2292
Toxic oil syndrome, 1459, 2587–2588
Toxins, 2584–2589. See also specific toxins.
  bronchiectasis due to, 2267
  inhalation of, acute bronchiolitis due to, 2335–2336
  pulmonary hypertension due to, 1902–1903
Toxocariasis, 1045–1046, 1753
Toxoplasmosis, 1036–1038, *1037, 1038*
  in HIV infection, 1675
Trachea. See also *Airway(s).*
  cartilage plates of, 12
    calcification of, 474, *476*
    development and growth of, 136
  descent of, during inspiration, in COPD, 2216
  deviation of, in aortic rupture, 2628, *2630*
  epithelium of, 5–12, *7, 11*
    response of, to injury, 9
  imaging of, 33–35, *34*
    on conventional radiographs, 211, 1251, *1252*
    interfaces of, in supra-azygos area, 219–223, *219–222*
  measurement of, 33–35, 2033
  metastasis to, 1398–1399, *1403,* 2036, *2040, 2041*
  morphology of, 5–17, *7, 11*
    postnatal changes in, 139
  neoplasms of, 2942. See also specific neoplasms.
    middle-posterior mediastinal mass due to, 3177t, *3180*
    upper airway obstruction due to, 2035–2036, *2037–2041*
  pressure/area behavior of, 34–35, *34*
  saber-sheath, 2036–2040, *2042, 2043*
  smooth muscle of, 13–14
  stenosis of, 2033–2035, *2034–2036*
    anomalous origin of left pulmonary artery with, 642
    congenital, 618
    in relapsing polychondritis, 1471
  trauma to, blunt, fracture due to, 2618–2622
    penetrating, 2653
    with endotracheal intubation, 2681
  tuberculosis involving, 831, *837*
Tracheal bifurcation lymph nodes, 179, *182*
Tracheal bronchus, 35, 626, *627*
Tracheal diverticulosis, 2047
Tracheal index, in saber-sheath trachea, 2036, *2043*
Tracheal stripe, posterior, 220–223, *221–222*
Tracheitis, 701, *701*
  acute bacterial, upper airway obstruction due to, 2021
  herpes simplex, *997*
Tracheitis chronica ossificans, 474, 2042, *2046*
Tracheobronchial glands, 14–16, *15*
  development of, 137
  hyperplasia of, in airway disease, 15–16

Tracheobronchial glands (*Continued*)
  in COPD, 2186–2187, *2187*
  in IgA production, 130
  neoplasms of, 1251–1259. See also specific
      tumors.
    general characteristics of, 1251–1253, *1252*
Tracheobronchial lymph nodes, 179–180,
    181–184
  in ATS classification, 184t, *185, 187*
Tracheobronchial melanoma, 1267
Tracheobronchial papilloma, 1262–1265,
    1262–1266
Tracheobronchial polyps, inflammatory, 1371
Tracheobronchial receptors, in respiratory
    control, *3050, 3051*
Tracheobronchial secretions, biochemical
    characteristics of, 60–61
  control of, 61–62
  defined, 60
  immunoglobulins in, 130–131
  nonbronchoscopic techniques for sampling of,
      in pneumonia diagnosis, 720–721
  physical characteristics of, 62–63
    cough effectiveness and, 130
  prenatal, 137
Tracheobronchial tree. See *Airway(s); Bronchial
    tree.*
Tracheobronchitis, acute pseudomembranous, in
    invasive aspergillosis, 701, *701*, 944, *946*,
    2022
  herpetic, 997, *998–999*
Tracheobronchomalacia, 2042–2046
  due to tracheostomy, *2034, 2035*
Tracheobronchomegaly. See *Mounier-Kuhn
    syndrome.*
Tracheobronchopathia osteochondroplastica, 474,
    2042, *2046*
Tracheoesophageal fistula, acquired, 2967
  congenital, 627–628, 2500
Tracheoesophageal septum, formation of, 136
Tracheoesophageal stripe, 221–223, *222*
Tracheomalacia, 2042–2046
  due to tracheostomy, *2034, 2035*
Tracheo-osteoma, 474, 2042, *2046*
Tracheopathia osteoplastica, 474, 2042, *2046*
Tracheostomy, complications of, 2674
  faulty placement of tube in, upper airway ob-
      struction due to, *2025*
  tracheal stenosis due to, 2033–2035, *2034,
      2036*
  tracheobronchial papillomas and, *1252*, 1262
Traction bronchiectasis, 2267. See also
    Bronchiectasis.
  in pulmonary fibrosis, 1591, 1599, *1600, 2271*
Traction bronchiectasis and bronchiolectasis,
    525, *526*
Traction diverticulum, 2966
Training, athletic, ventilatory response and,
    240–241
  of respiratory muscles, to increase strength
      and endurance, 259
Tram tracks, 483, *485*
  in bronchiectasis, *482*, 483, *2272, 2272, 2273*
  in chronic bronchitis, 2199, 2203
Transbronchial biopsy. See under *Biopsy.*
Transbronchial needle aspiration, 347–348
  in sarcoidosis diagnosis, 1571
Transcobalamin II deficiency, 726
Transdiaphragmatic pressure measurement, in
    diaphragmatic weakness detection, 3061
  in respiratory fatigue detection, 258
  in respiratory muscle performance assessment,
    419–420
Transfusions, pulmonary edema with, 2003
Transhilar-thoracic ratio, as indicator of
    pulmonary artery pressure, in diffuse
    interstitial disease, 1917

Transitional zone of lungs, 3, 17
Transmission electron microscopy, 351–354, *355*
Transmural pressure, of pulmonary vessels, 104
Transplantation, 1698–1734
  bone marrow. See *Bone marrow transplanta-
      tion.*
  bronchiolitis after, *2332, 2336–2337*
  heart-lung. See *Heart-lung transplantation.*
  liver, 1732–1734, *1734*
    pleural effusion after, 2764
    pulmonary edema after, 1974
  lung. See *Lung transplantation.*
  lung diseases treated by, 1699t
  lymphoproliferative disorder after, 1711–1713,
      1712–1715
  tuberculosis risk and, 803–804
Transthoracic needle aspiration, 345–347
  in pneumonia diagnosis, 721
  in pulmonary metastasis diagnosis, 1412
  in tuberculosis diagnosis, 846
Transthoracic needle biopsy, 370–371
  CT-guided, 315, 370
  of pleura, 372–373
  ultrasound-guided, 334, 370
Transthoracic pressure, pulmonary blood flow
    and, 275, *276*
Transthyretin, in amyloidosis, 2709
Transtracheal catheters, complications of, 2681
Transtracheal needle aspiration, 347–348
Transversus abdominis muscle, in expiration,
    247
  spinal levels of innervation of, 3055
Transversus thoracis muscle, on CT, 154, *156,
    260, 261*
Trapezius, in inspiration, 246
  on CT, 260, *260*
Trauma, adult respiratory distress syndrome
    after, 2005, *2005*
  cavities or cysts due to, 3104t
  chylothorax due to, 2768–2769
  fat embolism and, 1846
  head, hypoxemia with, 2647
    pulmonary edema due to, 1974–1976
  homogeneous consolidation due to, nonseg-
      mental, 3081t
    segmental, 3088t
  iatrogenic, 2659–2691. See also *Surgery;* spe-
      cific procedures.
  inhomogeneous consolidation due to, nonseg-
      mental, 3093t
  mediastinal, aortography in, 324–325
    CT in, 325, *325*
  mediastinal mass due to, in anterior compart-
      ment, 3172t
    in middle-posterior compartment, 3178t
  multiple masses or nodules due to, 3124t
  nonpenetrating, effects of, on chest wall,
      2644–2647
    on diaphragm, 2636–2644
    on lungs, 2611–2623
    on mediastinum, 2625–2636
    on pleura, 2623–2625
  nonthoracic, pulmonary effects of, 2647
  paravertebral mass due to, 3185t
  penetrating, 2647–2653
  pleural, pleural fluid eosinophilia with, 344
  pleural effusion due to, 2745t, 2761–2763,
      2763
  pneumatocele due to, 510, *510*
  pneumothorax due to, 2789–2790, 2789t
  pulmonary artery aneurysm due to, 1935
  solitary mass due to, 3118t
  solitary nodule due to, 3112t
Travel history, 390
Tree-in-bud pattern, 701, *702*
  in bronchiolitis, 2327–2330, *2330, 2331*

Tree-in-bud pattern (*Continued*)
  in cystic fibrosis, 2306
  in diffuse panbronchiolitis, *2352,* 2353
  in *Staphylococcus aureus* pneumonia, 745,
      746
  in tuberculosis, 827, *833*
Trematodes, 1047–1052. See also specific
    diseases.
Treponemataceae. See also *Syphilis.*
  classification and nomenclature of, 735t
  pulmonary infection due to, 776–778
Triangularis sterni, in expiration, 247
Trichinosis, 1043
Trichomoniasis, 1039
  empyema due to, 2752
Trichoptysis, 380
Trichosporon species infection, 952, 1753
Tricuspid valve, endocarditis of, septic
    pulmonary embolism with, 1829,
    1831–1832
Tricyclic antidepressants, thoracic disease due to,
    2539t, 2569
Trimellitic anhydride inhalation, 2528
Trimethoprim-sulfamethoxazole, thoracic disease
    due to, 2538t, 2558
Trimipramine, thoracic disease due to, 2569
Tripe palms, in pulmonary carcinoma, 1174
Tropheryma whippleii infection, 750
Trophoblast cells, in lung, during pregnancy, 132
Trophoblastic neoplasms, gestational, metastatic
    to lung, 1408–1409
Tropical eosinophilia, 1043–1045, *1044,
    1752–1753*
Tropical spastic paraparesis, 991
Trousseau's syndrome, 1779
Truncus arteriosus, persistent, 637, 3151t
Tube thoracostomy, complications of,
    2676–2677, *2677–2679*
Tuberculin skin test, 841–843, 841t–843t
  in HIV infection, 1652–1653
Tuberculoma, 813, *816*, 825–827, *830–832*
  central nervous system, 839
  solitary nodule due to, 3111t, *3113*
Tuberculosis, 799–848
  airway involvement in, pathologic features of,
      815–817, *823, 824*
    radiologic features of, 830–831, *836, 837*
  apical cap due to, 2795, *2798*
  bronchiectasis due to, pathologic features of,
      815, 816, 817, *823, 824,* 2269, *2270*
    radiologic features of, 830, *836*
  calcification in, 463–467, *476,* 805, 811, *812*
    pleural, 583, *584, 585*
  cavitation in, 3102t, *3106*
    disease transmission and, 800
    pathologic features of, 813–814, *813, 814,
        817–819*
    radiologic features of, *463,* 824, *829*
  centrilobular nodules in, *30,* 827–828, *833*
  chronic, airway obstruction due to, 2177
    fibrocaseous, 813, 814, *818*
  cicatrization atelectasis due to, *527*
  clubbing in, 396
  coal workers' pneumoconiosis and, 2418
  community-acquired pneumonia due to, 722
  consolidation in, homogeneous segmental,
      3087t
    inhomogeneous nonsegmental, 3093t, *3094*
  diagnosis of, 840–847
    bacteriologic investigation in, 843–846
    biochemical investigation in, 847
    closed pleural biopsy in, 373
    cytopathologic examination in, 846
    hematologic investigation in, 846–847
    skin testing in, 841–843, 841t–843t
  diffuse nodular pattern in, 3145t, *3146, 3147*

Tuberculosis *(Continued)*
  drug-resistant, 804
    in HIV infection, 1654
  endobronchial spread of, pathologic features
      of, 814, *819–821*
    radiologic features of, 828, *834*
  endotracheal, on spiral CT, *2030*
  epidemiology of, 799–804
    tests useful in investigating, 846
  extrapulmonary, 834–840, *838, 839*
    in HIV infection, 1652
  fibrosing mediastinitis due to, 835, 2856
  fibrosis due to, hilar displacement with, 533,
      533
  fungus ball in, 814, 817, *824, 922,* 923, *925,
      926, 3106*
  healed, linear shadow with, 483
  histoplasmosis vs., 811, 879
  in HIV infection, 803, 1648–1654
    clinical features of, 1651–1652
    diagnosis of, 1652–1653
    epidemiology of, 1648–1649
    HIV progression and, 1649, 1653
    pathogenesis of, 1649
    prognosis in, 1653–1654
    radiologic features of, 1649–1651, *1650–
      1652*
  incidental discovery of, 832–834
  laryngeal stenosis in, 2022
  lymph node enlargement in, sarcoidosis vs.,
      1545, 1547
  miliary, 713–715, *715, 716,* 3145t, *3146, 3147*
    clinical features of, 832
    in HIV disease, *1650, 1651*
    interstitial emphysema and pneumomediasti-
      num in, *2869*
    pathologic features of, 814–815, *822*
    prognosis in, 847–848
    radiologic features of, 447–453, *450, 452,*
      828–830, *835*
    time of appearance of, 3046
  nonreactive, 815
  nontuberculous mycobacterial infection vs.,
      853
  pleural boundary crossing by, 460
  pleural effusion due to, 2743–2747, 2744t
    asbestos-related effusion vs., 2435
    clinical features of, 2745–2746
    diagnosis of, 2746–2747
    epidemiology of, 2743–2745
    in HIV infection, 1652
    natural history of, 2747
    pathogenesis of, 2745
    rheumatoid effusion vs., 2754
  pleural fluid cytology in, 344
  pleural involvement in, pleural lymphoma and,
      2838
  postprimary, 811–834
    anatomic distribution of, 477, 811–812,
      820–821
    bronchiectasis in, pathologic features of,
      815, 816, 817, *823, 824*
      radiologic features of, 830, *836*
    bronchopneumonia in, pathologic features
      of, 814, *819–821*
      radiologic features of, 822, *827*
    cavitation in, pathologic features of, 813–
      814, *813, 814, 817–819*
      radiologic features of, 824, *829*
    clinical features of, 831–834
    consolidation in, homogeneous nonsegmen-
      tal, 3079t
      inhomogeneous segmental, 3097t
      radiologic features of, 821–824, *825–828*
    healing of, 813–814, *815–817*
    local parenchymal disease in, 813–814,
      813–818

Tuberculosis *(Continued)*
    nodular opacities in, 824–830, *830–835*
    of tracheobronchial tree, 830–831, *836, 837*
      pathologic features of, 815–817, *823, 824*
    pathogenesis of, 811–813, *813*
    pathologic features of, 811–818, *813–824*
      treatment-related, 818
    radiologic features of, 818–831
      interpretation of, 818–820
    vascular complications of, 817–818, *824*
  primary pulmonary, 804–811
    clinical features of, 811
    consolidation in, 807
      homogeneous nonsegmental, 3079t
    hematogenous dissemination of, 806
    lymph node involvement in, 805–806, *808,
      809,* 3164t, *3166*
      radiologic features of, 807–810, *810–812*
    pathogenesis of, 804–806, *806–807*
    pathologic features of, 804–806, *806–809*
    progressive, 806, *809*
    radiologic features of, 806–811, *810–812*
  prognosis in, 847–848
  pulmonary artery aneurysm due to, 817–818,
      1935
  pulmonary artery thrombosis in, 1774
  pulmonary carcinoma and, 848, 1080–1081
  pulmonary function testing in, 847
  radiologic features of, time of appearance of,
      3046
  reactivation. See *Tuberculosis, postprimary.*
  rib involvement in, 837–838, *839,* 3017, *3017*
  risk factors for, 801–804
  sarcoidosis and, 803, 1534–1535
  secondary. See *Tuberculosis, postprimary.*
  silicosis and, 803, 2408
  solitary nodule due to, 3111t, *3113*
  spinal, 837, *838,* 3023, *3025*
    paravertebral mass due to, 3185t, *3186*
  systemic lupus erythematosus and, 803, 1432
  transmission of, 800–801
Tuberous sclerosis, 686–690, *686, 687*
  diffuse reticular pattern in, 3134t
  Langerhans' cell histiocytosis vs., 1631
  lymphangioleiomyomatosis and, 679, 686
Tubular myelin, surfactant and, 56, *57*
Tubular shadows, 483, *485*
  in bronchiectasis, *482,* 483, *2272, 2272, 2273*
  in chronic bronchitis, 2199, 2203
Tuboreticular structures, in systemic lupus
      erythematosus, 1424
Tularemia, 766–767, *768,* 2749
Tumor(s). See *Neoplasm(s);* specific neoplasms
      and sites.
Tumor emboli, 1854
  with pulmonary metastasis, 1382, 1388–1389,
      1389, 1397, *1398, 1399*
Tumor markers, in pulmonary carcinoma, 1179
  prognosis and, 1200–1201
Tumor necrosis factor, in adult respiratory
      distress syndrome, 1983
  in *Pneumocystis carinii* pneumonia, 1657
  in rheumatoid disease, 1434
  thoracic disease due to, 2538t, 2556
Tumorlets, pulmonary, 1243–1245, *1244–1246*
Tumor-suppressor genes, in pulmonary
      carcinoma pathogenesis, 1082, 1083
Turbulence, airway resistance and, 59
Tussometry, 410
TWAR agent (*Chlamydia pneumoniae*), 722,
      1016–1017
Typhus, African tick, 1022
  scrub, 1020

Ulcer, gastrointestinal, pleural effusion with,
      2766

Ulcer *(Continued)*
  oropharyngeal, in histoplasmosis, 888
Ulcerative colitis, 1473–1475, *1474*
  pleural effusion in, 2766
Ultrasonography, 333–334, *333, 334.* See also
      Echocardiography.
  in assessment of chest wall invasion by pulmo-
      nary carcinoma, 1166
  in deep vein thrombosis, 1819–1820
  in diaphragmatic motion assessment, 2988–
      2989
  in diaphragmatic paralysis diagnosis, 2992–
      2993
  in diaphragmatic rupture diagnosis, 334, 2637
  in pleural effusion diagnosis, 333–334, *333,
      563, 564,* 578, 579
  transthoracic needle biopsy guided by, 334,
      370
Ultraviolet light, systemic lupus erythematosus
      and, 1424
Union Internationale Contre le Cancer, lymph
      node classification of, for lung cancer
      staging, 180–184, *185,* 188t, 1186, *1186,*
      1187t
Upper airway(s). See *Airway(s), upper.*
  obstruction of. See *Airway obstruction, upper.*
Upper airway resistance syndrome, 2069n
Upper paratracheal lymph nodes, in ATS
      classification, 184t, *185, 186*
  in classification for lung cancer staging, *185,*
      188t, *1186,* 1187t
Upper triangle sign, in atelectasis, *534*
Uremia, pleural effusion in, 2764
Urine specimen, in tuberculosis diagnosis, 844
Urinoma, pleural effusion with, 2764
Urinothorax, 2764
Urogenital tract. See also specific structures.
  cystic fibrosis involving, 2310–2311
  disease of, pleural effusion with, 2764
  tuberculosis involving, 835–837
  Wegener's granulomatosis involving, 1504
Urticaria, cholinergic, 2109
Urticarial vasculitis, hypocomplementemic,
      1432–1433
  emphysema in, 2243
Usual interstitial pneumonia, 1584. See also
      Pulmonary fibrosis, idiopathic.
  desquamative interstitial pneumonia and,
      1584–1585
Uterus, smooth muscle neoplasms of, metastatic
      to lung, 1409, *1410*
Uveoparotid fever, 1565

V sign of Naclerio, 2865
Vagus nerve, in pulmonary innervation, 145,
      146, 147
  pulmonary carcinoma invading, 1171
Valley fever, 893
Valsalva maneuver, 275n
  blood pressure measurement during, 396
  chest radiographs with, 305
    clinical utility of, 275, *276*
  pneumothorax and, 2789
Valves, in pulmonary lymphatics, 174, *174*
  in thoracic duct, 175
Vanishing tumor, due to interlobar effusion,
      579–581, *580*
  in hydrothorax due to heart failure, 2761,
      2762
Varicellavirus infection, 999–1004. See also
      Chickenpox; Zoster.
  diffuse alveolar damage due to, *713*
  epidemiology of, 1000
  laboratory findings in, 1003

Varicellavirus infection *(Continued)*
   pain due to, 387
   pneumonia due to, clinical features of, 1003
      epidemiology of, 1000
      laboratory findings in, 1003
      pathologic features of, 1001, *1001*
      prognosis in, 1003–1004
      radiologic features of, 1001, *1001–1003*
      remote, 1001, *1003*
   unilateral diaphragmatic paralysis due to, 2989
Varices, esophageal, 2967–2968, *2968*
   complications of sclerotherapy for, 2761,
      2968
   pulmonary vein, 645–647, *648–649*
Varicose bronchiectasis, 2268–2269. See also
   Bronchiectasis.
   bronchography in, *2279*
   CT findings in, 2275, *2275*
Vas deferens, congenital bilateral absence of,
   2283, 2299
Vascular cell adhesion molecule 1 (VCAM-1), in
   asthmatic airway inflammation, 2090
Vascular incisura, 205
Vascular malformations. See also *Arteriovenous*
   malformation.
   embolization therapy for, pulmonary acrylate
      glue embolism due to, 1865, *1867*
Vascular neoplasms. See also specific neoplasms.
   pulmonary, 1335–1343
Vascular pedicle, 227–228, *230, 231*
Vascular ring, congenital aortic, 2961
Vascular sarcoma, sclerosing interstitial. See
   Epithelioid hemangioendothelioma.
Vascular stents, complications of, 2674
Vasculitis, 1489–1525. See also specific
   disorders.
   classification of, 1490–1491, 1490t
   clinical features of, 1490
   hypocomplementemic urticarial, 1432–1433
      emphysema in, 2243
   in pulmonary hypertension, 1885, *1889*
   in sarcoidosis, 1541, *1542*
   large vessel, 1490t
   medium-sized vessel, 1490t
   pulmonary, hypertension in, 1912
      in rheumatoid disease, 1449–1451
      in tuberculosis, 817, *824*
      primary, 1489–1490
   small vessel, 1490t, 3130t
   systemic, bronchiectasis and, 2278
Vasculitis sign, in Wegener's granulomatosis,
   1499
Vasoactive intestinal peptide (VIP), 148
   actions of, in lung, 131
Vasoconstriction, in pulmonary hypertension,
   1880–1881, 1898
   in response to hypoxia, 106
Vasospasm, in progressive systemic sclerosis,
   1453–1454
VATS (video-assisted thoracoscopic surgery),
   371–372
Vegetable lipids, aspiration of, 2501, 2506
   embolization of, 1871
Vegetable wax storage disease, 2728
Vein(s), perforation of, with central venous
   catheter, 2683–2685, *2683, 2684*
Velcro rales, in idiopathic pulmonary fibrosis,
   1607
Venoarterial shunts. See *Shunting.*
Venography, contrast material for, venous
   thrombosis due to, 1778
   in deep vein thrombosis, 1819
      with spiral CT, 1820–1823
Veno-occlusive disease, pulmonary, 1930–1933,
   1931–1933
      after bone marrow transplantation, 1732

Veno-occlusive disease *(Continued)*
      pulmonary wedge pressure measurement in,
         1996
      pulmonary capillary hemangiomatosis vs.,
         1914
Venous admixture, calculation of, in ventilation/
   perfusion mismatch assessment, 112–113
Venous thromboembolic disease. See
   Thromboembolism; Thrombosis.
Ventilation, 51–60. See also *Respiration.*
   alveolar, 53–60
      determinants of, 53
      matching alveolar perfusion to, 108–111,
         109. See also *Ventilation/perfusion*
         entries.
   clinical assessment of adequacy of, limitations
      of, 3065
   collateral, anatomic pathways of, 31–33, *32*
      factors determining effectiveness of, 59–60
      resistance in, 59–60
      with airway obstruction, resorption atelecta-
         sis and, 514, *515*
   control of, 235–243. See also *Respiratory con-*
      trol system.
      disorders of, 3049–3056, 3049t
      during exercise, 241
      during sleep, 243, 243t
      in asthma, 2139–2140
      involuntary, *236,* 238–239, 3049–3051
      load detection in, 242
      voluntary, *236,* 239, 3049, 3051
   mechanical. See *Mechanical ventilation.*
   of acinus, 53–60
   pattern of, analysis of, in ventilatory control
      assessment, 419
      control of, 239
   pulmonary lymph flow and, 174–175
   regional, exercise and, 111
      gravity and, 110–111
   rhythm of, control of, 238–240
   with added load, compensatory mechanisms
      in, 241–242
Ventilation imaging, 327–330, *328,* 1800–1802.
   See also *Ventilation/perfusion scanning.*
Ventilation/perfusion heterogeneity, 108–111,
   109
   diffusing capacity measurement and, 415–416
   gravity and, 106, 110–111
   measurement of, 113–114, *113,* 416
Ventilation/perfusion mismatch, compensation
   for regional carbon dioxide retention in,
   3048
   exercise and, 107, 111
   hypoxemia due to, 115
   in adult respiratory distress syndrome, 1997
   in cardiogenic pulmonary edema, 1973
   in COPD, 2225–2226
   measurement of, 111–114, *113*
   mechanisms of, in disease, 111
   regional assessment of, 113
Ventilation/perfusion scanning, 326–331,
   327–329
   after radiation therapy, 2604
   in pulmonary hypertension diagnosis, 1891,
      1908, *1909*
   in pulmonary thromboembolism diagnosis,
      328–329, 330–331, 1800–1807
      diagnostic accuracy of, 330t, 1804–1807,
         1806t
      diagnostic criteria for, 1802–1804, *1802–*
         1804, 1805t
      technique for, 1800–1802
   indications for, 330–331
   technique for, 326–330
Ventilator. See *Mechanical ventilation.*
Ventilatory failure. See *Alveolar hypoventilation;*
   Respiratory failure.

Ventilatory response curves, 417–418, *417, 418*
Ventral respiratory group, in medullary control
   of ventilation, *236,* 239, *3050,* 3051
Ventricular function, in COPD, 2218
Ventricular hypertrophy, left, in hemodialysis
   patients, 1973
   right, electrocardiographic criteria for, 1934
      in COPD, 2218
Ventricular septal defect, clinical signs of,
   1895–1896
   pulmonary atresia with, 637
Ventriculoperitoneal shunt, migration of, pleural
   effusion due to, 2762
Verapamil, thoracic disease due to, 2538t, 2564
Vermiculite, pneumoconiosis due to, 2450, 2451
Vertebra. See *Spine.*
Very late activation antigen 4 (VLA-4), in
   asthmatic airway inflammation, 2090
Vibrio infection, 759
Video camera, film digitization using, 307
Video-assisted thoracoscopic surgery (VATS),
   371–372
Vinca alkaloids, thoracic disease due to, 2538t,
   2550–2551
Viral infection, 979–1010. See also specific
   viruses and groups.
   after bone marrow transplantation, 1730
   after lung transplantation, 1716–1717
   asthma provoked by, 2111–2112
   combined air-space and interstitial pattern of
      increased density in, 455
   COPD exacerbations and, 2176–2177
   dermatomyositis/polymyositis and, 1462
   diagnosis of, 981
   diffuse nodular pattern in, 3145t
   diffuse reticular pattern in, 3134t
   factors influencing severity of, 980
   idiopathic pulmonary fibrosis and, 1585–1586
   in childhood, atopy and, 2080
      COPD and, 2176
   in HIV disease, 1673–1675
   in infancy, asthma risk and, 2079–2080, 2112
   inhomogeneous consolidation in, nonsegmen-
      tal, 3093t
      segmental, 3097t
   long-term sequelae of, 980–981
   lymph node enlargement in, 3164t
   pathogenesis of, 980
   pleural effusion in, 2752
   pulmonary carcinoma and, 1079
   Sjögren's syndrome and, 1466
   systemic lupus erythematosus and, 1424
   with DNA viruses, 994–1010
   with RNA viruses, 981–994
Virchow's triad, in venous thrombosis
   development, 1777–1780
Virtual bronchoscopy, 311
Virus(es). See also *Viral infection;* specific
   viruses and groups.
   DNA, 994–1010
   respiratory, classification of, 981
   RNA, 981–994
Viscance, in work of breathing, 59
Visceral lymph nodes, 176–180, *179–184*
Viscosity, in respiratory mucus, 62–63
   cough effectiveness and, 130
Visual paraneoplastic syndrome, in pulmonary
   carcinoma, 1174
Vital capacity (VC), 406–407, *406*
Vitamin C, in defense against oxidant damage,
   2521
Vitamin D–binding protein, COPD and,
   2178–2179
Vitamin E, in defense against oxidant damage,
   2521, 2522
$V_{max_{25}}$, measurement of, 408, 409

Vmax$_{50}$, measurement of, 408, 409
  signal-to-noise ratio for, 410
Vocal cord paralysis, 2032
Vocal fremitus, 392
Voice sounds, 394
Volcanic dust, pneumoconiosis due to, 2466
Volvulus, colonic, with diaphragmatic paralysis, *2992*
  gastric, with diaphragmatic paralysis, 2990
    with hiatus hernia, 2996, *3001*
Von Recklinghausen's disease, *688, 689, 690–691, 690*
Voxel, defined, 309

Wacker's triad, in pulmonary thromboembolism, 1826
Waldenström's macroglobulinemia, 1290–1291, 2760
Water, aspiration of. See under *Aspiration (event).*
  in tracheobronchial secretions, 61, 62
Water intoxication, in asthma, 2137
Water loss, respiratory, bronchoconstriction in response to, 2109
Water-lily sign, in echinococcosis, 463, *467, 1056, 1056,* 2753, *2754*
Water-mist aerosol, mucus mobility and, 63
Weakness, respiratory muscle. See *Respiratory muscles, fatigue and weakness of.*
Weber fraction, load detection and, 242
Wedge filtration, for conventional radiographs, 302
Wegener's granulomatosis, 1491–1506
  clinical features of, 1499–1504
  defined, 1490t
  diagnostic criteria for, 1491, 1491t, 1505
  epidemiology of, 1491
  laboratory findings in, 1504–1506
  limited form of, 1491, 1499, 1506
  multiple masses or nodules in, 3123t, *3127*

Wegener's granulomatosis *(Continued)*
  pathogenesis of, 1491–1494
  pathologic features of, 1494–1496, *1494–1498*
  prognosis in, 1506
  pulmonary cavities in, 462, *466,* 1499, *1500,* 3104t, *3108*
  radiologic features of, 1496–1499, *1498–1503*
Weight. See also *Obesity.*
  body, adult respiratory distress syndrome prognosis and, 1998
  pulmonary function and, 405
Weight loss, in COPD, 2216
Weil's disease, 777
Welder's pneumoconiosis, 2453–2454, *2453–2455*
Westermark's sign, in pulmonary thromboembolism, *501,* 504, *506,* 1787–1788, *1792*
Wheezes, 394, 395
Wheezing, emotional laryngeal, 2032
Wheezing respirations, 395
Whipple's disease, 750
Whispering pectoriloquy, 394
White blood signal, 317
White plague, 799
Whooping cough. See *Pertussis.*
Williams-Beuren syndrome, 642
Williams-Campbell syndrome, 2285
Wilms' tumor, metastatic to lung, *1386*
Window settings, in CT, 312–313
Wiskott-Aldrich syndrome, 728
Wollastonite, pneumoconiosis due to, 2452
Wood dust exposure, idiopathic pulmonary fibrosis and, 1586
Wood pulp–worker's disease, 2363t. See also *Extrinsic allergic alveolitis.*
Woodchip fever. See *Organic dust toxic syndrome.*
Work of breathing, elastic recoil in, 53–58
  frictional resistance in, 58–60
Wrist actigraphy, in obstructive sleep apnea diagnosis, 2069

Wuchereria bancrofti infestation, 1043–1045, 1752–1753

Xanthogranuloma, mediastinal, 2925
Xanthoma, pulmonary, 1371
Xanthomatosis, cerebrotendinous, 2727
Xanthomonas maltophilia (Stenotrophomonas maltophilia) infection, 764
Xenobiotics, pulmonary metabolism of, 132
Xenon, for closing volume measurement, 413–414
  for ventilation imaging, 327–329, 1802
X-linked agammaglobulinemia, 724–725

Yellow nail syndrome, 2284–2285, *2285,* 2766
Yersinia enterocolitica infection, 758
  mesothelioma and, 2810
  sarcoidosis and, 1535
Yersinia pestis infection, 756–758
Young-Laplace relationship, for describing surface factors' role in elastic recoil, 58
Young's syndrome, 2283–2284
Yttrium, pneumoconiosis due to, 2456

Zellballen, in aorticopulmonary paraganglioma, 2942
Zenker's diverticulum, 2966–2967
  aspiration pneumonia secondary to, *2499*
Zeolites, mesothelioma and, 2809
  pneumoconiosis due to, 2452
Zinc chloride, inhalation of fumes from, 2527t
Zinostatin, thoracic disease due to, 2538t
Zirconium, pneumoconiosis due to, 2468
Zoster, 999. See also *Varicellavirus.*
Zuelzer-Wilson syndrome, 3052
Zygomycosis, 947–949, *948,* 2752

Vol. 1 ISBN 0-7216-6195-5

90071

9 780721 661957